A Dictionary of Psychological Medicine: Giving the Definition, Etymology and Synonyms of the Terms Used in Medical Psychology with the Symptoms, Treatment, and Pathology of Insanity and the Law of Lunacy in Great Britain and Ireland, Volume 2

Daniel Hack Tuke

Frontispiece. Plate I.

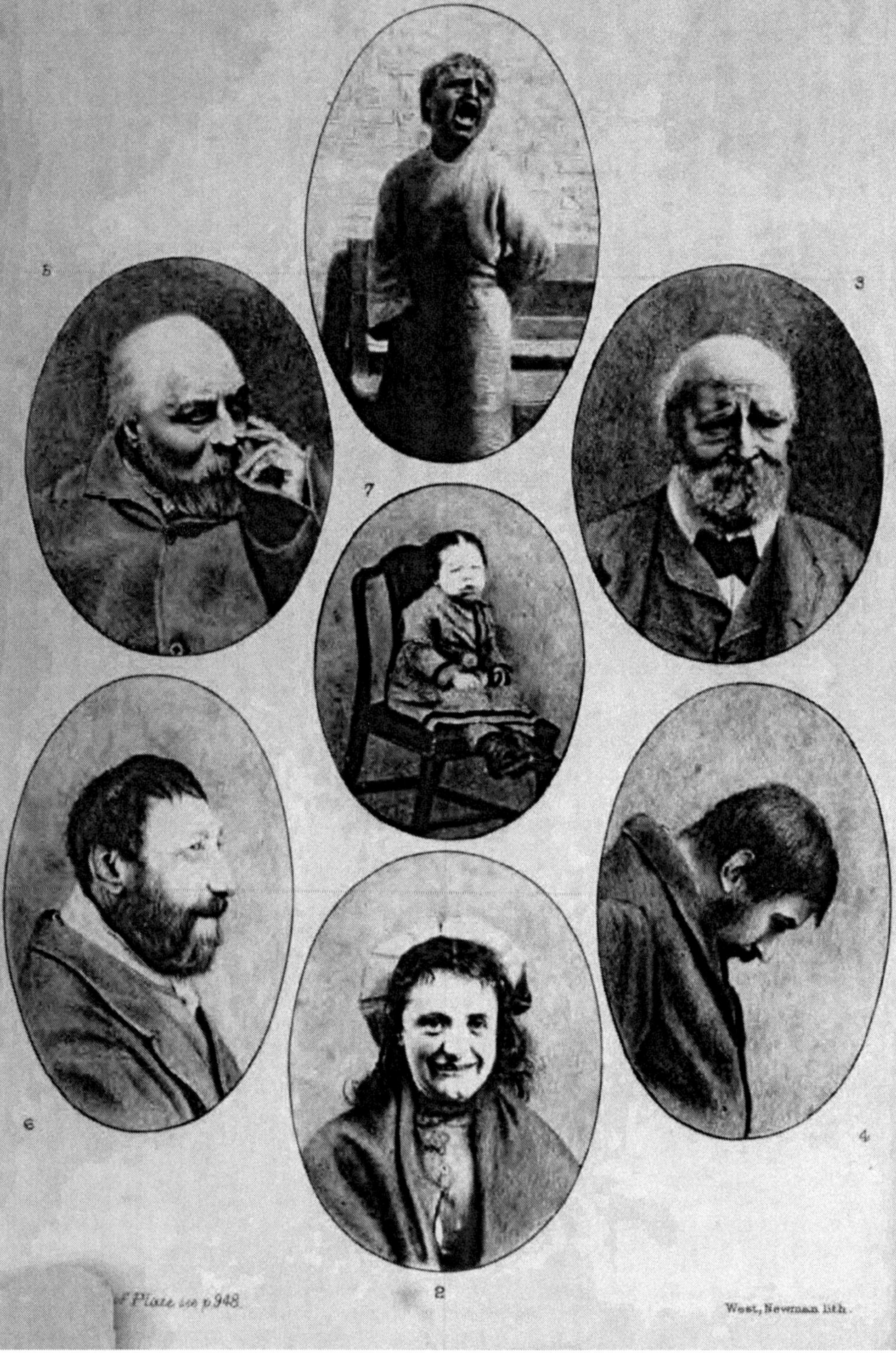

... of Plate see p. 948.

West, Newman lith.

A DICTIONARY

OF

PSYCHOLOGICAL MEDICINE

[illegible]

[illegible]

WITH THE

SYMPTOMS, TREATMENT, AND PATHOLOGY [illegible]

AND THE

LAW OF LUNACY IN GREAT BRITAIN [illegible]

EDITED BY

D. HACK TUKE, M.D.

[illegible]

VOL. II

LONDON

J. & A. CHURCHILL

11 NEW BURLINGTON STREET

1892

Frontispiece

Plate I.

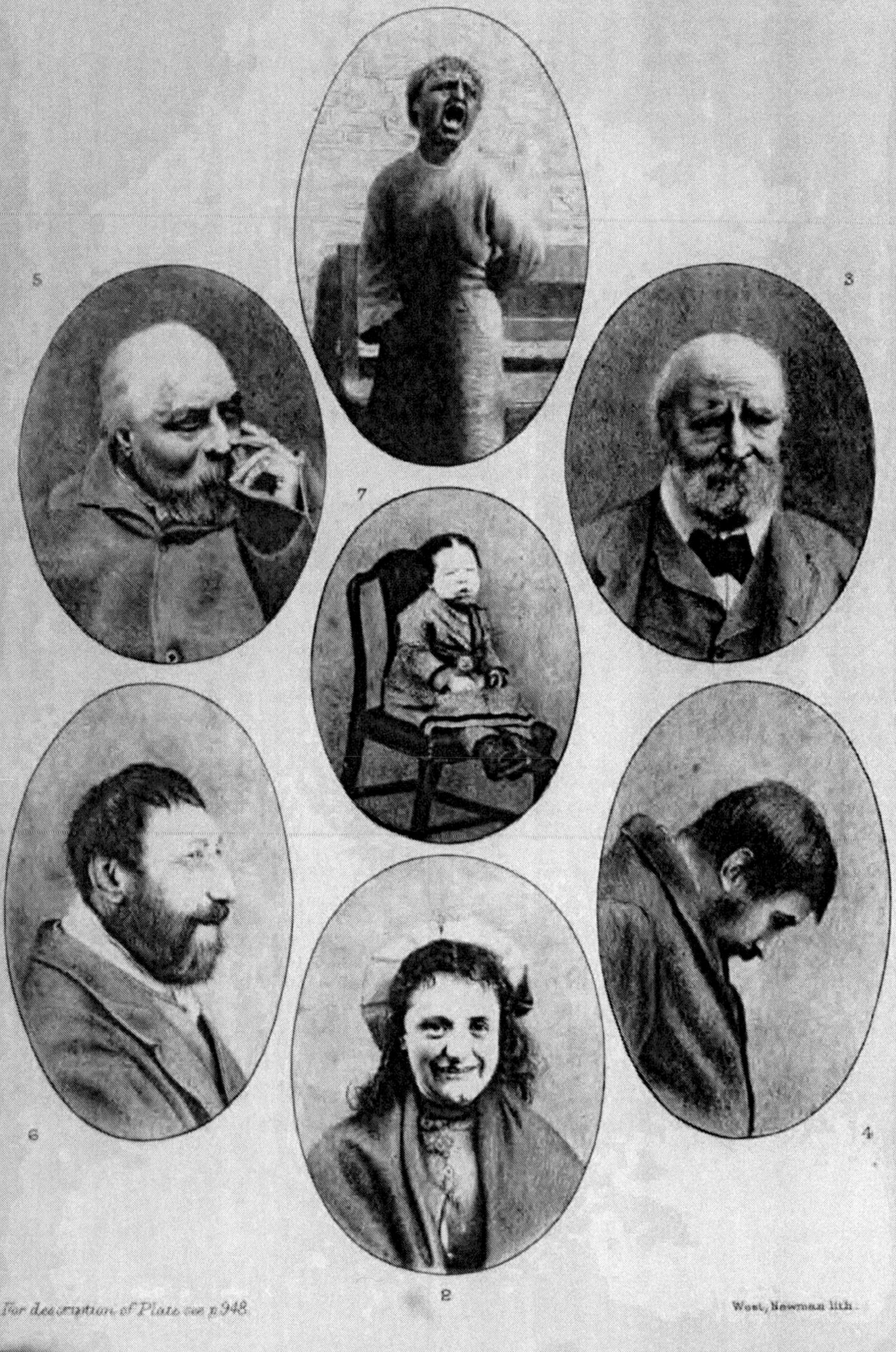

For description of Plate see p.948.

West, Newman lith.

[illegible] TION[illegible]

PSYCHOLOGICAL [illegible]

[illegible]

SYMPTOMS, TREATMENT [illegible]

[illegible]

LAW OF LUNACY IN GREAT BRIT[illegible]

[illegible]

D. HACK TUKE, M.D.

[illegible]

[illegible]

LONDON

J. & A. CHURCHILL

11 NEW BURLINGTON STREET

18[illegible]

Plate I

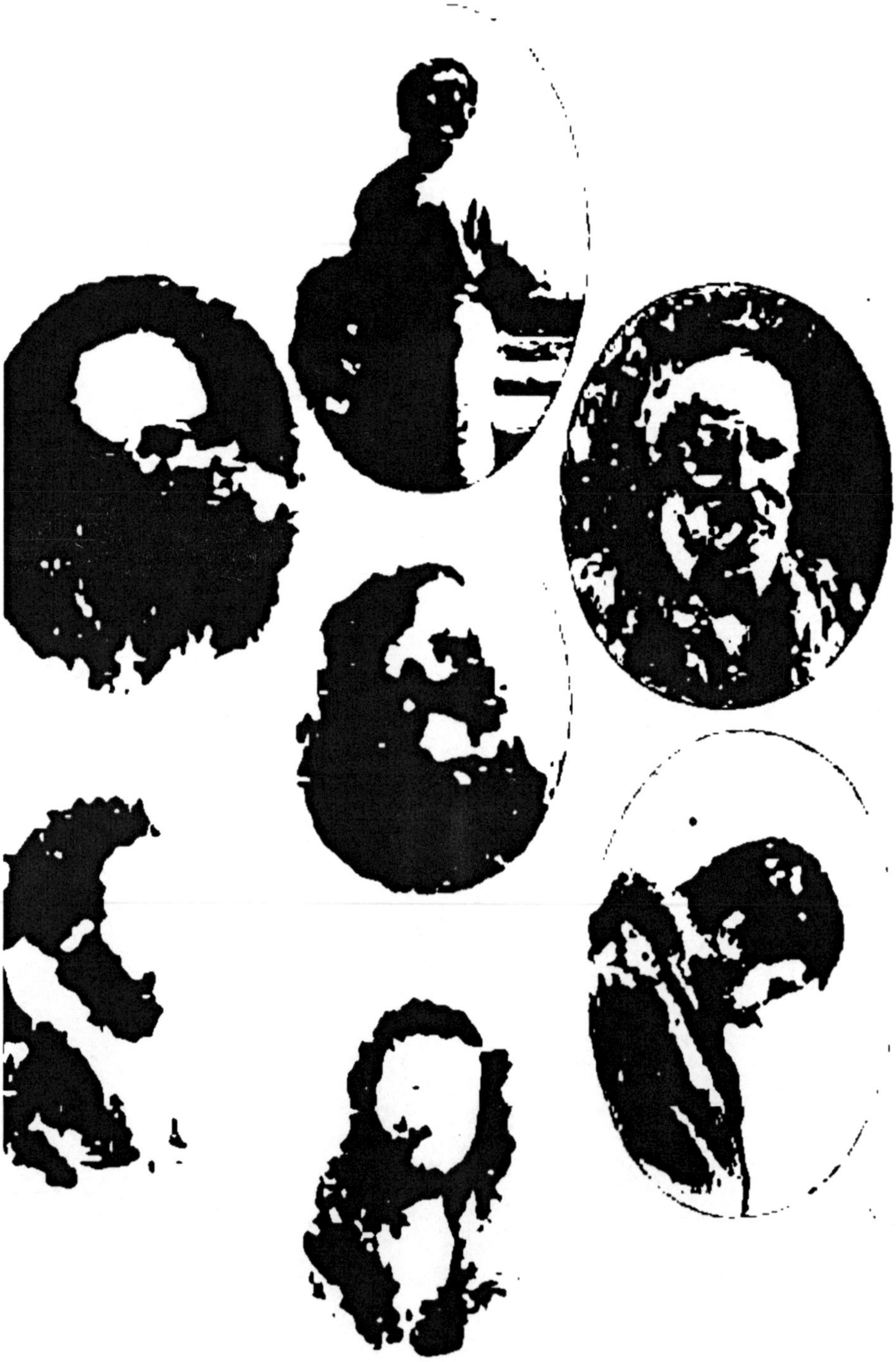

A DICTIONARY

OF

PSYCHOLOGICAL MEDICINE

GIVING THE DEFINITION, ETYMOLOGY AND SYNONYMS OF THE TERMS USED IN MEDICAL PSYCHOLOGY

WITH THE

SYMPTOMS, TREATMENT, AND PATHOLOGY OF INSANITY

AND THE

LAW OF LUNACY IN GREAT BRITAIN AND IRELAND

EDITED BY

D. HACK TUKE, M.D., LL.D.

EXAMINER IN MENTAL PHYSIOLOGY IN THE UNIVERSITY OF LONDON; LECTURER ON PSYCHOLOGICAL MEDICINE AT THE CHARING CROSS HOSPITAL MEDICAL SCHOOL; CO-EDITOR OF THE "JOURNAL OF MENTAL SCIENCE"

VOL. II.

LONDON
J. & A. CHURCHILL
11 NEW BURLINGTON STREET
1892

I

ICTUS EPILEPTICUS (*ictus*, a blow, from *ico*, I strike; ἐπιληψία, from ἐπιλαμβάνω, I seize upon). An old term for an epileptic fit which comes on suddenly without a premonitory aura. (Fr. *ictus epileptique.*)

IDEA (Lat. *idea*, from Gr. ἰδέα, form, look, or semblance of a thing). A distinct mental representation of an object of sense. A concept (*q.v.*).

IDEA, CHASE (Ger. *Ideenjagd*). A term used by German writers to denote the mental condition which often occurs in acute mania, when ideas chase each other through the brain with great rapidity, being excited by any desultory fancy and making but a feeble mental impression.

IDEA, FIXED (Fr. *idée fixe*). A form of monomania in which a dominant idea colours all thoughts and actions.

IDEA, VOLITIONAL.—A thought which arises in the mind owing to the voluntary direction of the mind thereto.

IDEALES.—One of Linnæus's three subdivisions of mental diseases—affections of the intellectual faculties.

IDEALITY. — The capacity to form ideals of beauty and perfection.

IDEAS, ASSOCIATION OF. — The recalling of one mental representation by the agency of another, either by reason of their habitually existing together, or by reason of a certain degree of similarity between them.

IDEAS, AUTOMATIC (αὐτόματος, spontaneous). Ideas that arise in the mind without any external stimulus.

IDEAS, INNATE.—Ideas which, according to one school of metaphysicians, originated without experience in the world. All that can now be admitted is that heredity supplies a strong tendency to certain ideas or trains of thought. (Fr. *idées innées.*)

IDEATION.—The formation of an idea or mental concept. The cerebral act by which an idea is produced. (Fr. *idéation.*) (*See* PHILOSOPHY OF MIND, p. 34.)

IDEATIONAL INSANITY. (*See* INSANITY, IDEATIONAL.)

IDENTITY, MISTAKEN.—The loss of the power to distinguish between oneself and another person.

IDENTITY, PERSONAL (*idem*, the same). The knowledge that one is the same person that he claims or is claimed to be.

IDEO-MOTOR MOVEMENTS (ἰδέα, aspect, also mode or manner; *moveo*, I move). Unconscious actions executed by reason of impulses emanating from the mind when fully occupied by some dominant idea (Carpenter).

IDEOPEGMA (πῆγμα, anything fastened together). A term used in the same sense as Idea, fixed (*q.v.*).

IDEOPHRENIA (φρήν, the mind). A term for delirium, characterised by anomalies of the ideas (Guislain).

IDEOPHRENIC INSANITY. (*See* IDIOPHRENIC.)

IDEOPLASTIC (πλάσσω, I mould). A term used for the stage of hypnotism in which the idea impressed upon the brain of the agent (suggestion) is converted into action.

IDEOSYNCHYSIA (σύγχυσις, confusion). A confusion of ideas. A term used for delirium. (Fr. *idéosynchisie.*)

IDIOCTONIA (ἴδιος, one's own; κτόνος, murder). Suicide, or self-murder. (Fr. *idioctonie*; Ger. *Selbstmord.*)

IDIOCTONOS (ἴδιος, κτόνος). A self-murderer or suicide.

IDIOCY, Accidental (ἰδιώτης, a private individual; also one who is illiterate or uneducated). Those cases of idiocy brought about by accidental circumstances, including the traumatic, inflammatory and epileptiform.—**I., Caucasian.** (*See* IDIOCY, FORMS OF.)—**I., choreic** (χορεία, a dancing). Either those cases of idiocy in which the chorea acts as a cause through the parent to the offspring, or those cases in which chorea occurs during childhood, and induces idiocy during development.—**I., congenital,** *congenitus*, born with). Idiocy commencing during fœtal life.—**I., cretinoid** (Cretin, *q.v.*; εἶδος, like). Idiocy developed in a cretinoid frame. The form in which the subjects are dwarfed, with stunted bodies, irregularly formed crania, and usually enlarged thyroids. (*See* CRETINISM.)—**I., developmental.** Idiocy due to a defect of cerebral development.—**I., eclampsic** (ἔκλαμψις, a shining forth). A name given to those cases of idiocy which follow and are due to infantile fits, some cerebral change having been induced which renders the brain incapable of higher development (Ireland).—**I., epileptic.** Idiocy dependent for its causation on the recurrence of epileptic fits.—**I., Ethiopian** (Ethiopia). (*See* IDIOCY, FORMS OF.)—**I., genetous**

(γένεσις, generation). A name given to those cases of idiocy which apparently commence anterior to birth (Ireland).—**I., hydrocephalic** (ὑδροκέφαλον, from ὕδωρ, water; κεφαλή, the head). Idiocy due to hydrocephalus (Ireland).—**I., hypertrophic** (ὑπέρ, excessive; τροφή, nourishment). Idiocy due to hypertrophy of all the cerebral structures, its cause being probably of an inflammatory nature. Mierzejewski (St. Petersburg) has described cortical hypertrophy in *Journal of Mental Science*, Jan. 1879.—**I., inflammatory.** Idiocy caused by a non-traumatic cerebral inflammation—*e.g.*, brain inflammation due to median otitis, rhinitis, or such as follows one or other of the acute specific fevers (Ireland).—**I., Kalmuc** (Kalmuc). A name given by Mitchell and Fraser to idiots who bear a facial resemblance to those described as Mongolian by Langdon Down.—**I., macrocephalic** (μάκρος, great; κεφαλή, the head). A synonym of congenital hydrocephalic idiocy; also those forms of congenital idiocy associated with enlargement of the head, due to hypertrophy of the intra-cranial structures.—**I., Malayan** (Malay). The form of genetous idiocy in which the face assumes a Malayan type. (*See* Idiocy, Forms of.)—**I., microcephalic** (μικρός, small; κεφαλή, the head). Terms for idiots whose heads are less than seventeen inches in circumference (Ireland). (*See* Microcephaly.) — **I., Mongolian.** (*See* Idiocy, Forms of.)—**I., Mongol-like.** The form of genetous idiocy in which the face assumes a Mongol type. (*See* Idiocy, Forms of.)—**I., Negro-like.** The form of idiocy in which the features are marked by a retreating forehead, and thick lips like a negro.—**I. of deprivation.** A name given to those subjects who have developed idiocy by being deprived of the several senses, the cerebral functions thus remaining undeveloped (Ireland).—**I., paralytic.** A name given to idiocy following infantile paralysis (Ireland).—**I., plagiocephalic** (πλάγιος, oblique; κεφαλή, the head). A name given to that class of idiots whose heads are so distorted that the features lie in an oblique plane (Shuttleworth).—**I., scaphocephalic** (σκάφος, the hull of a ship; κεφαλή, the head). That form of idiocy in which the head is keel-shaped.—**I., sensorial** (*sensorium*, the seat of the senses). The same as idiocy of deprivation, the deprivation being congenital.—**I., strumous** (*struma*, a scrofulous swelling). A congenital form of idiocy associated with the scrofulous or strumous diathesis.—**I., toxic** (τοξικόν, from τοξεύω, I shoot with an arrow and so slay; the meaning of τοξικόν became later anything deadly or noxious, and it finally acquired the special signification of any poisonous or deadly influence). A name given to that class of idiots in whom there is no bodily deformity, but mal-nutrition of the brain (Shuttleworth).—**I., traumatic** (τραῦμα, a wound). A name given to those cases in which idiocy has followed some injury to the head during or after birth (Ireland).

IDIOCY, Forms of.—The term idiocy has a very vague significance. It is associated in many minds with one type only of mental and physical condition, very often an imaginary type or one which rarely exists. It will be well to break down such contracted views and to efface the incorrect and distorted image. Looking round a large assemblage of children whose mental condition brings them under this generic term, it is very evident that they can be broken up into well-marked groups, and that instructive life pictures may be drawn of typical representatives of this interesting class. Looked at *en masse* they would give the impression of being heterogeneous to the last degree, but it will be found on closer investigation that it is possible to arrange them into groups with strong natural affinities among the constituents, and that in many cases a very remarkable family likeness may be traced. It is by reference to the variety of forms which such a process enables us to aggregate that light can be thrown on the probable ætiology as well as on the condition and forecast.

Ten per cent. of all cases of idiocy arrange themselves around a highly characteristic type which the writer has proposed to call the **Mongolian** variety. The members of this class are often the latest born of the family, and are connected with a phthisical ancestry. They are characterised by shortness of stature, their heads are brachycephalic, and there is often a remarkable deficiency in the posterior part of their crania. Their hair is usually sparse, and their eyes are obliquely placed, with small palpebral fissures and a great distance between their inner canthi. Their nose is depressed. Their ears are characterised by rounded pinnæ implanted rather far back. Their tongues are abnormally long and have a beef-steak appearance. They have speech, but it is deferred, and always of a guttural character. Their fingers and hands are dwarfed, the integument coarse, and having the appearance of a laundress's soddened hand, or in some cases as if the skin was too abundant. The ligaments of the joints are lax, so that undue mobility is permitted them. They walk and run with a stooping posture, and have [illegible] to adopt the tailor's position [illegible] rest. They are very grotesque, [illegible] humorous side of things, and [illegible] to their high appreciation of [illegible] by their very mobile face. They [illegible] characterised by strong self-will. [illegible] have wonderful imitative power, and [illegible] love of mimicry is very remarkable, [illegible] more so than their persistent [illegible]. They have a very defective [illegible], and have therefore a serious [illegible] to chilblains and frost-bite. [illegible] have little power of resisting acute [illegible]. Nevertheless they occasionally [illegible] the period of adult life. This [illegible] is drawn from a considerable [illegible] of whom it may be said that they [illegible] improvable cases, advantage [illegible] of their remarkable imitative [illegible].

[illegible] contrast to the picture delineated above is the case of the boy who [illegible] entered. Bright and intelligent [illegible] expression, with a well-formed [illegible] the features finely chiselled, the [illegible] planted, no adherent or defective [illegible] and the helix perfect in its contour. [illegible] and attitudes are very [illegible] and agile. He has well-made [illegible], and his finely tapered fingers are [illegible] motion, so that it requires [illegible] to prevent his doing [illegible] to articles of ornament about [illegible]. He hears perfectly, but gives no [illegible], living for the most part in a [illegible] his own, and has no power of [illegible]. He frequently sings and [illegible] picks up fragments of the music [illegible] and hymns he has recently [illegible], and warbles them with a pretty [illegible]. It is clear, therefore, that his [illegible] of speech is not the outcome of [illegible] or complete congenital deafness, [illegible] regard to the quickness of his [illegible], both of legs and arms that it [illegible] by any want of co-ordination. [illegible] a great deal that is said [illegible] when his attention can be fixed, [illegible] to amuse himself by touching [illegible] smelling objects around, or to get [illegible] of wood between his teeth, and [illegible] movements produce some [illegible] sensation of either sound or motion. [illegible] movements ever and anon be[illegible] in character, either bal[illegible] himself on alternate legs, or giving [illegible] motion to his body. When [illegible] observation he resists with all [illegible], and eel-like slips from one's [illegible]. He is impatient of restraint, and [illegible] beyond anything the physical [illegible] of his head. The history of [illegible] is in perfect harmony with clini[illegible] observation. He was the subject of meningitis from injury during the early months of his life, and may be regarded as a typical example of **accidental** idiocy. These facts and the assertion of his mother, leave no doubt that he was born with perfect faculties. With such a history and with such absence of physical deviation the prognosis is most unfavourable. The brain has received great injury, and the future will bear out the aphorism of the writer that "there is more hope from an ill-developed than from a damaged brain."

In strong contrast to this product of accidental origin is the one who now presents himself, and is a typical specimen of the **congenital idiots.**

He walks with a slouching and stooping gait, often breaking out into a tiptoe run. His head is narrow (scaphocephalic) and slightly asymmetrical. His hair is stubborn in its growth and refuses to adapt itself to the conventional form of hairdressing. His height is somewhat below the average of his age, and he manages his lower limbs maladroitly. His eyes are manifestly approximated, the inner canthi being closer together than normal, and he has well marked development of epicanthic folds. He has some amount of nystagmus, and is markedly hypermetropic. His tongue does not obey his will, and when he attempts to protrude it, a mutiny of the muscles carries it back into his abnormally narrow oral cavity. His teeth are decaying, and they are crowded in their jaws, the incisors overlapping one another. They are honeycombed in front from defective enamel, but there is no appearance of the peg-topped or notched varieties. The upper jaw is narrow like the lower, and has moreover a remarkably vaulted roof, the false palate falls down prematurely, and hides from view the posterior wall of the pharynx. The lower jaw besides being narrow falls very far short of reaching the projecting incisors of the upper jaw, so that a receding chin results, while the ascending ramus forms with the horizontal one a more obtuse angle than is usual. With a tongue so unwilling to obey his behests, and with a mouth so ill-formed it is not surprising that his speech is indistinct and halting, and that particular sounds such as the labials and sibilants are with great difficulty produced. His voice both in speaking and singing is discordant and unmodulated, and there is a tendency for the saliva to run over his chin, while he not unfrequently spits when making efforts at speech. His head is remarkably defective, posteriorly, so that his ears appear implanted far back on the cranium, giving a marked facial prominence. The ears are destitute of lobules, the pinnæ are large and flat as if ironed out, and are destitute of helices; moreover the pinnæ are unduly prominent. His hearing is slightly obtuse, but not to such a degree as to interfere with his hearing what is said to him or of catching up tunes. His trunk is bent forward slightly and he has a tendency to lateral curvature of the spine. His knees are flexed and his walk unsteady. His hands are defective as organs of prehension, and he is greatly amused by the automatic movements which he effects with them, while he sways his body backwards and forwards in a rhythmic way. His memory is extremely good for dates and persons, and he acquires arithmetical tables in a wonderful way, and yet is unable to apply the value of numbers in the slightest degree.

We will now select another boy for observation, he presents characters of much interest and is quite the type of his class. His head is markedly dolichocephalic, and when examination is made over the frontal region we are able to distinguish a very marked prominence along the situation of the medio-frontal suture. His expression is intelligent, his hazel eyes flit, however, from one object to another, and it is evident that his attention is readily diverted from what he has under his passing observation. He walks and runs with ease, and is busily employed between his impetuous runs in knotting and unravelling a piece of blind cord. It is very difficult to ascertain whether his hearing is perfect for he does not attend. Real conversation he has none, and if he does make use of words it is confined to the last word of one's sentence, and has the character of an echo of the latest sound. His activity is not confined to his lower limbs, his hands are constantly busy at mischief, and the mischief is the more enjoyed and repeated if it be attended by noisy results. There is slightly increased proximity of the inner canthi and he has very slight converging strabismus. His palate is not unduly arched, his teeth are small and show marks of early decay. His hands are well formed and his feet are quite normal in their structure and function. He is very impatient of restraint and rebels against the manipulations employed in the examination of his head. His ears are well formed, except that their lobules are adherent, and their implantation is normal. He is very self-willed, and screams with a shrill voice to obtain the object of his desire. He is intolerant of not being understood, and uses a sign language with great pertinacity. He bites his hands when in a temper and stamps with his feet to emphasise his wishes. The history of this case is that he was perfectly like a normal child up to the age of eighteen months, that he was interesting with his baby prattle and was able to walk with intelligent purpose. His parents are certain that as a baby he took the notice of people and objects usual to babies, and that in every way he showed no lack of intellectual power. When eighteen months old, however, eclampsic attacks took place, recurring at intervals for a period of three months, and the whole intellectual life of the child became changed. He ceased talking, he lost his inquiring look and gradually acquired a condition which has never ceased to give trouble and care. There is no history of hereditary taint, strict inquiry fails to discover any aberrant form on either side. The mother, about the seventh month of pregnancy, had been suddenly summoned on a long journey to attend the death-bed of her own mother and to take her share in an anxious nursing. There were many circumstances of a family nature which rendered her life a peculiarly embarrassed one, and a great deal of mental tension resulted. The case illustrates very well the class which the writer has proposed to call **developmental**, from the proneness of children who are subjected to such influences in the later months of pregnancy to break down at one of the developmental epochs. In this case it was evidently at the period of first dentition and the prow-shaped cranium, while differentiating it from that of *accidental idiocy*, indicates that the nutritive life of the embryo had been interfered with, resulting in a deferred synostosis of the medio-frontal suture, and in all probability a like arrest of development of the cerebral centres with consequent unstable equilibrium. Had the physical and emotional disturbance of the mother occurred during an early period of embryonic life it would have probably resulted in *congenital idiocy*, with the marks of deformation manifestly imprinted, while in this case taking place towards the end of intra-uterine life, a slight narrowing of the cranium and the prow-shaped frontal bone are the only outward signs of a condition of things which is full of anxiety as to the future intellectual life of the child. The prognosis is more grave than with external configuration more widely departing from a normal type.

Ethnic varieties of idiocy occur other than the *Mongolian* before described.

Negroid forms have been seen by the writer where the whole circumstances of the case precluded the possibility of Ethiopian impregnation. Moreover, the patients have not had a swarthy complexion, have had fair skins but with cranial and facial conformation of the negro. They have had woolly hair, prominent malar bones, puffy lips, and retreating chins, while their protruding eyes were still more exposed by the action of the occipital-frontalis muscle, leaving the forehead corrugated in transverse folds. They manifest great curiosity and acquisitiveness, and frequently are found hoarding pieces of valueless things for the mere sake of acquiring. The miscellaneous contents of their pockets are often very amusing.

Not less frequently specimens resembling the **Malay** family have been noted. They have had prominent upper jaws, large mouths, and long curly hair, their heads narrow, foreheads somewhat protuberant, and with widened noses. The writer has seen several examples where the Malay resemblance has been most marked, they have been free, however, from the ferocious traits which characterise the true Malay. The dolicho-cephalic cranium of the **American Indian** has not unfrequently its representatives among idiots. They are characterised by prominent cheeks, eyes deeply set, and simian-like nose. They have usually been met with in cases so low in type that moral and intellectual characteristics can scarcely be said to exist.

The boy, whose active and ever-restless movement and incessant talk betoken a comparatively bright intelligence, is a very good type of **microcephalic** idiocy. His cranium is small in all dimensions, the circumference not more than 15 inches. His eyes are bright and intelligent looking. The inner canthi are much approximated, and his nose is sharp and aquiline. He has a curious movement of his head from below upwards, with a somewhat sudden jerk. He runs with a stooping gait, and when he stops bears the weight of his body by resting his hands on his thighs a little above the knees. When running or walking he fails to bring his heels to the ground. He speaks in a chattering manner, repeating many of his short sentences over and over again. He reads easy words and can count, is fond of praise, and imitates the attitudes, movements, and sayings of those about him. About all he does and says there is a chirpy liveliness, and an apparent sageness in marked contrast to what would be expected from the contents of a cranium so diminutive. Although eighteen years of age he manifests no sign of puberty. He catches tunes very readily, and imitates with his mouth various musical instruments. His teeth are extremely small and regular, and there is no marked overcrowding, although his jaws are small.

In strong contrast to the microcephalic boy is the youth whose head has a circumference of 25 inches, with all the dimensions of his cranium in like proportion, but well formed. There is an absence of preternatural bosses, and the sutures give no indication that the size of the cranium is due to fluid. He walks circumspectly, and when in the act of prehension does it in a slow and deliberate manner, even the temptation of taking food to his mouth (and he is particularly fond of eating) does not induce him to feed himself in other than the most deliberate way. He talks, but it is in the same slow manner, and only in response to questions. His sentences are short, and their utterance tardy. Even when excited by the promise of reward he speaks with only slightly increased utterance. His progression is by slow walking, and no inducement makes him run. He is rather below the ordinary stature, has no deformity except that his fingers are shorter than normal. His face is largely developed, and his nose correspondingly so. When questioned he frequently makes feeble movements of his lips without utterance of sound, and only gives audible response when stimulated to do so. He is seventeen years of age, and the signs of puberty are not wanting. Though slightly dolicho-cephalic, the boy presents very typical features of *macrocephalic* idiocy, the outcome of hypertrophy of the white substance of the cerebrum. The last two cases illustrate in a very forcible way the truth that quality is as important a factor as quantity in cerebral organisation.

Very different is the child of ten years, whom we will now describe. His head is of greater size, reaching 30 inches in its circumference; it has a globular form, the fontanelle is raised, but there is no marked vaulting of the palate, the forehead is prominent, and the frontal and parietal bones are very large and thin. The face is small and pale, and in its size forms a marked contrast to the expanded cranium whose widened sutures are characteristic of *hydrocephalic* idiocy. He says a number of words, but does not construct sentences. He sings or rather hums simple airs which he has from time to time heard. His eyes are more distant from one another than usual, and they wander about when one speaks to him, so that it is difficult to determine whether he perceives. He is very affectionate and discriminates between those who wait upon him.

A form of idiocy which may be termed *cretinoid*, and is not unfrequently associated with an arrest of growth at either the first or second dentition. The child under observation is a female aged six years. Her height is 22 inches, her skin is of an earthy colour, dry and parchment-like. She is fairly well proportioned although diminutive. Her hair is scanty, and her eyes are somewhat obliquely placed. The areolar tissue generally is unduly developed, and above each clavicle there is a small tumour of a soft and yielding character. There is no evidence of the existence of a thyroid gland. Her forehead is wrinkled from the undue exercise of the occipito-frontalis muscle. The tongue is large and rugous, and a portion of it usually protrudes from the mouth. She understands all that is said to her, and sees the fun in humorous sentences. Her face is very mobile, and she takes great pleasure in making "faces" which give rise to laughter in others. She can say a few monosyllabic words, but is unable to construct sentences. She is vain and fond of clothing having a bright showy colour. She is very affectionate to those she likes, takes great objection to others, especially to those who have inadvertently passed some unflattering remark in her hearing. She is fond of music, but does not sing. She stands and walks by the aid of a sofa or chair, but cannot balance herself alone. The teeth have decayed prematurely. She is very self-willed and obstinate, is fond of dramatic exhibitions, and claps her hands if they please her. The writer has had several similar children under his observation, some living to be twenty-four years of age, but all retaining their infantile characteristics.

All the varieties of idiots enumerated above are subject to epilepsy in a far greater degree than those not the subjects of idiocy. There is, therefore, no characteristic class of epileptic idiots. The *developmental* variety is probably the most liable to attacks of epileptic convulsions, and the *Mongolian* the least. The time most liable to the occurrence of epilepsy is the developmental period of puberty. Of the gross number of idiots of all kinds as many as 25 per cent. may be regarded as ordinarily epileptic.

There is a class of feeble-minded people characterized by inco-ordinate movements of a chronic kind, and which by way of distinction may be called *choreic* idiots. When any voluntary effort is made the limbs assume a spastic rigidity. These cases are much more intelligent than outward appearance would lead one to believe. They are appreciative of shades of meaning, of plays upon words, they communicate by signs, and have no lack of the faculty of languages. They may be taught to hold a pencil, and are able with properly adapted arrangements to write letters. In spite of their maladroitness they have great happiness in their lives. They are the outcome of the use of instruments in parturition, but more frequently from the delay in calling them into use, and consequent prolongation of the birth. It should always be borne in mind that there is more danger from delayed instrumental assistance than from its early and expert employment.

The boy whom we have first under observation is quiet in repose, but directly he desires to express his pleasure, his wishes, or his fears, he is thrown into wonderful contortions. His history is that of instrumental birth. Another boy has the same contortion-producing state. He is one of twins, was the first-born of the family, was the subject of prolonged pressure at birth, and was born with suspended animation. His brother, whose birth was unattended by difficulties, is normal, both physically and mentally. Cases of this class have sufficient intelligence and appreciation of their condition to render it undesirable to express opinions respecting them, or sympathy for their condition, as they are extremely sensitive to such remarks.

Hemiplegia is occasionally met with associated with idiocy, but the connection is not markedly with any special class of idiots. Idiocy is also sometimes associated with pseudo-hypertrophic paralysis. Some of the most characteristic kinds of this disease have, in the writer's opinion, been allied to mental feebleness. Some time since three brothers came under observation, and in each the progressive disease was distinctly associated with well-marked mental weakness.

Idiocy is very rarely associated with disseminated sclerosis, probably from the rareness with which syphilis is a factor in idiocy. In one case only has the writer met with the combination of locomotor ataxia and congenital idiocy.

There is a very interesting class of children which is not at all similar to the classes previously described. They are full of vivacity, quick in their movements, quick in their perverted thoughts, and everlastingly in clever mischief. Unlike many others already discussed, they do not live in a world of their own, but interfere adroitly with all that goes on around them; they are observant, impetuous, cruel and destructive. They have no necessarily characteristic criminal conformation. They acquire languages readily, but in their case this is not an unmixed good, as they weary those around them with questions and inconveniently appropriate to their use the language of the gutter. They are so restless and mischievous that they need constant watchfulness, and have such a **mercurial** character that it does not seem an inappropriate name for this type.

Idiots, like sane people, are liable to mental perturbation, and are occasionally the subjects of acute mania or melancholia. Hallucinations of sense and delusions are occasionally met with.

In like manner, among idiots, are found special instances of extraordinary memory, of great calculating power, of histrionic ability, of musical art, or of great manipulative skill. They have been called **idiots savants**. They are to be found in most institutions devoted to idiots, and are usually members of the *congenital* kind. They are interesting as aberrant mental forms occurring in youths who are by no means intellectually strong in other particulars. They are to be regarded as exceptions from, not examples of, the classes which the writer has endeavoured faithfully to delineate from nature.

J. LANGDON DOWN.

IDIOCY, Pathology of.—It is desirable to remember with reference to this subject, that though much of it may be similar to that found in general medicine, yet there are differences and exceptions, which it will be the object of the writer to point out. The facts stated in this article are chiefly taken from the notes of autopsies made by him, aided in a few cases by published facts on the subject. It should also be borne in mind that the pathology is chiefly that of patients between five and twenty years of age.

Anæmia and Hyperæmia of the Brain.—Pure anæmia of the brain has rarely been found to exist, and uncomplicated hyperæmia is exceedingly uncommon. The hypostatic congestion occurring during the last few hours before death, and the hyperæmia which occurs after death are, of course, excluded. In the few cases in which uncomplicated pathological congestion was present, the vessels of the diploë in the calvarium were found congested, the veins of the dura mater and pia mater were loaded with blood, as were also the sinuses and choroid plexuses. The grey substance of the brain was of a dark-red colour, and there was an increase in the number and size of the drops of blood which are seen on making sections of the brain. In some cases, there was tortuosity of the vessels running transversely outward from the longitudinal sinus, a moist condition of the brain substance, and an increase in the amount of the sub-arachnoid fluid. In one case there was congestion of the right hemisphere of the brain, corresponding to a capillary nævus which occurred on the right side of the face during life. At the autopsy there was excess of sub-arachnoid fluid on this side, and the vessels were loaded with blood. The pia mater was exceedingly injected, especially over the frontal and parietal regions, less so over the superior temporo-sphenoidal convolution and occipital lobe. The excessive injection of the pia mater gave a pinkish hue to the whole of the right hemisphere.

Hypertrophy of the brain is a comparatively rare disease, but it is necessary that it should be considered, as, in the chronic stage, it is usually mistaken for chronic hydrocephalus. The cause of the affection, which may be general, or partial, is obscure. In general hypertrophy the process is not one of mere increased growth, but the nutrition of the organ is modified in character, as well as increased in activity. According to Virchow, the increased size of the brain is due to hyperplasia of the neuroglia. Rokitansky, on the other hand, thinks the augmented bulk is not produced by new fibrils, or by the enlargement of those already existing, but by an increase in the intermediate granular matter, most probably due to an albuminoid infiltration of the structure. Our own observations lead us to the opinion that the disease, as seen in imbeciles, is due to what appears to be granular matter, but whether this is due to an increase in the intermediate granular matter, or to an increased amount of connective tissue, which has broken down as the result of post-mortem change, we are at present unable to determine. Andral states that in two autopsies made by himself, the white matter resembled the white of egg hardened by boiling. In one post-mortem only have we noticed any peculiarity in the white matter, and in that case we find we have recorded that it is of "a peculiar whiteness." As a rule, the brain is found anæmic on section, but in some of our autopsies there was congestion of the membranes, a pinkish colour of the brain, an increased quantity of sub-arachnoid fluid, and some fluid in the lateral ventricles.

In these cases there was an increase in the number of blood-vessels, and the presence of a large number of leucocytes. On removing the skull-cap, which is sometimes increased in thickness, at others thinned, the convolutions are found to be flattened and so pressed together, that the sulci seem to be obliterated. The parts affected are the white matter of the two hemispheres, sometimes the corpus striatum and optic thalamus, rarely the pons and cerebellum. MM. d'Espine and Picot consider the affection to be a congenital one, and in this opinion we concur. They hold, however, that imbecility only results when hypertrophy of the brain is accompanied with sclerosis. Our experience does not lead us to this opinion, for in only one of the post mortems which we have made was sclerosis present. The principal symptoms are headache, at times intensified, excitement followed by coma, blunting or arrest of development of the intelligence, difficulty in walking, and convulsions. The symptoms are less marked in children than in adults, because the brain is less compressed, the cranial cavity increasing in size as the brain enlarges. Andral states that there are two periods in the disease. In the first, the chronic stage, the symptoms are slight; in the second, unless the patient has been previously carried off by the intervention of some other disease, those characterising an acute affection appear, and the patient dies of convulsions, of symptoms indicative of compression of the brain, or acute hydrocephalus. In the eight cases which we had under our care, four died of convulsions, two in a comatose condition, and the remaining two were carried off by diarrhœa or bronchitis. None of our cases presented signs of rickets.

As to the weights of the brains in such cases, the accompanying table gives the weights of eight hypertrophied brains, and a glance at it will show that there is a great difference between the weight of these and the average weight of brains of persons of the same age.

The diagnosis of hypertrophy of the brain from chronic hydrocephalus chiefly rests on the history of the case, and the form and size of the head. Dr. West remarks that "the symptoms of chronic hydrocephalus generally come on earlier and soon grow more serious than those of hypertrophy of the brain, and the cerebral disturbance is throughout more marked in cases of the former than in those of the latter." Our distinctive diagnosis of hypertrophy of the brain from chronic hydrocephalus rests on the following points.

Table showing Weight of Hypertrophied Brains and Average Weight of Brains of Individuals of the same Age.

Initials of Name.	Age.	Weight of Hypertrophied Brains.	Average weight of Brains (Dr. Sims' tables).	Average weight of Brains (Dr. Boyd's tables).	Average weight of Brains (Dr. Beach's tables).
A. H. S.	5	49½	39	40.23	40½
A. G. D.	8	53	40	45.96	39
T. J.	10	55	40	45.96	40
F. D.	11	49	44	45.96	41
P. D.	11	49½	44	45.96	41
W. J. E.	14	52	44	45.96	41
A. H.	15	62	44	48.54	42
A. C.	10	55	40	45.96	40

In hypertrophy of the brain, as a rule, the head does not attain so large a size as in chronic hydrocephalus.

In hydrocephalus the increase in the size of the head is most marked at the temples; in hypertrophy above the superciliary ridges.

In hypertrophy the head approaches the square in shape; in hydrocephalus it is rounded. In hydrocephalus there is often an elasticity over the late closed fontanelle; in hypertrophy there is none, and there is often a depression in that situation.

In hydrocephalus the distance between the eyes is increased from the fluid inserting itself between and distending the sutures formed by the frontal and ethmoid bones; in hypertrophy this is not the case.

Partial hypertrophy is even rarer than the general form, and some authors are of opinion that, in many of the cases which have been described as such, the enlargement was really due to gliomatous or other tumours.

Atrophy of the brain may be general or partial; it may be congenital or acquired some time after birth. The most common form of general atrophy is a small brain, such as is found in microcephalic idiots. We do not intend to enter fully into a description of this kind of brain, as it is treated of under MICROCEPHALY. In this form there is incomplete development, and it is usually congenital. The smallest brain we have seen weighed 7 ounces, yet a minute examination of it showed that nearly all the convolutions were present, though very small in size. In this brain, as well as in some others in our possession, there was great narrowing of the frontal portion, corresponding with the narrow forehead so often seen. The occipital convolutions were not well developed; in consequence, the brain was shortened and often being in the proportion of 1 to 3 or 4, the ordinary relation being 1 to 8.

Partial atrophy may be congenital or acquired. In the congenital form there is

FIG. 1.

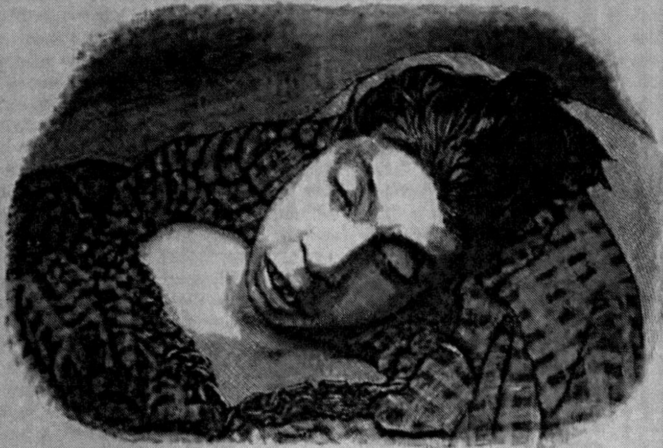

E. R., microcephalic idiot, from a photograph taken after death.

FIG. 2.

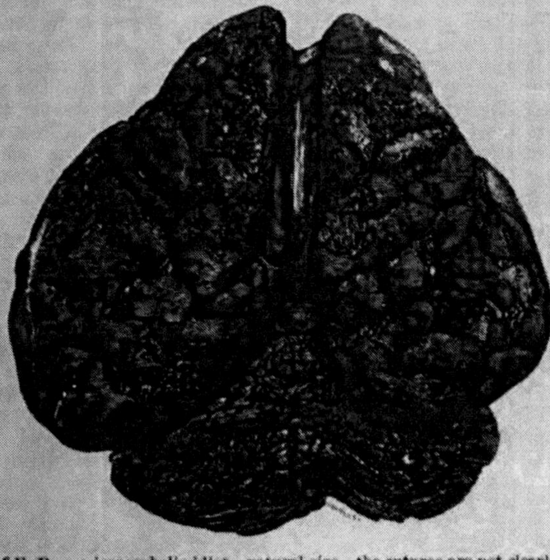

Brain of E. R., a microcephalic idiot—natural size—the sutures are not clearly shown, as the membranes have unfortunately not been removed.

the cerebellum was to a great extent left uncovered. As a rule, the nerves of special sense are well developed, and the ganglia of the base and the spinal cord are of normal size. The cerebellum is relatively larger than in the normal brain, non-development, or incomplete development, of certain portions of the brain. Cases are on record where there was absence or atrophy of the cerebellum; deficiency of the pineal gland; defects of the fornix; a rudimentary condition of the olivary bodies, optic thalamus, and corpus striatum; atrophy of the optic commissure; and atrophy or even entire absence of the corpus callosum. In none of our autopsies have we found the corpus callosum totally absent, but we have seen it incompletely developed in one case, a small and narrow body being present.

In the acquired form of atrophy there is a loss of nervous elements which had previously existed. This may occur during fœtal life or early childhood. In a case recorded by Dr. Warner and the writer there was intra-uterine wasting of the lower part of the ascending frontal and parietal convolutions, the whole of the supra-marginal with its lobule, and the superior temporo-sphenoidal. Cases of atrophy of one side of the brain, usually the left, with co-existent atrophy of the limbs of the opposite side of the body are not infrequent. An inflammation of the brain, meninges, or skull, occurring before birth, or coming on afterwards, will no doubt cause this disease. The paralytic form of idiocy seems to depend upon an atrophy of the brain, caused by chronic meningitis or inflammatory processes in the cortical substance. In one of the most marked cases of atrophy of the brain which has come under our notice the left diseased hemisphere weighed only 5½ ounces, while the right weighed 15½ ounces. The usual appearances found, post-mortem, are thickness of the cranium, opacity and thickness of the membranes, effusion of serum into the sub-arachnoid space, sometimes into the ventricles and atrophy of one hemisphere, including the corpus striatum, optic thalamus, and pons of the affected side. Since the fibres of the superior peduncles of the cerebellum undergo a complete decussation beneath the upper pair of the corpora quadrigemina, and those of the middle peduncles decussate in the pons Varolii, while the fibres of the pyramids of the medulla have their well-known crossed direction, there is atrophy of the cerebellum and of the spinal cord on the opposite side.

The course of events appears to be this: First, there is, as the result of chronic inflammation of the meninges, or of the cortical substance, wasting of one side of the brain. To compensate for this the skull becomes thickened, and serum is poured out beneath the arachnoid and into the ventricles. Then, since those parts of the brain which are connected with motion are wasted, the limbs whose action is governed by them are imperfectly nourished and become atrophied.

With reference to the microscopical appearances found in atrophy of the brain, a case is quoted by Dr. Major in the *Journal of Mental Science* for 1879, in which especial attention was paid to this point, with the following result.

The cortex of the convolutions of the affected side was seen to be reduced in thickness, and under a low power seemed to be made up of small round cells of uniform size, here and there only a pyramidal corpuscle being observable, in marked contrast with the appearances in the cortex of the opposite hemisphere. Examination with higher powers showed that the nerve-cell elements were extremely few, as well as small, ill-developed, and deficient in branches. The intercellular matrix of the neuroglia was denser and coarser than in the right hemisphere and under normal conditions. In the internal white matter the nerve-fibres were nearly absent in some places, the whole tissue being represented by numerous Deiter's connective tissue-cells with their dense intercommunicating network, naked nuclei and occasional vessels. The atrophied lobe of the cerebellum showed a condition of thickness and wasting of the outermost grey layer, few and ill-developed cells of Purkinje, and excess of connective-tissue corpuscles.

The spinal cord was not examined by Dr. Major, but was so by Dr. Taylor in a case related by him. There was shrinking of the anterior grey cornu and of the antero-lateral column of the affected side, but the number and size of the ganglion cells of the anterior cornua were almost identical. The cells on both sides were, after staining, identical in colour, in structure, outline, and processes, with those of the opposite healthy side. There was nowhere any degeneration of the nerve-fibres in the white columns, and the dorsal and lumbar regions were distinguishable in no respect from those of a healthy cord.

Softening of the brain may be general, or affect only certain parts. The usual seats are the corpus striatum, optic thalamus, central white matter of the hemisphere and the convolutions. The inflammatory form is not common; more often softening is due to a diminished supply of arterial blood, or to a feeble state of the circulation. As a rule, the affected portion of the brain is white in colour. The chief causes in our experience are the effusion of fluid into the ventricles and sub-arachnoid space, chronic hydrocephalus, thrombosis of the middle cerebral arteries and superior longitudinal sinus, tubercular or simple meningitis, and the presence of a tumour. When there is effusion of fluid in the lateral ventricles, which may be due to a feeble state of the circulation, leading to venous thrombosis, or to a diminished supply of arterial blood, as in the case of arterial thrombosis, the portions of the white matter of the brain surrounding the ventricles, the corpus callosum, optic thalamus, fornix and septum lucidum are the parts affected. They are also affected in chronic hydrocephalus, and were so in the cases of tubercular meningitis seen by the writer. The convolutions are often softened when there is excess of fluid in the sub-arachnoid space, or when the fluid is altered in character as the result of meningitis. On microscopical examination there is found only remains of nerve filaments, granular cells due to degeneration of the cells of the neuroglia or of nerve cells, granular fatty débris, particles of myeline and blood cells. The latter are usually changed in form, and their remains are often seen in the form of pigment or hæmatoidine crystals. The capillaries are usually dilated or present aneurysmal swellings.

Sclerosis of the brain is usually described as being diffuse or multiple. Diffuse cerebral sclerosis involves large portions; multiple cerebral sclerosis is disseminated in patches. Excluding acquired atrophy of the brain involving one hemisphere, as before described, which is an extensive diffuse sclerosis, the disease as a rule affects a considerable portion of one lobe or the whole of it. It is not distinctly circumscribed, and is said to involve the medullary substance chiefly and the grey matter rarely. So far as idiots and imbeciles are concerned, this cannot be said to be the case, for the grey matter was affected in five out of eleven autopsies in which diffuse sclerosis was found. It should however be said that in these five autopsies the medullary substance was also implicated. The white matter of the convolutions was affected in six, and that of the centrum ovale in five cases. Reduction in amount of substance was not equally marked, for in six cases the medullary and in two the cortical matter was so affected. The convolutions involved were the frontal in six, the ascending frontal in four, the ascending parietal in three, the parietal in four, the angular gyrus in one, and the occipital in five cases. The optic thalamus was sclerosed once. We have noticed that the affected portion of the white matter was sometimes like "white of egg," and in some cases it presented a honeycombed appearance. The increased hardness and density which the tissue acquires is due to an increased formation of the neuroglia with a disappearance of the proper nerve-tissue. In one case we found great increase in the number of the vessels, many of which were distended, and in addition there was extensive infiltration of the tissue with leucocytes, especially in the peri-vascular sheaths. In some cases there was an excess of fibrous tissue around the vessels. No doubt the sclerosis is due to a chronic inflammation of the meninges, as is seen in cases of inherited syphilis, or of the brain substance, and hence the microscopical appearances observed. It only remains to be said that this form of sclerosis is more common among males than females. The paralysis and atrophy of the limbs observed is of course due to the loss of the nerve-substance which controls their actions.

Multiple or disseminated sclerosis is not so common as the diffused form. It consists of numerous spots or nodules, scattered throughout the cerebrum, cerebellum, pons Varolii, medulla oblongata, and spinal cord. In the cerebral hemispheres the patches are found especially on the walls of the lateral ventricles (in one autopsy we found no less than five here), in the white substance of the cerebrum ovale, the septum lucidum, corpus callosum, and the basal ganglia. The cerebellum presents a few of these nodules and they are found in the central white matter. The convolutions of the brain and cerebellum are usually exempted. Many nodules are found in the pons, medulla oblongata, basal ganglia and the peduncles of the cerebrum and cerebellum. These lesions affect the whole of the spinal cord, and invade all the column, attacking the grey matter as well as the white. When seen through the pia mater, they appear as brown spots which change to a salmon colour on exposure to the atmosphere. They vary in size from a pin's head to a bean in the spinal cord, but in the brain they attain a larger size. They are usually circumscribed, and are tough or even cartilaginous in texture. The cranial nerves and the anterior and posterior roots of the spinal nerves have sometimes been found affected. The membranes of the brain and spinal cord are either normal or present signs of congestion and chronic inflammation. The cerebro-spinal fluid is increased, and is sometimes cloudy, and the ventricles are dilated. On examining the sclerosed patch microscopically, the trabeculæ of the neuroglia are seen to be thickened, the nuclei are swollen and increased in number, and Deiter's cells are large and well defined. The medullary sheath gradually disappears, but the axis cylinder remains. Finally the nodule consists of a wavy fibrillated structure, and all trace of nerve-tissue is lost. The walls of the vessels are thickened, the lumen diminished, and the adventitia is blended with the surrounding connective tissue. If the grey substance becomes involved, the nerve cells will become atrophied.

Hydrocephalus is frequently present, especially the chronic form. The acute affection will be described later on, when disease of the membranes is treated, and we confine ourselves now to chronic hydrocephalus. In this affection, there is an accumulation of serous fluid in the ventricles and in the arachnoid sac, so that the arachnoid membrane is often pushed upwards by it. The quantity varies from a few ounces to several pints. In one case we found as much as three pints present and both lateral ventricles were enormously dilated, extending from the posterior part of the occipital region to the anterior extremity of the frontal lobe. The openings by which the ventricles communicate with each other are dilated, and the septum lucidum, commissures, fornix and corpus callosum are stretched or even destroyed, while the surrounding brain substance is either softened, of normal consistence, or harder than usual. The cerebral hemispheres are flattened, the convolutions spread out, and the sulci obliterated. The parts at the base of the brain, including the nerves, are pressed downwards, flattened and sometimes distorted. The membranes are thin and softened, but the ependyma of the ventricles is usually thickened and rough, presenting the so-called "ice plant" granulations. The cranial bones in the autopsies we have made were thin and transparent, but they are sometimes thickened and spongy. Chronic hydrocephalus is said to be due to arrest of development of the brain, or to chronic inflammation of the ventricular lining membrane. According to Rokitansky, it results from repeated and continued active congestions of the ependyma of the ventricles and choroid plexus. The diagnosis between chronic hydrocephalus and hypertrophy of the brain has already been given, and it now only remains to mention that the hydrocephalic head is quite different from that found in rickets. In hydrocephalus the fontanelle is raised: in rickets it is depressed, and the head is elongated in the antero-posterior diameter. In hydrocephalus it approaches the globular form, and the antero-posterior, and transverse diameters are nearly the same. The widest circumference is often at the temples, where there is sometimes a perceptible bulging above the usual place of greatest width around the superciliary ridges.

Closely allied to chronic hydrocephalus is the condition named **porencephalus**, in which fluid takes the place of the brain in various parts. Generally the cavity is found on the surface of the cerebral hemisphere, and it may communicate on one side with the arachnoid sac, or be separated from it by the visceral arachnoid, and extend through a considerable extent of medullary substance. The defect may be acquired or congenital. In the following case, for which we are indebted to our friend Dr. Shuttleworth, a gap, four inches long, was found extending from the anterior part of the right frontal lobe nearly to the occipital, leaving the orbital plate uncovered, and disclosing part of the cavity of the lateral sinus. Internally, a narrowed ridge, marked by convolutions, separated this gap from the longitudinal sinus; and between it and the temporo-sphenoidal lobe was seen standing out, quite uncovered by convolutions, part of the caudal nucleus. The brain weighed 32½ ounces. The defect was probably of the nature of an arrest of development. There was no appearance of cicatricial tissue, and no descending sclerosis to be made out in sections of the spinal cord. The following cases we believe to be due to an acquired condition. In one case, the posterior half of the left and the posterior third of the right lobe were occupied by fluid; in another the anterior third of the right lobe, and the posterior halves of both lobes were filled with fluid; in a third case the right hemisphere consisted of a simple large sac, with thin walls of cortical substance. In five cases cysts were found, varying in size from a hazel-nut to a walnut. Some contained clear straw-coloured fluid; in others it was gelatinous in character. The parts affected were the third ventricle, the right lateral ventricle, the right occipital lobe, the convex surface of the right frontal region and the parietal lobe. In one case there were no less than six cysts. The spastic paraplegia so often seen in idiots and imbeciles, is no doubt often due to this condition of the brain.

The tumours of the brain chiefly found are tubercular, or gliomatous in origin. The former are the more common. In one autopsy there were no less than three tubercular masses present; one the size of a sixpence, situated half an inch in front of the fissure of Rolando; one as large as a shilling over the superior occipital convolution at its junction with the posterior parietal, and the third on the under surface of the cerebellum. They extended about half an inch into the substance of the brain. There was disease of the knee-joint in this case. Gliomata are said to vary in size from a cherry-stone to a closed fist. The largest one which the writer has seen was of the size of a small apple, and was situated in the right frontal region, half an inch posterior to the anterior border of the right lobe, the internal margin being bounded by the superior longitudinal fissure. Its lower surface was partly in front of and partly formed the roof of the right lateral ventricle. The convolutions directly over it were flattened out over a space about one inch and a half in length by one inch and a half in breadth. In one case a psammomum was found, growing from or attached to one of the choroid plexuses in the lateral ventricles. In another case a bony growth existed, which grew from the inner surface of the dura mater, in the position of the longitudinal sinus. The growth was a quarter of an inch in length, and was as large as a crow-quill.

Asymmetry of Hemispheres and Convolutions.—Excluding the asymmetry of the hemispheres and convolutions due to wasting disease, there is sometimes found inequality in size. In an autopsy made by the writer, the left hemisphere was larger than the right, the former being 6½ inches long, and 4½ inches broad, while the latter was only 5¾ inches in length, and 3⅞ inches in breadth. The difference in size appeared to be due to the convolutions, which were normal in size and arrangement on the left side, but on the right, while the frontal portion was normal, the convolutions of the parietal and especially of the occipital regions were very small. The convolutions of the ascending parietal region, according to the author's experience, are frequently asymmetrical; in one case there was a nest of very small convolutions which replaced it on the left side. General asymmetry of the convolutions on both sides is frequently found.

Alteration in Relation of Grey to White Matter of Brain.—When treating of sclerosis it was mentioned that there was reduction of both the grey and white substance, but an altered relation of the one to the other sometimes exists when sclerosis is not present. In all our cases of hypertrophy of the brain, the white matter was in excess, and in addition we have noticed that of six cases the white matter was in excess in five, and was reduced to a mere line in one case. This extreme reduction of the white matter was also found in four cases of sclerosis.

Simplicity of convolutions, both in size and arrangement, is often seen. It is not at all uncommon to find convolutions half an inch and sometimes nearly an inch in width. It is obvious that in such cases their arrangement must be very simple. On the other hand, convolutions smaller than normal are sometimes present. This was notably seen in a case of microcephalic idiocy. As a rule, when the convolutions are simple, all of them are more or less affected, but sometimes particular convolutions only are involved. On referring to our notes of autopsies, we find that the frontal convolutions were found to be simple in seven, the parietal in eight, the ascending frontal in four, the ascending parietal in seven, and the temporo-sphenoidal in five cases. In ten of these thirty-one autopsies there were combinations of convolutions affected. The angular gyrus is recorded as being simple once, and the island of Reil three times. The convolutions of the under surface of the brain were sometimes simple when those of the convex surface were normal in size. Generally the convolutions of certain regions of both sides were equally affected, but in four autopsies only those of one hemisphere were involved.

Thickening of the arteries is not often found, since, as we explained in the introduction to this article, the pathology does not refer to cases above twenty years of age. In one case, however, a boy aged sixteen years, there was seen to be thickening of the two vertebral and internal carotid arteries, and the right middle cerebral artery. The vertebral and internal carotid arteries were not only thickened, but when cut through remained patent.

Thrombosis may of course be arterial or venous, but as far as our experience goes, venous thrombosis is the more common. In seven autopsies where the condition was present, venous thrombosis was found five times, and arterial thrombosis only twice. The case mentioned under the heading of thickening of arteries was one of these, and the other was a boy aged thirteen years, in which the thrombus occurred in one of the branches of the right middle cerebral. It is curious that, in both these cases, the *right* middle cerebral artery contained the thrombus. In both there was excess of sub-arachnoid and ventricular fluid.

The superior longitudinal sinus was affected in all the five cases of venous thrombosis; the cavernous sinus also contained a thrombus in one case and the lateral sinus in another. In two cases the veins running into the longitudinal sinus were filled with thrombotic masses, and were so exceedingly brittle, that they snapped across when the dura mater was removed. In one of these five cases the brain was very soft; in the four others the lateral ventricles were dilated, and contained an excess of fluid. Embolism we have never seen.

Disease of the membranes of the brain is often found, and chronic meningitis is much more common than the acute form. Both affect chiefly the convex surface of the brain. The most frequent signs of the former disease are congestion and thickening of the dura mater; thickening and opacity of the arachnoid membrane, adhesion of the membranes to each other, of the dura mater to the skull, and of the pia mater, which is usually highly injected, to the brain, so that, on stripping it off, portions of the cerebral substances are torn away with it; increase of subarachnoid fluid, which is either clear, turbid, or converted into a soft purulent material; and an excess of clear or flocculent serum in the ventricles, which are usually dilated, and their lining membrane thickened and sometimes rough. Occasionally there is seen a thickened false membrane on the under surface of the dura mater, covering the convex surface of the brain, and extending for some distance along its base. This was found in five autopsies. In some cases, especially when syphilis is the cause, the brain is atrophied.

The acute form is either simple or tubercular. In simple acute meningitis the cerebral arachnoid is dry, opaque or greasy looking, and the pia mater is extremely vascular, with patches of opacity in places. A small quantity of generally turbid serum is found in the sub-arachnoid space, or there is a yellowish exudation, consisting of pus corpuscles and granular fibrin. This covers the surface, and is seen chiefly in the sulci between the convolutions and along the larger vessels. The cortical substance of the brain is sometimes softened and the ventricles are usually empty.

Tubercular meningitis we have only found in two cases, and in these the disease ran a lengthened course. The miliary tubercles are seen in the meshes of the pia mater, and are white or yellow in colour. In our cases they were found along the longitudinal and Sylvian fissures, the middle cerebral artery, and on the pons and medulla. The membranes at the base were thickened, opaque, and the meshes filled with yellowish exudation, especially about the optic chiasm and along the Sylvian fissures. In both, the ventricles were dilated and filled with serum, and the central parts of the brain much softened.

The diseases of the cerebellum most commonly met with are atrophy, tumours, and cysts of that organ.

Atrophy of the cerebellum is usually found in connection with atrophy of the brain, and when one side is affected, there is atrophy of the cerebellum on the opposite side. The reasons for this are given under the heading of atrophy of the brain.

Tumours of the cerebellum are usually tubercular in character. Cases of this kind are fully described by Dr. Ross. We have only seen tumours of the cerebellum three times; on two occasions the tumour was tubercular, and affected in one case the inferior vermiform process, and in the other the right lobe; in the third case it was fibrous, and was found in the substance of the left lobe. In this case there was great effusion into the lateral ventricles of the brain, and as a consequence the convolutions were flattened out and the sulci obliterated; both lobes of the cerebellum also were distended with fluid, and on examination the thin cerebellar substance gave way, and a thin-walled cyst came out of the left lobe, and collapsed as soon as it escaped. The cyst wall appeared to be of a fibrous texture. The fluid was examined to see whether a cysticercus was present, but with a negative result.

The chief affections of the spinal cord which are associated with idiocy and imbecility are, anterior acute polio-myelitis, giving rise to infantile spinal paralysis; congenital arrest of development of the pyramidal tracts, occurring in connection with porencephalus or a descending sclerosis of the pyramidal tracts, both giving rise to the spastic paraplegia of infancy; descending sclerosis of one side in connection with disease of the brain, and chronic myelitis. Pseudo-hypertrophic paralysis, though not a nervous disease, is said to be often associated with mental defect.

It is unnecessary to describe the appearances in infantile paralysis, further than by saying that the chief changes are found in the muscles and nervous system. The muscles have lost their normal striation, their contents are granular, and many are reduced in size; with reference to the nervous system, there is destruction of the ganglion cells of the anterior horns of the spinal cord.

Chronic transverse myelitis may end in softening, or be associated with ascending sclerosis of the columns of Goll and descending sclerosis of the pyramidal tracts of the lateral columns; sometimes the transverse myelitis is accompanied by central myelitis, which may extend forwards so as to destroy the ganglion cells of the anterior horns. In three autopsies we found the spinal cord softened, and in two, sclerosis of the columns of Goll and of the pyramidal tracts. Descending sclerosis of one pyramidal tract in the lateral column, on the side opposite to a cerebral lesion, is not infrequently seen.

As far as the membranes are concerned, we have found external spinal pachymeningitis, in connection with disease of the vertebral column, internal hypertrophic pachymeningitis, or thickening of the dura mater, and tubercular spinal leptomeningitis occurring together with cerebral tubercular meningitis.

Anomalies of the Convex Surface and Base of the Cranium.—The convex surface is often thinner than normal, and on holding it up to the light, it is seen to be diaphanous, especially in the region and neighbourhood of the anterior fontanelle, which sometimes is found to persist. Very often the arch of the cranium is not only thickened, but eburnated. In cases of unilateral atrophy of the brain, the skull is thickened on the same side to compensate for the wasting; at other times there is asymmetry, corresponding to the smaller size of one lobe of the brain. In a case where the right lobe was smaller than the left, the circumference of the right half of the calvaria measured 8½ inches, while that of the left half measured 9¾ inches. Sometimes there is asymmetry, due apparently to dilatations formed by the brain growing towards the side where there is least resistance. In one case the left side of the cranium was fuller and rounder than the right, but the right side of the forehead was squarer than the left, which receded gradually. In another case the forehead projected more on the right side than the left. In a case where rickets was present, the parietal bones overlapped the frontal, so that a ridge was present. When nearly all, or all the sutures of the convex surface become closed after birth, or when the patient is very young, a microcephalic skull is formed. In this kind of skull there is often great falling away of the front part towards the temporal region, which is found to correspond with an oval, and in some cases almost pear-shaped, brain. Sometimes the cranium is too narrow, owing to premature ossification of the sagittal suture. In these crania there is usually elongation in the antero-posterior diameter, by enlargement of the frontal and occipital regions, and thus a scaphocephalic skull exists. When there is too early ossification of the lambdoidal and coronal sutures, the skull is too short, and compensation often takes place in the region of the anterior fontanelle, and so conical or sugar-loaf heads are formed. In cases of chronic hydrocephalus and in hypertrophy of the brain, the skull is larger than normal. In hydrocephalus it is rounded in shape, in hypertrophy it is usually square; in hydrocephalus, the increase in the size of the head is most marked at the temples; in hypertrophy above the superciliary ridges.

Turning now to the base of the skull, the anomalies there found are supposed to be due to disorders in nutrition of the bone and cartilage. The most interesting deviation from the normal is that which is found in cretinism, where, according to Virchow, there is premature synostosis of the two parts of the sphenoid bone together and with the basilar process, and a steep descent of the clivus, or inclined plane formed by the union of the basilar process of the occipital bone with the sphenoid, reaching to the posterior clinoid processes. In all our autopsies there was ossification of the basilar process of the occipital with the sphenoid bone, but the bone in that situation was very thin and easily penetrated by the knife. The clivus was always very steep. Generally there was an elevated line round the foramen magnum, and often the sella turcica was narrowed from before backwards.

As far as the spine is concerned, there is usually posterior angular curvature and occasionally caries of parts of the vertebral column.

The pathology of idiocy would be incomplete if reference were not made to **sporadic cretinism** (Fig. 3). We are unable to say much about it, as the subject is treated of by Prof. Horsley,* but it is one in which we take great interest. Long ago, and previously to the publication of the report of the committee appointed by the Clinical Society to investigate the subject of myxœdema, we were convinced that there was a close relation between the two diseases, and that in fact myxœdema and sporadic cretinism were the same disease. We were led to this conclusion partly from the observation of cases of myxœdema kindly shown to us by Dr. Ord in the wards of St. Thomas's Hospital, and from an extensive acquaintance with the clinical signs of sporadic cretinism, many cases having been under our care; and partly from the fact that the intrinsic

* *See* CRETINISM.

pathological appearances are common to both. We had the opportunity a year or two ago to make a more extended examination than usual of a case of sporadic cretinism, and we found excess of mucin in the skin, and excess of fibrous tissue in the lungs, liver, spleen, and kidneys. More we cannot say, as the case will shortly be published. Usually, in sporadic cretinism, there is no thyroid gland, but cases are on record, and we have had one under our own care, in which a goîtrous condition was present. Concurrently with the usual absence of the thyroid gland is the presence of fatty tumours in the posterior triangles of the neck. The convolutions of the brain are simple in arrangement.

We close this article with a short account of the **microscopical appearances of the brain** in idiocy.

The cells as a general rule are not pyramidal or irregularly angular, but are round or pear-like in shape. The nucleus, which is either round or oval, is usually situated in the centre, with retracted protoplasm around, and externally there is either a clear space or faintly stained granular matter. Occasionally the nucleus is situated at the base, sometimes at the apex. The cells have few processes, and these are small and stunted.

FIG. 3.

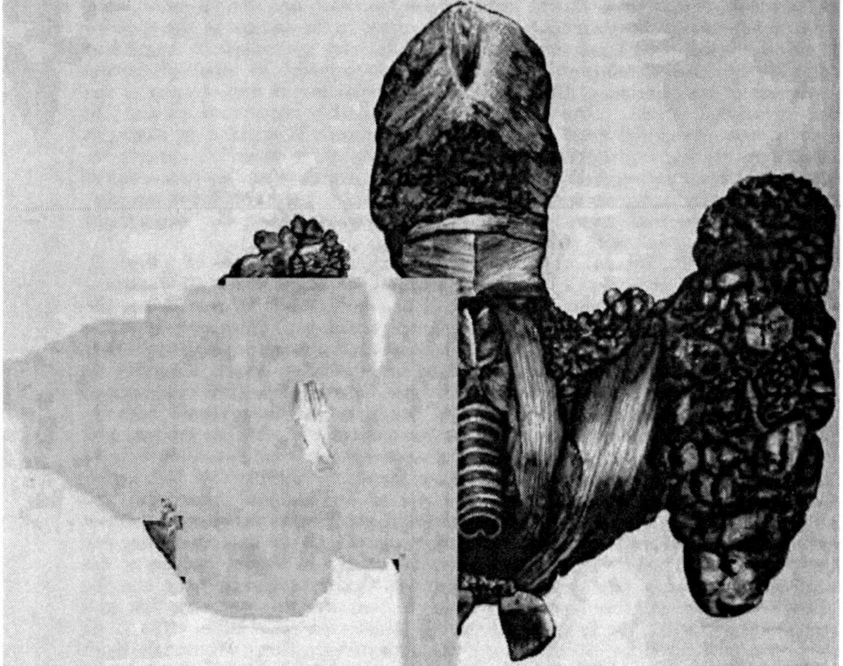

In the centre is seen the trachea with the sterno-hyoid and thyroid muscles turned aside. Outside these are the sterno-mastoid muscles and still externally are the fatty tumours.

The apical process is nearly always present. Now and then there are processes and no spaces, and then the cell is irregularly angular in shape. Sometimes a

FIG. 4.

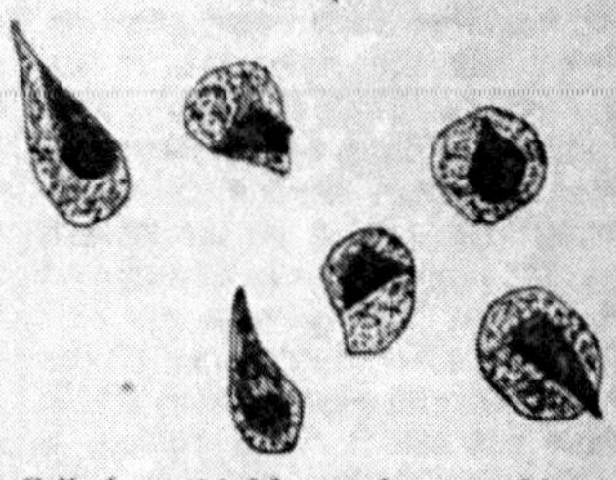

Cells from third layer of cortex of frontal convolution of a microcephalic idiot, showing nucleus, retracted protoplasm, and granular matter. The retracted protoplasm and granular matter are represented too dark in the woodcut.

curious honeycomb appearance is seen, from the accumulation of a number of cells with clear spaces. The above remarks apply to hardened sections. In frozen sections the nucleus is deeply stained, the protoplasm a little less so, and there are no clear spaces. The cells are of the same shape as above mentioned. Generally there is only one process, and at most only three or four. The apical process is always present; all stain deeply, and the secondary branches

FIG. 5.

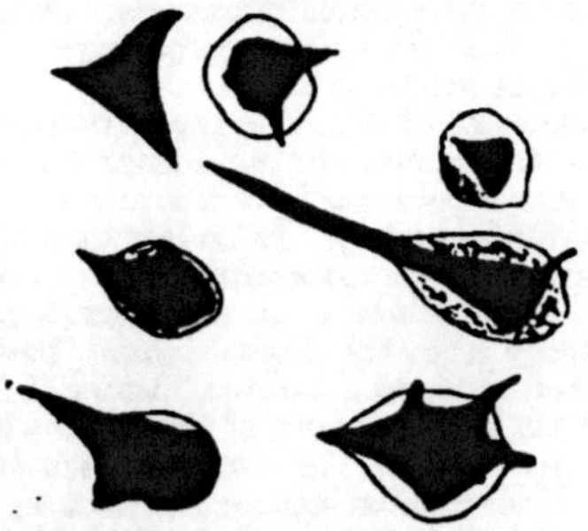

Cells from third layer of cortex of frontal convolution of a cretinoid idiot, showing nucleus, retracted protoplasm, and granular matter. The retracted protoplasm and granular matter are represented too dark in the woodcut.

are finely attenuated. The stunted appearance so frequently seen in hardened sections is not found.

In hardened as well as frozen sections, it is often difficult to make out more than five layers, and the third is the one chiefly affected. The nuclear vacuolation described by some authors we have not seen. FLETCHER BEACH.

IDIOCY AND IMBECILITY, ÆTIOLOGY OF.—In treating of the ætiology of idiocy and imbecility the joint authors of this article have endeavoured to combine their individual experiences (as set forth in their respective papers presented to the Annual Meeting of the British Medical Association in 1889), reference being also made to other published opinions on the subject.

The causes of idiocy and imbecility may be conveniently classified under three heads, according to the period at which their influence has come into operation, as follows:—

(1) Those acting before birth.
(2) Those acting at birth.
(3) Those acting subsequently to birth.

Class 1 will of course comprise causes dependent upon parentage, such as insanity, imbecility, epilepsy or other neuroses, alcoholism, syphilitic taint, tubercular and other morbid tendencies which the family history may disclose. Consanguinity of progenitors: old age or exhausted procreative powers of one or other parent; abnormal mental or physical conditions of the mother during gestation, are also included under this head; and the influence of illegitimacy may be considered in this connection.

Class 2 comprises: (1) Premature birth; (2) Difficult labour; (3) Instrumental delivery; (4) Accident at birth; (5) Asphyxia neonatorum. The relation of primogeniture and of twin birth to imbecility will also be discussed under this head.

Under **Class 3** we include: (1) Infantile convulsions (eclampsia); (2) Epilepsy and cerebral affections; (3) Febrile illnesses in childhood; (4) Paralytic affections; (5) Sunstroke; (6) Nervous shock; (7) Physical injury to head. The vexed question of overpressure at school comes in here for consideration.

It will be remarked that, as a rule, many causes combine together to produce imbecility. Most of the causes enumerated under Classes 1 and 2 may be looked upon as *predisposing;* whilst those in Class 3 are *exciting* causes. A congenital predisposition to nervous instability leads to an intellectual breakdown under the strain of some crisis of child-life, which under other conditions would be safely surmounted; and these cases Dr. Langdon Down classifies as *Developmental.*

Some few cases are clearly *accidental,* as those in which the head has been seriously injured in a fall; but in the great majority the influence tending to imbecility may be traced back previous to the child's birth, if only sufficient information can be gained. From this point of view the congenital far outnumber the non-congenital cases, though the statements of relatives would favour the opposite conclusion.

In estimating the ætiology of each case of idiocy and imbecility, it will be more scientific to sum up the various factors contributory to the condition than to attempt to discover a single cause. Taking those grouped under Class 1 we shall find that out of a total of 1180 cases taken from the Darenth Asylum case-books, intemperance was combined in 196 with the following causes:—phthisis, insanity, imbecility, epilepsy, syphilis, consanguinity, excitability, chronic neuralgia, abnormal conditions of the mother during pregnancy, premature labour, disease of the brain and paralysis. Further analysis shows that intemperance was combined with one cause alone in 90 cases, the most frequent associations with it being insanity, epilepsy, phthisis, and worry of the mother during pregnancy. Intemperance was combined with 2 other causes in 58 cases, with 3 in 25, with 4 in 18, with 5 in 4, and with no less than 6 in 1 case. On comparing the causes, we find that anxiety and worry of the mother during pregnancy were present in 33 cases, phthisis in 38, insanity in 24, and epilepsy in 24, while excitability was present in 13, fright of the mother during pregnancy in 16, imbecility in 13, and consanguinity in 10 cases. The least common combinations were ill-usage of the mother during pregnancy, disease of the brain, premature labour and syphilis.

Hereditary predisposition is a most potent predisposing cause, and accounts for a large number of cases. Confining our attention for the present to the combinations of the different factors, and remembering that the total number of cases from which the figures are taken is 1180, we find the following causes associated together—viz., insanity, epilepsy, imbecility, chronic neuralgia, excitability, extreme nervousness, disease of the brain and hysteria.

The most frequent combination of two causes is that of insanity with epilepsy, which accounts for 20 cases; insanity with epilepsy and other causes is present in 14 more cases; insanity occurring with imbecility alone is found in 6, and with imbecility and other causes in 3 cases. Insanity associated with the other causes accounts for 20, making a total of 63, or 5.3 per cent.

Then taking epilepsy, and excluding its combination with insanity, we find epilepsy with imbecility alone present in 6 cases, and with imbecility and other causes in 5, making a total of 11 cases; epilepsy with other causes accounts for 26 cases. If we add to these numbers those of epilepsy with insanity and other causes, we obtain a grand total of 71 cases, or 6.01 per cent.

Excluding insanity and epilepsy, imbecility is present in combination with other causes in 11 cases, and associated with epilepsy and insanity in 24, making a total of 35, or 3.0 per cent.

The most common combinations then are insanity, epilepsy, and imbecility with one another, or with other causes, and the total percentage of the combinations is 8.98. The other causes are also found associated together in a few cases, but it is not necessary to make special examination into them. Enough has been said to show that many causes act together in producing idiocy and imbecility.

Before proceeding further, it is advisable to mention that the facts which follow are, with few exceptions, the result of analyses of 2380 histories, of which 1200 are recorded in the Royal Albert Asylum case-books, and 1180 in those of the Darenth Asylum. The former asylum admits chiefly patients from the industrial and middle classes, a few being of wealthier parentage, while the latter only receives the children of paupers. A table on p. 664 shows the percentage under different heads.

Class I.—Taking the causes under this head separately, our experience leads us to give a prominent position to a *phthisical family history*. In no less than 28.31 per cent. of our cases such a history exists. Dr. Down, whose cases are taken almost entirely from the higher social classes, states he found a marked history of this disease in 25 per cent. of the fathers, and 20 per cent. of the mothers. We have not discriminated between the parents, nor have we reckoned the factor twice, when the taint exists in both. Dr. Grabham gives 22 as the percentage of phthisical history in the Earlswood cases. It is interesting to note that a family history of phthisis is frequent in imbeciles of the so-called "Mongol" type.

Next in order comes a history or indication of *inherited mental disease*. Our figures give a percentage of 16.47 with family history of insanity, and of 4.69 per cent. with family history of imbecility, equivalent together to 21.38 per cent. of inherited mental weakness. Dr. Down speaks of 16 per cent. on the father's side, and 15 per cent. on the mother's side; and Dr. Grabham refers to 18 per cent. of his cases in which hereditary taint is admitted. In addition to the number mentioned above, there were a few where the parents or ancestors were queer, dull, strange, peculiar, low and despondent, or eccentric.

Neurotic inheritance plays an important part as a cause. Epileptic patients are to a great extent excluded from the Royal Albert Asylum, but are freely admitted into the Darenth Asylum. Our figures give 8.69 per cent. with family history of epilepsy, and 11.30 per cent. with a history of neuroses other than epilepsy, making a total of 20 per cent., in which hereditary neurosis exists. These neuroses include—besides epilepsy—chronic neuralgia, excitability, extreme nervousness, hysteria, deaf-dumbness, disease of the brain and paralysis. Many of these causes are interesting, as they exemplify some of the metamorphoses of heredity.

Dr. Morel, in his "Traité des Dégénérescences," says, "We do not mean exclusively by heredity the very complaint of the fathers transmitted to the children, with the very identical symptoms, both physical and moral, observed in the progenitors. By the term heredity we understand the transmission of organic dispositions from parents to children." Moreau of Tours also says, "Just as real insanity may be hereditarily reproduced only under the form of eccentricity, so a state of simple eccentricity in the parents, a state which is no more than a peculiarity or a strangeness of character, may be in the children the origin of true insanity."

Dr. Maudsley mentions the case of a lady who suffered for some time from an intense neuralgia of the left half of the face; after the removal of a tooth suspected to be at the root of the mischief, the pain ceased, but an attack of melancholia immediately followed.

Menckel gives instances where the deaf-muteness of ascendants was transformed in their descendants into an infirmity of some other description, such as, hardness of hearing, obtuseness of the mental faculties, or idiocy. These causes are all forms of a neurotic diathesis, and therefore predispose to mental unsoundness in the children.

Parental alcoholism is, according to our experience, the fact next in order connected with family history, occurring in a percentage of 16.38 of our cases, according to the best information we have been able to obtain. This is rather in excess of the number given by Dr. Down, who states that in 12 per cent. of the fathers and in 2 per cent. of the mothers there was "avowed and notorious intemperance." No doubt the difference is due to the more frequent prevalence of drunkenness in the lower classes, for Dr. Shuttleworth's histories give a percentage of 13.25, which is nearly the same as that of Dr. Down, while at Darenth Asylum the percentage is found to be 19.57. If we were to push back our inquiries through the grand-parental generation and scrutinise the habits of six progenitors (as Dr. Kerlin, Superintendent of the Pennsylvania Institute for Feeble-minded Children, has done) our percentage would probably be not very different from the 38 per cent. which he gives in his ætiological table, published in the "Proceedings of the Association of Officers of American Institutions for Idiots." Dr. Beach found, on going through his histories, that there was a history of intemperance in the grand-parents in 22 cases, making a total of 253 patients with a history of intemperance, thus raising his percentage from 19.57 which was given above, to 21.44. He found that the intemperance was chiefly marked in the father, but in 12 cases the mother drank, and in seven cases both father and mother gave way to drink. In a few cases he found that intemperance was a family failing. Thus, in three cases the father's side of the family are described as intemperate, and in one of these the male side had been intemperate for many generations. In one case only was the mother's side given to drink, but here the result was very marked, for, not only was the patient in the Asylum an imbecile, but her two cousins were imbeciles also. In two cases sporadic cretinism was present in the children, and in one, three children in the family were microcephalic idiots.

The influence of a *syphilitic taint* in the causation of idiocy has been already discussed by us in papers communicated to the International Medical Congress at Washington in 1887. We stated that in our experience the characteristic signs of inherited syphilis were rarely met with amongst idiots, though, no doubt, with a more complete knowledge of parental histories, it might prove to be a more common factor in the arrest of cerebral development than at present appears. With special attention directed to this point, we have, however, so far been unable to ascertain the existence of syphilitic taint in more than 28 out of our 2380 cases, a proportion equivalent to 1.17 per cent. At the discussion which followed on the reading of our papers, Dr. Down stated that he agreed with the views we expressed, and that, not only from his clinical experience, but also from pathological investigation, he was of opinion that not more than 2 per cent. of idiots are the subject of congenital syphilis; this opinion was formed not only from his experience as an alienist, but as a physician to the London Hospital. In the majority of cases, the mental deficiency has not been noticed until the age of the second dentition, from which time gradual degeneration has ensued, probably from atrophic changes due to diminished calibre of cerebral arteries and thickening of membranes. That this is the true view is borne out by a well-marked case which came under the care of Dr. Beach, in which the pathological changes above mentioned were found at the autopsy.

With regard to *consanguinity* of progenitors as a cause of imbecility, various estimates of the proportion of consanguineous marriages have been made by Messrs. Boudin, Dally and Legoyt in France; and in this country by Dr. Langdon Down, Sir Arthur Mitchell, and Mr. George H. Darwin; but these estimates vary so much that it seems impossible to adopt, with any degree of certainty, a standard for comparison. We must be content with approximate guesses, and if we take the calculations of Professor Darwin, based upon the number of *same name* marriages, as most reliable, and also assume that consanguineous marriages are as fertile as those of strangers in blood, we shall find that the proportion of idiot children, who are the offspring of cousins, is not much in excess of the ratio of consanguineous marriages to marriages generally. In London, Darwin estimates the proportion of first-cousin marriages as 1.5 per cent.; Dr. Beach, whose cases are drawn from the London district, finds that 2.03 per cent. are the progeny of first cousins, a slightly higher proportion. In rural districts Darwin estimates the proportion at about 2.5 per cent., and in provincial towns at 2.0 per cent. Dr. Shuttleworth, whose patients are drawn from both these classes, states that 2.9 per. cent. of his cases are known to be children of first cousins. It is true that Dr. Down's statistics give a higher proportion—viz., from 4.75 to 5.4 per cent. of children of first cousins, but it must be remembered that his cases are derived from the higher social class, amongst whom marriages of consanguinity are more common than with the ordinary population.

The figures above given refer to first cousin marriages alone, in which presumably the influences at work attain their highest point; but if we include all consanguineous marriages, higher percentages will be obtained—viz., 2.54 by Dr. Beach, 5.83 by Dr. Shuttleworth, and 6.50 by Dr. Down.

Until legislative wisdom concedes some statistical information as to the frequency of cousin marriages, either in connection with the census or with the registration of marriages, we must continue to grope in the dark as to the comparative safety (*quâ* idiocy) of such marriages. We should, however, temper our purely statistical conclusions by such consideration of the facts of each case as may bring to light concurrent factors. In nearly all Dr. Down's cases, and in two-thirds of those of the authors of this article, causes for idiocy were discovered, in addition to the consanguinity of the parents, which would have been accepted as operative causes, had no consanguinity existed. No doubt morbid heredity, and especially morbid mental heredity, is likely to be intensified in the offspring of cousins; a notable case exemplifying this was one, where the father was intemperate, the grandfather intemperate and imbecile, and the mother's father was paralysed. On the whole, it does not seem probable that bad effects are produced otherwise than by the intensification of bad heredity common to both parents, and such is the conclusion of Dr. Bourneville and other authors who have inquired into the subject.

Passing now from causes connected with *family history* to those more *personal to the parents*, we have first to consider *abnormal conditions of the mother during gestation*.

Of course we must accept with caution much that mothers tell us on the subject, for they are apt to put down to this cause the idiocy and imbecility of their children, when other and more potent causes are present. Nevertheless, in a certain number of cases, we shall find good ground to believe that maternal debilities, either physical or mental, are truly responsible for the imperfections of the offspring. Dr. Shuttleworth's statistics give 21.41 and Dr. Beach's 38.47 as the percentage of such cases, mental abnormal states, such as worry, fright, &c., being about three times as numerous in Dr. Shuttleworth's, and 6½ times as numerous in Dr. Beach's cases, as depressing causes of a physical nature. The higher percentage given by Dr. Beach is probably due to the low physical and mental condition of many of the parents of his patients.

No doubt the *influence of the father's state*, both mental and physical, at the time of the procreative act resulting in conception, is an important factor in the production of idiocy, though it is one not easy to estimate. Instances have been noted in which the temporary mental condition of the father, arising from business anxiety and worry, seems to have been responsible for begetting an idiot child, and Dr. Down, as is well known, has adduced evidence in favour of one particular type—the sporadic cretin—being often associated with drunkenness in procreation. Later researches appear however to show that this is not such an influential cause as has been supposed, at any rate as regards the lower classes of society. *The old age of the father* in some few cases seems to be a cause of idiotic offspring; and the "Mongol type" of idiocy is frequently connected with the *advanced age* and impaired functions *of the mother*, more than half of such cases being the last children of a long family.

Sir Arthur Mitchell has laid some stress upon *illegitimacy* as a cause of idiocy. Statistics upon this point will necessarily differ considerably with the country and class from which the figures are drawn; our own notes give 1.76 per cent. of illegitimate children among the patients at the Royal Albert and Darenth Asylums. Of course, *emotional* causes will come specially into play in illegitimate cases. Kind says that in Hanover the percentage of illegitimate idiots is 9.5; whereas the general proportion of illegitimate to legimate births is 6 per cent.

Class 2.—We have included amongst "causes acting at birth" *premature birth.* Of course, this may be due to some of the causes already considered, such as maternal debility, or the presence of a syphilitic taint; but in some instances, probably, the bad start in life, consequent upon premature entrance into the world, may account for a backward condition of the intellectual powers, amounting in extreme cases to imbecility. Such cases have an aspect resembling that of idiots of the "Mongol type," and are often feeble physically as well as mentally. 3.52 per cent. of our cases were prematurely born. We notice that *attempts to procure abortion* are debited in certain American statistics with the production of idiocy, but we have been unable to obtain reliable evidence on this point.

Importance has been attached by Dr. Down and other authorities to the relative preponderance of *first-born children* amongst idiots; 24 per cent. of Dr. Down's cases being "primiparous." Dr. Grabham states that of 1100 cases at Earlswood, 23 per cent. of the males were first-born and nearly 25 per cent. of the females, a result contrary to what we should expect, were the cause simply due to pressure in parturition. We do not think that primogeniture is so perilous, *quâ* the production of mental defect, as has been suggested; other causes no doubt play a more important part.

Our cases furnish only 20.67 per cent. of first-born children, which exceeds but slightly the percentage to be expected, taking an average family as numbering five children.

Prolonged parturition is doubtless a considerable factor in the production of idiocy. Dr. Shuttleworth's statistics are admittedly imperfect on this point; but those of Dr. Beach give a ratio of 27.28 per cent. On combining the figures we obtain a proportion of 17.5 per cent. Of these the much larger number (14.24) are attributed to *protracted pressure without instrumental interference;* only 3.31 per cent. are attributed to *forceps delivery.* In comparatively few of the latter, however, were injuries noted due to the use of the forceps; and there is no doubt that prolonged parturition is more detrimental than delivery by forceps.

Prominence has been given to this subject during the last two years, in consequence of the statement of Drs. Winkler and Bollaan, who, in a paper published in a Dutch medical journal, said, that they were disposed to think that the use of forceps was much more frequently the origin of idiocy than is generally supposed. This statement was at once contradicted by Drs. Langdon Down and Fletcher Beach. Not only does prolonged compression of the head result in asphyxia, but a number of the cases, when born, are in a helpless condition, some having lost the use of their legs, others becoming subject to convulsions; moreover, the head is often crushed, distorted, or otherwise injured.

When death ensues early, meningeal hæmorrhage is found on the convexity of the brain, thickest over the central zone, and in some cases with actual cortical laceration. In the cases that suffer from convulsions, or spastic contractions of the limbs with inco-ordination and athetoid movements, atrophy of the convolutions in the central region is found.

On the other hand, in the cases which have been delivered by forceps, only a few are helpless or paralysed.

Asphyxia neonatorum was only stated in 153 of Dr. Beach's histories, a proportion of 12.96 per cent.; but there is no doubt that it was much more frequently present, for tedious or difficult labour is noted in 322 cases. Dr. Down states its frequency of occurrence as 20 per cent. amongst idiots generally, and 40 per cent. amongst those who are first-born children. Dr. Gowers has pointed out that of 26 cases of cerebral birth palsy, 16 were first-born children.

Occasionally idiocy is attributed to some *accident happening at birth,* such as injury to the head from the precipitate birth of the child into a chamber-pot in a sudden labour, or to hæmorrhage from the umbilical cord. Such accidents are alleged in 1.51 of our cases.

Twin birth is sometimes stated to be the cause of a child's idiocy, the mother pointing to the perfect twin as a proof that imbecility was not inherent to the conception. Of our cases 0.96 were twin-born and in many of these the other twin is also imbecile.

Class 3.—*Causes acting after birth* are more willingly alleged by the friends than congenital causes, owing to the stigma they consider attaches to congenital defect; in consequence caution is needed in accepting these statements. After going carefully through the information at our

Table of Causes of Idiocy and Imbecility in 2380 Cases Abstracted from the Royal Albert Asylum and Darenth Asylum Case Books.

—	Royal Albert Asylum—1200 cases.		Darenth Asylum—1180 cases.		Total—2380 cases.	
	Number of Times Recorded.	Percentage.	Number of Times Recorded.	Percentage.	Number of Times Recorded.	Percentage.
I. Causes acting before birth :—						
Family history of (A) Phthisis	291	24.25	383	32.45	674	28.31
" (B) Insanity	182	15.17 } 20.08	210	17.79 } 22.71	392	16.47 } 21.38
" (C) Imbecility	59	4.91 }	58	4.91 }	117	4.69 }
" (D) Epilepsy alone	41	3.41	116	14.06 } 36.86	207	8.69 } 20.0
" (a) Other neuroses	—	—	269	22.79 }	269	11.30 }
" (E) Intemperance	159	13.25	231	19.57	390	16.38
" (F) Syphilis	16	1.33	12	1.01	28	1.17
Parental or grand-parental :—						
(G) Consanguinity	70	5.83	30	2.54	100	4.20
Abnormal condition of mother during gestation :—						
(A) Physical	66 } 257	21.41	59 } 454	38.47	711	29.87
(B) Mental	191 }		395 }			
Old age of parents	3	0.25				
Illegitimacy	23	1.91	19	1.61	42	1.76
II. Causes acting at birth :—						
Premature birth	37	3.08	47	3.98	84	3.52
Primogeniture	228	19.00	264	22.36	492	20.67
Prolonged parturition :—						
(a) Protracted pressure	57	4.75	282	23.89	339	14.24
(b) Instrumental delivery	39	3.25	40	3.38	79	3.31
(c) Asphyxia	* —	—	153	12.96		
Accident at birth	27	2.25	9	0.76	36	1.51
Twin birth	17	1.41	6	0.50	23	0.96
III. Causes acting after birth :—						
Infantile convulsions (Eclampsia)	391	32.58	261	22.11	652	27.39
Epilepsy and cerebral affections	57	4.75	136 (epilepsy)	11.52	193	8.11
Paralysis (infantile)	15	1.25	7	0.50	22	0.92
Injury to head from fall, blow, &c.	99	8.25	48	4.06	147	6.17
Fright or shock (mental)	27	2.25	46	3.89	73	3.06
Sunstroke	8	0.66	5	0.42	13	0.54
Febrile illnesses—*e.g.*, scarlatina, whooping-cough, measles, typhoid fever, small pox	119	9.91	23	1.94	142	5.96
Overpressure at school	3	0.25	1	.08	4	0.16

* Owing to absence of this heading in earlier Case-books of Royal Albert Asylum, information is imperfect on this point, but *Asphyxia* is recorded in 20 out of 171 recently admitted cases, equal to a percentage of 11.7. It may be noteworthy that 15.3 per cent. were males, 5.0 per cent. females.

command we have come to the conclusion that about two-thirds of our cases are of congenital origin, and not more than one-third are accidental or acquired. As Dr. Down has pointed out, an innate tendency to brain defect may remain latent until some crisis of development, such as the period of second dentition or of puberty, and such cases he classes as *developmental.*

The most frequently alleged cause of idiocy and imbecility is no doubt *eclampsia* (*infantile convulsions*). To this cause about one-third (32.58) of Dr. Shuttleworth's, and more than one-fifth (22.11) of Dr. Beach's cases are attributed. The combined percentage is 27.39. In many, however, there are other contributory causes; and the consideration always suggests itself, that many children suffer from severe convulsions during teething, and yet escape being idiots. In one case, convulsions came on in consequence of a quantity of brandy being drunk by the child. Another case was very interesting; five weeks after the patient's birth the mother was suckling the child and fretting in consequence of the intemperate habits of her husband; the child, while at the breast, had a fit, and convulsions have occurred from time to time ever since.

Epilepsy and cerebral affections account for a percentage of 8.11. Dr. Shuttleworth's fifty-seven cases are due to brain disease of an active kind, such as acute hydrocephalus, and other forms of inflammation of the brain and its membranes; while Dr. Beach's 136 cases are entirely due to epilepsy.

As before mentioned, epileptic cases are to a great extent excluded from the Royal Albert Asylum, but in the Darenth Asylum one-third of the patients are subject to epileptic fits. The epilepsy was attributed to injury, a fall, fright, or masturbation. These are usually cases in which there is strong hereditary predisposition and the children are born with a very unstable brain. The presence of this predisposition is proved by the fact that no less than 338 (out of 1180 cases) of convulsions or disease of the brain occurred in other children of the family in which there was an idiot or imbecile child. After one of the causes above mentioned, epilepsy comes on, and imbecility is the result. Fortunately, under the influence of medicinal and hygienic treatment, the fits in a certain proportion of cases can be reduced in number and sometimes cease altogether; when the latter result is attained, the imbecility as a rule disappears. Such, at least, has been the experience at Darenth, though diverse views are held on this subject by various authorities.

In 147 cases (6.17 per cent.) there was a history of *severe injury to the head* from falls, blows, &c., the falls being often from the arms of a careless nurse, or down a flight of stairs. In estimating this cause it became necessary to exclude a large number in which epileptic fits followed, as the imbecility appeared to be more due to the epilepsy than the injury.

Fright is alleged as a cause in 73 cases (3.06), and what the parents call a *stroke*, in 22 cases, or 0.92 per cent.

Febrile illnesses, such as scarlatina, measles, typhoid fever, small-pox, and whooping-cough, are said to account for as many as 142 cases (5.96 per cent.) acute brain symptoms being associated with the majority, and in the rest general defect of nutrition apparently causing cerebral atrophy.

Sunstroke has been given as a cause in 13 cases (0.54 per cent.), many of these being children from India.

It is certainly remarkable that in these days of forced education, we have only met with 4 cases in which *over-pressure at school* has been alleged as the cause of the imbecility.

Mr. Galton tells us in his book on "Natural Inheritance" that "we appear to be severally built up out of a host of minute particles, of whose nature we know nothing, any one of which may be derived from any one progenitor, but which are usually transmitted in aggregates, considerable groups being derived from the same progenitor. It would seem that, while the embryo is developing itself, the particles more or less qualified for each new part, work, as it were, in competition to obtain it." If this be true, it would seem clear that a hindrance to the working of the particles qualified for the production of the brain would lead to imperfect development, and so would be the origin of idiocy and imbecility.

The law of retrogression by which, Mr. Galton says, the child is certain to reproduce not only some of the qualities of its father and mother, but also of remote ancestors, may account for the appearance of an idiot in a family, where the other children are healthy.

Geo. E. Shuttleworth.
Fletcher Beach.

IDIOCY IN ITS LEGAL RELATIONS.—The legal incidents of idiocy are now of comparatively little importance, owing (1) to the gradual displacement by modern scientific knowledge, and indeed by recent legislation,* of the old *presumptio juris et de jure*,† that idiots

* *Cf.* The Idiots Act, 1886, 49 Vict. c. 25.
† *See* Presumptions (Legal).

are incapable of being educated and trained, and (2) to the provisions of, and the practice under, the Lunacy Regulation Act, 1853, s. 47, now the Lunacy Act, 1890, s. 98, sub-s. 1, which limits the evidence admissible in proof of unsoundness of mind, upon a commission *de lunatico inquirendo*, to a period of two years before the date of the inquiry,* and raises an uniform issue—viz., the state of mind of the alleged lunatic at the time when the inquisition is being held.

A rapid sketch of the legal history of idiocy may still, however, be of interest and value. Fitzherbert† traces the origin of the royal jurisdiction over idiots to an assumed principle of the common law, which put every loyal subject under the king's protection, and therefore, *à fortiori*, charged him with the duty of caring for the estates and persons of those who were incapable of managing themselves.

This explanation, although rational, is unfortunately not historical, and the law of idiocy appears to have pursued the following course of development.‡

The incapacity of any feudal vassal to perform the services on which his tenure rested, entitled the superior to seize upon his rents and profits, and thus to procure a fulfilment of the condition upon which the estate had been granted. That this privilege existed with regard to *infancy* is indisputable; lunacy was perhaps treated as a mere temporary sickness, but idiocy seems to have been dealt with as permanent infancy. In consequence of the abuses which took place under this feudal *régime*, the custody of the persons and inheritances *idiotarum et stultarum à nativitate* was given to the Crown, probably in the reign of Edward I., by an Act, which is now lost, but the substance of which was repeated in the following reign, by the famous statute *de praerogativa Regis* (17 Edw. II. cc. 9 & 10). Under this enactment, the king was to have the rents and profits of an idiot's lands to his own use, during the life of the idiot, subject to an obligation to provide him with necessaries; and upon the idiot's death the lands were to be restored to his heirs. In the case of lunacy, however, the king was merely a trustee, holding the lands and tenements of the lunatic for his benefit and that of his family.

Neither the term *idiota* nor the term *lunaticus* was, however, made use of in this statute. The statutory distinction drawn is between the *fatuus naturalis* and him *qui prius habens memoriam et intellectum non fuerit compos mentis suae*. Now, although Coke defines an idiot as one "which from his nativitie, by a perpetual infirmitie, is non compos mentis," it is clear that the old writs* of inquiry, addressed to the king's escheators, recognised an idiocy which was not *a nativitate*, but had commenced subsequent to the birth of the party, and that the escheators themselves were eager to sweep as many forms of mental disease as possible within the category of those "natural fools," over whom the Sovereign had acquired under the statute such a lucrative jurisdiction. When persons *non compotes mentis*, however, says Collinson,† became distinguished into the two classes of idiots and lunatics, distinct writs were framed for each of them, one *de idiota inquirendo*, and the other *de lunatico inquirendo*. The former gradually fell into desuetude, partly perhaps from the generosity of the Crown,‡ but chiefly from the strong dislike evinced by juries to returning a verdict which was attended with such serious consequences.§ As has been already mentioned, the Lunacy Regulation Act, 1853, s. 47,‖ has made the old law of idiocy of little practical importance.

A. Wood Renton.

IDIOLOGISM (ἴδιος, peculiar; λόγος, a word). A term used by the late Ach. Foville, to denote the characteristic expressions employed by insane persons possessed by ideas of persecution.

IDIOPHRENIC (φρήν, the mind). A term used for that form of insanity due to disease of the brain itself.

IDIOSYNCRASIA OLFACTORIA (ἰδιοσυγκρασία, a peculiar temperament or habit of body; from ἴδιος, peculiar; σύγκρασις, a mixing together; *olfacio*, I smell an odour). Any perversion of the sense of smell.

IDIOSYNCRASY (ἴδιος, peculiar; σύν, together with; κρᾶσις, constitution). A term used in medicine to denote any peculiar and obviously non-correlated perversion towards certain external influences.

* Without special leave from the Master or Judge presiding at the trial.

† "Natura Brevium," edit. 1794, p. 232.

‡ Collinson's and Shelford's treatises on lunacy may be consulted on this subject with great advantage.

* See Collinson, vol. i. p. 117. *E.g.*, by one form, inquiry was to be made whether the party was *idiota et fatuus a nativitate sua an alio tempore*.

† Vol. i. p. 120.

‡ *Cf. ex parte Watson*, 1821 (Jacob's Reports, at p. 161).

§ Thus in Lord Wenman's case (cited 3 Atk. at p. 173) the jury refused to find him an idiot, but upon an inquisition of lunacy they found him lunatic without hesitation. In the reign of James I. (8 Jac. I.), it was under the consideration of Parliament to vest the custody of idiots in their relations, and to settle an equivalent on the Crown in lieu thereof.

‖ And *cf.* Lunacy Act, 1890, s. 98, sub-s. (1).

Such perversion may be psychical or physical, innate or acquired, permanent or temporary. The mind, emotions, or organic nervous system are usually affected simultaneously, but in a variable degree, by impressions received through the senses. Less frequently the higher nervous centres take no part, the phenomena being apparently of reflex production through the spinal centres (Ord).

IDIOSYNCRASY, IMAGINARY (ἴδιος, σύν, κρᾶσις; *imago*, an image). A species of false judgment in which the patients imagine that certain foods or medicines disagree with them, whereas if they are taken no ill results follow; there is usually a strong hysterical taint.

IDIOTIA (ἰδιωτεία, the condition of an ἰδιώτης). A state of idiocy or idiotism.

IDIOTIA ENDEMICA, IDIOTISMUS ENDEMICUS (ἰδιωτεία; ἔνδημος, pertaining to a people). Synonyms of Cretinism.

IDIOTS AND IMBECILES, THE AMELIORATIVE TREATMENT AND EDUCATIONAL TRAINING OF.—The means used for improving the condition of idiots and imbeciles may be considered under two practical heads:—

(1) Those directed to the Alleviation of Physical Defect and Infirmity.

(2) Those directed to the Improvement of the Mental and Moral Powers.

(1) In this article we can but cursorily allude to the correlation of physical and mental defect, which can be traced in every case of idiocy and imbecility. It must suffice to state broadly that bodily abnormalities, formative or functional, constitute an important element in the consideration of ameliorative treatment, and that without an improvement of the physical condition of the patient no mental progress can be reasonably anticipated. Consequently, we shall first consider the agencies of a physical character, including medical treatment, serviceable in combating physical defects and infirmities, and then pass in review the processes found useful in developing and strengthening the deficient mental powers.

The physical agents used may again be subdivided into (**A**) those of a **hygienic** character, and (**B**) those falling more appropriately under the head of **medical** treatment.

The physical exercises which form so important a part of the training of imbecile children, though of course directed to the improvement of the bodily powers, have so close a connection with mental training that it will be more convenient to consider these under the second of our main divisions.

(**A**) **Hygienic treatment** involves considerations which may conveniently be arranged under the following headings:—(1) Heredity, (2) Habitation, (3) Diet, (4) Clothing, (5) Cleanliness, (6) Exercise.

(1) *Heredity* is in this place referred to rather to point out the frequent inappropriateness of the care of an idiot child by its own parents than to protest against ill-assorted marriages which lead to the production of idiot children. It is obvious that those who have transmitted, in perhaps an intensified form, their own defects of character to their children, are not likely to be judicious in the treatment of these defects, and consequently the systematic training of defective children is, as a rule, best confided to a stranger. A neurotic mother will do well, both for her own sake and that of any future offspring, to obtain the aid of a kindly but judicious nurse to relieve her of some of the anxiety attaching to the care of her idiotic child. The administration of phosphorus to the pregnant woman has been advised as a prophylactic against idiocy in the offspring, but hygienic precautions on the part of the mother, anterior to the child's birth, are more likely to be productive of benefit. Above all the cultivation of an equable temperament in the pregnant woman is to be inculcated.

(2) *Habitation.*—There is no doubt that darkness and dirt in the dwelling tend to intensify bodily and mental enfeeblement. Nearly fifty years ago Dr. Güggenbuhl showed how much good resulted from the transference of cretins from the depths of Alpine valleys, shrouded for months in gloom, to the bright sunshine of the Abendberg. A similar experience has followed the gathering of idiots and imbeciles, whether from the slums of cities or from insanitary rural districts, into buildings, well-placed, well-lighted, well-warmed, and at the same time well-ventilated. Having regard to the proclivity of this class to tubercular affections, it is essential that such buildings should be on a dry soil, free from malarious influences, and exposed to the direct rays of the sun. The necessity for warmth, in view of the feeble circulation so common in this class, must be borne in mind; and a temperature of not less than 60° should be ensured both night and day.

(3) *Diet.*—Judicious feeding is of the first importance in the case of idiots, inasmuch as they are prone to a variety of digestive troubles. When the mother is decidedly neurotic or scrofulous, it may be advisable, when circumstances permit, to obtain the services of a strong-minded

and strong-bodied wet nurse, who will take entire charge of the idiotic infant. Failing this, some of the excellent malted foods now prepared for infants, will be found of service; and later, the value of oatmeal in the form of milk porridge, as a food rich in phosphates, should be borne in mind. Decorticated whole-meal bread is also of advantage. It is almost superfluous to dwell upon the importance of an ample supply of good milk; meat, in moderation, should be given, except in epileptic cases; and it is essential, when mastication is ill performed, that meat should be minced in a machine, and mixed with mashed vegetables, before being given to the patient. Regularity as to meal-times is most essential, and for feeble cases these should recur at moderate intervals. A cup of warm milk on first awaking, and a basin of bread and milk when the parents (or nurses) retire at night, may advantageously supplement the three regulation meals. A liberal allowance of sugar and other carbonaceous food is desirable; but it must be borne in mind that crude fat is not, as a rule, well assimilated. Diarrhœa and enuresis are often caused by an excess of watery vegetables, and the consumption of unsound fruit, however acceptable it may be to the patient, must be guarded against. As regards alcoholic drinks, the propriety of their use should be considered in each individual case: in the majority they may be dispensed with, but in some, malt liquor, especially porter, may advantageously be prescribed, whilst in others port wine is useful for its astringent as well as stimulant properties. Whilst a good diet will do much to abolish the depraved tastes which too often exist in idiots, great care should be taken to guard against gluttony, and especially against any tendency to eat garbage. The quantity of fluid taken at the evening meal must be limited in cases prone to enuresis.

(4) *Clothing.*—This demands in the case of idiots the greatest attention. In consideration of their feeble circulation it must be warm both summer and winter, and the body should be encased in flannel, Jaeger, or cellular cloth. Difficulties will arise in dirty cases with regard to flannel drawers, which wash badly: swansdown or cellular cloth may be substituted. In some cases a napkin arrangement like that of a young infant appears serviceable; but such expedients, even if they do not cause soreness, have a tendency to confirm habits which it is the object of training to correct. The hands and feet must be well guarded from the winter cold, or chilblains will inevitably occur. Soft boots lined with swansdown, and mittens, with woollen gloves, or handbags, are useful for this purpose. The style of clothing should be assimilated to that of normal children of similar age: it is undesirable to keep idiot boys in skirts (like girls) to avoid the initial difficulties of knickerbockers and trousers, these difficulties indeed often leading to efforts for the improvement of the habits, which otherwise would never be thought of. A kilted suit is an excellent transition from the dress of an infant to that of a boy. The fastening arrangements must be as simple as possible, and yet such as not to offer facilities for the morbid tendency to denudation which in some cases is a very troublesome trait. A still more troublesome practice is that of tearing the clothing, and this has to be combated by the use of closely woven material, carefully sewn and, if necessary, quilted. An external combination garment fastened only at the back is called for in extreme cases, but it is a mistake to keep the child constantly in such a dress.

With regard to beds and bedding, it may be stated that cribs are required for the younger cases and for epileptics, the sides being, if necessary, protected by padding. Wove wire or chain mattresses, thin horsehair, with bedding protected by mackintosh, are probably the most comfortable and convenient forms of beds. The pillows should not be too hard, but in epileptic cases there is an advantage in these being stuffed with horsehair rather than with feathers, in case of the patient turning on his face in a fit. The bedclothing must be warm and frequently tucked in: in restless and weakly cases the child may be placed in a flannel bag to ensure the limbs being covered; in other cases sleeping socks are useful.

(5) *Cleanliness.*—In the regeneration of an idiot, the inculcation of cleanliness is a cardinal point. In many cases the habits are disgustingly, and even viciously, filthy; in others they seem to be the result of a chronic babyhood. In the latter class, just such attention as is given to a baby when it begins to run about is necessary; the patient must be encouraged to indicate the calls of nature, and be trained to empty the bladder and the bowels at regular intervals. Soon after each meal there should be an adjournment for this purpose; and it will be necessary to raise the child once, twice, or even thrice during the night to prevent wetting the bed, and to place it on the commode upon awaking. In the grosser cases, emptying the bowels at intervals by means of an enema may be useful; and the regulation of the diet,

and especially of the drink, will sometimes have a good moral as well as physical effect. The wearing of india-rubber urinals and such-like mechanical contrivances is seldom serviceable, and they tend to foster negligence. Habits of cleanliness may, to a certain extent, be inculcated by a simple system of rewards and punishment.

Slavering is, in many cases, a habit to be overcome by teaching the child firmly to close its lips. A valuable means to this end is the practice of holding within the lips a small rod, such as a penholder. The provision of slavering cloths, made of quilted washing material, is called for in some cases.

The habit of *self-pollution* is unhappily not uncommon with imbecile boys even at an early age. Besides moral means, the affusion of cold water, and the careful removal from the glans penis of any irritating matter, may be of benefit. Circumcision is undoubtedly useful when there is a long foreskin.

Frequent *baths* are, of course, called for, and, judiciously given with appropriate frictions, serve to improve the superficial circulation and the cutaneous sensibility. Many idiots have a generic odour, and in their case a tepid bath, to which a little "Toilet Sanitas" has been added, may be advantageously given night and morning. The question of temperature of baths must be settled by considering the peculiarities of each case: cold is, as a rule, ill-borne, the powers of reaction being very feeble. Salt baths are serviceable in strengthening feeble limbs.

The condition of the skin must be carefully attended to, as, owing to defective nerve power, sores and sloughs are apt to form upon slight irritation. Emollient applications, such as vaseline, vinolia cream, and powders of zinc oxide or fuller's earth, are often useful.

(6) *Exercise* must be adapted to the physical condition of each case, but in all is essential, and, where spontaneous activity is deficient, may be administered in a passive form—that is, by massage and flexions of the limbs. The advantage of treatment by massage in the case of inactive idiots was insisted on by Édouard Séguin so long ago as 1846 ("Traitement, &c., des Idiots," p. 285), where he calls it "un agent précieux," giving rise to marked improvement, not only of the muscular, but of the nervous, system. A couple of hours at least daily should be spent in the open air whenever the weather permits, and in the stronger cases active play should be encouraged, as well as occupation of a useful kind.

(**B**) **Medical Treatment** will, of course, consist of the application of the ordinary principles of practice to the special morbid conditions of the idiot class. A deficiency of vital force, as evidenced by sluggish circulation, imperfect powers of digestion, and a tendency to tubercular disease, may be named as the most constant characteristic; and, consequently, the inappropriateness of all lowering measures is obvious. The scrofulous constitutions so frequently met with call for a liberal diet, and the administration of cod-liver oil and maltine, while the quality of the blood is improved by the use of some ferruginous tonic, such as Parrish's chemical food.

When an inherited syphilitic taint has been ascertained, the use of potassic iodide in combination with mercuric bichloride is sometimes of use in promoting absorption of adventitious deposits in the coats of cerebral arteries, and thus improving the condition of the brain. When the circulation is feeble, it is advisable to give stimulants in the form of porter or port wine, and hydrochloric acid with chloric ether is often of service in correcting digestive troubles. When diarrhœa is of the character of a mucous flux, an emulsion of castor oil with small doses of opium is useful; in other cases, astringents, such as sulphuric acid, kino, catechu, or sulphate of zinc may be tried. In the fermentative variety, with fœtid stools, the administration of small doses of carbolic acid has proved of service.

The spongy condition of gums frequently met with is best treated by the administration of chlorate of potash, and the aphthous condition of mouth by the local application of boracic glycerine. The various discharges from eyes, nose, and ears may be treated by astringent lotions of sulphate (or, in more severe cases, of chloride) of zinc. The skin eruptions so commonly met with in idiots demand the remedies appropriate to each variety. Ringworm and other parasitic affections find a congenial soil on the inactive skins of idiots, and are often difficult to cure. The liability to lice is a troublesome trait in some cases, and calls for careful combing, and the use of carbolic lotions. The tendency to chilblains is very marked, and the painting of the hands and feet with tincture of iodine is a good preventive. Frictions are of course not to be omitted; and when sores occur resin ointment is a valuable application.

Having regard to the feeble constitutional powers of idiots and imbeciles, prognosis as to the course of the exanthemata, and of acute disease generally, must be given with caution, especially when there is a liability to convulsions. Epilepsy is a frequent concomitant of idiocy, occurring probably in fully one-half of the cases. Bromides, combined with (or alternated with) ferruginous tonics, are beneficial in some cases if given in sufficient doses, and persevered with for long periods; but as epilepsy when combined with idiocy may usually be regarded as more than a functional disorder, the prospect of cure is not very encouraging. The shallow and irregular breathing which is met with in many cases renders the diagnosis of pulmonary disorder difficult: and the practitioner has to rely on general symptoms and on percussion, rather than on auscultatory signs, whilst expectoration is often absent. The characteristic temperature variations are perhaps the most valuable diagnostic indication of tubercular disease, which must of course be treated, as soon as suspected, with cod-liver oil, emulsion of hypophosphites or other approved remedies.

As regards surgical treatment the want of reparative power, and the difficulties which arise from the habits of the patient, render idiots, as a rule, bad subjects for operations. Where, however, constitutional irritation is caused by bone or joint disease it is quite legitimate to remove the diseased parts, and in scrofulous cases especially the results are often satisfactory. In cases of fracture much ingenuity has to be exercised to sufficiently secure the appliances so that the patient cannot tamper with them, and at the same time to avoid hurtful pressure, which in some instances will quickly produce gangrene. The persistently dirty habits of some patients will occasionally render it impossible to keep the skin sound, but much may be done by assiduous attention on the part of the nurse, and the use of spirit lotions, astringent powders,. and emollient unguents.

Recently, the operation of *craniectomy* (consisting of the removal of portions of cranial bones, either in lineal strips, or *à lambeaux*), has been recommended by M. Lannalongue (of Paris) and others, as serviceable in cases of microcephaly with premature ossification, as well as in cases where pressure is suspected from depressed or thickened cranial bones. In twenty-eight cases of craniectomy reported at the French Surgical Congress in 1891, there had been but one death, and it was claimed that in a large number of instances improvement followed, both in intelligence and in walking power. Craniectomies have been performed in America by Dr. Keen, and in this country by Mr. Victor Horsley, who, reviewing his own experience and that of others, concludes that craniectomy "should be carried out in all cases (of microcephaly), inasmuch as the condition is otherwise absolutely without hope, and interference has evidently secured notable improvement in some cases (see *British Medical Journal*, Sept. 12, 1891).

(2) Passing now to the second division of our subject (the means directed to the improvement of the mental and moral powers), we may consider the various methods of education and training as attracted to the following objects:—

(A) To develop and regulate the bodily activity in due relation to the higher co-ordinating power.

(B) To develop and exercise the senses and perceptive faculties.

(C) To train the hands to useful occupation.

(D) To cultivate the moral faculties.

As Dr. E. Séguin long ago pointed out, all efforts to train the feeble faculties of the idiot and imbecile, must, to be successful, proceed upon physiological principles. In other words, the education of these imperfect children must proceed upon the lines on which Nature herself proceeds in the development of normal children. In the normal baby we see from the first an abundance of spontaneous movement, apparently purposeless: as age advances and intelligence dawns, these movements are either intuitively, or under the mother's fostering care, brought into co-ordination, and by degrees subserve useful purposes. Of course the increase of intelligence in the normal child implies a gradual evolution of the senses, and a genesis of perceptive power. In the idiot, on the contrary, there is either deficiency of healthy movement or (it may be) an ill-regulated excess: whilst from central or peripheral defect, the senses are inactive, or obtuse, or there is such an absence of attention that sensations do not pass into perceptions. The first task of the trainer of idiots therefore will be to do what Nature and a judicious mother do for normal infants, viz.:—to develop (if need be) and to regulate the bodily activities, and to promote the discriminating exercise of the senses. These processes, though for convenience considered under separate headings, must of course go on simultaneously. It will be obvious that the regulation of the bodily activities implies the attainment of more or less co-ordination, and the gradual formation of will power. The training of the hand to useful occupation is but a later stage of the cultivation of purposive movements, aided by the progressive development of the senses and the intelligence; whilst the cultivation of the moral faculties, must, in any judicious system of education, proceed *pari passu* with that of the mental powers. We do not range, under the special modes of training peculiar to the circumstances of the idiot or imbecile, those educational processes which form a recognised part of the school education of every child, although it will be convenient to refer to certain methods of elementary instruction which seem peculiarly adapted to feeble intellects. The educational, as well as the hygienic, aspects of recreation must, moreover, not be lost sight of.

Under the first heading (**A**) then we consider **Methods of developing and regulating the Bodily Activities in due relation to the higher Co-ordinating Power.** These comprehend:—

(**1**) **Exercises to call forth Activity and at the same time awaken Powers of Attention and Imitation.**—In the case of apathetic idiots, bags filled with beans or maize are thrown by the teacher at the patient, who is encouraged to catch them and throw them back. In such cases a simple instinctive action may often be seen to pass by degrees into a purposive movement: the child first puts up his hands to guard himself from the missile, then grasps it, then returns it. Then follow simple muscular exercises, such as clapping the hands in time to music, simple movements of the arms (up, down, folded, behind the back, &c.); then movements of the legs; finally of the head. Marching in time to music follows.

It will be understood that individual infirmities have to be considered in devising drill appropriate to each case; and, where paralytic defects exist, the muscular powers of the teacher have to supplement the deficiencies of the pupil.

(**2**) **Exercises to regulate Abnormal Activities.** — In the restless, excitable class of idiots benefit is often derived from the soothing effects of music, which will arrest the attention when every other means fails. By slow degrees the movements of the patient will be brought into rhythm; and a judicious teacher will find means of transforming mere restless activity into exercises which may be dignified with the name of drill.

(**3**) **Exercises to promote Co-ordination.**—These are more especially useful in the large class of imbeciles who suffer from spasmodic or choreiform movements. A child who suffers from athetosis of the fingers is first set to pick up and place in their appropriate cavities the marbles on a "solitaire" board. Then comes what is called a "peg-board;" a flat piece of wood with perforations into which nail-like metallic pegs fit. The exercise is two-fold: first, the grasping of the pegs between thumb and finger, and secondly the insertion of them into the holes (in which they fit pretty tightly). Then come exercises in threading beads and perforating picture cards for Kindergarten work. The grasping of wooden blocks (ordinary children's bricks), and the building of them into various forms, are excellent exercises both for this class and for the restless children above adverted to. The lower limbs have also to be trained, and for this purpose a ladder lying upon the floor, with flat pieces for "rounds" is very useful. Over this ladder the children march, either stepping between the rounds, or upon them, as indicated by the teacher. Walking up and down steps is another useful exercise, promoting the due balancing of the body, and the alternate use of the feet. To such simple exercises as these gradually succeed others more commonly designated as "drill" (which should be set to music), and exercises with wands, wooden dumb-bells, gymnastic ladders, swings with foot-board, parallel bars and inclined planes, &c. It must, however, be borne in mind that the object to be attained is not athleticism, but due co-ordination of the muscles, the powers of attention, imitation, and of voluntary control being at the same time developed.

Logically, the muscular exercises requisite for speech-production, should be treated under this head, but having regard to the close relation of speech with hearing it will be more convenient to defer our remarks on this subject until we have considered the education of the senses.

(**B**) **Methods of developing and exercising the Senses and Perceptive Faculties.** — Whilst the muscular activities are being aroused and regulated, the senses must be quickened, the perceptions cultivated, and by these means the intellectual powers will be gradually brought into play. In the idiot, as in the normal child, it may be taken as an axiom "that the education of the senses must precede the education of the mind:" as Dr. Séguin has well remarked, "the organs of sensation being within our reach, and those of thought out of it, the former are the first that we can set in action." The normal child indeed sets them in action for himself; but for the abnormal, special sense-culture is needed. The senses of touch, of taste and of smell, as well as those of sight and of hearing, must be tested, and carefully trained by appropriate exercises, some few examples of which we give below:—

(1) **Touch.**—Let the child be made to handle rough and smooth surfaces, such as those of sand-paper and satin, to immerse the fingers in hot and in cold water by way of contrasting the sensations of heat and cold, to grasp spheres (such as large marbles) and cubes (such as those used in the Kindergarten system). Then come exercises like those previously described with the peg-board, with boards containing cavities differing in size and form, with beads which are at first picked up, and afterwards threaded. The handling of metallic spheres of equal size but different densities will arouse elementary ideas of differences of weight.

(2) **Taste.**—Salt and sugar, vinegar and similarly coloured syrups, milk and fluid magnesia, may be used in pairs for the purpose of contrasting tastes.

(3) **Smell.**—Coffee and snuff, soap and cheese, odorous, malodorous, and odourless flowers, may be offered for discrimination by this sense.

(4) **Sight.**—The initial difficulty with idiots is often to get them to fix their eyes steadily on anything. In some cases nystagmus, in others, crass dulness or incessant restlessness, not to mention optical defects, interfere most vexatiously with definite vision. The apt teacher will, however, know how to fix his pupil with his own eye: as Séguin quaintly puts it, "the main instrument in fixing the regard is the regard." Sparkling, attractive objects, such as mirrors, silvered balls, &c., are useful for this purpose; and bright coloured objects set in motion, such as the coloured glasses of the kaleidoscope, may also be of service. Exercises in the perception of colour come at a later stage: coloured balls and cups, cubes the faces of which are painted with six contrasting colours, are some of the means used. The child selects from the different coloured balls that of the same colour as the cup presented to him; or turns up on the cube the colour shown him by the teacher; it being understood that the exercise is in the perception of colours not in their names, which are, however, taught subsequently.

(5) **Hearing.** — Comparatively few idiots are deaf: they *hear*, but they do not *listen*. The skilful teacher will by the judicious use of his own voice make an impression on his pupil's auditory powers. Singing will often do this when simple speech does not suffice. Music, indeed, exercises a marked influence in arresting the attention of idiots; even those of low grade reproducing with fair correctness a tune which has made an impression on them, though destitute of speech. In music, then, we have an invaluable aid in the training of imbecile children: as we shall see presently, it often forms a stepping-stone to speech. In some cases the trial of notes of different pitch may be necessary; if the piano be not heard, try a mouth organ or a whistle. Trumpets, drums, harmonicons and other musical toys are often of service in the self-cultivation of this sense.

(6) **Speech.**—The cultivation of speech, a faculty defective in greater or less degree, in the majority of idiots and imbeciles, demands much ingenuity and perseverance on the part of the teacher. Hopelessly absent in a small minority of the cases (and these not always the least intelligent) articulation may in many instances be taught by processes consisting partly of lip and tongue gymnastics, partly of imitative exercises in simple sounds. Where deafness exists the former are of course alone applicable: but much may be done, as in the case of deaf mutes, by lip imitation. It is essential in every case of deficient speech first to examine carefully the condition of the vocal organs; in many we shall find a want of tonicity of the lips, attended with slavering, in others a flabbiness or abnormality of size of the tongue, in others a highly vaulted or cleft palate, in others again peculiarity of form of the lower jaw with irregular dentition. There may also be more or less paralysis of the vocal organs. In some cases (*e.g.*, in cleft palate) structural defects may be surgically amended: in others, functional weaknesses may be ameliorated by appropriate exercises. Thus in the case of the atonic lips, the patient should be made to hold between them a flat piece of boxwood, or a wooden penholder; opening and shutting the mouth as ordered by the teacher, protruding and drawing back the tongue, touching the lips and the palate therewith, are samples of the sort of preliminary drill to be gone through. The organs having been thus strengthened and brought under control, the teacher proceeds to show the child how to produce simple labial sounds—*e.g.*, "mam-ma, pap-pa, bab-ba." Then come the linguals "dad-da, tat-ta, &c.": labio-dentals, palatals, gutturals, nasals follow in due course. It will be observed that consonant sounds precede those of the vowels: the latter, indeed, must be taught in conjunction with a consonant either preceding

or following. From sounds which may be called simply phonetic, the child is led to pronounce the names of objects containing these sounds, the objects themselves being shown him. A table of speaking exercises constructed for the use of the schools of the Royal Albert Asylum is subjoined.

however imperfectly, for what it wants at table.

The defective functions having thus been developed and trained by the judicious exercise of the organs both of movement and sensation, the child no longer remains isolated (ἰδιώτης) from his surroundings and his fellows, but is prepared

Speaking Exercise.

I. *Consonants.*

Sound.	Phonetic.	Common Object.	Part of Body.	Part of Dress, &c.
M.	Mam-ma	Mat, Man, Miss	Mouth, Muscle	Muff, Muffler, Mitten
P.	Pap-pa	Pen, Pin, Pipe	Palm (of hand)	Pin, Pocket
B.	Bab-ba	Bell, Box	Bone, Bust	Bib, Bow
T.	Tat-ta	Table, Top, Tea	Toe, Tooth	Tie, Tape
D.	Dad-da	Door, Doll, Desk	Dimple	Dress
V.	Va-va	Velvet, View	Vein	Veil, Vest
F.	Fa-fa	Fan, Fire	Foot, Face, Finger	Fur, Frock, Flannel
L.	La-la	Lad, Lady, Lock	Lip, Limb, Leg	Lace, (E)lastic
R.	Ra-ree	Rag, Reel, Rail-road	Rib, (W)rist	Ribbon, Ring
S.	See-saw	Soap, Slate, Seat	Sole, Skin	Sock, Sash, Stocking
Z.	Za-zel	Zinc, Scissors	Hazel (Eyes)	Stays, Zone
Th.	The	Thimble	Thumb, Throat	Thread
Sh.	She	Shell, Shilling	Shoulders, Shin	Shoe, Shawl, Shirt
Ch.	Chick	Child, Chair	Chin, Chest, Cheek	Chain (of Watch)
J.	Jig	Ju-jube, Jug	Jaw, Joint	Jacket, Jewel
G (hard).	Gig	Girl, Gas	Gum	Garter, Gaiter
K.	Cake	Cat, Kite, Colour, Coat	Calf	Coat, Cap, Collar
N.	Nanny	Net, Nut, Knot	Nose, Nail, Neck	Necktie, Knot

II. *Simple Vowel Sounds.*

Vowel Sound.	Examples.	Vowel Sound.	Examples.
A open = (Ah)	Father	U (short) = Ŭ	Tun, Fun
A (broad) = (Aw)	All (*Aw*ful)	U (long) = Ū	Tune, Fume
A (short) = Ă	Cap, Tap	E (short) = Ĕ	Bed, Fed
A (long) = Ā	Cape, Tape	E (long) = Ē	Bead, Feed
O (short) = Ŏ	Cot, Knot	I (short) = Ĭ	Bit, Fit
O (long) = Ō	Coat, Note	I (long) = Ī	Bite, Fight
O͝O (short) = O͝O	Foot, Wood	Aspirate H	Hat, Hall
O͞O (long) = O͞O	Boot, Food	Double Letters, W. Y	Wall, You
		Diphthongs, O͡I, O͡W	Oil, Owl

So much for the methodical training of articulation. We have already remarked that music may be used as an aid to speech, and some of the old nursery rhymes (*e.g.*, Elliott's "National Nursery Rhymes"), set to catching music, and sung daily in class, will, by their easy repetition of sounds, help on the child in speech. At a later stage repetition of verses after the teacher, who must attend especially to the pronunciation, is an excellent exercise. As a rule, it is well to disregard signs, and make the child ask, to take part in the curriculum of school instruction. This must, of course, be reduced to its simplest form; though attention may be attained, abstract ideas will not be comprehended, and everything must be presented in a concrete form. Specially applicable to imbeciles is the Horatian maxim,

> Segnius irritant animos demissa per aurem
> Quam quæ sunt oculis subjecta fidelibus.

Objects and pictures must be constantly put before the pupil to render the teacher's words impressive. Reading is best taught by the "word-method"—*i.e.*, by associating pictures or objects with the printed names that designate them; and calculation must be taught by constant demonstration, whether on the abacus or the blackboard. The first steps of drawing and of writing are attained by making the pupil draw lines between points set him by the teacher; often a very creditable degree of proficiency is attained in these imitative arts. Mere parrot-like learning is to be eschewed,

> As in an idiot's brain remembered words
> Hang empty mid the cobwebs of his dreams;*

and the meaning of words learnt or read must always be made plain to the pupil. Some of the exercises of the Kindergarten system, more especially those known as "occupations," are well suited to form a link between sense-culture and intellectual and industrial training. It must, of course, always be an object to make instruction interesting, and not to strain the child's feeble intellectual powers by too long lessons. Singing and musical drill may well form a preponderating element in the educational course.

(C) Methods of training the Hands to Useful Occupation. — Many of the exercises mentioned as appropriate for promoting co-ordination, such as building with bricks and threading beads, perforating picture cards, &c., are first steps in this direction. Further steps may be taken in such occupations of the Kindergarten, as paper-folding, paper-weaving, card embroidery, and simple model-making, and the child's mechanical aptitudes may thus be trained and tested. Needle-work is neatly done by many imbecile girls; and some boys display special tastes for tailoring, shoe-making, or joinery. For both sexes some outdoor occupation is, during the period of training at least, highly desirable, and weeding in the garden is a valuable resource. The fondness for animals which exists in some cases should be fostered; many lads become useful assistants at the farm. The experience of the Royal Albert Asylum, where much stress has always been laid upon industrial training, is that about one-fourth of those tried at trades become proficient, while one-half of those put to outdoor work become more or less useful. Industrial training should, of course, in the younger cases at any rate, be alternated with school exercises, and the necessity of recreation must not be forgotten. The "dullard" must not be allowed to remain dull even in his leisure hours; and active outdoor games, such as cricket, croquet, &c., help in the training of the hand and eye. Musical entertainments are much appreciated, even by low-grade idiots; and simple dramatic representations, in which the patients can take part, are found of great value in institution-life, from their educational, as well as their recreational, aspects.

* Longfellow: "Tales of a Wayside Inn."

(D) Methods of cultivating the Moral Faculties. — Throughout the course of training hitherto described it is obvious that the character of the trainer must act and re-act upon the trained. If "love is the fulfilling of the law," it is the alpha and the omega of all efforts to improve the feeble-minded. Perfect confidence between the teacher and taught—that "love which casteth out fear"—is a condition indispensable to success. Coaxing, not coercion, must be the method employed. At the same time gentle discipline must be enforced; well-doing must be commended and rewarded; ill-doing reprehended and (if need be) punished. Whilst the axiom that "force is no remedy" is strictly adhered to, obedience must be insisted on, and the child taught to subordinate its will to that of its teacher. Even in the early stage of development an appeal to the moral sense may often be made through the stomach—*e.g.*, a few sweets as a pledge of commendation, the loss of pudding as an evidence of displeasure. Later it should be pointed out how harm inevitably results from evil-doing, and how necessary it is that one should do to others as one would be done by. God as the impersonation of good, and Christ as the impersonation of love, must be the fundamental notes of instruction of a religious character. Much interest is often evinced by feeble-minded children in listening to a simple recital of gospel narratives, and moral lessons may be judiciously evoked. It is most important that as the intelligence increases moral training should be enforced; of all imbeciles, the "moral imbecile" is the most unsatisfactory.

Dr. Auguste Voisin, physician to the Salpêtrière, has reported* cases of moral perversity, occurring in imbecile youths, distinctly benefitted by hypnotic suggestion, but this method does not seem to have been tested in this country.

Results of Training.—In conclusion, a few words as to results may not be inappropriate. During the fifty years over which efforts for the amelioration of the imbecile have now extended the sanguine prognostications of early enthusiasts may not have been realised, but nevertheless a large percentage of benefit has been recorded. An imbecile, however well trained, will always need some kindly aid and con-

* *Revue de l'Hypnotisme*, November 1888.

sideration from those with whom he is associated; it is not to be expected that he will, in the majority of instances, be able to manage his own affairs or compete in the labour-markets of the world. Placed in a niche, however, where he can without molestation exercise his acquired talents, he will in many cases turn out more or less remunerative work; and, failing this, he will, in consequence of having some resources within himself, cease to be a nuisance to his friends and surroundings. Even the improvement of habits by systematic training is not to be despised in relation to the comfort of the family; and it must ever be borne in mind that an idiot left untrained is pretty sure to deteriorate.

A review of twenty years' experience at one of the large English institutions furnishes the following results:—Of patients discharged after full training, 10 per cent. are self-supporting, whilst another 10 per cent. would be so if they had obtained suitable situations, and about 20 per cent. were reported as useful to their friends at home. This bears out in a remarkable manner the early estimate of Séguin, who says that "idiots have been improved, educated, and even cured: more than 40 per cent. have become capable of the ordinary transactions of life, under friendly control, of understanding moral and social abstractions, of working like two-thirds of a man; and 25 to 30 per cent. come nearer and nearer the standard of manhood till some of them will defy the scrutiny of good judges when compared with ordinary young men and women."

G. E. Shuttleworth.

IDIOTS SAVANTS. (Fr.) Feeble-minded children with a special development of some mental faculty, such as that of music, calculation, &c.

IDOLUM (εἴδωλον, an image). A name sometimes applied to a false idea, illusion or hallucination.

IDROMANIA (for Hydromania). Insane impulse to commit suicide by drowning.

IKOTA.—A Siberian form of religious insanity, occurring almost exclusively among married women. It is a hysterical psycho-pathological condition which in its milder forms is characterised by listlessness, with occasional outbursts of anger, the patient giving vent to inarticulate sounds when displeased; in its more intensely developed forms, outbursts of maniacal excitement of short duration are observed, in which the patient violently attacks those about her, or even lays hands on herself. (*See* Hysteria, Klikuschi, Lata.)

ILLUSION (*illusio*, a mocking). A deception, false appearance, or mockery; sometimes used synonymously but incorrectly for hallucination. In psychology, the term is used to denote the erroneous conception by the mind of some external object which is perceived by any one of the senses. (Fr. *illusion;* Ger. *Täuschung, Sinnestäuschung.*)(*Vide infra.*)

ILLUSION.—Illusion has been carefully distinguished since the time of Esquirol from hallucination, as being the false interpretation of a sensation actually perceived. We think that it is desirable to retain this distinction, although several able psychologists have recently insisted upon their essential identity—among them Prof. Ball. We have already expressed ourselves as follows: "No doubt the distinction is a very fine one in some instances. The question is not altogether unimportant, because while men easily, in even a perfectly sane state, convert a real object into something other than itself, they rarely perceive one externally projected, in the entire absence of a corresponding reality, without a more or less grave disturbance of the nervous system. It is maintained that an illusion is always a false interpretation, and therefore a purely psychical process—not an illusion of the senses at all. It must not be forgotten that an insane hallucination, as well as an illusion, may involve a false interpretation."

Certain hypnotic experiments tend to show how illusion runs into hallucination. Thus, in consequence of suggestion, a hypnotised subject may be made to see on a card a likeness which is not there. At the same time the central point around which the hallucination plays, is a dot actually there (*pointe de repère*). Sully defines illusion as any species of error which counterfeits the form of immediate, self-evident, or intuitive knowledge, whether as sense-perception or otherwise."* This, however—the popular signification of the term—is too wide for the alienist, who must restrict its use to sensory states. The above writer observes in reference to the separation between illusion and hallucination that "in the latter it is impossible in the majority of cases to prove that there is no modicum of external agency co-operating in the production of the effect" (*loc. cit.*).

It is hardly necessary to say that illusions like hallucinations are consistent with sanity. Few persons are not subject to visual and auditory illusions in the course of their lives. Expectant atten-

* "Illusions: A Psychological Study." By J. Sully. Second edition, p. 6.

tion at the moment an external object is perceived exerts a subtle influence upon the observer or auditor. It falsifies to an alarming degree the experiments of scientific and especially medical men. But these errors of personal equation are not symptoms of insanity.

An interesting illustration of the fact that the excitation of one of the special senses may increase or occasion the functional activity of another sense, is afforded by a circumstance recorded by Dr. Descourtis. He was seated at his desk, when a door in the storey below was slammed to, making a great noise. At that moment he perceived a smell which came from the other end of the apartment. A quarter of an hour afterwards there passed a carriage under his window, causing a loud sound, and the same odour returned. With the departure of the noise the smell also disappeared.

So much of what has been written in the article on hallucinations of the insane (*q.v.*), applies to illusions, that it is not necessary to enter into detail in this place.

Illusions arising from the exaggeration or perversion of internal sensations constitute the prominent symptoms of the hypochondriac, and are among the most striking examples of the serious effects of illusive sensations (*see* HYPOCHONDRIASIS).

THE EDITOR.

[*References.*—Esquirol, Des Maladies Mentales, Tome premier, p. 202. Brierre de Boismont, Hallucinations. Descourtis, Des Hallucinations de l'ouïe. Sully, Illusions, a Psychological Study.]

ILLUSIO SENSŪS (*illusio*, a mocking; *sensus*, the faculty of feeling). A synonym of Hallucination (*q.v.*).

IMAGE (Fr. *image*, from L. *imago*, a likeness). A term occasionally used in psychology for the mental representation of an object or sensation.

IMAGE, SUBJECTIVE (*imago*; *subjectum*, subject). An image perceived by the mind from changes independent of those produced by rays of light. Also a synonym of Visual Hallucination.

IMAGINARII.—One of Linnæus's three subdivisions of mental disease—affections of the sensory faculties.

IMAGINATION (*imaginatio*, a mental image; from *imaginor*, I picture to myself). The mental act or faculty of creating ideas or forming mental images either at will or involuntarily under the influence of strong emotion or other exciting cause, these ideas being of an order different from those formed by the judgment and ordinary reasoning. (*See* PHILOSOPHY OF MIND, p. 34.)

IMBECILE (Lat. *imbecillus*, weak). Feeble, weak; correctly applied to one of originally weak mental faculties.

IMBECILITY (*imbecillitas*, from *imbecillus*, weak). Weakness or helplessness of body or mind. In mental science used only in the latter sense. A term, strictly speaking, applied to a congenital defect of mental power, of the same kind as, but to a less degree than, idiocy. A condition of mental enfeeblement resulting from want of brain development. (Fr. *imbécillité*; Ger. *Geistesschwäche*, *Schwachsinn*.)

IMBECILITY, ACQUIRED.—Weakness of intellect which appears after a term, long or short, of apparent mental vigour. The term has also been used by some for dementia following acute psychic disturbances.

IMBECILITY, INTELLECTUAL.—A form of mental weakness in which the intellectual faculties are chiefly involved.

IMBECILITY, MORAL.—Imbecility affecting the moral faculties chiefly.

IMBECILITY, SENILE (*imbecillitas*; *senilis*, old). Senile dementia.

IMBECILLITAS INGENII (*imbecillitas*; *ingenium*, natural quality), **IMBECILLITAS MENTIS** (*imbecillitas*; *mens*, the mind). Terms used for idiocy and imbecility.

IMITATION (*imitatio*, from *imitor*, I copy). The act of doing anything with a view of making it like some other act. As a cause of disease it is to be found in certain hysteric and choreic states, and as a factor in the production of certain forms of insanity. (*See* CHOREA MAJOR, COMMUNICATED INSANITY, EPIDEMIC INSANITY, HYSTERIA, &c.) (Ger. *Nachahmung*.)

IMITATION; OR, MENTAL CONTAGION.—We have already trenched upon this subject under *Folie à Deux*, or Communicated Insanity, but more may well be said in regard to several important aspects of the effect of imitation. No one has more clearly analysed this tendency than M. Despine. He takes first the instinct of imitation, pure and simple—one more limited in its range than is generally supposed. It is principally observed in the young. As is well known, idiots are very susceptible to its influence. It is not characterised by any high or lofty motive. A monkey will imitate to the extent of self-destruction, as in an instance we know in which a medical man, annoyed with the imitative actions and grimaces of a monkey, placed a razor in its hand, and then went through the dumb show of drawing another across his own throat. The monkey immediately imitated the act, and with fatal consequences. A flock of sheep blindly follows their leader over hedge and ditch.

Then there is that form of imitation

which results from the law of self-interest. "There is first," M. Jolly observes, "a purely *instinctive*, and, so to say, passive immitation, and also an *intellectual* or active imitation; the former, common to us and the lower animals, and performed unconsciously, at all epochs and in all the conditions of material life; the latter, which belongs to the domain of mind, is concerned with intelligence and reflection, endeavouring to copy knowingly, and to faithfully and voluntarily translate everything that causes pleasure" (*L'Union médicale*, 1869). Intellectual imitation reproduces the master-pieces of art and genius, including the drama.

The third category includes that variety of imitation which determines moral contagion. It is scarcely needful to point out that this is of great importance to the psychologist and the social reformer. The principle underlies some of the most serious and lamentable events in society. On the other hand, it may favour noble acts, whether religious or political. In either case it may carry along in its train more or less mental derangement. Crimes are imitated, epidemics of particular forms of criminality are witnessed. The dreadful murders committed by Tropman in France, led to a crop of similar horrors in that country, Belgium, and England. Suicides are notoriously contagious. M. Despine complains of the confusion, avoided by Esquirol, between the imitation which is the outcome of moral imitation, and that which is the result of instinct. A man witnesses a certain act, and desires to commit it. In employing the same means to carry it out, he has been influenced by reasons which appeal to his intellect. It is no longer an unreflecting instinctive act. It is observed by Despine, that well-marked as it is with children and certain animals, instinct tends to become gradually effaced in adolescence and mature life, in the presence of more important and powerful motives and individual activity.

Lastly, imitation may be determined by nervous contagion. The morbid principle is contained in a neurotic condition liable to generate spasmodic phenomena, actual convulsions, and even abnormal moral manifestations, which cause in those who are susceptible to this contagion, a similar neurosis, and along with it bodily and mental phenomena of the same nature. Yawning is a familiar example. The epidemic convulsions which occurred in the cemetery of St. Médard are well known. Similar examples are given by M. Bouchut. One occurred in Paris in 1848, in a manufactory where 400 women were employed. One of the number became pale, unconscious, and convulsed. In a couple of hours 30 were affected in the same manner, and on the third day, 15; the same symptoms were present in all. A second epidemic of convulsions occurred in 1861, among the young women of the parish Montmartre, who were preparing for their first communion. In the first instance, 3 were taken in the church with loss of consciousness and general convulsive movements. The scene was repeated at the evening service. On the second day the same symptoms were developed in three other girls. The same happened on the third. On the fourth day, that of the first communion, 12 were seized with the same disorder. Twenty more were attacked in the evening. Lastly, on the following day, at the confirmation, no less than 15 were, as the archbishop approached, seized with convulsive tremors, screamed, and fell down unconscious, the hand being raised to the forehead. At this time 40 girls out of 150 presented nervous phenomena.

Women and children fall a prey to the influence of nervous contagion more easily than men, although the latter are by no means exempt. (*See* DEMONOPATHY; EPIDEMIC INSANITY; THEOMANIA.)

Despine asks, Ought we to attribute the frequent repetition of criminal acts (homicide, suicide, infanticide, incendiarism) exclusively to moral contagion? The reply is just: that we ought to do so, if acts are inspired by a physiological passion natural to man, as self-interest, hatred, jealousy, &c. In addition, however, to these causes, there may be in other instances a diseased condition of the brain, which is the essential factor. The passions which are in force are then pathological in their character; for example, murder is committed not from the desire of gain or even vengeance, but for the sake of killing; if suicide is committed, it is not from despair, but in consequence of an impulse. Of course those who witness such acts may be so affected by them, as to be disposed to imitate them.

M. Bouchut is stated to have attributed nervous contagion to a miasm formed in places where impressionable people are assembled together. It is, however, unnecessary to adopt this explanation when there is every reason to suppose that moral contagion amply suffices to produce it. M. Despine advances all that can be said in favour of the two hypotheses, and is unable to determine which possesses most probability; but he inclines to the doctrine of moral in contradistinction to miasmatic contagion. We regard the former as fanciful. Moral emotions may arrest mental epidemics, and therefore it is not remarkable, as Despine argues, that like emotions may cause nervous symptoms and convulsions.

The bearing of the doctrine of moral or psychical contagion upon the publication of the details of the crimes that are committed must be obvious. These are greedily read by the masses, and a fresh crop of crimes is the result. Unhappily, cheap newspapers, and the ease with which every fact is reported, have favoured the abuse of the liberty of the press. The morbid demand creates an unlimited supply of morbid literature; and as if there were not enough of actual crimes, novelists invent them and increase the evil. The air is full of real and fictitious crimes of the most revolting character. Moral contagion spreads the mischief far and wide without the action of any physical miasm.

THE EDITOR.

IMITATION, MORAL (*imitor; moralis*, relating to conduct). The reproduction in a person of the moral qualities of another, the passions or sentiments exhibited by others.

IMITATION, MORBID (*imitor; morbus*, a disease). The sudden onset of a convulsive or mental affection in a person who has recently witnessed the occurrence of such a disease in another—*e.g.*, chorea, hysteria, and certain forms of insanity.

IMPERATIVE IDEAS.—Synonyms.—French writers have employed the words *obsessions mentales* and *impulsions intellectuels*. The German synonym *Zwangsvorstellungen* is expressive.

Definition.—Morbid suggestions and ideas imperiously demanding notice, the patient being painfully conscious of their domination over his wish and will, and very frequently having a hereditary predisposition to insanity. Some of the French alienists extend the use of the term to actual delusion (*idée fixe*), as, for instance, ideas of persecution, but it is to be hoped that it will be carefully restricted to that intellectual tyranny which the individual deplores and is not deluded by.

For a considerable period alienists have felt the importance of differentiating between imperative ideas with the retention of sanity, and delusions or fixed ideas. That there is some derangement of the mental machinery in consequence of which certain thoughts or words dominate the wish and will of the individual cannot be denied; but there is a marked difference between the man who is conscious of the undue predominance of certain involuntary ideas, which do not amount to insane beliefs, and the man who holds delusive ideas and whose conduct is influenced by them.

A large number of words have been coined to express the special form which the obsession has assumed. Thus, we have *onomatomania* defined by Charcot and Magnan as a mental state in which a word or a name plays the chief part; they noted that such a condition frequently occurs in persons high in the scale of mental degeneration,* persons suffering from a loss of equilibrium. They maintained that it constitutes one of the so-called episodic syndromata of hereditary insanity, a certain soil being essential to such an obsession. Hence a most insignificant cause may determine the symptoms, the fall of a metallic body on the table having been known to excite an absurd horror of pins (*bélonéphobie*). The agonising search for a particular word may arise from a like apparently trivial exciting cause, and may become a verbal obsession so weighing on the mind as to cause an irresistible impulse to repeat it. The case is given of a man who met a former acquaintance, and, after they had parted, tried in vain to recall his name. It became a perpetual worry. He became quite ill, and paced the floor in intense distress. A fortnight after he suffered in the same way *àpropos* of another old friend, and relief came only when he succeeded in finding the name. He eventually experienced the like trouble in regard to the names of people totally unknown to him, and then of the number of articles (books, dishes, &c.) falling under his observation (*arithmomania*).†

Agoraphobia, the dread of large open spaces, is usually classed under imperative ideas or obsessions, although belonging to rather a different species of the genus. It was described by Westphal in 1872, who regarded it as a neurosis allied to epileptic vertigo. Often it is merely a nervous fear. A person may be conscious of the absurdity of the fear of walking across a field or square, but be unable to rid himself of it.‡

Claustrophobia, or *Clithrophobia*, the fear of closed spaces, belongs to the same division.

* The use of this word by the French conveys to an English psychologist a much greater loss of mental power than is intended by alienists in France. (*See* DEGENERATION.)

† *Cf.* "Archives de Neurologie," Sept. 1885.

‡ Legrand du Saulle employed the term *peur des espaces* and wrote articles upon it in the *Gazette des Hôpitaux*, 1877 and 1888. M. le Dr. Gros has contributed a number of cases to the *Annales Médico-Psychologiques*, 1885, p. 394. The term *Trichophobia* (fear of places), has been employed to comprise the fear of large and of confined spaces. *Acrophobia* has reference to the fear of heights, and so on, and so on, *ad nauseam*.

Acrophobia, described by Dr. Andrea Verga, means the dread of being in high places.

Astraphobia, the fear of an approaching storm, may be associated with unusual susceptibility to electrical conditions of the atmosphere.

Zoöphobia, the nervous fear of certain animals, as beetles, spiders, mice, toads, &c., is not uncommon.

Such terms may be multiplied almost indefinitely, as *topophobia* (Beard's name for agoraphobia) and *oikophobia* (morbid fear of home). There may be some convenience in this nomenclature, but the reader must not suppose that there is pathological justification for all the modern terms which have been added to psychological medicine in the realm of imperative ideas.

Coprolalia and the impulse to use blasphemous expressions (*manie blasphématoire*) without the slightest external cause, and frequently in women brought up in the most careful manner, occasion intense and prolonged mental suffering, often known only to a medical confidant, to whom the unhappy subject of the affection reluctantly reveals the intrusion of unsavoury words and the incipient ejaculation of unaccustomed and undesired epithets. The writer has for years been accustomed to label this variety as more especially an obsession.

In slighter degrees, every one is occasionally annoyed by the frequent recurrence of a line of poetry or of a tune in the course of the day; or a subject may haunt the memory for days which we would willingly get rid of, but cannot. A friend wrote to us after composing a poetical work: "I long to get it out of my brain and begin on 'fresh fields and pastures new,' but you know how difficult it is to make the vibrations cease when the intellectual chimes have been set to a particular tune."

The insanity of doubt may, when it has not developed so far as to involve the patient in a state of mind in which there is no longer a consciousness on his part of the morbid nature of his trouble, and an effort to resist it, be placed under imperative ideas as already defined (*see* Doubt, Insanity of).

The forms which imperative ideas assume while primarily mental may be either motor or sensory.

Many so-called eccentric habits belong to the motor division. As an illustration may be mentioned the harmless trick of always touching the same object in passing it during an accustomed walk, as happened with Dr. Johnson. Probably some motor acts may be explained by the influence of organic memory exerting itself after the cause of the particular movement has disappeared. If, for example, a piece of furniture, or a door, the presence of which has necessitated some action of the body in order to avoid it, be removed, the no longer required movement may continue, and in a nervous state of the system is likely to become an intolerable habit, and an imperative act, the outward and invisible sign of an imperative idea. Should its true character not be recognised, it may be attributed to occult agencies, and a belief in mysterious influences may be generated.

With regard to the sensory variety, which may assume a very definite character, sometimes so agreeable to the individual as to become a fascination, and at other times so intolerable as to be a torment, the explanation may, on analysis, be found in the association of a particular perfume with an occurrence with which it has no causal relation. This observation no doubt applies to all the organs of special sense. Certainly a particular colour in some persons has become associated with certain thoughts or feelings, the result being that the perception of the former may excite to an inconvenient and morbid extent a group of ideas which at last cannot be disassociated when the individual desires it, and at last constitutes an intolerable association from which there is no escape; or the order is reversed, and a particular thought or feeling induces sensory excitation, and suggests a colour, or scent, or taste, or even a vision of the object. Here, however, we invade the department of hallucination. But, although it may be difficult to draw a hard-and-fast line between sensory obsession and hallucinations, we do not now refer to the latter in their definite form, seeing that the individual is quite lucid and cannot properly be regarded as hallucinated. He who has perpetually a particular word brought within the range of consciousness does not hear it any more than we hear the words that ordinarily pass through our minds, and therefore he is not the subject of auditory hallucination.

Passing from the motor and sensory manifestations, we have the thoughts which are poured into the mind in opposition to the person's will, those imperative conceptions, or intellectual impulses, which are more especially recognised as falling under the title of this article. It is at this point that hypnotic suggestions throw considerable light upon those quasi-insane conditions which arise independently of hypnotism. That there exists a remarkable and instructive parallelism between spontaneous and artificially induced imperious suggestions we have satisfied ourselves by personal investigation.* They agree in this, that the individual is constrained to think, to speak, or to act, by an impression produced upon his mental organisation, from within or without, as the case may be, which excites the reflex action of the brain.

We have recorded several cases illustrative of the tyranny of imperative ideas. In one case, that of a lad of nineteen, a law student who had gained distinction at school and matriculated at the London University, met, in the course of his reading, with the expression, "*It was not incompatible.*" Soon afterwards he came across the German words, "*Ich liebe es nicht.*" Now, it struck him that the negative in the former sentence preceded, and in the latter succeeded the most important word. He then began to puzzle himself about negatives in general. Whatever he read raised the question in his mind as to the construction of sentences in which a negative occurred. It became an all-important, and absorbing problem. It interfered with his reading and working. The burden of his life was to place the negative in the right order, whatever that might be.

He himself was perfectly conscious of the erratic working of his mind in relation to this subject.

There was some insane inheritance. It would be very misleading to speak of this youth as insane. Such a mental condition would not interfere with a man's testamentary capacity, and were he to commit a crime, it would be impossible to prove his irresponsibility in the eye of the law.

In another case, that of a lady, the incessant tendency to count a certain number of times before performing the simplest acts of daily life, was the prominent and very distressing symptom. This imperious necessity occasioned great mental fatigue. It had lasted for some six years, and had become an intolerable burden. The process preceded turning over in bed, or removing her watch from under her pillow. At breakfast a considerable time would elapse before she could take up the teapot, the only means of accomplishing it being the enumeration of 10 or its multiples. The same course was pursued before opening the front door, or looking into the shop windows. It would be tedious to mention all the instances of this obsession, but it may be added that the trouble is experienced at times in regard to the number of inspirations, the number of steps she takes during a walk, and her foe does not leave her in peace when threading her needle or reading a book.

In a third case, the borderland between sanity and insanity cannot be said to have been preserved. In this instance the reading of a book frequently causes signs of irritation and disgust, and on investigation it is discovered that a particular word has been the source of the excitement—why is a mystery, until further inquiry discloses the fact that it occurs if a compound word happens to contain a syllable which is the name of a person to whom many years ago she took a great aversion. It is a long time since this person died, but she still dislikes to hear or see any word that has his name in it, even although in part only. When she objects, as she often does, to the touch of people with whom she comes in contact, it is found on careful investigation that this is part of the same invincible dislike to the individual in question. Hence she makes the demand to have certain things washed for her, and she always washes her hands and face on returning from a walk. She would ask questions again and again and again bearing on her fear of contamination, saying, "Let me say it again, Did So-and-so touch my dress?"

Intellectually she is regarded as perfectly sane, exceptional in wit, fond of science and music, and possessed of an excellent memory. There is, however, a great lack of patient application. There are no hallucinations of any of the senses.

Such a case illustrates the subtle morbid mental states which are associated with the dread of contamination with objects in themselves absolutely clean, but associated by some accidental circumstance or freak of our psychical constitution, with some individual or long past event in the patient's life. What the association may be can only be determined by skilful analysis in each case.

The **prognosis** is not as a rule favourable, but although the particular obsession may not be exterminated, the patient may pass during life for being sane in the society in which he moves. On the other hand, it may become so intolerable as to lead to suicide.

As to **treatment**, those who regard this mental condition as identical with neurasthenia, recommend the treatment which has been found useful in that state. At the same time, the Weir Mitchell treatment is only likely to be useful in rare cases. Régis advises, in addition to iron,

* "Artificial Insanity," *Journ. of Ment. Sci.* 1865.

phosphates, strychnine, &c., baths of various kinds, and especially electricity, either in the form of a powerful application, of galvanism to the head (Beard), or of Franklinism (Vigouroux). A few cases have been benefited by hypnotic suggestion.

Summary.—(1) Heredity has by some alienists been regarded as an essential part of the definition of imperative ideas, but we are unable to go to this length, although doubtless it will be very frequently found when carefully looked for.

(2) Common to all cases is the bondage under which the victim lies to pursue a certain trivial or disagreeable line of thought, often associated with vocal utterances, or motor acts, along with sanity in other respects. Hence, Esquirol's term, "reasoning monomania," apply to an allied mental condition. M. Ball's phrase —intellectual impulses—is an apt one, but we would observe—

(3) That if such cases are carefully analysed, they are generally found to arise out of emotional disturbance. Morel so fully recognised this, that he employed the words *délire émotif*, and referred the mental disorder to disease of the visceral ganglionic nervous system * (Régis).

(4) Closely associated with imperative ideas is the morbid tendency to doubt and to inquire wearisomely and endlessly into the most useless subjects. As persons who labour under this disorder ardently desire to be rid of the daily trial which torments them, it is very important to have distinct views as to the reply which ought to be made to their earnest entreaty for advice. It is a mistake to recommend them to do battle with the foe, and to make desperate efforts to eject it. By virtue of a psychological law, such a mental act serves to intensify a morbid impression. It is much better to smile at it, to affect not to care for the intruder, and to treat it with dignified indifference.

THE EDITOR.

[*References.* — Morel, Archives génerales de Médecine, 1866. Charcot and Magnan, Sept. 1885. Doyen, l'Encéphale, 1885. E. Régis, Les Neurasthénics Psychiques (Obsessions émotives ou conscientes), 1891. J. Falret, Congrès international de Médecino mentale de 1889. M. Ball, l'Encéphale t. i. 1881, p. 21. Trélat, Folie Lucide, 1860. Morel, Du délire émotif, in Archives générales de Médecine, 1866. Cullerre, Les Frontières de la Folie, 1888. *Idem*, Traité pratique des Maladies mentales, 1890. Krafft-Ebing, Lehrbuch der Psychiatrie, 1883. Emil Kraepelin, Psychiatrie, 1887].

IMPOTENCE, PSYCHICAL (*impotentia*, inability; ψυχή, the soul). Impotence due to mental disturbance.

* "Archives générales de Médecine," 1866.

IMPULSE (*impulsus*, from *impello*, I push against). An influence acting upon the mind, especially suddenly or involuntarily; a sudden thought, idea, determination or emotion. (Fr. *impulsion*; Ger. *Trieb, Antrieb.*)

IMPULSE, ANIMAL.—The uncontrollable desire towards purely animal acts—*e.g.*, rape, &c. Under this term Clouston includes perverted instincts, appetites and feelings.

IMPULSE, DESTRUCTIVE. — An uncontrollable desire to destroy, which may exist alone without much outward exaltation or depression, but which is usually found as one symptom of the general psychosis of mania, excited melancholia, and the first stage of general paralysis (Clouston).

IMPULSE, HOMICIDAL.—An uncontrollable desire to lay violent hands on, or kill persons indiscriminately; a common symptom in a minor degree at the outset of mania and even melancholia. (*See* HOMICIDAL MONOMANIA.)

IMPULSE, MORBID, EMOTIONAL. —An emotion prompting to an insane act, as in some forms of moral insanity (*q.v.*).

IMPULSE, MORBID, INTELLECTUAL.—An idea prompting to an insane act.

IMPULSE, ORGANIC. (*See* IMPULSE, ANIMAL.)

IMPULSE, SUICIDAL.—The sudden uncontrollable impulse to commit self-destruction. Impulsive suicide unaccompanied by marked mental depression or delusion. In rare cases the impulse is accompanied by unconsciousness. (*See* SUICIDAL INSANITY.)

IMPULSE, UNCONTROLLABLE.—A state of defective mental inhibition, in which an idea or emotion is transformed into action against the will or wish of the subject.

IMPULSES, EPILEPTIFORM. — Sudden impulsive acts, attended by unconsciousness, which are exactly the same in character as those that occur in epileptics, and yet the patients are not subject to ordinary epilepsy (Clouston).

IMPULSIONS, INTELLECTUELLES. (Fr.)—A term employed by Ball for Imperative Ideas (*q.v.*).

IMPULSIVE INSANITY. (*See* DESTRUCTIVE IMPULSES.)

IMPULSIVE MONOMANIA. (*See* MONOMANIA.)

IMPUTABILITY (*imputibilitas*; from *in*, *puto*, I think). The condition as to being of sound mind so as to be legally responsible for one's actions. (Ger. *Imputibilität, Zurechnungsfähigkeit.*)

INCAPACITY, TESTAMENTARY. (*See* TESTAMENTARY CAPACITY.)

INCOHERENCE (*in*, neg.; *cohæreo*, I stick to). A want or absence of cohesion or connection of ideas, language, &c., incongruity, inconsequence, inconsistency of diction. Also used by Prichard as a synonym of Dementia.

INCOMPETENCE, MENTAL (*in*; *competo*, I am capable; *mens*). A condition of mental disorder sufficient to prevent a person from managing his own affairs.

INCUBUS (*in*, on; *cubitum*, a couch). A synonym of Nightmare or Ephialtes.

INDECISION, MORBID (*in*; *decido*; *morbus*). An insane want of firmness or determination of the will, wavering of the mind, irresolution. (*See* ECCENTRICITY and MELANCHOLIA.)

INDIA.—To grasp the psychological characteristics of the Indian nation, we must remember that although the India of to-day consists of a vast mosaic of peoples, there are three great races—the primitive inhabitants, absolutely unmixed with others, and inhabiting mountains inaccessible to civilisation; the Hindoo, a fusion of the white race with the original black inhabitants; lastly, the Mussulman population drived from the Arab, Persian, Turcoman and Mongolian races.

The preponderance of castes is the corner-stone of all the social institutions of the Indian people and is of psychological interest. As it was three thousand years ago, so it is to-day—a striking contrast to the Jews.

The most religious person always establishes a division between the sacred and the profane, but it is not so with the Hindoos, to whom this distinction is absolutely unintelligible. Labour, meals, sleep, are religious acts. Implicit obedience to the orders of the innumerable hierarchy of their gods, to the laws of Menon, unchanged through two thousand years, has uniformly moulded their brains. Hence it happens that psychopathic manifestations are rare, and with difficulty distinguishable from that religious mysticism which still remains in spite of the intelligence and the artistic spirit found in these peoples in contrast with the primitive life of other races.

Those few endemic forms of mental disorder which do occur, reflect an entirely religious character, for when Indian civilisation under the impulse of Arabian science, is opened to intelligent speculations, their minds inevitably revert to their hereditary mysticism. The Arabian magic and astrology become, in the Indian people, supernatural speculations representing the fables of their ancestors, and enter into their very brain, which may be said to become a temple in which they get fixed, digested, and assimilated by the sacred flame of a limitless faith, and give birth to spiritualism and fakirism. India is in truth the country *par excellence* of spiritualism, and the fakirs are its priests. Moreover, the history of India in its psychological fixity, cramping as it does mental action and progress, affords no soil for the production of epidemics of insanity. In their place, we witness endemic manifestations, but, be it observed, always within the limits of superstition and faith. Hence it comes to pass that a population of 250,000,000 remains subject to the domination of 60,000 Europeans, and only prays to have its daily handful of rice, and to be permitted to obey the laws of Menon, all else being of little or no consequence. Another endemic feature is the prevailing fatalism, which can hardly be otherwise, since everything happens according to the preordained will of the gods.

If history, however, fails to show us cases of actual insanity in the form of epidemics, it nevertheless exhibits an important phenomenon of which we have already spoken, and which offers at the present day a living anachronism, not persons sane and insane, but all either sane or insane; that is, a people who cultivate their inheritance without exchange of ideas, preserving their own psychological ideas intact in spite of contact with other forms of thought, a people who have insanity within certain confined limits, and are content with the simple but good life of their ancestors.

We must not suppose that their intellectual level is superior to the average of that of the Europeans. In the arts and sciences, it is equal and often superior, but it possesses no creative power, and its genius is lost in mystic speculations. The immense number of monuments of Brahminism and Buddhism always indicate the confused modifications of the same primitive conception. The Indians were great in metaphysics, poetry, and theology, but in the exact sciences below mediocrity.

Another characteristic endemic which probably reflects the general habits of a people of primitive times, is the extraordinary habit of *seeing things as they are not*, to which could be applied (as Le Brun well expresses it in his learned work on Indian Civilisation) the term deforming psychology, by reason of which they entirely transform the facts in their three thousand years of civilisation, always under the ever-present influence of polytheistic mysticism.

(1) Thus there was the Vedic period about fifteen centuries B.C. The family and tribe were the basis of society, and the gods were confounded with their ancestors. The transmission of life to a son was only the passage of Agni, divine fire, fertile principle capable of perpetuating life, and making the spirits of the dead reappear—the first basis of spiritualism. The worship of woman was carried to the highest degree, as in feudal ages of chivalry, and this is important, because it explains how chivalry is strictly endemic, seeing that although not cultivated elsewhere, it is found in the race of the Rajpoots, the only one worthy of being compared with the cavaliers of the Holy Sepulchre. The principal aberration of this people, endemic to this day, consists in gambling away their own children, and even their personal liberty. They worshipped the forces of Nature, and their ancestors believed in the immortality of the soul, and in polytheism, subordinate to a belief in one god, master of all, and in the idea of bargaining between him and man.

(2) The Brahmin civilisation originated in the basin of the Ganges, where the laws of Menon were promulgated as they still exist. Brahminism dethroned woman; she became thenceforward almost a servant, and she was condemned to follow her dead husband to the funeral pyre.

(3) Buddhism, which prevailed from the fifth century B.C., exhibited fetishism at its highest point—the separation from the world, and, as a supreme hope, the destruction of form, that is to say, man's personality, and absorption into the state of Nirvana. As asceticism favoured its development, India was in time covered with monasteries and dervishes.

(4) Then, in the course of centuries, the Neo-brahmistic period was marked by the endemic renewal of that chivalry which the Brahmins had ultimately suppressed.

(5) During the Indo-Mussulman period, fertile in refinement and the sciences, the chivalric race of the Rajpoots flourished unchanged.

(6) The so-called modern period was characterised not only by the same chivalric organisations, but by endemic fatalism — the belief in unavoidable destiny.

Mental life passes in the masses without optimism or pessimism—the two extremes of feeling which in other races give rise to most disorders of the mind. The Indians suffer without complaint. Suicide—that gauge of human pessimism—is infrequent. The greatest sceptics will kiss Buddha's feet, and completely opposite dogmas exist in perfect harmony. Religious and intellectual revolutions are exceedingly rare. While, however, the results of spiritual excitement are wanting, there are chronic endemics crystallised under the form of numerous sects, along with perfect tolerance. True epidemics do not occur, or rather they are concealed by psychical customs, amidst which mental aberrations would only be noticed by comparison with the members of other races. If the Indians marry Europeans, the tendencies which in them are normal, but in us would be morbid, break out. Long ago the ancient Aryans understood this danger and forbade marriages with strangers. Thus the half-breeds resulting from such marriages constitute a race of a degenerate type. Similarly, the climate and soil of China are only adapted to the preservation of the mentality of its own children.

The priests of Baigns, when a tiger has eaten human flesh, think that the demon in it is mingled with the soul of the victim, and exorcise it in order to drive out the souls, and to this end begin to gesticulate, howl and whirl rapidly round, until thus intoxicated, they believe themselves transformed into tigers. They then throw themselves upon a goat, tearing its flesh with their teeth. They then show themselves covered with blood to the applauding public.

The belief in witchcraft exists among the Nilgerris, who see in the Karommbas, the inhabitants of marshy places, wizards gifted with supernatural power. These they implore to relieve them of their evils, which the Karommbas do by raving and whirling round and round until they fall to the ground.

On the whole, the Indians in their mosaic, offer to us a still unexhausted preserve of primitive psychical life, a mine for those who study folk-lore, but it has not as yet developed true endemic insanity, although we witness endemics of spiritualism, chivalry, and caste, which are influenced by preponderating religious colouring.

A. Tamburini.
S. Tonnini.

Note.—Hindoo medicine, as handed down to us in systematic works which were composed at an early period, probably dating from the tenth century to the third B.C., contains interesting references to madness. In the works of Charaka and Susruta, *Unmada* comprises madness and idiocy.* The causes of the disease are

* "Review of the History of Medicine," by Thomas A. Wise, M.D., from whose work this

recognised as they would be at the present day — improper food, over-work, powerful emotions, poison, &c. To these the derangement of the wind, bile and phlegm was attributed, and it was held that this disturbance affected the seat of the understanding and the heart, passing through the vessels and developing insanity. Six kinds of madness were enumerated, according as it was produced by one of the foregoing, by their combination, by violent passions, or by poison. When illusions are caused by the derangement of the wind the patient laughs, dances, and sings unreasonably, or cries without a cause. The skin becomes dry, rough, and of a dark-red colour, and emaciation follows. When bile is the cause, the symptoms are marked by impatience of control and anger, and he attempts violence; he removes all his clothes, and desires to live under the shade, or in water. In derangement of the phlegm, the symptoms are love of solitude, taciturnity, and anorexia. Madness caused by the combination of wind, bile, and phlegm, presents all the symptoms mentioned, and the disorder is very difficult to cure. Caused by strong emotions, as from fright or loss of money, the symptoms manifest themselves in talking, laughing, singing, and crying, and it is apt to terminate in dementia.

Treatment of these forms of insanity consisted in cleansing the body, anointing it with mustard oil, heated by the sun for two hours; giving *ghee* for some days, and then strong purgatives, emetics, errhines, and mustard oil. Prayers to God and advice to the patient were prescribed, as also exercise, studying the shastres, temperance, and the love of the gods. "Curious or wonderful exhibitions may be made before the patient, and he should be informed of the death of relatives and friends; or may be frightened by the alarm of robbers, by the approach of elephants, and harmless serpents. He should be threatened, and even beaten with a whip when he acts improperly, and should live on light food, such as barley and congee water, made agreeable by the addition of carminatives; *ghee* should be given with a concoction of vegetables" (p. 182). Notwithstanding the whipping recommended, it is advised that "during the cure the person should be generally treated, as much as possible, with kindness and consideration."

In cases in which poison causes mental disorder, the treatment must be varied according to the toxic agent.

Suicide is incidentally referred to in somewhat different terms from those employed at the present time, for it is observed that "when the patient has no sleep, *and is so courageous that he will throw himself from a height*, the disease will be fatal" (p. 183). THE EDITOR.

account is taken, kindly sent to the editor by the author for the purpose of preparing a work on the history of the insane in various parts of the world. See vol. ii. p. 179.

INDIAN HEMP. (*See* SEDATIVES.)

INEBRIETY, LAW OF.—The medico-legal questions that arise in connection with inebriety, may fairly be treated under the two heads of *contract* and *crime*.

As to the contractual capacity of the inebriate, three distinct theories have at different periods prevailed. The *first* is that of Lord Coke. "As for a drunkard, who is *voluntarius daemon*, he hath (as has beene said) no privilege thereby, but what hurt or ill so ever he doth, his drunkennesse doth aggravate it. *Omne crimen ebrietas et incendit et detegit.*" (Co. Litt. 247 *a.*) These remarks, although apparently applicable to the criminal law alone, are made by Coke with reference to the law of contract; and furnish him with a reason for extending to drunkenness the maxim of the common law with regard to lunacy, that no man of full age shall be allowed to disable or stultify himself. In the Year-Book of 39 Hen. VI. 42, it is said that a feoffment to one who is drunk or ill is good, but a feoffment to one of non-sane memory is bad. The distinction here pointed at between drunkenness and lunacy had disappeared by the time of Coke; drunkenness was itself regarded as a type of madness—*dementia affectata*—and the drunkard, like the lunatic, was not permitted to set up his incapacity as a defence to an action of contract.

The *second* theory, which governed the course of English case-law till the middle of the present century, may be stated thus: "If a man is so drunk . . . . as not to know what he is about, he cannot have that consenting mind which is indispensable to the formation of a contract, and his agreement is, therefore, merely void. But if his mind is only so confused or weak that he cannot be said not to know what he is about, but yet is incapable of fully understanding the terms and effect of his contract, and if this is known to the other party, then he may indeed contract, but the contract will be voidable at his option, on the ground not of his own incapacity, but of the other party's fraud in taking advantage of his weakness, though such weakness be short of incapacity." (Pollock "On Contract," p. 90.)

It will be observed that in this doctrine there are two branches, and that the drunkard's contract is either *void* for incapacity, or *voidable* for fraud, according to circumstances. Mr. Justice Buller, in his "Nisi Prius," said (p. 172), that under a plea of "no execution" (*non est factum*), the defendant "may give in evidence that they made him sign the bond when he was so drunk that he did not know what he did." This is an authority for the first branch of the doctrine under consideration. (*Cf. Pitt* v. *Smith*, 3 Camp. 33; *Cory* v. *Cory*, per Lord Hardwicke, 1 Ves. 19; *Gore* v. *Gibson*, 13 M. & W. 623.) *Lightfoot* v. *Heron* (3 Y. & Coll. 586) is conclusive as to the existence of the second. A. sold real property to B. At the completion of the purchase B. was drinking with C., A.'s solicitor, and acted without professional advice. The price, however, was fair, and it did not appear that either A. or C. had desired to prevent B. from employing a solicitor. Specific performance was decreed. It is clear that, if any advantage had been taken of B.'s position, the decision would have been different. Both branches of the theory are stated in the judgment of Sir W. Grant, in *Cooke* v. *Clayworth* (8 Ves. 12, 15): "I think," said his lordship, "a Court of Equity ought not to assist a person to get rid of any agreement or deed merely upon the ground of his having been intoxicated at the time; I say merely upon that ground, as if there was .... any unfair advantage made of the situation, or .... any contrivance or management to draw him into drink, he might be a proper object of relief in a Court of Equity. As to that extreme state of intoxication that deprives a man of his reason, I apprehend that even at law it would invalidate a deed obtained from him while in that condition."

The *third* and modern theory is that which was formally accepted in the leading cases of *Molton* v. *Camroux* (18 L. J. Ex. 68, 356),* and *Matthews* v. *Baxter* (L. R. 8 Ex. 132). It may be expressed in the following terms. A contract entered into by a person apparently sober, and not known, either actually or constructively, by the other contracting party, to be intoxicated, is valid if fair and *bonâ fide*, and especially if wholly or partly executed, so that the parties cannot be restored to their original position.

The facts in *Molton* v. *Camroux* are set out in the article on the CONTRACTS OF LUNATICS, to which it relates, and need not be recapitulated here.

In *Matthews* v. *Baxter*, A. had bought houses and land of B. at a public auction. A. was at the time, and to the knowledge of B., so drunk as to be incapable of transacting business. It was held by the Court of Exchequer that A.'s contract was not void, *but voidable only*, and that he might ratify it when sober.

The *ratio decidendi* in those cases is expounded by Sir Frederick Pollock, with his wonted elegance and force. "It is obviously reasonable that one who offers to contract with a drunken man (or a madman), knowing his condition, should do so at his peril. If the drunkenness (or lunacy) be not actually or presumably known to the other party, the contract is valid; for a man who is apparently (sane or) sober cannot be supposed absolutely incapable of knowing what he is about. But except in this case the other party must be able to see that it is at least doubtful whether the man is capable of understanding the effect of a contract; if he chooses to disregard that doubt, he cannot afterwards complain of being taken at his word. He is in a manner estopped from saying that by reason of the other's incapacity there is no contract which can be made binding on either of them. The law says to them: 'You offer to contract with a man whom you have every reason to believe impossible of contracting; and if he chooses to hold you to the bargain when he comes to his right mind, it does not lie in your mouth to say there was no contract, because he did not understand what he was about. If you thought he did understand it, you cannot complain of being in the same situation as if such was the fact. If you knew he did not understand it, then (when you meant to commit a fraud by taking an unfair advantage of his condition) you were careless enough to take the risk of his repudiating the contract, or you thought the mere chance of a ratification worth having. Still less can you complain in that case that the contract is ratified instead of being repudiated. And you have the correlative benefit of being able to sue on the contract if it is ratified, *or even if it is not repudiated within a reasonable time*.'" (Pollock "On Contract," pp. 446, 447.)

The law of England as to the criminal responsibility of the inebriate was practically settled on its present basis in the time of Coke. It has been tacitly modified in recent years, perhaps to a greater extent than most lawyers are aware, under the influence of advancing medical knowledge and criticism; but the *criteria* of

* See article on the CONTRACTS OF LUNATICS, *supra*. The doctrine of *Molton* v. *Camroux* had previously been accepted in Courts of Equity (*Niell* v. *Morley* 9 Ves. 478).

the sixteenth century are still propounded in legal text-books, and are nominally applied in the trial of criminal cases. It may be interesting, and in the light of the attention which the subject is now receiving it is most important, to trace the development of this branch of the criminal law. An admirable statement of Coke's theory as to the responsibility of inebriates to the criminal law will be found in Professor Gairdner's paper on "Drunkenness and Dipsomania," published in the *Birmingham Medical Review*, for January 1890. "A drunkard, according to Coke, is *voluntarius daemon—i.e.*, a man *possessed*, dominated by an evil spirit not his own, but whom he chooses, of his own accord . . . . to invite into possession, whereupon follows the strictly legal consequence that while the fact of possession, or, as we should say, of *insanity*, is admitted by implication, the privilege attaching to the fact is avoided or set aside; for, he adds, the drunkard *hath no privilege thereby but what hurt or ill so ever he doth, his drunkennesse doth aggravate*."

Sir Matthew Hale, in his "Pleas of the Crown," gives the following account of the legal theory:—

"The third sort of *dementia* is that which is *dementia affectata*—viz., drunkenness. This vice doth deprive men of the use of reason, and puts many men into a perfect but temporary frenzy, and therefore, according to some civilians, such a person committing homicide shall not be punished simply for the crime of homicide, but shall suffer for his drunkenness, answerable to the nature of the crime occasioned thereby, so that the general cause of his punishment is rather the drunkenness than the crime committed in it; but by the laws of England such a person shall have no privilege by this voluntary contracted madness; but shall have the same judgment as if he were in his right senses.

"But yet there seem to be two allays to to be allowed in this case.

"(1) That if a person by the unskilfulness of his physicians, or by the contrivance of his enemies, eat or drink such as causeth a temporary frenzy, as *aconitum* or *nux romica*, this puts him into the same condition in reference to crime as any other frenzy, and equally excuseth him.

"(2) That although the *simplex* frenzy, occasioned *immediately* by drunkenness, excuse not in criminals, yet if by one or more practices an *habitual* or fixed frenzy be caused, though this madness was contracted by the vice and will of the party, yet this habitual or fixed frenzy thereby caused puts the man into the same condition in relation to crimes as if the same were contracted involuntarily at first."

Other "allays" to the common law doctrine are now recognised.

(1) Drunkenness may properly be, and is, taken into consideration by a jury where the question for determination is whether an act was premeditated, or done with sudden heat and impulse.

Cf. Reg. v. *Grindley*, per Holroyd, J., 1819, MS. cited 1 Russ. *Crimes*, 115, n. (u). This dictum was declared not to be good law in *Reg.* v. *Carroll* (7 C. & P. 145); and it was said in *Reg.* v. *Meakin* (*ib.* 297) to be peculiarly erroneous in cases where a dangerous or deadly weapon was employed—by a prisoner. To formulate any such statement as this last, however, as an abstract portion of law is injudicious. Intoxication might be an extenuating circumstance where a drunken soldier used the bayonet, as well as where a drunken schoolmaster used the birch. The question is merely complicated by such hasty generalisations. The essence of the exception under discussion is the complete or partial inability of the accused to form the criminal intention which is necessary to constitute the criminal act; and the principle upon which his punishment is modified is the same, whatever may have been the instrument with which the act was committed.*

(2) Drunkenness may legitimately be considered where the prisoner acted in self-defence (*Reg.* v. *Gamlen*, 1 F. & F. 90), or under provocation (*Reg.* v. *Monkhouse*, 4 Cox, C.C. 55), and the question is whether the danger apprehended, or the provocation, was sufficient to justify his action. Other cases, explicable upon the same or similar principles, will be found in the law reports.

(3) In the case of *Wm. Rennie* (1 Lew. 76), it was laid down that drunkenness is no excuse for crime unless the mental derangement resulting therefrom is fixed and continuous (*Cf. Reg.* v. *Davis*, 1881, 14 Cox, C.C. 564, per Stephen, J.).

Mr. Justice Day, in the case of *Reg.* v. *Baines*, tried at Lancaster Winter Assizes in 1886, appears to have dissented from this view of the law. The following report is taken from the *Times* of Monday, Jan. 25, 1886: "Counsel for the prosecution . . . . submitted that a state of disease brought about by a person's own act

* *Cf.* Bacon, "Maxims of the Law," *Reg.* v. *Plowden*, Comm. 19.

* *Cf.* the following "charges" by Lord Deas, 5 Irvine, Justiciary Reports, 479; and *H. M. Advocate* v. *Granger*, 1878, *Scottish Law Reporter*, vol. xvi. p. 253.

—*e.g.*, *delirium tremens*—was no excuse for committing a crime, unless the disease so produced was permanent. His lordship remarked that . . . . it was immaterial whether the insanity was *permanent or temporary*, and added, I have ruled that if a man were in such a state of intoxication that he did not know the nature of his act, or that it was wrongful, he would be excusable."

(4) Involuntary drunkenness resulting from a temporarily diseased condition will exempt from criminal responsibility. *Cf. Reg.* v. *Mary R.*, 1887, per Palles, C.B. (cited by Norman Kerr, M.D., "Inebriety," 2nd edit., p. 395): "If a person," said his lordship, "from any cause—say long-watching, want of sleep, or depravation of blood—was reduced to such a condition that a smaller quantity of stimulant would make him drunk than would produce such a state if he were in health, then neither law nor common sense could hold him responsible for his acts, inasmuch as they were not voluntarily, but produced by disease."

It will be observed that this doctrine marks a decided advance on the second "allay" of Sir Matthew Hale *supra*.

(5) The law appears now to be the same where insane predisposition, and not actual physical disease, is the proximate cause of the intoxication. (*Cf. Reg.* v. *Mountain*, Leeds Assizes, April 1888, per Pollock, B.) A. Wood Renton.

INERTIA, MENTAL (*iners*, without skill, slothful). A want of functional mental activity, sluggishness of mental action.

INFLUENCE, UNDUE. (*See* Undue Influence.)

INFLUENZA, Mental Disorder following.—(I.) In no other allied disease is the nervous system attacked in so high a degree. Throughout the complaint nervous symptoms may occur and are sometimes so prominent as to form a nervous type. Such symptoms are headache, chiefly frontal, associated sometimes with vertigo, sometimes with marked hyperæsthesia of the sense organs, more rarely with nervous vomiting; sleeplessness which is obstinate; painful muscular sensations; lastly, pains in the course of the nerves, most commonly in the trigeminus, dependent probably on neuritis. After the subsidence of the fever, other nervous disturbances though they are less common, occur. Among these are severe affections, often incurable, of the sense organs, motor disturbances, especially well-marked pareses of the ocular muscles, paralysis of the extremities, referable to degenerative neuritis. Lastly, there have been recorded a few cases of severe organic changes in the central nervous system. Far more frequent and of much greater interest are the symptoms of intense nervous exhaustion, observed in the after-stages of influenza. These stand in no relation to the duration of the febrile stage, and such may persist for weeks. In other cases, hysterical and neurasthenic symptoms may ensue.

The psychical derangements are by no means new. They are as old as the influenza itself. In 1580, influenzal psychoses were observed, and again at the close of the last century. Bonnet (Bordeaux) reported a case of mania in 1837, and Crichton Browne in 1874, one of "acute dementia" following influenza. Recent observations show that psychoses after influenza are quite common.

Including our own and other reported cases, we reckon 54 cases, and on these we base our conclusions.

We divide the symptoms into those of febrile and post-febrile stages. Of the former fifteen cases were observed: Delirium—an acute transitory psychosis, associated with delusions and hallucinations, jubilant and noisy, or of a depressed character. From the onset this delirium is frequently adynamic. In some instances the very severe headache increases up to the height of the delirium, and is then followed by symptoms of meningitis, ending in coma and death. On post-mortem, hyperæmia of the brain and membranes is the rule; only in rare cases has meningitis been found.

The duration of the delirium may vary from a few hours to several days. It may be of remittent or intermittent type. It may be extremely difficult to differentiate between the psychosis of influenza and the delirium. Depression usually predominates. The expression of the patient points rarely to exaltation, religious ecstasy or erotomania, but more frequently to melancholia, with ideas of persecution, self-incrimination and hypochondriasis. Hallucinations are visual, auditory and tactile. Food is frequently refused in consequence of maniacal excitement, occasionally from the belief that the food has been drugged.

The temperature is as a rule raised more or less, and may reach 104 or more.

The prognosis is in general good, the mental affection disappearing in from one to a few weeks; more rarely its course is protracted. Death is to be attributed to a complication of pneumonia and cardiac weakness. Alcoholics attacked by influenza show symptoms of acute alcoholism.

The post-influenzal psychoses include all those cases (39) which appear on the cessation of the fever. The time of their appearance may vary from a few days to two or three weeks. The clinical features may be divided into three groups: (1) acute exhaustion; (2) melancholia; (3) mania.

(1) Acute exhaustion (11 cases), resemble essentially the delirium of collapse (Hermann-Weber) and the asthenic psychoses (Kraepelin). In the higher grades, the condition may be named acute hallucinatory confusion (Verwirrtheit). The bodily condition is marked by great weakness and anæmia. As a rule, health is restored in from three to six weeks. But rarely does it become chronic.

(2) Melancholia (22 cases); every degree of depression may occur. The form is in general simple, *i.e.*, without delusions. Many writers have drawn attention to the insomnia present in the convalescent stage of influenza as the starting-point of the morbid depression. It is often hypochondriacal in character.

(3) Mania. This is the least frequent of the mental sequelæ of influenza; only six typical cases have been recorded. Mania is as a rule without hallucinations and delusions. Severe mania with incoherence is very rare. The excitement begins in about a week after the invasion of the influenza, and rapidly culminates. Of the before-mentioned six cases, four recovered in from six to eight weeks, two ran a protracted course, and the prognosis was much less favourable.

Besides these principal types, there are a small number of cases on record in which hysterical and paralytic troubles as well as a few cases of paranoia followed the attack of influenza; but in all these cases the influenza seems to have been only an exciting cause, the predisposition being already there. It is advisable to name such cases *pseudo*-influenzal psychoses. Under this head would fall the acute alcoholic delirium after influenza.

The febrile and post-febrile mental affections thus differ very markedly from each other. The former differ in no wise from the ordinary effects of high temperature in the course of a fever. Predisposition plays no part. On the other hand, the post-febrile troubles assume definite types of mental disorder. Predisposition is here of the greatest importance. Of thirty-nine cases in this category, no fewer than twenty-one suffered from hereditary taint, *i.e.*, 54 per cent., a much larger proportion therefore than obtains in psychoses in general.

In the asthenic psychoses, it is the exhaustion produced by influenza which gives the character to the affection. In simple mental affections, the past history includes many chronic troubles (hysteria, anæmia, &c.) which have lowered the patient's vitality.

Although we have thus determined certain ætiological factors, we cannot in view of the short febrile stage of influenza, avoid the conclusion that a special toxic element plays an important part. In accordance with this conclusion, the psychoses may to some extent rank among those due to intoxication (toxic insanity).

To sum up:

(1) Influenza which affects more or less the whole nervous system, may easily be the cause of insanity.

(2) Such mental disorder is of frequent occurrence, as the recent epidemic (1890–91) proves, and is relatively of more common occurrence than in other acute febrile affections.

(3) The mental disorder may arise in the febrile stage, and present itself in the form of the ordinary delirium of fever, or much less commonly may appear as an acute febrile psychosis of more prolonged course, but of good prognosis as a rule.

(4) The mental disorder sets in on the cessation of the fever, and assumes, at one time an asthenic form, and at another, a simple psychosis in which melancholia predominates.

(5) All these disorders, presenting as they do no specific characters, run, in the majority of cases, a short course to recovery. A few, however, are more protracted in their course, and offer a graver prognosis.

(6) Besides the above, there are paralytic and hysterical psychoses; also cases of paranoia, occur as sequelæ.* L. Kirn.

INFLUENZA, Mental Disorder following.—(II.) There have been in our experience a number of cases in which, however true it may be that the fever of influenza is frequently followed by the same nervous disorders which any other febrile excitement might occasion, the mental affection is of a peculiar character. It is remarkable, for example, how the symptoms may simulate general paralysis. It is important to bear this in mind and to give a guarded opinion when post-influenzal.

We have seen a considerable number of cases of one form or other of mental disorder following influenza (although not always certainly caused by it), which have been admitted into Bethlem Hospital. The following short summary of 18 such cases

* The substance of this article has appeared in the *Allgemeine Zeitschrift für Psychiatrie*, Bd. xlviii. Heft 1 and 2.

will, it is hoped, assist the reader in the study of the relationship between the two factors.*

(1) Male, age 40, with insane inheritance. First attack. Date of influenza, May 3, 1890. Appearance of mental symptoms, May 17, the first being an epileptiform seizure; subsequently loss of memory, dirty habits, destructive, the symptoms being those of general paralysis—viz., unequal pupils, tongue-tremor, sluggish knee-jerks, loss of facial expression, writing very tremulous. Remains under treatment.

(2) Male, age 30. First attack; date of influenza, June 1891; mental symptoms early in August; depressed; suspected poison in his food; was excited two days before his admission, and said that God had visited him; admitted in a state of partial stupor, with refusal of food. It should be stated that before the influenza he was much reduced from over-work. Under treatment.

(3) Male, age 23. First attack; slight family history of insanity; date of influenza, April 22, 1891; he had delirium, and in the second week of May had pneumonia; mental symptoms appeared on the 22nd of this month, the form being that of acute mania; he recovered, and was discharged September 2, 1891.

(4) Male, age 27. No family history of insanity; first attack; had influenza in March 1890; was very weak afterwards and easily affected; the attack commenced almost immediately after the influenza; it assumed the form of melancholia with stupor; patient died in the hospital of acute peritonitis.

(5) Male, age 44. No insane inheritance; first attack; had influenza in the winter (1889–90), followed by bronchitis and abscess in the ear; business worry troubled him; appearance of mental symptoms in August; he had acute mania with marked exaltation; he recovered, and was discharged November 1890. In this case the influenza seemed to be the predisposing cause: the knee-jerk sluggish, as also the reaction of pupils to light. The diagnosis was (?) general paralysis.

(6) Male, age 41. No family history of insanity; influenza at Christmas 1889, and was ill with it a week; the mental symptoms appeared immediately afterwards; the symptoms being melancholia with idea of bowel obstruction, and hallucination of hearing, sight and smell; at first there were tremor of face, marked tremor of tongue, hesitation in speech; reflexes very lively; case diagnosed as (?) general paralysis; he was discharged well September 10, 1890.

(7) Male, age 46. Not reported to be hereditary; fourth attack; influenza at the beginning of January 1890; mental symptoms commenced shortly afterwards in the form of acute mania; the three previous attacks were of the same character; patient was discharged well in August 1890.

(8) Female, age 27. No heredity; fourth attack; influenza, February 1890; mental disorder end of April; admitted suffering from acute mania in September; the three previous attacks were marked by excitement; she was discharged well in August 1891.

(9) Female, age 28. Paternal aunt insane; first attack; influenza in December 1889; became mentally affected middle of August 1890; admitted in a state of acute mania; discharged recovered in February 1891.

(10) Female, age 46. Sister died insane; first attack; influenza in the beginning of October 1890; mental symptoms immediately after; admitted with acute mania; discharged well February 1891; she was re-admitted in April, labouring under melancholia, and remains under treatment (October 1891).

(11) Female, age 24. Brother insane; first attack; influenza, December 1889; hysterical excitement in the following March; admitted in June 1890 with acute mania; from July 1890 to January 1891 mental stupor; discharged recovered May 1891. It should be mentioned that the patient suffered from over-work as well as influenza.

(12) Female, age 24. No heredity history; first attack; influenza middle of December 1889; depressed and suspicious afterwards; admitted in February 1890, with melancholia and suspicion. Discharged in January 1891 relieved, and remained lethargic and defective memory.

(13) Female, age 31. No heredity; first attack; very severe influenza, November 1890; in December became irritable and forgetful; in May 1891 was very much depressed, with tendency to stupor; hallucinations of hearing and sight; to the Convalescent Home, October 13, 1891.

(14) Female, age 36. No insane history; second attack; influenza in May 1891; mental symptoms in July; acute mania; remains under treatment; the previous attack was in May 1883 (mania).

(15) Female, age 32. (Brother committed suicide two months after influenza in July 1891.) First attack; influenza in April 1891; depression came on after in-

* We have to thank Dr. Percy Smith for permission to publish these cases, and Dr. Corner, assistant medical officer, for reporting them.

fluenza; mental symptoms; delusional melancholia, with hallucinations of hearing, sight, taste (?) and smell; also strange feelings all over the body; remains under treatment.

(16) Female, age 46. Climacteric insanity in the mother; second attack; influenza beginning of March 1891; after the attack was depressed and despondent, and said she was going to die; in August, developed the idea of bowel obstruction, and the refusal of food; active melancholia; under treatment; twenty-one years ago had an attack of puerperal mania.

(17) Female, age 26. No heredity; first attack; influenza early in June 1891; immediately afterwards she became scrupulous and excitable; she was admitted labouring under melancholia, and remains under treatment.

(18) Female, age 68. Brother a dipsomaniac; first attack; influenza early in June 1891; symptoms of insanity immediately afterwards; admitted with melancholia, with refusal of food and idea of bowel obstruction; remains under treatment.

Reports of cases of mental disorder following influenza have appeared in a considerable number of the medical journals, at home and abroad.

Schweich in his work "Die Influenza," published in Berlin in 1836, refers on good authority to an epidemic of influenza in Germany so far back as 1580, in which mental symptoms were recorded.

A later epidemic occurred in 1737, in which the mental affection was much more severe, being in fact, raving madness. Death frequently intervened at an early stage.

Kraepelin (Dorpat) has reported eleven cases of insanity following influenza. He divides his cases into three classes: (*a*) Disorders with mental depression and fully developed melancholia. (*b*) Disorders which may be regarded in the light of delirium from exhaustion and which bear the stamp of so-called hallucinatory confusion. (*c*) Cases in which the mental disorder was apparently latent and was lit up by an attack of influenza (*Deutsch. Medicin. Wochensch.* 13 März 1891: "Ueber Psychosen nach Influenza").

Bartels has reported the case of a patient at Hildesheim, a paranoiac, who had almost recovered from his mental affection, when he had an attack of influenza, in consequence of which he relapsed and manifested acute symptoms of mental distress and confusion, apparently connected with hallucination. He sank rapidly and died. The post-mortem revealed pachymeningitis and leptomeningitis. (*Neurolog. Centralblatt*, No. 6: "Einfluss von Influenza auf Geisteskrankheit").

Becker, in the same journal, relates the case of a girl who, in good health but having a neurotic inheritance, was attacked with influenza and subsequently suffered from acute delusional insanity. The attack gradually subsided.

H. Fehr, of the asylum of Middelfort (Denmark) has published several cases of mental disorder following influenza. After the symptoms of the latter had passed away, the mental disorder appeared in the form of hallucinations and mental confusion. He agrees with Kirn, in comparing these psychoses to the mental disorders which follow febrile attacks.

A case is reported in the *Deutsche Reichszeitung*, No. 28, Jan. 29, 1890, of a young man of good family who became insane in consequence of a severe attack of influenza and killed his own mother with an axe.

Dr. Franz Mispelbaum, assistant medical officer at the Bonn Asylum, has written an article in the *Allgemeine Zeitschrift für Psychiatrie*, Bd. 47, 1 Heft 1891, entitled "Ueber Psychosen nach Influenza." In it he reports ten cases of mental disorder following influenza. He does not separate those with hereditary from those without hereditary history. He asks whether influenza is the only cause of the supervening insanity in any special way. He comes to the conclusion that it is not, but that it belongs to the same class as other post-febrile psychoses. It is an open question whether ptomaines are formed in the blood, or whether the streptococcus produces chemical decomposition. Whatever view is taken, it cannot be disputed that the exhaustion caused by influenza is not dangerous only to the pulmonary organs, but to the brain.

Schmitz, in an article in the *Allgemeine Zeitschrift* (Bd. 47, Heft 3), has reported eight cases of mental disorder following influenza, under his own observation. Among his conclusions are these:—That influenza is in the first place an epidemic nervous disorder; that in the study of this subject it is desirable to omit all cases in which there is a suspicion of the existence of any mental affection prior to the attack of influenza; that the psychoses resulting from influenza do not present any special characteristic unless it be the remarkably slow recovery from the attack; but in cases in which there was already some mental disturbance prior to the influenza the prognosis is very unfavourable, while on the contrary in other cases it is quite the reverse; that as regards treatment a generous diet, wine, and baths are indicated, and that no medicine is better than quinine, inasmuch as it is not only a tonic but destroys micro-organisms.

At the Edinburgh Royal Asylum, as many as 140 cases of influenza occurred in 1889-90, and have been reported by Drs. George M. Robertson and Frank L. Elkins, the assistant physicians. Frontal headache was almost always present, accompanied by giddiness, or lightheadedness. Usually there was considerable mental depression. Among the sane inmates of the asylum there was a want of attention and concentration of thought. Disagreeable dreams disturbed the sleep, and in four cases there was delirium. In patients labouring under delusional insanity, especially with suspicion, there was aggravation of the mental symptoms.

We do not observe any statement of beneficial effect upon the mental condition of the patients, nor do we note any report of lasting insanity among the sequelæ in the sane population of the institution who were attacked by the epidemic.

The number of patients affected by the outbreak of influenza, which was severe in character, amounted to 817, and of the officials there were 175, making a total of 992.

THE EDITOR.

[References.—Prof. Arnold Pick, Prague, Ueber Geisteskrankheit nach Influenza. Mendel's Neurolog. Centralblatt, 1890, No. 4. See also Wien. klin. Wochenschr., 1890, s. 349. Dr. van Deventer, Centralblatt für Nervenheilkunde und Psychiatrie, N.F. vol. i., Ueber Influenza verbunden mit Nerven- und Geisteskrankheiten. Ewald, Deutsche Med. Wochenschr., 1890, No. 4. Senator, Berlin. klin. Wochenschr., 1890, No. 9. Metz, Neurologisches Centralblatt, April 1, 1891. Weber, Medico-Chir. Trans. (London), 1865. Christian, Archives Générales de Méd., Sept. 1873. Pétriquin, Gaz. Médicale de Paris, No. 31, 1837. Revilliod, Medical Brief, St. Louis, March 10, 1891. Kraepelin, Deutsch. Med. Wochenschr., March 13, 1891. Kirn, Allgem. Zeitschr. f. Psych., 1886. Wille, Archiv f. Psych., 1888. Bartels and Becker, Neurolog. Centralblatt, March 15, 1890. Dr. A. Leledy, L'Influenza et l'aliénation mentale, 1891. Savage, Influenza and Neuroses, 1892.]

INHIBITION.—Definition.—Any influence which retards, controls, restrains, or prevents the activity of nerve elements is termed inhibition.

Inhibitory action is exercised in two ways: (1) By a superior nerve-centre acting on an inferior, as for instance, when the action of coughing, which is actuated by a centre of inferior rank, is inhibited by the superior regions whose action is accompanied by the feeling of willing. (2) By an influence carried to the region to be inhibited by an afferent nerve. The inhibition of the cardiac movement by stimulation of the vaguses is a case in point.

It may now be taken as an accepted doctrine that the entire hierarchy of the nerve-centres, from the lowest up to the highest, is continually subject to inhibition. Upon each of them acts a restraining influence which prevents it from breaking out into action except upon the reception of an appropriate stimulus, and which produces its return to quiescence when the stimulus is withdrawn, and the occasion for activity has passed away. It appears that there is nothing in the constitution of the nerve-centres themselves to bring about their subsidence to rest after stimulation, but that the exercise of a continuous control is needed to bring them to rest and keep them at rest. Upon all the strata of nerve-centres except the highest of all, this controlling influence is exerted by centres of higher rank than themselves, each centre or region inhibiting those below, and being in turn inhibited by those above. In the case of the very highest, which of course cannot be inhibited in this way, the control is exercised in the second of the two ways mentioned, that is to say, by incoming currents arriving along afferent nerves from all parts of the body.

The **consequences** and **implications** of this doctrine are very far-reaching and important. If all the centres of which the nervous system is composed are subject to and exercise control, then it appears that the destruction of any one centre will necessarily liberate from control some other; and that damage to any one centre will weaken the control that it has exercised on its inferiors. Hence every destruction or damage to nerve-tissue; must necessarily have a twofold effect. It must be followed by loss or diminution of the function that was exercised by the destroyed or damaged tissue; and it must be followed by over-action of the parts that were controlled by the tissue now damaged or weakened. It is not necessary here to examine the various losses in the various regions of nerve-tissue, and to show how universally true is this law, but one corollary of the law must be insisted on. It is well known that if a nerve-muscle preparation be subjected to a constant stimulus, as to a continuous current of electricity passed through the nerve, no contraction takes place in the muscle; but that if the stimulus be removed, a contraction takes place, and this is the important point—the vigour of the contraction depends on the *suddenness* of the removal. It is possible to diminish, and at last to arrest, the current, by steps so gradual that no, or scarcely any, contraction takes place in the muscle, but at each inequality or irregularity in the process, a jerk of the muscle takes place. What is true in this low level of nervous action is equally true in the high level of the nerve-centres. The amount of over-action depends in every case on the suddenness with which the control is removed. When the centres destroyed or placed out of action are the very highest, the exaggerated action of the centres immediately below them produces the manifestations of mania; and the more sudden the removal of the highest regions, the more exaggerated the maniacal manifestations. Hence it is that outbreaks of acute mania usually occur with great rapidity, and hence also no doubt it is that tumours of the brain, whose encroachment is of necessity gradual, are seldom or never attended by outbreaks of mania.

While the intensity of the over-action depends on the suddenness with which removal of the inhibiting regions takes place, the quality of the over-action—its degree of elaborateness—depends on the level or rank of the region which is lost. The more elevated the region that is over-acting, the more highly elaborate, the more complex and intricate, are the activities that are excessive; while the lower down in the nervous hierarchy the loss extends, and the more inferior therefore the rank of the centres that are freed from control and allowed to over-act, the simpler, grosser, and more fundamental the nature of the activities whose over-action takes place. Thus, if we trace a progressive malady, such as general paralysis of the insane, in which the loss progresses steadily downwards, involving at first only the very highest strata of all, and at last all but the very lowest, we find that in the early stages, while the activity is excessive, it is of so elaborate a character that it is very difficult to lay the finger upon any single act as being erroneous. There is a general excess of activity, the movements are too rapid, too energetic, the letters written are too numerous, the conversation is too continuous, but we cannot say of any one act that it is erroneous or unadapted to the circumstances, of any one letter that it is improper, or of any one verbal expression that it is redundant. It is the *ensemble* that is excessive. As the malady progresses, and as the strata are successively deleted from above down, so we find that not only are the more elaborate or more complex activities lost, but that what remain, the simpler and more fundamental, are present in excess. When the patient can no longer write letters in excess he will eat and drink to excess. When he can no longer walk to excess he will tear up his clothing.

To how great a degree the excess of action in any particular case of insanity is due to loss of control, and how far it is due to direct over-stimulation and over-action of nerve elements beyond what the normal amount of inhibition can restrain, is a question on which different observers will differ considerably in the interpretation of the same case. At the present time the tendency appears to be less and less to consider outbreaks of any kind as due to direct stimulations breaking down normal control, and more and more to regard them as owing to the "letting-go" of nervous action by removal of the control to which it is normally subject.

C. A. Mercier.

INHIBITION, MENTAL (*inhibeo*, I hold in; *mens*). The restraining influence of mental states over any reflex or automatic action. Also the restraining influence of one mental condition over another.

INHIBITORY INSANITY. (*See* Abulia; Moral Insanity.)

INNOCENT (*innocens*, harmless). An old term for one who is an idiot.

INQUISITIONS OF LUNACY. (*See* Chancery Lunatics.)

INSANE (*insanus*, not healthy). Affected with insanity.

INSANE, ATTENDANTS ON.—It is a happy circumstance that the *status* of attendants in asylums has been distinctly raised in recent times. There cannot be any difference of opinion as to the onerous duties which fall upon this class, the large amount of power which they necessarily possess, and the extreme importance of securing men and women who have the qualities essential to the right performance of the service upon which they enter. Much is expected of them, and therefore everything ought to be done to educate them for the post which they fill, and to render it as little irksome as possible. The systematic training of attendants has been carefully considered and reported upon by a committee of the Medico-Psychological Association in the autumn of 1890. This committee considered it advisable that the Association should institute a scheme for this purpose. The following were the recommendations of the committee in regard to training.

(1) That a period of three months' probation be required before the attendant is considered to have formally entered training.

(2) That a period of two years' training and service in the asylum (including the period of probation) be required before an

attendant is allowed to become a candidate for examination.

(3) That the system of training be by:—

(*a*) *Study of text-books*—the committee recommending the handbook for attendants prepared by a sub-committee of the Association in 1885. Other books at the direction of each superintendent.

(*b*) *Exercises*, under head, and ward attendants, to be arranged, at the discretion of the superintendents.

(*c*) *Clinical instruction* in the wards by the medical staff.

(*d*) *Lectures* or *demonstration* (other than ward instruction) given by the medical staff, at least twelve of which shall be attended by each attendant during his two years of training.

(*e*) *Periodical examination* to test progress left to the discretion of the superintendent.

(4) Scope of training should be limited to the ordinary requirements of nursing and attendance on insane patients, combined with instruction on the general features of mental disease, together with general ideas of bodily structure and function, sufficient to enable nurses under training to understand such instruction and to qualify them to render them "first aid," especially in the case of accident or injury that may arise in asylums.

With regard to **examination** it was recommended—

(1) That examinations be held twice yearly.

(2) That they should be held at individual asylums wherever there may be candidates.

(3) That they should be partly in writing, and partly *vivâ voce*.

(4) That the papers should be set by the examiners of the association who are appointed from time to time for examining medical candidates for the diploma of the association.

(5) That the examination be conducted as follows:—

The papers to be answered on the day fixed, under the supervision of the superintendent, and to be examined and valued by the superintendent and an assessor. The practical part to be conducted by the superintendent and the assessor on as early a day after the fixed day as can be conveniently arranged by the superintendent and assessor.

(6) That the assessor be the superintendent of a neighbouring asylum, the consent of the council of the association to his acting as such, having been obtained.

(7) That the candidate obtains a certificate of morality and suitability from his or her superintendent before being admitted to the examination, and that this certificate shall be sent by the superintendent and assessor to the secretaries when application is made to them for the form of certificate to be given to the candidate.

Certificates.—(1) The certificate to be in the form appended.

(2) The certificates to bear consecutive numbers, to bear the seal of the association, and to be issued and countersigned by the secretaries of the association for the division of the kingdom where they are granted.

(3) Certificates to be granted and signed by the examining superintendent and his assessor.

(4) The superintendent to send to the general secretary a list of successful candidates after each examination.

Register.—(1) That a register of candidates who have passed the examination be kept by the general secretary of the association.

(2) That in the case of misconduct on the part of a holder of a certificate, a superintendent (or, in private nursing, the medical man in charge or the employer) should be requested, by a notice on the back of the certificate, to at once transmit a report of the circumstances to the general secretary, who will lay the same before the council for consideration. The council, will, if it thinks fit to do so, direct the secretary to erase the name of the delinquent from the register.

(3) That each candidate, before receiving the parchment certificate, shall sign the appended agreement.

(4) That superintendents and other members of the association on engaging attendants who profess to be on the register should satisfy themselves that such is the case, by inquiring of the secretary.

(5) That the register be published annually in the journal, together with the names (if any) that have been erased by direction of the council.

Form of Certificate.—This is to certify that ______ ___ has, after examination by us, shown to our satisfaction that (he *or* she) has attained proficiency in nursing and attendance on insane persons. Before this certificate is granted, it has been testified to us by____________, under whom (he *or* she) has been trained for two years, that ____________'s character, conduct and aptitude have been such as to entitle (him *or* her) to be admitted to examination for this certificate.

Signed

____________, Examiners.

A paper must be signed by the successful candidate before receiving the certificate.

Dr. Clouston, in a paper read before the Medico-Psychological Society (1876), made a number of practical suggestions in addition to the training of attendants, among which were, the increase of pay, the maximum in ten years to be not less than £50 per annum; pensions to all who become ill or serve long, as in the Civil Service; making provision for changing attendants from one asylum to another, the pay and pension counting as if no change had been made; receiving diplomas from the asylums where they were trained; providing facilities for the marriage of at least one-half of the male attendants; making their lives as pleasant as possible by good accommodation, days off duty, annual holidays, social gatherings, means of amusement and instruction, and, above all, reasonable facilities for satisfying the social cravings of human nature.*

Dr. Clouston appeals in this paper to the chaplains in asylums to take some interest in the moral welfare of attendants. The following passage might with advantage be hung up on the walls of every chaplain's house in the asylums of Great Britain:—"I am certain that the chaplain should be a more valuable official in an asylum than he commonly is. How many asylum chaplains preach to the attendants, now and then speaking to them in a direct and real way as to their special temptations, and setting before them a high ideal of duty?"

THE EDITOR.

[*References.*—Dr. Luther Bell, Directions for Attendants. Conolly, Teachings for Attendants. Report of the Commissioners in Lunacy for England and Wales, 1859. Sisterhoods in Asylums, Journal of Mental Science, April 1866. Dr. Clouston, On the Question of Getting, Training, and Retaining the Services of Good Asylum Attendants, Journal of Mental Science, Oct. 1876. Dr. W. A. F. Browne, The Training of Asylum Attendants, Journal of Mental Science, January 1877. Dr. A. Campbell Clark, Digest of Essays on Hallucinations by Asylum Attendants, Journal of Mental Science, April 1884. Handbook for the Instruction of Attendants on the Insane, prepared by the Sub-Committee of the Medico-Psychological Association, appointed at a Branch Meeting held at Glasgow, February 21, 1884: Authors, A. C. Clark, C. M. Campbell, A. R. Turnbull, A. R. Urquhart. London: Baillière & Co. 1885.]

INSANE DIATHESIS. (*See* DIATHESIS, INSANE.)

INSANE EAR. (*See* EAR, HÆMATOMA AURIS, and OTHÆMATOMA.)

INSANE TEMPERAMENT (*in*, neg.; *sanus*, sound; *temperamentum*, disposition). The mental constitution which tends to the development of insanity and allied neuroses. (*See* DIATHESIS, INSANE.)

INSANIA (*insania*, madness; from *in*, neg.; *sanus*, sound). Insanity.

INSANIA CADIVA (*cado*, I fall). A synonym of Epilepsy.

INSANIA GRAVIDARUM (*gravidus*, pregnant). A synonym of Insanity of Pregnancy or Gestation.

INSANIA LACTANTIUM. (*See* INSANITY, LACTATIONAL.)

INSANIA LUPINA (*lupus*, a wolf). A synonym of Lycanthropia (*q.v.*).

INSANIA OCCULTA (*occulo*, I hide or conceal). (*See* INSANITY, CONCEALED.)

INSANIA POST PARTUM. (*See* INSANITY, PUERPERAL.)

INSANIA PUERPERARUM (*puerpera*, a lying-in woman). A synonym of Puerperal Insanity (*q.v.*).

INSANIOLA (dim. of insania). A minor degree of insanity, extreme eccentricity. (*See* ECCENTRICITY.)

INSANITAS (*in*, neg.; *sanitas*, health). Disturbance or defect of health, improperly used for insanity.

INSANITIES. (*See* EPILEPSIES AND INSANITIES.)

INSANITY.—Synonyms.—Lat. *Insania*; *insanitas*, from *insanus*, unsound. Fr. *folie*, *insanité de l'esprit*, *aliénation mentale*. Ital. *insania*, *follia*, *alienazione mentale*. Sp. *insania*, *locura*. Ger. *Irrsinn*, *Irresein*, *Wahnsinn*, *Verrücktheit*. **I., acquired.** Insanity occurring after a longer or shorter period of life of apparent sanity.—**I., adolescent.** The mental disturbance which occurs at the period between puberty and full development, usually between the ages of 18 to 25, notably between 20 and 25, when the function of reproduction is attaining its full development, and the body is arriving at its full growth (Clouston). (*See* DEVELOPMENTAL INSANITIES.)—**I., affective** (*affectio*, feeling). A synonym of Insanity, Moral. Used for those forms of mental derangement in which the passions or emotions are principally perverted.—**I., alcoholic** (alcohol, from Arab *al*, the; *kohol*, anything very fine or subtle). A term employed by some to denote any mental derangement due to alcohol, by others limited to acute alcoholism or delirium tremens, chronic alcoholism, mania à potu, and dipsomania. (Fr. *folie par intoxication alcoolique*; Ger. *Verfolgungswahnsinn der Trinker*.) (*See* ALCOHOLISM.)—**I., alternating.** A synonym of Circular Insanity (*q.v.*). (Fr. *folie à formes alternes*; Ger. *circuläres Irresein*.)—**I., ambitious.** The form of insanity in which ideas of grandeur and personal exaltation are marked

* *Journal of Mental Science*, Oct. 1876, p. 388.

characteristics. Used as synonym of General Paralysis of the Insane, and the Monomania of Grandeur. (Fr. *folie ambitieuse.*) — **I., amenorrhœal** (ἀ, neg.; μήν, a month; ῥοία, a flow). Skae's term for insanity produced by the suppression of the menstrual flow. (*See* MENSTRUATION AND INSANITY.)—**I., anæmic** (ἀν, neg.; αἷμα, blood). Mental disease due to pure anæmia of the brain from starvation, chlorosis or prolonged indigestion, or other causes of anæmia. Most of these cases of melancholia are of a mild type, but cases of acute mania may occur.—**I., arthritic.** (*See* ARTHRITIC INSANITY.)—**I., cataleptoid** (κατάληψις, a seizing; εἶδος, likeness). A form of insanity in which there is an ecstatic abstraction with more or less rigidity of the limbs. (*See* CATALEPSY, and STUPOR, MENTAL.)—**I., choreic.** A form of insanity commonly met with in children and young people, in which choreiform movements, often of an exaggerated type, prevail. In the acute stage of chorea there may be delirium of an inco-ordinated jerky kind (Maudsley); in cases of chronic chorea the mental affection is often depression at first, then mania with impulsive acts of violence or suicide, and in the end dementia. (Fr. *folie choréique.*) (*See* CHOREA AND INSANITY.)—**I., circular.** (Fr. *folie circulaire, folie à double forme*; Ger. *Circuläres Irresein of Krafft-Ebing.* (*See* CIRCULAR INSANITY.) — **I., climacteric.** (*See* CLIMACTERIC INSANITY.)—**I., communicated.** (*See* COMMUNICATED INSANITY.)—**I., concurrent** (*con*, together, with; *curro*, I run). Insanity caused by other diseases or diseased conditions which continue to exist—*e.g.*, from syphilis, epilepsy, chorea, alcoholism, &c. — **I., confusional primary.** The form in which there is a rapidly developed fever with mental confusion, incoherence, slight delirium, and hallucinations, but no definite melancholia or mania.—**I., congestive.** Insanity supposed to be due to congestion of the brain substance. (Fr. *folie congestive.*)—**I., consecutive.** Insanity following and due to fevers, visceral inflammations and other internal affections.—**I., constitutional.** Insanity the result of a pre-existing physiological or pathological condition. — **I., delusional primary** (*deludo*, I play false with). That form of insanity in which there is little primary mental impairment, the mental affection being as it were naturally evolved in early life through the original constitution of the brain, which gradually develops an unsound state of mind without much preliminary explosion or brainstorm, in the shape of an attack of mania or melancholia (Clouston). (Fr. *folie systematisée*: Ger. *primäre Verrücktheit.*)—**I., delusional secondary.** A chronic incurable form of insanity, the sequel of some acute types; persistent delusions being often present. (Ger. *secundäre Verrücktheit.*) — **I., demonomaniacal.** (*See* DEMONOMANIA.) (Fr. *folie démonomaniaque.*)—**I., depressive** (*depressus*, weighed down). A synonym of Melancholia. (Fr. *folie dépressive.*)—**I., deuteropathic** (δεύτερος, second; πάθος, an affection). Insanity caused by disorder of, or developmental changes in other organs than the encephalic centres.—**I., developmental** (*développer*, to unfold). A synonym of the Insanities of Puberty and Adolescence. — **I., diabetic** (διά, through; βαίνω, I run or move). The occurrence of mental disturbance in a patient suffering from diabetes mellitus. The association of insanity and diabetes has by some been regarded as merely a fortuitous one, while they at the same time deny that it can act as a causative influence; others recognise this form, but as of rare occurrence. The general form of mental disorder found with diabetes is melancholia. (*See* DIABETES AND INSANITY.)—**I., diathetic** (διάθεσις, a placing in order). A name given to any form of insanity which arises out of a morbid diathesis. (Fr. *folie diathésique.*)—**I., doubting.** A form of insanity, generally melancholia with suicidal tendencies, in which there is a morbid doubting and inability to make up the mind to action, even for the most trivial every-day duties. (Fr. *folie du doute*; Ger. *Grübelsucht.*) (*See* DOUBT, INSANITY OF, and GRÜBELSUCHT.) —**I., egressing** (*egredior*, I pass out of, or come out of). Insanity growing out of the former disease, of which it is an exaggeration—*e.g.*, egressing from hysteria, ecstasy, hypochondriasis, &c. (Bucknill.)—**I., emotional** (*e*, from; *moveo*, I move). Mental derangement chiefly exhibited with regard to the emotions. (*See* MORAL INSANITY.)—**I., epidemic** (ἐπί, upon; δῆμος, a people). Insanity generally of a hysterical type, occurring usually in women, especially in places where they are congregated in large numbers—*e.g.*, convents, hospitals, &c. The psychosis as a rule is a hysterical development of religious enthusiasm, and marked by ideas of demoniacal possession. Epidemics of this nature are recorded by Hirsch as having occurred in Sweden in the seventeenth century, in which paroxysms of acute excitement were observed, the patients throwing themselves on the ground with the most marvellous contortions, uttering inarticulate cries and howls. Another development of this nature was the practice of naked dances at the meetings of the converted (Wretholm). In England "the Jumpers" of Cornwall in 1760, and in America "the Barkers" in the early part of the present century, are also to be classified under this neurosis. (*See also* IKATO, KLIKUSCHI, LATA, TEGRETIER, &c.) (Fr. *folie épidémique.*) (*See* EPIDEMIC INSANITY.)—**I., epileptic** (ἐπιλαμβάνω, I seize upon). Various forms of mental disorder associated with epilepsy, or preceding it, or following its development. (Fr. *folie épileptique.*) (*See* EPILEPSY AND INSANITY.)—**I., erotic** (*q.v.*) (ἐρωτικός, relating to love). Insanity with symptoms tending towards special sexual excitement, as occurs in satyriasis. May be only sentimental.—**I., exophthalmic** (ἐξ; ὀφθαλμός; exophthalmic goitre). A form of insanity recently recognised, in which the symptoms are mainly restlessness, irritability and even violence, with dirty habits and refusal of food, occurring in patients suffering from Graves' disease—exophthalmic goître. (*See* EXOPHTHALMIC GOÎTRE AND INSANITY.)—**I., febrile** (*febrilis*, feverish). Insanity which occurs as the result of an acute inflammation or a specific fever. It may be the initial delirium of the fever starting the morbid process, and passing from delirium into mania, or it may be the direct consequence of a febrile attack occurring in a neurotically predisposed subject (Savage).—**I., feigned.** Insanity simulated for any definite reason—*e.g.*, in the hysterical or hypochondriacal, to excite sympathy and pity; in prisoners, to escape the punishment for a crime; or in mendicants, for the purposes of charity. (*See* FEIGNED INSANITY.)—**I. from deprivation of the senses.** The mental aberration, generally melancholia, which is sometimes observed to follow either total or partial blindness or deafness. Such cases frequently suffer from hallucinations of sight or hearing, their subjective experiences becoming objective realities to them (Clouston).—**I. from intoxication.** The Anglicised term for Morel's *folie par intoxication.*—**I., furious.** A term for the disease Agriothymia (*q.v.*).—**I., gastro-enteric** (γαστήρ, the belly; ἔντερον, an intestine). The form of insanity, caused by disorder of the gastro-intestinal tract, such as catarrhal conditions, constipation, pressure of a tumour, &c., and usually melancholia (Clouston's visceral or abdominal melancholiacs).—**I., gouty** (Old Fr. *goute*, *goutte*, from Lat. *gutta*, a drop). The various forms of insanity accompanying the gouty diathesis, or occurring after the cessation of the acute joint affection. Deep melancholia is a common accompaniment of the gouty diathesis, and Garrod has described the acute delirious or "gouty mania" as a post-podagrous phenomenon. Attacks of acute mania have been described as depending on undeveloped gout, and as passing off with the development of acute gout, and gouty degenerations of various kinds may tend to ideas of dread, persecution, and to senile weak-mindedness, or in the end to apoplexy (Savage). (*See* GOUT AND INSANITY.)—**I., hereditary** (*hereditarius*, relating to an inheritance). Insanity produced by hereditary weakness of the nervous system, occurring usually at some period of physiological activity, puberty, childbirth, climacteric, &c., and not induced by any other apparent exciting cause. (Fr. *folie héréditaire*; Ger. *erbliche Geisteskrankheit.*) (*See* HEREDITY.)—**I., homicidal.** A term applied either to homicidal mania or melancholia, or the homicidal impulse; implying any mental aberration, one of the symptoms of which is a homicidal tendency. (*See* HOMICIDAL MONOMANIA.)—**I., hypochondriacal.** The extreme stage of hypochondriasis. (Fr. *folie hypochondriaque.*) (*See* HYPOCHONDRIASIS.)—**I., hysterical.** The form of insanity which occurs chiefly in women, as an extreme form of hysteria. (*See* HYSTERIA.)—**I., ideal** (Lat. *idea*, from Gr. ἰδέα, form; the look or semblance of a thing). One of Arnold's two divisions of insanity, as according to him the objects of sensation are represented in the mind by ideas or images, while the mental states which arise from the exercise of the faculties in reflecting upon sensible objects, or the operations of the mind may be called notions. Mania was comprised under this division.—**I., ideational.** Those forms of insanity in which perversion of the reasoning powers is the chief characteristic.—**I., idiopathic** (ἴδιος, peculiar; πάθος, an affection). Group IV. of Morel's classification, which includes (1) progressive weakening or abolition of the intellectual faculties resulting from chronic disease of the brain or its membranes, and (2) general paralysis.—**I., imitative.** The form of communicated insanity in which the mental affection has been copied from an insane companion. (Fr. *folie imitative.*)—**I., imposed** (*in*; *pono*, I place on). A form of communicated insanity in which the person affected imposes as it were his insane conceptions on another morally and intellectually weaker than himself. (*See* FOLIE À DEUX.)—**I., impulsive** (*impulsus*, from *impello*, I drive on). A term similar to instinctive insanity. Also and more generally applied to those forms of insanity in which the will and judgment appear paralysed, and in which an uncontrollable impulse drives to acts of an insane character, such as homicide, suicide, violence, &c.—**I., infantile.** (*See* CHILDREN, INSANITY IN.)—**I., inhibitory** (*inhibeo*, I arrest). Clouston's term for the forms of insanity in which the loss of power of inhibition is the chief, and by far the most marked symptom. (*See* DIPSOMANIA; IMPULSIVE, DESTRUCTIVE, HOMICIDAL, SUICIDAL; KLEPTOMANIA; LYCANTHROPIA; MORAL INSANITY; NECROPHILISM; NYMPHOMANIA; PLANOMANIA; PYROMANIA; SATYRIASIS, &c.) — **I., instinctive** (*instinctus*, an instigation). The form of insanity of acts rather than words, of impulse rather than reflection. There is a propensity to commit wrong acts—*e.g.*, theft, suicide, homicide, &c. (Fr. *folie instinctive.*)—**I., intellectual** (*intelligo*, I choose between). A term used in the same sense as ideational insanity. Also those forms of insanity in which the chief manifestations of mental derangement relate to the intellect, being of the nature of false conceptions or delusions.—**I., intermittent.** Insanity apparently caused by exposure to miasm, and one of the class of post-febrile insanities. Sydenham has described a peculiar form of mania that used to follow ague, occurring in the quotidian, tertian, or quartan forms. (*See* AGUE AND INSANITY.)—**I., ischæmic** (ἴσχω, I keep back; αἷμα, blood). A synonym of Anæmic Insanity. Prof. Ball classes general stupor under ischæmia of brain, due to spasm of capillaries. (Fr. *folie ischémique.*)—**I., katatonic** (κατατείνω, I stretch tightly.) Kahlbaum's term for the group of motor and mental symptoms present in *melancholia* attonita, preceded, if typical, by simple melancholy, and a period of excitement (melancholic or maniacal). Lastly, it may end in dementia. These alternations are rarely well-marked. (*See* KATATONIA.) — **I., lactational** (*lac*, milk). A form of insanity due to the physical prostration following prolonged nursing. (*See* PUERPERAL INSANITY.) — **I., limophoitic** (λιμός, hunger; φοιτάω, I roam about in frenzy). Insanity caused by hunger or starvation.—**I., lucid** (*lucidus*, clear). A synonym of Moral Insanity. (Fr. *folie lucide*).—**I., maniacal.** (*See* ACUTE MANIA.)—**I., melancholic.** (*See* MELANCHOLIA.)—**I., menstrual** (*menstrualis*, monthly). The mental disturbance which occurs at the menstrual period only. (*See* MENSTRUATION AND INSANITY.)—**I., metastatic** (μετάστασις, change). Any form of insanity which appears and disappears with the disappearance or appearance of certain physical affections—*e.g.*, asthma, gout, erysipelas, &c.—**I., monomaniacal.** (*See* MONOMANIA.)—**I., moral** (*moralis*, relating to conduct). Prichard's term for those cases of insanity in which there is uncontrollable violence and depravity of the instincts and emotions, without any impairment of the intellectual faculties. (Fr. *folie morale*; Ger. *moralisches Irresein.*) (*See* MORAL INSANITY.) —**I., notional** (*notio*, a becoming acquainted with, a taking cognisance of, from, *nosco*, I know). One of Arnold's two divisions of insanity. (*See* INSANITY, IDEAL.) Under this division he places delusive insanity.—**I. of acts.** The Anglicised term for the French *folie des actes* (*q.v.*). (*See* MORAL INSANITY.)—**I. of asthma** (ἆσθμα, heavy or laborious breathing). Insanity occurring in the subjects of, or alternating with attacks of spasmodic asthma. (*See* ASTHMA AND INSANITY.)—**I. of Bright's disease.** A variety of mental derangement, half delirium and half mania, which results from uræmic poisoning. (*See* BRIGHT'S DISEASE AND INSANITY.)—**I. of cardiac disease.** The various forms of mental disorder occurring in the subjects of cardiac disease, especially the post-rheumatic forms. (*See* CARDIAC DISEASE AND INSANITY).—**I. of childbirth.** The insanity which comes on in the puerperal month. (*See* PUERPERAL INSANITY.)—**I. of childhood.** Insanity occurring in children before the age of puberty. It is most commonly a congenital condition, but acute mania, melancholia, delusional insanity, and dementia have been observed as primary disorders in children. (*See* CHILDREN, INSANITY OF.)—**I. of cyanosis** (κυανός, dark blue). Mental disorder due to cyanosis from bronchitis, cardiac disease, and asthma. A form of delirium with confusion, hallucinations of sight, sleeplessness, sometimes suicidal impulses and vague fears. The symptoms are usually worst at night, and end in mental stupor, passing into coma. It is more commonly seen in persons of advanced age than in the young (Clouston).—**I. of delivery.** A temporary but true mental derangement occurring during labour, or at the moment of birth of the child, and probably caused by the pain or agony of the labour. There may be suicidal inclinations or desire to injure the offspring. The attack subsides when the labour is over.—**I. of gestation** (*gestatio*, pregnancy). (*See* INSANITY OF PREGNANCY.)—**I. of grandeur.** A synonym of General Paralysis of the Insane; also a term used for the monomania of grandeur. (*See* MEGALOMANIA.) —**I. of lead poisoning.** A variety of mental disease described by Rayner, Savage and others, associated with lead poisoning, or the impregnation of the system with lead-salts. (*See* LEAD POISONING, MENTAL DISORDER FROM.)—**I. of masturbation** (*masturbo*). The distinct form of mental disorder produced by excessive self-abuse. (*See* MASTURBATION AND INSANITY.)—**I. of myxœdema** (*μύξα*, mucus; *οἴδημα*, a swelling). The maniacal and melancholic attacks occurring in the subjects of myxœdema; also the mild form of dementia into which many myxœdematous cases lapse. (*See* MYXŒDEMA AND INSANITY.)—**I. of oxaluria** (oxalates; *οὖρον*, urine). A form of melancholic insanity occurring in those suffering from oxaluria. (*See* OXALURIA AND INSANITY.) — **I. of persecution.** The form of insanity in which there are delusions of persecution. (PERSECUTION MANIA.) (Fr. *folie des persécutions.*)—**I. of phosphuria, I. of phosphaturia** (phosphates; *οὖρον*, urine). A form of melancholia occurring in those suffering from phosphatic deposits in the urine. (*See* PHOSPHATURIA AND INSANITY.)—**I. of pregnancy.** The form of insanity, generally of a melancholic type, which occurs during pregnancy. (*See* PUERPERAL INSANITY.)—**I. of puberty.** The insanity occurring at the age of puberty. (*See* PUBESCENT INSANITY.)—**I. of self-abuse.** (*See* MASTURBATION AND INSANITY.)—**I., ovarian.** A term used by Skae to denote the mental affection occurring in unmarried women approaching the climacteric, the symptoms being usually of a sexual character, with delusions of an amatory nature. (*See* OLD MAID'S INSANITY.)—**I., paralytic.** A synonym of General Paralysis of the Insane. Also used to denote the mental disturbance that accompanies and results from gross brain lesions—*e.g.*, apoplexies, ramollissements, tumours and chronic degenerations affecting the convolutions and their functions, either primarily or secondarily. (*See* POST-APOPLECTIC INSANITY.)—**I., paroxysmal** (*παροξυσμός*, the height of a disease). A form of cerebral disturbance, in many cases of an epileptic character, in which attacks of madness come on suddenly, last for a short time, and then entirely pass off, the interval being of variable length and quite free from maniacal symptoms. They may be of a furious, destructive or dangerous nature, or consist of quiet but ridiculous actions. (*See* EPILEPTIC INSANITY.) — **I., partial** (*pars*, a part). A term applied to those cases of chronic mania known as monomania (*q.v.*).—**I., pathetic** (*παθητικός*, susceptible of emotion or suffering). One of Arnold's subdivisions in the classification of mental disorders; it included the varieties of melancholia.—**I., pellagrous.** (*See* PELLAGRA.)—**I., perceptional** (*perceptio*, a receiving). The group of insanities in which there are derangements of one or more of the perceptions, but the term is of little practical value.—**I., periodic** (*περιοδικός*, coming round at certain times). The form in which attacks of insanity, usually mania or melancholia, recur at more or less regular intervals, but in which the remission is not accompanied by complete restoration to mental health.—**I., phthisical** (*φθίσις*, consumption). Clouston's term for the form of insanity which arises occasionally at the same time as the occurrence of phthisical symptoms. It may be of the maniacal, melancholic, or monomaniacal type, and the symptoms of a morbid mental suspicion run through all the cases. (*See* PHTHISICAL INSANITY.) **I., podagrous** (*πούς*, the foot; *ἄγρα*, a seizure). (*See* GOUT AND INSANITY.)—**I., post-connubial** (*post*, after; *connubialis*, pertaining to marriage). The form of insanity which occurs directly after marriage, due to mental or sexual excitement. (*See* MARRIAGE AND INSANITY.) — **I., post-epileptic** (*post*, after; *ἐπιλαμβάνω*, I seize upon). Insanity occurring after the onset of epilepsy, or after a single epileptic fit. (*See* EPILEPSY AND INSANITY.)—**I., post-febrile.** Insanity occurring during the decline of a specific fever.—**I., post-puerperal.** The form of puerperal insanity which occurs after delivery. (*See* PUERPERAL INSANITY.)—**I., preparturient.** (*See* PUERPERAL INSANITY.)—**I., pre-puerperal.** (*See* PUERPERAL INSANITY.)—**I., primary.** The form of insanity which develops in childhood and puberty with the development of the body. It may be congenital, or arise in consequence of injury or disease of the brain occurring in early life, or at puberty; it is often marked by the presence of uncontrollable impulses to commit foolish or criminal acts; intercurrent attacks of great excitement may occur, and the higher faculties of the mind are ill-developed. (*See* VERRÜCKTHEIT; PARANOIA.) — **I., primordial.** A synonym of Primary Insanity, Primary Delusional Insanity, and Primäre Verrücktheit.—**I., protopathic** (*πρωτοπαθής*, affected by a primary affection). A term sometimes used as a synonym of Schröder van der Kolk's Idiopathic Insanity. Also the insanity caused by disorder of, or developmental changes, in the encephalon.—**I., pubescent.** (*See* DEVELOPMENTAL INSANITIES.)—**I., puerperal.** (*See* PUERPERAL INSANITY.)—**I., reasoning.** (*See* MORAL

Insanity.) (Fr. *folie raisonnante.*)—I., recurrent. (*See* Recurrent Insanity.)—I., religious. The forms of insanity in which delusions of a religious nature occur.—I., rheumatic. A synonym of Choreic Insanity, from its frequent association with a rheumatic diathesis. (*See* Rheumatic Fever and Insanity.) — I., saturnine (*saturnus*, an old name for lead). A synonym of Insanity from Lead Poisoning. (*See* Lead.) — I., scheming (*schema*, appearance, demeanour, bearing). Arnold's term for those cases of mania in which the delusions bear on the reformation of society and amelioration of mankind.—I., senile. The form of insanity which occurs in old age. (*See* Old Age.) — I., sensorial. The forms of insanity in which illusions or hallucinations are predominant symptoms. (Fr. *folie sensorielle.*)—I. sequential (*sequor*, I follow). Insanity caused by other diseases which have subsided—*e.g.*, fevers, inflammations, &c.—I., simulated. (*See* Feigned Insanity.) — I., simultaneous. A variety of communicated insanity (*q.v.*) in which two or more persons hereditarily predisposed contract the same kind of insanity at the same time. (Fr. *folie simultanée.*) — I., stuporous. (*See* Stupor, Mental.)—I., suicidal. The form of insanity, whether impulsive or not, in which the patient makes determined efforts at self-destruction. (*See* Suicidal Insanity.)—I., symbolising (*symbolon*, a sign or token). A form of delusional insanity in which the patient imagines everything happening to him or about him has special reference to himself, and in which the most roundabout arguments are adduced to connect such occurrences with his special delusion.—I., sympathetic (*συμπαθητικός*, affected by like feelings). The forms of insanity in which there is an apparent or real sequence of mental disturbance on certain visceral affections—*e.g.*, of the heart, lungs, kidneys, &c., or where the insanity appears to be induced by the presence of a foreign body—*e.g.*, a calculus, intestinal worm, &c. (Fr. *folie sympathique.*) — I., symptomatic (*σύμπτωμα*, an occurrence). Insanity which is the symptom of some visceral affection other than of the brain. (Fr. *folie symptomatique.*)—I., syphilitic. The form of mental disease which depends on the actual presence of the syphilitic poison in the system. Also used to denote hypochondriasis produced by the dread of syphilitic disease. (*See* Syphilis and Insanity.)—I., toxic (*τοξικόν*, *lit.*, pertaining to archery; also anything deadly). Those forms of insanity apparently caused by the introduction of some organic or inorganic poison into the system—*e.g.*, alcohol, lead, &c.; also lithic acid, urea, bile, &c.—I., transitory. Krafft-Ebing's term for that form of insanity which lasts for a very short period, three or four hours to six days. It is generally caused by some sudden shock occurring in a mind already physiologically or organically affected—*e.g.*, in one suffering from prolonged grief; in one addicted to alcoholic excess, &c.—I., traumatic (*τραυματικός*, relating to wounds). Insanity caused by some external violence. (*See* Traumatic Insanity.)—I., uterine. Insanity apparently due to some disease or displacement of the womb. (*See* Climacteric Insanity and Menstruation.)—I., visceral. Insanity due to some disease or disorder of the abdominal or thoracic viscera. (*See* Sympathetic Insanity.)—I., volitional. Insanity characterised by derangement of the will, either by its excess or by its inertia (*abulia, q.v.*).—I. without delusion. A synonym of Moral Insanity (*q.v.*).

INSANITY, CONCEALED.—Cases from time to time occur in which sufferers from mental alienation succeed in concealing their real state of mind, and difficulties are presented not dissimilar to those which surround the diagnosis of feigned insanity. The fact that a patient is able to keep his symptoms in the background implies a considerable amount of self-restraint, and the impossibility of applying a test independent of the patient's will, may occasionally lead even experienced observers astray. Certain forms of insanity, of course, do not admit of being hidden. Such are general paralysis and simple dementia. It may be questioned, in the latter condition, whether the degree of weak-mindedness which exists, justifies the treatment of the sufferer in such and such ways, but the weakness cannot itself be concealed. The same is true of all forms of dementia from so-called organic brain diseases and also of senile dementia. In the last-named affection the mental state is often disputed, but the essence of the contention is really under what category the patient should be classed. That there is some failure of mind is rarely denied by the disputants, and it is obvious that the unfortunate patient is incapable of concealment.

In those forms of insanity in which expansive emotional disturbance is the most prominent feature concealment is difficult to maintain. Emotional instability does not usually permit of such exercise of will power as is necessary for dissimulation. Hence maniacal excitement is not to be repressed. The mere fact that the patient is able continuously to restrain himself proves that he is at least convalescent. The difficulty with these cases arises in distinguishing how far a certain excitability may be consistent with sanity or in judging what degree of instability may permanently remain after an attack of acute mental disease without precluding the return of the patient to society. These may be very difficult problems, but they are not connected with concealment properly so called.

It is otherwise, however, with melancholia. With this condition, even at its worst, there is often relative intellectual integrity and great fixity of purpose. Delusions may be retained and concealed, or delusions may have disappeared, or may have never distinctly existed, and the patient may remain extremely depressed, and even intensely suicidal. Cheerfulness is often temporarily assumed at the height of a melancholic attack to facilitate suicide. No doubt a more lasting deception is often attempted with the same object, and sometimes, perhaps, successfully. The difficulties here may be considerable. The very nature of *melancholia passiva* is such that the symptoms tend to escape attention. Some melancholiacs court sympathy, and are glad to fortify themselves by confession; in others the mental hyperæsthesia takes the form of extreme sensitiveness as to their own weakness, and they shrink from talking of their state. This reticence may exist when convalescence is well established.

The best indications that depression or depressive delusions are not concealed are—

(1) After an attack of insanity, a return to the *status quo ante* as to spirits, &c. Here, unfortunately, the physician has generally to depend upon the statements of others as to his patient's previous state.

(2) The healthy interest shown by the patient in his business and his surroundings. This is hard to feign persistently when the mind is pre-occupied either by delusions or by depressive emotion.

The manifestation of insanity which is most readily concealed is delusion occurring in an indifferent emotional state. Hence cases of concealed insanity are most frequently cases of paranoia. It was maintained by Heinroth that lunatics never deny a delusion, though they may refrain from giving expression to it. This is not an absolute rule, but it is nevertheless generally true. It will occur in the majority of cases that delusion is not denied when the patient is directly questioned about his beliefs. It is therefore of the greatest value to have a clue in doubtful cases, such as can usually be furnished by relations or friends. In a certain proportion of cases no preliminary information is forthcoming. Where there is a doubt, it is important, if possible, to see the patient at his own home. His mode of life, his surroundings, his dress, the evidences of his habits, &c., will often afford valuable indications of his mental state. Thus a patient, whose condition was disputed, who made his living by literary work, and who exhibited extreme shrewdness in evading inquiries, was found when visited at his own house to be in the habit of writing seated in the middle of his room surrounded by a sort of paper tent. It turned out that he had made this contrivance to prevent his enemies from stealing his ideas while he was writing them down.

In conversing with a patient in whom insanity is suspected, and concealment appears to be attempted, great tact and patience are required. It is well to lead the conversation according to some definite plan. In the absence of any decided clue, it is best to begin by inquiries about the health. This, besides being the natural mode of beginning for a physician, is specially useful in these cases as giving an opportunity for complaints of improper influences, injurious treatment, &c. Proceeding to the state of his affairs, his relations to his family and friends, his occupation and business, his religious sentiments, &c., we usually come upon some trace of delusions. It is important as far as possible to let the patient himself talk uninterruptedly. A maladroit question will often stop instead of urging the flow of his confidence. Ball reminds us that a similar phenomenon occurs in the delirium of fevers. The fever patient left to himself mutters on incoherently, but replies sensibly when addressed. There is probably only an analogy between the states, but the observation holds good in both cases. It should always be remembered that the majority of patients who conceal their delusions belong to the class who believe they are watched or persecuted or conspired against. They are the most suspicious of all people. They are always apt to think that any person who questions them closely is among those who are in a conspiracy against them. They will not satisfy him by recounting what they believe he is already privy to. This feeling is heightened when the questioner unskilfully betrays a knowledge of the patient's affairs, the possession of which he does not frankly account for. It has been very truly said that the method of the cross-examining lawyer should always be present in our mind, but never apparent in our manner.

We must recollect that lunatics who make an effort to conceal their insanity do so either in order to be released from restraint, or to avoid being placed in restraint, or because believing themselves to be persecuted they think it will be somehow worse for them if they speak of their torments. In any of these cases they know what their questioner wishes to come at. Therefore, to try and baffle them logically only produces reticence, or point-blank denial. On the other hand, kindliness, frankness, and sympathy will win confidence, while a familiarity with the phenomena of mental disease by rendering us alive to the importance of slight indications, and showing us how various symptoms are associated together, will enable us in most cases to elicit what is required without producing irritation.

In doubtful cases the patient must often be seen many times. Notes should be made of each interview. One can thus go back on any trifling indication thrown out on a former occasion, and can also observe the subjects about which the patient is most ready to converse. Either persistent return to or persistent avoidance of one topic may point to delusion.

The patient should be induced to write. Many patients refer freely on paper to delusions which they will hardly communicate in conversation. Little peculiarities of written language will sometimes betray the reticent patient, and when followed up we shall find that they indicate that he attaches special meanings of his own to particular words, a symptom of advanced paranoia. When possible it is of great value to have continuous watch maintained upon a case. In this way insane habits can be discovered and manifestations which are reactive to sensory hallucinations, or which are dictated by delusion, can be observed and investigated. Careful inquiry should be made as to sleep, and the conduct at night observed. It is well known that many patients have hallucinations only at night.

How far it is possible for an individual suffering from delusions to conceal them from the observation of a skilled and careful observer may be questioned, but cases occasionally come under notice in which delusions undoubtedly exist for protracted periods undiscovered by those among whom the sufferer lives. Too much importance must not be attached in all cases to the retrospects of the insane, which sometimes indicate only the state of mind at present subsisting; yet, taking the acts of certain patients for years, together with the delusions which they eventually openly exhibit, one can have no doubt that delusive beliefs have existed long before they were suspected. Thus, every experienced alienist will have met cases (most frequently in females) in which a singular restlessness, a perpetual change of residence and unwillingness to reside for any length of time in one place, have existed for some years before they were found to be due to the idea of persecution. The patient is followed and tormented. He or she moves to another locality. The change is probably really beneficial at the time; at any rate, there is freedom from persecution for a period. The persecution recommences, however, in the new place, and is soon followed by another move. All this time the true motive is concealed. A curious illustration of this condition is given in a case described under the misleading title of "Larvated Insanity," in the *Journal of Mental Science*, April 1886. The same observer has noted a case in which a man of great intellectual attainments, who had led an active life, was compelled to relinquish his employment in consequence of being lamed by an accident. In his retirement he was surrounded by friends who saw no change in his mental faculties, but noticed that he had acquired the odd habit of never going to the same church twice running, and also that he spoke sometimes with a curious bitterness of Jews. After some years, during which nothing was suspected, he revealed in confidence to his wife that the Jews had been annoying him ever since he gave up business, and that when he went to church, Jews came into some part of the same building and made grimaces so as to attract his attention from his prayers. Shortly afterwards a note-book was found in which he had from Sunday to Sunday recorded the annoyances to which he was subjected. Histories like this lead one to suspect that cases of successful concealment of delusion may be not infrequent.

CONOLLY NORMAN.

INSANITY, CONCEALMENT OF. (*See* INSANITY, CONCEALED.)

INSANITY, EROTIC; OR, EROTOMANIA (*folie érotique*, *délire amoureuse*, nymphomania, satyriasis, love melancholy, *Liebeswuth*), does not constitute a special form of mental disorder having its cause and its symptoms and development always in the same manner, but it is a pathological condition which presents itself in the course of various forms of mental disease as an intermediary stage of variable duration. According to Morel we ought not to take in a too rigid sense the description of Esquirol, when he says that persons suffering from nymphomania and satyriasis are victims of a physical disorder, whilst an erotomaniac is the toy of his own imagination; and when he adds that erotomania is to nymphomania and satyriasis what vivid but chaste and honest affections are to wild libertinism. In the case of erotomania, Esquirol considered merely the amorous passion which is regarded as the cause of the derangement, whilst in the case of the two other disorders, he maintained that we are always able to recognise some lesion or derangement of the sexual organs as the starting-point of the mental malady; the brain and spinal cord become implicated later on during the course of the affection.

It is of no interest to examine whether this interpretation is Esquirol's or, rather, Morel's own; the only point which cannot be disputed is that brain, spinal cord and sexual organs all take part in erotomania, although not equally; but it is not always possible to determine which of the organs was attacked first or affected most profoundly; sometimes the insane ideas predominate, sometimes the morbid impulses of an irresistible nature. In erotomania the will is generally powerless, the sentiments are perverted, the intellect is deranged, and the genital organs are excited. It would often be rash to decide whether there is over-excitement of one function or depression of another. The solution of this problem is very difficult, because both kinds of phenomena may develop in a very variable manner. Erotomania appears only as an episode in the course of a mental disorder, as vesania, hypochondriasis, epilepsy, and general paralysis. If we consider these affections as forming separate classes, we might study erotomania as a species having two sub-species —nymphomania and satyriasis. In this way it would be easier to find some links which unite all the forms of derangement mentioned above. By creating too many types the mind becomes confused.

The ætiology of erotomania is very complicated; heredity plays an important part, but the diseases also of early childhood, the affections of adult age (insanity or not), and other causes serve to favour its development. We also remind the reader of the predisposition relative to the race and the condition of the surroundings, of education and of other factors. We know that every nation regulates in its own particular way the relations between the two sexes. The appetites are different in the manner heredity and observation have formed them. The control which the individual exercises over himself differs according to family and nation; the derangement modifies and transforms the original disposition, but it does not suppress it completely.

Many individuals of degenerated and unbalanced mind present temporary or permanent erotomania until they arrive at the last stage of exhaustion consequent on their habits of masturbation; the same is the case with idiots and patients suffering from dementia. Sometimes erotomania is only transitory, appearing at the commencement of certain forms of insanity; in general paralysis it may present itself in spite of complete sexual impotency. Other patients fall in love with an inanimate object, with a being which has disappeared, or with an historical personage; sometimes, if brought into the presence of the being they love, they even manifest a disgust, which cannot be overcome.

Every individual obeys a more or less irresistible impulse, according to the integrity of his reason and will-power; for a number of years religion may effectively arrest the impulse and raise a sufficiently strong barrier to the patient's instincts (religious celibacy, sects of various kinds, philosophical doctrines). Suppressed nature, however, demands its rights, and the unnatural life of monks often leads to erotic insanity; in such cases we see in the same individual mystic ideas associated with irresistible sexual appetite provoking wild excesses; mysticism and morbid moral perversion are often met with in mental disorder, and especially in individuals with defective mental equilibrium. Such individuals pass rapidly from an excess of conscience into an excess of depravity. They are unable to do anything in moderation. The most contradictory morbid impulses meet in this class of patients, and their insanity not being recognised exposes them to grave responsibilities.

Marriage is harmful for such patients, as entailing unhappiness and misery on the other party, without calming the excitement of the patient. An individual with unbalanced mind will masturbate day and night although he has a wife, and very often never desires or finds any satisfaction in married life; the same patient, irresponsible from an intellectual and moral point of view, will disappear among the crowds of the large towns to give himself entirely to masturbation, hiding his [illegible] from others, and seeking satisfaction of his insane ideas in touching the [illegible] of his passion without their knowledge; he imagines himself to have actual [illegible] with ladies of high extraction, [illegible] princesses, the photographs of which he has been gazing at; complicated [illegible] ideas are united in him. He is unable to control himself, and ought to be [illegible] in his own interest and for the security of others.

An individual with weak intellect has a great tendency to imitation; a child with perverted instincts ought to be separated from others in order not to contaminate them. Society ought to provide for this necessity in the different systems applied to children who are predisposed to do evil. It will suffice to remind the reader of the great epidemics observed in the course of past centuries in the midst of human agglomerations (convents, prisons, schools); in almost all cases it has been sufficient to take several very active individuals, whose minds were disordered, away from the community, where their presence encouraged the contagion, in order to suppress the epidemic immediately. Certain forms of insanity and of disorder of the nervous system spread by imitation among predisposed individuals, and this law applies also to erotomania.

In our opinion, there is no interest in detailing the gestures, words and actions of individuals labouring under erotomania. The talents of great novelists and of clever [illegible] have in these latter years been only too much exercised in depicting these sad subjects without benefit to any one; they have only served to propagate vices which fortunately would have remained unknown. True cases of sexual perversion are certainly exceptional, but in many cases it is an acquired habit; the morbid tendency cannot always be appealed to. Often hysterical patients will, under the influence of their morbid condition, lie at every opportunity, but nevertheless telling lies may be an acquired habit. It would be contrary to truth and science to say that all vicious habits depend on an irresistible morbid impulse, innate since childhood; instruction, education, *régime*, and treatment modify morbid tendencies; there are individuals who are rebellious against every discipline, and refractory to any treatment, but they are not so numerous as some extremists would have us believe. An attentive and impartial study of insanity will testify to the truth of our opinion.

Temporary erotomania is curable; in idiots and dements it becomes permanent and incurable, from physical exhaustion.

As regards therapeutics, two rules must be followed—treatment of the original disorder, vesania, hysteria, or general paralysis; suppression of the sexual excitement and strengthening of the weakened physical powers.

GUSTAVE BOUCHEREAU.

[*References*.—Esquirol, Des maladies mentales. Morel, Traité des maladies mentales. Foville, Nouveau dictionnaire de médecine et chirurgie pratiques. Bucknill and Tuke, A Manual of Psychological Medicine. Ball, Folie érotique.]

INSANITY OF ADOLESCENCE. (*See* DEVELOPMENTAL INSANITIES AND PSYCHOSES.)

INSANITY OF DOUBT. (*See* DOUBT, INSANITY OF.)

INSANITY OF LACTATION. (*See* INSANITY, LACTATIONAL; and PUERPERAL INSANITY.)

INSANITY OF PUBESCENCE. (*See* DEVELOPMENTAL INSANITIES AND PSYCHOSES.)

INSANITY, POST-APOPLECTIC. (*See* POST-APOPLECTIC INSANITY.)

INSENSÉ. (Fr.) A French term for one of unsound mind; a lunatic.

INSIPIENTIA (*insipientia*, want of wisdom, from *in*; *sapientia*). An old term used by Hildanus Centur, Ep. 41, for dementia.

INSIPIENTIA INGENITA (*ingenitus*, inborn). An old term for imbecility.

INSOLATIO. (*See* SUNSTROKE.)

INSOMNIA.—Loss of sleep has been classified under various heads by writers on wakefulness. Thus, Germain-Sée has made no less than nine divisions: (*a*) Dolorous insomnia; (*b*) digestive insomnia; (*c*) cardiac and dyspnoeal insomnia; (*d*) cerebro-spinal, neurotic, insomnia, comprising lesions of encephalon, general paralysis, acute and chronic mania, hysteria, hypochondriasis; (*e*) psychic insomnia (emotional and sensorial); (*f*) insomnia of cerebral and physical fatigue; (*g*) genito-urinary insomnia; (*h*) febrile, infectious, autotoxic insomnia; (*i*) toxic insomnia (coffee, tea, alcohol).

Among the causes of insomnia those of a predisposing character are: the female sex, old age, nervous temperament, intellectual pursuits.

Of exciting causes may be enumerated organic or functional diseases of the brain, worry, anxiety, grief, and bodily pain; noise, if not monotonous; fever; coffee, tea, &c.

Among the insane, insomnia is one of the most frequent symptoms, except in chronic dements. In melancholia it is the most distressing accompaniment of the disorder, and is especially marked in the early morning.

A careful analysis of the conditions or

causes of insomnia has been made by Dr. Folsom (U.S.), based on notes of his own cases. The principal ones may be briefly enumerated as follows:—Habit, reflex causes, as indigestion, genito-urinary disorders; autotoxic causes, as gout, lithæmia, syphilis, habitual constipation; anæmia, vaso-motor changes, neurasthenia, hallucinations of sight or hearing, astigmatism—the strain of the eye which in health may be unnoticed, producing "in states of debility, headache, dizziness, spasmodic muscular action or wakefulness"; and the neurotic temperament.

Under SEDATIVES will be found an exhaustive article which will convey to the reader a large amount of information as to the character of the most important drugs used for the purpose of procuring sleep.

[*References.*—Dr. A. Marvaud, Le Sommeil et l'Insomnie, Étude Physiologique, Clinique et Thérapeutique, 1875. Dr. Folsom, Insomnia, Disorders of Sleep, 1890.]

INSTINCT.—The present writer understands by the word "instinct" "a generic term, comprising all those faculties of mind which are concerned in conscious and adaptive action, antecedent to individual experience, without necessary knowledge of the relation between means employed and ends attained, but similarly performed under similar and frequently recurring circumstances by all individuals of the same species."* Since he wrote on the origin and development of instincts,† the question has been very seriously raised whether characters of any kind which are acquired during the lifetime of the individual can be transmitted by heredity. The bearing of this question on the whole science and philosophy of instinct is clearly both direct and profound. Therefore it is well to begin the present article with a few words upon this side of the subject.

Prior to the publication of Prof. Weismann's papers on heredity, it was the generally accepted doctrine of evolutionists that, while the main cause or factor in the process of evolution is natural selection or survival of the fittest, this main factor is more or less largely assisted in its operation by the inherited effects of use and disuse of organs, as well as by the direct action of the environment in causing adaptive changes of structure and habit. Be it observed, there can be no question touching the efficacy of these factors, so far as the individual is concerned; the only question is whether the adaptive changes which they produce can in any case or in any degree be transmitted to progeny, and thus serve to assist natural selection in its work of adapting species to their various conditions of life.

This is not the place to argue such a question; but, as regards the special case of instinct, it certainly appears to the present writer that natural selection alone is demonstrably inadequate as a theory to account for all the facts. In other words, it appears not only incredible, but inconceivable, that a large proportional number of instincts could ever have come into existence at all, if in their origin and throughout their development they were dependent only on natural selection, waiting, or, as it were, watching, for congenital variations of habit which might happen to occur in the required directions. For the large proportional number of instincts in question are of so complicated and refined a character that in our opinion (which here follows that of Mr. Darwin) they can only be ascribed to intelligent and intentional adjustments of action on the part of the ancestors of the animals which now present them—adjustments which, although thus intelligent and intentional in their origin, afterwards become mechanical or automatic in the species, owing to their continued repetition in successive generations. It is well known that in the lifetime of the individual highly complicated adjustments, which in the first instance require intelligence and intention for their performance, become by frequent repetition mechanical or automatic; and, therefore, if acquired characters admit of being inherited, we have at once an easy explanation supplied both of the origin and development of the class of instincts in question. On the other hand, if acquired characters do not admit of being inherited, instincts of this class become almost obnoxious to the theory of descent. In order to render this perfectly clear, we will take two parallel examples.

Caterpillars which in form and colour resemble the twigs of trees on which they habitually live, present the instinct of "posturing" in a way which completes the resemblance, standing up stiffly and motionless, so as to give themselves the best possible chance of being mistaken for twigs by their enemies, the birds. Now, in such a case there is no difficulty at all in ascribing the development of an instinct to the unaided influence of natural selection, because the instinct is here of so simple a kind that congenital or fortuitous variations of habit in the directions required may always have been of a proproportional number sufficient to furnish

* "Mental Evolution in Animals," p. 154.

† "Animal Intelligence," "Mental Evolution in Animals," and article "Instinct," in "Encyclopædia Britannica."

natural selection with its necessary material, just in the same way as similar variations in form and colour must have been of sufficient frequency to furnish natural selection with its material for slowly perfecting the resemblance of the caterpillars to the twigs. But it is the greatest of possible fallacies to argue, as has been argued, from such a simple instinct as this to the causation of instincts in general. This particular instance is, indeed, a very good one to prove the competence of natural selection as the sole cause of a simple instinct, seeing that throughout the whole course of its development no single caterpillar can ever have had an opportunity of "learning by experience" the advantages of imitating the position of a twig; in so far as any caterpillar failed to imitate that position adequately, it must have failed fatally. Now, however, let us take the second of our two parallel instances. Several different species of Sphex display the instinct of stinging spiders, insects, and caterpillars in their chief nerve-centres, in consequence of which the victims, though not killed outright, are effectively paralysed; they are then conveyed to a burrow previously formed by the Sphex, and, continuing to live in this motionless state for several weeks, are at last available as food for the larvæ of the Sphex when these are hatched. Now, of course, the remarkable fact with regard to this instinct is that the Sphex only stings its prey in the nerve-centres; and, in the case where the prey is a caterpillar, no less than nine successive nerve-centres require to be successively pierced. Apparently, then, we have here an instinct of so astonishingly peculiar and specialised a kind that, if all instincts are due to natural selection acting upon congenital variations alone, this is an instinct which ought never to have come into existence; the chances must always have been infinity to one against a merely fortuitous variation conferring a tendency to sting a caterpillar in its nine nerve-centres, and nowhere else. But, in accordance with Mr. Darwin's own theory of the origin and development of instincts (which recognised the effects of "hereditary habit" in co-operating with natural selection), the difficulty presented by such cases is to a large extent mitigated. Here, for example, is his opinion on the particular case in question:—

"Please take the trouble to read on perforation of the corolla by bees, p. 425 of my 'Cross-fertilisation,' to end of chapter. Bees show so much intelligence in their acts that it seems not improbable to me that the progenitors of pompilius originally stung caterpillars and spiders, &c., in any part of their bodies, and then observed by their intelligence that if they stung them in one particular place, as between certain segments on the lower side, their prey was at once paralysed. It does not seem to me at all incredible that this action should have become instinctive—*i.e.*, memory transmitted from one generation to another. It does not seem necessary to suppose that when pompilius stung its prey in the ganglion, it intended or knew that its prey would keep long alive. The development of the larvæ may have been subsequently modified in relation to their half-dead, instead of wholly-dead, prey, supposing that the prey was at first quite killed, which would have required much killing," &c.*

It is not without remembering the special objects of the "Dictionary of Psychological Medicine" that we have rendered this brief statement of a great issue in purely biological science. For we take it that the most important of possible questions in psychological medicine, have been raised by the raising of this issue in biological science. Whether or not the study of mental pathology in connection with heredity is henceforth to be exclusively restricted to variations, and therefore to aberrations, that are congenital; whether or not qualities of mind which are acquired by ancestral experience or individual education are in any degree transmitted to posterity; whether or not diseases of mind which have been superinduced by worry, undue strain, alcoholic or sexual excess, &c., exercise any predisposing influence of a pathological kind upon the offspring of parents thus afflicted—these are surely questions of first-rate importance to the student of psychological medicine. And if this is the case, there is no direction where his studies may be turned with so much advantage for a fair consideration of the basis of such questions as that which has been briefly indicated in the above paragraphs. Within the range of morphological science it is not at all easy to find any definite evidence to prove that natural selection has *not* been the sole cause of organic evolution, and, therefore, that congenital variations are *not* the only kind of variations which admit of being inherited. The reasons why it is very difficult to obtain such evidence from morphological sources become sufficiently apparent when we bear in mind certain general considerations,

* "Mental Evolution in Animals," pp. 301–2. See also another letter on the same subject and to the same effect, "Life and Letters of Charles Darwin," vol. iii. p. 245.

which the limits imposed by the present article forbid us to enter upon. But, as we have endeavoured to indicate, the phenomena of instinct furnish much more crucial tests as between the Darwinism of Darwin himself and the ultra-Darwinism of the school of Weismann. These tests uniformly support the former, and, therefore, offer the most serious difficulties against the latter. And, in our opinion, until these difficulties shall have been surmounted by the ultra-Darwinian school in question, mental pathologists will continue to be justified in holding their traditional doctrines touching the transmissibility of acquired mental characters.*

The only other point where the facts of instinct appear at all to touch the subject-matter embraced by this dictionary is that having reference to instincts as diseased. Unfortunately, however, very little attention has been paid to this topic by mental pathologists; and, therefore, it is but very little that we are now in a position to say about it. Indeed, the remarks we have to offer can be of small value beyond indicating the lines in which observation may be profitably directed.

Seeing that all the other faculties of mind are liable to pathological impairment, or even destruction, we should be prepared to expect that such should also be the case with instinct. But here, as elsewhere, it is of importance to draw a distinction between imperfection and aberration. We should not regard a man as intellectually deranged (*i.e.*, insane) because he is intellectually deficient (*i.e.*, stupid as distinguished from idiotic). And, similarly, we ought to distinguish between instinct as healthy and abnormal; even though highly imperfect, it need not therefore be deranged. Imperfection of instinct is, indeed, a phenomenon of frequent occurrence, often leading to fatal mistakes on the part of individuals presenting it.† Moreover, the mechanism of many instincts is easily thrown out of gear by any small deviations in the normal converse of an animal with its environment.‡ Thus, for instance, according to the late Mr. Spalding, "a chicken that has not heard the call of the mother until eight or ten days old then hears it as if it heard it not." But even such cases, although undoubtedly derangements of instinct, are scarcely entitled to be regarded as insanities of instinct. To make good this distinction by analogies drawn from physiology, we may say that an instinct thus deranged resembles a limb, the neuro-muscular co-ordinations of which have been impaired by a want of appropriate use during the time of its development; whereas an instinct smitten by insanity may be likened to a limb which is affected by locomotor ataxy—*i.e.*, it exhibits phenomena of a pathological order, springing from some neurotic disturbance, as distinguished from any lack of external conditions required for its suitable development. As an example of insanity affecting an instinct, we may quote the following:—

"A white fantail pigeon lived with his family in a pigeon-house in our stable yard. He and his wife had been brought originally from Sussex, and had lived, respected and admired, to see their children of the third generation, when he suddenly became the victim of the infatuation I am about to describe. . . . . No eccentricity whatever was remarked in his conduct until one day I chanced to pick up somewhere in the garden a ginger-beer bottle of the ordinary brown stone description. I flung it into the yard, where it fell immediately below the pigeon-house. That instant down flew paterfamilias, and, to my no small astonishment, commenced a series of genuflexions, evidently doing homage to the bottle. He strutted round and round it, bowing and scraping and cooing and performing the most ludicrous antics I ever beheld on the part of an enamoured pigeon. . . . . Nor did he cease these performances until we removed the bottle; and, which proved that this singular aberration of instinct had become a fixed delusion, whenever the bottle was thrown or placed in the yard, no matter whether it lay horizontally or was placed upright, the same ridiculous scene was enacted: at that moment the pigeon came flying down with quite as great alacrity as when his peas were thrown out for his dinner, to continue his antics as long as the bottle remained there. Sometimes this would go on for hours, the other members of his family treating his movements with the most contemptuous indifference, and taking no notice whatever of the bottle. At last it became the regular amusement with which we entertained our visitors, to see this erratic pigeon making love to the interesting object of his affections, and it was an entertainment which never failed, throughout that summer at least. Before next summer came round he was no more."

G. J. Romanes.

* For a full discussion of the origin and development of instincts, see the works already alluded to in a previous foot-note (p. 704).

† For example see *loc. cit.*, p. 167 *et seq.*

‡ *Ibid.*, pp. 169–70.

INSURANCE AS AFFECTED BY SUICIDE. (*See* Life Insurance in Relation to Suicide.)

[illegible] FACULTIES. A [illegible] faculties which communi[illegible] and animals knowledge of [illegible] internal sensations, and also of [illegible] world; their object is to know [illegible] perceive qualities and rela[illegible] (See FACULTIES, INTELLECTUAL.) [illegible] *intellectuelles*; Ger. *Ver*[illegible].) (See PHILOSOPHY OF MIND, [illegible].)

[illegible]. (See HABITUAL [illegible] and INEBRIETY.)

[illegible].—The depriving of [illegible] affected with mental disorder of [illegible] rights, preventing his managing [illegible] affairs. May be voluntary or not.

[illegible] SPEECH (*inter*, [illegible] *jacio*, I throw). The expres[illegible] of the emotions by inarticulate sounds, [illegible] with or apart from ordinary speech [illegible].

[illegible]. (See CONSAN[illegible].)

[illegible] INSANITY.—[illegible] recognised daily, tertian, quartan, [illegible], and annual intermissions. Even [illegible] the interval covered several years, he [illegible] the term intermittent. "When [illegible] is regular or periodic, [illegible] season, the same period of [illegible], the same physical and moral [illegible] bring back a disorder having the [illegible] character, the same crisis, and the [illegible] duration. When, on the other hand, [illegible] intermission is irregular—and variable [illegible] are usual—the attack is provoked [illegible] causes, it does not assume the [illegible] form, while its duration and crisis [illegible] different. The attack sometimes [illegible] out suddenly, but more frequently [illegible] indicated by symptoms similar to [illegible] which ushered in the first illness" ("[illegible] Mentales," vol. i. p. 79).

[illegible], MORBID (*intro*, [illegible]; *specio*, to look at; *morbus*, a dis[illegible].) The unnatural dwelling on and [illegible] into one's own acts, the morbid [illegible] weighing of one's personal worth, [illegible] criticism of one's own conduct. ([illegible].)

[illegible] ACTS. (See FOLIE [illegible].)

[illegible], Provision for the Insane. [illegible] the condition of the insane [illegible] in former days a melancholy [illegible].

[illegible] the Report of the evidence given [illegible] Select Committee of the House of [illegible] of the Lunatic Poor in Ireland, [illegible] early part of this century, a mem[illegible] the Committee said:—"There is [illegible] so shocking as madness in the [illegible] of the peasant, where the man is [illegible] labouring in the fields for his bread, and the care of the woman of the house is scarcely sufficient for the attendance on the children. When a strong man or woman gets the complaint, the only way they have to manage is, *by making a hole in the floor of the cabin*, not high enough for the person to stand up in, with a crib over it to prevent his getting up. The hole is about five feet deep, and they give this wretched being his food there, and there he generally dies. Of all human calamity I know of none equal to this, in the country part of Ireland, which I am acquainted with."

Superstition played a large part in the olden treatment of those afflicted with madness, nor can we censure this, when we consider that the crude condition of medical science offered no substitute. Holy wells, sacred relics, herbs over which masses had been sung, the prayer of the priest, exorcism, exerted at any rate some influence upon the mind in a certain number of cases, and were well intentioned, although based on the false assumption of the malignant action of a demon. When they failed to inspire hope, they did not inflict so much injury upon the constitution of the patient as frequent and copious venesection, repeated purges and depressing emetics. Both systems, the ecclesiastical and the medical, were equally removed from scientific therapeutics, and resulted in a condition of the insane which was a disgrace alike to religion and medicine. In Kerry, near Tralee, was situated, centuries ago, Glen-na-galt—*i.e.*, valley of the lunatics. Here were two wells, called Tober-na-galt, or "Lunatics' Wells." To these, madmen resorted, passing through a stream in the glen, the spot acquiring the name of Ahagaltaun or the "Madman's Ford." They drank of the waters, and eat the cresses hard by, both being regarded as possessed of supernatural powers in the cure of lunacy. A few years ago we visited this famous locality, which we found to be about nine Irish miles south of Tralee, the traveller passing Camp on the Dingle road. The driver was well aware of the old tradition that madmen were irresistibly attracted to the glen to be cured of their malady, just as the Island of Valencia was formerly supposed to possess a certain fascination for the sea-fowl which flocked there. On descending into the valley we called to our aid a labourer in a field who readily gave us all the information in his power. He remembered a poor lunatic resorting thither, some thirty years ago, and he was sure that none had been there since, with the exception of a priest who had escaped from the Killarney Asylum, and was brought back by the police. The place where the sacred pool was visited is now a bog, but the water-cresses, once so valued for their special properties, grow luxuriantly, as also rag-wort, which owes its name to the belief dear to herbalists, that it was curative of rage or madness. Within a short distance, on the other side of the road, remains the stone, imbedded in the grassy bank amidst ferns and brambles, to which those afflicted in mind made their pilgrimage. The stone is hollowed out into a basin about a foot in diameter, and was full of water, in fact it is rarely dry in this wet climate. Here it was that the madman stooped down to drink of the healing water. The worn stone on either side of the basin tells of the numbers who have visited it, and left the impress of their hands.

The origin of the ancient belief in the wonderful virtue of Glen-na-galt is thus accounted for. In the Fenian tale called "Cath Finntraglia, or the battle of Ventry," there landed on this spot Daire Dornmhar, the monarch of the world, to conquer Erin. Finnmac-Cumhail and his warriors marched forth to stay their progress, and gained the victory. Gaul, the son of the King of Ulster, who had gone to the help of Finn, entered so eagerly into combat that his excitement ended in an attack of mania. In this frenzied condition he fled from the battle-field, never resting till he plunged into the valley. We are left to infer that he was cured, and thus revealed to others the miraculous character of the valley in which the pool and the water-creasses were ever at hand, for distempered souls who were drawn there by an invisible influence (*see* "O'Curry's Lectures," p. 315).

The Dean of St. Patrick's, the renowned Swift, left his money to found an asylum for the insane, which was opened in 1745, being the first institution for the insane in Ireland. The subsequent history of St. Patrick's Hospital was not one which rendered it an example of the humane treatment of the insane; even in the Report of the Lunacy Inquiry Commission of 1879, it is described as "one of the most defective institutions for the treatment of the insane which we have visited."

The Cork Asylum, built some years later, was well conducted, being highly spoken of in evidence before the House of Commons in 1817.

The Richmond Lunatic Asylum in Dublin, opened in 1815, gained considerable reputation, but neither it nor the other institutions then in operation provided for more than a very small proportion of the mass of Irish lunacy. It was not until the year 1821 that the Lord-Lieutenant was authorised to erect a number of district asylums in Ireland, and these were not occupied to the full extent before 1835. In the carrying out of this scheme certain commissioners had been appointed who now were succeeded by the Board of Works, who acted until 1861, when two members of the Board, the chairman included, and the two inspectors of the insane who had been appointed as a Board by an Act of Parliament, passed in consequence of the report of the Select Committee of 1817 already mentioned, were constituted commissioners.

The number of lunatics and idiots in Ireland on the 1st of January 1891, that is to say, the total number under official cognisance, and their distribution, were as follow:—

In *District Asylums*: M. 6194, F. 5294, Total 11,488.

In *Private Asylums*: M. 253, F. 368, Total 621.

In *Gaols*: M. 2.

In *Poorhouses*: M. 1566, F. 2395, Total 3961.

In *Central Criminal Asylum*, Dundrum, M. 150; F. 29, Total 179; making a grand total, M. 8165, F. 8086, Total 16,251.

The **total number of insane and idiots in the United Kingdom**, January 1, 1891, was:—

England and Wales: M. 39,162, F. 47,633, Total 86,795; Scotland: M. 5894, F. 6701, Total 12,595; Ireland: M. 8165, F. 8086, Total 16,251.

Grand Total for Great Britain and Ireland: **M. 53,221; F. 62,420; Total, 115,641.**

THE EDITOR.

IRELAND, THE LUNACY LAWS OF.—There does not appear to have been any legislation in Ireland on behalf of the insane until 1787, excepting in the case of the private institution erected by Dean Swift in Dublin in 1745, which was recognised by a charter granted in the reign of Geo. II. (in which various regulations under Swift's will were embodied), and by Parliamentary grants of money from the legislatures of both countries. The Irish statute of 27 Geo. III. c. 39, passed in 1787, was an amendment of an Act passed in the previous year, which dealt with the regulation of the gaols and prisons in the Kingdom, but which contained no lunacy clause. The amendment included among its provisions sec. 8, which enacted that the Grand Juries of the several counties should provide the necessary money for supporting wards in the county infirmaries for the reception and support of idiots and the insane, who were to be recommended and certified to by two or more magistrates of such county: sec. 12 gave the Inspectors-General of Prisons power and authority to visit and inspect all madhouses and idiot asylums, as well as gaols and prisons. Prior to this enactment no provision had been made for the maintenance of lunatics, though the County Infirmary Act had been in existence twelve years. Owing to the defective working of these clauses, we find that in 1810 the first lunacy legislation in respect to the criminal insane took place by the Act (50 Geo. III. c. 103) repealing the laws relating to prisons in Ireland, and re-enacting such provisions as had been found useful. Sec. 2 provided that every prison be furnished with rooms or cells according to its size for the reception and solitary confinement of persons of unsound mind. Sec. 69 provided that any Judge of the Superior Courts, or any two Justices of the Peace, might examine on oath into the condition of any person on his becoming insane, empowering them to issue a warrant to the keeper of the prison to detain such person "during the continuance of such insanity, in such room, cell, or other place within the precincts of the prison as he or they shall think proper, or as shall have been specially provided for the purpose." Power was also granted the keeper of a prison on his own authority to confine persons becoming insane while in prison, in any such room, cell, or place.

It was not till 1795 that we find attempts made for the adequate accommodation of the lunatic poor of Ireland. Institutions sprang into being known as Houses of Industry, two of which were located in the cities of Cork and Dublin, and the Act 55 Geo. III. c. 107, passed June 22, 1815, provided for the separate control by a distinct body of Governors of the Richmond Asylum, then being built in Dublin under the control of the Governors of the House of Industry there. These Governors were to be appointed by the Lord-Lieutenant, were not to exceed fifteen in number, and could make bye-laws, appoint and remove officers, &c. An Act 11 Geo. IV. c. 22 made it a District Asylum, and enacted that not more than 150 patients were to be received, a provision abrogated by 1 Gul. IV. c. 13. In 1817 the first General Act (57 Geo. III. c. 106), for the establishment of district asylums throughout all Ireland, was passed. No provision was made in the Act whereby sites might be acquired whereon to build these asylums, and a special Act (1 Geo. IV. c. 98) had to be passed for this purpose in 1820. Important considerations had in the meantime presented themselves, and both Acts were accordingly repealed in the ensuing year, and their essential provisions, with others, embodied in "An Act to make more effectual provision for the establishment of Asylums for the Lunatic Poor, and for the custody of Insane Persons charged with offences in Ireland" (1 & 2 Geo. IV. c. 33), under which the existing asylums have in fact been erected. Its principal provisions were—power granted to the Lord-Lieutenant and Privy Council to erect any number of asylums for the lunatic poor for such districts as should seem expedient, these districts including one or more counties, or counties of cities, but not parts of a county or county of a city: each asylum was to contain not less than 100 nor more than 150 inmates where the district consisted of more than one county, and less than 100 and not less than 50 if of one county only; (this provision was expressly repealed by 8 & 9 Vict. c. 107 sec. 13): the funds for erecting these asylums were to be advanced out of the growing produce of the Consolidated Fund arising in Ireland, and after completion sums were to be supplied by the grand juries at the several ensuing assizes for repayment of money so advanced: power granted to the Lord-Lieutenant and Privy Council to appoint governors of such asylums as well as commissioners of general control and correspondence, not more than eight of these latter, whose duties were to be, the superintendence of erection, establishment, and regulation of all these asylums; they were chosen from the governors, and the posts were honorary: power to the Lord-Lieutenant on recommendation of these Commissioners of Control, to frame and authorise rules and regulations for the management of these asylums—these were known as the Privy Council Rules, and were to have the force of law: the sites purchased for the erection of asylums, and the asylums themselves, were to be vested in the Commissioners of Control: the grand juries of the several counties were to present at the next ensuing assizes such sums as might have become payable for maintenance, &c., this if refused could be enforced by order of Court: provision for the annual audit of accounts by the governors; returns of number of patients admitted and discharged, and number and names of the officers and servants of each institution—these returns were to be signed by the secretary or chief officer and countersigned by three of the governors.

Under this Act the Commissioners of Control were under no obligation to consult the grand juries, or any other local authority, and the friction that ensued between these bodies necessitated some years later the institution of a Commission of Inquiry, with the result that the Board of Control was superseded and a new Board established, consisting of four commissioners only, the then medical superintendents of lunatics being two of these, while the other two were the chairman and another member of the Board of Public Works.

At the date of the first Act of 1817, the Richmond Asylum at Dublin and the Cork Asylum were already in occupation, and nine other asylums were ordered to be erected by the Lord-Lieutenant (population of Ireland in 1817, 7,000,000), at Armagh, Belfast, Londonderry (in the province of Ulster); Carlow, Maryborough (in the province of Leinster); Limerick, Clonmel, Waterford (in the province of Munster); and one at Ballinasloe (for Connaught). The Armagh Asylum (at first for counties Armagh, Monaghan, Fermanagh, Tyrone and Donegal, later on Tyrone and Donegal were relegated to the Londonderry District Asylum) was the first completed, three years after the passing of the Act; Limerick Asylum (for Counties Limerick and Clare) was opened in 1827; Belfast (for Antrim and Down) and Londonderry (for Derry, and later on for Tyrone and Donegal) in 1829; Carlow in 1832; Maryborough and Ballinasloe in 1833; Clonmel in 1834; and Waterford in 1835. These asylums provided accommodation for 980 patients and were erected at a cost of £204,000. An Act (7 Geo. IV. c. 14) in 1826, to enable the Lord-Lieutenant to provide for the erection of additional asylums, was passed, but not acted on for 17 years. In 1830, by the Act 11 Geo. IV. c. 22, the Richmond Asylum in Dublin (for counties Dublin, Louth, Meath, and Wicklow), and by 8 & 9 Vict. c. 107 the Cork Asylum (for its county), were constituted District Asylums. In 1852 Kilkenny and Killarney provided asylums for their districts, Tyrone in 1853 obtained one near Omagh, Sligo Asylum (for counties of Sligo and Leitrim in the province of Connaught) and Mullingar Asylum (for Meath and Westmeath) were built in 1855; Letterkenny (for Donegal) in 1865; Castlebar (for Mayo) in 1866; Ennis (for Clare) and Enniscorthy (for Wexford), in 1868; while Downpatrick (for Down) and Monaghan (for Monaghan and Cavan) were built in 1869.

The principal rules and regulations of the Privy Council for the government of District Asylums now in force (amended in 1855) are as follows: The appointment of a Board of Governors to which certain duties were assigned (secs. 1 *et seq*): Persons labouring under mental disease for whom papers of application are filled up in the prescribed forms to the satisfaction of the Board, and who shall be certified as insane by a registered physician or surgeon . . . . shall be admissible into district asylums after having been examined by the medical superintendent or in his absence by the visiting physician (sec. 11). The medical superintendent is to make a return, to the inspectors, of the vacancies and admissions (Form F.) within one week from the date of every meeting of the Board at which orders for admission have been made and sanctioned (sec. 14). The friends of a patient or the signatory of the application for admission to sign a form (Form G.) for the removal of any patient when necessary (sec. 15). A person transferred from a gaol to a district asylum (sec. 2, Act 1 & 2 Vict. c. 27) and who shall not have been certified of sound mind may, after expiration of his sentence, be regarded and treated as if he had been admitted as an ordinary patient (sec. 12); a person under remand when certified to be insane may be removed by warrant of the Lord-Lieutenant to the asylum of the district in which he is confined, remaining there till certified sane, when by a similar warrant he shall be remitted to his former place of confinement (sec. 13). Clause 23 deals with the discharge of patients, this to be effected by an order from the Board, and a certificate signed by both medical officers; the inspectors, too, may order the discharge at the request of the superintendent in the interval between the meetings of the Board; expenses may be allowed patients without means by the Board on their discharge (sec. 24). Clause 25 enacts that persons confined in the Central Criminal Asylum and removable therefrom under sec. 12, 8 & 9 Vict. c. 107, shall, if insane at the expiration of their term of imprisonment, and if paupers, be transmitted, after due inquiry by the inspectors, to the asylum of their particular district, or if this cannot be ascertained, to the asylum of the district in which their offence was committed. Clause 26 deals with the admission into district asylums of poor paying patients, and the scale of payment; this has been supplemented by sec. 16 of 38 & 39 Vict. c. 67, which enacts that the property of any person confined in a district asylum, if more than sufficient to maintain his family (if any), may be made applicable for his maintenance in the asylum by order of a Court of Summary Jurisdiction, and persons liable for the maintenance of such patients will be liable for their support on application of the medical superintendent. The adoption of a system of education in asylums, the appointment of schoolmasters and mistresses to such, at the option of the Board of Governors, is authorised by secs. 73-77.

The officers of the asylum service are appointed under the provisions of the Act 30 and 31 Vic. c. 118, and are as follows: The Lord-Lieutenant has power to determine, increase or diminish the staff of male and female officers and servants of any district asylum, as well as to appoint their salaries and duties (sec. 2); the appointment of medical superintendent rests with the Lord-Lieutenant, and other officers are appointed by the Board with his approval (sec. 3); the appointment of officers by the Board is to be at first probationary, to be confirmed by them at a meeting from three to six months after such appointment—if not so confirmed, the officer ceases to hold the post, which after six weeks is to be declared vacant (sec. 4): the Lord-Lieutenant assumes the right of appointment if this be neglected by the Board within two months (sec. 5): the medical superintendent holds office during pleasure of the Lord-Lieutenant; all the other officers may be removed by the governors with the Lord-Lieutenant's approbation, and all servants by the Governors absolutely (sec. 6): superannuation allowances may be granted by the governors with the approval of the inspectors as per Superannuation Act of 1859 (sec. 8).

The administrative heads of asylum service in Ireland—the two inspectors of lunatics—originate from the appointment (Act 7, Geo. IV. c. 74) of the Inspectors General of Prisons to the supervision of lunatics in asylums and gaols. By 5 and 6 Vict. c. 123, sec. 1, the Inspectors-General of Prisons were constituted Inspectors of Lunatic Asylums, and by 8 and 9 Vict. c. 107, sec. 23, the Lord-Lieutenant was empowered to appoint in their place, and with the same functions, one or two duly qualified and experienced persons to act as inspectors of lunatics.

There are three modes by which an insane person can be admitted into a district asylum: (1) In the case of urgency the governors or the medical superintendent, or in his absence the visiting physician, may admit on their or his own authority, stating their reasons for this step, and submitting the case to the Board at its next meeting (the formal certificates are in this instance necessarily dispensed with). (2) The ordinary form of admission—in which formal application is made to the Board by the friends of the patient. A declaration must be made by some one before a magistrate on behalf of the patient, alleging his insanity and destitution; a magistrate and a clergyman, or Poor Law Guardian, must certify that they have personally inquired into the case; a medical certificate, which need be signed by only one physician, must be produced; and an engagement must be signed by the applicant to remove the patient when pronounced no longer a fit subject for the asylum. For the admission of a paying patient into a district asylum the forms are the same, with the addition of an undertaking by the applicant to pay a certain sum (which may be modified by the inspectors); an additional signature to the medical certificate; the signature of a magistrate and clergyman only (not a Poor Law Guardian) to the certificate that the case has been inquired into; and the sanction of one of the inspectors after the Board has approved of the application. (3) A process adopted in the case of dangerous lunatics; information sworn before two magistrates, who, after examining the patient, and on certificate from a physician, may order the committal of the lunatic to the district asylum. This has grown up out of the power entrusted to magistrates under 1 Vict. c. 27, to commit to gaol persons apprehended under circumstances denoting a derangement of mind, and it is at present adopted under the sanction and provisions of the Act 30 and 31 Vict. c. 118, secs. 9 and 10. The latter section also provides that any relative or friend may nevertheless take such person under his own care, if he shall enter into sufficient recognisances for his peaceable behaviour, before two justices of the peace.

Inquests are held in every case of death in the Central Criminal Asylum.

Clause 14 of 8 and 9 Vict. c. 107, contemplated and authorised the gradual enlargement of district asylums under Order in Council of the Lord-Lieutenant; such has, however, never been accomplished, and the Union Workhouses, which now serve the functions of the former houses of industry, always have a number of idiots and insane among their inmates. An important provision, 8 and 9 Vict. c. 107, sec. 15, by which the Lord-Lieutenant could order the erection of an asylum for the reception of particular classes of lunatics, or could order an asylum for each of the provinces, in addition to the district asylums already erected, to be built for the reception of chronic and incurable cases, has up till now received no recognition.

We come now to consider the various Acts of Parliament dealing with criminal lunatics, and with the erection of a special asylum for their detention. The Act 1 & 2 Geo. IV. c. 33, provided for the procedure in the cases of persons charged with offences, and (*a*) found to be insane when the offence was committed, and thereupon acquitted—in these cases the jury should add to their finding a statement to this effect, and whether their acquittal was on that account; (*b*) found to be insane and incapable of pleading when charged; and (*c*) appearing to be insane if brought up and not so charged—in these latter cases the prisoner was to be found insane by a jury specially empannelled. The clerk of the Court was in all cases to make an order that the person was to be confined as the Court might direct for the time being, and the Lord-Lieutenant was subsequently to give such order for his detention and custody as might seem fit; but if a lunatic asylum was already in maintenance in or for the county wherein the prisoner was tried, then he was to be removed to this asylum and there detained. The Act passed for Ireland, 1 Vict. c. 27, expressly conferred on magistrates in Ireland the power (which had been taken away from magistrates in England and Wales by 1 Vict. c. 14) of committing dangerous lunatics to gaol. The passing of this Act, and its difference from that applying to England and Wales, was due to the murder in the streets of Dublin of a gentleman of high position, by a lunatic, who, on the previous day, had been refused admission into the district lunatic asylum in consequence of lack of accommodation. Sec. 1 made it lawful for any two justices on being satisfied from medical testimony, and on view and examination of the person, *or other proof*, that the person is a dangerous lunatic, to commit such person to the gaol of the county, whence he might be discharged by order of the justices (one of whom signed his committal warrant), or by superior judges, or until removal of the prisoner to a lunatic asylum by order of the Lord-Lieutenant, which last-named power was conferred by secs. 2 and 3. The provisions of this Act being unsatisfactory, inasmuch as the removal of a patient from the gaol to an asylum was purely a matter of choice and not of necessity, and that it omitted to require sworn depositions to testify that the lunatic entertained a purpose, or seemed to do so, of committing an indictable offence, the Act 8 and 9 Vict. c. 107, was passed, sec. 10 of which enacts that it shall not be lawful for such justices to commit such person to gaol unless information on oath should have been made before such justices, stating facts which would lead to the belief that the person contemplated a crime, or was a dangerous lunatic or idiot. The person swearing such information might also, if the justices saw fit, be bound to appear at the next assizes or quarter sessions to support his information, the presiding judge being empowered to examine into the case and report to the Lord-Lieutenant. Ultimately the power of justices was abrogated by 30 and 31 Vict. c. 118, secs. 9 and 10 of which provide that such lunatics were to be committed by the magistrates to their district asylums; sec. 11, as in the former Act of 1 Vict. c. 27, provided that the Lord-Lieutenant might order the discharge of such person, on its being duly certified that he was of sound mind, or had ceased to be a dangerous lunatic. The evils attendant on the association of the criminal with the non-criminal insane, and of the close intercourse of the criminal lunatic with the insane criminal, were not remedied until 1845 by the Act 8 and 9 Vict. c. 107, by which "the establishment of a central asylum for insane persons charged with offences in Ireland" was passed. The Commissioners of Public Works in Ireland were constituted trustees for the purchase of site, and the erection, maintenance and furnishing of a suitable building. The Lord-Lieutenant (sec. 8) could, on completion of the asylum, order all criminal lunatics then in custody in any asylum or gaol, or who should thereafter be in custody, to be removed to the Central Criminal Asylum. The entire staff was to be appointed by the Lord-Lieutenant, and rules and regulations were, with the advice of the Privy Council, to be established (sec. 9). Persons removed to the asylum by order of the Lord-Lieutenant were to remain under confinement therein so long as they should respectively be legally detained in custody, or until it should be certified that they were of sound mind, they were then to be remitted to prison or discharged. The Inspectors of Asylums practically form the Board. Clause 22 makes it lawful for the medical superintendents of all asylums, including the Central Criminal, to hold and deliver clinical lectures.

The Rules and Regulations of the Privy Council for the Central Criminal Asylum have under this Act the force of law. The principal of these are the following: The inspectors are to visit this asylum at least once a month, separately or together (sec. 1), and at each monthly visitation shall make note of the health, &c., of the patients for Government information (sec. 2); all complaints are to be investigated by them, officers may be suspended if necessary, and a report sent to the Lord-Lieutenant (sec. 3); an annual report is also to be sent by them to the Lord-Lieutenant, as to the general state of the institution, &c., and on the recovery of a lunatic they are to submit a full report of the case to the Chief or Under Secretary (sec. 4). Lunatics charged with minor offences, and transferred from district asylums to the Central Asylum, shall, at the discretion of the Lord-Lieutenant, and on the report of the inspectors, be liable to be sent back to the institutions from which they came.

The Act regulating Private Lunatic Asylums in Ireland is the 5 & 6 Vict. c. 123, amended in some few particulars, and made perpetual, by 38 & 39 Vict. c. 67, and also amended as to the office of inspectors by 8 & 9 Vict. c. 107. By its provisions it is unlawful for a person to keep a house for the reception of two or more insane persons without a licence for every house so kept (sec. 3), which licence is for each county to be issued by the justices of the peace of that county assembled in Quarter Sessions (sec. 4). A new licence may be granted to another person, or for another house, in the same county in the event of licensee's ill-health, destruction of the house by fire, or other event, under the same provisions as in the case of granting a licence, notice of the cause of change being given to the Clerk of the Peace within seven days after its occurrence (sec. 12). A licence may be revoked by the Lord Chancellor on recommendation of the inspectors, notice of such revocation having been made in the *Dublin Gazette*, and coming into effect within three calendar months, the inspectors being bound to give seven days' notice to the licensee before transmitting the recommendation to the Lord Chancellor (sec. 13). For the purpose of receiving a patient into a licensed house, an order in the prescribed form, and a medical certificate signed by two medical practitioners, also in the prescribed form, are necessary. If signed only by one and not by two medical men, the reason must be given, and the patient may be admitted, but a second medical signature is necessary within fourteen days of the first signature. The Act 5 & 6 Vict. c. 123, s. 18, provides for the proper medical visitation of every licensed house not kept by a medical practitioner; this must take place once a fortnight (but by sec. 19 permission may be obtained in case of a house licensed to receive less than eleven patients, for this visitation to be made once in four weeks), and the medical officer, whether resident or visiting, shall once in every fortnight at least, make and sign a statement in a medical journal according to prescribed form (Schedule G.), which is to be laid before the visiting inspectors for inspection and signature. One of the Inspectors of Lunatics is authorised to visit every licensed house in Ireland once at least every six months (sec. 20), to inspect every part of the house included in the licence, and to see every patient, inquire into restraint exercised, inspect the certificates of admissions since last visit, and enter in a book kept for the purpose a minute as to such investigation and inspection, and if the visit is the first after the granting or renewal of a licence, the licence is to be seen and signed.

Fraudulent concealment of any part of a licensed house, or of a patient therein, from the inspector or medical visitant, constitutes a misdemeanour (sec. 24). If the inspector doubts the propriety of detention of any patient, he may specially inquire into his mental state, and if further consideration be requisite he shall make a minute thereof in the patients' book (sec. 27), and make a special visit accompanied by the principal medical officer of the nearest district asylum; and if after two such special visits (a period of not less than fourteen days elapsing between each, and a notice being posted to the proprietor fourteen days before the second visit, and, if possible, to the person who signed the order, or the notice being entered in the patients' book at the first visit), they shall come to the conclusion that the patient is unnecessarily detained, they may order his discharge, the result of their visits and the order of discharge being entered in the patients' book and signed (secs. 28–30). This power of liberation by the inspector does not extend to Chancery patients, patients confined by order of the Lord-Lieutenant, or of any criminal court, a report to the Lord Chancellor or the Chief Secretary being all the power he has in such cases (sec. 31). The statutory certificates are requisite where a single patient is received into a house, excepting in the case of a lunatic residing with a guardian or relative who derives no profit from him, or with the committee of the person or his nominee (sec. 36); these exceptions are, however, no bar to the visitation and examination by the inspectors, by order of the Lord Chancellor, of such patient (sec. 38). Public hospitals and charitable institutions not kept for profit, or institutions maintained by Grand Jury presentment or Parliamentary grant, are not affected by this Act, except in regard to visitations ordered by the Lord Chancellor or of the inspectors, and in regard to certification (sec. 49).

The Lunacy Regulation Act, 34 Vict. c. 22, deals with Commissions in Lunacy, and the management of the property and visitation of persons found lunatic by inquisition. The following is a short summary of its principal clauses. By this Act the office of Registrar in Lunacy is established, he receives copies from the inspectors of the medical certificates, &c., of patients admitted into any licensed house, and copies of the same when a patient is sent by justices as a dangerous lunatic to a district asylum; any person receiving a lunatic into his care is to transmit to the registrar within one week a prescribed statement, similar notice being given on cessation of custody or change of place of custody. The confinement, detention of, or interference with, the property of any lunatic entails a like notice to the registrar. Wilfully false returns are accounted as perjury, and wilful neglect entails a penalty. By the direction of the Lord Chancellor medical visitors are to visit lunatics and report, and an inquiry may be ordered on such report, which may stand as a petition for a commission to inquire as to the alleged lunacy, and the lunatic is to have a notice of this report as well as of the presentation of the petition for inquiry, when he may demand a jury; if he so demands the Lord Chancellor shall order it, unless on examination he deems the lunatic incapable of forming such a wish, in such a case, or if he do not demand it, the jury may be dispensed with. If the case goes before a jury it may be sent to a Common Law court, and an order of the Lord Chancellor, or certificate of a Judge or Recorder declaring a person of unsound mind, shall be deemed an inquisition. The Lord Chancellor may issue a special commission, and inquiry by legal visitors may be directed as regards the person's property before he is declared of unsound mind. Evidence may be taken orally, witnesses cross-examined orally, and oaths administered by the Lord Chancellor and masters. Secs. 30–48 deal chiefly with the powers and duties of the masters and registrar. The Lord Chancellor's control over the estates of a lunatic continues after his death, and in such event the committee of the estate is to make a statement to that effect to the master, who reports to the Lord Chancellor. The visits, inquiries, &c., of the medical and legal visitors are controlled by the Lord Chancellor, and they are to visit all lunatics personally four times in each year, except where they are resident in licensed houses or asylums, when they need not be visited more than once a year; they report to the Lord Chancellor as to the mental and bodily state of the patients, and such reports are filed by the registrar, kept secret, and on the death of patient or in case of supersedeas, destroyed. The Lord Chancellor may, where the property of the lunatic does not exceed £2000, or £100 a year, apply it for his benefit without inquisition. Committees of estate need not be appointed where the Lord Chancellor is of opinion that the lunacy is but temporary; he may dissolve partnerships, and through the committee of the estate dispose of property belonging to the lunatic, and act in every legal capacity for him. A petition for traverse must be presented within three months after the day of the return of the inquisition, and the trial of the traverse within six months of the date of the Lord Chancellor's order thereon; persons not petitioning or not proceeding to trial within the prescribed times are barred of their right to traverse. The Lord Chancellor may order one or more new trials on traverse, but he may notwithstanding such traverse make order for the management of the person and estate. Traverse of an inquisition made by a Judge of the Superior Courts and jury cannot be granted, but the Lord Chancellor may order a new trial. With the consent of the lunatic he may also order the commission to be superseded, and may appoint a guardian to a person of weak mind, whose powers are given in secs. 103 *et seq.* The remaining clauses provide for the Lord Chancellor's powers as to fees, annuities, salaries, &c., and his right to make general orders for regulating forms and proceedings, duties of office, &c., to be laid before the Houses of Parliament.

I. Ashe.

[The following are the statutes relating to lunatics in Ireland:—1 & 2 Geo. IV. c. 54; 6 Geo. IV. c. 54; 7 Geo. IV. c. 14; 11 Geo. IV. and 1 Will. IV. c. 65; 1 & 2 Vict. c. 27; 5 & 6 Vict. c. 123; 8 & 9 Vict. c. 107; 14 & 15 Vict. c. 81; 16 & 17 Vict. c. 70, sec. 52; 18 & 19 Vict. c. 109; 19 & 20 Vict. c. 99; 19 & 20 Vict. c. 120, sec. 36; 29 & 30 Vict. c. 109, secs. 68, 80; 30 & 31 Vict.

c. 109; 31 & 32 Vict. c. 97; 34 & 35 Vict. c. 31; 35 & 36 Vict. c. 74; and 38 & 39 Vict. c. 67.]

IRRENANSTALT; IRRENHAUS.—German terms for a hospital for the insane, a lunatic asylum.

IRRESEIN; IRRSINN. German equivalents for unsoundness of mind; insanity.

IRRITABILITY (*irrito*). Mental restlessness, agitation and impatience, resulting from a loss of inhibitory power consequent on nervous exhaustion.

ISRAELITES.—The history of the Israelites, a people who have played so great a part in the civilisation of the world, offers an infinity of subjects in the domain of psychopathic manifestations. This race presents a strange mixture of great truth and its opposite, of heroism and servility, arrogant revolt and excessive idolatry. The psychical constitution of the Jewish people is well marked. In their early history we see what may be called an epidemic of scepticism and moral insanity. The destruction of Sodom and Gomorrah was the punishment of the corruption of a limited number, characterised by sexual inversion. Men and women, as Moses tells us, reversed their natural instincts. Again, it is distinctly stated in the sixteenth chapter of Genesis that, at the time of Joseph, sorcerers and magicians existed and were held in esteem by the people. These must not be confounded with witches, in whom only the spirit of evil predominates. They should not be regarded as a Christian transformation of sorcery, for we find witches co-existing with sorcerers before the Christian era, under the form of evil genii, demons, and satyrs, who had their opposites in the good genii from the time when the existence of both good and evil was recognised.

We note in passing, the peculiar mental condition into which the inhabitants of Asia were thrown by divine decree, a deep sleep—stupor—in which they no longer understood how to read, and all characters were to them "as a sealed book."

The mental depression under which the daughters of Zion laboured may well have passed the boundary line of sanity in some instances. "They sit upon the ground and keep silence, covering their heads with dust, while their expression, we are told, became darker than darkness itself" (Lamentations). The Ninevites, who sprinkled ashes on their heads, remained speechless and wept continually. Although they acted in accordance with Eastern custom, they were certainly examples of contagious sympathy.

Cases of anthropozoic insanity occur sporadically.

Leprosy was a plague causing much trouble to the people of Israel, and manifested itself on the mental side by profound melancholia, and even rapid decay of the intellectual powers.

We know little of cases of simple convulsive neuroses unmixed with other disturbances. There are, however, examples of hysterical dancing.

Epilepsy is a very old disease. It was not regarded as a simple nervous malady, but as an example of damoniacal possession. From the days of Abram, according to tradition, it was the custom to wear a ring in the nose in order to escape from malignant spirits and lunacy. The annulus *varium* subsequently became the annulus *aurium*. This ring in Hebrew was called *Nesem*, and it was with the *nesems* of the women that Aaron made the golden calf. (*See* HISTORICAL SKETCH OF THE INSANE.)

A. TAMBURINI.
S. TONNINI.

ITALY, Historical Notes upon the Treatment of the Insane in.—Although, owing to political vicissitudes, Italy has not long regained her greatness and unity, yet she, like other great and civilised nations, has always turned her attention to the study of mental diseases, and the foundation of lunatic asylums. In a very short space of time, in comparison to that occupied by her historical political revival, there arose in many of her hundred cities, beside those buildings devoted to the fine arts and industry, others of a sterner type, owing their origin to philanthropy enlightened by psychological science.

Clinical institutions soon flourished in her renowned centres of learning, as well as certain other scientific institutions which have done great honour to this lovely country, and the new and daring "laws of criminal anthropology," which are now the world's property, had their first, most inspired, and most hearty advocates in Italy.

Relative to the history of psychological study, Italy retains traditions so worthy of remembrance that they have descended to us through the gloom of the Middle Ages; while in earlier centuries she possesses some truly glorious records, which take us back to the days of the greatness of ancient Rome.

Asclepiades, who lived in Rome about 100 B.C., introduced a genuine psychological system of treatment for melancholia and "forme stuporose," and was thus the first to lay the foundation of the modern moral treatment of mental disease.

During the first centuries of our era

Cælius Aurelianus wrote "De Morbis Acutis et Chronicis." In this treatise he is the first to describe the classic paralysis of the brain and the delirium of exaltation. He attacked the inhuman modes of treating lunatics at that time in vogue, and was the true champion of an ancient "no restraint" theory.

But this was a dying flicker of the lamp of that grand civilisation. After this period, the history of Europe can only be read with astonishment at the general decay which took place during the Middle Ages. During this epoch, not only is the loss of most of the rational principles of ancient times to be deplored, but also the substitution of more irrational methods for them. Everything fell a prey to mysticism; superstition, fostered by the priesthood, became a dogma of religious belief, so that it is useless to surmise what witches, demoniacs (the "possessed"), and vampires really were (*see* EPIDEMIC INSANITY). Such beings were common to all the countries in Europe during this wretched period. Secular teaching did not begin to make way in Italy until the fourteenth century. Not before the early part of the fifteenth did Antonio Guarnerio, professor at the University of Pavia, begin to turn the tales about witches to ridicule, and to caricature the prophecies of hysterical and epileptic persons.

Yet mediæval Italy may boast of having been among the first of European countries to establish asylums for the insane. The oldest (Italian) asylum was built in Rome about A.D. 1300. Another was founded at Bergamo in 1352, and St. Boniface's at Florence in 1377. These institutions, however, only served as places of confinement, for, even in the last century, hardly any notion existed of giving them the character of hospitals.

After the Middle Ages, if Italy was not the first to start along the path of reformed psychological treatment, she nevertheless speedily countenanced every rational innovation. Amongst those who must be associated with the glorious name of Wier, the German, we must not omit to mention the Italians, J. B. Porta and Paolo Zacchia. Porta published his "Magia Naturalis" in 1569; while Zacchia, as Papal Archivist (Archiatre) dared to maintain that demoniacs were only persons suffering from melancholia, with delirious fancies and delusions.

When, in the course of last century, asylums, which had previously been considered in the light of prisons or places of restraint, assumed the character of hospitals, Italy was one of the first to adopt this reform. Three years after the foundation of the Charité at Berlin, the first true lunatic asylum in Italy was established at Turin.

Nor did Italy remain behind in the progress of psychological science at that revival in European civilisation which marks the end of the eighteenth century. Among the most brilliant names connected with this revival is that of J. B. Morgagni. In his work "De Sedibus et Causis Morborum," he clearly indicated that the brain was the seat of mental diseases, and proposed a mild and rational treatment. The name also of Vincenzo Chiarugi is connected as closely with this psychological revival, as are those of Pinel in France and Tuke in England.* Chiarugi, as did Daquin in Savoy, commenced reforming the Florentine Asylum, some years before Pinel began his work in France, and substituted a humane and judicious treatment in place of systems based on superstition and cruel ignorance. "Labour" or "work" was his special introduction, a method now employed in well-organised asylums as the principal means of cure. His publications mark a real advance in psychological science. At the close of last century Chiarugi was the leader in a reorganisation of the Asylum of San Servolo in Venice, an institution which had not benefited by the recent reforms, though it had been some years in existence.

The commencement of the nineteenth century was most auspicious, and psychological science advanced with rapid strides, whether viewed from a philanthropic and practical, or from a scientific standpoint. In 1813, the fine and beautiful Asylum of Aversa was built in the province of Caserta; it is now under the excellent supervision of Prof. Virgilio. In 1818 a portion of the hospital of St. Ursula, at Bologna, was transformed into a lunatic asylum. In the same year the asylum of St. Nicholas was opened in Siena. In 1827 Pisani founded the Palermo Asylum. The Asylum of St. Benedict was commenced at Pesaro in 1827, and the Genoa Asylum in 1841. Asylums at Perugia and Ancona were already in existence.

During the second half of the century, Italy was endowed with many other asylums. Some of these will bear comparison with the most important establishments of this kind in Europe or America, both as buildings and as scientific institutions.

* Although Conolly was so many years later his name ought to be included in any record of the reform in the treatment of the insane.—ED.

Omitting mention of the smaller asylums, we must notice those at Reggio-Emilia, Imola, Voghera, Mombello, Como, St. Clemente, Novara, Verona, and, lastly, that at Florence. Thus, Italy, though she has not yet reached the ideal of seeing all her provinces provided with asylums, has gradually established a very large number of them, especially in her northern and central districts. The scientific study of psychology naturally developed beside the perfected institutions for lunatics. In 1830 the first Italian treatise on psychology was written by Dr. G. B. Fantonetti, while a similar work by Dr. Luigi Ferrarese appeared in 1823. At this time is to be noticed the opening of the first clinical institution in Italy, at Florence in 1840, under the supervision of Bini, and of another at Turin, in 1850, under Stefano Bonacossa. The first publications of Andrea Verga, whose beloved and well-known name is a great honour to the study of psychology in Italy, appeared in 1841. The merit of having originated the "Record of Mental and Nervous Diseases" at Milan belongs to him, as well as that of having founded the "Societá freniatrica Italiana." Nor must the name of Castiglioni and his "system of anatomy" be forgotten. The name of Biagio G. Miraglia, director of the Aversa Asylum since 1842, also became famous in Italy, although this scientific man had a system of phrenology not altogether in accordance with recent psychological discoveries. The well-known names of Porporati and Balardini also deserve mention, especially the latter, who, in 1844–5, waged war against the harsh enactments against "la pellagra" in Lombardy. In 1846, Biffi, now a celebrated doctor of the insane, commenced his career with excellent physiological writings.

During the second half of the century, while Italy was being provided with fine asylums, the activity of scientific men in the department of psychology continued to increase.

By the middle of the century clinical institutions were already in existence at Florence and Turin. To these establishments others were soon added, one, at first under the management of Livi, at Siena; another at Bologna, in 1860; then one under Lombroso at Pavia, and another at Naples in 1863, which was suppressed at the end of one year, only to be re-opened some years later under Professor Buonomo. Professor Andrea Verga lectured on psychology at the Ospedale Maggiore, in Milan, from 1866 until a few years ago. In 1867 a clinical institution in charge of Professor Tebaldi, was started at Padua; and shortly afterwards Girolami assumed the control of one in Rome, and Livi of another at Modena in 1874, which was annexed to the Reggio Emilia Asylum. This establishment has the universally admitted honour of having largely contributed to the development of experimental psychology in Italy. The college at Reggio soon became the laboratory for those experimental studies, where men, who have been an honour to Italian science, attacked the most difficult problems with research and objective observation. First among these was Professor Tamburini. He not only continued Livi's work at Reggio Emilia, but also perfected it, both in the asylum by clinic teaching, and (outside) by the publication of that important psychological record "La Rivista sperimentale di freniatria e di Medicina legale." This work, thanks to the labours of Tamburini himself, and of his colleagues Seppilli, Riva, Buccola, Amadei, Tanzi, Marchi, Belmondo and others, is one of the first in Europe. Turin, at the same time, became another important centre for psychological study, partly owing to the assistance of a clinical institution there under the control of Morselli for some years, but especially because it afforded an opportunity to Lombroso and his colleagues to show what Italy could afford as the propounder of the newest laws of sociology and criminal anthropology.

The clinical institution at Pavia became another important centre, for it has always been fortunate in possessing celebrated professors of clinical psychology; Lombroso first, then Tamburini, and lastly Raggi.

During the early stages of the study of psychology in Italy, this progress and activity of scientific men were almost exclusively confined to the northern and central provinces. However, in the last decade, a remarkable advance is noticeable even in southern Italy and Sicily. Asylums have sprung into existence at Naples, Nocera Inferiore, Girifalco, Teramo, as well as the private Villa di Salute at Palermo, and other private asylums of less importance.

The clinical institution at Naples is worth notice. Reformed by Buonomo in 1883, it became a scientific institution of the first rank; Professor Bianchi under Buonomo's guidance became the leading spirit there, and has since succeeded him as its chief.

We now proceed to give a brief account of Italian asylums, and of the methods of treatment employed in them, regretting that space does not allow us to give a detailed account of each.

There are 83 establishments in Italy devoted to the care of lunatics, including provincial asylums, institutions, supported by charity, private asylums, and special wards in hospitals; in about ten of these, the number of patients varies from four to twelve. Thirty-five out of the sixty-nine provinces are provided with establishments for the care of lunatics; the rest send their lunatics to the asylums of other provinces, either as joint supporters, or in some cases by special arrangements. Seventeen out of the thirty-five provinces thus provided own and manage their asylums themselves. In eighteen provinces the asylums belong to charitable bodies, which also manage them. Five provinces, Bologna, Venice, Naples, Cremona and Palermo have two asylums each. Five others, Florence, Turin, Genoa, Caserta, and Bergamo, possess, in addition to the central asylum, one or two more or less distant branch institutions. Only thirty-nine of the eighty-three Italian asylums are really public institutions, twelve are private, and the remainder consist merely of hospital wards reserved for lunatics.

The number of lunatics under treatment in asylums, as well as the proportion of the former to the population of Italy are shown in the following table, which has been compiled from the last census of the insane made by Professor Andrea Verga.

An average taken from the above gives the following results:—

Number of Insane to every 100,000 Inhabitants.		
Males.	Females.	Total.
78.1	70.1	74.1

Number of Inhabitants to each Insane Person.		
Males.	Females.	Total.
1280	1428	1350

In every former census the number of insane in Emilia had been the greatest. But in the present census Liguria has the misfortune of heading the poll.

Next, dividing Italy into three great districts we get the following result:—

District.	Number of Lunatics.
Upper Italy	10,431
Central Italy	8,364
Southern Italy and Islands. .	3,629
Total . .	22,424

The great predominance of patients in Upper and Central over those in Southern Italy is clearly evinced by these figures, and this difference becomes more striking, when we remember that population is denser in the south than in the rest of the country. This disproportion, as Tamburini justly observes ("Les Institutions Sanitaires en Italie," Milan, 1887, p. 168), is due less to the fact that there are fewer lunatics in the southern provinces than that few institutions exist there because so many difficulties stand in the way of their foundation.

Italian asylums may further be classified according to their organisation and the date of their construction. We have:—

(1) Those reconstructed since 1871—Macerata, Imola, St. Clemente, Novara, Voghera, Mombello, Como, Cremona, Florence.

(2) Old institutions partly reconstructed, and much improved—Reggio, Siena, Rome, Ferrara, Pesaro, Lucca, Aversa, Perugia.

(3) Asylums made out of buildings designed for other purposes—Bologna, Parma, Racconigi, Verona, Girifalco, Naples, Turin, Palermo, Alessandria.

(4) Old asylums left in their primitive condition—Genoa, St. Servolo, Ancona, Bergamo, Brescia, and others.

By classifying asylums according to their organisation we obtain three groups.

(1) Asylums composed of detached buildings—Mombello, Reggio, Rome, St Servolo, Siena, Macerata, Perugia, Florence.

(2) Asylums composed of small separate buildings, communicating with each other—Imola, Voghera, Como.

(3) Asylums built as single buildings, comprising the rest.

Those of class 1 are usually formed by various separate buildings, grouped around a large central structure, in which the functions common to all are performed.

In those of class 2 the detached buildings communicate with each other by one-storeyed galleries; they are all of more or less recent date.

Those of class 3 consist of single buildings, divided into wards and yards for different classes of patients.

Though Italy has not yet reached the same point that England and other nations have, with regard to criminal lunatic asylums, she is now seeking to solve this problem. There are already institutions partly devoted to this purpose at Ambrogiana, Montelupo, Fiorentino, and Aversa. Beltrani Scalia is at the head of the Government department which regulates Italian prisons. He is an enlightened philanthropist, who devotes much of his time to the study of anthropological and social questions. He has calculated that out of every 1000 males confined in Italian prisons, 12.25 are insane, whilst it is known that out of every 1000 males at large of fifteen years old and upwards, 1.24 are inmates of lunatic asylums.

The treatment practised in Italian asylums is most rational and humane.

The management of asylums is studied with the greatest care. All the light of modern science is being brought to the assistance of the insane. There are scarcely any institutions where infirmaries, departments fitted up for treatment by electricity and hydropathy, workshops, &c., do not exist.

As it is now universally recognised that work is the principal factor to be employed in a system of moral treatment, the chief asylums are now endeavouring as far as possible to afford their patients conditions suitable for those occupations with which their inmates are familiar, and have formerly practised.

The history of the lunatic asylum at Reggio-Emilia records among its most important undertakings, the formation of a real agricultural colony, initiated by Zani. It contains about 100 inmates, and possesses more than 50 "ettari" of land, in great part worked by lunatics. Imola, Macerata, Aversa, St. Servolo, Florence, and Turin all possess farms, but of less importance.

A special department for idiots in the Siena asylum is worth mentioning here, as a practical institution on a scientific basis, and almost the sole attempt of this kind which has been made in Italy up to the present time. For some time past the need of an enlightened institution of this description has been felt in Italy. The opening of the first small idiot asylum at Chiavari in Liguria, must be mentioned to complete our record.

Food and general service leave nothing to be desired. Kitchens and laundries in which steam has triumphed over older systems, give our asylums the cheerful appearance of factories.

All Italian asylums do not possess that scientific system of study which should always be our guide in the art of healing. The "no restraint" method is partially applied, but is scarcely anywhere rigorously enforced. Only Professor Tamburini has, for some years, practised it successfully at the Reggio-Emilia asylum.

The branch of benevolence which concerns lunatics may, on the whole, be said to be vigorous and flourishing in Italy. We may add that "Societá di Patronato" for lunatics have already been successfully introduced, an expression of the most enlightened civilisation.

Italy as yet possesses no laws respecting lunatics and asylums, but an excellent Bill, in accordance with the amendments proposed by the alienists assembled at Milan in October 1890, is about to be discussed in our Parliament.

Departments.	Italian Population, calculated Jan. 1, 1888.			Number of Patients in different Asylums and Hospitals Jan. 1, 1889.		
	Males.	Females.	Total.	Males.	Females.	Total.
Piedmont	1,614,289	1,617,661	3,231,950	1,270	1,114	2,384
Liguria	461,877	467,859	929,736	628	599	1,227
Lombardy	1,988,869	1,928,963	3,917,832	2,063	1,924	3,987
Venice	1,522,093	1,495,296	3,017,389	1,266	1,677	2,943
Emilia	1,174,543	1,128,452	2,302,995	1,567	1,462	3,029
Tuscany	1,191,247	1,148,850	2,340,096	1,301	1,262	2,563
Marche	495,126	504,080	999,206	598	521	1,119
Umbria	315,336	296,785	612,121	297	182	479
Lazio	507,271	452,918	960,189	630	444	1,074
Naples	3,975,452	4,062,734	8,038,186	1,558	910	2,468
Sicily	1,610,413	1,582,086	3,192,499	626	382	1,008
Sardinia	374,938	348,918	723,856	91	52	143
Whole of Italy	15,231,454	15,034,602	30,266,056	11,895	10,529	22,424

APPENDIX.

List of the Principal Italian Lunatic Asylums.

	Inmates.
Piedmont—	
Alessandria Asylum	368
Cuneo "	475
Novara "	426
Turin "	1018
(with branch at Collegno)	
Liguria—	
Genoa Asylum and branch	747
Dell' Incoronata Cornigliano	352
Lombardy—	
Astino (near Bergamo)	349
Brescia	335
Como	737
Cremona	179
Mombello	1168
Biffi (Milan)	121
Voghera	418
Venice—	
St. Servolo (Venice) for males	1001
St. Giacomo di Tomba (Verona) new	—
Emilia—	
Reggio-Emilia (most important in Italy)	773
Bologna	494
Imola	982
Ferrara	309
Colorno	310
Tuscany—	
Bonifazio and Castelpulci (Florence)	819
(The old Bonifazio Asylum is now suppressed, and a fine large new one is to be opened shortly at St. Salsa. It has been built under the direction of Prof. Tamburini, and a clinical institute of psychology will be annexed to it. This is also an entirely new building.)	
Fregionaira (near Lucca)	612
St. Nicolo (Siena)	1028
Marche—	
Ancona	328
Macerata	315
St. Benedict (Pesaro)	345
Fermo	131
Umbria—	
Perugia	485
Lazio—	
St. Maria della Scala (Rome)	1074
Naples—	
Aversa	752
Sales and Madonna dell' Arco (Naples)	671
Teramo	242
Nocera dei Pagani (interprovincial)	695
Catanzaro (in Girifalco)	180
Sicily—	
Palermo	1005
Villa di Salute (Mezzomorreale)	200
Sardinia—	
Cagliari (near the town hospital)	143

SILVIO TONNINI.

J

JACKSONIAN EPILEPSY. (*See* EPILEPSIES and INSANITIES.)

JACKET, STRAIT. (*See* STRAIT JACKET.)

JACTATION, JACTITATION (*jactatio*, a tossing to and fro). A restless and anxious tossing to and fro from one posture to another; a symptom of conscious or unconscious distress, observed in all severe mental affections.

JAPAN, The Insane in.—We are not in possession of any recent information in regard to the provision made for the insane in Japan. From a pamphlet entitled "A Visit to the Yedo Poor House," by Mr. Edward B. Paul, H.B.M.'s Legation, written in 1877, we learn that in 1873 a Poor House was established in Uyéne for the purpose of caring for distressed persons requiring medical attendance, and other objects. It was intended to admit the insane, for whom separate apartments and an attendant were to be appointed. In the account of the establishment, it is stated that "lunatics are frequently brought out of their rooms for the purpose of bathing or exercise, and are treated according to the nature of their mental aberration."

Mr. Paul makes the following statement in regard to the building set apart for this class:—

"Some distance apart from the buildings described above are a series of long, low sheds which contain the insane inmates of the establishment. I regret not being able to give such good account of this department of the Yoiku-in as the rest of the house. The sheds above mentioned are very roughly constructed, and bear a striking resemblance to a row of dens in a menagerie. They are divided into compartments of about 6 ft. by 4 ft. in size. These have a frontage of strong wooden bars, communicate with the latrines behind, and are separated from each other, laterally, by wooden partitions, which allow every sound made in one cell to be distinctly heard in those adjoining. A space of about three feet separates the front of the cells from the true frontage of the building, which is closed at night by ordinary shutters, and in winter days probably by paper slides. These sheds face the South, and in addition to the discomfort arising from the extremely circumscribed space allotted to him, the patient must find the heat in summer intolerable, and at night when the shutters are closed outside he must be nearly stifled, as there is no proper provision for ventilation. The building is heated in cold weather by charcoal braziers, the fumes of which must, in the absence of good ventilation, combine with the waste products of respiration and transpiration to produce a highly poisonous condition of atmosphere. The patients must, moreover, suffer terribly from colds and draughts on windy days, owing to the improper character and hasty construction of the building. The most tractable of the patients are taken out for exercise every morning and evening, and to walk in a large open space in the compound. Those patients who are very violent are treated with the douche, the apparatus for which stands at the rear of the sheds. They are also tied up with ropes till the paroxysm is over. There is accommodation for fifty patients in the asylum, which is always full, the superintendent having had to refuse several applications for admittance. I was told that the mortality in this department is very high."

The foregoing of course relates to a period of transition in Japanese progress, and it is only fair to add that we are assured on good authority that lunacy has since received its due share of the attention which has raised Japanese medical science in general to the high position it has won with such phenomenal rapidity during the last fifteen years. Unfortunately there is no available information that enables us to offer details as to the present methods of care and study of the insane, and neither the periodical reports of the Central Sanitary Bureau nor the calendars of the Tokyo University allude to the subject. THE EDITOR.

JEALOUSY as a Symptom of INSANITY.—Jealousy is primarily associated with the sexual passion, and is a compound of fear of loss of a possession, associated with a feeling of depression due to wounded self-love.

It is a natural feeling, and stimulates the males to fight, and thus has aided in the struggle for existence, leading to the survival of the fittest. Like the other normal feelings, it may become disordered in degree or in relation, being unreasonable in amount, or arising altogether from false ideas.

It may occur alone as a symptom of insanity, or combined with other evidences of mental disorder.

It is more common in women than in men, and may occur in them in connection with marriage engagements, under puerperal conditions and at the menopause.

Insane jealousy may be aroused in relation to the marriage partner, to children, or to friends.

We shall now proceed to discuss it in more detail under the above heads.

It occurs in young and unmarried women and widows often without any grounds. A single woman dwells upon her singleness and wishes she were married; she then fixes her regards on some man, and is at once in an attitude of expectant attention, which induces her to see in every indifferent act a meaning or a suggestion which was never intended. If the man happens to be married or engaged, the jealousy may lead to serious social troubles, and may give rise to attempts at murder. The famous case of a lady now at Broadmoor is an example. She believed a doctor wished to marry her, and she found that his wife was fond of chocolate creams, and most ingeniously managed to introduce poisoned creams into the stock from which the doctor's wife bought her sweets, and poisoned several children, though the intended victim escaped.

False accusations may be made as to seduction and the like in these cases. Such cases are allied to hysteria. With widows similar ideas may arise.

During pregnancy and after delivery, ideas of the same kind may occur; during pregnancy it is common for the lower animals to shun the males, and in woman a like feeling may arise. Then, as so often occurs in the neurotic, the feeling of personal aversion is transferred, so that the wife believes that the coldness is on the part of her husband. She then seeks for evidence, and again expectancy conjures up the thing she dreads. A servant or a sister is suspected, and misery and suicide, or attempts at homicide may follow.

In some such cases and in those belonging to the next section, mothers may murder all their children to spite a father, or to spare them from contamination.

After delivery, there may occur various perversions of the sexual instincts, so that in one case erotic desire is manifested, and in another dislike to husband, or suspicion or dread of him arises. The development of this insane jealousy resembles that in the cases of pregnancy. Though insane jealousy in married women may occur at any age, we believe it is most common about the climacteric. At this period there may be a revival of desire (and also of reproductive power), which is not easily satisfied, and which may cause the wife to believe that she is neglected for some other woman, or a feeling of antipathy to the husband may arise, which becomes misinterpreted for dislike on his part, just as to the reeling man the earth seems to stagger.

In either case the woman becomes suspicious and is on the look-out for evidence, when trifles light as air suffice to satisfy her. One woman searches her husband's pockets, while another puzzles over his blotting-pad; one watches the governess and opens her letters, while another declines cohabitation, but watches the bedrooms of the servants. When once the false idea has got fairly established, reason is of no avail to disturb it. The wife's life is more and more solitary, her interests are narrowed, and she becomes unmotherly and indolent, her whole character is often perverted, and her friends are alienated; she may take to vicious habits of drink or masturbation. Frequently there is moral perversion, and we have met with patients during this stage who became kleptomaniacs.

Hallucinations, especially of hearing, are common, and the *voices* usually are insulting.

During this stage of insane jealousy acts of violence and destructiveness are common. We have met with instances of wanton destruction of valuable property belonging to the husband with the idea of thus preventing the mistress from enjoying the rights of the wife.

It is common for the wife to write injurious letters and post-cards, and thus to cause general scandal.

It must be remembered that the jealousy may have grounds, and may only be unreasonable in degree; and again that it may be associated with reasonable conduct in other social relationships. Thus, a man may have a wife who suspects his every act, and searches and doubts, yet she may do no harm and conduct her home affairs well; in such cases the man has no relief, for though unreasonable she is not to be treated as a lunatic, and the husband must submit to the moral defect, as he would have to a physical one.

If the symptoms are directly related to the menopause, there is a fair prospect of recovery with time, but this probably will be two or three years.

We believe that removal from home is necessary while the wife is definitely told that she is suffering from a well-recognised disorder, for which she will have to be kept away as long as she harbours these false ideas. She needs generally some bodily treatment, and hypnotics for a time may be required. She should have a sensible middle-aged companion of her own social station to occupy and amuse her. She should see her husband from time to time, the visits being regulated by her behaviour. She may be tried at home after six months' absence, but if any signs of the old symptoms recur she must be sent off again, this time for a shorter period, and thus she may be tested. This treatment is tedious and costly, but if properly carried out and begun early enough, the result is often good.

Under similar conditions, with the addition of alcoholic excess, precisely similar ideas may arise. In some cases the malaise of the climacteric period leads to the intemperance. In these patients also, good results may follow a similarly carefully arranged seclusion or separation.

Vindictiveness is common among the jealous, and on the Continent vitriol throwing may give rise to legal trouble.

In man, jealousy is less frequent, but may arise under similar conditions. Some young men, mostly masturbators, get false ideas as to the love of certain girls, and make foolish offers of marriage, and will not be discouraged; they may murder the girl in a fit of insane jealousy, generally shooting her.

In married men the insane jealousy is frequently associated with feelings of loss of desire or of impotence, and may occur in diabetes, locomotor ataxy, and alcoholism. We have met elderly men who for a time have told the most circumstantial tales of the perfidy of their wives, these tales being wholly groundless, and being denied on recovery.

But once start the idea as in the mind of Othello, and no one can tell how, under favouring conditions of mental instability, the unreasonable growth may develop.

In our experience alcoholic excess is not an uncommon cause of insane jealousy in men, which may also be associated with ideas that poison is being administered for their removal; thus mania of persecution may appear, and end in chronic mania.

It is essential to seclude the insanely jealous man in nearly all cases, as he is homicidal, and probably suicidal. We do not think men recover so frequently as do women; in them the treatment must depend on general conditions.

Insane jealousy in relationship to children may be associated with the other forms of the disorder, and may lead to serious consequences, or it may slowly grow out of a feeling of loss of affection and loss of interest in the children, such as is commonly met with in cases in which there is menstrual irregularity. The jealousy may be directed against the husband, the nurse or the governess, and may be associated with fancies that the children's affection is being alienated from the mother.

In some cases strongly infanticidal impulses arise. We have never met a man insanely jealous of his offspring.

The last form of insane jealousy to which we refer is that in reference to friends. Here again the disorder is mostly a feminine one.

Women believe that influences are at work to loosen the bands of established friendship; they dwell on the slightest signs of want of affection and magnify them. These cases are more frequent in middle-aged, single women who have poured out their affection upon some female friend. These women-friendships have something peculiar in them, the relationships being often emotional and associated with unhealthy mutual self-analysis. A gradual change in this relationship may lead to passionate jealousy, with fancies that the once loved one has become influenced against, and believe all sorts of moral evils of, her friend.

Such jealousy may lead to violent hatred and to acts of passion. We have known the idol attacked and seriously damaged.

To sum up. Jealousy as a symptom of insanity may occur in men and women, and may be the chief among other symptoms of mental disorder; or it may be the residuum of a more or less acute attack of insanity, a form of monomania.

It may affect the marital, the parental, or the social relationships.

It may occur in the single or married; it is more common in women; it may be connected with age and loss of power, or with the climacteric period. It is a frequent accompaniment of alcoholic intemperance. It has no special import as a symptom, but it often leads to homicidal or suicidal acts.

The treatment depends on general conditions, but must generally be of the so-called moral kind, such as change of surroundings and companionship, rather than medicinal. GEO. H. SAVAGE.

JERKS, JERKERS.—A name given to the hysterical form of maniacal excitement in which the patients went through a pantomimic performance, jerking, twisting, and contorting their bodies into all manner of shapes. It was due to the religious enthusiasm prevalent in some of the American States in 1798–[illegible], consequent on the extravagances of revival preaching.

JEWS. (*See* ISRAELITES.)

JOINTS, HYSTERICAL AFFECTIONS OF.—A mimicry of severe disease of a joint, described by Charcot, generally the knee or hip, occurring in a person of hysterical disposition. The main symptoms complained of are pain and difficulty of movement; the former is always described as most acute, and with it there is associated an abnormal degree of cutaneous hyperæsthesia. There is no heat, redness or swelling of the part, and the concurrent deformity, though simulated, shows a marked difference from the ordinary abnormal conformation of the joint seen in hip disease, &c. Occasionally there is some cutaneous hyperæmia and some crepitation on passive movement of the joint, but there is never any rise of temperature, or effusion into the joint-cavity. (*See* HYSTERIA.)

JUDGES (INSANITY OF).—A *non compos* ought not to sit as a judge; but it is laid down in Brooke's "Abridgement" (fo. 258, 7) that should such a case occur, the fines, judgments and other records taken before him would be good; but it is otherwise as regards matters *in fait* (*i.e.*, by deed or writing), which might be avoided by a person of non-sane memory. Since the Act of Settlement, the judges of the Superior Courts hold office *quamdiu se bene gesserint* and are not removable except upon an address to the Crown by both Houses of Parliament. A. WOOD RENTON.

JUDGMENT (Fr. *jugement*, from *juger*, to judge; from Lat. *judico*, I decide). An intellectual operation, by which the characteristics of ideas or facts presented to the mind are valued or compared so that opinion or action may be guided by the result. (Ger. *Urtheilskraft*).

JUMPERS.—A name given to those hysterical fanatics who in their devotional exercises worked themselves into a state of frenzy, and began to jump about in a strange, uncontrollable manner. They appeared in Cornwall in 1760. The name has also been given to a family in Maine, U.S.A., which has evinced a like psycho-pathological condition, a sudden and peremptory order compelling immediate response on their part. The affection appears to have spread among the members of the family by imitation, and thus evinced a spurious hereditary character.

JURISPRUDENCE, MEDICAL. (*See* CRIMINAL LUNATICS, EVIDENCE, PLEAD, &c.)

JUVENILE INSANITY. (*See* DEVELOPMENTAL INSANITIES.)

K

KAKOSMIA SUBJECTIVA (*κακός*, bad; *ὀσμή*, a smell; *subjicio*, I cast under). A disturbance of the olfactory centre in some hysterical, epileptic, insane, or syphilitic subjects, which causes the perception of a bad odour. (*See* SMELL, HALLUCINATIONS OF).

KALMUC IDIOTS. (*See* IDIOCY, FORMS OF.)

KATALEPSIA. Catalepsy (*q.v.*).

KATATONIA (*κατατείνω*, I stretch tightly; *Spannungs Irresein*, Ger.) is a disorder which Kahlbaum was the first to describe in 1874 as a special form of mental disease in a monograph,* illustrated by numerous examples.

Typical cases of this kind pursue their **course** according to the following scheme: There is at the commencement a condition of depression, melancholia, and of mental uneasiness and distress. After a longer or shorter time this is succeeded by a phase of excitement, of the maniacal kind, or it assumes the character of *melancholia agitata*. This second stage is followed—often very soon — by a condition of rigidity and immobility, to which the term *attonita* (Attonitität) is applied. After this, the patient may recover, or, in an unfavourable case, the disease terminates in general confusion, and at last in actual dementia.

There are, however, many deviations from this general scheme, and we may distinguish two varieties, *katatonia mitis* and *katatonia protracta*. In the former the *attonita* is not fully descriptive, for only the principal symptoms are present; in the latter the various phases frequently follow each other.

The **prognosis** of the disorder is favourable in cases of *katatonia mitis;* and even in protracted cases, after, it may be, a duration of several years, the patient may recover.

The various stages of the disease, which we have described above in general, are distinguished by a series of characteristic symptoms, and in addition to the actual mental phenomena we have specially to mention anomalies of the psycho-motor sphere, after which the disorder has received its name.

The most conspicuous **symptoms** are those of the stage called *attonita*. We are particularly struck by the absence of any spontaneous movements and by more or less complete immobility. In the more advanced phases of this condition the movements of inspiration and expiration are very slight, and those of the eyelids are very rare. However, as soon as we attempt to produce passive movements of any part of the patient's body, we meet almost always with a powerful resistance; the groups of muscles antagonistic to the attempted movement commence to contract energetically—this has been termed the symptom of negativism. The negative muscular contraction is not equally strong in all parts of the body, but appears to be strongest in movements of the shoulder-joint and in attempts to extend the head or to raise it when flexed upon the chest. If the muscular resistance in passive movements is but slight, and if we succeed in overcoming it, the parts often remain for some time in the position given them; in this way we may force the patient into the most uncomfortable positions: this has been called the symptom of *flexibilitas cerea*. Even the ordinary position of the patient in this stage is not a comfortable one; with relaxed muscles he seems to have become rigid in the most *bizarre* attitudes; specially frequent is the position in which the thighs flexed at the hip-joint are drawn up close to the abdomen (the legs being flexed on the thighs), and the head is flexed on the chest, so that the whole body appears to be rolled up into one mass. As a partial symptom of this tendency to muscular contraction, we have to mention specially the condition in which the lips are protruded like a snout (*Schnauzkrampf*).

Not unfrequently this rigid immobility is interrupted by monotonous movements incessantly repeated in an automatic manner: such have been called stereotyped movements (*Bewegungsstereotypie*).

Another most important symptom is the so-called mutism (*mutacismus*), a pathological tendency to be silent. In a slight manner this symptom is present in every case, and in many cases it exists fully developed for months and even for years. We have, however, to add that in some cases there seems to be a desire to speak, so that in such instances at least, the mutism may be considered as a consequence of the general motor inhibition.

Just as the immobility is frequently

* *Die Katatonie*, August Hirschwald, Berlin, 1874.

interrupted by stereotyped movements, so the mutism may be interrupted by the monotonous utterance of incessantly repeated words—verbigeration (*q.v.*).

We have also to mention that patients of this kind often refuse to take food; on the other hand, boulimia is not unfrequently observed, and we differ decidedly in our opinion from some authors, who have stated that the latter symptom is a sign of commencing dementia, and therefore unfavourable with regard to the prognosis of the case.

Among the vaso-motor and trophic derangements, we have specially to mention a tendency to cyanosis of the peripheral parts, and salivation which may attain a high degree and last a long time. In a case described by Arndt there was also polyuria present.

Among the other stages of the disorder, that of excitement is of a specially peculiar form. We frequently find a certain pathos and a tendency to declamatory and sermon-like speaking; the gestures are stiff and theatrical; speech shows indications of verbigeration, or it may be fully developed. The monotony of the whole behaviour is quite distinct from typical mania.

The stage of commencement is the least characteristic one; there are almost without exception hallucinations, especially of vision, and not unfrequently the patient's ideas run on religion. In well-developed cases we are struck, even in this first stage, by the motor inhibition.

Kahlbaum states that sometimes the commencement of the disorder is marked by a convulsive attack of a varying kind.

Also the last stage, the terminal dementia, is often characterised by the continuation of the stereotyped movements.

In order to fully understand katatonia it is necessary to know the points of view which Kahlbaum has given in his thoroughly original treatise on "Die Gruppierung der psychischen Krankheiten" (Kafemann, Danzig, 1863). This is not the place to go deeply into this question; however, we must mention that Kahlbaum's scheme has been rejected by many renowned authors. There are undoubtedly cases which do not pursue their course according to the scheme, and there is also such a number of mixed and transitional forms that it may even be an open question whether we are justified in considering katatonia a special disorder. However this may be, the lasting merit of Kahlbaum's treatise is that he has given an excellent description of a series of morbid conditions which up to his time, and unfortunately, by many authors even in our times, were considered from a very superficial and merely psychological standpoint. The purely psychological interpretations, upon which is founded, *e.g.*, the name of "*melancholia attonita*" (*Erstarrung im Seelenschmerz*), are, when considered from the standpoint of the motor system, nothing but empty words and *à priori* conclusions. Kahlbaum was the first to give us an objective and clinical symptomatology.

CLEMENS NEISSER.

[*References.*—De la Catalepsie, Arch. de Méd., Août, 1857, J. Falret. Allg. Zeitsch. f. Psych., 1877, Bd. xxxiii. p. 602, Hecker. Kahlbaum's Katatonie, Allg. Zeitsch. f. Psych., Bd. xxxiv., 1878, s. 731, Tigges. Alienist and Neurologist, 1882, Kiernan. Beitrage zur Lehre der Katatonie, 1882, Konrad. Ueber Katatonische Verrücktheit, Laufenauer, 1882. Ueber Normale und Kataleptische Bewegungen, Arch. für Psych. und Nerv., Bd. xiii. Heft 2, 1882, Rieger. Amer. Journ. of Neur. and Psych., 1883, p. 343, Spitzka. Ueber Ætiologie und Behandlung der Katatonie, Nied. Ver. für Psych., 1883, Dunkerloot. Specielle Pathologie und Therapie des Geisteskrankheiten, 1886, Schüle. Die Katatonie, Allg. Zeitsch. f. Psych., 1887, Bd. xxxiii.; Brosius. Ueber die Katatonie, 1887, Clemens Neisser. In addition to Kahlbaum's Mémoire, La Catatonie, par J. Séglas et Ph. Chaslin, Paris, 1888. Katatonia, Brain, 1891, Dr. Mickle. Ueber Tetanie und Psychose, Allg. Zeitsch. für Psych., Bd. xxx. s. 28, R. Arndt.

MM. Séglas and Chaslin, to whom we are indebted for many references, conclude that the attempt which Kahlbaum has made to differentiate katatonia, is not justified by clinical observation, and repeats J. Falret's opinion that in the description of this disorder facts more or less dissimilar have been confounded together, and that Kahlbaum has given the history of a symptom or a group of symptoms rather than a genuine and distinct form of mental disease. Considering that on the physical side the predominant symptom is the presence of disorders of the motor system, and on the psychical side a state of melancholia, the other symptoms not being in any way special, the authors think that katatonia ought not to be separated from mental stupor, of which it is only a variety related to degeneration and, especially, hysteria.]

KATZENSUCHT.—The German term for Galeanthropy (*q.v.*).

KAWA.—The resin of *Piper methysticum* which has been macerated and allowed to mix in a vessel with saliva gives a kind of extract, which, mixed with water or cocoa-nut milk, furnishes an intoxicating drink, which is used habitually by the inhabitants of Tahiti, but which is now being replaced by alcohol. It produces a condition of intoxication, a blunting of the senses, with ecstasies and elation. The controlling centres are in abeyance; the individual is absorbed in a train of ideas, on which he ruminates, and which occupy all his attention. Then the subject falls into a state of torpor from which he cannot be aroused without inducing violent excitement. He enjoys this torpor, which, according to Bourra, resembles the ecstasies of a prolonged siesta in hot countries, although the conceptions are of a more melancholy and painful nature. M. LEGRAIN.

KENOPHOBIA (κενός, empty, vacant; φοβός, fear). A synonym of Agoraphobia (*q.v.*).

KENOSPUDIA (κενοσπουδέω, I am eager for trifles; from κενός, empty; σπουδή, zeal). A term formerly used to express mental abstraction, or what is commonly known as "brown study." It is also used as a synonym of Somnambulism.

KIDNEYS (see BRIGHT'S DISEASE).—Dr. Thomas Ireland, of the Berbice Asylum, British Guiana, has recently stated that Bright's disease is very common among the patients there. During 1890, there were thirty-five deaths from this cause, confirmed by post mortem. The patients were mostly dements, and when admitted were obtuse, without any clear history of previous acute mental disorder. Occasionally delusions or hallucinations were present.

KLEPTOMANIA (κλέπτω, I steal).

Synonyms. — Monomanie du vol, or kleptomaniaque; Cleptomanie (Fr.); Stehlsucht (Ger.).

Definition.—In the strict sense of the term, an irresistible impulse to steal.

The diseased manifestations of such isolated propensities as stealing, fire-raising, &c., were viewed by some of the older writers on psychology as distinct varieties of monomania, and elevated by them into special insanities; thus a morbid tendency to acts of theft received the name of kleptomania.

The term was employed by Marc, who observes, that this condition—the impulsive form—is doubtless very singular and inexplicable, as are so many of the intellectual and physical phenomena of life; but it is not the less real on that account, as is proved by numerous examples. He remarked a tendency to this affection in pregnant women, as likewise have Jöng and Tardieu.

Marcé states that many observations on the subject of kleptomania quoted by Esquirol are evidently cases of incipient general paralysis; but independently of such cases, and in those noticed in imbeciles and dements, others are recorded which present an isolated intellectual lesion, and an irresistible impulse to steal.

Lasègue, in an able article entitled "Le vol aux étalages" (Shop-lifting), demonstrates the existence of this affection, but regards it as due, not so much to irresistible impulse as to cerebral defect.

A desire to acquire is natural to every one. This feeling in persons of well-regulated minds and honest conceptions is kept under control of the will; not so, however, in the case of the professional thief, who regards all property as legitimate spoil, and with whom desire is soon followed, if possible, by possession. There is a growing disposition amongst the rising school of criminal anthropologists to regard the majority of criminals as persons of unsound mind, having a special neurosis, to look upon them as drawn to crime by instinct. Our own observation leads us to believe that the professional thief, setting aside those of weak mind, is not a criminal by instinct, but rather from the force of bad example and a criminal education. But it is not of him we would speak, the opinion of the expert is not called for in his case, the interest of the question lies with those individuals whose thefts, as Lasègue states, are the result of intellectual disturbance.

It is by no means an uncommon occurrence for men, but especially women, of respectable family, who move about in society, and who are able to satisfy their wants and tastes, to be arrested on a charge of stealing articles of different value. The position of the accused, their correct mode of living in the past, the nature of the theft, and the inconsiderable value of the articles stolen, compared with the risk of detection and subsequent exposure, all tend to make us inquire, how far mental disease is or is not the cause of the crime.

These cases are difficult, the plea of irresistible impulse is not unfrequently adopted in extenuation of the offence, but unsupported by any other evidence of mental disturbance it is indefensible. As a rule, the theory of irresistible impulse is incompatible with the conduct of the accused; generally a favourable moment has been seized to execute the theft, art and precaution have been employed in concealing it, and either a denial of the act when detected or some evasive excuse has been made. These circumstances do not remove the possibility of insanity, and any inquiry into the mental state ought to be directed, as Lasègue has pointed out, not so much to the greater or lesser degree of the impulse, but to the degree of intellectual confusion or weakness that may exist. To determine this, various points require consideration; as regards the object, the inducement to steal, and the nature and value of the articles stolen; as regards the subject, whether there was a perfect consciousness of the act and its illegality. In addition, it is of considerable moment to inquire into the family history and antecedents, to establish if possible the existence of hereditary disease, the occurrence of fits in childhood or any evidence of mental derangement prior to the development of the propensity. Symptoms which indicate the commencement of general paralysis ought to be particularly noted. The complications of puberty and pregnancy, the presence of physical disorders, a history of head injury, are all worthy of attention; nor must the effect of alcohol on a neurotic temperament be overlooked in these cases. We are cognizant of the particulars of a case where a lady was detected stealing in a shop, and in addition to various articles of wearing apparel, a quantity of brandy was found in her possession. There was a family history of insanity, and she was addicted to drink. All these circumstances are of importance in attempting to decide the existence of a morbid mental condition which might have limited the intellectual liberty of the individual, and which alone should determine the irresponsibility of the accused.

It has been stated that pregnancy exerts some influence in the development of this monomania. Marc alleges that a propensity to steal shows itself in women labouring under disordered menstruation, and in those far advanced in pregnancy, the motive being a mere wish for possession. There is no doubt that pregnant women manifest desires, or, as they are termed, longings for various things, but a distinction ought to be made between those longings, which have for their object articles of food, and those which centre on dress, jewels, &c. On the one hand it is known that utero-gestation brings about sympathetic disturbances in the whole digestive system, and causes not only such gastric disturbances as sickness and vomiting, but sometimes also an excessive or depraved appetite. The cravings resulting from this morbid state of the appetite may, according to Dr. Playfair, prove altogether irresistible; to appease them theft of articles of food may be resorted to. Marc details the case of a wealthy lady of high rank in society, who, being pregnant, stole a roast chicken from a pastry-cook's shop, in order to satisfy the keen appetite which the sight and smell of this dish had developed within her. On the other hand, when the longing has for its object articles of dress or jewels, no such physiological explanation is forthcoming. Jöng states that pregnant women do not steal such objects as the result of their pregnant condition, but from bad instinct or gross error. He further remarks that women of the lower orders, who willingly indulge in longings for certain aliments, know very well how to abstain from stealing from fear of generating in their children a like predisposition, thus proving that pregnant women retain possession of their moral liberty. Marcé endorses Jöng's view; Tardieu also agrees with him on the whole, but makes the reservation that pregnancy may in some very rare instances determine in women a true irresistible impulse to theft. When a pregnant woman pleads pregnancy in excuse for crime, the fact of pregnancy should be regarded as a secondary consideration, and not accepted as direct proof. The mental condition ought to be examined, because the true bearings of the case are much more likely to be elucidated from the circumstances accompanying the deed, than from the consideration that she is pregnant.

The child will appropriate what does not belong to it; the fascination of a new toy or the appetite aroused by a favourite food may prove too strong. There is inability to resist a sudden temptation. In young children judicious care and timely punishment will invariably eradicate the failing. There are certain children, however, of a morally perverse nature, in whose case kindness and punishment are alike useless. They are thieves and liars, and are cruelly disposed, because it is in their nature to be so. They frequently possess a hereditary neurosis; they are morally insane. Such are to be found at a later age in schools; they pilfer the property of their companions. Self-respect, duty towards others, reputation and interest are forgotten, and it is a bad omen in a growing lad when he gives way to such practices, for sometimes the evil, if persisted in, becomes incurable.

There are certain weak-minded individuals who are natural criminals, and amongst them petty thieving is very common. They are to be found in all classes of society. They are intellectually, morally, and physically degenerate, and when uncared for and left to themselves, invariably sink into the dregs of the criminal classes. Such are more or less intellectually weak, yet not so weak that their mental state excites particular attention, unless, perchance, they commit some crime involving the risk of life; their moral nature is low, and their physical state below par. In twenty-five such instinctive criminals undergoing sentence, mostly for repeated acts of petty larceny, we found a low receding forehead, a weak lower jaw, a contracted high-arched palate, weakly developed mammæ and deficient sensibility, the most general marks of physical degeneracy. Even when protected from want, and well cared for by their friends, a natural propensity to theft will betray itself. Take the case of M.; he had been at school but never acquired much knowledge; his intellect was limited. He possessed three different lodgings in Paris. He was in the habit of visiting his friend's houses, and it often happened that some small article of value was missing subsequent to his visit. Yet he was never detected, and frequently servants were brought into trouble and disgrace owing to his pilferings. This system continued for years. After his death, which happened suddenly, in each of his lodgings a miscellaneous assortment of articles was found, which he had purloined during his lifetime. He came of a neurotic stock, two brothers died of convulsions in childhood, and an uncle was hypochondriacal.

Amongst the insane kleptomania is of most frequent occurrence in imbeciles, general paralytics, and epileptics; apart from those three classes, it may also result from delusions.

Theft is by no means infrequent amongst idiots and imbeciles. As a rule, they steal without reflection, and merely to satisfy an animal instinct. They will purloin whatever takes their fancy. Sometimes they display a considerable amount of ingenuity and low cunning in their methods of procedure.

It is an important point, and should always be borne in mind, that acts of stealing occur, and are amongst the first noticeable symptoms in the initiatory stages of general paralysis. When a man in apparent health attaches undue importance to some article of no great value, and finally carries it away surreptitiously, it is more than probable that his conduct is the result of cerebral disease. In the *Journal of Mental Science*, January 1873, Dr. Burman has related six interesting cases. All were convicted of stealing and sent to prison, and in all of them general paralysis became manifest soon afterwards.

The same propensity is observed in the later stages of the same disease. The patients steal under the delusion that everything belongs to them. They appropriate all sorts of articles, hoard and conceal them, and immediately afterwards lose all recollection of them. To satisfy their gluttonous appetites they will steal food, and in their hurry and eagerness to devour it, disastrous consequences sometimes ensue; suffocation has been known to take place in such circumstances. We can remember one patient, in Dundee Royal Asylum, who snatched a piece of meat from a plate which an attendant was carrying, bolted it, and died before assistance could be rendered, the meat having become impacted in his throat.

Again, theft may be the unconscious act of an epileptic. Of 128 epileptics admitted into Broadmoor Asylum during the twenty-three years (1864–1887), twenty-three had been charged with larceny. Legrand du Saulle has recorded a number of instances where acts of stealing were committed by vertiginous epileptics. One case in particular is noteworthy. The patient was a young man who experienced curious sensations in the epigastric region about three or four times a year. This aura was invariably followed, for a period varying from a few hours to three days, by confusion of the intellect. During this time, and when in his confused state, he displayed a strong propensity for stealing, although at other times he was scrupulously well behaved. When his intellect became clearer he was questioned with reference to his strange conduct, but declared he remembered nothing. Legrand du Saulle, in summing up the case, states that, taking into consideration the aura, the supervening mental disturbance, the amnesia, and the invariably similar character of the acts committed, it was clear that larvated epilepsy was the sole cause of this unusual vesania and abnormal criminality.

In conclusion, we find that genuine kleptomania does not proceed from irresistible impulse so much as from a morbid mental condition. This latter is in many instances difficult to establish. In every case it is important to investigate the antecedents of the individual. The plea of irresistible impulse alone is indefensible, and, unless sufficient data are forthcoming to establish a pathological state of intellectual weakness, the accused person ought to be held responsible.

The state of pregnancy cannot be held as an exculpatory plea in cases of stealing unless supported by other evidence of mental derangement.

Acts of theft may be due to the presence of moral insanity in certain children.

The weak-minded are prone to commit petty acts of larceny. Their mental state ought to be inquired into whatever the nature or magnitude of the offence. They are intellectually and physically degenerate.

Imbeciles and idiots steal without reflection and merely to satisfy an animal instinct.

The importance of the occurrence of acts of theft as one of the symptoms in the early stages of general paralysis cannot be over-estimated. It has happened that men have been convicted and im-

punished for stealing, who soon afterwards developed most marked symptoms of this disease. Were the evolution of the symptoms of mental diseases more generally recognised and understood an improvement might be looked for in dealing with such cases.

Theft may be the unconscious crime of an epileptic, or the unmeaning act of a dement.

J. Baker.

[References.—Bucknill and Tuke, Psychological Medicine. Taylor, Medical Jurisprudence. Marcé, Traité de la Folie des Femmes Enceintes, and Maladies Mentales. Trélat, La Folie Lucide. Tardieu, Sur la Folie. Legrand du Saulle, Gazette des Hôpitaux, Nov. 1876. Lasègue (abstract by Motet), Journal of Mental Science, Jan. [illegible]]

KLIKUSCHI.—A hysterical psychopathy of an epidemic and endemic character, occurring among the females of Kursk and Orel. The attacks have been described by some as pure hysteria, others give evidence of phenomena of a hystero-epileptiform type, while some writers describe attacks of such severity as to [illegible] paroxysms of acute mania. The [illegible] called Klikuschi ("screaming [illegible] possessed") and the attacks are mainly influenced by religious emotion; they last usually for a short time only, but they may continue for a whole day or more in a succession of paroxysms. It resembles in its features the "Ikota" of the Samojeds (*q.v.*).

KLOPEMANIA (also Clopemania) (κλοπή, theft; μανία, madness). A synonym of kleptomania (*q.v.*).

KOPIOPIA HYSTERICA (κόπος, weariness; ὤψ, the eye; hysteria, *q.v.*). A term applied to the nervous phenomena associated with weakness of vision in a hysterical person. The symptoms are described as hyperæsthesia of the fifth and optic nerves, with loss of power of accommodation and inability to maintain a persistent effort of fixation on any object.

KREMDLINGS, KRETINS. (*See* Cretin.)

KUTUBUTH (Arab). An old term for a form of melancholia which was said to affect people chiefly in the month of February. It was characterised by great restlessness, the patients wandering to and fro continually, quite unconscious whither they were going.

L

LACTATIONSIRRESEIN. The German term for lactational insanity.

LAGNEIA FUROR (λαγνεία, lust; *furor*, madness). Insanity with unbridled appetency, including nymphomania and satyriasis (Mason Good).

LAGNESIS; LAGNEIA (λάγνος, lustful, or λαγνεία). A term for an excessive or morbid venereal appetite.

LAGNOSIS (λάγνος, lustful). A synonym of Satyriasis.

LALOPATHY (λάλος, talkative; πάθος, a disease). A synonym of Aphasia. Also any disorder or defect of speech.

LALOPLEGIA (λάλος, talkative; πληγή, a stroke). Paralysis of speech from whatever cause.

LARVATED EPILEPSY. (*See* Épilepsie larvée.)

LARYNGISMUS (λαρυγγίζω, I vociferate). Besides the ordinary meaning of this word—spasm of the laryngeal muscles only—Marshall Hall has applied the term to express a symptom or group of symptoms occurring in convulsive diseases—*e.g.*, infantile eclampsia, epilepsy, hysteria, and hydrophobia—in which cases the larynx is sometimes partially, sometimes completely, closed.

LARYNX, HYSTERICAL AFFECTIONS OF.—The laryngeal developments of hysteria are chiefly aphonia and a short dry cough. (*See* Hysteria.)

LASCIVUS (*lascivus*, unrestrained). A Paracelsian term for chorea, in allusion to the character of the motor symptoms.

LATA.—The Malay name under which a form of religious hysteria is known in Java. It is chiefly found among the native women, both of the higher and lower social ranks, and is marked by paroxysmal outbursts which take the form of rapid ejaculations of inarticulate sounds and of a succession of involuntary movements; there is temporary loss of consciousness, but the mental powers remain quite intact except during the paroxysm. The disease is propagated by imitation (Hirsch).

LATAH. (*See* Miryachit.)

LATHYRISM. (Lathyrisme médullaire spasmodique. Lathyrismus.)—Catani proposes this name for a disease presenting the same form as spastic spinal paralysis, caused by poisoning with several kinds of lathyrus, which is the name of a leguminous plant cultivated in the centre and the South of France ("gesses"), in Italy and Algeria ("djilbee"), used partly as food for cattle, and partly, under certain conditions, as food for man.

The first accounts of this disease were handed down from antiquity. "At times, those who continuously lived on leguminous plants were attacked by weakness in the loins, which remained; but also those who lived on peas (ὄροβος), had pains in their knees." (Hippocrates.)

In more recent times we have reports of large numbers being attacked by lathyrism from some districts of France (Département Loire et Cher), from Italy (Abruzzo, Latium), from India (Allahabad), and from Algeria. The best account of it we have is that by Bouchard and Proust, who observed the disease in Kabylia (Algeria, province of Palestro).

The poisoning was always produced by mixing the corn-flour for the preparation of bread with flour prepared from lathyrus (in equal parts or more), in cases where corn could not be obtained in sufficient quantity on account of poverty, famine, bad soil, climate, or unfavourable weather.

It seems that Lathyrus cicera and L. clymenum are especially poisonous; it has been maintained that only the crops of certain years produce lathyrism. The poison is contained in the healthy seed, unlike to ergotism and pellagra, where the poisoning is produced by diseased corn or maize respectively.

The disease attacks people of any age, who for some time (at least several weeks) have been living exclusively or mostly on lathyrus, generally during the rainy season; a cold is often stated as the exciting cause. The disease mostly breaks out suddenly, often during the night with pains in the lumbar region, with a girdle sensation, pains in the legs, and paralysis of the lower extremities, which after a while develop into spastic paraplegia. The patients on awaking feel weakness and tremor in their legs, so that they can rise and walk only with difficulty. Afterwards stiffness in the legs comes on with a considerable resistance to active and passive flexion. Walking becomes impossible, or is possible only with the help of a long stick, grasped with both hands and put down in front of the feet. The legs, which are in a state of rigid extension with the thigh adducted, are dragged forwards with flexion of the knee, with the toes flexed, the heel raised up, and the foot slightly rotated inwards; and on advancing one leg the whole body is thrown forwards. Only the toes touch the ground, and they collide with every obstacle, so that the patient easily stumbles and the dorsal surface of the toes becomes sore through constant friction.

The tendon reflexes of the lower extremities are greatly increased, including ankle clonus.

The exaggeration of the myotatic excitability can also be seen in spontaneous clonic action of the foot in standing, walking, or sitting with the heel raised, and this is imparted to the whole body in the form of vertical oscillations.

The upper extremities are perfectly free from motor derangements. The sensibility and reflex excitability of the skin do not show any constant disturbances, not even in the lower extremities. Some reports, however, mention insensibility of the lower extremities and paræsthesia (formication).

There is generally no atrophy of the muscles nor are there vaso-motor derangements, but retention and incontinence of urine as well as sexual impotence are constantly among the first symptoms. Cerebral symptoms and general derangements of nutrition are absent.

When the patients abstain from taking the infected food, the disease terminates after some weeks or months in recovery. In other cases, spastic phenomena in the lower extremities remain permanently and sometimes genuine contractures may develop. We do not know of any case in which the disease has terminated fatally, and therefore there has not yet been any post-mortem examination of lathyrism. Although we do not know anything yet about the condition of the nervous system, all the symptoms seem to point to a disease of the lateral columns of the spinal cord, so that lathyrism would have to be placed in one class with ergotism which affects the posterior column, and with pellagra which affects the lateral and posterior columns combined.

The chemical nature of the poison is also quite unknown to us (alkaloid? Marie). Paralysis of the lower extremities has been produced in animals (rabbits) by poisoning with lathyrus and by an injection of an extract of the seed of Lathyrus cicera. Farmers have sometimes lost all their cattle and horses through lathyrus poisoning.

The treatment follows from the ætiology.

F. Tuczek.

LAW OF LUNACY, 1890 and 1891.—An abstract of the law relating to the reception of lunatics into asylums, hospitals, or licensed houses, and into private houses as patients under single care, together with the law bearing upon their care and treatment, and their removal and discharge.

The space at our disposal will not permit of more than a condensed account of the law as it stands especially with regard to the duties imposed upon medical practitioners in carrying out its various provisions. The forms which are necessary for the reception, discharge, or removal of patients are given, and these are deemed sufficient for the purposes of this abstract. The Lunacy Act, 1890, which came into operation on May 1, 1890, includes the Lunacy Amendment Act, 1889. It is intended to consolidate certain of the enactments respecting lunatics, and will now be the standard for regulating all matters connected with the care and treatment of the insane in England and Wales.

Provisions for Placing Lunatics under Care and Treatment.—Under the provisions of this Act:

(Sec. 9) No person can be placed under care and treatment or be received and detained in an institution for lunatics, except upon "judicial authority" or when found lunatic by inquisition. The powers of this judicial authority shall only be exercised by a justice of the peace specially appointed, or a judge of County Courts, or a magistrate.*

(Sec. 10) Justices so appointed shall be selected with regard to the convenience of the inhabitants of each petty sessional division of the county and the appointments shall be made annually by the justices of a county at the Quarter Sessions held in October, and all such appointments shall be published in each petty sessional division.

Urgency.—(Sec. 11) In cases of urgency, however, any person (but if possible a relative of the alleged lunatic) who is twenty-one years of age, and who has seen the alleged lunatic within two days of the date of the order under which a person may be detained as a lunatic, may sign an "urgency order" (see Form 4) if "it is expedient either for the welfare of the person (not a pauper) alleged to be a lunatic or for the public safety that the alleged lunatic should be forthwith placed under care and treatment;" such order must be accompanied by one medical certificate and shall remain in force for seven days from its date. It may be made before or after a petition is presented; if a petition is pending it remains in force until the petition is finally disposed of.

The medical practitioner signing the certificate shall have personally examined the patient not more than two clear days before his reception and shall state the date of such examination in the certificate (*see* Forms 8 and 9).

Reception Order.—(Sec. 4) To obtain an order (Form 3) for the reception of a person (not a pauper or criminal lunatic) a petition (Form 1) must be presented to a judicial authority, if possible, by the husband, wife, or relative of the alleged lunatic, or if not so presented it shall contain a statement of the reasons why it is not so presented, and of the connection of the petitioner with the alleged lunatic. The petition must be accompanied by two medical certificates on separate sheets of paper as to the mental condition of the alleged lunatic (Form 8).

(Sec. 5) The petitioner must be twenty-one years of age, he must have seen the alleged lunatic within fourteen days before presenting the petition, and shall himself undertake to visit the patient twice every six months, or appoint some one to do so. (Sec. 31) Whenever practicable, one of the medical certificates accompanying the petition shall be signed by the usual medical attendant of the alleged lunatic; if it is not practicable to obtain a certificate from him the reason must be stated in writing by the petitioner, and such statement shall be part of the petition. Each of the two persons signing the medical certificates shall separately from each other personally examine the patient not more than seven clear days before the presentation of the petition. If upon the presentation of the petition the judge or justice is satisfied with the evidence of lunacy he may make an order forthwith, or appoint a time (sec. 6), not more than seven days after the presentation of the petition, for the consideration thereof. The judge or justice if he think necessary may visit the alleged lunatic. The petition shall be considered in private, and no persons but those interested shall be present without the permission of the judge or justice, and he may make an order, dismiss the petition or adjourn the consideration of it for any period not exceeding fourteen days; all persons admitted to be present shall be bound to secrecy. (Sec. 7) If the petition is dismissed the judge or justice shall deliver to the petitioner in writing his reasons for dismissing it, and send a copy to the commissioners, who may give such information as they think proper to the alleged lunatic or other proper person, and if a second petition is presented the person presenting it shall state the facts concerning the first petition and its dismissal.

Authority for Reception.—(Sec. 35) A reception order thus obtained shall be suffi-

* An order for the reception of a patient shall not be invalid if signed by a J.P. other than one specially appointed, if the order is subsequently signed within 14 days by a "judicial authority."

cient authority to take the lunatic to the place mentioned in the order for his reception and detain him there. All the necessary documents shall be delivered to the petitioner and shall be sent by him to the person receiving the lunatic. (Sec. 36) Where a lunatic has been temporarily placed in a workhouse he may be received in the institution for lunatics named in the order any time within fourteen days. And if his removal has been suspended by a medical certificate of unfitness for removal he may be received in the institution for lunatics mentioned in the order within three days after date of a medical certificate that he is fit to be removed. The reception order lapses if the lunatic is not received under it before the expiration of seven clear days.

Right of Lunatic to be seen by a Justice.—(Sec. 8) If a lunatic has been received as a private patient under a judicial order without seeing a judge or justice he shall have the right to be taken before or visited by one unless the medical superintendent sign a certificate within twenty-four hours of the patient's reception that such right would be prejudicial to the patient (*see* Form 5). Subject to such certificate, the person receiving the patient shall give notice of his right in writing to the patient (*see* Form 6) within twenty-four hours after his reception, and if within seven days he wishes to exercise the right shall get him to sign a notice to that effect (*see* Form 7), and shall post it to the judge, or justice, or justices' clerk of the petty sessional division or borough where the lunatic is, and the judge or justice shall arrange as soon as conveniently may be to visit the patient or have him brought before him. The judge or justice shall be entitled to see all documents, and after personally seeing the patient shall report to the commissioners. Any person having charge of a lunatic omitting to perform any duty in connection with such right of a patient to see a judge or justice shall be guilty of a misdemeanour.

Reception Order after Inquisition.—(Sec. 12) A lunatic so found after inquisition may be received in an institution for lunatics, or as a single patient upon an order signed by the committee of the person of the lunatic and having annexed thereto an office copy of the order appointing the committee; or, if no such committee has been appointed, upon an order signed by a master.

Lunatics not under Proper Care and Control, or cruelly treated or neglected.—(Sec. 13) Every constable, relieving-officer, and overseer of a parish who has knowledge that any person within his district or parish, *who is not a pauper and not wandering at large*, is deemed to be a lunatic, and is not under proper care and control, or is cruelly treated, or neglected, by any relative or other person having care or charge of him, shall within three days of obtaining such knowledge give information thereof upon oath to a justice specially appointed under this Act, who receiving such information upon oath, from any person whomsoever, that a person within the limits of his jurisdiction is so cruelly treated or neglected, or not under proper care and control, may himself visit the alleged lunatic. Or without visiting him, authorise two medical practitioners to examine him and certify as to his mental state, and shall proceed in the same manner as if a petition for a reception order had been presented to him by the person giving the information with regard to the alleged lunatic. If the justice is satisfied after such inquiry that the alleged lunatic is a lunatic and is neglected, or cruelly treated by any relative or person having charge of him, and that he is a proper person to be detained under care and treatment, the justice may order him to be received into any institution for lunatics, to which if a pauper he might be sent under this Act, and the constable, relieving-officer, or overseer upon whose information the order has been made, or any constable whom the justice may require to do so, shall forthwith convey the lunatic to the institution named in their order.

(Sec. 14) The medical officer of a union, if he knows that a pauper in his district is a lunatic, and a proper person to be sent to an asylum, shall, within three days of such knowledge, give notice thereof to the relieving-officer or overseer, who shall give notice within three days to a justice, who shall order the pauper to be brought before him and some other justice within three days.

Lunatic Wandering at Large.—(Sec. 15) Every constable, relieving-officer, and overseer of a parish who has knowledge that any person (whether pauper or not) wandering at large within their respective districts is deemed to be a lunatic, shall immediately take the alleged lunatic before a justice, who, upon the information of *any person*, may cause the alleged lunatic to be brought before him, and shall call in a medical practitioner, and shall examine the alleged lunatic, and make such inquiries as he thinks advisable. And if the justice (sec. 16) is satisfied that the alleged lunatic is a proper person to be detained, and the medical practitioner signs a medical certificate with regard to the lunatic, the justice may by order direct the lunatic to be conveyed to, received, and detained, in an institution for lunatics named in the order. (Sec. 17) Such justice may examine the alleged lunatic at his own house or elsewhere.

(Sec. 18) Unless a justice is satisfied that a lunatic is a pauper, he shall not sign an order for his reception into an institution for lunatics or workhouse. A person visited by the medical officer at the expense of the union shall be deemed a pauper.

(Sec. 19) A justice making an order for the reception of a lunatic otherwise than upon petition, in this Act called "a summary reception order," may suspend the execution of the order for such period, not exceeding fourteen days, as he thinks fit, and in the meantime may give such directions or make such arrangements for the proper care and comfort of the lunatic as he considers proper.

If a medical practitioner who examines a lunatic as to whom a summary reception order has been made, and certifies in writing that the lunatic is not in a fit state to be removed, the removal shall be suspended until the same or some other medical practitioner certifies in writing that the lunatic is fit to be removed. Any medical practitioner who has certified that the lunatic is not in a fit state to be removed shall, as soon as in his judgment the lunatic is in a fit state to be removed, be bound to certify accordingly.

Removal of Lunatic to Workhouse in Urgent Cases.—(Sec. 20) If a constable, relieving-officer, or overseer is satisfied that it is necessary for the public safety and the welfare of an alleged lunatic that he should be at once placed under care and control, such constable, officer, or overseer may remove the alleged lunatic to the workhouse, and the master of the workhouse shall (unless there is no proper accommodation in the workhouse for the alleged lunatic) receive, relieve, and detain him therein, for not more than three days, and before the expiration of that time the constable, relieving-officer, or overseer shall take such proceedings with regard to the alleged lunatic as are required by this Act.

(Sec. 21) Any justice, if satisfied that it is expedient for the welfare of the lunatic or for the public safety, may make an order for the reception of such lunatic into a workhouse, if there is proper accommodation. In any case where a summary reception order might be made, such order may be made to provide for the detention of the lunatic until he can be removed, but not for a period beyond fourteen days.

(Sec. 22) In the case of a lunatic as to whom a summary reception order may be made, nothing in this Act shall prevent a relation or friend from taking the lunatic under his own care, if a justice having jurisdiction to make the order, or the visitors of the asylum in which the lunatic is intended to be placed, shall be satisfied that proper care will be taken of him.

Reception Order by two Commissioners.—(Sec. 23) Any two or more commissioners may visit a pauper or alleged lunatic not in an institution for lunatics or workhouse, and may, if they think fit, call in a medical practitioner, and if he signs a medical certificate with regard to the lunatic, and the commissioners are satisfied that the pauper is a lunatic, they may send him to an institution for lunatics.

(Sec. 24) If the medical officer of a workhouse certifies that a person therein is a lunatic or a proper person to be allowed to remain, and that there is accommodation sufficient for his care and treatment, such certificate shall authorise his detention against his will for fourteen days pending a justice's order. (Sec. 25) A pauper discharged from an asylum not recovered may also be detained in a similar manner in a workhouse.

Requirements of Reception Orders and Medical Certificates.—(Sec. 28) A reception order shall not be made upon a medical certificate founded only upon facts communicated by others.

(Sec. 29) A reception order shall not be made unless the medical practitioner who signs the medical certificate, or where two certificates are required, each medical practitioner who signs a certificate, has personally examined the alleged lunatic in the case of an order upon petition not more than seven clear days before the date of the presentation of the petition, and in all other cases not more than seven clear days before the date of order.

Where two medical certificates are required, a reception order shall not be made unless each medical practitioner signing a certificate has examined the lunatic separately from the other: and in the case of an urgency order, the lunatic shall not be received unless the certifying medical practitioner has seen the patient not more than two clear days before his reception.

Persons disqualified from signing Medical Certificates.—(Sec. 30) A medical certificate accompanying a petition for a reception order, or accompanying an urgency order, shall not be signed by the petitioner or person signing the urgency order, or by the husband or wife, father or father-in-law, mother or mother-in-law, son or son-in law, daughter or daughter-in-law, brother or brother-in-law, sister or sister-in-law, partner or assistant of such petitioner or person.

Patients not to be received under Certificate by Interested Persons.—(Sec. 32) No person shall be received in any institution for lunatics or as a single patient where any certificate accompanying the reception order has been signed by (a) the manager of the institution or person who is to have charge of the single patient; (b) any person interested in the payments on account of the patient; (c) any regular medical attendant of the institution; (d) the husband or wife, father or father-in-law, mother or mother-in-law, son or son-in-law, daughter or daughter-in-law, brother or brother-in-law, sister or sister-in-law, or the partner or assistant of any of the foregoing persons, &c. Neither of the persons signing the medical certificates shall bear a similar relationship to each other; no person shall be received as a lunatic in a hospital under an order made on the application of or under a certificate signed by a member of the managing committee of the hospital.

Commissioners and Visitors not to sign Certificates.—(Sec. 33) A medical practitioner who is a commissioner or a visitor shall not sign any certificate for the reception of a patient into a hospital or licensed house unless he is directed to visit the patient by a judicial authority under this Act or by the Lord Chancellor, or Secretary of State, or a committee appointed by the judge in lunacy.

Amendment Orders and Certificates.—(Sec. 34) Orders and certificates, if in any respect incorrect or defective, may be amended within fourteen days next after the reception of the patient, with the sanction of one of the commissioners and (in the case of a private patient) the consent of the judicial authority by whom the order for the reception of the lunatic may have been signed, and if the commissioners deem any such certificate to be incorrect or defective, if it be not amended to their satisfaction within fourteen days, any two of them may, if they think fit, make an order for the patient's discharge.

Order and Certificate to remain in Force in Certain Cases.—(Sec. 37) Although a patient may be admitted as a pauper, and afterwards be found entitled to be classed as a private patient, the same order shall hold good. Also an order for the reception of a private patient shall authorise his detention if he afterwards appear to be a pauper. In the case of a patient temporarily removed, or transferred from one place of confinement to another, the original order and certificate or certificates shall remain in force.

Duration of Reception Orders.—(Sec. 38) Every reception order dated after or within three months before the commencement of this Act, shall expire at the end of one year from its date, and any such order dated three months or more before the commencement of this Act shall expire at the end of one year from the commencement of this Act unless continued as provided by the Act.

In the case of any institution for lunatics the commissioners may order that the reception orders of patients detained therein shall expire on any quarterly day next after the days on which the orders would expire under the last preceding subsection. Transfers are not to be considered reception orders under this section. A reception order shall remain in force for a year after the date by this Act or by an order of the commissioners appointed for it to expire, and thereafter for two years, and thereafter for three years, and then for successive periods of five years, if not more than one month nor less than seven days before the expiration of the period of one, two, three and five years respectively, a special report of the medical officer of the institution or medical attendant of a single patient as to the mental and bodily condition of the patient with a certificate that he is still of unsound mind, and a proper person to be detained under care and treatment, is sent to the commissioners. If, in the opinion of the commissioners the special report does not justify the accompanying certificate in the case of a patient in a hospital or licensed house, they shall make further inquiry, and if dissatisfied, they may order his discharge. If the patient is in an asylum the commissioners shall send a copy of the report to the clerk to the visiting committee of the asylum, and the committee, or any three of them, shall investigate the case, and may discharge the patient, and give such directions respecting him as they think fit.

The manager of an institution for lunatics or person having charge of a single patient shall be guilty of a misdemeanour if he detains a patient after he knows the order for his reception has expired. The special reports and certificates under this section may include and refer to more than one patient. A certificate of the secretary to the commissioners that a reception order has been continued shall be sufficient evidence of the

... This section does not apply to lunatics so found by inquisition.

Care and Treatment.—Report of Mental and Bodily Health to be sent to Commissioners.—(Sec. 39) At the expiration of one month from the reception of a private patient, the medical officer of every institution, and the medical attendant of every single patient, shall send a report to the commissioners as to the mental and bodily condition of the patient and in the case of every house licensed by the justices a copy of such report shall be sent to their clerk. In the case of a licensed house within the immediate jurisdiction of the commissioners, one of them shall visit the patient as soon as convenient, and report if his detention is proper. Where the house is licensed by justices, they shall arrange for the medical visitor to visit and report to the commissioners if there is any doubt as to the propriety of detaining the patient. The commissioners shall satisfy themselves whether the patient is properly detained, whether he should be discharged, or whether an inquisition should be held upon his case. Similar arrangements for visiting a single patient shall be made by the commissioners, and the commissioners may, with the consent of the Treasury, pay the medical visitor for his services. Private patients in asylums shall also be visited in the same manner and reported upon. In any case under this section the commissioners may order a patient's discharge. This section shall not apply to lunatics received under a removal order or to lunatics so found by inquisition (sec. 8, 1891).

Mechanical Restraint.—(Sec. 40) Mechanical means of restraint, which shall be such appliances as the commissioners may by regulation determine, shall not be applied to any lunatic except for the purposes of surgical or medical treatment, or to prevent him from injuring himself or others. Where restraint is applied a certificate must be signed by the medical officer of the institution, or medical attendant of a single patient giving the reason for it. A full record is to be kept from day to day, and a copy sent to the commissioners at the end of every quarter. In the case of a workhouse the copy to be sent to the clerk to the guardians.

Patient's Letters.—(Sec. 41) All letters written by any patient shall be forwarded unopened by the manager of every institution for lunatics, and every person having charge of a single patient, if addressed to the Lord Chancellor, any Judge in lunacy, Secretary of State, Commissioners, or a commissioner, or to the person who signs the order for his reception, or on whose petition such order was made, or to any Chancery visitor, or any other visitor, or to the visiting committee, or any member of it. Every such manager or person having charge of a single patient shall be liable to a penalty of £20 who makes default in carrying out the obligations of this section.

(Sec. 42) In every institution for lunatics where there are private patients the commissioners have power to direct that notices shall be posted up, so that every private patient can see them, setting forth the right of patients to have such letters forwarded; and the right to request a personal and private interview with a visiting commissioner or visitor. The commissioners or visitors shall direct where these notices shall be posted, and any manager of such institution shall be liable to a penalty not exceeding £20.

The Medical Practitioners certifying shall not attend the Patient professionally.—(Sec. 33) A medical practitioner upon whose certificate a reception order for a private patient has been made shall not be the regular professional attendant of the patient whilst detained under the order, nor shall a medical practitioner who is a commissioner or visitor professionally attend a patient in a hospital or licensed house, unless he is directed to visit the patient by the petitioner upon whose application the reception order was made, or the Lord Chancellor, Secretary of State, or committee appointed by the judge in lunacy.

(Sec. 44) The commissioners shall control the visiting of a single patient not found lunatic by inquisition by a medical practitioner not deriving profit from the charge of the patient; and (sec. 45) they may require him to report upon the case and give any information they may direct.

More than One Patient in Unlicensed House.—(Sec. 46) The commissioners have power to give permission for more than one patient to be received in an unlicensed house as "single patients."

Order to Visit Lunatic.—(Sec. 47) One commissioner or one justice may give an order to a relative or friend of a patient in an institution for lunatics or a licensed house to be admitted to see him. This order may be for admission generally, or for a stated number of times, with or without restriction as to the presence of an attendant. If the manager or principal officer refuses, prevents, or obstructs such admission, he shall be liable to a penalty not exceeding £20.

Commissioners may appoint Substitute for Petitioner.—(Sec. 48) The commissioners may appoint any person as a substitute for the person upon whose petition a reception order was made if such person is willing to undertake the duties and responsibilities of the petitioner.

Order to examine detained Lunatic.—(Sec. 49) Any person may obtain an order from the commissioners to have any person who is detained as a lunatic examined by two medical practitioners who satisfies the commissioners that it is proper for them to grant such an order. If after two examinations with seven days intervening between them the medical practitioners certify the patient may be discharged without risk or injury to himself or the public, the commissioner may order his discharge at the expiration of ten days.

Inquiry as to Property of Lunatic.—(Sec. 50) The Lord Chancellor and the Commissioners are empowered to make inquiry as to the property of any person detained as a lunatic.

Order to Search Records.—(Sec. 51) Any person applying to a commissioner or visitor may, if the commissioner or visitor think fit, have an order to search whether a particular person is, or has been, detained within the last twelve months as a lunatic, together with date of his admission, removal or discharge. The applicant shall pay to the person appointed to search a sum not exceeding 7*s*.

Diet of Lunatics.—(Sec. 52) The visiting commissioners may determine and regulate the diet of the pauper patients in a hospital or licensed house, and the visitors of a licensed house shall have the same power subject to the direction of the visiting commissioners.

Males not to have custody of Female Lunatics.—(Sec. 53) Males shall not be employed in the personal custody of female patients except in cases of urgency which must be reported to the visitors or commissioners at their next visit.

Diet and Accommodation of Workhouses.—(Sec. 54) The visiting guardians shall enter in a book to be kept by the master of the workhouse a quarterly report upon the diet, accommodation, and treatment of any lunatics or alleged lunatics in the workhouse, and the book shall be laid before the commissioners at the next visit.

Leave of Absence.—(Sec. 55) Any two visitors of an asylum or licensed house, or a commissioner, or in the case of a hospital, two members of the managing committee may, with the advice of the medical officer, permit a patient to be absent on trial as long as they think fit. In the case of a pauper they may make an allowance not exceeding the cost of his maintenance in the asylum. The manager of any hospital or licensed house may also, with such permission, take or send under proper control, one, two, or more patients to any specified place or to travel in England (sec. 9, 1891) for the benefit of their health or allow a private patient to be absent on trial. The medical officer of a hospital or licensed house may on his own authority permit any patient to be absent for forty-eight hours. Such patient may be brought back to the asylum with fourteen days of the expiration of the term of his leave of absence, unless his detention is medically certified to be no longer necessary.

Removal of Single Patients.—(Sec. 56) Any person having charge of a single patient may remove him to any new residence in England or Wales, seven days' previous notice having been given to the commissioners and the person on whose petition the reception order was made or who made the last payment for him. With the previous consent of a commissioner leave of absence may also be obtained (sec. 10, 1891).

Pauper Lunatic may be delivered up to Friend.—(Sec. 57) The visiting committee of an asylum may order a pauper lunatic to be delivered up to a relative or friend, and the authority liable for his maintenance shall pay to the person taking charge of the lunatic an allowance not exceeding his rate of maintenance in the asylum.

Removal of Lunatics.—(Sec. 58) A person having authority to discharge a private or a single patient may, with the previous consent of a commissioner, remove the patient to any institution for lunatics or to the charge of another person named by the commissioners in their consent; (sec. 59) two commissioners may order the removal of a lunatic from one institution to another. Upon the death of a person having charge of a single patient the commissioners may direct the patient to be removed to the charge of another person or may also at any time order the patient's removal to the care of another person or to any institution for lunatics: (sec. 60) two commissioners may in a like manner order the removal of a lunatic or alleged lunatic from a workhouse to an institution for lunatics if they think the case unsuitable for the workhouse. The guardians have power of appeal against the commissioners' order to the Secretary of State, who shall employ another commissioner to visit the workhouse, and report specially to him, and his decision shall be final; (sec. 61) the authority liable for the maintenance of [illegible] lunatic in a hospital or licensed house may order his removal; (sec. [illegible]) the guardians may order the removal of any lunatic from a workhouse; (sec. [illegible]) any two members of the committee of an asylum may order a pauper patient who has been delivered to the custody of a relative or friend to be removed to the asylum; (sec. 64) any two visitors of an asylum may order a pauper lunatic belonging to the county to be removed into the asylum from any other institution, or they may order him to be removed from the asylum to some other institution for lunatics; (sec. 67) in both cases the medical officer of the institution must certify that the lunatic is in a fit condition to be removed; (sec. 70) all removal orders signed by the commissioners must be in duplicate, one shall be given to the manager of the institution from which the lunatic is removed and the other given to the manager who receives him, together with a copy of the original reception order and other documents; (sec. 71) an alien may be removed to his own county upon the order of a Secretary of State, after inquiring into the case and report by the commissioners.

Discharge of Lunatics.—(Sec. 72) A private patient may be discharged from an institution by the person on whose petition the reception order was made, or, if there is no person qualified to direct his discharge, the commissioners may do so; (sec. 73) the authority liable for the maintenance of a pauper lunatic may order his discharge, but in the case of either a private patient, a single patient, or a pauper, if the medical officer of the institution or the medical attendant of the single patient certifies that the patient is dangerous and unfit to be at large, he shall not be discharged unless two visitors of the asylum, or the commissioners visiting a hospital or licensed house, or a commissioner in the case of a single patient, consent, in writing, to his discharge; (sec. 75) a legal and a medical commissioner visiting a patient may, within seven days of their visit, discharge him if they think he is detained without sufficient cause; (sec. 77) any three visitors of an asylum may order the discharge of any person detained therein, whether he is recovered or not, and any two visitors may do so with the advice of the medical officer; (sec. 78) two visitors, one of whom must be a medical practitioner, after two visits with not less than seven days' interval between them, may discharge any patient from a licensed house if it appears to them that he is detained without sufficient cause.

(Sec. 79) On the application of a relative or friend of a pauper lunatic confined in an asylum, two visitors may discharge the lunatic upon the undertaking of the relative or friend that he shall no longer be chargeable to any union, and shall be properly taken care of, and prevented injuring himself or others.

(Sec. 80) When the visitors of an asylum intend to order the discharge of a pauper patient, except upon the application of a relative or friend, they may send notice of their intentions to a relieving-officer of the union to which the lunatic is chargeable, and the relieving-officer may remove the lunatic to the workhouse.

Discharged Patient may have a Copy of the Documents upon which he was confined.—(Sec. 82) The secretary of the commissioners shall, upon the discharge of a person who considers himself to have been unjustly confined as a lunatic, furnish to him, upon his request, free of expense, a copy of the reception order and certificate or certificates upon which he was confined, and if the order was made upon petition, also of the petition, and statement of particulars upon which the reception order was made.

(Sec. 83) When a private patient in a hospital or licensed house or detained as a single patient recovers, the manager or medical attendant, as the case may be, shall notify the same to the person on whose petition the reception order was made, and in the case of a pauper, to the guardians of his union, and if the patient is not removed within seven days he shall be forthwith discharged.

Inquests.—(Sec. 84) The coroner shall summon a jury to inquire into the cause of death of a lunatic within his district if he considers it necessary.

Recapture of Escaped Lunatics.—(Sec. 85) If any person detained as a lunatic escapes, he may be retaken within fourteen days without a fresh order or certificate.

(Sec. 86) A person lawfully detained as a lunatic in England and Wales escaping into Scotland or Ireland, or *vice versâ*, may be brought back.

Voluntary Boarders.—(Sec. 229) Any person who is desirous of voluntarily submitting to treatment may, with the consent of two commissioners or justices, be received and lodged as a boarder in a licensed house, and any relative or friend may also be received. Consent shall only be given upon the application of the intending boarder. Notice of the reception of a boarder must be given to the commissioners within twenty-four hours. The commissioners may order the manager to remove a boarder or take steps to obtain an order for his reception as a patient if they consider his mental state renders such a step necessary (sec. 20, 1891).

(Sec. 338) It shall be lawful for the commissioners, with the approval of the Lord Chancellor, by rules, to prescribe the books to be kept in institutions for lunatics and houses for single patients, the entries to be made therein, and the returns, reports, extracts, copies, statements, notices, plans, and documents, and information to be sent to the commissioners or any authority or person.

T. OUTTERSON WOOD.

Section 339.

THE SECOND SCHEDULE.

FORM 1.

Sections 4, 5.

Petition for an Order for reception of a Private Patient.

In the matter of *A.B.* a person alleged to be of unsound mind.

To a justice of the peace for

[*or*

To His Honour the judge of the county court of *or* To stipendiary magistrate for .]

The petition of *C.D.* of [1] in the county of .

1. I am [2] years of age.

2. I desire to obtain an order for the reception of *A.B.* as a lunatic[3] in the asylum [*or* hospital *or* house *as the case may be*] of situate at [4]

3. I last saw the said *A.B.* at on the [5] day of

4. I am the [6] of the said *A.B.* [*or if the petitioner is not connected with or related to the patient state as follows:*]

I am not related to or connected with the said *A.B.* The reasons why this petition is not presented by a relation or connection are as follows: [*State them.*]

The circumstances under which this petition is presented by me are as follows: [*State them.*]

5. I am not related to or connected with either of the persons signing the certificates which accompany this petition as (*where the petitioner is a man*) husband, father, father-in-law, son, son-in-law, brother, brother-in-law, partner or assistant (*or where the petitioner is a woman*), wife, mother, mother-in-law, daughter, daughter-in-law, sister, sister-in-law, partner or assistant.

6. I undertake to visit the said *A.B.* personally or by some one specially appointed by me at least once in every six months while under care and treatment under the order to be made on this petition.

7. A statement of particulars relating to the said *A.B.* accompanies this petition.

If it is the fact add:

8. The said *A.B.* has been received in the asylum [*or* hospital *or* house *as the case may be*] under an urgency order dated the

The petitioner therefore prays that an order may be made in accordance with the foregoing statement.

[Signed]

full Christian and surname.

(Section 23, 1891). Date of presentation of the petition

[1] Full postal address and rank, profession, or occupation.
[2] At least twenty-one.
[3] or an idiot or person of unsound mind.
[4] Insert a full description of the name and locality of the asylum, hospital, or licensed house, or the full name, address, and description of the person who is to take charge of the patient as a single patient.
[5] Some day within 14 days before the date of the presentation of the petition.
[6] Here state the connection or relationship with the patient.

FORM 2.

Sections 4, 5, 11.

Statement of Particulars.

STATEMENT of particulars referred to in the annexed petition [or in the above or annexed order].

The following is a statement of particulars relating to the said *A.B.* [1]:—

Name of patient, with Christian name at length.

Sex and age.

†Married, single, or widowed.

†Rank, profession, or previous occupation (if any).

†Religious persuasion.

Residence at or immediately previous to the date hereof.

[1] If any particulars are not known, the fact is to be so stated. [Where the patient is in the petition or order described as an idiot omit the particulars marked †.]

†Whether first attack.
Age on first attack.
When and where previously under care and treatment as a lunatic, idiot, or person of unsound mind.
†Duration of existing attack.
Supposed cause.
Whether subject to epilepsy.
Whether suicidal.
Whether dangerous to others, and in what way.
Whether any near relative has been afflicted with insanity.
Names, Christian names, and full postal addresses of one or more relatives of the patient.
Name of the person to whom notice of death to be sent, and full postal address if not already given.
Name and full postal address of the usual medical attendant of the patient.

[Signed]

When the petitioner or person signing an urgency order is not the person who signs the statement, add the following particulars concerning the person who signs the statement.
Name, with Christian name at length.
Rank, profession, or occupation (if any).
How related to or otherwise connected with the patient.

Section 6.

FORM 3.

Order for reception of a private patient to be made by a Justice appointed under the Lunacy Act, 1890, Judge of County Courts, or Stipendiary Magistrate.

I, the undersigned *E.F.*, being a Justice for specially appointed under the Lunacy Act, 1890 [*or* the Judge of the County Court of *or* the Stipendiary Magistrate for], upon the petition of *C.D.*, of[1] in the matter of *A.B.* a lunatic,[2] accompanied by the medical certificates of *G.H.* and *I.J.* hereto annexed, and upon the undertaking of the said *C.D.* to visit the said *A.B.* personally or by some one specially appointed by the said *C.D.* once at least in every six months while under care and treatment under this order, hereby authorise you to receive the said *A.B.* as a patient into your asylum.[3] And I declare that I have [*or* have not] personally seen the said *A.B.* before making this order.

Dated

[Signed] *E.F.*
A Justice for appointed under the above-mentioned Act, [*or* The Judge of the County Court of *or* a Stipendiary Magistrate.]

To[4]

[1] Address and description.
[2] Or an idiot or person of unsound mind.
[3] Or hospital or house or as a single patient.
[4] To be addressed to the medical superintendent of the asylum or hospital, or to the resident licensee of the house in which the patient is to be placed.

Section 11.

· FORM 4.

Form of urgency Order for the reception of a private patient.

I, the undersigned, being a person twenty-one years of age, hereby authorise you to receive as a patient into your house[1] *A.B.*, as a lunatic,[2] whom I last saw at on the[3] day of 18 . I am not related to or connected with the person signing the certificate which accompanies this order in any of the ways mentioned in the

[1] Or hospital or asylum or as a single patient.
[2] Or an idiot or a person of unsound mind.
[3] Some day within two days before the date of the order.

margin.[4] Subjoined [or annexed] hereto[5] is a statement of particulars relating to the said *A.B.*

[Signed] Name and Christian name at length.
Rank, profession, or occupation (if any).
Full postal address.
How related to or connected with the patient.
[If not the husband or wife or a relative of the patient, the person signing to state as briefly as possible:—1. Why the order is not signed by the husband or wife or a relative of the patient. 2. His or her connection with the patient, and the circumstances under which he or she signs.]

Dated this day of 18 .

To superintendent of the asylum [hospital *or* resident licensee of the house].

[4] Husband, wife, father, father-in-law, mother, mother-in-law, son, son-in-law, daughter, daughter-in-law, brother, brother-in-law, sister, sister-in-law, partner, or assistant.

[5] *See* Form 2.

Describing the asylum, hospital, or house by situation and name.

Section 8.

Form 5.

Certificate as to Personal Interview after Reception.

I certify that it would be prejudicial to *A.B.* to be taken before or visited by a justice, a judge of county courts, or a magistrate.

[Signed] *C.D.*,
Medical Superintendent of the Asylum *or* Hospital *or* Resident Medical Practitioner *or* Attendant of the , *or* Medical Attendant of the said *A.B.*

Section 8.

Form 6.

Notice of Right to Personal Interview.

Take notice that you have the right, if you desire it, to be taken before or visited by a justice, judge of county courts, or magistrate. If you desire to exercise such right, you must give me notice thereof by signing the enclosed form on or before the day of

Dated [Signed] *C.D.*
Superintendent of the Asylum or Hospital *or* Resident Licensee of [*or as the case may be.*]

Section 8.

Form 7.

Notice of Desire to have a Personal Interview.

Dated

[*Address*]

I desire to be taken before or visited by a justice, judge, or magistrate having jurisdiction in the district within which I am detained.

[Signed]

FORM 8.

Sections 4, 11, 16, 23, 24.

Certificate of Medical Practitioner.

In the matter of *A.B.* of[1] in the county[2] of , [3], an alleged lunatic.

I, the undersigned *C.D.*, do hereby certify as follows:

1. I am a person registered under the Medical Act, 1858, and I am in the actual practice of the medical profession.

2. On the day of 18 , at[4] in the county[5] of [separately from any other practitioner],[6] I personally examined the said *A.B.*, and came to the conclusion that he is a [lunatic, an idiot, or a person of unsound mind] and a proper person to be taken charge of and detained under care and treatment.

3. I formed this conclusion on the following grounds, viz.:—

(*a*) Facts indicating insanity observed by myself at the time of examination,[7] viz.:—

(*b*) Facts communicated by others,[8] viz.:—

[*If an urgency certificate is required it must be added here. See* Form 9.]

4. The said *A.B.* appeared to me to be [*or* not to be] in a fit condition of bodily health to be removed to an asylum, hospital, or licensed house.[9]

5. I give this certificate having first read the section of the Act of Parliament printed below.

Dated

[Signed] *C.D.*, of[10]

Extract from section 317 *of the Lunacy Act*, 1890.

Any person who makes a wilful misstatement of any material fact in any medical or other certificate or in any statement or report of bodily or mental condition under this Act, shall be guilty of a misdemeanor.

[1] Insert residence of patient.
[2] City or borough, as the case may be.
[3] Insert profession or occupation, if any.
[4] Insert the place of examination, giving the name of the street, with number or name of house, or should there be no number the Christian and surname of occupier.
[5] City or borough as the case may be.
[6] Omit this where only one certificate is required.
[7] If the same or other facts were observed previous to the time of the examination, the certifier is at liberty to subjoin them in a separate paragraph.
[8] The names and Christian names (if known) of informants to be given, with their addresses and descriptions.
[9] Strike out this clause in case of a private patient whose removal is not proposed.
[10] Insert full postal address.

FORM 9.

Sections 11, 28.

Statement accompanying Urgency Order.

I certify that it is expedient for the welfare of the said *A.B.*, [*or* for the public safety, *as the case may be*] that the said *A.B.* should be forthwith placed under care and treatment.

My reasons for this conclusion are as follows: [*state them*].

FORM 10.

Section 24. *Certificate as to pauper Lunatic in a Workhouse.*

I, the undersigned medical officer of workhouse of the Union hereby certify that I have carefully examined into the state of health and mental condition of *A.B.*, a pauper in the said workhouse, and that he is in my opinion a lunatic, and a proper person to be allowed to remain in the workhouse as a lunatic, and that the accommodation in the workhouse is sufficient for his proper care and treatment separate from the inmates of the workhouse not lunatics [*or*, that his condition is such that it is not necessary for the convenience of the lunatic or of the other inmates that he should be kept separate].

The grounds for my opinion that the said *A.B.* is a lunatic are as follows:

Dated

[Signed]

Medical Officer of the Workhouse.

FORM 11.

Section 24. *Order for detention of Lunatic in Workhouse.*

I, the undersigned *C.D.*, a justice of the peace for , being satisfied that *A.B.*, a pauper in the workhouse of the is a lunatic [or idiot or person of unsound mind] and a proper person to be taken charge of under care and treatment in the workhouse, and being satisfied that the accommodation in the workhouse is sufficient for his proper care and treatment separate from the inmates of the workhouse not lunatics [*or*, that his condition is such that it is not necessary for the convenience of the lunatic or of the other inmates that he should be kept separate] hereby authorise you to take charge of, and, if the workhouse medical officer shall certify it to be necessary, to detain the said *A.B.* as a patient in your workhouse. Subjoined is a statement of particulars respecting the said *A.B.*

[Signed] *C.D.*,
A justice of the peace
for

Dated
To the Master of the
Workhouse
of the

Statement of Particulars.

Name of patient and Christian name at length.
Sex and age.
Married, single, or widowed.
Condition of life and previous occupation (if any).
Religious persuasion as far as known.
Previous place of abode.
Whether first attack.
Age (if known) on first attack.
When and where previously under care and treatment.
Duration of existing attack.
Supposed cause.
Whether subject to epilepsy.
Whether suicidal.
Whether dangerous to others.
Whether any near relative has been afflicted with insanity.
Name and Christian name and address of nearest known relative of the patient and degree of relationship if known.
I certify that to the best of my knowledge the above particulars are correct.

[To be signed by the relieving-officer.]

FORM 12. Section 16

Order for reception of a Pauper Lunatic or Lunatic wandering at large.

I, *C.D.*, having called to my assistance *E.F.*, of , a duly qualified medical practitioner, and being satisfied that *A.B.* [*describing him*] is a pauper in receipt of relief [*or* in such circumstances as to require relief for his proper care and maintenance], and that the said *A.B.* is a lunatic [*or* an idiot, *or* a person of unsound mind] and a proper person to be taken charge of and detained under care and treatment, *or* that *A.B.* [*describing him*] is a lunatic, and was wandering at large, and is a proper person to be taken charge of and detained under care and treatment, hereby direct you to receive the said *A.B.* as a patient into your asylum [*or* hospital, *or* house]. Subjoined is a statement of particulars respecting the said *A.B.*

[Signed] *C.D.*,
A justice of the peace for

Dated the day of one thousand eight hundred and .

To the superintendent of the asylum for the county [*or* borough] of [*or* the lunatic hospital of ; *or E.F.* proprietor of the licensed house of ; describing the asylum, hospital, or house].

Note.—Where the order directs the lunatic to be received into any asylum, other than an asylum of the county or borough in which the parish or place from which the lunatic is sent is situate, or into a registered hospital or licensed house, it shall state, that the justice making the order is satisfied that there is no asylum of such county or borough, or that there is a deficiency of room in such asylum; or (as the case may be) the special circumstances, by reason whereof the lunatic cannot conveniently be taken to an asylum for such first-mentioned county or borough.

Statement of Particulars.

STATEMENT of particulars referred to in the above or annexed order.

The following is a statement of particulars relating to the said *A.B.*[1]:—

Name of patient, with Christian name at length.
Sex and age.
†Married, single, or widowed.
†Rank, profession, or previous occupation (if any).
†Religious persuasion.
Residence at or immediately previously to the date hereof.
†Whether first attack.
Age on first attack.
When and where previously under care and treatment as a lunatic, idiot, or person of unsound mind.
†Duration of existing attack.
Supposed cause.
Whether subject to epilepsy.
Whether suicidal.
Whether dangerous to others, and in what way.
Whether any near relative has been afflicted with insanity.
Union to which lunatic is chargeable.

Names, Christian names, and full postal addresses of one or more relatives of the patient.

Name of the person to whom notice of death to be sent, and full postal address if not already given.

[Signed] *G.H.*
To be signed by the Relieving-Officer or Overseer.

[1] If any particulars are not known, the fact is to be so stated. [Where the patient is in the order described as an idiot omit the particulars marked †].

Section 38.

FORM 13.

Certificate that patient continues of unsound mind.

I, , certify that *A.B.*, the patient [*or A.B., C.D.*, &c., the patients] to whom the annexed report relates, is [*or* are] still of unsound mind, and a proper person [*or* proper persons] to be detained under care and treatment.

[Signed]
Medical superintendent *or* resident medical officer of the asylum, *or* superintendent of the hospital *or* resident medical practitioner *or* medical attendant of the house situate at , *or* medical practitioner visiting the said *A.B.*

Dated

Section 229.

FORM 14.

Consent to the admission of a boarder.

We hereby sanction the admission of *A.B.* as a boarder into for the term of from the day of in accordance with the provisions of the statute and in terms of *A.B.'s* application.

[Signed]
Two of the Commissioners in Lunacy.
[*or* Two of the justices for .]

Dated the day of 18 .

Section 13.

FORM 15.

Order for Reception of a Lunatic not under proper care and control, or cruelly treated or neglected, to be made by a Justice appointed under the Lunacy Act, 1890.

I, the undersigned *C.D.*, being a Justice for specially appointed under the Lunacy Act, 1890, having caused *A.B.* to be examined by two duly qualified medical practitioners, and being satisfied that the said A.B. is a lunatic not under proper care and control [*or* is cruelly treated or neglected by the person having the care or charge of him], and that he is a proper person to be taken charge of and detained under care and treatment, hereby direct you to receive the said A.B. as a patient into your asylum [*or* hospital *or* house]. Subjoined is a statement of particulars respecting the said A.B.

(Signed)
A justice of the peace for appointed under the above-mentioned Act.

Dated

To the Superintendent of the Asylum for , or of the lunatic hospital of , or the resident licensee of the licensed house at .

Note.—Where the order directs the lunatic to be received into any asylum, other than an asylum of the county or borough in which the parish or place from which the lunatic is sent is situate, or into a registered hospital or licensed house, it shall state, that the justice making the order is satisfied that there is no asylum of such county or borough, or that there is a deficiency of room in such asylum; or (as the case may be) the special circumstances, by reason whereof the lunatic cannot conveniently be taken to an asylum for such first-mentioned county or borough.

Statement of Particulars.

STATEMENT of particulars referred to in the above or annexed order.

The following is a statement of particulars relating to the said A.B.[1] :—

Name of patient, with Christian name at length.

Sex and age.

†Married, single, or widowed.

†Rank, profession, or previous occupation (if any).

†Religious persuasion.

Residence at or immediately previous to the date hereof.

†Whether first attack.

Age on first attack.

When and where previously under care and treatment as a lunatic, idiot, or person of unsound mind.

†Duration of existing attack.

Supposed cause.

Whether subject to epilepsy.

Whether suicidal.

Whether dangerous to others, and in what way.

Whether any near relative has been afflicted with insanity.

Union to which lunatic is chargeable.

Names, Christian names, and full postal addresses of one or more relatives of the patient.

Name of the person to whom notice of death to be sent, and full postal address if not already given.

[Signed]

To be signed by the relieving-officer, overseer, or other person on whose information the order is made.

[1] If any particulars are not known, the fact is to be so stated. [Where the patient is in the order described as an idiot omit the particulars marked†].

LEAD POISONING, MENTAL DISORDER FROM.—The **toxic effects of lead on the nervous system** have been recognised from the very earliest date of medical literature, Paul of Ægina referring to epilepsy and convulsions caused by lead poisoning, while Dioscorides mentions delirium produced by lead.

Aretæus speaks of epilepsy following colic, and several writers in the Middle Ages describe colic terminating in delirium, which they do not appear to have recognised as being the result of lead intoxication.

In the nineteenth century the effects of lead on the brain have been fully recognised; so that Tanquerel des Planches in 1836, described them under the term "lead encephalopathy," as being divisible into four classes. These he described as (1) delirious, (2) comatose, (3) convulsive, and (4) a delirious, comatose and convulsive form.

The conditions described by Tanquerel were those produced by very obvious, coarse intoxication, in which the association of the lead poisoning and the cerebral results was obvious; but in a paper printed in the *Journal of Mental Science* for 1880, the writer drew attention to cases in which mental disorder, of a more obscure and chronic kind, seemed to have resulted from a minute and protracted toxic action; the mental disorder taking the form specially of chronic hallucination. Drs. Savage, A. Robertson, and Ringrose Atkins (*Journal of Mental Science*, 1880), published cases of a confirmatory character.

Dr. Bartens (*Zeitschrift*, xxxvii. Band. 1 Heft) has recorded cases collected from French and German literature.

The physiological action of lead is such as to warrant the conclusion of its special action on the nervous system.

In small, medicinal quantities (Lauder Brunton) it appears to "cause contraction of the muscular walls of the arteries, to raise arterial tension, and to slow the heart." It produces mental depression and thirst.

It checks the elimination of uric acid, and so probably produces gout. It is cumulative in the system, being found largely in the nervous tissues.

It is eliminated to a slight extent by the kidneys, in which it tends to produce cirrhotic changes, but is chiefly eliminated in the mucus of the intestinal canal.

Single poisonous doses, even when very large, would seem, from the cases recorded by Woodman and Tidy, to be rarely fatal; convulsions being the principal nervous symptom remarked.

In experimental cumulative poisoning of animals by Harnack (Wynter Blyth On Poisons), in rabbits, heart paralysis occurred, in dogs, chorea. Henkel, in dogs observed shivering, paralysis and convulsions, while Dr. Blyth, in accidental poisoning of cows, noted paralysis and delirium. Paralysis has also been noticed in cats, rats, mice, and other animals in lead factories.

In man it would seem to have special action on the optic nervous apparatus; optic neuritis, amaurosis and blindness being very frequently recorded (four of six cases recorded by Dr. Robertson were totally or partially blind).

The tendency of lead to affect the nervous tissues is further shown by the calculations made by Blyth on Henkel's researches, showing the proportion of lead to the dry matter, in

Liver	.03 to .10 per cent.
Kidney	.03 to .07 „
Brain	.02 to .05 „
Bone	.01 to .04 „
Muscles	.004 to .008 „

Dr. Blyth obtained (*Lancet*, 1887) one grain and a half of sulphate from the cerebrum only, in a fatal case of cumulative poisoning.

The pathologic results on the nerve tissues, have been studied by various observers. Gombault ("Archiv de Physiologie," 1873) found a granular condition of the medullary substance of some of the peripheral nerves, and Westphal ("Archiv für Psychiatrie," 1874) found a similar condition in the radial nerve. Kussmaul and Maier ("Deutscher Archiv für Klin. Med.," Band. ix. Heft 2) found sclerosis of the cœliac and superior cervical ganglia, in a case in which there had been colic, vomiting, diarrhœa and collapse. Monakow ("Review," *Journ. Ment. Sci.* 1881) found wasting of the frontal and temporal gyri, effusion in the membranes, but no adhesions, the brain solid, the scalp thickened, and pigmentary deposits in the nervous tissue.

In a case in which delirium was followed by coma and death in an employ of a lead factory (*Lancet*, 1887), the appearances were summarised as those of "serous apoplexy" only.

The presence and toxic action of lead on the body generally, are evidenced by the blue discoloration of the gums around the teeth (if these exist), the metallic taste, offensive breath odour, constipation, yellow tint of skin, emaciation, look of premature senility (a marked wrinkling of face in very chronic cases), as well as by the well-known colic, palsies, arthralgias, anæsthesiæ and gout.

The palsies are probably due to affection of the nerves, the muscles not contracting with the faradic, but only with the primary, current.

Vulpian and Raymond have also described cases of ataxia with left anæsthesia and right hyperæsthesia.

Absorption of the poison by inhalation would seem to lead to the most rapid and violent action on the nervous system; the most acute cases occurring in those working in an atmosphere impregnated with the dust of lead compounds; but severe and rapid effects result from it in a potable form; the slowest and most insidious from mere contact.

Predisposition to mental defect may probably be ascribed to this toxic agency, since Dr. Royer (Woodman and Tidy) has recorded that lead poisoning either in the father or mother produces miscarriages, and causes epilepsy, eclampsia, idiocy and imbecility in the offspring. Further inquiry into the results of such nerve degeneration in the families of workers in lead would be very desirable.

Mental disorder from lead intoxication, does not occur without an antecedent period of premonitory symptoms.

These consist of headache, wakefulness, disturbed sleep, and some terrifying dreams; with sensory derangements, especially tinnitus aurium and flashes of light, together with slowness of ideation and depression of spirits.

These may endure for a day or two only, or for longer periods, varying with the intensity of the toxic action or the neurotic predisposition.

The slighter and most acute forms of lead encephalopathy assume the form of delirium. Three cases of this form are described as having occurred under the observation of Dr. Langdon Down (*Med. Times and Gazette*, Aug. 1860). In these the delirium occurred only at night, the patients being merely dull intellectually by day. Dread was the striking characteristic of the delirium, with visual hallucinations of black animals, &c. The striking likeness of this delirium to that produced by alcohol was noted, and Laurent has also dwelt on this similarity.

Rapid remission and recurrence of the delirium is a marked characteristic, and it yields very readily to treatment on removal of the cause.

Beyond these conditions in which the toxic action on the brain is more or less overcome by the stimulus of the daily life, Tanquerel describes others in which there is a state of melancholy, tremor or stupor, with tranquil melancholic delirium (especially nocturnal), these conditions interchanging rapidly in a few hours. These more severe cases usually show some muscular difficulties, especially awkwardness of movement of the limbs, with trembling of the face and arms.

Furious delirium of a maniacal type, accompanied by marked affection of speech with hallucinations in which those of sight predominate and associated with amaurosis, would seem to be next in the order of intensity of toxic action.

This maniacal delirium may be complicated with convulsions. Dr. A. Robertson (*Journ. Ment. Sci.*, 1880) reports such a case, the delirium lasting four days; on recovery there was complete amaurosis from atrophy of the optic disc and other retinal changes. Hammond ("Dis. of Nerv. Sys.," 1876) describes a case in which, after a few days of maniacal delirium, convulsions occurred.

Tanquerel describes cases of a comatose form, occurring suddenly without antecedent mental disturbance, especially in persons who already have some lead palsy. The coma is incomplete, as the patients can be roused momentarily.

He also describes a state of sub-delirious coma.

These states, unless they rapidly pass away, become complicated by convulsions, and this comatose convulsive form is the most dangerous. He describes limited convulsions, like those produced by electric shocks and general or epileptiform attacks.

The more gradual degeneration of the brain, by less extensive poisoning, may produce various conditions.

Dr. MacCabe (*Journ. Ment. Sci.*, 1872, p. 233) records a case of "monomania" with "depressing visceral symptoms and a fixed idea that people were whispering about her."

Dr. Monakow (*Journ. Ment. Sci.*, 1881) describes the case of a painter, aged fifty-six, who for thirty-five years had suffered from attacks of lead colic: five children, born of a healthy wife, died of convulsions. During the last ten years there was paralysis of extensors, disorder of articulation, dulness of hearing. Then ataxia, left anæsthesia (incomplete) and right hyperæsthesia. The train of mental symptoms was weakness of intellect, loss of memory, sleeplessness, maniacal disturbance, confusion of thought, delirium in which he was destructive, dirty and aggressive.

Then emaciation, loss of strength and of articulation, and death by coma in five months.

The course of the disease had in this case some resemblance to general paralysis.

In the cases recorded by the writer (*Journ. Ment. Sci.*, 1880) of the gradual evolution of hallucinations and chronic insanity, these did not differ from similar disorder produced by alcoholic tippling, except in the marked wrinkling of the face in two of the cases (a symptom dwelt on by Tanquerel) and by the greater persistence and predominance of visual hallucinations and motorial troubles (startings and tremors).

Lastly, the writer recorded (*op. cit.*) two cases in which the lead first caused gout, and in conjunction with this in one man produced symptoms closely resembling general paralysis; in the other, complicated by alcohol, there were epilepsy and anæsthesia, such as seen in profound alcoholic poisoning. Both improved with the recurrence of gout.

The **prognosis** in lead encephalopathy has been to a great extent indicated in the order of description. The cases of nocturnal delirium may recover at once; the continuous delirium, if arrested within three or four days, convalesces in a week or two; but if more protracted, convalescence may occupy two or three months, as in Dr. Savage's case (*Journ. Ment. Sci.*, 1880).

The comatose and convulsive forms are very unhopeful of mental recovery, whilst in those in which there are delirium, coma and convulsions, there is great danger of a fatal termination.

The rapid nerve degeneration produced by this poison, as illustrated in its action on the optic nerve, makes the prognosis much more grave than in similar mental states arising from other causes.

The **diagnosis** of cerebral disorder due to plumbism primarily rests on the history of exposure and of the special symptoms already enumerated.

Lead intoxication, like alcohol, follows the law of dissolution of the nervous system, from the least organised to the most organised as described by Dr. Mercier ("Coma," *Brain*, 1887), and formulated by Dr. Hughlings Jackson (*Brit. Med. Journ.*, 1889), but besides this general degeneration there are localised affections and tendency to degeneration, such as the affection of optic and motor nerves probably determined by the local functional activity in the individual, which markedly distinguish the special action of lead from alcohol, in acute poisoning.

In chronic poisoning the lead cases may present the extreme wrinkling of the face described by Tanquerel and present in two of the writer's cases.

The rapidity of permanent irrecoverable degeneration is a noteworthy characteristic of lead action, and the sudden variation in intensity of symptoms in the acute stages is also striking.

The mental symptoms do not offer any pathognomonic characteristic.

The action of lead on the brain, from the symptoms and pathology recorded, is certainly not inflammatory, but degenerative, its primary effect probably producing anæmia, by its action on the vessels, and on its further direct action on the nervous tissue first arresting nutrition and then inducing degeneration.

The blood, although on analysis it contains so little poison, is doubtlessly the vehicle of its conveyance to the tissues, and these are found to contain it, very much in the proportion of their blood supply. If this is so, the localisation of toxic action may be determined by local functional activity (increasing local blood supply), and it would be desirable to bear this in mind in the case of persons exposed to or suffering from toxic action.

The prevention of lead poisoning and its treatment are fully described in every work on medicine, and little that is special to the cerebral affection can be advanced here.

Elimination of the poison must be the primary object of treatment. For this purpose copious diluents with increasing doses of the iodide of potassium are most efficacious, aided by profuse sweatings, from hot air or vapour baths.

Sulphur baths have also been strongly recommended, and after their use a blackish discoloration of the skin and nails has been observed, ascribed to the "formation of a sulphide" (Fagge).

The slighter forms of delirium, if special treatment is indicated, demand stimulation rather than sedatives; in the more violent delirium, ice to the head is beneficial, while in coma and convulsions, active counter-irritation by blisters, and derivation by sinapisms to the extremities appear to be indicated.

A nutritious diet, with an excess of fat, is advised, as a preventive and as aiding elimination.

H. Rayner.

[*References.*—Tanquerel des Planches, Lead Encephalopathy, 1836. Journ. Ment. Sci. 1872, MacCabe; 1880, Drs. Rayner, Savage, Robertson, and Atkins. Bartens, Zeitschrift, Band xxxvii. Heft 1. Winter Blyth, On Poisons, Lancet, 1887. Woodman and Tidy, Forensic Medicine. Gombault, Archiv. de Psychologie, 1873. Westphal, Archiv für Psychiatrie, 1874. Kussmaul and Maier, Deutsch. Arch. f. Klin. Med. Monakow, Review, Journ. Ment. Sci., 1881. Langdon Down, Med. Times and Gaz., 1860. Laurent, *ibid.* Hammond, Dis. Nerv. Sys. Mercier, Brain, 1887. Hughlings Jackson, Brit. Med. Journ., 1889. Lauder Brunton, Pharmacology. Fagge's Medicine, 1891.]

LEAPING AGUE.—A variety of the dancing mania observed some time since in Scotland. (*See* Choromania; Epidemic Insanity, &c.)

LE RAGLE.—A name given by d'Escayrac de Lauture in 1885 to hallucinations, mostly visual, more rarely auditory, olfactory, gustatory, or tactile, which not unfrequently happen to travellers in the desert, especially to such as are in a debilitated state from previous illness, or who have suffered from great fatigue, want of food, anxiety, terror, &c. Combined with these hallucinations there are illusions of sight and hearing. They usually occur in the hours between midnight and early morning, frequently recur at about the same time in the twenty-four hours for each individual, and are of sudden onset and fleeting duration. (Hirsch).

LEREMA (λήρημα, silly talk). The silly childish talk of senile dementia. (Fr. *lérème;* Ger. *Geschwätz.*)

LERESIS (λήρησις, silly talking). Talking nonsense; the garrulousness of an imbecile.

LEROS (λῆρος, silly talk). An old term for a slight delirium.

LESCHENOMA (λέσχη, gossip). A term for garrulity or loquacity; the idle or useless talkativeness symptomatic of certain mental affections as well as hysteria.

LETHARGIC STUPOR (ληθαργικός, drowsy; *stupor*, insensibility). A synonym of Trance (*q.v.*).

LETHARGY (λήθη, forgetfulness; ἀργία, idleness). A condition of prolonged semi-unconsciousness partaking of the character of profound sleep, from which the patient may be momentarily aroused, but into which he immediately lapses again. (*See* Trance.)

LETHE (λήθη). Oblivion, or total loss of memory. (Fr. *oubli;* Ger. *Absterben, Vergessen.*)

LETHEOMANIA (λήθη; μανία, madness). The morbid or insane longing for narcotics or anæsthetics.

LEUCOMORIA (λευκός, white, wan; μωρία, folly). A term for restless madness, restless melancholia. (Fr. *leucomorie;* Ger. *unruhiger Wahnsinn, unruhige Melancholie.*)

LIEBESWUTH; LIEBESWAHNSINN. The German equivalents for erotomania.

LIFE INSURANCE, Suicide in relation to.—The question how far suicide is an indication of insanity in the contemplation of law is considered in the article upon Evidence. It is here proposed to deal with the *suicide provisos* in policies of life insurance, whereby the insurers are exempted from liability in case the assured should "die by suicide," "commit suicide," or "die by his own hand." The construction of this proviso has sharply divided judicial opinion both in England and in America; but it is thought that the English law upon the subject may be accurately stated as follows:—

(1) When a person who is assured commits suicide in a sane mind, neither his representatives nor his assignees have any claim under the policy, even although the insurer has, by an express condition, undertaken the hazard of the suicide of the assured. Such contracts are void on grounds of public policy. (*Cf. Amicable Society* v. *Bolland*, 4 Bligh, N.S. 194, reversing *Bolland* v. *Disney*, 3 Russ. 351; *Cleaver* v. *Mutual Reserve Fund Life*, 39 W. R. 638, and see *Law Quarterly Review*, vol. vii. pp. 306–7.)

(2) When the assured commits suicide while in a state of unsound mind, the policy is not, *in the absence of any special condition*, rendered void thereby. (*Horn* v. *Anglo-Australian and Universal Family Life Insurance Co.* 1861, 30 L. J. Ch. 511.)

(3) But, when there is a condition in a life policy exempting the insurers from liability in case the assured should "commit suicide," "die by suicide," or "die by his own hand," and the assured does *voluntarily* kill himself, the policy is void whatever may have been the mental or moral state of the deceased at the time, and even if the policy has been assigned to the insurers themselves. (*Cf. White* v. *British Empire &c., Co.*, 1868, L. R. 7 Eq. 394. This proposition will be most easily justified by a rapid survey of the cases on which it is based. In *Borrodaile* v. *Hunter* (1843, 5 M. & G. 639), the policy contained a proviso terminating the risk in case the assured should die by his own hands, or by the hand of justice, or by duelling. The insured had been observed for some time to be labouring under dejection of spirits, though he performed his various duties as usual. Without any apparently direct cause, he flung himself from Vauxhall Bridge into the Thames. The defendants refused to pay the policy money, on the ground that the case came within the terms of the suicide proviso. The jury found that the deceased leaped from the bridge *voluntarily—i.e.*, knowing that the result of his act would be death, and intending to bring that result about —*but* that at the time he did so, he was not in a state of mind capable of judging between right and wrong. Erskine, J., entered judgment for the defendants, and this ruling was supported, on appeal, by a majority of the Court of Common Pleas. Chief Justice Tindal, however, dissented on the ground that the words "die by his own hands," being associated in the proviso with the words "die . . . . by the hands of justice or by duelling," the principle *noscitur a sociis* applied, and the condition must be construed as extending to criminal acts of self-destruction alone.

The point of law that was settled in *Borrodaile* v. *Hunter* cannot be better stated than in the language of Erskine, J. "It seems to me that the only qualification that a liberal interpretation of the words with reference to the nature of the contract requires is, that the act of self-destruction should be the voluntary and wilful act of the man, having at the time sufficient powers of mind and reason to understand the physical nature and consequences of such act, and having at the time a purpose and intention to cause his own death by the act, and that the question whether at the time he was capable of appreciating and understanding the moral nature and quality of his purpose is not relevant to the inquiry, further than as it might help to illustrate the extent of his capacity to understand the physical character of the act itself."

In *Cliff* v. *Schwabe* (1846, 3 C. B. 437) the facts were as follows: Louis Schwabe effected a policy with the *Argus Assurance Co.* on his own life, subject *inter alia* to a condition that "every policy effected by a person on his or her own life should be void if such person should *commit suicide* or die by duelling or the hand of justice." Schwabe died in consequence of having voluntarily—*i.e.*, for the purpose of killing himself—taken sulphuric acid, but under circumstances tending to show that he was at the time of unsound mind. In an action by his administratrix upon the policy, the defendants pleaded that Schwabe *did commit suicide* whereby the policy became void; and at the trial Mr. Justice Cresswell directed the jury "that in order to find the issue for the defendants it was necessary that they should be satisfied that Louis Schwabe died by his own voluntary act, *being then able to distinguish between right and wrong, and to appreciate the nature and quality of the act he was doing, so as to be a responsible moral agent*, that the burthen of proof as to his dying by his own voluntary act was on the defendants; but, that being established, the jury must assume that he was of sane mind, and a responsible moral agent unless the contrary should appear in evidence." Upon a bill of exceptions it was held by the Court of Common Pleas —not, however, without the dissent of two strong judges—Pollock, C.B., and Wight-

LOGOMANIA (*μανία*, madness). A form of insanity in which there is great talkativeness.

LOGOMONOMANIA (*μόνος*, single; *μανία*, madness). A term for a form of insanity characterised only by great loquacity (Guislain).

LOGONEUROSES (λόγος, reason; *νεῦρον*, a nerve). Another term for mental affections. In the singular, used to denote a derangement or impediment of speech.

LOGOPATHY (*πάθος*, a disease). A morbid affection of speech due to cerebral disease.

LOGOPLEGIA (*πληγή*, a stroke). Inability to pronounce certain words as a result of paralysis. A synonym of Aphasia.

LOGORRHŒA (*ῥοιά*, a flow). The same as logodiarrhœa (*q.v.*).

LONGINGS (A.S. *longen*, to desire earnestly). The name given to the mental symptom observed in pregnant women, and in those suffering from suppression of the normal uterine discharges, by which peculiar and whimsical desires are expressed. (Fr. *envie*; Ger. *Gelüstung*.)

LOQUACITY (Fr. *loquacité*, from *loquacitas*, talkativeness). Excessive talkativeness, volubility of speech, frequently a symptom of mental disease. (Ger. *Geschwätzigkeit*.)

LOVE-MELANCHOLY.—A popular term for true erotomania.

LUCID INTERVAL (Fr. *intervallo lucide*). An interval between the paroxysms of insanity, during which the mind appears clear, and the patient is apparently capable of conducting himself sanely. (Ger. *heller Zwischenraum*.)

LUCIDITY (*lucidus*, clear). A state of clearness or freedom from delusions or mental disorder.

LUCOMANIA. (*See* LYCOMANIA; LYCANTHROPIA.)

LUES DEIFICA; LUES DIVINA (*lues*, a spreading or contagious disease; *deifica*, making into a god; *divina*, godlike). Old terms for epilepsy.

LUKE'S, ST., HOSPITAL OF. (*See* REGISTERED HOSPITALS.)

LUNACY (*luna*, the moon). The legal term representing those deviations from a standard of mental soundness, in which the person, property, or the civil rights may be interfered with, when incapacity, violence, or irregularities threaten danger to the lunatic himself or to others. (Fr. *folie*; Ger. *Wahnsinn*, *Mondsucht*.)

LUNACY LAW, ENGLISH. (*See* LAW OF LUNACY.)

LUNACY LAW, IRISH. (*See* IRELAND, THE LUNACY LAWS OF.)

LUNACY LAW, SCOTTISH. (*See* SCOTLAND, THE LUNACY LAWS OF.)

LUNATIC (*luna*, the moon, from its supposed influence in causing mental disease). (1) A term applied to those diseases considered to be under the influence of the moon's phases, as epilepsy and insanity. (2) Also those affected by such diseases. (3) Also an insane person, one affected by lunacy. Act 16 & 17 Vict. c. 97, declares that the term lunatic shall mean and include every person of unsound mind, and every person being an idiot. (Fr. *lunatique*; Ger. *Wahnsinniger*.)

LUNATIC ASYLUMS. (*See* ASYLUMS, ENGLAND AND WALES, &c.)

LUNATICS, CRIMINAL. (*See* CRIMINAL LUNATICS.)

LUNATISMUS (*luna*, the moon). A name given to those somnambulists who only walk about at the time the moon shines.

LUNE (*luna*). A fit of insanity.

LYCANTHROPIA (λύκος, a wolf; ἄνθρωπος, a man). A species of insanity in which the patient is under the delusion that he is a wolf or some wild beast, having been changed into such by the agency of the devil.

LYCANTHROPY.—The most classic form of endemic insanity really Greek, if the case of the Prœtides cannot be so considered, is that of lycanthropy, upon which we will make a few remarks, because it is a subject somewhat obscure and but little discussed in treatises on mental disorders. While upon this theme we shall pass the boundaries of the country (Arcadia), and the period of its origin, and follow it in Europe up to the mediæval epoch.

We note especially that the wolf was a constant companion of Mars in Greek and Roman mythology.

We see in this the adoration of divine scourges, such as still exists in the worship of snakes and tigers in southern India.

Lycosura, a mountainous city of Arcadia, specially worshipped wolves, and it would appear that before Lycaon, Osiris was transformed into a wolf.

A bronze she-wolf was sacred to the oracle of Delphos, to commemorate the transformation of Latona into this animal, in order that she might more securely give birth to Apollo and Diana.

The fable of Romulus and Remus is well known.

The Greeks worshipped a Zeus Lycæus (from λύκος, a wolf).

In its primitive meaning lycanthropy probably alluded only to the transformation into wolves, but subsequently the word was used to signify transformation into other animals. Thus, in the period of fully developed lycanthropy when men, transformed into wolves, wandered through the forests, Citeus, son of Lycaon, laments the metamorphosis of his daughter into a bear, and Iphigenia at the moment of sacrifice was changed into a fawn.

But the meaning of lycanthropy continued to degenerate until more recent times, when it is known by the common people as a most mischievous, bad spirit that roams the earth at night; this is the *loup garou* of the French, called in Italy also *lupo manaro*,* *versiera*.

The native country of lycanthropy, therefore, seems to have been Arcadia, but in some sort it was endemic in other mountainous countries where there were many wolves.

For instance, Virgil (Ecl. viii. 95) speaking of another region says :—

> Has herbas atque haec Ponto mihi lecta venena
> Ipse dedit Mœris; nascuntur plurima Ponto;
> His ego sæpe lupum fieri et se condere silvis
> Mœrim, sæpe animas imis excire Sepulcris,
> Atque satas aliò vidi traducer messes.

This is the fable: Lycaon, King of Arcadia, son of Titan and the earth, founder of Lycosura on Mount Lyceo, was one of the founders of the important Pelasgian race. He was the first to sacrifice human victims to Jove and was, therefore, changed into a wolf, and wandered in the woods with many others likewise transformed. Ovid says of him,

> Territus ipse fugit, nactusque silentia ruris
> Exululat, frustraque loqui conatur.—
> Met. i. 232.

The members of Lycaon's and Antheus's families, who passed a certain river and gained the forest, became wolves, and when they recrossed this river regained their human forms. Others believe that Lycaon is the constellation of the wolf, and this may result from the existence of the constellation of the bear into which Lycaon's niece was transformed.

However this may be, in Lycaon we find three united qualities, those of wolf, king, and constellation.

Perhaps the character of wolf was a divine attribute, where the wolf represented brute force as seen in the destruction of herds in a mountainous country, and was in reality given to him who appears to have consolidated the Pelasgians and formed their first laws, inasmuch as we see his name stamped on the firmament.

We have enlarged on the mythology of lycanthropy because it affords a striking example of the *superstructure of psycdopathy on fable*.

It is not only in the legend of Lycaon that lycanthropy is mentioned. Homer speaks of the sorceress Circe who changed Ulysses' companions into swine.

Sanctified by the lupercalian feasts of the Romans, enriched by the story of Circe, of Nebuchadnezzar, of Jonah in the oriental history, lycanthropy, however modified, found much nutriment in Christianity and forms an interesting page in the important psychological phenomenon of witchcraft.

A propos of this we refer to Bodin (" La Démonomanie ou traité des Sorciers," Paris, 1587), who connects lycanthropy with witchcraft and sorcery, from the fact that the word "ram" is used for demon, because the ram is as offensive in its habits as a demon.

Michael Verdun and Pierre Burgot, tried at Besançon in 1521, were changed after dances and sacrifices to the devil into two agile wolves, who rejoined others in the forest and coupled with them.

Bodin also mentions the lycanthrope of Padua, the famous *lupo manaro*, whose arms and legs were cut off, and were found to be covered with a wolf's skin.

The witches of Vernon often met together in 1566 under the form of cats and were dispersed and wounded. Certain women suspected of being witches were examined and found to bear the same wounds which were inflicted on them while in the form of cats.

Pierri Mamor and Henri di Colonia were undoubtedly transformed into wolves, according to the same Bodin.

Greece and Asia have always been more infested with lycanthropy than the West.

In 1542 under the reign of the Sultan Soliman there were so many *lupi manari* at Constantinople that the Sultan with an armed force drove off 150!

The Germans called them Werwolf (Währwolf). *Wer* was derived from the Teutonic word signifying *man;* in Gothic *weir*. The French termed them, *loups garous*, the Picardians, *loups carous*. The Latins called them *varios et versipelles* (*Vir*, man).

In Livonia at the end of December the devil called together the witches, beat them and transformed them into wolves who threw themselves on men!

For Bodin this is quite possible. Some contemporary doctors spoke of lycanthropy as a mental malady, but he shields himself behind Theophrastus, Paracelsus and Pomponius, and deems that it is absurd to attempt to compare natural with supernatural phenomena, and bravely concludes

* The *lupo manaro* of the Middle Ages was a witch dressed as a wolf. It was also a hobgoblin peculiar to the City of Blois that frightened children. The *lupo marino* was regarded as a most ravenous fish.

that if this malady existed as the doctors said, it could only be in the individual affected with lycanthropy, and how could the fact be explained of others having assisted *de visu* at the transformation? "Now that silver can be changed to gold and the philosopher's stone fabricated, it ought not to seem strange that Satan transforms persons." St. Thomas Aquinas says, "*Omnes angeli boni et mali ex virtute naturali habent potestatem transmutandi corpora nostra.*"

Gervais of Tilbury, *temp.* Hen. II., says, "Videmus enim frequenter in Anglia per lunationes homines in lupos mutari, quod hominum genus *gerulfos* Galli nominant. Angli vero *werewolf* dicunt, *were* enim Anglice virum sonat, et *ulf* lupum." "Otia imp. ap. Scriptt. Brunsv.," p. 895.

A curious work translated from the French in 1350 encouraged the spread of this delusion; this was the romance of "William and the Werewolf; or, William of Palermo." As to this history, a king of Apulia had a fair son named William. The king's brother, wishing to be heir to the throne, bribed two ladies to murder the child. What follows shows a mixture of popular belief with what in other cases became actual mental disease. While the child was at play a wild wolf caught him up, ran away with him to a forest near Rome, taking great care of him. But while the wolf went to get some food, the child was found by a cowherd, who took him home. The writer then says: "Now you must know that the wolf was not a true wolf, but a werewolf or manwolf; he had once been Alphonso, eldest son of the King of Spain, and heir to the crown. His step-mother, Braunde, wishing her own son Braundinis to be the heir, so acted that Alphonso became a werewolf."

In the sequel, the Emperor of Rome, while hunting, met the boy William, and, being much pleased with him, took him from the cowherd, placing him behind him on his horse. At Rome he was committed to the care of his daughter Melior to be her page, and, of course, they fell in love with one another.

The emperor, however, designed her for some one else. A friend provides for their escape by sewing them up in the skins of two white bears, and they concealed themselves in a den. There the werewolf finds them and supplies them with food; they are pursued, but escape to Palermo. An opportunity occurs for William (a werewolf was painted on his shield) to fight against the Spaniard, and he takes the king and queen prisoners, and refuses to release them until the wicked Queen Braunde agrees to disenchant the werewolf. This she does, and Alphonso is restored to his right shape, and is warmly thanked for his kindness to William, who is happily married to Melior, and becomes Emperor of Rome.*

A typical case of lycanthropy was admitted into the asylum of Maréville under the care of M. Morel, and reported by him in his "Études Cliniques."

"The patient, after residing for a time in a convent, returned home, where he became the victim of fearful mental agony and terror. He was not only absorbed in dwelling upon his bodily ailments, but dreaded everlasting torture, merited, as he believed, for crimes, which, however, he had not committed. He trembled in all his limbs, imploring the help of Heaven and his friends. Soon after, he repelled their sympathy, and, concentrating all his delusional activity on his own sensations, became a terror to himself, and endeavoured to inspire every one else with the same sentiment. '*See this mouth*,' he exclaimed, separating his lips with his fingers, '*it is the mouth of a wolf; these are the teeth of a wolf; I have cloven feet; see the long hairs which cover my body; let me run into the woods, and you shall shoot me.*' All that human means could adopt to save this unfortunate patient was done, but unhappily in vain. He had remissions which gave us some hope, but they were of short duration. In one of these he experienced great delight in embracing his children, but he had scarcely left them when he exclaimed, 'The unfortunates, they have embraced a wolf.' His delusions came into play with fresh force. '*Let me go into the woods*,' said he again, '*and you shall shoot me as you would a wolf.*' He would not eat. '*Give me raw meat*,' he said, '*I am a wolf.*' His wish was complied with, and he ate some food like an animal, but he complained that it was not sufficiently rotten, and rejected it. He died in a state of marasmus and in the most violent despair" (vol. ii. p. 58).

Such is the graphic account given by M. Morel. It will suffice to illustrate the terrible suffering which the delusion of being transformed into an animal occasions.

A. TAMBURINI.
S. TONNINI.

[*References.* — Böttiger, Beitr. zur Sprengel's Geschichte der Medizin, Bd. ii. pp. 3-45. Paulus Ægineta (Syd. Soc.), vol. i. p. 389. Aëtius, vi. u. Oribasius, Synops. viii. 10. Actuarius, Meth. Med. i. 16. Psellus, Carm. de re med. Avicenna (who calls it *cucubuth*), iii. 1, 5, 22. Haly Abbas, Theor. ix. 7. Pract. v. 24. Albucasis,

* See translation by Sir Humphrey de Bohun, A.D. 1350, edited by the Rev. Walter W. Skeat, M.A. 1867.

Ægypt. l. 11, 28. Rhazes, Divis. 10, Cont. i. Nicander, Theriaca (Schneider's ed.) Rhanæus, Supplement 3. Cur und Neue Anmerk von Natur und Kunstgeschichten, 1728. Majolus Dier Canicul., t. 2, colloq. iii. Wier, De Præst. Dæm., lib. vi. ch. xi. Fincelius, De Mirabil. lib. xi. 1541. Bodin, Démonomanie. Collection Dros, sur la Franche-Comté Melanges, i. 4. folio 267. Bibliothèque royale; also vol. xxii. folio 257. De la Folie, par L. F. Calmeil, tom. i. p. 279, who states that the Parliament of Franche-Comté ordained in 1573 that the *loups-garoux* should be hunted down. Art. by Dr. N. Parker, on Lycanthropy, or Wolf-madness, a Variety of Insania Zoanthropica, in Journ. Ment. Sci., 1854, p. 52. Morel, Études Cliniques, 1852, tom. ii. p. 58. Burton, Anatomy of Melancholy, 1651. St. Augustine, De Civitate Dei, cap. v. Mizaldus, cent. v. 77. Schenckius, lib. i. Forestus, lib. x., De morbis cerebri. Vincentius Bellavicensis, Spec. Met., lib. xxxi. c. 122. Pliny, lib. viii. c. 22. Ovid, Met. I. i.]

LYCOMANIA. Lycanthropia.

LYCORREXIA; LYCORREXIS (λύκος, a wolf; ὄρεξις, a longing after). A name given to the morbid wolfish appetite observed in some forms of mental disease. A synonym of Bulimia (*q.v.*).

LYPE (λύπη, sadness). Mournfulness.

LYPEMANIA.—A synonym of Melancholia (Esquirol). (Fr. *lypémanie.*)

LYPÉMANIE RAISONNANTE (Fr.). Esquirol's term for what is known as reasoning melancholia, where the patient is aware of the absurdity of his fears, but is unable to escape from them.

LYPÉROPHRÉNIE (Fr.) (λυπηρός, distressing; φρήν, mind). Melancholia.

LYPOTHYMIA (λύπη; θυμός, disposition). A synonym of Melancholia. (Fr. *lypothymie.*)

LYSSA (λύσσα, rage). A synonym of Madness, mania; also used for Hydrophobia.

LYSSAS (λύσσας, raging mad). A maniac.

LYSSETER (λυσσητήρ, one who is raging mad). A madman. (Fr. *lyssétère.*)

LYSSOPHOBIA (λύσσα, rage; φόβος, fear). A synonym of Hydrophobophobia.

M

MACHLOSYNE (μαχλοσύνη, lust); **MACHLOTES** (μαχλότης, lust). Terms used as synonyms of Nymphomania. (Fr. *machlosyne.*)

MACROCEPHALIC IDIOCY (μακρός, large; κεφαλή, head). (*See* Idiocy.)

MACROMANIACAL (μακρός, large; μανία, madness). A term for that form of insanity in which the insane person conceives things, especially parts of his own body, to be larger than they in reality are.

MACROPSIA HYSTERICA; MACROPSY, HYSTERICAL (μακρός, large; ὄψις, sight; hysteria, *q.v.*). A visional defect found in hysterical subjects, and usually associated with monocular polyopia. Objects held very close to the affected eye appear enormously magnified, while, if removed a few feet from the observer they diminish in size more rapidly than normal. With this there is also to be found concentric lessening of the field of vision, with reduction or transposition of the colour-field (Charcot). (*See also* Micropsy, Hysterical.)

MAD (A.S. *gemád*). The popular term for one who is insane.

MÄDCHENSCHNEIDER (Ger.) A man who has an insane desire to cut or wound girls. A "Jack the Ripper."

MADNESS (Sax. *gemaad*). Professor Wilson in his lexicon (p. 30), states that this word may be recognised in several Indo-European languages; that Madah is the Sanskrit for madness, and Madayati for "he drives mad, or insane." Prichard adopts this statement. For Hebrew equivalent *see* page 3 of this Dictionary. Gr. Μαργοσύνη; Μάργη; Μαργότης. Lat. *Insania, Vesania, Vecordia.* Lyssa was employed by the Greeks not only for rabies, but for madness in man. (*See* Mania.)

MADNESS, CONGENITAL (*congenitus*, born with). A synonym of Idiocy.

MADNESS, DEMENTIAL (*dementia*, madness). A term used as a synonym of Dementia.

MADNESS, FURIOUS (*furiosus*, enraged). A synonym of Acute Mania.

MÆEUSIOMANIA. (*See* Maieusiomania.)

MÆNAS (μαινάς, one frenzied or inspired). Mania, fury. (*See* Mainas.)

MAGNETISM, ANIMAL (μάγνης, a magnet, first found near the city of Μαγνησία). Properties attributed to the influence of a particular principle which has been compared to that which characterises the magnet. It is supposed to be transmitted from one person to another, and to impress peculiar modifications on organic action, especially on that of the nerves. (*See* Hypnotism; Braidism; &c.)

MAGNUS MORBUS (*magnus*, great; *morbus*, a disease). An old name for epilepsy.

MAIEUSIOMANIA (*μαίευσις*, delivery of a woman in childbirth; *μανία*, madness). Insanity attendant upon parturition; a synonym of Puerperal Mania. (Fr. *méeusiomanie*.)

MAINAS (*μαινάς*, from *μαίνομαι*, I rage). Derangement, or an excited state of the mind.

MAISON D'ALIÉNÉS (Fr.). A lunatic asylum.

MAISON DE SANTÉ (Fr.). A private lunatic asylum.

MAISPSYCHOSEN.—The German term for psychoses connected with pellagra.

MALACIA (*μαλακία*, softness, weakliness). A term generally used to denote morbid softening of a tissue or part, but it has also been used by some authors to indicate the depraved or fanciful appetite observed in hysteria, pregnancy and insanity, such as dirt-eating, &c.

MALADIE DU PAYS.—A French synonym of Nostalgia.

MALADIE DU SOMMEIL.—The French term for what is popularly known as the sleeping sickness.

MALADIE LUNATIQUE.—A term used in France either for mania or epilepsy.

MALADIES MYSTIQUES.—A general name given in France to affections of a hysteric type such as ecstasy, trance, catalepsy, &c.

MALADY, ENGLISH.—A term used abroad for hypochondriasis.

MALARIA and INSANITY.—Malaria is sometimes assigned as the cause of mental disorder. An attack of malaria may be attended with, or followed by, extreme collapse, coma or delirium, epileptiform or tetanoid convulsions, or mental symptoms of various degrees and kinds. In many cases the occurrence of insanity may be a chance coincidence, and not dependent upon an attack of malaria as a cause. Simple uncomplicated attacks of malaria are rarely followed by mental disturbance; but when the nervous system has been weakened by syphilis, alcohol, and various excesses, not only is some neurosis likely to supervene, but it is likely to be of a serious and intractable nature. Simple cases, where no cause beyond the malaria has been ascertained, generally recover.

Some neuroses appear to be forms of ague, and may be recognised as being malarious, partly by their periodic nature, partly by their supervention on a more or less distinct cold stage, partly by their occurrence in a malarious district, and partly by the fact that the patient has already been the subject of ague.*

In the *Medical Times and Gazette* (vol. i. p. 217, 1865), Dr. Handfield Jones reports that "in a situation exposed to malaria and never free from its diseases, while the other members of a family had the intermittent fever under different but ordinary forms, the two younger ones were attacked with paralytic affections suddenly, the one in the leg and thigh, the other in the arm. The palsy disappeared almost spontaneously in both, and was succeeded by the regular quotidian." He further states that "perhaps nothing is more proving as to the depressing effect of malaria on nervous power than the diminution of the intellect, often proceeding to perfect idiotism, which sometimes follows severe or long-continued intermittents." Sir R. Martin says: "I have seen a complete but temporary prostration of the mental powers result from a residence in our terais and jungly districts in India, as in the Gondwana and Aracan, but especially after the fevers of such districts." In the *Indian Annals of Medical Science* (vol. vii. p. 76), Dr. Beatson states that "after repeated attacks of intermittent fever, in addition to general muscular weakness, a partial paralysis of one or more limbs is not an uncommon occurrence," and this he ascribes to congestion of the nervous centres, inducing a chronic degenerative type.

The occurrence of paralysis of certain groups of muscles after malaria is not uncommon. Dr. Manson, in his medical report on the health of Amoy, quotes a case of gradual impairment of sight following an attack of dengue fever. Amongst the Chinese he also noted many instances of dyspepsia, debility, rheumatism, "paralysis of certain groups of muscles, and even insanity," as consequences of dengue.

Pinel has recorded a case of recurring suicidal tendencies after an attack of tertian fever, and Baillarger considers that intermittent fevers predispose to insanity in two ways, first by acting like all nervous affections, and secondly by producing anæmia. Sullivan, writing on the endemic diseases of tropical climates, states that in one patient the effect of miasma produces prostration, in another it produces over-excitement, or increased muscular sensibility; one man may be seized with delirium, another falls into a state of stupor. On exposure to the poison of malaria, some are seized with local paralytic affection, or general hyperæsthesia, while others do not complain of pain.

* Bristowe, "Principles and Practice of Medicine," 7th edit. p. 290.

Neuralgic affections of one or other branches of the fifth pair, as in that involving the supra-orbital, and constituting one form of the malady known as "brow-ague," is adduced as an example of a neurosis being a distinct form of ague. Several authors have described intermittent paroxysmal mania or maniacal delirium occurring in the place of an attack of ague, or as its principal symptom.

Of the form which follows ague, Sydenham, who first described it, states that acute mania tending to pass into chronic, occurs chiefly after protracted *quartans*. Sebastian, however, states that insanity occurs as frequently after attacks of *tertian* or double quartan type, and that, in these cases, it is more commonly of an acute delirious character, whilst after quartan it takes on a more chronic form, and tends to pass into stupidity or melancholia (Greenfield).

During an attack of intermittent fever there may be delirium in persons predisposed thereto, and this delirium is not always in proportion to the intensity of the fever (Lemoine and Chauminer, *Annales Med. Psych.* 1887), or there may be a condition with exhaustion analogous to the typhoid state of other acute disorders. In severe and prolonged cases of malarial disease there is a tendency to intermittent mental affections, or chronic insanity with or without paralysis. The more important mental conditions are met with as sequelæ, in persons who have passed into convalescence after a very acute or prolonged attack of malaria. These symptoms at such period may be transitory and curable, in the form of quiet delirium, melancholia with or without stupor, or simple mania with or without impulsive tendencies, or occasional outbursts of excitement. These conditions are generally considered curable. The pseudo-general paralytic type has been frequently observed. It sometimes presents most of the features of general paralysis, with mental and physical symptoms, which, although difficult to distinguish from those of general paralysis, are, nevertheless, somewhat different in their course and duration. Mentally there is frequently weak-mindedness or slight exaltation, with or without marked delusions. In one case admitted to Bethlem there was partial dementia with confusion, and in another melancholia with confusion and hallucinations of hearing. The physical symptoms may be those of nervous debility with tremors, alteration of the reflexes, or even definite symptoms of a system lesion in the spinal cord.

Dr. Osborne has described a peculiar appearance of the margin of the tongue after attacks of malaria. This condition is termed the "malarial margin." Its colour is faintly blue, and there is marked transverse indentation or crimping, apparently confined to the submucous tissue, while the superficial integument continues smooth, moist and transparent.

The **prognosis** in such cases is unfavourable. They seldom terminate like general paralysis, but go on for years and die of some complication, or succumb to the advance of a degenerative lesion. Sometimes when alcohol has formed an additional factor in the causation, the case may do well. When syphilis forms a complication, recovery is rare. In one case, under observation at present (with a history of malaria and syphilis), there is partial dementia, with hallucination of hearing and lateral sclerosis of the cord. The mental symptoms on the one hand are of an intermittent type, and do not appear to advance in severity, although the disease is of four years' duration; whilst, on the other hand, the lesion in the cord is progressing unfavourably. The mental disorders occurring during an attack of malaria are generally transitory and curable, unless the malaria is of undue severity, when there is apt to be permanent instability, or a chronic form of insanity.

The **diagnosis** is often difficult. The periodic or intermittent nature of the mental attacks may be a guide. Sometimes one may have to distinguish between the pseudo-general paralysis following malaria, insanity with paralysis, and general paralysis.

The **pathology** is vague. Suggestions have been made as to the presence of micro-organisms in the blood, and the existence of pigment in the blood and vessels, but their relation to mental disorder is quite unknown.

The occurrence of a large amount of pigment granules in the blood has long been known. Meckel, Virchow, and Herschel have described them as frequently occurring after intermittent fevers. For accounts as to the mode in which the pigment is formed, the reader is referred to the paper by Virchow, "Die Pathol. Pigmente," in *Archiv für Pathol. Anatomie and Physiologie*, vol. i. art. 9; and to the work of Rokitansky, "Pathological Anatomy," *Sydenham Soc. Trans.*, vol. i. p. 204; also to the works of I. Vogel, Bruch, Hensauger, Lobstein, Andral, Trousseau and Leblanc.

Breschet and Cruveilhier seem to have been the first (in 1821) to detect pigment in the blood-vessels in the form of black, sharply-cut masses ("Considérations sur une altération organique appelée Dégénérescence Noire"). In 1823 Dr. Halliday published a case of melanosis, in which he found black pigment in the vessels at the base of the brain, and in those of the choroid plexus (*London Med. Repos.*). In 1825 Billard and Baily observed capillaries of the brain to be obstructed by pigment. In 1852 Zervin, in a contribution on the "Treatment of Ague by Arsenic," throws doubt upon the researches of Heschl (*Deutsche Klinik*, Nos. 40, 41). Bright described and figured the brain of a man who had died from cerebral paralysis, which appeared to have resulted from an attack of fever. The cortical substance was of a dark colour like black-lead. In 1874 Hammond had a patient suffering from deafness, pains in the head, and epileptic convulsions, in whom an ophthalmoscopic examination showed the existence of double optic neuritis, with pigmentary deposit. There was a history of malarious fever in the case, and recovery from these symptoms, including the deafness, followed the use of arsenic. Planer (*Wien Zeitschrift*, February 1854) found that in cases in which there were cerebral symptoms, the pigment in the blood was found in the state of black, or more commonly of brown-yellow, brown, or (very rarely) red granules, many of which were united together by a clear hyaline substance, which was soluble in acids and alkalies. Meckel observed pigment cells very rarely; Virchow more frequently. Planer never saw in the pigment masses anything like a nucleus. The aggregation of the pigment grains sometimes formed black or brown flakes of the most variable form; these flakes were sometimes considered to be constituted by a hyaline substance, in which black pigment was imbedded. Planer found two hæmatoidin crystals adhering to this clear substance. The relative number of the pigment masses as compared to the blood globules, was not determined. In some cases the capillaries seemed almost choked up with them. He did not find that the colourless corpuscles of the blood were more numerous.

The cerebral substance was often found affected by the pigment change, and it appeared certain that the pigment was in the vessels. Meckel describes a case in which there were numerous punctiform hæmorrhages in the grey substance, produced by blocking of vessels through pigment, and since then several cases of the same kind have been seen by Planer. In some cases the flakes, already referred to as seen in the blood in the heart and large vessels, were in the cerebral capillaries, and of such size that it seemed impossible they could pass. In fact, Planer conjectures that the extreme abundance of pigment granules in the cerebral vessels must have been caused by the fact that they could not pass through the cerebral capillaries, which (especially in the grey matter) are the finest in the body (Kölliker).

From this account it is evident that the pathology of the affection is very indefinite, and we have yet to learn whether in these cases excessive pigmentation occurs in the nerve-cells of the brain and spinal cord, and if so, in what way does the degeneration differ from the pigmentary changes found in ordinary conditions of functional hyperplasia, as in severe attacks of acute mania, epileptic insanity or general paralysis? THEO. B. HYSLOP.

MALARIAL EPILEPSY (Italian, *mal'aria*, from *malo*, bad; *aria*, air; ἐπιληψία, the falling sickness). The occurrence of epileptic seizures in persons resident in malarious districts. The actual fit is preceded by a great rise of temperature, followed in the intervals by facial neuralgia, and the attacks are said to cease when the subjects are removed from malarial influences.

MALAYAN IDIOTS. (*See* IDIOCY, MALAYAN; IDIOCY, FORMS OF.)

MAL DE LAIRA (Fr.). The barking disease, a form of hysterical epidemic which occurred in the seventeenth century in some of the German convents.

MAL DE TERRE, MAL DE SAINT-JEAN, MAL DIVIN, MAL CADUC, MAL INTELLECTUEL, MAL SACRÉ, MAL SAINT, MALADIE COMITIALE, MALADIE HERCULÉENNE, MALADIE SACRÉE. French synonyms of Epilepsy.

MALFORMATION. (*See* MICROCEPHALY; IDIOCY; &c.)

MAL GRAND, MAL HAUT (Fr.). Terms employed both in England and on the Continent to denote the typical and fully developed epileptic seizure.

MALLEATION (*malleus*, a hammer). A name given to a symptom which may occur in hysteria, chorea or insanity, when the hands, one or both, act convulsively in striking as if with a hammer. (Fr. *malléation*; Ger. *Hämmern*, *Schmieden*.)

MAL PETIT (Fr.) A form of epilepsy in which there is only a momentary loss of consciousness. A term in general use in England and on the Continent.

MALUM CADUCUM (*malum*, an evil; *caducus*, falling). A synonym of Epilepsy. The "falling sickness."

MALUM HYPOCHONDRIACUM (malum; hypochondriasis) (*q.v.*). A synonym of Hypochondriasis.

MALUM HYSTERICUM (*malum*; hysteria) (*q.v.*). A synonym of Hysteria.

MALUM MINUS (*malum*; *minor*, less). The lesser sickness; the form of epilepsy unaccompanied by convulsions; the *petit mal* of the French.

MANDRAGORA and MANDRAGORINE.—Mandragora officinarum. *Linn.* Common Mandrake. (Radix.)

Μανδραγόρας μῆλα. Dioscorides, lib. iv. cap. 76. Mandragora, Pliny, Hist. Nat. lib. xxv. cap. 94; ed. Valp. Atropa Mandragora, Linn. South of Europe. Mandrake is an acro-narcotic poison; when swallowed it purges violently. The roots from their fancied resemblance to the human form were called *anthropomorphon*, and were supposed to prevent barrenness. Dr. Sylvester has drawn attention to the ancient uses of this plant as an anaesthetic.

Avicenna employed it as a soporific.

"Mandragora," says Pliny, "may be used safely enough to procure sleep, if there be proper regard to the dose, that it be answerable in proportion to the strength and complexion of the patient. Also it is an ordinary thing to drink it against the poison of serpents; likewise before the cutting, cauterising, pricking or lancing of any limb to take away the sense or feeling of such extreme cases. And sufficient it is in some to cast them into a sleep with the smell of mandragora." ("Natural History," bk. xxv. ch. 13.)

Iago soliloquises:—

> Not poppy, nor mandragora,
> Nor all the drowsy syrups of the world,
> Shall ever medicine thee to that sweet sleep
> Which thou ow'dst yesterday.
>
> (*Othello*, act iii. sc. 3.)

In ancient times those who took mandragora, or mandrake, were named "mandragorites." It is a very interesting fact, pointed out by Dr. B. W. Richardson, that "as on recovery from its effects there was wildness of the senses, and fear, the saying of 'shrieking like mandrakes' became applied, by a strange perversion, to the plant instead of the person:

> And shrieks like mandrakes torn out of th' earth,
> That living mortals, hearing them, run mad."

This physician, some years ago, cut up the root of mandragora, and attempted to make a tincture from it with alcohol. He found that this preparation did not bring out the active principle, it being most soluble in water. It appears that the ancients were aware of this. He then made a weak tincture, using one-sixth part of alcohol, and letting the root (in fine powder) macerate for four weeks. The statements of ancient writers were now fully justified. Narcotism, dilated pupils, motor and sensory paralysis, and then mental excitement were observed. He concluded that its action was purely upon the nervous centres. "The whole of the facts, indeed, lead clearly to the acceptance of the belief that the medicinal use of mandragora in ancient times has been correctly recorded" ("The Asclepiad," vol. v. No. 18, 1888, p. 182). Its anaesthetic properties were found by him to be of the most potent kind. It is conjectured that Banquo referred to mandragora in the question, "Or have we eaten of the insane root that takes the reason prisoner?"

A reference to the plant occurs in "Antony and Cleopatra":—"Give me to drink Mandragora."

It was regarded as possessing aphrodisiac properties. It is employed, according to Littré and Robin, in the form of the powdered root, the average dose being $8\frac{1}{2}$ to 9 decigrammes. THE EDITOR.

[*References.*—Pareira, vol. ii. pt. 2, p. 227. The Mandrake, sold by herbalists. White Bryony (Bryonia dioica).]

MANIA. (Lat. *mania*; from Gr. *μανία*, madness; from *μαίνομαι*, I rage; from Aryan root *man*, to think; derivation according to Esquirol, from *μήνη*, the moon). Insanity characterised in its full development by mental exaltation and bodily excitement. The term is also sometimes used for acute mania. Popularly it is used for the delusions of the insane. (Fr. *manie*; Ger. *Wuth*, *Raserei*, *Tollheit*, *Tollsucht*.)—**M., acute** (*acutus*, sharp). An intense mental exaltation with great excitement, complete loss of self-control, with at times absolute incoherence of speech and loss of consciousness and memory (Clouston.)—**M., acute delirious** (*acutus*; *deliro*, I am insane). A psychosis of sudden onset, attended with increased bodily temperature, and marked by delirium with sensory hallucinations, marked incoherence, restlessness, refusal of food, loss of memory, and rapid bodily wasting, terminating frequently in death. (*See* ACUTE DELIRIOUS MANIA.)—**M., alcoholic.** (*See* ALCOHOLISM.)—**M., amenorrhoeal** (*ἀ*, neg; *μήν*, a month; *ῥοία*, a flow). A term employed by Skae in his causation classification of mental affections. (*See* AMENORRHOEAL INSANITY.)—**M. a pathemate** (*a*, from; *πάθημα*, a calamity or catastrophe.) (*See* EMPATHEMA.)—**M. a potu** (*a*, from; *potus*, drink). Madness following, or due to alcoholic abuse. Also a synonym of Delirium Tremens (*q.v.*).—**M., asthenic** (ἀ, neg.; σθένος, strength). Mania in which there is a general anæmic state with nervous debility and consequent irritative excitement.)—**M. a temulentia** (*a*, from; *temulentia*, drunkenness). A synonym of Delirium Tremens.—**M., cardiac** (καρδία, the heart.) A form of insanity occurring in the course of heart disease (Fr. *manie cardiaque.*) (*See* CARDIAC DISEASE IN THE INSANE.)—**M., chronic** (χρονικός, pertaining to time). A condition of mental exaltation in which the acute symptoms have run into a chronic course, and in which exacerbations of restlessness, excitability, and destructiveness may occur without any marked physical objective symptoms.—**M., congestive** (*congestus*, heaped up). A form of insanity characterised by marked impairment of the intellect from the beginning, with confusion of ideas and incoherence of language; the delusions are sometimes of an exalted, and at other times of a depressed, nature; there is muscular weakness and perceptive dulness. (Fr. *manie congestive.*)—**M. contaminationis** (*contaminatio*, defilement). (*See* MYSOPHOBIA.) —**M. crapulosa** (*crapula*, drunkenness). A synonym of Dipsomania.—**M., dancing.** A psychopathy of hysterical origin spreading like an epidemic, being induced by imitation and sympathy, in which dancing of the most grotesque and extravagant character formed the most prominent symptom. It arose in Germany in the twelfth century, spreading thence to Aix-la-Chapelle, and from that city to the Netherlands. Occurring generally among women, the attack usually commenced with convulsions of an epileptiform character, on recovery from which the patients commenced singing and leaping about, contorting their bodies most violently, until they fell down completely exhausted, their senses all the while being apparently dead to surrounding impressions. A tympanitic distension of the abdomen accompanied by pain followed the attack, which in mild cases then terminated. In the more severe attacks a species of temporary furor would then seize the patients who dashed themselves against walls, or flung themselves into rivers. Similar quasi-maniacal attacks have been recorded as occurring among the ancients, and were subsequently common in Italy (Hirsch). (*See* EPIDEMIC INSANITY; JUMPERS; &c.)—**M., delusional** (*deludo*, I mock at). The form of mental affection in which maniacal conduct is associated with some fixed delusion.—**M. embriosa** (*ebriosus*, given to drinking). A synonym of Dipsomania.)—**M., ephemeral** (ἐφήμερος, living only a day). A rare form of mental exaltation which is sudden in its onset, acute in its character, and accompanied by incoherence, partial or complete unconsciousness of familiar surroundings, sleeplessness, and frequently a tendency towards homicide. An attack may last from an hour up to a few days. It occurs mostly in the subjects of epilepsy, or in such as are subject to the Jacksonian form of epilepsy; others are examples of the *epilepsie larvée* of Morel, the mental explosion taking the place of an ordinary epileptic fit; others are young persons with a strong neurotic heredity, and it is therefore found among hysterical girls and youths (Clouston). (*See* TRANSITORY MANIA.)—**M., epileptiform.** (*See* INSANITY, EPILEPTIC.)—**M., erotic.** (*See* INSANITY, EROTIC.) — **M., feigned.** (*See* FEIGNED INSANITY.)—**M., furious** (*furiosus*). A synonym of Acute Mania. The fully developed or violent stage of mania.—**M. gravis** (*gravis*, heavy, serious). A synonym of Acute Delirious Mania.—**M. hallucinatoria** (*q.v.*) (*hallucinari*, to wander in mind). A form of mania in which visual, auditory, olfactory, and other sense hallucinations predominate.—**M., histrionic.** (*See* HISTRIONIC MANIA.)—**M., homicidal.** (*See* INSANITY, HOMICIDAL; INSANITY, IMPULSIVE.) — **M., hysterical.** (*See* MANIA, HYSTERICAL.)—**M., incomplete.** A synonym of Manie Raisonnante.—**M., incomplete primary.** An abnormal state of the emotions and sentiments without marked intellectual affection.—**M. intermittens** (*intermitto*, lit., I send between; I leave off for a while). Mania which presents a succession of attacks during the intervals of which the patient appears well. (*See* MALARIA AND INSANITY.)—**M., joyous.** Mental exaltation with hilarious lightheartedness. (Fr. *manie gaie*; Ger. *Chäromanie*). (*See* CHÆROMANIA.) — **M. lactea** (*lacteus*, milky). A name given to puerperal insanity in allusion to the idea that it was caused by a metastasis of milk to the head. Also used as a synonym of Lactational Insanity. (*See* PUERPERAL INSANITY.) — **M. melancholica** (*melancholia*). A synonym of Melancholia. — **M. menstrualis.** (*See* MENSTRUATION.) — **M. metaphysica** (τὰ μετὰ τὰ φυσικά). A term for a form of mental disease characterised by a fidgety questioning of the why and wherefore of everything. (Ger. *Grübelsucht.*)—**M. metastatica** (μετάστασις, a being transformed or changed). Insanity following the arrest of an accustomed discharge, or the suppression of a rash.—**M., moral.** (*See* MORAL INSANITY.)—**M., partial moral.**

The intense activity of some one passion or propensity and its predominance or complete mastery over every other. (*See* KLEPTOMANIA; INSANITY (EROTIC); PYROMANIA; DIPSOMANIA; &c.)—**M. pellagria.** (*See* PELLAGRA.)—**M. periodica** (περιοδικός, coming round at intervals). A form of mania which returns at intervals. The term has also been used as a synonym of Folie circulaire. (*See* INSANITY, PERIODIC.)—**M. postmenstrualis** (*post*, after; *menstrualis*, the monthly flow). The form of insanity which occurs just after the menstrual period. (*See* MENSTRUATION AND INSANITY.)—**M. potatorum** (*potator*, a toper). A synonym of Delirium Tremens.—**M. praemenstrualis** (*prae*, before; *menstrualis*, the monthly flow). The form of insanity which occurs just before the menstrual period. (*See* MENSTRUATION AND INSANITY.)—**M., puerperal.** (*See* PUERPERAL INSANITY.)—**M. puerperarum acuta** (*puerpera*, a lying-in woman; *acutus*, sharp). A synonym of Insanity, Puerperal.)—**M., reasoning** (Fr. *raison*). A synonym of Insanity, Moral. (Fr. *folie raisonnante*.)—**M., recurrent** (*re*, back again; *curro*, I run). The form of mania indistinguishable in its symptoms from ordinary mental exaltation, which shows a tendency towards relapse without, as in *folie circulaire*, the intervention of some other mental disturbance. Also used by some as a synonym of Folie Circulaire.—**M., senile** (*senilis*, pertaining to an old man). Mania, the result of senile arterial degeneration and brain changes, or the mental exaltation, whatever its cause, occurring in the aged.—**M., simple** (*simplex*). A state of mental exaltation of mild character marked by restlessness, loquacity, partial loss of self-control, foolishness of conduct, &c., persisting for some time, and unattended with incoherence or marked excitability.—**M. sine delirio** (*sine*, without; *delirium*, madness). A synonym of Moral Insanity. (Fr. *manie sans délire; folie raisonnante*).—**M., sthenic** (σθένος, strength, vigour). Mania in which there is a general hyperæmic condition with an excess of nervous energy.—**M., suicidal.** (*See* SUICIDAL INSANITY.)—**M., symptomatic** (σύμπτωμα, an occurrence). The form of mania caused by some other disease, of which it is as it were a symptom.—**M., systematised** (σύστημα, an organised whole). A synonym of Monomania. (Fr. *manie systématisée*.)—**M. transitoria** (*transitorius*, having a passage). (*See* TRANSITORY MANIA.)

MANIA (Gr. *μανία*) is a term which appears to have been in use from the earliest period in the history of medicine. It has borne throughout very much its modern significance, expressed briefly in the old English synonym of furious madness. It is true that it has from time to time, most recently by Skae, been used in a sense covering every variety of insanity, but this usage has never been regarded as quite defensible, and the modern tendency certainly is to restrict the meaning of mania to a form of acute insanity having more or less definite limitations, and exhibiting certain groups of symptoms more or less distinctly marked. In this sense we use the word.

Mania calls for detailed study as one of the great types of mental disease. Not only is mania itself a common condition, but states resembling it occur as intercurrent (episodic) phases of almost every other mental affection.

Definition.—Mania may be defined as being an affection of the mind characterised by an acceleration of the processes connected with the faculty of imagination (perception, association, and reproduction), together with emotional exaltation, psychomotor restlessness, and an unstable and excitable condition of the temper.

The typical maniac presents a rapid flow of ideas, with inability to fix the attention, producing apparent or perhaps real incoherence. He exhibits unmeaning gaiety, passing into uproarious hilarity; he is constantly in motion; his temper, though variable, always tends towards excitement, and is easily roused to the extreme of fury.

The older notion that mania is a, so to speak, sthenic disease, and that its phenomena correspond to a genuine increase of functional activity, must be regarded as incorrect. The restlessness, mental and motor, of mania is rather the analogue of a discharging lesion, and is no more to be considered a sign of strength than are the perhaps forcible movements of a limb affected with spasm. Dr. Clouston has pushed this analogy to the length of calling mania psychlampsia. Without pursuing the comparison too far, it may suffice to point out that the highest faculties of the mind as regards intellectual matters are judgment and the power of fixing the attention. As regards affective matters, the highest faculty is what we may briefly call balance. These mental powers are essentially of the nature of inhibition, and they are precisely the powers that are in abeyance in mania. The faculties that are exalted are faculties of the lower order. The result is the characteristic loss of control, together with an unstable and excitable emotional state, and extreme mobility in the imaginative sphere.

Analysis of Symptoms of Mania.

A. *General Bodily Symptoms.*—The general nutrition is markedly affected, especially in cases of a severe type or of any considerable duration. In cases that never pass beyond maniacal exaltation (*vide infra*), and sometimes in the earlier stages of mild mania, the muscular tone appears to be really increased, and the patients assume a bright, sharp intelligent look which may perhaps not be natural to them, and which fades out on recovery. But this condition is usually very temporary, and in severe cases never appears. The patient in the early stage tends to rapidly lose flesh and remains meagre. The skin often becomes dry and shrivelled, which partly accounts for the aged appearance that cases of mania soon put on. Or the skin is more rarely greasy and clammy. It is observed that the violent exertions of the maniac are not accompanied by an abundant flow of perspiration, and that it is difficult to get the sweat glands to act. In very many cases the hair becomes rough and bristling. In unfavourable cases there is a tendency of the nails to become brittle, and there is a great liability to the occurrence of othæmatoma. The appetite is capricious. In very early conditions there may be little care for food, and meals may be neglected, but the general tendency is towards voracity, increasing if the case become chronic. In spite, however, of a ravenous appetite, the patient does not gain flesh as long as his state remains purely maniacal. The tongue is rarely healthy; usually coated with white fur in the early stages; it either remains foul or assumes a red irritable appearance, and often presents glazed patches. It is generally stated that the bowels are confined. This is not so as a rule. In some early cases, especially in women, and in cases of a distinctly hysterical type, there is a tendency towards extreme constipation, and frequent purgation may be required; but in a very large number of cases of mania the bowels tend to be rather more active than in health.

In women the menstrual functions are almost always disordered. The menses are often absent during the continuance of an attack of acute mania, and are usually scanty and irregular. In very many cases the menstrual period is always associated with an exacerbation of mental trouble. Violent, dangerous, destructive, and indecent tendencies are aggravated at that time, and a large number of women then show a liability towards insane impulse, absent at other times. Self-mutilation, which is so generally associated with sexual disturbance in both sexes, is most apt to occur in women who are menstruating. The return of the menstrual function, after its suspension, may be either a good or bad prognostic sign according as it is or is not accompanied by amelioration of mental symptoms. If not speedily followed by mental improvement, restoration of the menses removes one element of hope, and often precedes the passage into chronic alienation.

In many cases salivation is a well-marked symptom, passing off when there is a temporary improvement in the mental state, and returning with an exacerbation of mental excitement.

The pulse in very early states may be full and bounding, but it tends to become small, and often remains remarkably slow even though the patient is incessantly restless.

Temperature is normal, or in severe cases subnormal. Elevation of temperature in mania means either the setting up of gross cerebral mischief with passage into acute delirium, or the approach of an intercurrent inflammatory affection.

Early maniacal cases exhibit a proneness to contract acute intercurrent diseases. Whitlow and other acute suppurations often follow trifling injuries or occur without apparent exciting cause. Anthrax is not unfrequent. Erysipelas, if prevalent, is specially apt to attack such cases. It has been frequently observed that the occurrence of an illness accompanied by much pain or fever, or suppuration, will sometimes cut short, or appear to cut short, a maniacal attack. Whether this phenomenon results from altered conditions of the circulation (and perhaps of the blood itself), or whether it is a mere effect of "shock," may be questioned.

Insomnia is always a marked feature in mania. In many cases there appears to be hardly any sleep for almost incredible periods, and that although the patient is at the same time wearing himself out by every form of restlessness. Without a doubt, absence of sleep contributes to bring about the characteristic wasting, and is an element of danger through its liability to lead to exhaustion.

B. *Special Nervous and so-called Psychical Symptoms.*—Exaltation shows itself in the sensory sphere by an apparent hyperæsthesia. How far this is real may be questioned. The general sensibility in many cases no doubt seems increased in early stages of mania, but later on there are indications that a degree of bluntness of this sense, and also of smell and taste supervenes. Thus the patient, whose skin seemed at first so sensitive that he found his clothes irksome, will afterwards endure the cold of a winter's night while he roams his room naked, or will smear himself with irritating and loathsome substances in a manner that a person with normal senses hardly could endure. Occasionally one meets with instances in which the acute maniac seems indifferent to pain, moving a broken limb or an inflamed joint in a manner that would be impossible to a sane person. Now and again one finds traces of that singular perversion of sense which a recent German teacher calls *Freudenschmerz*, wherein a patient seems to find a distinct pleasure in inflicting severe injuries upon himself. It is probable that this condition is by no means unknown in hysteria.

With regard to the senses of hearing and sight, increased acuity in the perception of sense impressions certainly exists. Attention is lively and sharp though entirely unstable. The acute maniac appears to see and hear better than a sane person because every impression tells upon him. As regards capacity for perception, he is continually in a state similar to that of the sane man who is intently looking or listening with a purpose. Everything attracts his notice. In the ordinary lives of all of us thousands of impressions are daily made upon our senses which never reach the higher centres, or, if they do, make so little impression there that they can only be recalled by an effort or imperfectly, or for a very short time after the perception is registered. This, of course, is in some degree accounted for by pre-occupation, but not altogether, for the absent-minded sane person does not exhibit the apparent increase of sensibility shown by the maniac, while, on the other hand, anger sometimes, and mental perturbation or anxiety frequently, will develop temporarily in the sane, a similar condition to that which is so markedly produced in the earlier conditions of alcoholic and other intoxications.

The filling of the mind with an enormous number of sense impressions, the blurring as it were of the mental canvas by the superposition of a crowd of details without the due and normal foreshortening and proportional distribution account in a great degree for the confusion of memory which is one of the ordinary phenomena of an attack of mania.

This sharpness of perception, together with abandonment of the usual restraints on the expression of whatever thoughts or feelings are called up by surrounding objects, produces occasionally an appearance of wit and smartness which is, however, very superficial. The maniac is incapable of any sustained mental effort, because he cannot fix his attention. He is unable to add anything to his stock, and his mind runs in a very narrow groove. The talk of such a man, if he have been clever and educated may, in case it remain tolerably coherent, seems sparkling at first, but it soon wearies. There is no real production, and no genuine mental activity. Together with increased perceptive power and inability to fix the attention, there is a marked increase of rapidity in the association of ideas. This, in mild cases, heightens the notion of wit which the conversation may produce. Sometimes the ideas tend very decidedly to arrange themselves along lines of mere verbal assonance: a word calls up another of similar sound, the latter, again, another more or less alike, and so on. This condition may perhaps be related to a state of special activity of the centre for perception of sound. In other cases objects seen appear to serve chiefly as the starting-point of trains of ideas which change rapidly with slight changes in the visual surroundings. But in most cases no special form of association predominates.

Incoherence in conversation is a very striking and important symptom in cases of mania. It depends chiefly on accelerated association of ideas. Thought is always so much more rapid than speech that in communing with ourselves we habitually use a species of mental shorthand. People who talk to themselves aloud probably always seem incoherent to those who hear them and who are unable as one usually would be to supply many apparently dropped links in the chain, for we can seldom know what lines of association connect diverse ideas in the mind of another person. In mania, association is much accelerated, the attention is unfixed, sensory impressions are acutely perceived, and a strong tendency exists to give immediate utterance to every passing thought; therefore apparent incoherence naturally results. This is the form of incoherence common in acute mental disease. If one is sufficiently interested to listen carefully, one will often be able to discover the clue to much which at first seemed entirely disconnected. Absolute incoherence of ideas is certainly very much rarer. It is a phenomenon not easily intelligible, since to the sane a succession of ideas without any connection is probably impossible, but it does seem to occur in severe cases of primary mania, as well as in cases of secondary mania (*i.e.*, acute mental disease that has passed into a state of chronic excitement with dementia).

Combined with motor restlessness and accelerated association rate, and closely connected with increased sensory receptivity, there is found the symptom of garrulity. Thereby incoherence is emphasised, and the hurrying flow of ideas is betrayed. The maniac is almost always talkative, nay, almost always talking. Gaiety, indignation, anger, find their vent in constant speech. The tendency to give voice to every emotion and every idea is, of course, in strict conformity to the general mental exaltation. Garrulity is often the earliest indication of the oncome of an attack, whether of primary or of recurrent mania. That vague term "excitement," so frequently used in describing the condition of the maniac, generally resolves itself into garrulity with motor restlessness.

Exaltation in the emotional sphere, though a symptom of varying intensity, is important as being very constant and as giving its special tone to the maniacal state. Emotional exaltation shows itself in two forms, which may be, and generally are, associated together. One is exhibited in gaiety, varying from mere levity to the most unbounded hilariousness; the other in irritability of temper, which similarly varies from the mere mood in which a man conceives that he does well to be angry up to a state of ungovernable fury. However the older descriptions of mania may have been tinctured with results of mismanagement and inhumanity rather than with the true colours belonging to the disease, there can be no doubt that furious madness is not altogether a misnomer as applied to acute mania. Yet in this state we do not see the outbursts of utterly blind destructive fury with profound engagement of consciousness which occur in epileptic insanity. In average cases the temper is more irritable than constantly exalted; it is, as it were, vigilant. The patient is hyperæsthetic, trifling excitation produces undue discharge. To use Dr. Savage's apt phrase, it is a word and a blow with him, and the blow comes first. In some cases bad temper and quarrelsomeness so far predominate as to be a special feature in the ailment. Usually they are somewhat less prominent than the accompanying hilarity. The association of these two states is in itself a morbid indication. In health, good humour and high spirits are associated. All things please the man who is pleased with himself, and irritability of temper subsides when the mood becomes gay.

With regard to the emotional exaltation of the maniac, it has been questioned whether this is a primary condition or whether, according to Mendel, it is merely the result of increased rapidity of thought and lack of control, producing a joyous feeling of freedom, strength, and well-being.

Though the emotional exaltation and the acceleration of the functions of mental reproduction seem in many cases to be merely opposite sides of the medal, yet it is to be noted as against Mendel's view that the former is often out of all proportion to the latter, and that in the worst cases, when excitement, imaginative bustle, and the rush of ideas are constant, there is often little trace left of the earlier emotional exaltation. The feelings are probably comparable in such a case to those of a man in a feverish dream, conscious indeed of perpetual movements and incessant thought, but finding therein only weariness and irritation, not by any means joy.

A case of mania may run through its course without the appearance of hallucination. Usually in the typical form, however, hallucinations of vision or of hearing occur at one time or other. More rare are hallucinations of the other senses. Illusions are common. Delusions connected with hallucination, or originating spontaneously, occur. The general characteristic of these phenomena is that they are conformable to the emotional state. Hallucinations are in the main of a pleasurable nature, and delusions are usually of the exalted type. In fact, the genesis of the delusion often appears to be an effort of the mind to account, as it were, for the exalted emotional state, a typifying or allegorisation in definite form of the essential maniacal condition. Delusions occurring in mania are to be distinguished from those of paranoia (delusional insanity) by the absence of systematisation, and of that peculiar fixity and limited range which give its special character to the latter affection. On the other hand, the exalted ideas of the maniac have neither the exuberance, the constant variability, nor the essential incoherence which betray the entire mental breakdown of general paralysis of the insane.

A very common symptom in maniacal conditions is erotic excitement. This varies from a mere coquetry, a somewhat extended application of the command "love one another," an undue attention to the opposite sex, and so forth, up to the extreme of salacity, when the mind is wholly occupied by the urgent sexual appetite, and all restraint is abandoned (*see* NYMPHOMANIA; SATYRIASIS; &c.). It is needless here to dwell upon the well-marked signs of sexual excitement, but it is of some importance to recognise the lesser conditions of this state. In milder cases a little more fondness for dress and ornament than usual, a tendency to talk on questionable subjects, and a smirking, affected manner will often give the clue to the existence of these feelings. So will, in women, a tendency to excessive love of scandal, a liability to suspect every one about them of misbehaviour, complaints of the misconduct of other women, and so forth. A tendency to protestations of the patient's personal purity, together with an over-energetic and often dirtily expressed abhorrence of uncleanness points in the same direction. In more marked conditions nestling in the hair, peeping through the fingers, and peculiar restless movements form the transition to downright indecency of gesture and act.

Closely connected with salacity, particularly in women, is religious excitement. For obvious reasons many maniacs are fond of talking of religious matters, and exalted delusions naturally often take a religious form. But, besides this, there is a large class of cases in which religious emotion occupies or seems to occupy the entire imagination. Ecstasy, as we see it in cases of acute mental disease, is probably always connected with sexual excitement if not with sexual depravity. The same association is constantly seen in less extreme cases, and one of the commonest features in the conversation of an acutely maniacal woman is the intermingling of erotic and religious ideas.

Many cases of mania exhibit a strong tendency to masturbation. The whole subject of this vice occurring in the insane is elsewhere dealt with (*see* MASTURBATION). It suffices here to say that the occurrence of self-abuse in acute cases is not necessarily of bad prognostic import, nor indication of any special ætiological factor. It seems in such cases to depend on a temporary exaltation of the sexual sensations and appetites with loss of control, or it is perhaps to be regarded as a primary perversion of instinct. In this light we may also probably regard certain other dirty acts of the maniacal. Most lunatics are untidy in personal habits from loss of the finer sense of propriety. Many again are dirty from negligence, but there are also cases of pseudo deliberate filthiness, which are not easy to account for unless on the supposition that the natural instincts are perverted. Such patients will eat their own fæces, or smear their bodies and their rooms with excrementitious substances. The tendency to these disgusting forms of filthiness is often combined with sexual excitement and masturbation. This combination is particularly likely to occur in young hysterical women.

Many patients suffering from acute mania are apt to undress themselves. This habit appears to be in some cases connected with uneasy sensations in the skin (hyper- and paræsthesiæ), in some with more or less definite sexual notions (exposure, solicitation, &c.), in others it is a mere form of general restlessness. It is apt to be accompanied by a tendency to destructiveness (*see* DESTRUCTIVE IMPULSES).

Course of the Disease.—A so-called prodromal stage of melancholia has been described by many authors as always preceding mania, at least in cases of first attack. It is probable that the importance of this symptom has been exaggerated. No doubt we very often find a state of mental depression with or without hypochondriacal dreads occurring as a precursor to acute mania. But this is certainly in many cases the mere physiological expression of the fact that the patient is conscious of a certain illness which he may or may not recognise as chiefly affecting his mind. The consciousness of increasing loss of mental control must necessarily be an exceedingly depressing feeling. Excluding such a condition, the cases are comparatively few in which prodromal melancholia is a well-marked stage in the inception of mania.

Digestive troubles, with loss of sleep, are usually the first symptoms that attract notice. In the early stage there is very often headache. The temper becomes irritable, the patient grows restless, and after a brief period true maniacal exaltation appears. Rarely, this remains the condition throughout. More often excitement rapidly increases into typical mania, which may then, or later, pass into grave mania. These phases require brief individual consideration. In maniacal exaltation, though there is wasting, there is less bodily disturbance than in other conditions of mania. The characteristic acceleration of mental processes is present, but in a minor degree. The patient sleeps little, is restless, changeable, full of plans and projects, unable to settle down to anything, bustling, talkative, noisy, but only slightly if at all incoherent. All his acts are dictated as he imagines by distinct motives, and he is capable of giving a plausible reason for his most foolish actions. Episodically, he is highly passionate, and he is easily moved to indignation and tears. His restlessness often shows itself in strange acts of vagabondage, for which he finds ingenious reasons. He is lavish in expense, often benevolent in an extravagant way, furious if he is thwarted, but full of self-satisfaction throughout. He interferes in matters in which he has no concern, or formerly had no interest. He expresses with exuberant energy the most exaggerated opinions about everything. Opposition or laughter may infuriate, they never suppress him. In minor matters he disregards the ordinary rules of society, or believes himself to be superior to their consideration. He often engages in wild matrimonial projects, or exhibits marked amatory tendencies with little restraint. He frequently also indulges in intoxicants with very undue or unwonted freedom, and thereby precipitates the course and aggravates the symptoms of his disease. Such patients in modern times are the eager though turbulent followers of every "crank" who has a crazy view or project to promulgate; they often throw themselves into politics, and many of them expend incredible energy in writing to the newspapers, or to people high up in the political and social world, to secure the redress of grievances, personal or public, and to generally aid in reforming society.

This, or a similar condition, seems to be almost permanent in some cases, forming one of the phases of *folie raisonnante*. It is also common in recurrent insanity. In acute primary mania it is rare save as a stage in the beginning, or towards the end of the affection.

The general symptoms of typical mania have been already discussed. It is only necessary now to say that it differs from maniacal exaltation by presenting an engagement of consciousness. The typical maniac is not merely restless and talkative with a supposed motive, he is restless or noisy for mere noise and motion's sake. In other words, excitation passes into movement without the intervention of the reasoning ego. These are the cases also in which incoherence, real or apparent, is marked. These cases exhibit hallucinations and delusions. They are liable to variations of temper and emotional state partly through the influence of delusions. They sometimes exhibit an almost constantly furious state of temper. In typical mania sleep may be absent for lengthened periods, and it is always profoundly disturbed. After an attack of maniacal exaltation it usually occurs that the patient's memory for the events of his illness is perfect. In typical mania, on the other hand, the memory is commonly lost from an early period of the attack, and the patient remembers only what occurred from a date corresponding to the subsidence of maniacal symptoms. Or the recollection may exist but only in a vague summary way.

In grave mania consciousness is more profoundly clouded, movements are more entirely objectless, and the mental state approaches that of acute delirious mania (*q.v.*), to which *mania gravis* seems to form a transition, and into which it sometimes passes. The patient has lost the distinctive emotional tone of ordinary mania. He is indifferent when left to himself, but may be passionate and intensely violent if disturbed. He lives seemingly in the passing moment. His whole mental field is filled with hallucinations and delusions. He does not know where he is, nor always who he is. He answers without seeming to attach any significance to his words, and probably when asked a question several times answers each time differently, and quite from the purpose. He babbles to himself sometimes noisily, sometimes more quietly with little or no traceable coherence. He is dirty, destructive, and regardless of all that goes on around him. His nutrition is profoundly interfered with (*vide supra*) and he wastes rapidly. When this state gradually develops from typical mania it usually goes on to death by exhaustion. The other terminations of mania are:—

(1) **Recovery.** This is most hopeful in cases of typical mania; less so in maniacal exaltation, and in the latter case specially liable to be followed by relapse. *Mania gravis* is always of serious prognostic import, yet perfect recovery does occasionally occur. It is usually found that recovery from any form of mania is preceded by a state of dulness. The patient passes from excitement into a state resembling mild dementia before he begins to return to his original condition. This appears to be due to mere exhaustion. Occasionally one sees a state of mild melancholic depression following a favourable case of mania, but this is not nearly as common as dulness. Recovery may take place with a certain permanent mental enfeeblement (the *Heilung mit Defekt* of Neumann). The patient is fit to rejoin society, and is sane, but he is not the man he was. He is on a lower level, be it intellectually, emotionally or morally, and he never regains the *status quo ante*.

(2) **Passage into Chronic Weak-mindedness.**—Patients who do not recover, and who do not die early either of exhaustion or of some intercurrent affection, tend to fall into chronic dementia (*q.v.*), or into what is called chronic mania. With the latter affection there is associated a considerable degree of permanent loss of mental power, so that it is really a state closely akin to chronic dementia. However, it may for descriptive purposes be differentiated by the retention of delusion. The delusions of this state are unsystematised and highly incoherent. The emotional state has ceased to be active. Patients of this class, though often noisy and sometimes passionate, are very frequently tractable, able to do simple work, and when under proper supervision are much saner in their acts than in their words.

Conolly Norman.

MANIA A POTU. (*See* Delirium Tremens.)

MANIA HALLUCINATORIA (Mendel).—Under the name "mania hallucinatoria" Mendel describes a tolerably well marked variety of insanity, the clinical recognition of which is of some importance. It is usually comparatively sudden in its oncome. It is the most frequent form in which insanity appears after acute diseases, fevers, child-birth, &c. It is common in acute alcoholism. The writer has also found this type of disease occurring with phthisis, and other wasting affections, and has noted its association with nostalgia.

Symptoms.—The affection, according to Mendel, is ushered in by a brief period of insomnia, or disturbed sleep. Then the patient becomes restless, cries and laughs unmeaningly, wanders aimlessly about, has usually a sudden outburst of violence or destructiveness, and rapidly passes into incoherence with lively and varying hallucinations of one or more senses, accompanied by and giving rise to delusions of grandeur or of persecution, or more commonly of both mixed. Hallucinations of taste and smell in the earlier stage very commonly originate the ideas that there is poison or dirt in the food, that suffocating vapours are being applied, &c. Hallucinations of sight are the most prominent in the fully developed stage, and are often of a terrifying nature. The emotional state is not exalted, it is variable, confused, a prey to hallucination and delusional impressions, but without any persisting tendency to elevation. Superficially it would seem as if the hallucination gave colour to the emotional state, and not *vice versâ*, as in other forms of mania. Of course, both phenomena being subjective have essentially the same origin, and are not to be separated any more than the two sides of a coin. The real point is this, that in the condition under consideration the mental state is constantly varying. There is a continual activity of a sort, but without a set in any special direction.

Naturally, the concomitant of this state, or rather it would be more correct to say a portion of this state, is confusion in the intellectual sphere. Incoherence results in this affection, not so much from mere want of attention or over-rapidity of association, as from exuberant hallucinations perpetually breaking connection. German authors who have written since the appearance of Mendel's memoir, have generally inclined to treat confusion, and not hallucination, as the characteristic phenomenon. Under the name "verwirrtheit" (confusion) Meynert describes an affection which includes *mania hallucinatoria*. The "confusional stupor" of Dr. Hayes Newington is closely akin to the latter affection, and no doubt must be grouped as a sub-division of the former. Krafft-Ebing, by the name he gives to a group of cases (*Wahnsinn*), emphasises the prevalence of delirium, but in his description of the state he attributes more importance, and ascribes more generality, to confusion as a symptom. No doubt the mania hallucinatoria of Mendel belongs to a large class of cases which connect typical acute mania with stupor on the one hand and with delusional insanity on the other.

Prognosis and Course.—A case of well marked mania hallucinatoria, is, on the whole, hopeful, but exception must, of course, be made for those cases in which the disease is associated with serious or incurable general illness (phthisis and so forth). Attacks are sometimes very brief, menstrual cases occasionally approaching to *mania transitoria*. Rarely, cases pass into a state resembling grave mania or acute delirious mania and terminate in death.

Mendel draws attention to the fact that patients suffering from this affection are just those in whom most frequently there remains after recovery, or during episodes of partial lucidity, an accurate recollection of their numerous hallucinations.

Conolly Norman.

MANIA, HYSTERICAL. — The phrase "hysterical mania" has been used to denote insanity associated with disturbance of the reproductive organs in women, and has also been applied to the forms of insanity that follow long-continued hysteria; in neither case very correctly. Insanity which accompanies sexual affections is often not maniacal, and alienation following long-continued hysteria more commonly belongs to the paranoiac type. But there is a form of mania characterised clinically by certain features which justify us in using the term in a merely descriptive sense.

Symptoms. — Weakness, with irritability, is the fundamental note of the hysterical character. Irritable weakness, long recognised as the basis of many functional nervous affections, has become more comprehensible by the aid of recent theories of brain action. The higher centre is weak: the lower unduly active, perhaps from direct irritation, perhaps merely because the controlling (higher) centre is enfeebled. Hence the tendency to convulsion, the emotional instability, the sensitiveness, the desire for imitation, and the other well-known symptoms of hysteria. All forms of mania seem to have, in common with hysteria, the element of irritable weakness. It is, therefore, not to be wondered at that some cases should present features common to both conditions.

The sufferer from hysterical mania, in our sense of the word, is exceedingly emotional. The pain of melancholia is unknown, the appearance of depression is very shallow. A trifling and passing depressive emotion is responded to by instant tears, perhaps with loud outcry, and by a great display of grief, but the feeling is quite temporary. There is a certain hyperæsthesia showing itself by a too quick response to every emotional irritation, without any permanent substratum of painful feeling. In a similar way there is a sharp irritability of temper without the constant state of anger which will sometimes occur in other forms of mania. The entire emotional state is unstable in the extreme, and the expression of emotion bears a peculiar whimsical and uncertain character, such as is also seen in the entire conduct of the patient. Impulse is very apt to be translated into action with alarming rapidity. Impulse and whim sometimes rise almost to the dignity of ruling motives in a mind incapable of forming any fixed resolution.

Connected with impulse is the so-called imperative concept. The phenomenon is very common in hysterical cases. It takes the form either of a sudden feeling that such and such an act must be performed, or of a more or less abstract idea invading the mind without apparent associative connection, and interrupting the ordinary train of thought. In many of these imperative ideas there is evidently, however, an association of which the patient is unconscious, which we might call the association of opposition. Thus, a patient of Obersteiner's could not behold the elevation of the host without the instant intrusion into his mind of a certain disgusting idea; and a young male patient of mine, an onanist of extremely hysterical character, complained that when he prayed he was tormented by imperative thoughts as to whether or not the B.V.M. obeyed natural calls like other people.

The association of opposites, to some degree, but not wholly, explains many acts of the hysterical maniac. Such cases, if the attack is not of a very mild type, are apt to be extraordinarily filthy. The dirtiness does not arise from mere carelessness, nor seemingly, as in many lunatics, from mere perversion of the natural instinct to cleanliness, but the hysterical patient often appears to be possessed of a passion for the dirty both in the moral and physical sense, and takes a special delight in nastiness of every sort. Here we find coprophagous patients, patients who smear themselves with fæces, urine, or menstrual fluid; patients who masturbate incessantly, or who sometimes adopt fantastic methods of self-abuse.

Intense egotism and an ever-wakeful self-consciousness are characteristic features of the condition under consideration. In everyday life the selfish egotism of the hysterical woman is well enough known. The morbid introspection and self-consciousness which lead to continual watching of physical and mental processes no doubt contribute to functional disturbance in both spheres. The self-consciousness of hysteria not only gives its peculiar note to many cases of mania, but has a very practical bearing on their treatment. If we can rouse the patient from the morbid state of introspection, &c., we have fulfilled the most important indication for cure. In a large number of cases thoughts and feelings connected with the activity of the sexual organs chiefly occupy the mind. In women the function of menstruation is very frequently interfered with. In men, irritable weakness of the sexual organs (or centre) is very common, leading to frequent pollutions, and so forth. The influence of masturbation in producing these conditions, and the mental disturbance accompanying them, has been probably exaggerated. No doubt self-abuse often exists in such cases, but it may be questioned which factor stands in a causal relation to the other. Certainly the brooding self-conscious state which is so characteristic of the hysterical is dangerously apt to lead to masturbation in persons who are not strong-minded. When the thoughts, especially of the young, are entirely turned inwards, the sexual element is certain to appear, and as the sexual function is eminently an altruistic one, the mere secret brooding and watching over it are in themselves morbid and injurious. There is no function so easily disturbed by attention as the sexual. Again, the activity of the sexual organs is probably in both sexes fundamentally periodic. The concentration of the attention on the genitalia, &c., by keeping up a constant, even though slight excitement, interferes with the rhythm and disturbs the action.

Other indications of morbid egotism are the love of notoriety and of histrionic display. Even when self-esteem assumes the guise of self-sacrifice and benevolence, the truly egotistical feelings which lie at the basis cannot be concealed. Not infrequently the hysterical maniac identifies himself with the Saviour of the world or some martyr or saint, and talks of sacrificing himself for the sins of others, of doing some great penance, or the like. Hysterical patients rarely commit suicide, and then more often from whim or love of attracting attention than from depression or in obedience to delusion. Much more frequent is the tendency to mutilation, which, indeed, should always be borne in mind in cases of this class. Mutilation is attempted with the idea of expiation, in the glow of religious excitement, under the notion that the flesh is being sacrificed, or some saintly example or scriptural precept is being followed, also with the view of attracting notice or exciting sympathy, and finally, from mere whim. The pudenda, for obvious reasons, are a frequent point of attack.

In milder cases, the feigning of illnesses which do not exist, and the concealment of existing ones are common. The same subtlety and deceitfulness which occur in the hysterical who are sane, are unfortunately not unknown among the class of hysterical maniacs.

Religious excitement is usually a prominent symptom, and is not uncommonly associated with a disgusting salacity. This combination is probably in part due to the mere association of opposition.

Religious excitement, with or without delusion, more commonly the former, often passes into ecstatic conditions which are sometimes ushered in by convulsions; or more rarely the period of ecstasy terminates in a convulsion. Ecstasy may pass into stupor (miscalled "acute dementia"), which may again pass off, giving way to maniacal symptoms.

Hysterical cases, though liable to impulsive outbursts of destructiveness and violence, do not exhibit the same degree of motor excitability as other maniacal patients. They are rather distinctively noisy and talkative than restless. The perpetual motion of the typical maniac only extends to the tongues of the hysterical. Their talk is particularly incoherent. It is apt to be chopped up into short sentences, often repeated over and over again with unmeaning persistence. It very often takes the interrogative form. A peculiar silliness is very common; a repeating over of childish words or sentences; a deliberate mal-position of the words of a sentence; a reckoning over of names, numbers, colours in a sort of catalogue, and so forth. Very often the semblance to the feigning of incoherence is very striking. A patient, who from her acts evidently understands what is said, will reply with silly sentences or exclamations entirely from the purpose, laughing and grimacing, then perhaps replying sensibly for a moment and passing again into the same state of silly incoherence or verbigeration. Some patients feign various emotions, fear, delight, &c. in quick succession. Others indulge in unmeaning attitudes and gestures, which become more marked when the patient perceives that they are observed. This attitudinising and histrionic display adds much to the odd appearance of not being in earnest, just referred to.

With regard to facial expression, traces of sexual excitement are generally very evident, especially in women.

Hysterical cases are particularly liable to suffer from constipation. On the whole their sleep is less disturbed than in proportionately severe cases of other forms of mania.

Hysterical symptoms may give their characteristic tone to cases of very varying degrees of severity, from maniacal excitement up to grave mania: but speaking generally, the graver cases are rare, and cases which are typically hysterical very seldom pass into that form of mania which is dangerous to life.

With regard to **ætiology**, the influence of sexual affections has been over-estimated. In many women a history of uterine disturbance is really only a history of hysteria. Nevertheless, sexual affections in both sexes sometimes seem to lead to this condition. Sexual excess is no doubt occasionally a cause, and incomplete sexual intercourse is specially liable to produce hysterical mania. Its relations to masturbation have been already dealt with. The writer has seen some exquisite cases in young men whose minds had given way under the terrors held over their heads by advertising quacks. Sudden fright and shock not uncommonly appear to be the immediate exciting cause in women. Seduction, and more particularly indecent assault, are often followed by insanity of this particular form.

In view of **prognosis**, and with reference to the course of the disorder, there is nothing specially unfavourable in hysterical mania occurring in a young woman or in an adolescent. In the former case, indeed, it is perhaps one of the most favourable as it is one of the commonest forms in which insanity appears. In later life hysterical symptoms form an element in a serious prognosis as to mental recovery. CONOLLY NORMAN.

MANIAC (Mid. E. *maniack*, from Lat. *mania*; Gr. *μανία*, madness). One suffering from mental exaltation. Also popularly one who is insane. (Fr. *maniaque*; Ger. *Tobsüchtig.*)

MANIACAL DELIRIUM (*deliro*, I am crazy); **MANIACAL FURY** (*furiosus*). Synonyms of Acute Mania.

MANIAS, FASTING.—From time to time a fasting mania attracts public attention, and the medical psychologist, if he is wise, will profit by the spectacle, so far as he can eliminate mere imposture.

> There is some soul of goodness in things evil.
> Would men observingly distil it out.

In 1890 and 1891, such manias occurred and were witnessed in London. We have looked back on our medical experience to see what knowledge it might afford on the question of fasters and fasting. We find from this review of the past that we have met with two clear examples of death by voluntary fasting. The latest of these is too near the present to allow me to give the details. The other, having occurred so far back as 1848, and having been recorded already in part, may now be rendered in the following report.

A Fast of Fifty-five Days.—A gentleman, about thirty-three years old, had often been subject to fits of depression and melancholy. He was a man of good social position, had somewhat distinguished himself in his scholastic life, and was always considered as extremely good-natured and thoughtful, though from his earliest age obstinate and self-willed. He was one of those of whom it is said that if "he took anything into his head nothing would turn him." He was not subjected at any time to much restraint; and, as he was comfortably provided for by a business which demanded but little personal attention, he really had as small occasion for anxiety as most men we have known. He read a great deal, cared nothing for out-door or athletic amusements, and was somewhat listless about the course of events, though he could usually be interested in political controversy, and up to his death was wont to speak on the state of political parties. He was not the only man of his turn of mind, in our experience, who, whilst brooding over his own infirmities, has been inclined to political discussion; but he perhaps showed this tendency more than others of his class. He was always nervous about himself, as we were told, and yet, at the same time, was ready-minded and even courageous in the face of sudden danger. In religion he was not enthusiastic, and his melancholy was untouched by any saddening religious sentiment; but he brooded over imaginary physical evils, which he almost invariably referred to the stomach, and he sought advice from men of all kinds who professed to practise medicine, having just as much faith in a pretentious quack or in the veriest old woman, as in the most regular professor, so long as his whim for liking them lasted. In a word, he became, as his friends said, a confirmed hypochondriac, a man to be pitied, and beyond hope of amendment.

In stature this gentleman was tall, we should say near upon six feet. In figure he was, naturally, very slight, and he was at all times a small eater. To the best of our recollection, he took no wine nor other alcoholic drink; if he took any, it was the smallest quantity; so that, though he would be under no pledge, nor connected with the total abstinence movement—which at the time was little considered—he was, practically, a total abstainer.

For many years the condition of this gentleman had continued the same. He was induced to try the effects of change of air and scene; but this he declared wearied him too much, and finally he settled down a confirmed invalid of the *malade imaginaire* type, pure and simple. In seeking one day advice from a professor of a schismatic school of physic, he gathered what he supposed to be an entirely new light as to the cause of his malady. The professor, very learned and imposing, detailed to the sufferer the ideas then prevailing as to the cause of primary digestion, from the experiments which Dr. Beaumont had conducted on that most interesting of physiological instructors, Alexis St. Martin. The history of the accidental shot which made St. Martin such a figure in history, the account of the opening into his stomach, and the notes that had been made from visual inspection of the process of digestion; the description of the gastric juice that was extracted; and the further explanation as to the solvent action of the gastric juice on food, became a perfect fascination for the anxious invalid;

and when the learned expositor improved the occasion by telling his patient that all this demonstrative argument was but a prelude to the grand inference he drew as to the patient's condition, the inference being no more nor no less than that the unfortunate patient could not possibly digest food because he produced no gastric juice, the impression produced was positive and unanswerable.

From that day, by a kind of logical determination which was, we may say at once, impossible to combat, so as to carry conviction to the mind of the sufferer, he maintained that, as he had no gastric juice, it was utterly useless for him to take nutriment of any kind except water, which required no digestion. The idea implanted in his mind held its place, and was never uprooted. Unfortunately, it was confirmed by the effects of a first attempt at reduction of food. The stomach, no doubt very feeble and irritable, was relieved by a reduction of food, and therewith the depression of mind was signally relieved, an occurrence by no means unusual, and perhaps a natural consequence.

Soon after his first attempt to reduce food to a minimum, there succeeded another stage, in which the desire for food appeared to pass away altogether. Then when, by a great effort and with much repugnance, food was taken, it caused pain, disturbance, and a greater depression than usual of mental power, with a more determined dislike to the process of feeding, and a firmer and deeper conviction of the truth of the hypothesis that he failed to produce digestive fluid.

In time there seemed to be an entire failure of desire for food; a loss of sense of taste; a loathing at the odour of food; an irritable objection to have the subject of feeding even spoken about; and, finally, a resolute determination not to take any more food at all unless appetite or desire for some particular kind or quality of food revisited him. From that moment the rigid fasting commenced. Of water he would partake readily, but not largely; for he said that in quantity it was heavy and cold, and caused painful distension. He would take it to allay thirst, and nothing more. For ten days, under this *régime*, he went about the house, and walked occasionally in the garden, refusing medical advice. After this he took to his bed, and declined to rise except to have the bed made. He now wished for medical attention, but was as resolute with his medical advisers against taking food as he was with the members of his family. Once an effort was made to feed him, perforce, with milk; but he resisted so determinately, and subjected himself to such danger by his resistance, that the attempt was not made a second time.

A great reduction of bodily weight occurred during the earlier stage of the process of fasting. He sank into the extremest state of emaciation during the first three to four weeks of his trial, after which he did not seem to us to undergo rapid change, although we saw him almost daily. He slept a great deal and at times he tried to read; but the effort of reading soon became wearisome and painful, and was never more than a mere listless occupation. He was not at any time irritable, except when pressed to take food, and he was fond of hearing the current topics of the day; but he soon became weary with conversation, and would drop off into a semi-somnolent state while conversing. We never heard him complain of any pain or discomfort; he did not seem to express or feel desire to live, and he certainly never expressed any desire to die.

As the last days of his life drew near he became much feebler rather suddenly, and his mind, we thought, was inclined to wander for brief intervals. But he quickly recovered himself, and on the day before his death he was unusually clear in his mind. He was painfully shrunken in feature; his voice was low, and almost bleating; his colour was leaden dark; his lips were blue and cold; his limbs were cold; and his breath was cold and offensive, having the odour of newly-opened clayey soil. On the morning of his death he, for the first time from the commencement of his fast, said that he would eat, and that which he wished for was fruit or raw vegetable, with cream. An attempt was made immediately to pacify his desire, under the hope that if he once recommenced to take food of one kind, he might be tempted to take more promising support; but it was of no avail, and in fact nothing was swallowed. Soon after this he sank into unconsciousness, and so succumbed. He died on the fifty-fifth day of his fast, having abstained from all food and partaken of no other drink than water for seven weeks and six days.

We had the opportunity of taking part in the post-mortem examination of this gentleman on the day immediately following upon his death. The emaciation was so extreme that he might almost be said to be a skeleton clothed in semi-transparent flesh. The outline of almost every bone could be traced. On opening the chest the lungs were found collapsed, and so shrunken that they looked like small and half-dried sponges, and divided by the knife rather like soft leather than pulmonary tissue. The heart was reduced to quite half its natural size, was empty of blood in all its cavities, and had its ventricles so attenuated that they resembled auricles rather than ventricles; whilst the auricles were mere shrivelled appendages that could not easily be separated from the ventricles as distinctive structures. The abdominal viscera were attenuated to the last degree; the stomach was reduced to a straight tube, and was with difficulty distinguishable from the duodenum. The intestinal canal was empty through its entire length; it was free of redness, abrasion, or ulceration, but the inner surface of the colon and the peritoneal surface presented a few dark spots, melanotic in type. The liver was reduced to half the normal size, and the gall bladder was empty and collapsed. The pancreas and spleen were so reduced in size they could hardly be made out, and the kidneys, although they showed no obvious sign of organic disease, were atrophied quite as much as the liver, and were separated, by shrinkage, from their capsules. The bladder was empty and shrunken.

Not a trace of fatty matter was found at any part, not even in the orbits. The muscles were flaccid, wasted, dry, and leathery to the touch.

On opening the skull cavity, the dura mater was found collapsed, dry, and loose, wanting entirely in tension; the arachnoid and pia mater could not be defined, and the sinuses were empty of blood. The cerebrum and cerebellum, like the other organs, were much shrunken; they were white and firm, resembling the same structures after long immersion in spirit. Between the grey and white matter there was no difference of tint.

The brain, which was dissected very carefully, yielded no obvious trace of acute organic mischief. The bulb of the olfactory nerve was reduced to a line on each side, and the optic nerves were atrophied; as were also the globes of the eyes themselves.

Altogether there was universal atrophy of structure, with dryness of every texture and absence of blood.

We have narrated the above details because they indicate most clearly the length of time during which fasting may be carried on in man under favourable circumstances, and the condition to which the body is reduced by fasting before it ceases to carry vitality.*

Lessons.—Bringing these facts to bear on the starvation ordeals which were commenced publicly in America by Dr. Tanner, and which have been continued in London, we may assume (1) *that a forty or forty-two days' fast with continuance of life is well within the order of natural phenomena*, and that the human body has a possible power of endurance from ten to eleven days beyond what has recently been attempted, *the extreme limit being fifty-three to fifty-five days.* It is right to dwell on this point, because the technical opinion on fasting that will have to be given in our coroner's courts, and in courts of justice, as well as the opinion that will have to be written in our technical and standard works of medical jurisprudence, must in future be considerably modified in many particulars. It has been accepted that, after a certain degree of starvation—a degree comparatively short after what is now known—any act requiring much physical exertion is impossible. A once famous medical jurist, whose lectures were always sound and practical, Dr. Cummin, related that a girl eighteen years of age was confined in the depth of winter in a closed room for twenty-eight days. She had with her a gallon of water, some pieces of bread, amounting to about a quartern loaf, and a mince pie; and she was said to have subsisted on this small quantity of food for the twenty-eight days without fire, and to have ultimately escaped from her prison by breaking down a window-shutter that had been nailed up, getting out of a window on to a roof below, and walking several miles, from Enfield Wash to Aldermanbury. In commenting on this feat, one of our most eminent authorities, the late Dr. Guy, expressed his disbelief; and he was confirmed in this opinion by Drs. Woodman and Tidy, who considered that while it is possible life might be prolonged, "in all the recorded cases the muscles have become so weak before half the time mentioned, that the sufferers could not even help themselves to water, much less walk this distance."

This opinion bearing on starving persons may apply to persons who would succumb easily; and it might possibly apply more distinctly to persons who have been subjected to starvation by force rather than to those who permit themselves voluntarily to undergo the infliction; but we must henceforth so far change the usually accepted canon as to admit a wide range of capacity for starvation amongst the various specimens of human kind. It seems clear that, where the disposition to

* In the Transactions of the Albany Institute for 1830 Dr. McNaughton reported a case of a precisely similar kind in a man named Kelsey, who died from self-starvation on the fifty-third day. Kelsey took more exercise than the patient we have referred to, and died, therefore, a little earlier, or rather existed a little shorter time.

starve goes with the starving, the powers of endurance are immensely prolonged. Nor is the psychology of this phenomenon peculiar. When the disposition for the starvation is present, when the will goes with the experiment, and when faith, by whatever it may be fanned, keeps hope and courage alive, the chances of continuance of life must be greatly increased. There is then neither wasting worry nor feverish desire for life; there is then none of that corroding fear and dread of death which so materially—we use the term in its physical meaning—favour dissolution.

Thus we should expect that men or women who voluntarily submit to starvation, and that men and women who in days of enforced starvation have most courage to endure, will endure the longest, and will recover with the greatest facility, if the chances of recovery be offered.

Fasting girls of the hysterical type, whether they succeed in secretly obtaining a small supply of food or not, are examples of this.

(2) *Sustaining Power of Water.* — A second lesson is that life may be long sustained by water alone, and that, in instances where a long period of existence is maintained on mere aqueous fluids, it is the water that sustains. In short, in a sense, water becomes a food. The knowledge of this truth is corrective of some of the most grievous and mischievous errors. Persons undergoing severe privation and fatigue, persons suffering from disease, persons suffering from repugnant dislike to animal and vegetable foods, have for long seasons been supplied with drinks of wine or of spirits and water. Forgetting the water altogether, or treating it as a thing of no consideration, they have declared—and others, even medical men, have declared for them—that they were sustained on alcohol, and therefore the alcohol was largely diluted with water. It was vain to urge that the Welsh miners, who, some years ago, were buried alive without solid food, were able to live ten days on water alone. It wanted such proofs as these we have now got to demonstrate the actual nature of the sustaining agent, and to exclude the agent alcohol, which, often obtaining all the credit, does more evil than good.

(3) *Treatment.*—A third lesson relates to the practice of treating patients who have long abstained from food. Here we may be guided by the experience gained in districts where famines most commonly prevail. Mr. Cornish, in his admirable report on a great famine in India, takes the utmost care to explain that the danger of the deficient food supply was comparatively small when there was any sufficient quantity of moisture. So long as fruits and herbs and plants of a succulent and wholesome kind could be obtained, so long there was strictly no famine. But when the juices of fruits and other succulent vegetable supplies of water were cut off, then indeed the people were famine-stricken with a vengeance. Mr. Cornish also refers to another fact—briefly, it is true, yet still with sufficient effect to show his meaning—that when the famine-stricken had passed a certain period of time without food or drink, when they had to a large extent lost the desire for food and drink, they frequently died even when the relief came and food was carefully supplied to them. He relates that in one instance he took a sufferer to his own home, and there, with the most scrupulous care, tried to restore life and health, but without avail; and he is led to explain that there is a period in a famine when all the foods that may come in are practically useless to the persons who are in hunger and athirst, and yet do not at first sight appear likely to die. This is the secondary effect of famine on the body; but, be it observed, it only occurs when, in addition to deprivation of solid food, there is also deprivation of fluid. Let the fluid be supplied in even small quantity, and, though the emaciation may be extreme, death may be averted, and the subjection of the stomach to new and proper aliment may lead to perfect restoration of life. For insane patients who have refused food it is most important to bear this in mind.

(4) *Lessons in Economy.*—Fourthly, a lesson is rendered to economic science. When we know how little food is really required to sustain life, we may the more readily surmise how very much more food is taken by most persons than can ever be applied usefully towards sustainment. We have no compunction in asserting that, while fasting enthusiasts are subjecting themselves to considerable danger from abstinence, hundreds of thousands of persons are subjecting themselves to a slower but equal danger from excesses of foods and drinks. These keep up their experiment, and, with every vessel in their bodies strained to repletion and seriously overtaxed, continue to replete and to strain the more. If we could induce, therefore, such persons to contemplate their proceedings, and to strike a fair comparison between their own foolhardiness and that of the faster, the moral they would easily draw would not be without its worth. Unfortunately, the comparison cannot be made with effect, because the feat of excess is in the swim of fashion, while the feat

of fasting is very much out of it. The first is a vice which, by familiarity, begets favour and competition; the second is a madness which must be treated as a disease, or folly, which, by its oddity, begets only curiosity, compassion, and contempt.

(5) *Physiological Lessons.*—From a physiological point of view, a good many lessons are to be learned from fasting manias. That during a fast of forty days the temperature of a man should to the end remain steady is of itself an important bit of evidence. We have been led to believe that in a very few days the process of abstaining from a sufficient supply of food, to say nothing about abstaining from food altogether, is a certain means of reducing the animal temperature. It was never surmised that water alone would lead to conditions in which the vital warmth would for many weeks remain practically sustained. That the respiration should remain so little affected is a second equally remarkable fact; and that the muscular power should be kept up so as to enable a starved man to walk, talk, and compress the dynamometer to 82° for forty days is beyond what any physiologist living would have admitted as possible previously to the events that declare the possibility. These results, coupled with unquestionable waste of tissue, and with the painful and frequent disturbance of the stomach, are quite sufficiently remarkable to demand the attention of the thoughtful physiological scholar.

(6) The most striking lesson of all remains, namely, that *during the whole of the fasting period the* mind *of the faster is unclouded*, and, taking it all in all, *his* reasoning powers *are good*. Whoever remembers what depressions of mind, what lapses of memory, what stages of indecision and vacuity come on when for a few hours only the body is deprived of food, will wonder not a little that any human being could remain self-possessed and ready for argument and contention during a fast of over six weeks. Yet, from the examples supplied, the possession of mental is even more conspicuous than that of physical endurance. Suppose it be urged that the excellent sleeping faculties of the fasters kept their minds in good balance, we do but move the difficulty one step farther back, since to sleep in a state of fast, and to wake again refreshed, is itself a strange order of phenomenon. In sleep there is in progress the repair of the body. How shall there be repair when the food material out of which the repair is secured is not supplied? For a starving man to sleep and die we might be prepared; for a starving man to awake in the shadow of semi-consciousness or dementia, or for a starving man to wake in the terror and excitement of delirium and rage, we might be prepared; but for such a man to wake up refreshed and, at the worst, no more than irritable, is a new revelation affording unsuspected evidence of the grand part which water plays in the economy of life. The physiologist himself will wonder how water sustains life for such long periods. He will see that under its influence a kind of peripheral digestion is established in the body itself, by which, independently of the stomach, the body can subsist for a long time on itself; first on its stored-up or reserve structures, and afterwards on its own active structures. He will infer that, by the influence of the water imbibed, the digestive juices of the stomach are kept from acting on the walls of the stomach. He will discern that by the steady introduction of water into the blood, the blood-corpuscles are retained in a state of vitality, and in a condition fitted for the absorption of oxygen from the air. He will note that the minute vesicular structures of the lungs and of all the glandular organs are kept also vitalised and physically capable of function; and he will understand how that water-engine, the brain, is sustained in activity, its cement fluid, and its cell structures free.

The act of the professional faster, of taking some undescribed powder as a sustainment, is, in our opinion, either a self-delusion or a pretence, but it may, as a fancy or placebo, give faith, support the mind, and strengthen the will; or it may be a mere pretentious discovery. Whichever it be, the evidence is certain that the ordeal can be borne without it by those who can undertake the ordeal, a class of men who are specially constituted to starve, and who, by the speciality, are led to undertake what to the ordinary constitution would be impossible, and which under compulsion would often end in death in the second quarter of a trial of forty days. B. W. RICHARDSON.

MANICOCOMIUM (μανικός, insane; κομίζω, I care for). A hospital or asylum for the insane. (Fr. *manicome*; Ger. *Irrenhaus manicomio.*)

MANIE.—The French term for mania or mental exaltation.

MANIE AIGUË (Fr.). Acute mania.

MANIE BIENVEILLANTE (Fr.). Mental exaltation with benevolence of disposition.

MANIE CALME (Fr.). A mild form of mania. Simple mania.

MANIE CONTINUE. The French term for mental exaltation of long standing, as opposed to manie aiguë.

MANIE GAIE (Fr.). (*See* CHAEROMANIA; CHAIROMANIA.)

MANIE HALLUCINATOIRE (Fr.). (*See* HALLUCINATIONS.)

MANIE INCENDIAIRE (Fr.). (*See* PYROMANIA.)

MANIE INTERMITTENTE (Fr.). Maniacal attacks with short intervals of apparent mental health.

MANIE MALFAISANTE (Fr.). Mania with freaks of mischievousness; mental exaltation with a malevolent disposition.

MANIE RAISONNANTE (Fr.). Pinel's term for what was subsequently called moral or emotional insanity.

MANIE SANS DÉLIRE (Fr.). (*See* MORAL INSANITY.)

MANIE SYSTEMATISÉE (Fr.). (*See* MONOMANIA.)

MANIE TRISTE (Fr.). A synonym of Melancholia.

MANIGRAPH; MANIGRAPHY (*μανία*; *γράφω*, I write). One who specially studies insanity. Also a description of or work on insanity.

MANIODES (*μανιώδης*, mad). The same as maniacal.

MANIOPŒOUS (*μανία*; *ποιέω*, I make). Anything causing or inducing insanity. (Fr. *maniope*; Ger. *rasendmachend*.)

MANUSTUPRATIO (*manus*; *stupro*). Masturbation.

MARRIAGE AND INSANITY, Association between; and POST-CONNUBIAL INSANITY.—There are three distinct heads under which this needs to be considered.

(1) **Those who are slightly insane before marriage**, but who become markedly so after.

(2) **Those with some slight mental disorder like hysteria before marriage, though with complete recognition of their surroundings**, who marry and then develop insanity.

(3) **Those in whom neurosis was in no way suspected before marriage.** Of these there are two classes: (*a*) Those in whom the symptoms come on very shortly after the marriage, and (*b*) those in whom the insanity develops as the result of nervous exhaustion from sexual excess at a later period.

In all the above cases there is commonly a history of neurosis in the family or in the individual. The disorder may occur in men or in women, but it is much more common, in our experience, among the latter. It may occur at any age. We have seen it in very young persons, and also in women who have married after forty-five. We believe it is predisposed to in some cases by prolonged and intimate courtship, in which there is a frequent stimulus to the passion with no gratification.

As will be seen, the symptoms may vary, there being nothing which is specially characteristic of the cases as a whole; they are fairly curable, and are of great medico-legal interest.

(1) In the first group are a few cases of insanity with delusions, but with quiet self-control, which enables the patient to pass muster as only a little "cold" or odd. Such patients will in some instances follow the wishes of a mother and allow the marriage ceremony to be completed without any active objection, but they rarely allow the marriage to be consummated, and it is then that the husband finds out the terrible accident of his wife's insanity. In some the word *hysteria* has been so used as to mislead the mother into believing that marriage will cure the disorder. We can speak from experience when we say that the prospect of relief being thus afforded is extremely small, too small to justify the risk involved. This form of disorder is more common among women, but we have met one man who was suffering from true insanity when he married, and who has never recovered since. He showed his insanity on the day of his marriage, though his friends recognised that he was full of extravagant ideas even earlier. We have known patients contract marriage, both in the excited stage of general paralysis of the insane and also in early locomotor ataxy, who later developed marked insanity; in these latter probably there was loss of sexual self-control, but no true insanity before the marriage.

In speaking of the cases under this head it is necessary to remark that some weak-minded women have been made to marry men for pecuniary reasons, and in some such cases nullity has been decreed.

(2) The second group is nearly allied to the one just considered, but in it the mental disorder preceding marriage is of very slight degree and is very generally considered to be hysteria, and nothing more. There is a certain number of young persons of both sexes who, at the onset of the engagement or during its progress, suffer from a temporary revulsion of feelings or at least a change in feeling. Some say they have an antipathy, while others say they have ceased to have any real human feeling at all. Some, again, will say calmly that they have none of the feeling or sentiment necessary for marriage,

and these people often break off their engagements. In one case, at least, such a change in feeling led to an action for breach of promise of marriage. These cases differ somewhat in the two sexes. Thus, young women more often speak of loss of affection, while young men think of the loss of power and fear that they are impotent. In both sexes it is not uncommon to hear that there has been the habit of masturbation, but we do not think this is the general cause in all the cases of this kind; absolute chastity is in some cases quite as much a cause. If marriage is completed during this stage, the wife, as a rule, refuses marital rights, and thus trouble is started. The wife in one case for which nullity was declared objecting and resisting. In several similar instances we have had the same history of refusal and repugnance. If the husband is violent and forces his wife to yield, the result is likely to be even worse, and permanent estrangement may arise.

On the man's part the idea of impotence may have become so dominant that no congress is possible, and it is such cases in which true obsession arises. Instead of the fear of impotence, some idea connected with the wife, either as to her purity, or as to her local physical formation, may completely prevent congress, and this may lead to suicidal attempts. Probably most of the suicides which take place soon after marriage are due to ideas of impotence. There is an almost endless chain of these ideas of obsession which may prevent for a time or for ever virile acts in relation to one woman. The best treatment is to recommend abstinence from marriage as long as morbid feelings exist, and if they arise after marriage, to suggest general measures, and *command* that no attempts at connection be made. Thus the benefit of the desire to break a commandment may come to your aid.

(3) In this group are some very important cases from a medico-legal point of view. For, if in the former groups it can be shown that there was mental disorder of a kind which affected the marriage contract, a decree of nullity may be obtained; but in the last group, if the completion of marriage is the cause of the mental aberration, no such relief can be obtained.

In most of the cases which have come under our notice there has been marked instability before marriage, and in some cases there have been previous attacks of insanity or of grave hysteria which may have been concealed from the husband. It is possible that at some future period the concealment of such important facts may be considered sufficient to enable the contract to be adjudged invalid. In some cases the day after marriage the bride is found to be in a kind of stupor from which it is impossible to rouse her. This state of partial dementia may continue, or it may pass into dementia of a more active type, or it may give place to wildly maniacal excitement, in which eroticism is common, so that the coy bride assumes all the airs of the courtesan. There often appears to be some terrible dread at the bottom of the mental feeling, and this may follow though there has been no active resistance to the completion of the marriage. Separation from home and husband for a time will generally lead to recovery, and ultimately there may be return to home and domestic life, but this must be tried with great caution, as the memory of the first illness will persist.

The shock of marriage in some instances has been sufficient to start acute delirium which has ended fatally, but we have so far not met with such a case ourselves.

The second set of cases following marriage result from exhaustion. This may arise from great actual excess or from what we would call relative excess, for, under certain conditions, the indulgence of the sexual passion is more exhausting than under others. There seem too to be certain women who produce much more exhaustion than do others. The disorders due to this form of weakness occur most commonly in men, women not suffering nearly so frequently from the results of sexual excess. These men begin by losing the little self-control they have, and seek a continuance of their gratification, and often take alcoholic or other stimulants to assist them.

They become restless, sleepless, irritable, and later may attack their wives. Jealousy may spring up with fancies that the wife has carried on some intrigue or that she was not virtuous before marriage. It is common for acute mania to develop. The patient when placed under control is thin, with a worn aspect with widely dilated pupils which react feebly. There is general excitability, appetite is bad, the tongue moist, tremulous, often furred. There is often aversion to friends, and both homicidal and suicidal tendencies are common. Rest, tonics, and liberal diet are the means to be used, and the result is generally favourable. Geo. H. Savage.

MARRIAGE IN RELATION TO INSANITY, The Law of.—This difficult and important subject may be considered most conveniently under the following heads:—

(1) **The Effect of Insanity upon the Capacity to Marry**; and

(2) **The Effect of Supervening Insanity upon a Valid Contract of Marriage, and upon the Rights, Duties, and Legal Remedies of the Contracting Parties.**

(1) **The Effect of Insanity upon the Capacity to Marry.**—The development of the present law of England as to the competency of the insane to marry is a study of peculiar interest. It seems at one time to have been held, contrary to the civil law,* but in conformity to the opinion of some of the civilians,† that the marriage of an idiot (and *a fortiori* of a lunatic) was valid, and that his children were legitimate.‡ By the middle of the 18th century a more rational rule had been clearly established. It was settled § that idiots, being incapable of giving the consent which is the basis of marriage, were *ipso facto* incapable of marrying, and that the marriage of a lunatic was absolutely void, unless it had been contracted during a lucid interval. The statute 15 Geo. II. c. 30—extended to Ireland by 51 Geo. III. c. 57—carried the reaction against the early common law doctrine to a somewhat extreme length. It provided that the marriages of lunatics and persons under frensies (if so found by inquisition or committed to the care of trustees by any Act of Parliament) contracted before they were declared of sound mind by the Lord Chancellor or the majority of such trustees, should be totally void,‖ by the operation of the statute alone, and without the necessity of any proceedings for declaration of nullity being taken in the Ecclesiastical Courts.¶ The practice which prevailed during the subsistence of this statute was thus clearly and concisely stated by Sir William Scott in *Turner* v. *Meyers*. "When a commission of lunacy has been taken out, the conclusion against the marriage will be founded on the statute; where there has been no such commission, the matter is to be established on evidence. The statute has made provisions against such marriages, *even in lucid intervals*, till the commission has been superseded. In other cases, the Court will require it to be shown by strong evidence that the marriage was clearly held in a lucid interval if it is first found that the person was generally insane." 15 Geo. II. c. 30, was however repealed by the Statute Law Revision Act, 1873 (36 & 37 Vict. c. 91); the lunatic so found, and the lunatic not so found, by inquisition were placed as regards their capacity to marry, on the same footing before the law, and no further legislation has occurred to complicate the subject.

By the time of Lord Stowell it was clearly recognised, and indeed insisted upon, by the Ecclesiastical Courts that marriage being a *consensual* contract* could be entered into by those persons only who were capable of *consenting*;† but till recent years, somewhat hazy and even contradictory notions have prevailed as to the nature and degree of the consent which would validate this particular contract.

It may be interesting to consider a few of these dicta in chronological order.‡ In *Turner* v. *Meyers* (1808, *ubi supra* at p. 418) Sir William Scott said: "We learn from experience and observation all that we can know; and we see that madness may subsist in various degrees, sometimes slight, as partaking rather of disposition or humour, which will not incapacitate a man from managing his own affairs, or making a valid contract. It must be something more than this, *something which*, if there be any test, *is held by the common judgment of mankind to affect his general fitness to be trusted with the*

* *Furor contrahentis matrimonium non sinit, quia consensu opus est* (Paulus, D. 23, 2, 16, 2).

† Sanchez, lib. 1. disp. 8, num. 15 *et seq.* In *Turner* v. *Meyers* (1808, 1 Hagg. Consist. Rep. 414), referring to this point Sir William Scott (afterwards Lord Stowell) said: "It is true that there are some obscure *dicta* in the earlier commentators on the law that a marriage of an insane person could not be invalidated on that account, founded, I presume, on some notion that prevailed in the Dark Ages of the mysterious nature of the contract of marriage, in which its spiritual nature almost entirely obliterated its civil character."

‡ "Un Ideot à nativitate poet consenter en marriage, et ses issues serout legitimate. Trin. 3 Jac., B.R., enter Stile and West adjudge sur un speciall verdit, pur un pettit question." Rolle's Abridg., 357, 50 (7).

§ *Morison* v. *Stewart*, 1745; *Cloudesley* v. *Evans*, 1763; *Parker* v. *Parker*, 1757; cited 1 Hagg. Consist. Rep. 417.

‖ This Act is stated to have been passed to meet the case of Mr. Newport, the natural son of the Earl of Bradford, who left him a very large fortune, with remainder to another person.

¶ *Ex parte Turing*, 1812, 1 Ves. & Beam, 140 and note.

* *Consensus non concubitus facit matrimonium* was the rule of the civil law. It is laid down in some of the old books (*e.g.* Collinson, 1, 555), that a marriage by a *non compos*, when of unsound mind, might be rendered valid by consummation in a lucid interval.

† *Harford* v. *Morris*, 1776, 2 Hagg. Consist. Rep., 423, 427; *Turner* v. *Meyers*, *ubi supra*.

‡ It is not here contended that our law on the question of the competency of the insane to marry can be divided into precise chronological periods; still less is it suggested that the cases in which vague or erroneous *dicta* were laid down, were wrongly decided. On the contrary there is, perhaps, no case upon the *civil* capacity of the insane under the old law, which would be disposed of differently at the present day.

management of himself and his own concerns." In *Browning* v. *Reane* (1812, 2 Phill. E. R. 69, 70), the test of capacity is stated a little more precisely, but it is mixed up with the test of competency applied in inquisitions *de lunatico inquirendo.* "*If the incapacity,*" said Sir John Nicholl, "*be such .... that the party is incapable of understanding the nature of the contract itself, and incapable from mental imbecility to take care of his or her own person and property,* such an individual cannot dispose of her person and property by the matrimonial contract any more than by any other contract."

In *Harrod* v. *Harrod* (1854, 1 K. & J. at pp. 14, 16), the modern theory was foreshadowed by Page Wood, V.C., in the following passages: "The contract itself, in its essence, independently of the religious element, is *a consent on the part of a man and woman to cohabit with each other, and with each other only.* .... When the hands of the parties are joined together, and the clergyman pronounces them to be man and wife, they are married if they understand that by that act they have agreed to cohabit together, and with no other person."

In *Hancock* v. *Peaty* (1867, 1 P. & D. 335, 341), Sir J. P. Wilde (afterwards Lord Penzance) made use of the following remarkable expressions:—"The Court here has not, as in many testamentary cases, to deal with varieties or degrees in strength of mind with the more or less failing condition of intellectual power in the prostration of illness or the decay of faculties in extended age. *The question here is one of health or disease of mind; and if the proof shows that the mind was diseased,* the Court has no means of gauging the extent of the derangement consequent upon that disease, or affirming the limits within which the disease might operate to obscure or divert the mental power."*

The doctrine of Lord Penzance in *Hancock* v. *Peaty* has now been impliedly overruled. In *Durham* v. *Durham* (1885, 10 P. D. at p. 82), Sir James Hannen said: "It appears to me that the contract of marriage is a very simple one, which (it) does not require a high degree of intelligence to comprehend. It is an engagement between a man and woman to live together and love one another as husband and wife to the exclusion of all others. This is expanded in the promises of the marriage ceremony by words having reference to the natural relations which spring from that engagement, such as protection on the part of the man and submission on the part of the woman. .... A mere comprehension of the words of the promises exchanged is not sufficient. The mind of one of the parties may be capable of understanding the language used, but may yet be affected by such delusions, or other symptoms of insanity as may satisfy the tribunal that there was not a real appreciation of the nature of the engagement entered into."

It may now be possible to formulate, and briefly illustrate, a few propositions which will give an accurate idea of the law as to the competency of the insane to marry, at the present day.

(1) Marriage is the voluntary union for life of one man and one woman to the exclusion of all others. (*Cf. Hyde* v. *Hyde*, 1 P. & M., 133; in *Re Bethell*, 1888, L. R. 38 Ch. D. 294, per Stirling, J.).

(2) The contract of marriage can be entered into by such persons only as are capable, at the time, of understanding its nature and comprehending its effects, as above described.

An analysis of this proposition, with a few illustrations of its constituent parts, may be useful.

The capacity to marry means in law a capacity to understand the nature and effects of the contract of marriage. No other evidence of capacity is necessary or sufficient. In *Harrod* v. *Harrod* (1854, 1 K. & J. 4), the question at issue was the validity of the marriage of a woman named Harrod. She was deaf and dumb and extremely dull of intellect, had never been taught to read or write, and understood the signs and gestures of those persons only who were constantly living with her, and was unable to tell the value of money. Upon the other hand, the evidence showed that she *did* understand the nature of marriage. "She had been residing previously," said Page Wood, V.C., "with a married couple and must have known that they lived together in a manner differently from unmarried persons like herself. She remained up to the time of her own marriage perfectly respectable and chaste: she went through the solemnity in which the hands of herself and her husband were joined. A child was born of the marriage in due time and not before. .... That shows she was aware she had performed a solemn act, imposing new duties, and she was constant to her husband during the rest of her life—a period of nearly thirty years." His lordship, held, therefore, that the marriage was valid.

* These observations should be compared with the remarks of the same learned judge in *Smith* v. *Tebbitt* (1867, 1 P. and D., 421), and with those of Lord Brougham in *Waring* v. *Waring*, 1848, 6 Moo. P. C., pp. 348-353.

Again, the capacity required by law must exist at the time of marriage. "The law," said Sir John Nicholl in *Portsmouth* v. *Portsmouth* (1829, 1 Hagg. E. R. at p. 359) . . . . "admits of no controversy. . . . . When a fact of marriage has been regularly solemnised, the presumption is in its favour; but then it must be solemnised between parties competent to contract, capable of entering into that most important engagement, the very essence of which is consent." Two recent cases *Hunter* v. *Edney* (1881, 10 P. D. 93) and *Cannon* v. *Smalley* (1885, 10 P. D. 96) must be referred to in this connection. In *Hunter* v. *Edney*, the parties were married on March 17, 1881. There was clear evidence that the wife, whose mental state was in question in the suit, was in an abnormally excited and troubled condition on the morning of the marriage. She received her future husband coldly, at first refused to go to church, and was continually rubbing her hands. After the ceremony, she was with difficulty persuaded to change her dress to go away. When the newly married couple reached their apartments in London, she refused to have supper, and said that she did not want to get married and that she was false. She lay down on the bed in her clothes, and for three hours refused to undress. The marriage was not consummated. In the morning, she asked her husband to cut her throat. A medical man was called in who pronounced her to be insane, and this view was subsequently confirmed by Dr. Savage, who reported, and gave evidence at the trial, that in his opinion the patient was suffering from melancholia, owing in the first instance to hereditary insanity excited by the idea of marriage. Sir James Hannen, after carefully reviewing the facts, gave judgment as follows: "I come to the conclusion that the evidence which has been given of her manner preceding the marriage, establishes that that excitement had been set up by the idea of her approaching marriage, and *that she was not able to know and appreciate the act she was doing at that time, but that she took an entirely morbid and diseased view of it.*"

In *Cannon* v. *Smalley*, on the other hand, the respondent, who was married to the petitioner on January 1, 1884, and who was clearly insane ten days afterwards, was shown to have performed her usual duties until the day before the marriage, and to have written a perfectly sensible letter to the petitioner on the 28th of December 1883. Sir James Hannen said: "She was then suffering in her physical health, and it might be in this case that physical had something to do with mental health, and that even at that date the balance of the respondent's mind was unsettled and likely to be upset; *but the question to be decided is whether it is shown to have been upset on the 1st of January* 1884, *the date of the marriage.*" His lordship was of opinion that the balance of the evidence was in favour of the respondent's capacity.

Durham v. *Durham*, the facts of which are too well-known to need recapitulation, was decided upon the same principles. Sir James Hannen held that the circumstances, which threw doubt upon the soundness of mind of the respondent, were capable of being explained, consistently with the assumption of sanity, by her natural shyness, by the fact that her affections had been given to another person, and in some measure by the conduct of the petitioner himself. His lordship also held that the inference of incapacity to which the subsequent insanity of the respondent gave rise was rebutted by the methodical and rational manner in which she made arrangements for her approaching marriage.

Without discussing the merits of these particular cases, it may be permissible to point out that the principles on which they were determined are clear. A marriage is presumed to be valid. Upon the party who alleges incapacity rests the burden of proving his assertion. The proof required is that legal capacity to marry did not exist at the time of the marriage. Supervening insanity is by no means conclusive evidence of such incapacity, even in the absence, and *à fortiori* in the presence, of positive proofs of sanity at or about the critical period. But where marked symptoms of mental unsoundness appear at the time of marriage, and shortly afterwards develop into undoubted incapacity, the Court both may and will consider whether the party whose competency to marry is in dispute was able to know and appreciate, free from the influence of morbid ideas or delusions, the nature of the contract into which he or she was entering. It is thought that these sentences contain an accurate statement of the present law of England upon this point.*

(3) Whenever from natural weakness of intellect or fear—*whether reasonably entertained or not*—either party is actually in a state of mental incompetence to resist

* The fact that, after an engagement to marry, a defendant discovers that *before* the engagement was entered into the plaintiff had for a short time been insane, is no answer to an action for breach of promise, *Baker* v. *Cartwright*, 1861, 30 L. J. (N. S.) C. P. 364.

pressure improperly brought to bear, such party cannot enter into a valid contract of marriage—there being no more consent here than in the case of a person of stronger intellect and more robust courage yielding to greater pressure or more serious danger.

In *Scott* v. *Sebright* (1886, 12 P. D. 21), from which this proposition is, with slight modifications, taken, the petitioner, a young woman of twenty-two years of age, entitled to the sum of £26,000 in actual possession, and a considerable sum in reversion, had become engaged to the respondent, and shortly after coming of age was induced by him to accept bills to the amount of £3325. The persons who had discounted these bills issued writs against her, and threatened to make her a bankrupt. The distress caused by these threats seriously affected her health and reduced her to a state of bodily and mental prostration in which she was incapable of resisting threats and coercion, and being assured by the respondent that the only method of evading bankruptcy proceedings and exposure was to marry him, she reluctantly went through a ceremony of marriage with him at a registrar's office. In addition to other threats of ruining her, the respondent immediately before the ceremony threatened to shoot her, if she showed that she was not acting of her free will. The marriage was never consummated, and the petitioner and the respondent separated immediately after the ceremony. It was held by Butt, J., that there was not such a consent on the part of the petitioner as the law requires for the making of a contract of marriage, and that the ceremony before the registrar must be declared null and void.*

A suit for declaration of nullity of marriage on the ground of insanity should be brought (1) by the contracting party himself on the recovery of his reason; (2) by the guardian, where the contracting party is a minor; (3) by the committee of the estate of a lunatic so found by inquisition; (4) by a curator or guardian *ad litem*, where the contracting party is *sui juris*, but still insane, though not found lunatic;† (5) where the contracting party is dead, by one of the next-of-kin, or any one having interest;‡ (6) by the sane contracting party.§

In *Hancock* v. *Peaty* (1867, 1 P. & D. at p. 336) the Court being satisfied by the evidence that the petitioner was not of sound mind at the date of her marriage with the respondent, postponed pronouncing its decree in order to give the respondent an opportunity, if so advised, of establishing the fact of the petitioner's recovery, and intimated that if satisfied of her recovery, *it would not pronounce a decree of nullity except at her instance.*

(2) The Effect of Supervening Insanity upon a Valid Contract of Marriage, and upon the Rights, Duties, and Legal Remedies of the Contracting Parties.

The points arising under this head are chiefly points of practice.

(*a*) Divorce proceedings are not criminal, and may therefore be instituted by a husband or wife against a wife or husband who is insane at the time of such proceedings, and continued, in spite of such insanity, at any rate when it is incurable (*Mordaunt* v. *Moncrieffe*, 1874, L. R. 2 Sc. & Div. App. 374).

The case of *Mordaunt* v. *Moncrieffe* deserves a somewhat careful examination.

On April 28, 1869, Sir Charles Mordaunt presented to the Divorce Court a petition for the dissolution of his marriage with Lady Mordaunt on the ground of her adultery. Two days afterwards, the citation was duly served on Lady Mordaunt, whose solicitors entered an appearance for her, but on a representation, supported by affidavit, that she was insane, the Court, on July 27, 1869, appointed her father, Sir Thomas Moncrieffe, to act as guardian *ad litem*. Upon the plea of Lady Mordaunt's alleged insanity, issue was joined, and the question was tried by a special jury who, on Feb. 25, 1870, found that Lady Mordaunt "was, on 30th April, 1869 (the day on which the petition for divorce had been served upon her), in such a state of mental disorder as to be unfit and unable to answer the petition; and that she had ever since remained and still remained so unfit and unable." On March 8, 1870, Lord Penzance ordered that no further proceedings should be taken in the suit until Lady Mordaunt had recovered her mental capacity, and the order was confirmed, on appeal, by the full Court of Divorce—Lord Chief Baron Kelly dissenting. On March 12, 1872, Dr. Harrington Tuke having made an affidavit that the recovery of Lady Mordaunt had become hopeless,

* See art. UNDUE INFLUENCE. *Cf.* also *Portsmouth* v. *Portsmouth*, 1828, 1 Hagg. Eccles. Rep. 355.

† It seems that a guardian *ad litem* will not be appointed where there is a substantial dispute as to the unsoundness of mind of the person to whom it is proposed to assign the guardian. *Fry* v. *Fry*, W.N. 1890, 34.

‡ *Cf.* Pope on "Lunacy," pp. 249-251, where this subject is minutely discussed.

§ Mr. Pope's statement that the sane contracting party had in no case successfully petitioned for declarator of nullity is no longer accurate. *Cf.* *Durham* v. *Durham*, *Hunter* v. *Edney*, *Cannon* v. *Smalley*, *ubi supra*.

Sir Charles Mordaunt applied to the Court to dismiss his petition for divorce so that he might appeal to the House of Lords and thereby open the real question requiring adjudication. The petition was accordingly dismissed, and on July 1, 1873, the case was argued at the Bar of the House, the following Common Law judges attending to assist, Kelly, C.B., Martin, B., Keating, J., Brett, J., Denman, J., and Pollock, B. At the close of the argument, on the motion of Lord Chelmsford, the following question was propounded for the opinions of the Common Law judges:—*Whether under the statute 20 & 21 Vict. c. 85, proceedings for the dissolution of a marriage can be instituted or proceeded with, either on behalf of or against a husband or wife who, before the proceedings were instituted had become incurably insane?*

The majority of the judges—Kelly, C.B., Denman, J., and Pollock, B. (Martin, B., had retired before the opinions were delivered), concurred in holding that divorce may be asked and decreed on behalf of, or against, a lunatic, the Court appointing a guardian *ad litem* for his protection. But Keating, J., and Brett, J., held that the insanity of either husband or wife is an absolute bar to divorce. In the House of Lords, Lord Chelmsford and Lord Hatherley adopted the view of the majority of the Common Law judges, and held that the wife's insanity ought not to bar or impede the investigation of the charge of adultery brought against her.*

A summary of the opposing contentions in *Mordaunt* v. *Moncrieffe* may be of interest and value.

Against the divorce it was argued (1) that divorce proceedings are quasi-penal, that in the criminal law every step against a prisoner is arrested by his becoming a lunatic, and that by analogy the same rule should be applied to suits for the dissolution of marriage; (2) that the Divorce Act clearly intended that the new Court should not act upon a petition until it had investigated the countercharges (if any) of condonation, connivance, or recrimination, and that for the proper determination of these charges the evidence of the respondent was indispensable; (3) that the judgment of Sir Cresswell Cresswell in *Bawden* v. *Bawden* (2 Sw. & Tr. 417, 31 L. J. P. M. & A. 94) was a distinct authority upon the point; and (4) that "it was so obviously unreasonable that one so incapacitated (as Lady Mordaunt) should be proceeded against for adultery and convicted, and her marriage dissolved, that it could not have been intended or contemplated by the legislature."

On the other hand, *in favour of Sir Charles Mordaunt's* petition, it was contended (1) that adultery was not by the law of England a crime, that the Act conferred no criminal jurisdiction on the Divorce Court, and that therefore the assumed analogy, above mentioned, failed; (2) that under the Divorce Act the Court *was bound* to dissolve a petitioner's marriage if satisfied that his case was proved unless some countercharge was established against him; (3) that *Bawden* v. *Bawden* must be overruled; (4) that the evidence of the respondent was not necessarily indispensable to the proof of a countercharge, and (5) that the possibility of hardship to individuals was equally unavoidable, in whichever way the case might be decided. The language of Kelly, C.B., on the last point may be referred to, L. R. 2 Sc. & Div. at p. 381.

Within the limits of the present article it has of course been impossible to give a *complete* account of the respective arguments in *Mordaunt* v. *Moncrieffe*, but it is hoped that the above synopsis may assist students of this very complicated decision.

It cannot be too clearly pointed out and remembered that *Mordaunt* v. *Moncrieffe* is merely an authority for the proposition with which we have prefaced our analysis of the case.

It *does not decide* that the insanity of a respondent to a petition for divorce, existing at the time *when an alleged act of adultery was committed*, would be no defence to the petition,* and the question of how far insanity affords an answer to a charge of adultery, would in all probability be determined by "the rules in *Macnaghten's case*," applied in the emasculated form in which they now do duty in criminal cases.

(*b*) The lunacy of a husband or wife is not a bar to a suit by the committee for the dissolution of the lunatic's marriage (*Baker* v. *Baker*, 1880, 5 P.D. 142, 6 P.D. 12). But if the lunatic died after obtaining a decree *nisi* for the dissolution of the marriage, the legal personal representative could not revive the proceedings for the purpose of applying to make the decree absolute. (*Stanhope* v. *Stanhope*, 1886, per Cotton, L. J., 11 P. D., at p. 107.)

The supervening insanity of a husband

* Sir Charles Mordaunt was left at liberty to proceed with his suit for a divorce, which he in fact did. Lord Chelmsford declined to determine the question whether a lunatic can be a petitioner for a divorce. See, however, *Baker* v. *Baker*, 1880, 5 P. D., 142; 6 P. D., 12.

* We are not able to refer to any reported case in which this question has in fact arisen.

or wife is no ground for a dissolution of their marriage,* and is no answer to an action for the restitution of conjugal rights. In *Hayward* v. *Hayward*† Sir Cresswell Cresswell said: "A husband is not entitled to turn his lunatic wife out of doors. He may be rather bound to place her in proper custody, under proper care, but he is not entitled to turn her out of his house. He is less than ever justified in putting her away if she has the misfortune to be insane." Again, a judicial separation will not be granted upon the ground of cruelty arising from positive mental disease. "An insane man," said the Judge Ordinary in *Hall* v. *Hall* (1864, 3 S. & T., at p. 350), "is likely enough to be dangerous to his wife's personal safety, but the remedy lies in the restraint of the husband, not the release of the wife." This principle is, of course, inapplicable where the misconduct complained of is unconnected with, or is shown to have been itself the exciting cause of, the respondent's insanity (*White* v. *White*, 1 S. & T. 592). A. Wood Renton.

Marriage on the Ground of Insanity, The Plea of Nullity of.—There are several aspects from which this subject has to be viewed; first, there are the women who may have been forced into marriage, they being either at the time only, or permanently, insane. An idiot or imbecile might be forcibly married for the sake of her property, though this is only likely to occur when the imbecility is of a mild form, or only partial, so that with a certain amount of brilliancy there may be marked intellectual defect. In some of these cases it is possible that the contract might be held to be good, while in others it would clearly be seen that the marriage was null and void. Several such cases have been tried and are referred to by legal authorities.

In the following remarks we shall not enlarge upon the possibilities of the future but only speak of what is at present the law and its practical outcome. This will be best done by referring to certain cases which have within recent years been before the Courts. There seems to be no chance of setting aside a marriage because one or other of the contracting parties has had former attacks of insanity, though it can be shown that these attacks have affected the mind, and are likely to recur. The onset of insanity following immediately on marriage will not be admitted as a plea for nullity, even though the marriage have not been consummated at the time; it seems, too, that though the person who becomes insane have all sorts of false ideas before marriage, yet, unless these affect the mind in direct relationship to the marriage itself, it is doubtful whether they would be accepted as a ground for declaring nullity.

It is, as might be expected, a much more common thing to meet with cases in which the question is raised as to the sanity of the wife rather than as to the mental capacity of the husband. The general course of cases in which the question is raised is as follows: the symptoms may be maniacal or melancholic; a woman after her engagement becomes, as her friends think, hysterical, and they honestly believe and are often supported in their belief by medical men, that this hysteria will pass off with the marriage and with the usual sexual intercourse; the marriage may even be hastened to effect this, but instead of any good following the woman from being simply fanciful and depressed becomes markedly melancholic, developing strongly suicidal ideas and strong feelings of disgust against her husband. In such cases, there is little doubt, but that the woman was not in a fit state to enter into a contract of marriage, and if her friends admit this it is possible that a judge may allow it also; but it is very likely that the judge may require more proof of insanity affecting the contract than is forthcoming, and so the plea may be set aside.

In the second group of cases a woman instead of being depressed may suffer from erotic insanity, or from weakness of mind with eroticism, and may be willing to marry any one who may offer himself, and here again it will be found to be very difficult to establish the fact that she was too insane to understand the nature of her act.

To return to the first class. A case was tried in London before Mr. Justice Hannen; *Hunter* v. *Hunter*, otherwise *Edney*, and in this nullity was decreed. The young woman was the daughter of an insane father, she herself during the courtship wished to break off the engagement as she was "not fit for marriage," she was kept away from her lover for a time, he seeing her after an interval only shortly before the marriage. Stimulants had to be given to get her to go to church; she went away with her husband, but would not undress, and did not get into bed, she would not allow marital congress, and the next day her husband sent her home to her mother's, where we found her suffering from simple melancholia.

* The usual incidents of marriage arise, therefore, in spite of supervening insanity. This subject is too technical to be pursued here.

† 1856, 1 S. & F., at p. 84.

She herself was wishful for the divorce, and gave evidence in the Court, or rather made a statement which satisfied the judge, and nullity was decreed. In another case tried later *Cannon* v. *Cannon*, the nullity was not granted, though in nearly every particular the cases were alike, but in this case the depression was followed by a period of exaltation, during which she returned to her husband, and consummation took place without in any way relieving her symptoms, and though it seems to us that this should not make any difference in law, yet it appears that if the woman is still *virgo intacta* there would be a better chance for obtaining a nullity decision.

In a third case, differing in many particulars, namely the "cause célèbre" of Lord Durham, there were shown to have been peculiarities in the lady before marriage, but these were not considered sufficient to cause her friends to take any really active steps for her protection. She passed placidly through her engagement, and seems to have been married without causing any anxiety, but there was great objection to consummation, and very shortly after, though the husband and wife cohabited, the mental symptoms developed rapidly, passing into the most violent mania, and from that time to this there has been no restoration to health. It was decided that the lady was sufficiently sane at the time of marriage to complete the contract, and so the marriage must stand, though there is now no doubt that the insanity was developing at the time of marriage. We must recognise that certain unstable women are upset more or less completely in mind by the mere consummation of marriage, and we have seen several well-marked instances of insanity following marriage in both men and women within a few days.

This is one of the accidents which must be accepted with marriage contracts.

From the cases already tried it will be seen that there must be brought very clearly into evidence that the person was insane at the time of the marriage, neither only before nor directly after; the facts of its being both before or after are important, but would not suffice without the proof as to its existence on the actual day of marriage. Though such insanity is most common in women, we have seen one case in which a doctor was undoubtedly of unsound mind when he married. The marriage being in Scotland, and taking place in a private house, allowed many things to be passed over which would not have been tolerated in a place of worship; in this case the wife elected to suffer, and would not try to get a decree of nullity.

In the second group of cases in which excitement is the chief symptom, considerable anxiety may be caused by the eroticism of a patient who was formerly staid and proper. In several such cases trouble has arisen in this way. A patient in this state manages to escape from an asylum, and may at once give herself up to prostitution, and cause great scandal and distress to all concerned. In several cases we have known such patients really try to get married, but as far as our experience goes these attempts have failed, the patient either being taken back to an asylum or being otherwise cared for.

Yet there is a very real danger that a person in the earlier stage of acute mania may be still able to control his actions sufficiently to mislead those who do not already know him into the belief that he is sane, and capable of entering into a contract, though within a very short time it is clear that he is maniacal. We have already said that it will be very difficult to prove that the patient was not capable of entering into the marriage, but we believe it is quite worth a trial, rather than to allow without a struggle the mad marriage to continue.

In the earlier stages of general paralysis of the insane, it is very common to find patients wishful to enter into marriage, and we have met with several instances in which during the earlier periods of nervous degenerations, strongly marked eroticism has led men to marry. This has occurred in early mania, in early general paralysis, in locomotor ataxy, and in senile dementia; the old men's marriages providing a number of such cases. But as yet we do not know of any case in which the marriage has been upset on this ground, but it is pretty certain that such cases will occur.

To complete the subject, it should be noted that certain persons, women especially, commit acts of adultery which lead to divorce suits, while they are of unsound mind; so far the plea has not, we believe, been successfully raised, but we have met with several instances in which previously modest and virtuous women have, as the result of insanity, generally of a maniacal form, formed illicit connections which have led to divorce. It seems to us that in these cases the insanity would be a defence to the action, but the point has not yet been raised in any reported case. *Mordaunt* v. *Mordaunt* relates solely to procedure. GEO. H. SAVAGE.

MASSAGE. (*See* NEUROSES, TREATMENT OF FUNCTIONAL.)

MASTURBATION is the artificial excitement and gratification of sexual passion. It is most frequently practised by lads about or after the period of puberty, but it has its victims in both sexes, and at all ages, and in persons of neurotic temperament it produces most baneful results.

(1) Masturbation **may be a mere vice** which the youth has been taught by some prurient companion at school or has accidentally learned in the awakening of his own sexual feelings, and which he discontinues when old enough and wise enough to realise its nature. It leaves a sense of shame and regret, but, unless the practice has been long and greatly indulged, no permanent evil effects may be observed to follow. It is needful to say this plainly, not in order to minimise the evils of the vice, but because the after-lives of such youths are often made miserable through their falling into the toils of the lying "specialists" and "nerve doctors" whose advertisements defile our walls and newspapers. These impostors trade upon the fears of their victims in order to empty their pockets. They paint in the strongest colours the frightful results of masturbation, asserting the loss of manhood and suggesting the approach of permanent insanity, but they "dare to hope that a cure may yet be possible" if the victim will only pay for their unparalleled skill and experience and for the priceless medicine which they alone can supply. This foul trade requires to be exposed, for its extent and its evil results are little realised, and shame shuts the mouths of its victims.

(2) **Consequences.**—If years do not bring wisdom, and if the vice be still secretly indulged, the baneful consequences cannot be escaped.

This habit, when long and often indulged in defiance of reason and conscience, seems more than any other to acquire a mastery over its victim, and the nervous exhaustion which by its very nature it produces makes him less and less able to resist it. Gradually the appearance, manner, and character become altered, and the typical signs of habitual masturbation are developed.

The face becomes pale and pasty, and the eye lustreless. The man loses all spontaneity and cheerfulness, all manliness and self-reliance. He cannot look you in the face because he is haunted by the consciousness of a dirty secret which he must always conceal and always dreads that you may discover. He shuns society, has no intimate friends, does not dare to marry, and becomes a timid, hypersensitive, self-centred, hypochondriac.

(3) **Moral and Mental Degeneration.**—Too often, and especially in neurotic subjects, the results grow darker still, and involve moral and mental shipwreck.

The whole nature is deteriorated and demoralised, and the victim of confirmed masturbation becomes a liar, a coward, and a sneak. His mental faculties become blunted, his energy and power of application fail, and his only shadow of enjoyment is in the filthy habit which has so debased and degraded him. Even that palls, and the miserable wretch would commit suicide if he dared, but he rarely has the courage thus to close the life he has wasted, and sinks into melancholic dementia, relieved only by occasional excitement due to a temporary revival of his jaded passions.

This, the extremest form of the insanity of masturbation, may be greatly modified in different cases. Its subjects are usually of markedly neurotic temperament, and the nervous exhaustion and weakened will make them an easy prey to any form of neurotic disturbance.

Temporary attacks of maniacal excitement, or of obstinate resistive melancholia, or of dreamy stupor may occur, and the prevailing mood may be one of querulous discontent or of vain self-satisfaction.

(4) Masturbation **may be merely a symptom manifested during an insanity which has been quite otherwise induced.** In acute mania it is very often observed, and is merely a phase of the nervous excitement and an indication that the ordinary and normal self-control is lost for the time. In general paralysis, too, it is frequent, and has the like significance.

In epileptic insanity it may be at once a cause and a result. Some epileptics are habitual masturbators, and some invariably have a fit at or after the sexual orgasm. The religious sentiment, often so strong in epileptics, does not prevent the vice; and, indeed, masturbators are often religiously disposed persons who would never resort to fornication, and compromise with conscience by indulging the solitary vice.

(5) Masturbation **may be purely the result of perverted innervation** in persons who never previously practised the habit, and who utterly loathe it even while yielding to it. Such cases are rare, but they certainly do occur, and are allied, as instances of perverted innervation, to nymphomania occurring in perfectly chaste persons or to the storms of sexual feeling sometimes observed during lactation.

(6) Masturbation, so-called, is sometimes practised by very **young children,**

and has usually been taught by a prurient nurse, or provoked by phimosis, or, in either sex, by neglect of cleanliness. Some kind of sexual orgasm seems to be thus inducible long before puberty, and this early vice powerfully predisposes to habitual masturbation in after years. Mothers cannot be too vigilant in detecting and correcting such practices.

(7) Masturbation in **women** is more frequent than is commonly supposed. It is associated not rarely with the nervous irritability, wayward fancies, and nondescript ailments of hysterical girls, and the habits, amusements, and literature of certain classes of society are too apt to encourage the vice. About the age of thirty-three, when the chance of marriage is getting faint, and again about the climacteric period, some women experience great sexual instability, of which this practice is too often the result.

While possibly less exhausting and injurious than in the other sex, it may be more frequently and easily indulged, mere friction of the thighs often sufficing to produce the erotic spasm; and it is impossible to prevent the practice by any mechanical or surgical interference. To tie the hands or enclose them in a muff sometimes answers well, but in bad cases it is futile, as friction is made against the bed, or the furniture, or even by the patient's own heel.

(8) The **treatment** of masturbation must be at once moral and medical.

First and chiefly the moral sense must be awakened to the evil and the danger of the practice, and the will must be strengthened to resist the temptation which habit has intensified, and which inclination and opportunity make so strong. Tonic treatment, local and general, is required to correct relaxation and restore normal energy, and lastly other interests and occupations must banish the prurient fancies and impulses by which the patient has been enthralled.

It is easy to lay down these clear general principles, but few tasks are more difficult than their effectual application in actual practice.

The co-operation of the patient is, of course, essential to recovery, but to secure and maintain it is the great difficulty. If he really desires to conquer himself and honestly tries to aid his cure, the old habit is apt to prove stronger than his good resolutions, his weakened will is overcome, and he falls just when victory seemed near. This pitiful experience is so often repeated that the struggle seems vain, and it is difficult to inspire new hope and new effort in one who has so often failed.

If he does not really wish to conquer and forsake his vice, help and encouragement are alike in vain. He chooses and seals his own fate, and makes mental and moral shipwreck.

When honest efforts fail, and the patient declares in pitiful despair that he cannot forsake the vice which he deplores, or argues that his nature absolutely demands and requires the relief it affords, some direct operative interference, which shall prevent masturbation and show him that he can live without it, may be of much service. The best form of such interference is so to fix the prepuce that erection becomes painful and erotic impulses very unwelcome. To accomplish this, the prepuce is drawn well forward, the left forefinger inserted within it down to the root of the glans, and a nickel-plated safety-pin, introduced from the outside through skin and mucous membrane, is passed horizontally for half an inch or so past the tip of the left finger, and then brought out through mucous membrane and skin so as to fasten outside. Another pin is similarly fixed on the opposite side of the prepuce. With the foreskin thus looped up any attempt at erection causes a painful dragging on the pins, and masturbation is effectually prevented. In about a week some ulcera- of the mucous membrane will allow greater movement and with less pain, when the pins can, if needful, be introduced into a fresh place, but the patient is already convinced that masturbation is not necessary to his existence, and a moral as well as a material victory has been gained.

For cases so extreme that there is no wish to discontinue the practice, or so long continued that the power of erection is almost lost, this mode of treatment is unsuitable and of little service.

Blistering and cauterising are sometimes used to prevent masturbation, but they are only effectual for the time, and the itching which follows them tends to aggravate the evil. An irritable condition of the valve at the junction of the seminal and urinary tracts is believed by some to be a great cause of secret vice, and the local application of nitrate of silver is said to be followed by excellent results.

Castration and ovariotomy have been urged as radical cures, but it is doubtful if they deserve the title. Sexual desires are not destroyed, and their prurient indulgence would not be prevented, although impregnation were made impossible. Clitoridectomy still has its advocates, but the whole of the sensitive surface cannot

WILL conquer

be removed, and in this country at least the operation is generally deemed ineffectual and unsatisfactory.

To allay local irritation and excitement, a prolonged sitz bath as hot as can possibly be borne is probably the most effectual remedy, while the cold sitz bath night and morning is very helpful as a tonic. Of the medicines which are said to be calmatives of sexual excitability, not one can be really depended on, and even the bromides seem to act by virtue of their calmative power over all forms of nervous excitement rather than by any special action as sexual sedatives. Many deem salix nigra a specific, and it well deserves trial. Seminal emission is certainly controlled by gokeroo, but it has failed to correct masturbation. Of general tonics, strychnine and quinine are the most serviceable.

All treatment is likely to fail unless the solitary habits which so favour the vice are broken and unless the prurient imaginings be dispelled by new interests and healthful occupation. The patient should take to cricket, or golf, or volunteering, or cycling, or any other pursuit which implies healthy exercise and free intercourse with others.

He must avoid everything that suggests debasing thoughts, he must shun the society, amusements, and novels which favour them, and he must by patient effect conquer his inclinations and regain the self-control he had thrown away. We may give the most earnest counsel and the wisest prescriptions, but the patient's recovery depends after all mainly on himself.

To prescribe sexual intercourse as a certain cure for masturbation, which is too often done, is wrong both morally and medically. Marriage is, of course, the natural remedy for strong sexual feeling, but some of the worst masturbators are married persons, of both sexes, who continue to practise their vice notwithstanding full opportunities for normal intercourse. Entire continence is quite compatible, in both sexes, with perfect health, and sexual excess does not cease to be baneful although indulged naturally and under the shelter of marriage. Such excess entails its own penalty, not seldom in the form of general paralysis, just as certainly as confirmed masturbation.

The duty of parents as to warning their children against secret vice is delicate and difficult. There is the risk of suggesting what had never been thought of, but this risk seems small compared with the danger of allowing a child to contract, for want of warning, a habit so baneful and degrading. D. YELLOWLEES.

MATTOID (Ital. *mattoide*, mad-like). On the border line of insanity. A crank. (Lombroso and Havelock Ellis.)

MATURITY, INSANITY OF. The various forms of mental disturbance peculiar to, and occurring at the age of, full vitality—*e.g.*, general paralysis of the insane, &c.

MECHANICAL RESTRAINT. (*See* TREATMENT.)

MEDICAL CERTIFICATES. (*See* CERTIFICATES, MEDICAL.)

MEDICO - LEGAL. (*See* INDEX — RENTON, A. WOOD.)

MEDICO-PSYCHOLOGICAL ASSOCIATION OF GREAT BRITAIN AND IRELAND.—This Association originated in a circular dated Gloucester, June 19, 1841, addressed to medical men officially connected with the Public Lunatic Asylums of Great Britain and Ireland. It was signed by Dr. Samuel Hitch, at that time medical officer of the Gloucester Lunatic Asylum.

It proposed the foundation of an "Association of Medical Officers of Hospitals for the Insane"—the original title. On July 27 of the same year the Association was instituted, having for its object the inter-communication of all matters calculated to improve the treatment, care, and recovery of the insane, the management of institutions for this class, and the acquirement of a more extensive and correct knowledge of insanity.

It was decided to hold annual meetings at which papers should be read and discussed bearing on the subject.

Among the original members of the Association were Sir A. Morison, Dr. Prichard (Bristol), Dr. Conolly, Mr. Gaskell, Dr. Monro, Dr. Stewart (Belfast), Dr. W. A. F. Browne, Dr. Hitch, Dr. Hutcheson, Dr. Shute, Dr. Davey, Dr. de Vitré, Dr. Charlesworth, Dr. Begley, Dr. Sutherland, Dr. Poole, Dr. Kirkman, Dr. Corsellis, Dr. Thurnam, Dr. (afterwards Sir Charles) Hastings, Dr. Mackintosh, and Dr. McKinnon.

The first annual meeting was held at the Nottingham Asylum, November 1841.

In 1844, the Association held its annual meeting at the York Retreat, Dr. Thurnam being president. It was on this occasion that the idea was suggested of a Journal, as the organ of the association, in consequence of a letter received from Dr. Damerow (Halle), who was the editor of the *Allgemeine Zeitschrift für Psychiatrie.* He expressed the hope, writing on behalf of the corresponding Society in that land, that their English brethren would follow their annals" by publishing a periodical devoted to the same important object, by which means a mutual exchange of publications might take place, highly beneficial to both nations." A resolution was cordially adopted declaring the proposal to be "deserving of the best consideration of this Association." At subsequent meetings the subject was discussed, and in 1852 (July 20), at the Annual Meeting held at Oxford, it was resolved on the motion of Mr. Ley (the Treasurer), seconded by Dr. Thurnam, that the Journal should be undertaken. Dr. Bucknill was elected editor. Mr. Ley's proposition was cordially supported by Dr. Conolly. The first number of *The Asylum Journal* was issued on November 15, 1853. This name was changed to *The Asylum Journal of Mental Science* in 1855, and to *The Journal of Mental Science* at the Annual Meeting in 1858.

The title of the Association itself was changed in 1853 to "The Association of Medical Officers of Asylums and Hospitals for the Insane"; and in 1865 to "The Medico-Psychological Association."

In 1887 the words were added "of Great Britain and Ireland."

The Jubilee of the Association was held at Birmingham on July 23, 1891, only one original member having survived, Dr. Davey, formerly one of the Medical Superintendents at the Hanwell Asylum. Mr. E. B. Whitcombe, M.R.C.S., Medical Superintendent of the Borough Asylum (Winson Green), Birmingham, occupied the presidential chair.

It may be stated that whereas the Association numbered 44 members at its foundation, there are now (October 1891) on the roll 474.

The Association has carried out and amplified the original purpose of its founders.

It has introduced a pass examination, successful candidates in which receive a Certificate of Efficiency in Psychological Medicine. Combined with this, the Gaskell Prize is offered annually to those who, having passed the above, and complied with certain conditions, present themselves for the Honours Examination.

The Association has, moreover, instituted examinations of attendants, male and female, and grants certificates to those who satisfy the examiners.

A medal and ten guineas are offered annually for the best essay on a clinical subject contributed by an Assistant Medical Officer of an Asylum. THE EDITOR.

[*Reference.*—Dr. Blandford's Index to the first twenty-four volumes of the Journal of Mental Science, with Historical Sketch of the Association, by Hack Tuke, M.D. Also Journ. Ment. Sci. Oct. 1881.]

MEDICO-PSYCHOLOGY (*medicus*; ψυχή, the mind; λόγος, a discourse). That branch of medicine dealing with the symptoms, pathology, and treatment of mental affections.

MEGALOMANIA (*μεγάλος*, from *μέγας*, great; *μανία*, madness). This word has been, and still is, employed in reference to two distinct mental disorders, or rather to the same symptom occurring under very different psychological conditions. Formerly, the term was applied to the exaltation or delirium of grandeur which usually accompanies general paralysis of the insane. French alienists have restricted its use to cases in which this symptom is present without paralysis, and this is the practice generally adopted at the present day. From this point of view it is a systematised delusion—a monomania—and by those who adopt the term "paranoia," it is regarded as a frequent characteristic of this form. (*See* EXALTATION.) An article by the late Dr. Foville on "Megalomania" will be found in the *Transactions of the International Medical Congress*, 1881. (Fr. *Mégalomanie*, *Monomanie des grandeurs*, and *Monomanie ambitieuse*; Ger. *Grössenwahnsinn*.)

MEGALOPIA HYSTERICA; MEGALOPSIA HYSTERICA (*μέγας*, great; ὤψ, the eye or vision; hysteria). A visual defect occurring in hysterical subjects in which some objects appear larger than they in reality are. (*See* MACROPSY, HYSTERICAL.)

MEGRIMS (*migraine*, from hemicrania). Besides its ordinary meaning, a term sometimes applied to epilepsy and epileptic seizures.

MELANCHOLIA. — **Definition.** — A disorder characterised by a feeling of misery which is in excess of what is justified by the circumstances in which the individual is placed.

Symptoms.—(1) The cardinal symptom of melancholia is indicated by the definition; it is the expression of a feeling of misery for which no sufficient justification exists in the circumstances of the individual. Associated with this cardinal symptom are two other groups of symptoms; (2) defects of nutrition and of other bodily processes; and (3) defect of conduct. Commonly there is present, (4) the expression of a delusion.

(1) The feeling of misery is expressed (α) by the face, (β) by attitude, (γ) by gesture, (δ) by verbal expression.

(α) The expression of the face in melancholia is very characteristic. The jaws are not firmly closed, the lower jaw falls away from the upper, with or without parting of the lips, and thus gives the face an elongated appearance. The forehead is puckered by several parallel transeverse wrinkles, which extend high up on the forehead, and, beneath these, at the middle of the forehead, are several vertical wrinkles. The eyebrows are drawn upward at their inner ends, and are approximated to one another, so that the direction of each is downward and outward. The fold of skin between the brow and lid participates in this movement, and gives to the opening of the eyelids a triangular outline, the base of the triangle being horizontal, and the inner and shortest side perpendicular. The corners of the mouth are drawn downwards, the under lip is sometimes thrust forward and upward, at others hangs away from the teeth.

(β) The attitude in melancholia is one of general flexion. An erect figure is never seen in this malady. The head is bowed, the back is bent, in severe cases the legs are bent at the knees. The tendency of the thumb is to lie, not opposed to the fingers, but parallel with and alongside them.

(γ) Among the gestures expressing misery, the most prominent and characteristic is that of weeping, which is common in its full expression. But when not fully expressed, the eyes in melancholy patients are commonly full of tears. Very loud obtrusive uproarious weeping does not appear to be associated with deep melancholy. Wringing of the hands may be either constant, frequent or occasional. A succession of slow nods of the head, the first of which is the most emphatic, and the remaining three or four of much less and of decreasing emphasis, is a striking and characteristic gesture expressive of melancholy. Sighing and groaning, striking the head with the fists, sitting with the face buried in the hands, tearing the hair, standing for a considerable time in one attitude, sitting and rocking the body backwards and forwards, are all gestures expressive of misery.

(δ) The verbal expressions of misery in melancholia are, apart from the expression of delusion, not numerous, and, belonging chiefly to the emotional division of language, may be looked upon in the light of verbal gestures. Such an utterance as "Oh dear!" is scarcely more articulate, and no more expressive, than a groan. The peculiarity of the verbal expressions of misery is mainly the frequency of their repetition. A man will repeat such a phrase as "Oh dear!" or "Oh God!" hundreds of times in the course of an hour.

It should here be stated that the expression of misery is not always proportionate to, nor a measure of, the degree of misery that is felt. The training of civilized man, especially in this country, is so much directed towards the suppression of the display of emotion, that in the early stages of melancholia, when control is but little impaired, the expression exhibited before other people, and especially before strangers, may fall far short of indicating the degree of feeling experienced. On the other hand, when misery has been severely felt and freely expressed for long periods, a habit of complaining by face, gesture and utterance has grown up, which continues after all real intensity of feeling has passed away; and thus, in the later stages of the malady, the expression is frequently in excess of the feeling.

(2) In true melancholia—that is to say, in cases in which there is not merely an expression, but an actual experience of misery — there is defect of nutrition throughout the whole body, and this defect is always of the nature of a slackening, weakening, diminution of activity in the process of nutrition. In all the parts of the body that are open to observation, the nutritive defect shows itself conspicuously. The skin is dry, and is often of an earthy, muddy, unwholesome tint; the hair is dry, harsh and staring; the nails grow unusually slowly, and rarely want cutting. The mouth is dry, the tongue is furred, the bowels are constipated, the urine is loaded, the pulse is slow, the body-temperature is lowered, the whole consensus of symptoms goes to show that every bodily process is slackened, lowered, wanting in vigour.

(3) The conduct in melancholia exhibits a defect which is strictly comparable with the defect in the nutritive processes. It is wanting in energy and vigour. When the feeling of misery is not very great, the defect in activity of conduct may be but small. The patient takes less exercise, is prone to sit indoors rather than to exert himself by walking abroad or by games of activity; but when the misery is great, the inactivity becomes very marked. The patient does not go out at all, but shuffles up and down his room, or sits in his chair all day, and cannot be induced by any amount of urging to take even the exertion necessary to keep his person neat and tidy, nor even clean. His hair becomes unkempt and matted, his linen dirty, his skin filthy.

(4) Delusion is a very frequent, though not an invariable accompaniment of

melancholia. Many cases begin with a simple feeling of misery without delusion, and, in trifling and mild cases, delusion may not occur, or may not become conspicuous in the whole course of the malady. But, as a rule, the disorder of feeling is accompanied with more or less evidence of disorder of thought, and actual delusion accompanies the melancholia. Not only does delusion usually accompany the melancholia, but as a rule the gravity of the delusion has some relation to the depth of the feeling of misery, so that if the circumstances were as the patient deludedly believes them to be, they would go far to justify the feeling that he experiences. It would serve no useful purpose to enter at large here upon the character of the delusions entertained by melancholiacs. They are extremely numerous and diverse, and belong to all the varieties of delusion enumerated elsewhere (*see* DELUSION), except of course those of increased consequence and welfare. A list of those already observed, to be exhaustive, would well-nigh occupy the whole of this volume, and it is improbable that the next case that occurs would repeat any one of those so enumerated.

Course and Terminations.—Melancholia differs from other varieties of insanity in that it commonly arises *de novo* in a healthy person. It is very far less common for a person who already exhibits some other form of insanity to become melancholic than to become maniacal, demented or epileptic. Usually the onset of melancholia is gradual. A patient does not suddenly sink into deep melancholia, as he suddenly becomes maniacal or epileptic. He is noticed to be somewhat dull, somewhat lethargic, somewhat uneasy, and in less than his usual spirits, but usually these slight beginnings of the malady attract no notice, and it is not until the disorder has become fully established that it is remembered for how long the symptoms have been gradually increasing. At length the degree of misery and the other symptoms reach a grade at which the limits of the normal are unmistakably exceeded, and it becomes manifest that the patient is suffering from a morbid depression.

The subsequent course of the case may vary within wide limits. A large proportion of patients who are young, and who are taken in hand at an early stage of the malady, recover rapidly and completely; and there is scarcely any class of patients that comes under the care of the alienist that shows results so satisfactory as this one. The recovery is often rapid, and may sometimes be even sudden, a person who was last night plunged in misery, being this morning cheerful and contented. More commonly the first step in the improvement is a long stride, and occurs upon a definite date, and thereafter follows a period of slower and more gradual improvement, attaining at length to recovery. Not uncommonly it happens that improvement may be gradually gained until a certain degree of nearness to recovery is reached, and at that point the ameliorative process comes to a standstill, and the final stages of recovery are extremely difficult to bring about.

Melancholia is a malady which is very liable to relapse, and the relapse may take place at almost any period in the life history of the patient. Thus it may take place during the period of recovery, and the course of recovery may be interrupted and delayed by the occurrence of one or two or several relapses. Or the relapse may occur at a longer or shorter period after recovery—at the end of a few months, or a few years, or of half a lifetime.

On the other hand, melancholia may terminate rapidly in death. The patient may become thinner, weaker, more dejected, more incapable of assimilating food, more incapable of exhibiting energy, until he dies of exhaustion; and death in this way may occur very rapidly, in a few weeks, or may be the termination of many months of illness.

Instead of terminating either in recovery or death, melancholia may merge into mania of more or less acuteness, of which it then appears to have been the initial stage. Indeed, the frequency with which this occurs has led a very thoughtful alienist—Dr. Sankey—to the conclusion that all cases of insanity, save of course general paralysis, begin in melancholia; or at least that the ordinary and normal succession of events is melancholia, mania, dementia, a succession which may be interrupted at any stage by recovery or death. Be this as it may, it is certain that melancholia is often a step to mania, and still more often a stage on the road to dementia. These observations lead us directly to the consideration of the

Varieties of melancholia, which the industry of clinical alienists has rendered perhaps unnecessarily numerous, no fewer than thirty varieties having been described by various authors. It will not be necessary to consider all these in detail here, especially as some of the varieties are dealt with at length in other articles in this volume (*see* FOLIE CIRCULAIRE; MELANCHOLIA ATTONITA), but certain well-marked varieties may well be described.

Simple Melancholia is that variety of the malady in which the depression of feeling is unattended by delusion. Most cases of melancholia exhibit this phase at the outset, when the depression is not severe; and a few cases, which never attain a great degree of severity, remain throughout free from manifestation of delusion. But the great majority of cases show, at one time or another of their course, evidence of the existence of delusion, and probably in no case does the feeling of depression attain great intensity without the appearance of delusion.

Melancholia with delusion is the complement of simple melancholia, and includes all cases which are not included in the previous class.

Cases of melancholia are again divided into *acute* or *chronic* according to their duration. Any case which culminated in a few weeks would come under the former category. Cases of really chronic melancholia, that is to say, cases in which an unjustifiable feeling of misery is experienced, for many months or for years together, are far from common. Doubtless there are many cases in which the expression of misery has become habitual, and is maintained long after the actual feeling has passed away, but it is very doubtful whether there is any real feeling of misery in many of the cases classed as chronic melancholics.

Melancholia has again been divided into *active* and *passive*, according as the manifestations of the feeling of wretchedness consist of exaggerated gestures, loud cryings and moanings, &c., or as the patients are listless, lethargic and languid. An extreme degree of passivity with depression of spirits constitutes the variety known as *melancholia cum stupore* or *melancholia attonita* (*q.v.*).

Intervals of melancholy occur in the course of other forms of insanity, as in mania, dementia, epilepsy, and general paralysis, and when so occurring it has been designated by a special title; but there is nothing in the symptoms or manifestations of melancholy occurring under these circumstances which is different from those of ordinary melancholy, and although its manifestations may be mingled with those of the other maladies or their results, there is no need to consider such cases separately.

Suicidal Melancholia. — A separate variety of melancholia has been erected under this title, and in it would be included any case in which there is a tendency to suicide. The tendency to self-destruction is by no means always in proportion to the depth of the depression, some cases, in which the manifestations do not indicate severe depression, being most determined and persistent in their attempts to commit suicide, while to others, in whom the feeling of misery is evidently profound, the idea of suicide never seems to present itself. Often, it may be said usually, the attempt at suicide is made in the same way in the same case, and a man who is bent upon destroying himself by shooting, will neglect opportunities of compassing his end by drowning or hanging, and will use only the one particular method which commends itself to him. The tendency to suicide having once exhibited itself in any case, renders that patient for ever after a source of anxiety to those who have the care of him; for in consequence of the want of proportion between the tendency to suicide and the manifestations of depression, it becomes impossible to infer, with any safety, from the disappearance of the latter, that the former also has disappeared. Many cases are on record in which patients, who have apparently recovered from melancholia, have committed suicide on being freed from restraint. When once a person has fully determined to commit suicide, it is well-nigh impossible to prevent him from carrying out his intention. The ingenuity with which he will construct lethal weapons out of the most harmless implements, out of the materials of clothing, the secrecy with which he will carry out his preparations, and the suddenness and determination with which he will carry them into effect, are such as, if persisted in over a long period, to render futile the most stringent watchfulness and precaution. The sharpening of bits of barrel hoop, of nails and bits of wire, into deadly instruments, is a matter of daily occurrence in large asylums. Female patients will pull threads out of their sheets until they have got enough to twist into a cord wherewith to strangle themselves. One man will hang himself from a post three feet high, another will drown himself in a basin of water, a third will stuff a lump of meat into his throat and suffocate himself.

Pathology.—The nature of the change in nerve-tissue that underlies melancholia is obscure. Whatever change may be assigned as the efficient cause of the symptoms must be one which will account for the whole of them. When we find the alteration of feeling, the alteration of conduct, and the alteration of nutrition invariably concomitant, and invariably exhibiting certain common features, we cannot reasonably ascribe them to separate lesions of nerve-tissue, but must admit that any valid explanation must account for all by the occurrence of a single change. The nature of this change is indicated by the nature of the modification that affects all these processes. The characteristic alteration of conduct is its diminished activity. The characteristic alteration of the nutritive processes is their diminished activity. The characteristic alteration of consciousness is the diminution of the feeling of well-being; and we now know enough of the nervous accompaniment of consciousness to know that the feeling of well-being is dependent for its existence on a high state of activity of the nerve-tissue, on a high degree of tension of the nerve energy existing therein. But a high degree of activity of the nerve elements produces great activity of conduct; and a high tension of nervous energy produces great activity of all the nutritive processes. Hence, when feeling is depressed, conduct diminished, and nutritive processes inactive, we must infer that the opposite condition exists—that the nervous elements are unduly inactive, and the tension of the nervous energy is reduced below the normal. Any lowering of the vigour of the motor currents going to the muscles will have the effect of reducing the energy of the muscular contractions; and when the vigour of the nerve-currents is lowered throughout the whole of the hierarchy of the nerve-centres, not only will muscular contractions be weakened, by affection of the lowest rank of centres; not only will movements be rendered less frequent and less vigorous, by affection of the middle rank of centres; but, by affection of the highest ranks, the whole phenomena of conduct will be diminished, weakened, attenuated and impaired. The muscular system is not the only recipient of motor nerve-currents. Similar currents have been demonstrated to regulate the activity of glands, and the disturbances of nutrition that invariably follow section of nerves, indicate with equal certainty that the nutrition of every tissue in the body is dependent on and is regulated by "motor," that is to say, outgoing, currents from the central nerve regions. When the vigour of these motor currents is great, the nutritive processes in the tissues are active, the various bodily processes exhibit an abounding vitality, secretions are copious, visceral movements vigorous, the skin is clear and tense, the eyes are bright, the hair and nails grow rapidly and evenly, the whole body exhibits evidence of activity and vigour. When the motor currents are feeble and attenuated, the opposite state of affairs obtains; secretions are scanty, excretion is inefficient, visceral movements are languid, the skin is lax, and is opaque and earthy looking, the eye is dull, the muscles are lax, the hair and nails grow slowly and irregularly, and the whole of the bodily processes exhibit evidence of languor, feebleness and inactivity. Thus, the defect of conduct, the passivity, the indolence, the lethargy of melancholia are dependent upon precisely the same alteration of nerve action as the constipation, the loaded urine, the foul tongue and the other physical symptoms; and hence it appears no longer extraordinary that the one set of symptoms should invariably accompany the other. That precisely the same nervous defect underlies the feeling of melancholy does not appear to need very urgent insistence, for it is found generally that the feeling of well-being bears a regular proportion to the manifestations of activity of nerve elements. Generally, when there is a high degree of spontaneity of movement, and a high degree of activity of bodily processes, the consciousness of self is highly pleasurable; and when movements are languid, and bodily processes slackened, the consciousness of self loses its buoyancy and becomes depressed. This concomitance of the variations of the feeling of well-being with the variations in the other signs of nervous activity is shown in many ways. It is shown in the diurnal fluctuations, the general feeling of well-being attaining its height at mid-day when activity is greatest; and being at its ebb in the small hours of the morning when activity, both of movement and of nutrition, is at its minimum. It is shown in the phenomena of illness, and the fluctuations that occur from time to time in the course of all lives; and it is shown conspicuously in the contrast between youth and age, one full of abounding vigour and with exalted feeling of well-being, always in high spirits and happy; the other placid alike in body and in mind, physically inactive, and mentally no more than content.

Ætiology.—If such be the pathology of melancholia, the search for its ætiology is considerably simplified, for whatever will produce a lowering in the tension of the nerve energy, and an inefficiency or slackening in the mode of working of the nerve-elements, may produce melancholia. Of all the conditions upon which this modification of nervous action may depend the most important is undoubtedly that of hereditary disposition (*see* Heredity).

While some individuals are born with nervous systems of great vigour, containing so great a store of energy, so easily and rapidly renewed, that they are capable of powerful and sustained exertion, are with difficulty fatigued, require little sleep, rapidly recuperate the energy that they expend, exhibit a high degree of vigour in all their bodily processes, and maintain throughout all vicissitudes of circumstances a buoyant, hopeful, eager and confident mind; others are so constituted from birth that their nervous systems contain but a poor accumulation of force, an accumulation which is easily depleted, is slow to recuperate, so that they are capable of but little and brief exertion, are easily fatigued, require much sleep, but obtain perhaps little, exhibit the signs of feebleness and languor in all their bodily processes, are easily and profoundly depressed in mind by slight reverses of fortune, and even in their best moments are rather content than happy, rather placid than in good spirits. Persons of the first class of constitution are proof against the attacks of melancholia, while persons of the second class require but little solicitation or provocation from circumstances to sink into a slough of despond.

An hereditarily acquired tendency to undue feebleness of nerve action may be aggravated into activity by several different provocative agents. Any unusual demand upon the powers of the organism, any occasion requiring the expenditure of large draughts of energy, may so deplete the activity of the nervous system as to bring about melancholia. Occasions of this nature may arise from circumstances either within or without the organism. Thus, at the period of puberty, when large re-arrangements in the distribution of nerve energy are being made, and when copious draughts of energy are being called for in order to satisfy the new functions and new activities that are then arising, melancholia frequently appears, mingled usually in more or less intricate combination with hysteria, the special product of that time. At the time of the other momentous changes, of pregnancy, childbirth, suckling, and the climacteric, all of which deplete the activities of the nervous system by making large draughts upon its energies, melancholia may appear. After exhausting attacks of bodily disease, after exhausting exertion, either physical or mental, after the prolonged exertion of climbing a mountain, or after the prolonged exertion of preparing for an examination, melancholia may supervene. Similarly, untoward circumstances, the loss of friends, or of fortune, or of character; any circumstance which is calculated to produce sorrow, grief, uneasiness, anxiety, in an ordinarily constituted person, may, if it act upon a person of less than ordinary stamina, produce melancholia; and the more severe the stress, the greater, naturally, is the chance of melancholia occurring.

Diagnosis.—The nearest allies to melancholia, and the maladies for which it is most likely to be mistaken, are dementia, hypochondriasis, and hysteria. To *dementia* it is allied, not merely in appearance, but in nature, for the melancholy feeling never reaches a morbid degree without some general weakening of the mental powers, which constitutes a slight degree of dementia, and, in well marked cases of melancholia, in which the amount of depression is great, the weakening of the mental power becomes very marked, and constitutes of itself a veritable dementia. If in such cases we have regard to the conduct alone, and neglect the manifestations of misery, we shall have no hesitation in recognising the considerable degree of dementia, or impairment of mind, that exists. Melancholia differs, then, from dementia in the superaddition to the symptoms of the latter of evidence of depression of mind; this evidence being, in many cases, so much the more prominent symptom as to throw into the shade the co-existing dementia, which then remains unrecognised. On the other hand, there are cases in which the dementia is by far the more prominent of the mental peculiarities, and the depression of mind is not conspicuous; in such cases the melancholic element may be overlooked, and the case be considered one of simple dementia. Such errors of diagnosis are not of great importance, the two conditions being sufficiently alike in nature to need the same treatment and to warrant the same prognosis.

Hypochondriasis is distinguished from melancholia, to which it is very nearly allied, by the persistence with which the patient assigns his malaise to bodily disease, and by the degree to which his thoughts are enthralled and engrossed by his bodily condition. Between hypochondriasis and melancholia there is every possible gradation, from the patient whose only peculiarity is his persistent and too much absorbed attention to some real or half imaginary local disorder, to him who is sunk in misery which he ascribes to the judgment of God upon his sins. In the former case the patient is distinguished by his enthusiastic acceptance of remedy after remedy, and his eager pursuit of one medical practitioner after another. Throughout all the dread and wretchedness of his career he clings fast to the faith that he will at length discover the man who shall administer the drug that will cure him. The melancholy man has no such hope. No ray of comfort brightens the gloom of his life. So far from entertaining hopes of recovery or confidence in treatment, he rejects with something like contempt the advice that is tendered for his welfare.

The distinction of *hysteria* from melancholia is in the different degrees to which the attention of others is sought and claimed in the two cases. In hysteria the whole aim and end of the display of symptoms by the patient will be found to have regard to the attraction of notice, of interest, and of sympathy from others. In melancholia, on the other hand, the patient is quite indifferent to the way in which her actions and symptoms may impress other people. She is too much absorbed in the misery that she suffers to bestow a thought upon the way in which her conduct is regarded.

One other condition is necessary to bear in mind in the diagnosis of melancholia. The malady has been defined as "a feeling of misery in excess of what is justified by the circumstances in which the individual is placed;" and, in order to say with any confidence that the malady exists, it is necessary to know the circumstances of the individual in order to judge whether the misery experienced is justified by them or no. It may be that the misery is so profound that scarcely any circumstances, however adverse, would be a justification for it, and in such cases the diagnosis is not difficult; or it may be that the feeling of misery may be accounted for by a reason which is palpably and manifestly the outcome of a delusion, as that the patient has been deprived of his wings, or has had another person's brains substituted for his own. But there is a large class of cases in which the reason alleged may possibly be true, and, if true, would justify the feeling of unhappiness. If a patient appears afflicted with melancholy, and declares that he is on the brink of ruin; that his wife is unfaithful; that he is a wicked and dishonest man; that he is liable to arrest; it is necessary to be very cautious in regarding his statements as unfounded. It may be that they are true, and that his feeling of misery is only the normal and natural feeling that such circumstances ought to inspire.

Treatment.—The treatment of melancholia is indicated very obviously by the account of the pathology that has been given. If the defect which underlies the whole malady is a weakening and slackening of the nerve-action, and a diminution of the tension of the nerve-currents, then the treatment must be directed to arousing a more intense activity, and restoring the tension to its normal height. There is no reason to doubt that the process of storing energy in the nerve-elements is a part of the general process of nutrition, nor that if we can by any means increase the activity and vigour of the nutritive processes generally throughout the body, we can compel the nerve-elements to take a share in the increased activity, and may by degrees restore them to their normal state. The whole of the treatment of melancholia is therefore directed to stimulating and increasing the activity of the processes of nutrition. First among the restorative measures is the administration of food. It is usually found, when a melancholic patient comes under care, that for a considerable time he has not taken a sufficiency of food. Owing to the slackening of the nutritive processes, sufficient pabulum has not been assimilated by the tissues, and owing to the same reason the representation in consciousness of the needs of the body has been obscure and insufficient. Hunger has not been felt, and hence food has not been taken in sufficient quantity. The subjects of melancholia are often emaciated, usually thin, and always are less well nourished than they are wont to be in their normal condition of cheerfulness. Always there is want of inclination for food, often there is positive distaste for it, and not unfrequently there is complete and obstinate refusal to take it. Hence the first necessity in the treatment of a melancholy patient is to insist on the ingestion of abundance of aliment, and if necessary to employ force for the purpose.

Dr. Blandford has pointed out that in some cases food is withheld in consequence of the dyspepsia which so frequently coexists with the mental depression; but this is a mistake, and may easily become a fatal mistake. Food, abundance of food, must always be administered, no matter what the state of the patient's digestion may appear to be, no matter how directly contrary it may be to his inclination. It is not enough to give slops and concentrated essences of meat and peptic fluids. Solid food of varied nature and considerable bulk must be given if the greatest benefit is to be obtained.

In order that the food thus given may be digested and assimilated, the next point of importance is to see that plenty of exercise be taken. Some care will be necessary here to graduate the exercise to the patient's strength, for it is probable that before he has come under care he has for long taken but little exercise, and the sudden undertaking of strenuous exertions may have a very deleterious effect; but some exercise should be insisted on, and, as strength returns, it should be gradually and somewhat rapidly increased. In prescribing exercise two points are to be attended to. The exercise should bring into play as far as possible the large muscular masses. The patient should not stand at a bench manipulating with his hands. If nothing better offers he should be made to walk, but better than walking is some exercise which employs in strenuous exertion a larger number of muscles, including the bulky muscles of the back. Rowing, riding, and cycling are indicated if there be no suicidal tendency, while, if such a tendency exist, excellent exercise may be got from such work as using a cross-cut saw, working a chaff-cutter, or turning the homely mangle. In very severe cases, in which emaciation is great, weakness extreme, and disinclination to exertion profound, the employment of massage may be of great benefit to start the processes of nutrition, and make them recommence their forgotten task, but such methods do not commonly need to be employed for long.

It will always be difficult to carry out the measures indicated so long as the patient is in his own home, and surrounded by his familiar environment; and for this reason an important part of the treatment is the removal of the patient to new surroundings. But this is not the only reason why such a change is beneficial. The mere fact of change, of living in different rooms, in a different locality, among different people, in a different physical, mental and moral atmosphere to that which is customary, is itself a powerful provocative of increased tissue metamorphosis. In customary surroundings, the organism becomes habituated to certain sets of impressions arriving at more or less regular and expected times; and the more thorough the habituation the less the change produced by the impressions. All are familiar with the fact that a slight noise which is new and unaccustomed will awake them from the profoundest sleep, while sleep may continue throughout a deafening uproar if only the organism has become accustomed to the noise by long habituation. The value of removal to new surroundings is in the much more vigorous tissue-changes that are brought about by impressions of ordinary intensity. A third reason for the beneficial action that is always found to result from change of surroundings, when the change is to the interior of an asylum, is in the habits of order, discipline, and obedience that are there found to prevail. In the patient's own home he has been accustomed to freedom of action, and the influence of others by persuasion or otherwise has been discontinuous and feeble. But in an asylum he lives in an atmosphere of order and discipline; and finding that all around him submit with cheerfulness to rule and governance, he is insensibly influenced by the contagious example of the rest to subordinate his own inclinations to the desires of those with whom he is placed. Of course the surroundings should be made as cheerful as possible. Every effort should be made to engage the patient's attention, to cause him to interest himself in some occupation, to get his mind as well as his body to work; but efforts in this direction will be for the most part futile until the nerve-elements have been compelled by physical means to resume their function of storing and expending energy.

With regard to drugs, it was for many years customary to treat melancholic patients by routine with opium; but this treatment has of late years dropped almost entirely out of practice. Every now and then we meet with a patient who appears to be benefited by opium, but the cases are not frequent, and the drug is now seldom used. Of much more avail are drugs, such as iron, quinine, arsenic, and strychnine, which tend to simulate the processes of digestion and of nutrition generally; and in the writer's experience the most valuable drug in the treatment of melancholia has been the syrup of the phosphates of quinine, iron, and strychnine, known as Easton's syrup.

Of the symptoms that have to be dealt with, the most frequent and troublesome are dyspepsia, with its attendant constipation, and sleeplessness. The constipation appears to be often largely due to the fact that the bowels are empty or nearly so, and that nothing passes *per anum*, because there is nothing to pass, or at any rate the intestines do not contain enough solid matter to arouse them to the performance of their normal movements. It is found that in many cases the bowels are freely relieved without the use of aperients, when a systematic course of copious feeding is entered on and maintained. When it becomes necessary to give aperients, the best form is one of the many aperient mineral waters given fasting in the morning.

What has been said of constipation applies also in great measure to sleeplessness. It is a frequent experience of the most healthy people that sleep and hunger are incompatible, and that it is a hopeless task to endeavour to sleep with an empty stomach. In melancholia the amount of food taken is habitually less than normal, and less than the body needs, and it is for this reason, as much as for any other, that sleep is so rare and so difficult to obtain. In the great majority of cases it will be found that the best soporific is a bellyful of food, and it not unfrequently happens that patients who have not slept, or have scarcely slept, for weeks in spite of the administration of enormous doses of opium, of bromides, of chloral and other hypnotics, will fall asleep immediately, and sleep long and soundly, after being compelled to eat a hearty and copious meal. Where food alone will not produce sleep, it will usually be found that the addition to the food of some stimulant will produce the desired effect. A bottle of stout, or a glass of stiff hot grog, on the top of a good supper will produce a drowsiness which is very hard to resist. More especially is this the case when the meal comes at the end of a day of tiring exercise in the open air. When the patient is not strong enough to take much exercise, and, indeed, often when he is, it will be found that a long drive in an open carriage produces a remarkably soporific effect. All these measures should be well tried before recourse is had to drugs, and the cases will be rare indeed in which their combined action will be ineffectual. Of course, in very severe and very acute cases, several of the measures cannot be taken, and it may then happen that recourse must be had to drugs. In that case it is best to give the drug hypodermically, after the patient has had a meal, and it is important that the patient should be already undressed, in bed, and quiescent before the drug is given. After its administration, absolute stillness should be enjoined, and in this way the effect is most likely to be obtained. When it is necessary to give a drug the dose should be a full one. If morphia, not less than ½ gr.; if chloral, not less than 30 grs.

Under the head of treatment should be mentioned the precautions that it is necessary to take in suicidal cases. These precautions may be summed up in two words—incessant watchfulness. When a patient has once manifested a suicidal tendency, he should never be left alone, waking or sleeping, day or night, until he is quite cured and fit again to take his place in society. Of course all weapons and appliances that could be used for a suicidal purpose should be removed from his reach. He should not be allowed razors, knives, scissors, glass, crockery, or anything that can be made into a weapon. But no amount of precaution of this character is of the slightest avail if the patient is allowed to be alone. He must be watched incessantly; an attendant must be always with him. He must be watched while dressing and undressing, taken to the closet, watched while on the seat, and brought away. Even with all this precaution, it is not always possible to prevent a patient from destroying himself. He may run head forwards against a wall, and fracture his skull; or he may throw himself headlong downstairs. But unless such precautions as have been mentioned are taken, the patient may as well be left to himself.

When the measures of treatment here described have been followed, when abundance of food has been administered, and a sufficiency of exercise taken, the waste of the tissues that exercise involves, the activity of tissue that it necessitates, predisposes the tissues to absorb nourishment, and stimulates them to resume their neglected function of assimilation. The process of assimilation, once begun, is a stimulus to the innumerable nerve-endings that are distributed among the tissues, and initiates a constant tide of nerve-currents that flow upward to the brain. Stimulated by these currents, the elements of the nerve-tissue in their turn begin to resume their activity both of function and of nutrition. They begin once more to absorb energy, and to expend it through the channels of nerve-fibre. The energy thus distributed enters the tissues of the body at large, and, acting as "motor" currents, reinforces their molecular activity, re-invigorates their nutrition, and is a cause of still more energetic currents returning to the brain, there to act as stimuli to nutrition and activity. Once the process is started, it continually reinforces itself, and hence we find that in the cure of melancholia it is the first step only which gives trouble. Once we can bring about a slight amelioration we need as a rule have little anxiety for the result.

Not unfrequently it happens, however, that the process is started in the way indicated, and is successfully pursued up to a certain point, but that when the patient is nearly well he comes to a standstill, and the final stage, the finishing off of the cure, is very difficult of attainment. In such cases an entire change of scene and surroundings will sometimes complete the recovery.

Prognosis.—In the majority of cases of melancholia the prognosis is favourable. The majority of cases recover. The character of the prognosis is influenced by the following considerations: (1) *The acuteness of the case.* Moderately acute cases are the most favourable. Extremely acute cases, in which the patient almost suddenly falls into extreme depression, rapidly wastes, early becomes wet and dirty, and neglectful of decency, are less hopeful. It is not always possible to arrest a process so headlong in character. But cases of moderate acuteness, in which the progress of the case has been rapid without being sudden, are favourable; chronic cases, in which there is merely an exaggeration of a state of depression which is usual, are much less hopeful. (2) *The period at which treatment is begun* is an important factor in the formation of prognosis. Every day that is lost in beginning vigorous treatment retards recovery, and renders it less probable; and prolonged neglect to enforce the measures already described, prolonged dependence on moral suasion, is disastrous. (3) *The degree to which the bodily health and condition are affected.* The more completely the affections of bodily health and condition correspond with the mental depression, the more hopeful the case. When the mental depression is severe, but the patient eats pretty well and sleeps pretty well, the prognosis is less favourable. In *youth* the prognosis is almost always favourable, and the more advanced the age the less favourable the prospect. A strong *hereditary tendency* is not as a rule an unfavourable element in a case. It is not unfavourable to recovery, although it increases the chances of subsequent recurrence of the malady. Termination in death does not as a rule take place except in the very acute cases; and on the other hand the more chronic the case the more is it likely to terminate in dementia. CHARLES MERCIER.

MELANCHOLIA, active (μελαγχολία; *ago*, I do or perform). A condition of mental depression occurring most frequently in women and men of middle age, characterised by a restless agitated state of misery, with occasional outbursts of aggressiveness, the result of some prominent delusion.—**M., affective** (*affectio*, feeling). The form of melancholia in which the affections or emotions only are concerned.—**M. agitata or agitans** (*agitatus*, from *agito*, I disturb, excite, &c.). Those instances of acute melancholia in which there is an active expression of the internal anguish by voice, behaviour, and gesture.—**M., alcoholic** (*alcohol*). The form which occasionally results after long-continued alcoholic abuse from the sudden stoppage of the stimulant when combined with insufficient food.—**M. anglica** (*anglicus*, English). A synonym of Suicidal Insanity.—**M. a potu** (*a*, from; *potus*, a drinking, or tippling.) Mental depression due to alcohol.—**M. attonita** (*attonita*, thunderstruck). A term used by Bellini, Sauvages, &c., for melancholy with stupor.—**M. autochirica** (αὐτός, self; χείρ, the hand). A synonym of Melancholia, Suicidal.—**M. canina** (*caninus*, pertaining to a dog). A synonym of Lycanthropia (*q.v.*).—**M., cataleptic** (καταλαμβάνω, I seize). A condition of mental depression chiefly occurring among the young, in which the mental stupor is associated with a plastic rigidity of the muscles.—**M., chronic** (χρονικός, pertaining to time). Melancholia in which the acute symptoms, somewhat modified, have persisted for any great length of time.—**M. complacens** (*complaceo*, I am well liked). The form in which there is self-complacency and satisfaction.—**M., convulsive** (*convello*, I tear). Clouston's term for a state of mental depression of an extreme type accompanied by muscular agitation and excitement and usually by great obstinacy, complicated by convulsive seizures of an epileptiform character, which occur seldom, are prolonged in character, and are succeeded by a rise of temperature (Clouston).—**M., delirious** (*deliro*, I rave). A psychosis the analogue of acute delirious mania, in which the mental symptoms are of a melancholic type, coloured at times with those of hysteria. A condition of typho-melancholia as opposed to typhomania or acute delirious mania.—**M., delusional** (*deludo*, I deceive). A term for that variety of mental depression in which delusions, many being what are known as fixed delusions, remain throughout the disease of the same character and are from the beginning the most prominent mental symptom.—**M., epileptiform** (epilepsy). A synonym of Melancholia, Convulsive (*q.v.*).—**M. erotica** (ἐρωτικός, pertaining to love). (*See* INSANITY, EROTIC.)—**M. errabunda** (*erro*, I roam about). A synonym of Kutubuth (*q.v.*).—**M., excited** (*excito*). A condition of melancholia in which the muscular expression of the prevailing emotion is strong and uncontrollable by volition (Clouston).—**M. flatuosa** (*flatuosus*, from *flatus*, wind). A synonym of Hypochondriasis.—**M., general.** The form of melancholia in which the depression extends to all the faculties and intellectual manifestations. (Fr. *mélancolie générale*).—**M., homicidal** (*homicida*, a manslayer). The condition of melancholia usually associated with suicidal tendencies, in which, under the influence of some delusion, a patient harbours homicidal intentions.—**M., hypochondriacal** (hypochondriasis, *q.v.*). A condition of mental depression in which hypochondriacal symptoms colour the melancholic state.—**M., hysterical** (hysteria, *q.v.*). A condition of mental depression occurring principally in young girls, in which symptoms of a hysterical type predominate. — **M. malevolens** (*malevolens*, evilly disposed). The form in which mischievous acts and propensities prevail. — **M. metamorphosis** (*μεταμόρφωσις*, a transformation). A form of melancholia in which the patient imagines he has been tranformed into some animal, or that he is some inanimate object —*e.g.*, a building, a glass utensil, &c.—**M. misanthropica** (*μισάνθρωπος*, hating men). The form of mental depression in which the patient hates and shuns the society of his fellowmen.—**M., misanthropical** (*μισανθρωπία*, hatred of mankind). Melancholia with aversion to human society, a desire for solitude, and a repugnance to the pleasures of life. — **M. moralis** (*moralis*, pertaining to morals). Mental depression with moral perversion or with moral delusions. — **M. nervea** (*nervus*, a nerve). A synonym of Hypochondriasis.—**M. of lactation.** (*See* PUERPERAL INSANITY.)—**M. of pregnancy.** (*See* PUERPERAL INSANITY.) — **M. of puberty** (*pubertas*, marriageable age). A form of mental alienation occurring at puberty in which the patient often evinces a listless and moody apathy and perverseness of conduct. (*See* DEVELOPMENTAL INSANITIES.) — **M., organic** (*ὄργανον*, arrangement). The mental depression, usually of a simple type, accompanying gross organic brain disease, such as tumours, ramollissements, &c. — **M., passive** (*patior*, I suffer). A form of melancholia allied to melancholia cum stupore, in which the delusions and hallucinations of ordinary melancholia are combined with passivity and apparent listlessness to surrounding sense impressions. (*See* MELANCHOLIA CUM STUPORE.) —**M. periodica** (*περιοδικός*, coming round at intervals). A name given to the melancholic stage of folie circulaire.—**M. persecutionis** (*persecutio*, a following after). The form of mental depression in which the patient has the delusion that he is followed or persecuted by enemies ; it is generally associated with auditory hallucinations and suicidal tendencies. — **M. pleonectica** (*πλεονεκτέω*, I strive to gain more). Insanity with desire for gain; morbid covetousness. — **M., puerperal.** (*See* PUERPERAL INSANITY.)—**M., reasoning.** (*See* LYPÉMANIE RAISONNANTE.)—**M., recurrent** (*re*, back again; *curro*, I run). The form of mental depression in which there is an irregular alternation of melancholic symptoms and recovery, extending over a great many years, and resulting in most cases in permanent dementia.—**M. religiosa** (*religio*, piety). The form of melancholia in which the patient has great despondency as to his future salvation, or in which a morbid religious emotionalism tinges the mental aberration.—**M., resistive.** Melancholia accompanied by obstinate resistance to any form of interference, generally purposeless and independent of delusion, but also frequently the direct result of some present delusion. — **M. saltans** (*salto*, I dance). A synonym of Chorea.—**M., senile** (*senilis*, old). The mental depression occurring in the aged, and usually associated with arterial degenerative change. — **M., sexual** (*sexualis*, from *sexus*, the male or female gender). The mental affection in which delusions as to the sexual organs or powers predominate. (*See* MASTURBATION, and INSANITY.)—**M., simple** (*simplex*). The form of mental depression in which the melancholia is mild and uncomplicated, and where the affective depression and pain are more marked than the intellectual or volitional aberrations (Clouston). — **M. simplex** (*simplex*, simple). Heinroth's term for melancholia without delusions or hallucinations.—**M. sine delirio** (*sine*, without; *delirium*, raging madness). Etmüller's term for an abortive form of melancholia in which there is only mental depression without delusion.—**M., stuporous, M. cum stupore** (*stupor*, unconsciousness). A state of mental depression accompanied by a morbid condition of mental lethargy or torpor. (Fr. *mélancolie avec stupeur.*) —**M., suicidal** (*sui*, himself; *caedere*, to kill). The form of mental depression in which ideas of, or a longing after, self-destruction, dependent on or independent of delusion, are present.—**M., sympathetic** (*συμπαθητικός*, affected by like feelings). A mental depression primarily produced by an affection of some other organ than the brain.—**M. transitoria** (*transitorius*, having a passage through). A condition similar to mania transitoria or mania ephemeral, in which a mental depression takes the place of a mental exaltation.—**M. uterina** (*uterinus*, pertaining to the womb). A synonym of Nymphomania.—**M. zoanthropia** (*ζῶον*, an animal; *ἄνθρωπος*, a man). A species of monomania in which the patient believes himself transformed into an animal. (*See* CYNANTHROPIA; LYCANTHROPIA.)

MELANCHOLIA CUM STUPORE. (*See* STUPOR, MENTAL.)

MELANCHOLIC DIATHESIS.—A hereditary brain constitution, consisting of a melancholic temperament with a nervous diathesis. The subjects are persons wanting in emotional balance and resistive power, have strong unreasoning likes and dislikes, are morbidly introspective and gloomily imaginative, and very often irritable (Clouston).

MELANCHOLIC, MELANCHOLICUS, MELANCHOLODES, MELANCHOLUS. (*See* MELANCHOLIA.) A labouring under mental depression or melancholy. One of a gloomy, morose disposition. Also that which belongs to or relates to melancholy.

MELANCHOLY (μελαγχολία). (*See* MELANCHOLIA.) A state of mental depression in which the subject experiences a feeling of mental pain with listlessness, weariness, and a sense of ill-being, but which differs from melancholia in that there are no morbid sense perversions, no irrationality of conduct, no morbid loss of self-control, no sudden or determined impulse towards suicide or homicide, and where surrounding events and occurrences still afford a certain amount of interest, though lessened in degree, and where the power of application to ordinary duties is still present.

MÉLANCOLIE AVEC DÉLIRE, MÉLANCOLIE DÉLIRANTE (Fr.). Melancholia with disturbance of the intellectual faculties. Delusional insanity of a melancholic character.

MÉLANCOLIE SANS DÉLIRE.—Etmüller and Guislain's term for simple melancholia.

MEMORIA (*memoria*, memory). The cerebral faculty by which past impressions are recalled to the mind.

MEMORY. (*See* PHILOSOPHY OF MIND, p. 27.)

MEMORY, Disorders of.—Disorders and alterations of the memory are so frequent, so various and so conspicuous, that it is not surprising to find them mentioned from early times. Greek physicians were occupied with them from a practical, other authors, among whom was St. Augustine, from a speculative point of view. The subject, however, has only recently been studied scientifically and in detail. Several conditions were necessary to achieve this, among which the most important was the predominance of the physiological method in psychology. As long as the memory was considered a "faculty," a sort of independent entity of the organism, it was impossible to look for or even to conceive the immediate cause of its derangement. In addition to this, the study of the cerebral functions, although still imperfect, has opened quite a new field of research. Anatomy, physiology and pathology have led us to consider the brain not so much a single organ as a congeries of organs, each of which has its function and is comparatively independent of the others. Nothing but this doctrine, known under the name of "cerebral localisation," renders intelligible that most frequent disorder, partial loss of memory, which for a long time was an inexplicable mystery.

With so rich a material, the investigation of which is but of recent date, we are able to undertake only a provisional classification, founded on the principal symptoms and intended only to put in some order the pathological phenomena of the memory. From this standpoint the classification may be made into three fundamental groups, comprising (1) loss (*amnesia*), (2) exaltation (*hypermnesia*), and (3) illusions of the memory (*paramnesia*).

(1) **Amnesia** represents by far the most important group of diseases of the memory. A subdivision may be made into classes, according as amnesia is total or *partial*.

Total amnesia affects the whole memory in all its forms. It divides our mental life into two or more pieces, thus leaving gaps which cannot be bridged over. These gaps made by the absence of the memory, may be of very variable duration and may extend over from two seconds to several weeks and months. Such temporary amnesia appears and disappears, as a rule, very suddenly.

The shortest, most distinct and most common cases of this form are met with in epileptic vertigo. The suicidal and homicidal attempts, robbery, unreasonable or ridiculous actions, accomplished during this period, which Hughlings Jackson styles "mental automatism" are so well known and so numerous, that it suffices to recall them here. It is probable that in certain short cases of epileptic vertigo there is momentary loss of consciousness, so that in order to be quite exact, we ought to say, that there is loss of *consciousness* and not loss of memory, but in cases of longer duration, in which the patient conceives and performs actions, which are complicated and nevertheless well adapted to their purpose, it is difficult to assume loss of consciousness; some of the patients even say "that they seem to awake out of a dream," so that it is really the impression upon the memory which fails.

Temporary amnesia is also frequent in cases of cerebral excitement, and then represents a *retro-active* character, that is to say, the patient, when recovering from unconsciousness, has lost not only the recollection of the accident he met with (fall from a horse or a carriage, blow on the head, &c.), but also the recollection of a more or less long period of his life before the accident. Dr. Frank Hamilton has reported twenty-six cases of this kind, which he communicated to the Medico-legal Society of New York (1875) and upon the forensic importance of which he lays stress. According to his opinion amnesia of events *before* the cerebral shock may extend over a period varying from five minutes or more to two or three seconds. It seems, therefore, that in order that a recollection may organise and fix itself, a certain time is necessary, which in consequence of the cerebral excitement does not suffice.

The forms of amnesia which we intend to mention, represent suppression of only a short period in the mental life of the patient; there are also many cases of long duration, as, *e.g.*, that of a woman who in consequence of her delivery forgot the period of her life between her marriage and the birth of the child, and never recovered the recollection of it. She did not believe she was married and the mother of a child until those around her had borne witness of the fact. She remembered accurately the rest of her life (*Lettre de Villiers à G. Cuvier*). More recently Sharpey has published in *Brain* (October 1879) curious observations of total amnesia, which necessitated complete re-education of the patient, which was very soon effected.

Lastly, we have in the group of total amnesia to mention the *alternating* memory, which is met with in the changes of personality (cases of Macnish, Azam, &c.). This pathological condition may be artificially produced in individuals who have often been hypnotised, in which case there are two memories, one comprising the facts of normal life, the facts of hypnotic life being excluded; the second comprising the facts of the whole life, normal as well as hypnotic. The individual thus passes through two conditions: in the former he possesses a partial memory only, composed of all the fragments of his normal life, which he links together; in the latter he retains the memory of his whole life.

As an hypothesis about the causes of this alternating memory, we should say, that there are two different physiological conditions, which, by their alternation, produce two cœnæsthesiæ, which on their part produce two different forms of association of ideas, and consequently two memories.

Partial amnesia is represented by the most frequent and best known forms of the pathology of memory. The isolated loss of one distinctly limited group of recollections appears at first sight *bizarre* and inexplicable, but if we consider the exact meaning of the word "memory," partial amnesia, far from being surprising, seems but the natural and logical consequence of a morbid influence. The word "memory" is actually a general term, meaning a property common to all feeling and thinking beings, but this general term is reducible to particular, concrete cases; in one word, the memory is broken up into *memories*, memory of sight, hearing, muscular sensations, taste, smell, &c.), and therefore it is natural that there should be partial amnesia.

The study of aphasia, pursued with such ardour and success for the last twenty years, affords us an excellent example of partial amnesia. Taking the word aphasia as a *generic* term to denote disorders of the *facultas signatrix*, it is necessary to distinguish different species: word-blindness, word-deafness, aphemia (verbal aphasia) and agraphy. These morbid conditions are so well known that it will be sufficient to recall their general features and to show that they depend on partial amnesia.

Word-blindness is the loss of the memory of the graphic images of words. The patient is able to see and distinguish figures, colours and objects, but letters and syllables are incomprehensible to him, and he is reduced to the condition of a man unable to read; he has lost one group of recollections. Moreover, this disorder has again varieties, thus it may be confined to the loss of memory of only musical signs (notes, flats, sharps, &c.).

Word-deafness is amnesia of auditory images. The patient is not deaf; he is able to hear noises, the striking of clocks, or the ticking of a watch, but words sound to his ear as a noise without meaning. He resembles a man who has gone into a country where speech is not known.

Aphemia (the most frequent case), that is to say ordinary aphasia (Broca's type), consists in the loss of the motor memory of articulation. There is neither paralysis of the tongue nor of the lips, nor of the organs of articulation in general, but the patient does not know how to articulate, and is reduced to the condition in which we all were before we were able to speak; the motor memory of speech has been lost or severely injured. This condition comprises a larger number of varieties than the others, from the loss of all words to the loss of a small number only.

Agraphy has been ingeniously defined as "aphasia of the hand" (Charcot); it consists in the loss of motor graphic representation. Many agraphic patients move their hands and arms easily, and hold the pen or pencil correctly, but it is impossible for them to recall any co-ordinate movements, which allow of writing letters and words. These patients also resemble those who have never learned writing. There are numerous varieties of this form of disorder; some patients are able to draw, to copy, &c.

If we keep in mind that each of these forms corresponds to a definite cerebral lesion (the third left frontal convolution in aphemia; the inferior parietal lobule in word-blindness, the first temporal convolution in word-deafness, and probably the lower part of the second frontal in agraphy) we come to the conclusion, that the images—our recollections—are localised in certain parts of the cerebrum, and that partial amnesia depends on organic causes.

It remains to mention amnesia of *progressive form*, which consists in a slow but continuous dissolution leading to complete abolition of the memory, as in paralytic and senile dementia. The dissolution of memory seems to follow a *law*, not in the rigorous sense of the word. We can only say what takes place in the majority of cases. The progressive destruction of the memory descends from the unstable to the stable recollections. Recent impressions not sufficiently fixed, and rarely repeated, represent the weakest degree of recollection and disappear first of all; old impressions, well fixed—automatic habits—in short all impressions which represent the stable form of recollections, disappear last. In the same way the recollection of proper names (individual terms) disappears before that of the common nouns and of the adjectives (general terms). This is however nothing but a particular instance of the biological law, that the structures formed last are the first to disappear.

(2) **Hypermnesia,** or exaltation of the memory, about which we have little to say. General exaltation of the memory is difficult to determine, because the degree of exaltation is quite a relative matter; we should have to compare the memory of one and the same individual with itself; it seems to depend exclusively on physiological causes, especially on the rapidity of the circulation. Hypermnesia may also be divided into *general* and *partial*.

General over-activity of the memory is produced in many individuals in danger of being drowned, who after having been saved from an imminent death, say that "at the moment when the asphyxia commenced, they seemed to see in one instant the whole of their life with even the smallest incidents spread out before them." It may also be due to the ingestion of toxic substances (haschisch and opium): De Quincey, Moreau (of Tours), and many others have given detailed descriptions of this general hypermnesia.

Partial hypermnesia is by its nature strictly limited; the most frequent cases, and the easiest to prove, consist in the recollection of languages, long completely forgotten, which returns in fever, in chloroform-narcosis, &c. Coleridge, Abercrombie, Hamilton, and Carpenter, have reported a great number of cases. Still more curious is the *regressive* recollection of several languages, or the recollection of the native language long forgotten, in the hour of death. Dr. Rush observed that an Italian, who had lived for a long time in America, and been attacked by yellow fever, spoke *English* at the commencement of his malady, *French* in the middle, and *Italian* the day of his death. A great number of similar cases have been reported by careful observers; the last sentences spoken in the hour of death were in the native language, which the patients had neglected for a great many years.

(3) **Paramnesia,** the term applied to certain illusions of the memory, which consist in the fact, that an individual believes that he has before experienced circumstances which are actually new to him. This illusion may be produced while a person is awake, but more frequently in dreams. Wigan, in his "Duality of the Mind," seems to have been the first who reported a case. Being present at the funeral service of a princess at Windsor, he all at once had the feeling as if he had been present at a similar occasion before. Sander (*Archiv f. Psychiatrie*, 1883, iv.) and A. Pick (*ibid.* 1876, vi.) have since published similar observations. This phenomenon, however, has been studied more recently, and more in detail by Kraepelin (*ibid.* xvii. and xviii.), who has grouped these false recollections in three classes:—

(*a*) Simple paramnesia, a simple image which appears as a recollection. Thus Kraepelin, who had never smoked, dreamed that he was having his fourth or fifth cigar. These illusions are very frequent in general paralytics, who fatigue those around them with accounts of voyages or adventures, which are not true.

(*b*) Paramnesia by identification; a new experience appears as the photography of a former one. Some lunatics brought for the first time into an asylum have the feeling as if they had been there before and had seen the same persons, &c.

(*c*) Associated or suggested paramnesia: an actual impression suggests an illusion of the memory—a pseudo-recollection of something similar in the past. Among others Kraepelin cites the case of a young man, with whom everything that he imagines seems to have occurred in the past.

Several theories have been proposed for the explanation of these illusions, but none have succeeded in accounting for them in a satisfactory manner. TH. RIBOT.

[*References*.—Sir Henry Holland, Mental Physiology, 1852. Hering, Ueber das Gedächtniss als allgemeine Function der Organisirten Materie, 1876. Carpenter, Mental Physiology. Wundt, Grundzüge der Philosophischen Psychologie. Ribot, Les Maladies de la Mémoire, 1881. Sully, Outlines of Psychology, 1884. Dr. Savage, Case of Acute Loss of Memory, Journ. Ment. Sci. April 1883. Dr. Creighton, Unconscious Memory in Disease, 1886. Forel, Das Gedächtniss und seine abnormitäten, 1885. Fouillée, La Survivance et la Sélection des Idées dans la Mémoire, Rev. des Deux Mondes, 1885. A. Pick, Loss and Recovery of Memory, Archiv f. Psychiatrie, Bd. xvii. Heft 1. Kraepelin, Ueber Erinnerungsfälschungen, Archiv f. Psychiatrie, 1887, Bd. xviii. 199, 395. H. Verneuil, Memory from the Physiological, Psychological, and Anatomical Point of View, 1888. Burnham, Memory Historically and Experimentally Considered, Amer. Journ. 1888-9, ii. 431-464.]

MENINGITOPHOBIA (*meningitis*; φοβέω, I fear). Symptoms of cerebrospinal meningitis, produced from fear of the disease. (*See* HYSTERIA.)

MENOPAUSE. (*See* CLIMACTERIC INSANITY.)

MENSTRUATION and INSANITY.—Esquirol has said that the derangements of menstruation form one-sixth of the physical causes of insanity, and Morel exactly agrees with him.

The following general conclusions have been arrived at by the writer after careful inquiry into the condition of the menstrual function in 500 lunatics.

(1) That in idiocy and cretinism puberty is usually delayed or absent.

(2) That in epileptic insanity the fits are generally increased in number, and that the patients frequently become excited at the catamenial period.

(3) That in mania exacerbations of excitement usually occur at the menstrual period, and that a state of intense excitement is almost continuous in patients suffering from menorrhagia.

(4) That in melancholia a large proportion of patients suffer from amenorrhœa.

(5) That in dementia the patients usually menstruate in a normal, healthy manner.

(6) That in general paralysis the change of life frequently occurs early.

(7) That, very rarely, the catamenia reappear in aged insane women after a prolonged cessation.

Amongst thirteen idiots and imbeciles menstruation was delayed beyond the normal time in half the number of cases. "In extreme degrees of cretinism the reproductive powers are never developed at all; and in less degrees menstruation appears late and continues scanty and irregular through life; whilst even in cases of the slightest description the average date of the first menstruation is as late as the eighteenth year." *

Amongst fourteen idiots, imbeciles, and cretins, seven, aged respectively 14, 16, 16, 18, 19, 22, and 22, had not begun to menstruate.

In mania, it is agreed by Esquirol, Greissinger, and Morel that increased excitement is observable at the catamenial period. On the other hand, we occasionally find instances in which mania is associated with more or less suppression of the menses. The mischief in these cases may be due either to congestion of the brain in consequence of the blood usually discharged by the normal channel being retained, or the amenorrhœa may be due to the general condition of anæmia which often accompanies an attack of asthenic insanity.

It cannot fairly be stated that in cases of recovery from mania the return of the catamenia always precedes the cure of insanity in cases where the discharge has been suppressed. Frequently the order is reversed, the patient becomes sane and is discharged from the asylum, but the monthly flux does not occur regularly for some weeks or months afterwards. A reappearance, however, of the catamenia cannot but be regarded as a favourable sign during an attack of insanity, and in many cases is followed by recovery. In puerperal insanity also the outlook becomes brighter on the return of the menstrual flux.

In insanity with menorrhagia, erotic actions and obscene language are frequent accompaniments.

Out of one hundred and sixty-two cases of mania, no less than ninety-nine, or about two-thirds of the total number had attacks of excitement which could be distinctly referred to the catamenial period.

Of these ninety-nine, in eleven instances the maniacal excitement was observed to

* Report on "Cretinism," presented to the Sardinian Government, 1848.

occur at periods varying from one day to a week before the accession of the catamenia. In the remaining eighty-eight, the mania appeared to occur, and to be at its worst, during the period of the catamenial discharge.

An increase in the number of fits and maniacal excitement occurred in many epileptics at the monthly periods.

Eighty-nine cases were made the subject of inquiry. The mental condition was in most cases that of dementia with excitement, but in a few instances dementia and melancholia were represented. In twenty-seven cases out of these eighty-nine the epileptic fits were either more numerous or occurred only at that time; in eleven cases maniacal excitement alone occurred; and in twenty-eight cases there was an exacerbation both of the epileptic seizures and of the maniacal condition at the menstrual periods. Four epileptics had amenorrhœa; and of these four, three had ceased to menstruate from old age. This last fact is remarkable as showing the effect of epilepsy in shortening life, since only three in eighty-nine epileptics had reached the menopause.

In melancholia "the uterine functions are more or less disordered, and are suspended in the large majority of cases."* In such patients the general condition of anæmia may produce amenorrhœa, and hence asthenic melancholia, but amenorrhœa and melancholia are also sometimes the result of a plethoric condition of the system. "Many patients, in consequence of plethora uteri, imagine themselves pregnant, and lament the disgrace which they thereby incur, but this delusion vanishes with the return of the period." †

The recurrence of menstruation in melancholia, if coincident with an improvement in the mental symptoms, justifies our giving a favourable prognosis.

In dementia, if the bodily health improves or remains good and there is no amelioration of the mental condition, the prognosis as to the recovery of mental health is most unfavourable, but such patients live to a great age. The catamenial function, as well as those of other organs, is discharged with great regularity.

Amongst forty-two cases of dementia, exclusive of epileptics, no less than thirty-two were regular in every respect, and eight had amenorrhœa.

Sixteen cases of delusional insanity were investigated. Thirteen were regular, one had menorrhagia, and two amenorrhœa. This form of insanity is compatible with healthy function in most of the organs of the body.

In two cases of moral insanity both were regular.

One case of monomania was regular.

Of four convalescents, three were regular, one had amenorrhœa.

Five cases had been in the asylum less than a month. Condition of function unknown.

Suppression of the catamenia in general paralysis at an early age was found in a large proportion of instances.

We venture to offer two suggestions in explanation of this abnormality.

In the first place, one of the theories of the pathology of general paralysis assumes that this disease is due to diminution of the calibre of the vessels of the brain. If this diminution exists in the vessels of that organ, why should it not also be present in the vessels of the uterus?

Hence a smaller quantity of blood would proceed to the ovaries, and these bodies being already predisposed to a sluggish performance of their function by the general state of depression of the whole system, amenorrhœa would naturally be the consequence.

In the second place, it has been found by the writer and others that in general paralysis of the insane there is a large increase in the white corpuscles of the blood at the expense of the red globules, which undoubtedly shows that a condition of anæmia exists. Amongst the sane anæmia is frequently the cause of amenorrhœa, and there is no reason why the same cause should not operate just as forcibly in constitutions already lowered and depressed by a disease which is almost universally acknowledged to be slowly but surely fatal.

Thirteen cases of general paralysis were inquired into. Of these thirteen, three, aged respectively, 46, 53, and 55, were considered too old to menstruate.

Excluding these three, ten remain, of whom four only menstruated regularly, being aged respectively, 31, 29, 34, and 32.

The remaining six, or three-fifths of the number who had not arrived at the change of life, never menstruated. Their ages, respectively, were, 34, 40, 30, 33, 40, and 35.

Three of these six cases were aphasic.

Amongst 158 old women* whose cases were inquired into, four were found in whom the catamenia had reappeared late

* Bucknill and Tuke's "Psychological Medicine." See also Falret's work, p. 300, and Morel, p. 194.

† Van der Kolk, on "Mental Diseases," p. 144.

* Menstruation returning in old women is not true menstruation. The ovaries and uterus are in senile atrophy. Hæmorrhage simulating menstrua-

in life. Two of these were more than 60 years old, and two were over 70.

A curious case was also under the care of the writer in which an insane patient, who had long passed the change of life, was under the delusion that she was pregnant. Her efforts to expel the supposed fœtus had the effect of bringing on the catamenia, which continued for several months, and then ceased suddenly.

The above remarks apply only to healthy or disordered uterine functions and their connection with the various forms of insanity. The reader is referred to an able and exhaustive work ("La Femme pendant la Période menstruelle," Dr. Icard, 1890) for a record of cases of organic disease of the womb, and their effects upon the intellectual faculties of the female. In this work it is affirmed that Rossignol (1856) has stated that out of 1236 prostitutes 980 were troubled with some uterine affection, which in many cases produced more or less mental aberration.

The idea that menstruation is a disgrace to a woman has long since disappeared with the advance of civilisation. We no longer say "Mulier speciosa, templum œdificatum super cloacam." We try rather to alleviate the symptoms of painful but healthy function by modern therapeutical appliances.

The importance of avoiding all emotional disturbance at the menstrual period has been insisted on by the authors of all ages.

The Levitical law prohibited connection with a woman at this crisis. Ezekiel considered such an act equivalent to adultery. A council of Nice ordered that Christian women should not enter a church during the catamenial period.

The Talmud affirmed that a child conceived during the flux was subject to every vice and disease. He would become a drunkard, insane, epileptic, or homicidal.

The Koran declared that a woman was impure eight days before and eight days after her courses.

Michelet believes that out of 28 days a woman is suffering from the effects of the monthly period for not less than 20.

Moreau states that the negroes shut up their women in huts during the time of the menstrual discharge.*

The medico-legal aspect of the effects of menstruation upon the emotional centres cannot be over-estimated. Krugelstein says: "Amongst all the female suicides it has been my lot to see, the act was committed during the catamenial period."*

Dr. Icard truly says: "The menstrual function can by sympathy, especially in those predisposed, create a mental condition varying from a simple psychalgia, that is to say, a simple moral malaise, a simple troubling of the soul, to actual insanity, to a complete loss of reason, and modifying the acts of a woman from simple weakness to absolute irresponsibility. The tribunal cannot appraise with any certainty the disposition of a woman who is the subject of menstrual disturbance."†

The following morbid mental phenomena have been observed by Icard to occur at the menstrual periods: Kleptomania, pyromania, dipsomania, homicidal mania, suicidal mania, erotomania, nymphomania, religious delusions, acute mania, delirious insanity, impulsive insanity, morbid jealousy, lying, calumny, illusions, hallucinations, melancholia; of which he reports cases at great length in his admirable work.

In the writer's experience, kleptomania is met with more frequently at the climacteric, pyromania being associated with puberty; dipsomania is also chiefly a disorder of the change of life. Erotomania is found at all ages, morbid jealousy at the menopause, lying in young women, calumny in moral insanity; and the other forms of mental aberration mentioned by Icard, which are not symptoms but diseases, are met with at all ages.

H. SUTHERLAND.

[*References.*—Sutherland, H., The Change of Life and Insanity, West Riding Asyl. Med. Reports, vol. iii. p. 299. Sutherland, H., Menstrual Irregularities and Insanity, West Riding Asyl. Med. Reports, vol. ii. p. 54. Merson, J., The Climacteric Period in Relation to Insanity, West Riding Asyl. Med. Reports, vol. vi. p. 85. Bucknill and Tuke, Catamenia in Prognosis, 3rd edit. pp. 148, 150. Mayer, Die Beziehungen der krankhaften Zustände in den Sexualorganem des Weibes zur Geistesstörungen. Marie, Etudes sur les Causes de la Folie puerpérale, Ann. Méd.-psych. 1857, t. iii. p. 577. Bruant, De la Mélancolie survenant à la Ménopause. Brouardel, Etat mental des Femmes enceintes. Petit, Des Rapports de la Paralysie générale avec certains Troubles de la Menstruation. Marcé, Traité de la Folie des Femmes enceintes. Brierre de Boismont, De la Folie puerpérale, Ann. Méd.-psych. 1851, p. 587. Ricard, Etude sur les Troubles de la Sensibilité génésique à l'Epoque de la Ménopause. Berthier, Des Névroses menstruelles. Schroter, Die Menstruation in ihren Beziehungen zur den Psychosen. Reikel, De la Folie puerpérale.]

MENTAL ABERRATION, MENTAL ALIENATION (*mens*, *alieno*, I alter in nature from). Synonyms of Insanity.

MENTAL EPIDEMICS. (*See* EPIDEMIC INSANITY.)

tion may be due to disease of uterus or of distant organs.

* "La Femme," Icard.

* *Op. cit.* p. 179.

† P. 266.

MENTAL EXPERTS. (*See* EXPERTS, MEDICAL.)

MENTAL PHYSIOLOGY.—Mental physiology is one division of the great department of physiology. It seeks to discover the bodily organisation with which mental operations are connected. Seeing that the brain is admitted to be the organ of mind, it endeavours to trace their correlation in detail. Unconscious no less than conscious mind falls within its range. The student of mental physiology makes the functions of the nervous system his special object of study, employing for this end all the means within his reach. He endeavours to discover the laws by which mental operations are governed, and to classify their phenomena, but he is not concerned with speculative metaphysics in the usual sense of the term. Mental physiology embraces the modern psychological methods of research which are instituted to determine the relation between the action of external stimuli on the sensory end-organs, and the resulting sensation or motion, as well as the reaction time of mental phenomena generally.

Sir Henry Holland, the first to write a work entitled "Mental Physiology" (1852), defined it as "that particular part of human physiology which comprises the reciprocal actions and relations of mental and bodily phenomena as they make up the totality of life." His book comprised chapters on the effects of mental attention on bodily organs, on mental consciousness in its relation to time and succession, on time as an element of the mental functions, on sleep, on the relations of dreaming, &c., on the memory as affected by age and disease, on the brain as a double organ, on phrenology, on instincts and habits. Hypnotic phenomena and doctrines were also included in his survey.

Dr. Carpenter adopted the same title for his work which appeared in 1874. He included in his range of subjects the general relations between mind and body, the functions of the nervous system, attention, sensation, perception and instinct, ideation, ideo-motor action, the emotions, the will, habit, memory, common sense, imagination, unconscious cerebration, reverie and abstraction, sleep, dreaming, and somnambulism (spontaneous and induced), and the influence of mental states on the organic functions.

Both Sir Henry Holland and Dr. Carpenter travelled beyond the strict boundary of mental *physiology*, and entered upon the consideration of mental *pathology*, because the latter throws light upon the former. Following these lines, the University of London introduced in 1886 the subject of "Mental Physiology, especially in its relations to Mental Disorder."

Professor Ladd's text-book adopts the expression "physiological pyschology" as the equivalent of mental physiology, and he defines it as "the science of the phenomena of human consciousness in their relations to the structure and the functions of a nervous system." In other words, he regards the mind as standing in peculiar relations to the bodily mechanism. Its object is to bring mental phenomena and those of the nervous system "face to face."

THE EDITOR.

MENTAL SCIENCE. (*See* PHILOSOPHY OF MIND, p. 27.)

MENTALISATION (*mens*, the mind). The physiological act of exercising the functions of the brain for thought, reasoning, perception, judgment, or other mental acts.

MENTE CAPTI (*mens*, the mind; *capio*, I seize or lay hold of). The term applied in Roman law to those deficient in intellect.

MERANÆSTHESIA (*μερίς*, a part or portion; *ἀναισθησία*, want of feeling). The condition of partial anæsthesia. (*See* HYSTERIA.)

MESMERISM (Mesmer, Anthony, the promulgator of the doctrine of animal magnetism). The process whereby the mesmeric sleep or trance was induced. This condition is identical with what is now known as hypnotism, induced hypnotism, induced somnambulism, the hypnotic state, &c. (*See* HYPNOTISM.)

MESMERO-PHRENOLOGY (mesmerism; *φρήν*, the mind; *λόγος*, a discourse). The name formerly given to that condition of a mesmerised person in which when any phrenological organ, so called, is touched, its functions are manifested. (*See* HYPNOTISM; SUGGESTION.)

METALLOPHAGIA (*μέταλλον*, a mineral; *φαγεῖν*, to eat). A name given to a kind of insanity in which the patient exhibits a desire to swallow pieces of metal. (Fr. *metallophagie*; Ger. *Metallschlucken*.)

METAPHYSICAL MANIA. (*See* DOUBT, INSANITY OF; MANIA METAPHYSICA.)

METASTATIC INSANITY. (*See* INSANITY, METASTATIC; MANIA METASTATICA.)

METHILEPSIA (*μέθη*; *λῆψις*, a seizing); or **METHOMANIA** (*μέθη*, intoxication; *μανία*, madness). An irresistible desire for intoxicating substances or alcoholic stimulants. (*See* DIPSOMANIA.)

METHYLAL. (*See* SEDATIVES.)

METROMANIA (*μήτρα*, the womb; *μανία*, madness). A synonym of Nymphomania. (Fr. métromanie; Ger. Mutterwuth.)

MICROCEPHALY.—Microcephaly means abnormal smallness of the head. What makes this condition interesting is that the diminished size is principally in the brain. We should call any head microcephalic which measures less than 17 inches—431 millimetres—in circumference.

As a general rule, the heads of idiots are somewhat smaller than those of ordinary people. But this observation is of little use in dealing with individuals; for, save in the case of hydrocephalic and of microcephalic idiots, the difference in the size of the head from normal people is never considerable, and it is not uncommon to meet with imbeciles who, without any hydrocephalus, have heads larger than those of people of ordinary intelligence.

Charles Vogt wrote a book ("Mémoire sur les Microcéphales ou Hommes-Singes") to show that these diminutive heads indicate a stage of development of the original simian ancestors of man. This thesis, though supported by descriptions of a painstaking collection of cases with comparative studies of the brains of a few monkeys, was not confirmed by more careful inquiries. There are brains of human microcephales which weigh even less than the full-grown brain of the ourang or chimpanzee; but when one leaves cubic capacities and weights to examine the anatomical structure, it soon appears that the brain of the microcephale is human in its characteristics. All the typical fissures and convolutions are there, though diminutive in size and simple in form. It is a small rudimentary human brain which does not resemble that of any monkey that exists, or indeed could have existed. The variations in the convolutions of the microcephale sometimes indicate the period when the arrest of development began. Though microcephalic brains cannot be reduced to one type, they are often asymmetrical in their convolutions, much more so than those of the highest ape. The corpus callosum is often shortened in proportion to the hemispheres, and the occipital lobes arrested in growth so that they do not completely cover the cerebellum. Gratiolet has observed that in the brain of the ape the temporo-sphenoidal convolutions appear first, and the frontal lobe last; whereas in man the frontal convolutions appear first and the temporo-sphenoidal last. From this it follows that no arrest of development can make the human brain to resemble more nearly that of the ape than the human adult brain does. Evolutionists also sought to find in other parts of the organism of the microcephale vestiges of arrested development of the simian type, but here they were even less successful. The peculiarities which they noted, such as elongation of the forearm, or the body being covered with shining hairs, were inconstant in their occurrence. There were also other peculiarities found in various microcephales, such as want of the testicles, or the non-appearance of the incisors, which could in no way be explained by the theory of atavism.

On the other hand, Bischoff, Asby, and Giacomini, who, in the most painstaking manner, examined and measured every part of the bodies of microcephales, have declared that their inquiries afford no arguments for the simian origin of man, and that the deficiency in microcephales is generally localised in the cranium and its contents.

Though not the reappearance of an atavistic type, microcephaly seems to be a very ancient malformation. Microcephalic heads are portrayed in the Egyptian monuments, both in sculpture and painting. One such figure is evidently intended to represent a lunatic or a man of small intellect. A mummified skull has been engraved by Dr. Morton, in which the head is abnormally small and low in the forehead with prognathous jaw. Two microcephalic statues have been found at Rome.

In microcephalic brains the deficiency is proportionally most marked in the hemispheres, especially in the upper gyri. The basal ganglia and the cerebellum are not diminished in the same proportion. The forehead generally slants rapidly; the head is cone-shaped or oxycephalic, giving the creature a bird-like appearance. The base of the skull, as well as the cerebrum, is sometimes asymmetrical in microcephales. The palate is generally flat, though in some cases it is arched or vaulted. The face is large in proportion to the cranium. Microcephales are generally short of stature, sometimes mere dwarfs.

The causes of this deficiency are obscure. Though in a considerable number of microcephalic skulls the sutures have been found closed, the cases in which the sutures still remain open are so numerous that it is now impossible to hold that closure of the sutures can be anything more than an occasional cause of microcephaly. Possibly the closure of the sutures is simply a process accompanying the cessation of the growth of the brain. The theory of Klebs that microcephaly is owing to hour-glass contraction of the uterus on the fœtal head does not seem to have received confirmation of late. There is, however, no doubt that early morbid processes, such as inflammation or the pressure of fluid within the cranium, are sometimes the cause of the premature arrest of the growth of the brain. It has been recently shown that microcephaly is sometimes accompanied by micromyelia. The spinal cord shares in the abnormally small development of the brain: it is shortened and smaller. The diminution in size has been found to be most marked in the pyramids, the columns of Goll, the ganglia of the anterior horns, and to a lesser degree in the direct lateral cerebellar tract. As this deficiency in development is unaccompanied by any traces of local disease, it would appear that the diminution of bulk in the cord comes in correspondence with the diminished brain.

No doubt the cerebral tissues are sometimes more or less diseased. Fletcher Beach in one case found in microscopic sections from the frontal lobe that few of the nerve cells had processes, and these were small and stunted. Alexandra Steinlecher found the nerve-cells in the microcephalic brain less in quantity. The same scarcity of large cells was found in the shortened spinal cord. Further studies of these brains are much to be desired.

Though this is a rare form of idiocy, it has been noted that microcephales have frequently brothers and sisters with the same deformity. A villager in Holland had fourteen children, of whom four were microcephalic; and in the Becker family there were four microcephalic children, one of whom was described at length in the monograph of Professor Bischoff on Helene Becker. Fig. 1 is a side view (left) of her brain.

All persons with heads less than 17 inches in circumference are of feeble intelligence. With heads of 12 inches in circumference and less the mental manifestations are very faint. The smallest human brain which we ever saw was shown to us by Dr. Fletcher Beach. It belonged to a girl of twelve years of age who died at the Clapton Asylum. It weighed only seven ounces. There is an engraving of this brain in the *Transactions* of the International Congress, vol. iii. p. 618, London, 1881.*

This child never could stand or walk. She had to be fed with a spoon, she never spoke a word; and her highest accomplishment was shaking hands. We have many other brain weights on record, from 300 grammes, the weight of a new-born child's brain, up to 610 grammes with a circumference of 16¾ inch = 426 millimetres.

* See also Idiocy (by Dr. Beach, p. 651).

The mental power and energy of microcephales are not always commensurate with the volume or weight of the brain, some have more intelligence than others who have larger heads. This disparity is often owing to the brain tissues in the microcephales being more or less diseased. Nevertheless, dealing with larger weights, the rule becomes apparent that the mental powers mount with the size of the brain.

Fig. 1.

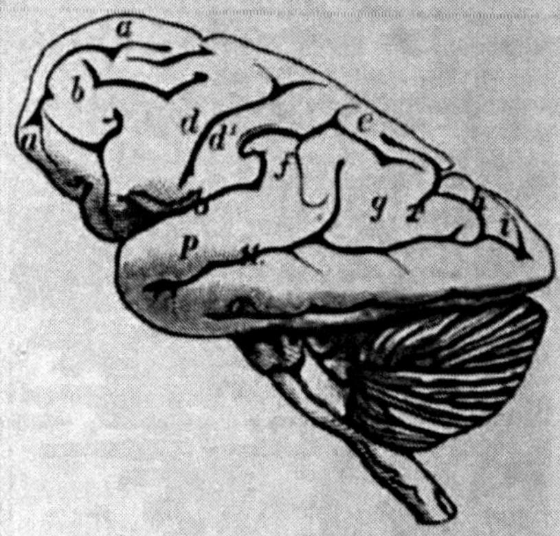

1. The central fissure (of Rolando) runs between *d* and *d*¹.
2¹. The unfinished fissura occipitalis perpendicularis externa.
6. Posterior branch of Sylvian fissure.
11. The parallel fissure.
a. The superior frontal gyrus.
b. The inferior frontal gyrus.
d. Anterior central gyrus.
*d*¹. Posterior central gyrus.
c. Præcuneus.
f. Lobulus supra marginalis.
g. Gyrus angularis.
h. Undetermined.
i. Cuneus.
p. Gyrus temporalis superior.
o. Gyrus temporalis medius.

From Dr. Berkhan's statistics* it appears that in Germany microcephales stand to other idiots as one to a hundred. We are sure that for Scotland this proportion would be much too high.

* Dr. Berkhan, of Brunswick, has made valuable contributions to the study of idiocy and imbecility. Herr Kielhorn, of the same place, is the excellent master of an "Auxiliary School" for the borderland cases which we have visited. We have described his work, and suggested the establishment of similar institutions in England, in the *Journal of Mental Science*, Jan. 1888. This course has been also urged by Dr. Shuttleworth (*Journal of Mental Science*, April 1888). Much has been done since then, mainly through the indefatigable exertions of Dr. F. Warner, to render the adoption of this scheme, or a modification of it, probable.—Ed.

There are always about a dozen microcephales in the large asylum of Darenth for the pauper idiots of London. Many of them are wretched little creatures who cannot even execute any voluntary motions, save perhaps to follow with their eyes the spoon which feeds them. On the other hand, some microcephales are active and energetic. The impressions of the senses are lively, but they have little power of continuous attention. They are generally restless, imitative, and inclined to fly into a passion. Few of them can speak. Their mental capacities differ little from idiots of other types, though in general they have more use of their limbs and better health. Their command of the muscles is perhaps due to the better development of the cerebellum.

Under a special system of education, microcephales improve like other idiots, though perhaps not so much as might be expected. The spontaneous mental activity, in their case, is more vivacious than the power of receiving knowledge through systematic lessons. Some writers have stated that there is found in the mental characteristics of microcephales a strong resemblance to those of monkeys. Microcephales are a deal stupider than normal human beings, and so are monkeys; but here the resemblance ends. The microcephale has less energy than an ordinary child, hence he is less fond of climbing, he has human affections and human sympathies; he laughs at what amuses him, and weeps when in pain. A microcephalic boy, a pauper boarder from the north, whom we had at Larbert, was a cunning and calculating thief. He was very imitative and observing, but never uttered a word. In general when microcephales remain mute, we believe it is owing to the low sum of their mental faculties, not to deficiency in any particular convolution of the brain.

In the lower grades of microcephaly the sexual instinct is either very faint or wanting. In the higher grades the testicles become developed, though later than with normal males, and the female microcephales menstruate later than ordinary women. One microcephale aged twenty-five years conceived, but the embryo was born dead. This is the only instance on record of the reproductive function coming into exercise in one of these creatures.

As generalisations drawn from beings so abnormal are apt to be misleading, let us consider some particular cases of microcephales which have been carefully studied. The two Aztecs who have been exhibited for many years in America and Europe are fair examples of microcephales. They have been often examined and described. Originally brought from Mexico, they are obviously of Indian origin. They have curious heads of black crisp-looking hair which stands out like a broom, starting up after being depressed. Professor Dalton who saw them when they were seven and five years of age, says that the boy was 2 feet 9¾ inches high, and weighed a little over twenty pounds. The girl was 2 feet 5½ inches high, and weighed seventeen pounds. Their bodies were tolerably well proportioned, but the heads were extremely small. The antero-posterior diameter of the boy's head was only 4½ inches = 114 millimetres; the transverse diameter less than 4 inches = 100 millimetres. The antero-posterior diameter of the girl's head was 4⅓ inches = 111 millimetres; the transverse diameter only 3¾ inch = 94 millimetres.

They were described as very vivacious, restless, and excitable, but unable to speak anything save a few isolated words. In manners they were soft and gentle. We saw these creatures twice, the last time in Glasgow in 1880 where they were being exhibited for a penny. They were publicly married in London in 1867, and cohabited, but had no offspring. The female showed jealousy of the male by shaking her finger at him "when he paid attention to other ladies." She was playing with a toy. They said that she was not fond of children. They seemed gentle and good-natured, and spoke a few isolated words, such as, when we asked the male what he would do with some money? he answered, "cigar," being fond of smoking. The female said "cold," when the showman exposed her neck to let me see how well nourished she was. They were both of low stature. The male had, for an Indian, a tolerable beard. He was said to be forty-six, the female several years younger. We could see no grey hairs. The male had $\frac{18}{14}$ teeth, some of which were decayed. They had both vaulted palates. The male wanted a metacarpal bone in each little finger, and the big toe overlapped the others on each foot. Deformities of the toes are common with idiots. We measured the head of the male microcephale as well as we could for his bushy hair.

The following were noted:

	Mill.		Inch.
Antero-posterior (from glabella to occipital protuberance) .	216	=	8½
Circumference	381	=	15
Transverse (from tragus to tragus)	240	=	9½

A boy named Freddy, with a very small head, has been carefully observed and described by Dr. Shuttleworth, under whose care he has been for eighteen years. He is short of stature, but well built, vigorous, and active. The following are some of the head-measurements:

		Inch.		Mill.
Antero-posterior .	in 1875	$8\frac{1}{2}$	=	215
Circumference . .	in 1871	$14\frac{1}{8}$	=	358
"	in 1875	$14\frac{1}{2}$	=	368
"	in 1881	15	=	381
Transverse . .	in 1875	10	=	280

Other comparative measurements showed a slow growth of the head between 1871 and 1875.

When seventeen years of age he was four feet six inches in height. In the first years of his residence in the asylum Freddy was difficult to manage, biting and kicking when angry. As a result of his discipline he became better behaved, and fairly sociable. He is still quick and irritable. He has good use of his limbs, joins in the drill, and is observant of external changes and new objects. He uses a few words such as "look," come," and "see," which he does with a meaning. His mental processes are very simple, and he learns little with the passing years. His portrait is given below, from a woodcut used in the writer's book on "Idiocy," at p. 93.

FIG. 2.

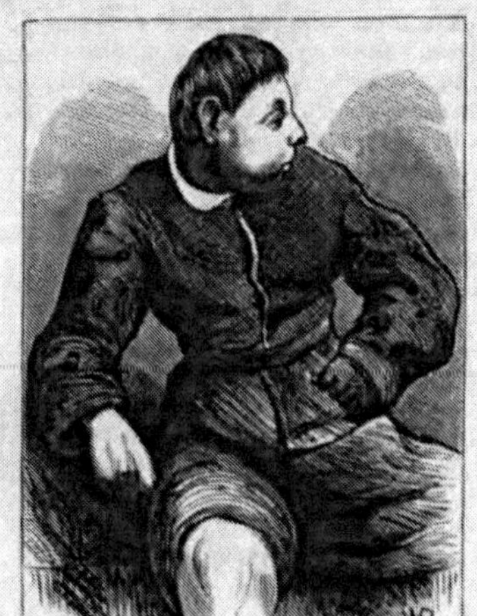

The case of Antonia Grandoni has been described by Professor Cardona and Dr. Adriani, of Perugia. Antonia died in 1872, aged 41 years. She was 52 inches in height, and weighed 66 pounds. Two of her portraits (Figs. 3 and 4) are given from other woodcuts in the writer's work, at pp. 104–5.

FIG. 3.

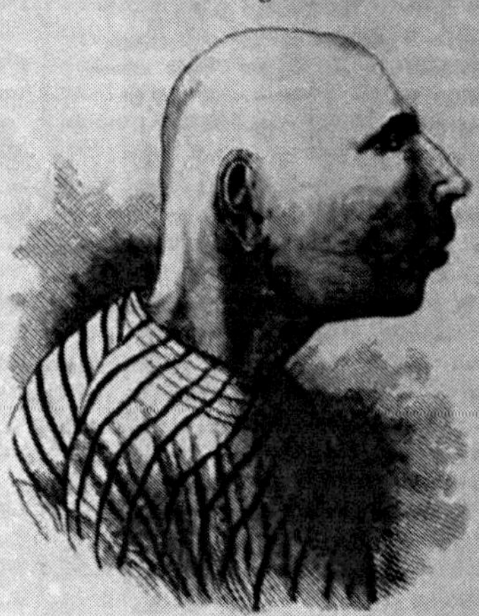

FIG. 4.

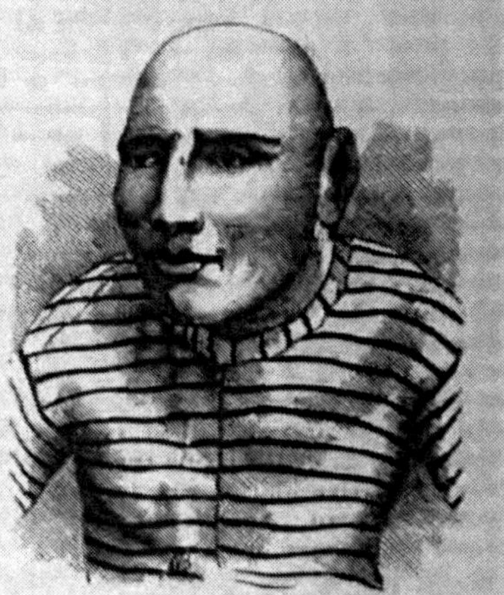

Amongst the head measurements were:

	Mill.		Inch.
Antero-posterior	135	=	5.4
Circumference	380	=	15
Transverse	105	=	4.2

The encephalon weighed 289 grammes; the cerebrum, 238 grammes; the cerebellum, pons, and medulla, 51. The cerebrum was not only absolutely small, but small out of due proportion to the other parts.

On comparing these ascertained facts with the brains of other microcephales, it appears that, while with brain weights nearly corresponding, the mental manifestations in all other cases were those of the lowest grades of idiocy, in Antonia they did not sink below weakmindedness. She could dance, play well on the cymbals, was fond of being noticed, especially by the other sex, had a good memory for the names of places and persons, but no memory of time. She learned to do easy work in the house, and to go out to buy provisions. Indeed Cardona goes so far as to say that the poverty of the brain of Grandoni in the small size accorded to it by Nature could admit of a sensibility, an intelligence, and an education, which has not fallen much short of the average of her countrywomen.

A longer description of Antonia and of Freddy will be found in the writer's book above mentioned. In Antonia's case one might expect the brain tissues to be healthy, and this was fairly borne out by a careful microscopical examination.

Dr. Lannelongue has tried an operation for the relief of microcephaly, which consists in the removal of strips of the frontal and parietal bones along the lines of the sutures. Though he does not hold that the closure of the sutures is the cause of microcephaly, he believes that there is often compression or arrest of the growth of the brain. Professor Horsley, and Dr. Keen of Philadelphia, have performed similar operations on microcephalic children. So far as we can gather, in twelve such operations there were four deaths, and decided improvement is specified in only two cases. These surgeons consider that the hopelessness of any considerable improvement in the mental power of the microcephale justifies the risk of the operation. We should be inclined to restrict the operation to children under five years in whom there were some proofs of compression. W. W. IRELAND.

[*References.*—Gratiolet, Mémoire sur la Microcéphalie considérée dans ses rapports avec la question des Caractères du Genre humain, Journal de la Physiologie de l'Homme et des Animaux, Paris, 1860. Vogt, Mémoires sur les Microcéphales, Geneva, 1867. Bischoff (Th. L. W.), Anatomische Beschreibung eines Microcephalen 8 Jährigen Mädchens, Munich, 1873. Aeby, Beiträge zur Kenntniss der Mikrocephalie, Archiv für Anthropologie, sechster und siebenter Band, Brunswick, 1874-5. Ireland, On Idiocy and Imbecility, London, 1877. Bucknill and Tuke's Manual, 4th edit. 1879. Beach, Morphological and Histological Aspects of Microcephalic and Cretinoid Idiocy, Transactions of International Medical Congress, vol. iii., London, 1881. Giacomini's Cervelli dei Microcefali, Turin, 1890; at the end of this complete monograph there is a list of the literature of microcephaly filling fourteen pages. Horsley, V., On Craniectomy in Microcephaly, Brit. Med. Journ., September 12, 1891.]

MICROMANIA (*μικρός*, small; *μανία*, madness). The form of insanity in which the patient imagines that his body or some part of it has become small. Delusion of belittlement. (Fr. *délire des petitesses.*)

MICROPSY, HYSTERICAL (*μικρός*; *ὄψις*, signs; hysteria, *q.v.*). The visual defect found in hysterical subjects, in which objects at a certain distance appear smaller than they really are, associated as a rule with functional monocular polyopia and hysterical macropsy (*q.v.*).

MIND. (*See* PHILOSOPHY OF MIND, p. 27.)

MIND-BLINDNESS.—Mind-blindness represents a form of visual disturbance in which the capability of *seeing* and perceiving objects is preserved, but in which the capability of *recognising* them, save through the other senses, is lost.

The term "mind-blindness" has been chosen by Munk for a certain condition in the dog, which he was able to produce by an operation on the occipital lobe. The dogs are able to see, but they are not able to recognise by means of the visual sense persons, localities, and objects familiar to them. The operation—extirpation of the cortex at a certain part of the occipital lobe—is said to extinguish the memory of all visual images. The science of mind-blindness in man has not yet been brought to a definite conclusion. The results of the experiments on animals cannot without reserve be transferred to human pathology. In a series of cases the condition which has been described as mind-blindness has also been observed in man.

In these cases perception of the impressions of light, simple optical perception as such, continues to exist; the patient sees, but he is not able to interpret the impressions which he receives through the retina, he is not able to make any use of them mentally, he does not connect any ideas with them. The memory of visual images is entirely lost. In several instances colour-blindness was found associated with mind-blindness, but we cannot decide whether this is constant. It is important to note that in one and the same case hemianopsia can be present with mind-blindness, as has been observed several times. Remarkable is the occurrence of mind-blindness in connection with aphasic derangements of speech. It has been already attempted to make a distinction between certain forms of mind-blindness. We may be allowed to separate from pure mind-blindness in the sense as stated above, the word-blindness—*i.e.*, the inability to recognise writing or print, because there have been cases in which word-blindness existed without mind-blindness. Whether we are also allowed to separate from mind-blindness other cases in which there is aphasia—the so-called optical aphasia—is not certain.

We must take care not to compare mind-blindness with a similar visual derangement, as represented by diminution of the acuteness of vision and by monochromasia. This condition can be produced in man experimentally, by means of coloured light and the use of limned spectacles. For the decision of the question whether there is in a given case genuine mind-blindness, the consideration of these factors is of great importance, because, in order to produce an optical image in our perception, a certain degree of acuteness of vision and the capability of distinguishing colours are necessary. The anatomical cause of mind-blindness, which is a disturbance of vision, originating in the cortex, lies in a disease of the occipital lobe. Supposing that the optical field of perception lies in the cuneus, and has its centre in the first occipital convolution, we have to place the field of the memory of visual images in the remaining part of the cortex of the occipital lobe, without being able to say whether it covers only a part, and in that case which part, of the remainder of the cortex of this lobe.

E. Siemerling.

[*References.*—H. Munk, Ueber die Funktionen der Grosshirnrinde, Berlin, 1881. H. Wilbrand, Die Seelenblindheit als Herderscheinung und ihre Beziehungen zur homonymen Hemianopsie, zur Alexie und Agraphie, Wiesbaden, 1881. Nothnagel und Naunyn, Ueber die Localisation der Gehirnkrankheiten, Wiesbaden, 1887. Wernike, Lehrbuch der Gehirnkrankheiten, Bd. ii. p. 544. Fuerstner, Sehstörung bei Paralytikern, Arch. fuer Psych. und Nervenkr. Bd. viii. p. 162, und Bd. ix. p. 90. Stenger, Die Cerebralen Sehstörungen der Paralytiker, Arch. fuer Psych. und Nervenkr., Bd. xiii. Zacher, Beitraege zur Pathologie und Pathologischen Anatomie der progressiven Paralyse, Arch. fuer Psych. Bd. xiv. Reinhard, Beitraege zur Localisation im Grosshirn., Arch. fuer Psych. Bd. xvii. and xviii. Luciani und Sepilli, Die Functionslocalisation auf der Grosshirnrinde, 1886. Bernheim, Contribution à l'étude de l'aphasie, de la cécité psychique des choses, Rev. de Méd. viii. p. 185. Jastrowitz, Centralblatt fuer practische Augenheilkunde, 1887, p. 254. Ross, On Aphasia, London, 1887. Thomsen, Charité-Annalen, x. Jahrgang, p. 573. A. Pick, Zur Pathologie des Gedaechtnisses, Arch. f. Psych., Bd. xvii. Charcot, Un cas de suppression brusque et isolée de la vision mentale des signes et des objets (formes et couleurs). Mauthner, Centralblatt fuer Augenheilkunde, 1880, p. 288. Schoeler-Uhthoff, Beitraege zur Pathologie der Sehnerven und der Netzhaut bei Allgemeinerkrankungen, Berlin, 1884. Freund, Ueber optische Aphasie und Seelenblindheit, Arch. f. Psych. Bd. xx. Brandenburg, Arch. f. Ophthalmologie, xxx. 3. Batterham, Brain, 1888. Bruns und Stoelting, Neurol. Centralbl 1888, No. 7. Lissauer, Ein Fall von Seelenblindheit nebst einem Beitrage der Theorie derselben. Wernicke, Die neueren Arbeiten ueber Aphasie, Fortschritte der Medicin, 1886, p. 371. Siemerling, Ein Fall von sogenannter Seelenblindheit nebst anderweitigen cerebralen Symptomen, Arch. f. Psych. Bd. xxi. p. 284. Hughlings Jackson, Neurol. Centralbl. 1884, 47.

MIND-DEAFNESS.—A term employed by Munk to denote the condition in which the power of recognising familiar words and terms is lost, the auditory apparatus being unimpaired. In animals it is caused by destruction of the first temporal convolution.

MIND, DEPRAVED. (*See* Cacothymia.)

MIND, FACULTIES OF THE. (*See* Philosophy of Mind, p. 27.)

MIND, PHILOSOPHY OF. (*See* Philosophy of Mind, p. 27.)

MIND, SCIENCE OF. (*See* Philosophy of Mind, p. 27.)

MIND, UNSOUNDNESS OF.—A term first used by Lord Eldon to denote a condition of intellect, not marked by delusions or idiocy, but which unfits the person for the management of himself and his affairs.

MISANTHROPIA (*μισέω*, I detest; *ἄνθρωπος*, a man). A term for hatred of men or their society, or dislike of human companionship or conversation; it was ranked by old writers as the second stage of melancholia and hypochondriasis, in which men show an aversion towards friends and acquaintances, shun their presence and seek seclusion.

MISOGAMOS, MISOGAMUS (*γάμος*, marriage). An abnormal mental condition in which a person shows an unreasoning and morbid hatred of wedlock. (Fr. *misogame*; Ger. *Heimathschen.*)

MISOGYNOUS (*γυνή*, a woman). An unreasoning and morbid dislike of the female sex. (Fr. *misogyne*; Ger. *Weiberfeind.*)

MISOLOGIA (*τά λόγια*, literary matters). An unreasoning hatred of intellectual or literary matters.

MISOMANIA (*μῖσος*, hatred, detestation, persecution; *μανία*, madness). A synonym of Delirium, or Delusion of Persecution.

MISOPÆDIA (*παῖς*, a child). An insane hatred of one's own children.

MISOPSYCHIA (*ψυχή*, life, the soul). A term for hatred or weariness of life; melancholia with disgust of life. (Fr. *misopsychie*; Ger. *Trübsinn mit Lebensüberdruss*).

MISOZOETICUS, MISOZOIA (*ζωή*, life). Hatred or disgust of life. Melancholia with suicidal inclinations.

MISSMUTH (Ger.). Melancholy, sadness.

MISTAKEN IDENTITY.—A term used in mental disease for the delusion exhibited by some insane persons, who deny their identity, claiming to be kings, potentates, deities, &c.

MNEME (*μνήμη*, recollection). A synonym of Memory.

MNEMONICA (μνημονικός, pertaining to memory). The art of memory or of remembering.

MOGILALIA (μογιλαλία, from μόγις, λαλέω, I speak with difficulty); **MOLILALIA** (μόλις, for μόγις, *v.s.*) Old terms for any difficulty of speech either from physical or mental defect. Also a synonym of Stammering (*q.v.*).

MOLYBDENEPILEPSIA (μόλυβδος, lead; epilepsy). A synonym of Saturnine Epilepsy, or Epilepsy induced by Lead Poisoning. (Fr. *molybdépilepsie;* Ger. *Bleifallsucht.*)

MONATSREITEREI.—The German equivalent for Nymphomania or Satyriasis.

MONDKRANKHEIT. — A German term for madness; insanity.

MONDSUCHT.—A German term for lunacy; also a synonym of Somnambulism.

MONGOLIAN IDIOTS. (*See* IDIOCY, FORMS OF.)

MONOCULAR POLYOPIA HYSTERICA (μόνος, one; *oculus*, eye; πολύς ὤψ, many-eyed; hysteria, *q.v.*). A term employed for the monocular diplopia or triplopia occurring in hysterical subjects. It may also occur as a natural defect corrected in the healthy condition of the normal action of accommodation, and due to the segmentary structure of the crystalline lens, occurring in the aged, commencing cataract, astigmatism, &c. Parinaud ascribes its occurrence in hysteria to the contraction of the muscle of Brücke (*m. ciliaris oculi*). It embraces the conditions known as hysterical macropsy and micropsy (*q.v.*) (Charcot).

MONODIPLOPIA HYSTERICA (διπλόος, ὤψ, hysteria). A synonym of Monocular Polyopia Hysterica.

MONOMANIA. — The essential element of the definition of monomania is *partial* insanity. Those who have logically maintained its existence hold that the morbid mental state is restricted to one subject, the patient being of sound judgment and healthy feeling on all others. Employed in this sense it must be discarded as untrue to clinical experience, and as the term is sure to be misunderstood when employed in a broader sense, its use is to be regretted. At the same time there is truth in the doctrine that the range of mental aberration in some instances is by no means co-extensive with the mental faculties, and the subjects upon which they may be engaged. No one who has anything to do with the insane, doubts that a man who labours under a terrible delusion or hallucination or an uncontrollable impulse, may be able to prepare an elaborate balance-sheet, or if a lawyer, might give trustworthy advice to his client. Partial insanity in this sense must therefore be admitted.

The term monomania has a history which cannot be passed over without a brief notice. No less than one hundred and thirty pages of Esquirol's "Maladies Mentales" are devoted to this form of mental disease. He invented the word. He described it as a chronic cerebral affection without fever, characterised by a partial lesion of the intelligence, the affections, or the will.

Intellectual monomania was defined as based on illusions, hallucinations, morbid associations of ideas, or delusions, concentrated upon a single object or a circumscribed series of objects, outside of which the patient feels, reasons, and acts like sane people.

Affective monomania (corresponding to the *manie raisonnante* of previous authors) was defined as a state in which without defect of reason the affections are perverted, and the character changed.

Instinctive monomania (or *monomanie sans délire*) was regarded by Esquirol as a lesion of the will, the patient being driven to perform acts of which his reason and conscience disapprove.

These varieties of partial insanity may be associated with exaltation or depression, but if the latter, Esquirol applied to them the term lypemania, while he resolved to restrict that of monomania to partial insanity of a joyous character. He observes, "writers have confounded" monomania with melancholia because in both the delusion is fixed and partial.

Under monomania Esquirol placed:—(1) M. *érotique* (*see* INSANITY, EROTIC), (2) M. *raisonnante*. Under this head he discusses the moral insanity of Prichard, and expresses a doubt whether he has quite sufficiently distinguished it from another variety of insanity free from intellectual disorder, the *manie sans délire*. "The moral insanity of Prichard, or the *manie raisonnante* of Pinel, is a true monomania. Patients labouring under this variety of insanity certainly have a partial mental disorder." (*Op. cit.* ii. 70.) (3) M. *d'ivresse*, (4) M. *incendiare*, (5) M. *homicide*.* It must be remembered that

* "A la fin du quinzième siècle, Marescot, Riolan et Duret, chargés d'examiner Marthe Brossier, accusée de sorcillerie, terminèrent leur rapport par ces mots mémorables: *Nihil a demone; multa ficta, a morbo pauca.* Cette décision servit depuis le règle aux juges qui eurent à prononcer sur le sort des sorciers et des magiciens. Nous nous dirons, en caractérisant le meutre des monomaniaques-homicides: *Nihil a crimine, nulla ficta, a morbo tota.*" (*Op. cit.* ii. 843.) Esquirol's defence of homicidal monomania is one of the ablest chapters

this form is also an example of reasoning mania. Esquirol observes that nearly all the facts of *manie sans délire* belong to monomania or to lypemania, being characterised by a fixed and exclusive insanity. There are irresistible impulses. (6) M. *suicide*, (7) M. *hypochondriaque*.

A thoughtful contribution * to the subject now treated of has been made by Dr. Bannister (of the Kankakee Asylum, Illinois), who is disposed to defend the continued employment of the term. "That there may be and are cases in which a single delusion or imperative conception forms the whole of insanity, either at one of its stages, or during its whole course, I have very little doubt." He argues that we admit that there may be a single hallucination, and if this be true, it may be a starting-point for an equally limited delusion. The case is given of a female patient, who had a certain delusion in regard to a family living next door to her, who were constantly tormenting and injuring her and her friends. She talked reasonably upon every subject but this. She had auditory hallucinations which she referred to the evil influence of this family. She also charged them with injuring her lungs, and appeared from her grimaces and semi-convulsive movements to be in acute pain. Her disposition was excellent, and she never expressed a wish to do her imaginary enemies harm. We, however, can hardly agree with Dr. Bannister, that "the defect of judgment that permitted a patient to accept the hallucinations as realities, and to build up upon them the delusions, does not necessarily imply any general defect of intelligence." Other cases are recorded in support of the writer's opinion, but we scarcely think that they justify the scientific use of the term, although they justify its employment in a general sense, and it is probable that it will pass current as a practically reasonable word. Although it would be unsafe to employ it in a Court of Law, there are occasions on which a medical witness may truthfully contend for a partial insanity, which allows of a patient exercising his judgment in some matters, while admitting that there are others on which his opinion would be warped by his delusions. THE EDITOR.

MONOMANIA, AFFECTIVE (*monomanie affective*). Esquirol's term for emotional insanity in which the subject is not deprived of reason, but in which affections and dispositions are perverted. (*See* MORAL INSANITY.)

MONOMANIA, INSTINCTIVE (*monomanie instinctive*). Esquirol's term for emotional insanity marked by perverted moral sense or by destructive impulses. In this form the actions are involuntary, instinctive and irresistible.

MONOMANIA, INTELLECTUAL (*monomanie intellectuelle*). Esquirol's term for monomania with delusions of an exalted nature.

MONOMANIA OF GRANDEUR, MONOMANIA OF PRIDE (μόνος, alone, single; μανία, madness). That form of monomania in which the patient believes himself to be some great or noble person or deity, or one endowed with extraordinary talents, beauty, grace, attributes, &c.

MONOMANIA OF SUSPICION.—That form of monomania in which the patient believes himself to be the victim of some enemy who has evil designs against him.

MONOMANIA OF UNSEEN AGENCY.—That form of monomania in which patients believe that they are influenced by some agency, unnatural, unseen or impossible.

MONOMANIACUS, MONOMANIAC. — Terms for one labouring under monomania.

MONOMANIE ANTHROPOPHAGIQUE (Fr.). The species of insanity in which the patient shows a longing for human flesh or food.

MONOMANIE BOULIMIQUE (Fr.). A term synonymous with Bulimia (*q.v.*).

MONOMANIE DES RICHES (Fr.). A term for monomania of great riches or possession.

MONOMANIE DU VOL (Fr.). A synonym of Kleptomania (*q.v.*)

MONOMANIE ÉROTIQUE (Fr.). A synonym of Erotomania (*q.v.*).

MONOMANIE EXPANSIVE, MONOMANIE GAIE. French terms used in the same sense as amenomania (*q.v.*).

MONOMANIE INCENDIAIRE (Fr.) A term for pyromania (*q.v.*).

MONOMANIE MEURTRIÈRE.—A French term for homicidal insanity.

MONOMANIE ORGUEILLEUSE (Fr.). A synonym of Megalomania (*q.v.*).

MONOMORIA (μόνος, alone, single; μωρία, folly). A synonym of Melancholia.

MONONŒA (νόος, the mind). Thought or concentration of mind on one subject as in monomania.

MONOPAGIA (πάγιος, fixed, established). A synonym of Clavus Hystericus.

MONOPATHOPHOBIA (πάθος, an affection; φόβος, fear). A term synonymous with Hypochondriasis. A morbid

of his remarkable work, which it is impossible to read without surprise and admiration.

* *The American Journal of Neurology and Psychiatry*, vol. iii. No. 1, 1884.

fear or dread that one is about to suffer from some definite disease.

MONOPLEGIA, HYSTERICAL (πληγή, a stroke; hysteria, *q.v.*); **MONOPLEGIA, HYSTERICAL TRAUMATIC** (hysteria; τραῦμα, a wound). The occurrence in a hysterical subject of paralysis or paresis of one limb, either following or independent of traumatic injury. With it may be associated anaesthesia, either total, partial, or irregular in distribution, while other phenomena of hysterical type may accompany the affection, such as retraction of the visual field, monocular polyopia, diminution of the sense of hearing or smell on the affected side. Charcot has noticed rapidly ensuing and persistent amyotrophy of the affected limb.

MONOPSYCHOSIS (ψυχή, the mind or soul). Clouston's term for monomania or delusional insanity.

MOON.—The belief in the influence of the moon in causing insanity is of great antiquity. Hence the Greeks employed the word σεληνιάζω to denote the production of madness and epilepsy.

Reference is made by Giraldus Cambrensis in his "Topographia Hibernica" to the influence of the moon: "Hinc est quod lunatici dicuntur, qui singulis mensibus pro lunæ augmento cerebro excrescente languescunt." He reports the observation of an "expositor" on Matt. chap. iv. 24, that the sick are here called lunatics, not because their insanity comes from the moon, but because the devil, who causes insanity, avails himself of "lunaria tempora" in order that he may disgrace the creature into blaspheming the Creator, and sensibly adds: "Potuisset autem, ut arbitror, salva quadam venia, non minus vere dixisse, propter varios humores in plenilunio nimis enormiter excrescentes, valetudinariis hæc accidere" (Dymock's Op. Girald. Camb. v. p. 79).

Esquirol, in his day, stated that the Germans and the Italians believed in lunar influence as a cause of mental disorder, and he refers to the use of the word "lunatic" by the English as an evidence of their holding the same belief. He cites Daquin, of Chambery, among his own countrymen, as holding this opinion, and supporting it in his "La Philosophie de la Folie," published in 1804. Esquirol himself writes thus cautiously and wisely: "Certain isolated facts—the phenomena observed in some nervous affections—would seem to justify this opinion. I have not been able to satisfy myself that this influence is real, notwithstanding all the care I have taken to ascertain the truth. . . . At the Salpêtrière, where practical truths are studied by those who reside there, the influence of the moon is not believed in. I may say the same of the Bicêtre and certain private asylums in Paris." He, however, adds, with an open mind, that an opinion which has been held for centuries and is consecrated by popular language, merits careful observation ("Des Maladies Mentales," t. i. p. 29).

No observations which have been made since the time of Esquirol have shown, conclusively, any relationship between the moon and lunacy. Medical men have endeavoured to erase the words descriptive of insanity in the insane which orginated in the popular belief, but custom has proved too strong, and the last Lunacy Act has continued to employ the terms in question, both in the title of the Act and in the medical certificate, where "an alleged lunatic" appears in the printed form.

The employment of words derived from the "moon," as applied to the insane, is sufficiently frequent in English literature, whether prose or poetry, to indicate the general belief in the old doctrine.

THE EDITOR.

[*References.*—Rush, Med. Inquiries, 1815, p. 170. Mead, De imperio solis et lunæ in corpore humanâ et morbis. Dr. Allen, Cases of Insanity, 1821, pp. 76–104; Manual of Psychological Medicine, 1879, 4th ed., p. 79. MM. Leuret and Mitivié, De la fréquence du pouls chez les aliénés, Paris, 1832. Dr. S. B. Woodward, Report of the Worcester Asylum (U.S.), 1841. Dr. Laycock, On Lunar Influence, *Lancet*, 1842–3. Dr. Thurnam, The Statistics of the Retreat, 1845, pp. 113–117].

MOONED; MOONSTRUCK.—Popular terms for one of unsound mind. A lunatic.

MORAL CONTAGION.—The engendering or engrafting of some moral perversion on a subject of weak moral character by some abnormality in the moral conduct of another. (*See* COMMUNICATIVE INSANITY; CONTAGION, MENTAL; EPIDEMIC INSANITY; HYSTERIA; and IMITATION.)

MORAL INSANITY.—**Syn.** Emotional or Affective Insanity. Fr. *Folie raisonnante* or *folie lucide raisonnante*, *monomanie affective*; Ger. *Moralisches Irresein*; Lat. *Mania sine delirio*.

Definition.—A disorder which affects the feelings and affections, or what are termed the moral powers, in contradistinction to those of the understanding or intellect (Prichard).

A form of mental disease, in regard to which so much difference of opinion exists among mental physicians—a difference of opinion doubtless held with equal honesty by each party—calls for dispassionate consideration, and a mode of treatment altogether free from heated assertion and dogmatism. We have no doubt that, to a very considerable extent, the divergence of sentiment among medical men equally competent to arrive at a conclusion, is due to the want of definition of the terms employed in discussing the question. Probably those who entertain different views on moral insanity would agree in their recognition of certain cases, as clinical facts, but would label them differently.

To come then to the root of the difficulty which has arisen—we meet with a certain number of persons who grow up presenting a marked contrast in their moral nature to the other members of the family, although they have all been subjected to the same influences, social, educational, and religious. The theologian may be satisfied to explain the phenomenon, by attributing to such member of the family a double dose of original sin, but those physicians who are opposed to the doctrine of moral insanity would not adopt this explanation. Severity and kindness may alike fail to elicit the moral feelings or to check immoral tendencies. The child in spite of parental and scholastic training may remain an incorrigible liar or thief; may exhibit premature depravity; may be cruel to other children and to animals; and, having grown to man's estate, may break the laws of the land, and be convicted of a criminal act. The examination of the mental condition of the person may show no defect of the intellectual faculties, and yet the mental expert may feel confident that the alleged criminal is not responsible for his actions. Or again, an individual who has betrayed no strangeness in his youth may receive a shock which is followed by a change of character including moral perversion, terminating it may be in a homicidal outburst. Now in these examples it may occur that a careful investigation into the past history fails to reveal any lack of mental power, in the direction of memory and facility in acquiring ordinary knowledge. What then is the position taken by those who have studied the subject and refuse to admit the presence of moral imbecility or insanity, although granting that such persons are not morally guilty of the crime? It is this: In the vast majority of the cases of alleged moral insanity, very careful inquiry proves that there is congenital or acquired intellectual weakness. Hence it is safe to infer that such mental disorder would be found in all cases whatever, provided a thorough investigation were carried out by competent experts. This, however, is an inconclusive argument—something very like a *petitio principii*. At any rate one thing is perfectly certain, that it may be practically impossible to detect the intellectual flaw, and yet a physician may be driven to decide that a person is insane. The really important clinical fact remains that cases arise in which the stress of the disease falls on the moral nature while those faculties which are generally regarded as reasoning and perceptive, are so little, if at all, deranged, as not to attract attention. It has naturally happened that moral insanity has become associated with questions of crime, but it would be a very great mistake thus to limit the range of this term. Cases occur in which there is a simple feeling of intense mental depression for which the sufferer can give no explanation, and which is in no degree associated with a delusion. Here there can be no doubt that the clinical fact would be admitted by all experienced alienists, but those who are unable to regard it as a disorder of the emotions only would hold that the inability to recognise the groundlessness of the depression is in itself an intellectual defect.

It would seem, as we began by saying, to resolve itself into a question of words. At the same time it appears unscientific to confound together a state of simple emotional depression with that of delusional melancholia.

There can be no doubt that in a number of cases of seeming moral insanity, there develop, in course of time, definite delusions, especially of suspicion. But what if a man commits a crime in the preliminary stage of the disorder of the emotions, prior to the development of intelligential disorder? It is not sufficient to predict what will eventually be developed—the fact remains that the disorder has not advanced beyond moral insanity. If it be preferred to call moral insanity the incipient stage of a form of mental disease which involves the intellectual as well as the moral faculties, enough is conceded to permit both parties in the debate to agree. Just as mental frequently precede motor symptoms in coarse brain disease (tumours, syphilitic disease, arterial degeneration, atrophy, &c.), so may mental symptoms first marked by moral perversity be followed by delusional insanity. In a young man under Dr. Clouston's care, this was the sequence of events, while a third stage was marked by motor disturbance—convulsions with partial paralysis of one side. Likewise there are instances of senile insanity in which moral lapses first attract attention, then distinct mental weakness, and lastly apoplexy and paralysis. There may be even in these cases occurring in advanced life, a predisposition to insanity which is brought to the surface by a moral or physical shock; this so far affects the question of moral insanity now under consideration that there may be underlying the apparently coarse causation of the attack an instability of nerve-tissue which is the factor in immediate relation to the moral disorder.

It is highly important to bear in mind that many cases of moral insanity are complicated with epilepsy.

This fact does not appear to us to remove the case from the category of moral disorders. Epilepsy may surely affect one part of the mental constitution in preference to another. It may, and generally does, seriously injure the memory, but it may pervert the moral nature so as to induce homicidal attacks, and leave the memory intact.

On the whole, it appears to us, while fully granting that a searching inquiry into the mental condition present in such cases of alleged moral insanity, would very frequently reveal intellectual disorder—that clinical observation cannot be satisfied without distinguishing between the cases which are, and those which are not, markedly complicated with intellectual defect or disorder. To obliterate distinctions, however fine, between these conditions, does not seem the way to advance the scientific study of insanity.

We would now refer to the bearing of mental science on the form of insanity under consideration. We have elsewhere recorded how Herbert Spencer would meet a legal opponent of the doctrine of moral insanity who should base his argument on the statement that as intellect is held to be evolved out of feeling, and as cognitions and feelings are declared by him to be inseparable, there cannot be organic or acquired moral defect without the intellect being involved. Spencer's answer does not militate against anything maintained in the present article. Indeed,* he finds an indication of such structural deficiency as may lead to results alleged to be present in moral imbecility and insanity, in the fact that every complex aggregation of mental states is the outcome of the consolidation of simpler aggregations already established. This higher feeling is merely the centre of co-ordination, through which the less complex aggregations are brought into proper relation. The brain evolves under the co-ordinating plexus which is in the ascendency, an aggregate of feelings which necessarily vary with the relative proportions of its component parts. But in this evolution it is obviously possible that this centre of co-ordination may never be developed; what Spencer calls the higher feeling, or most complex aggregation of all, may never be reached in the progress of evolution, and moral imbecility may result, or such waywardness of moral conduct from youth upwards as we maintain occurs without marked disorder of the intellect. When in the absence of congenital defect, the moral character changes for the worse under conditions which imply disease rather than mere vice, Spencer finds a clue to a probable cause in so simple an occurrence as fretfulness, which arises, as we all know, under physical conditions, such as inaction of the alimentary canal. Fretfulness is, as he justly says, "a display of the lower impulses uncontrolled by the higher." This is essentially a moral insanity. So is the irascibility of persons in whom the blood is poor, and the heart fails to send it with sufficient force to the brain. Spencer puts it in terms which bear directly upon the question we are discussing, when he says, "irascibility implies a relative inactivity of the *superior* feelings. . . . . The plexuses which co-ordinate the defensive and destructive activities, and in which are seated the accompanying feelings of antagonism and anger, are inherited from all antecedent races of creatures, and are therefore well organised—so well organised that the child in arms shows them in action. But the plexuses which, by connecting and co-ordinating a variety of inferior plexuses, adapt the behaviour to a variety of external requirements, have been but recently evolved, so that, besides being extensive and intricate, they are formed of much less permeable channels. Hence, when the nervous system is not fully charged, these latest and highest structures are the first to fail: instead of being instant to act, their actions, if appreciable at all, come too late *to check the actions* of the subordinate structures." (*Op. cit.* p. 605.)

Hence, although "no emotion can be *absolutely* free from cognition" (p. 475), it is allowed by Spencer that there may be "a relative inactivity of the superior feelings," and therefore moral insanity, by whatever name it may be called, is in full accord with the principles of mental evolution and dissolution, as laid down by this great psychologist.

The following propositions appear to be warranted by a careful consideration of the psychological, as well as the clinical, facts:

(1) The higher levels of cerebral de-

* These views are also expressed in the "Principles of Psychology," vol. i. p. 575.

velopment which are concerned in the exercise of moral control—*i.e.*, "the most voluntary" of Hughlings Jackson, and also "the altruistic sentiments" of Spencer—are either imperfectly evolved from birth, or having been evolved have become diseased and more or less functionless, although the intellectual functions (some of which may be supposed to lie much on the same level) are not seriously affected; the result being that the patient's mind presents the lower level of evolution in which the emotional and automatic have fuller play than is normal.

(2) No doubt it is difficult to lay down rules by which to differentiate moral insanity from moral depravity. Each case must be decided in relation to the individual himself, his antecedents, education, surroundings, and social status, the nature of certain acts, and the mode in which they are performed, along with other circumstances fairly raising the suspicion that they are not under his control.* THE EDITOR.

[*References.*—For a series of cases supporting the position taken in this article, see the writer's paper on Moral Insanity in the Journal of Mental Science, July and October, 1885; also, Prichard and Symonds, with chapters on Moral Insanity, by Dr. Hack Tuke, 1891. Consult the works of Maudsley and Clouston. Jules Falret, De la Folie morale, 1866. C. H. Hughes, A Case of Moral Insanity, Alienist and Neurologist, 1882, No. 4. Wright, The Physical Basis of Moral Insanity, Alienist and Neurologist, 1882, No. 4. A. Holländer, Zur Lehre von der "Moral Insanity," 1882. Brancaleone Ribaudo, Contributo sull' esistenza della follia morale, Palermo, 1882. Salemi-Pace, Un caso di follia morale, Palermo, 1881. Tamburini and Seppilli, Studio di psico-patologia criminale sopra un caso di imbecillità morale con idee fisse impulsive, Reggio, 1883, 2nd edit. 1887. G. B. Verga, Caso tipico di follia morale, Milano, 1881. Virgilio, Delle malattie mentali, 1882. Legrand du Saulle, Les Signes physiques des Folies raisonnantes, Paris, 1878. Mendel, Die moralische Wahnsinn, 1876, No. 52. M. Gauster, Ueber moralisches Irresinn, 1877. Motet, Cas de Folie morale, Ann. Méd.-psych. 1883. Reimer, Moralisches Irresinn, Deutsche Wochenschrift, 1878, 18, 19. H. Emminghaus, Allgemein. Psycho-pathologie, &c., Leipzig, 1868. Todi, I pazzi ragionanti, Novara, 1879. Grohmann, Nasse's Zeitschrift, 1819, 162. Heinrich, Allgem. Zeitschrift f. Psychiatrie, i. 338. Morel, Traité des Dégénérescences, 1857. B. de Boismont, Les Fous criminels de l'Angleterre, 1869. Solbrig, Verbrechen und Wahnsinn, 1867. Griesinger, Vierteljahrschrift f. ger. u. öffentl. Med., N.F. iv. No. 2. Krafft-Ebing, Die Lehre von moral Wahnsinn, 1871. Stoltz, Zeitschr. f. Psychiatrie, 33. H. 5 und 6. Livi, Revista sperimentale, 1876, fasc. 5 et 6. Gauster, Wien. med. Klinik, iii. Jahrg. No. 4. Mendel, Deutsche Zeitschr. f. prakt. Med. 1876, No. 52. Wahlberg, Der Fall Hackler, Gesammelte kleinere Schriften, Wien, 1877. Bannister, Chicago Journal, Oct. 1877. Palmerini, Bonfigli, Revista sperimentale, 1877, fasc. 3 et 4, &c. Bonvecchiato, Il senso morale e la follia morale, Venice, 1883. Dagonet, Folie morale, 1878. Lombroso, L'uomo delinquente, 4th edit. 1889. Laurent, Les Habitués des Prisons, 1890, ch. vi. Tamburini and Guicciardini, Ulteriori studi su un caso d' imbecillità morale, Archivio di Psichiatria, 1888, fasc. i. Sighicelli and Tamburini, Pazzia morale ed epilessia, Revista sperimentale, 1888, fasc. iv. D' Abundo, Un caso di pazzia morale, Archivio di Psichiatria, 1889, fasc. i. Marro, I caratteri dei delinquenti, Turin, 1887, part ii. ch. 18.

* Dr. Goldsmith, "Case of Moral Insanity," *Amer. Journ. of Insanity*, Oct. 1883.

MORAL TREATMENT OF INSANE. (*See* TREATMENT.)

MORBUS A CELSI (Celsus). A synonym of Catalepsy.

MORBUS ASTRALIS (*morbus*, a disease; *astralis*, pertaining to the stars). A synonym of Epilepsy.

MORBUS CADUCUS (*cado*, I fall); **MORBUS COMITIALIS** (*comitia*, the assemblies for the election of magistrates); **MORBUS DÆMONIACUS** (*daemon*; Gr. δαίμων, an evil spirit); **MORBUS DÆMONIUS** (*daemon*); **MORBUS DIVINUS** (*divinus*, holy, belonging to the gods). Synonyms of Epilepsy.

MORBUS ERUDITORUM (*eruditus*, learned); **MORBUS FLATULENTUS** (*flatus*, wind). Synonyms of Hypochondriasis.

MORBUS FOEDUS (*foedus*, horrible). A synonym of Epilepsy.

MORBUS GESTICULATORIUS (*gesticulatio*, expression by signs). A synonym of Chorea.

MORBUS HERACLEUS (Ἡρακλῆς, *Hercules*); **MORBUS HERCULEUS** (*Hercules*); **MORBUS INFANTILIS**; **MORBUS INTERLUNIS** (*inter*; *luna*, between the moon's phases); **MORBUS LUNATICUS** (*lunaticus*, belonging to an insane person); **MORBUS MAGNUS**; **MORBUS MAJOR**; **MORBUS MENTALIS** (*mentalis*, pertaining to or affecting the mind). Synonyms of Epilepsy.

MORBUS MIRACHIALIS (*mirachialis*, adjectival form of *mirachulum*, corruption of *miraculum*, a miracle). A synonym of Hypochondriasis.

MORBUS POPULARIS (*populus*, the people); **MORBUS PUBLICUS** (*publicus*, the people); **MORBUS PUERILIS** (*puer*, a youth). Synonyms of Epilepsy.

MORBUS RESICCATORIUS (*re*; *sicco*, I exhaust); **MORBUS RUCTUOSUS** (*ructo*, I eructate). Synonyms of Hypochondriasis.

MORBUS SACER (*sacer*, holy). A synonym of Epilepsy.

MORBUS SALTATORIUS (*salto*, I dance). A synonym of Chorea Major.

MORBUS SANCTI JOANNIS.—A synonym of Epilepsy.

MORBUS SANCTI VALENTINI.—A synonym of Chorea Major, also of Epilepsy.

MORBUS SCELESTUS (*scelestus*, infamous); **MORBUS SELENIACUS** (*selene*, the moon); **MORBUS SIDERATUS** (*sidera*, the stars); **MORBUS SONTICUS** (*sonticus*, dangerous); **MORBUS VIRIDELLUS** (*viridellus*, from *viridis*, young, youthful); **MORBUS VITRIOLATUS** (*vitrum*, anything clear or transparent). Synonyms of Epilepsy.

MORDMONOMANIE.—The German term for homicidal mania.

MORIA (*μωρία*, folly). A synonym of Idiotism, also Dementia.

MOROSIS (*μώρωσις*, dulness of the senses). Fatuitas, idiotism.

MOROSITATES (*μώρωσις*, dulness of the senses, silliness). A term applied by Linnæus to certain forms of mental aberration under which he includes pica, bulimia, polydipsia, antipathia, nostalgia, panophobia, satyriasis, nymphomania, tarantismus, hydrophobia, &c. (*q.v.*).

MOROTROPHIUM (*μωρός*, foolish; *τροφή*, that which nourishes or sustains). An insane establishment, lunatic asylum or madhouse.

MORPHIA. (*See* Sedatives.)

MORPHINOMANIA, MORPHIOMANIA, MORPHOMANIA (morphia, morphine; *μανία*, madness). The morbid uncontrollable desire for morphia. The morphia habit. (Fr. *morphéomanie*; Ger. *Morphiomanie*.) (*See* Art.)

MORPHIOMANIA, or **MORPHINOMANIA** (morphia habit, opium habit, morphinism, *Morphiumsucht*, *morphinismus chronicus*, *morphinisme*).

Definition. — By morphiomania we understand the diseased craving for morphia as a stimulant, together with the clinical aspect of the disease, which is produced by morphia-intoxication. Morphiomania is similar to alcoholism, in which also the diseased craving for drink is connected with somatic and mental derangements, produced by the continuous taking of alcohol.

The history of morphiomania begins with the year 1864. Great Britain has contributed very little indeed to the literature of this subject, which is very extensive.

As causes of morphiomania, all those conditions have to be mentioned for which morphia is used on account of its narcotic effects; conditions of bodily pain and mental distress. To the former belong all kinds of neuralgia, migraine, and headache; pains at the commencement of tabes dorsalis and in cerebral diseases, gout and rheumatism, hepatic colic and dysmenorrhœa, asthma, nausea of pregnant women, and nocturnal emissions, &c. To the latter belong the mental depression of hypochondriasis and melancholia, grief over the loss of a dear relative or friend, mental excitement caused by over-work, anxiety in agoraphobia, neurasthenia, hysteria, &c. Among other causes we may mention imitation and falling a victim to temptation. Mental causes alone induce morphiomania much more rarely than somatic ones. Between mental and somatic causes stands—often belonging to both—sleeplessness, which is of great importance because of its frequency. Not every one who gets morphia injected becomes a morphiomaniac; a certain disposition, a neuropathic constitution, is required, which is characterised by weakness of will, inability to resist mental impressions, and an abnormal excitability. If morphiomania is produced by these, it is a *disease*; if this disposition is not present, it is a vice.

There is no **pathological anatomy** of morphiomania because the changes which have been found to have taken place in the bodies of morphiomaniacs cannot be brought into distinct connection with morphia, and have therefore to be taken as accidental changes.

The **symptoms** of morphiomania have, for the sake of a better view, to be considered under several groups. We ought to take into this chapter the symptoms of intoxication only, but it is practical to treat here also of those symptoms which are produced by leaving off morphia, and which are called symptoms of abstinence or deprivation.

A. Intoxication.—First we shall enumerate the symptoms of intoxication, and we distinguish these as (*a*) *somatic* and (*b*) *mental symptoms*. In every morphiomaniac symptoms of abstinence can be observed during the period of intoxication, because the effect of one dose of morphia ceases, and therefore produces symptoms of abstinence before another dose is injected.

Among the (*a*) *somatic symptoms* of intoxication have to be mentioned—

(1) *Motor Disturbances.* — These are paresis, ataxy, and tremor, represented by the decrease of peristaltic motion of the intestines, incontinence of the bladder, ataxic gait, and tremor on writing. The knee-jerks are not at all influenced by morphia; if they are absent, we have to suspect tabes dorsalis; if they are increased, we have to think of neuritis or of spastic spinal paralysis.

(2) *Derangements of the Organs of Secretion:* Partial or complete impotency in men. There is not only no *libido*, but also no erections, and the seminal secretion ceases, although ex-

ceptions are not rare. In women, amenorrhœa and sterility develop, but here also we have exceptions. The children of mothers who suffer from chronic morphia poisoning have in the first days of their life to pass through a stage of abstinence similar to that of adults, during which often dangerous collapses occur, and in which the life of the children can only be saved by an injection of morphia or by opium. In women the secretion of milk, and *fluor albus* cease. The secretion of saliva decreases, and that of sweat increases. Often also the quantity of urine is increased. The functions of the sebaceous glands of the skin are lessened, and the skin becomes dry and brittle.

(3) *Derangements of Nutrition.*—Loss of appetite, foul tongue, no sense of satiety, slow digestion, sluggishness of the bowels. General loss of nutrition; anæmia begins to develop itself.

(4) *Various Derangements.* — Trophic derangements of the nails of the fingers and toes (dry and brittle), of the hair (becomes grey, white, and comes off), and of the teeth, the enamel of which becomes soft and falls off. Healthy teeth become loose and are very often observed to fall out. Contraction of the pupils produced by morphia-taking is sometimes unilateral—consequently unequal pupils and decrease of the range of accommodation (hypermetropia). Cutaneous eruptions occur in consequence of the increased diaphoresis. Fever is mostly a consequence of abscesses caused by the injections. The occurrence of *febris intermittens ex morphinismo* is doubtful. If morphia is injected into a vein, the vaso-motor system is greatly irritated, the temperature rises, congestions are produced in the head and lungs (dyspnœa), and the frequency of the pulse is greatly increased. That albumen and sugar appear in the urine of persons who suffer from chronic morphia poisoning, as a sole consequence of intoxication by morphia, has not been proved with sufficient certainty. Neuralgia is rarely a consequence of the morphia habit.

(*b*) The *mental symptoms* of INTOXICATION have to be divided into *temporary* and *permanent*. To the (1) *temporary symptoms* belong attacks of anxiety, hallucinations of vision, and drowsiness. *The* (2) *permanent* effect on the mind is represented in a decrease of its general functions, which, however, develops in most cases only after large doses have been taken for years. It includes weakening of the intellect, loss of memory, deadening of all sensation, and an extraordinary injury to the *morale*. This last point is of the greatest importance, and we have to keep it well in mind in treating a patient. The whole nature of the man undergoes a moral revolution. Truth, right, and honour lose for him their meaning, and the mental state of such patients can, without straining the interpretation, be called a kind of moral insanity. Morphiomaniacs forge prescriptions, deceive their relations and the doctor, become negligent, hardened in conscience, and dissolute, and show morbid impulses of various kinds; they acquire an extraordinary artfulness in trying to hide and to excuse things which relate to their abuse of morphia. Chronic morphia-poisoning produces mental weakness, and therefore belongs to the causes of insanity. We are not allowed to speak of "morphia-insanity" in general, because intoxication, as well as abstinence—two conditions contrary to each other—can produce forms of insanity which differ as regards symptoms and prognosis. The most frequent form of insanity produced by intoxication is monomania (mania marked by delusions as to persecution, and mania with exalted views, together with mental weakness). This form is mostly incurable. Very frequent also in morphiomaniacs are abnormal mental conditions which do not present a fully developed form of insanity. We may well say that such persons are not in a normal mental state, but it is often very difficult to refer the symptoms to any special form of insanity.

B. SYMPTOMS OF ABSTINENCE. — It is practicable to distinguish between the (*a*) *symptoms of sudden* and of *slow deprivation*. The most important, because the most dangerous, symptom is collapse, which, however, only occurs after sudden deprivation, and which may cause death by paralysis of the heart. Another symptom of sudden deprivation is the excitement which bears the character of *delirium maniacale;* in women it often assumes a somewhat hysterical form. It is well known that every delirium may be followed by albuminuria, a fact which we do well to bear in mind.

(*b*) *Slow deprivation.*—We shall first treat of *the somatic* and then the *mental symptoms*. *To the* (1) *somatic symptoms* belong: Contractions of single muscles, local and general, tremor, sense of weakness and debility, ataxic gait, paresis of the muscles of the eye, inequality of the pupils, disturbance of accommodation, neuralgia and neuralgic pains, especially in the calves of the legs, hemicrania, all kinds of paræsthesia, sense of heat and cold, pains in the stomach, the intestines, anus, and bladder, dysmenorrhœa, hyperæsthesia of all the senses, derangements of the vaso-motor and respiratory system, paralysis of the vessels, which can be proved by the sphygmograph, and which can be changed by a full dose of morphia into normal tension; besides this, reflex disturbances, as paroxysmal sneezing, yawning, singultus, choking, vomiting, and general convulsions. Of anomalies of the secretory system we must mention: coryza, lacrymation, diarrhœa, sweating, nocturnal emissions, and menorrhagia. General nutrition fails, and the body loses weight. We have to mention among *the* (2) *mental symptoms* of abstinence: general restlessness, sleeplessness, depression of mind, loss of memory, slight mental disturbance (a quiet and an excited form), great craving for morphia, wine and other narcotic and alcoholic stimulants. Among other symptoms of abstinence, forms of insanity (one lasting a short time and another chronic) and attacks of hysteria have been observed. After the patients have become weaned from morphia, some of the before-named symptoms still continue, and we have to watch very carefully over the *morale* of the patient.

(c) Under *secondary symptoms of abstinence*, or, better, under secondary conditions of debility, we include symptoms of general weakness which appear some weeks or months after the period of deprivation, if the patient is not very careful; it is a breaking down resulting from too early and too great exertion.

(d) We have no sufficient *explanation of the symptoms of abstinence;* we have still to accept the explanation that the nervous system is deprived of a customary stimulant. It is impossible to explain the symptoms chemically, as has been tried by supposing that oxide of morphia, which is said to be formed in the organism, causes the symptoms of abstinence as soon as no more morphia, which is an antidote to oxide of morphia, is introduced into the system.

The **diagnosis** of morphiomania is generally easy, because the patient himself confesses his abuse, and because the marks of the injections confirm his statements. It is more difficult if the patient is suspected to be in the habit of taking morphia but he himself denies it. This may happen if morphia is during or after the period of deprival secretly introduced into the system. It is impossible to prove it as certain, and we have therefore to try to find it out in any possible way. To analyse the urine, saliva, fæces, and the contents of the stomach in search of morphia is, apart from the complexity of this process, far from being reliable. It is best to inspissate the urine of the patient suspected to take morphia secretly, and to inject the residue subcutaneously into an animal. If the urine contains morphia, the animal will show symptoms of acute morphia poisoning. But this experiment is only successful if large doses have been taken secretly. We also can examine the pulse with a sphygmograph. For a short time after the period of deprival there is paralysis of the vessels. If we find during this time signs of tension of the arteries, we must be suspicious. However, this is not a certain proof.

Treatment.—A. Methods of Deprivation.—(*a*) *Slow Deprivation, Laehr-Burkardt Method.*—This is the oldest method, but also the worst of all. It reduces slowly the daily doses, but, as even in the slowest process the symptoms of abstinence cannot be avoided, the sufferings of the patients are very much prolonged, and, as the patient is not kept under control, he mostly succumbs to the temptation to take morphia secretly. This method does not require any special arrangements as regards a locality for the patient to stay in, but can be applied at any place.

(*b*) *Sudden Deprivation, Levinstein Method.*—The patient is at once deprived of all morphia, but, as it always causes a maniacal delirium, special arrangements have to be made. This method can only be applied in an asylum, where the patient can be isolated. It is apt to cause collapse and paralysis of the heart, and therefore it must be rejected, although apart from this danger it helps the patient in the quickest way over the sufferings of deprivation.

(*c*) *Quick Deprivation, Erlenmeyer Method.*—It is the best and most rational method, and is highly esteemed. It avoids all the dangers of sudden abstinence, and deprives the patient of the customary dose in from three to eight days with the greatest care and under proper supervision. The patient is kept in bed, and is surrounded by experienced attendants; female attendants are to be preferred, even in the case of male patients.

B. The Place most Suitable for undergoing Treatment by Deprivation.—It must not be at the patient's own house or in his family, neither at a bathing-place, because these do not give the slightest chance of success. Better is a hydropathic institution, an institution for nervous diseases, or even an asylum, but the most suitable place is a house specially established for and restricted to this one purpose of cure of morphiomania by deprivation. Of the greatest importance, however, in all such institutions is the personality of the physician himself. A patient who suffers from morphia poisoning should never be placed under the care of a doctor who has been or is a morphiomaniac himself, because this does not give the slightest guarantee for the success of the treatment.

C. The Treatment of Individual Symptoms during the period of deprivation can not be gone into here, because there are too many of them, and a description of their treatment would exceed the space of this article. We will only draw attention to two important points: First, that collapse has always to be considered as a symptom dangerous to life, even in its commencing stage, and that a full dose of morphia is the only means to save the life of the patient; secondly, that it is entirely wrong to try to lessen the suffering of the period of deprivation by substituting for morphia another drug or another medicine. The lamentable consequences of the treatment of morphiomaniacs with cocaine are an instructive example hereof. Codeine, which lately has been very much recommended, must be absolutely rejected, and it is contrary to experience to maintain that people cannot become accustomed to codeine, and that the deprivation of codeine does not cause any symptoms of abstinence. In fact, there exists a codeine mania, and its withdrawal causes severe symptoms of abstinence.

D. Prevention of Relapses.—We have to keep in mind that morphiomania is a secondary disease which has been produced by another disease preceding it (ætiology). Under the intoxication by morphia the symptoms of the first disease disappear, but return after the patient has left off taking morphia. Therefore, to prevent the patient returning to morphia, the first disease has to be treated, and everything depends on the success of this treatment. The chronic intoxication by morphia, as well as the deprivation of it, have very much weakened the patient. We have to be careful not to be deceived by an increase of weight, which is often astonishing, and which takes place in consequence of the patient's large appetite after the period of deprivation is over. This is only the laying on of fat, which is of no importance whatever as regards the general strength. For months after, the patient must remain without mental or bodily work which requires effort; he must be placed in pleasant surroundings, and must be kept away from every temptation.

E. General prophylaxis would be possible by making laws by which the sale of morphia to the public would be regulated; also, by public instruction and warning, and lastly by the exercise of great caution on the part of medical men. Such laws are in force in many countries, but the avarice and the passions of men succeed in making them void.

The prognosis of morphiomania as a disease is most unfavourable; it terminates sooner or later fatally by general marasmus. A certain number of patients become insane, while others commit suicide. The prognosis of deprivation is good. If done cleverly, the treatment by deprivation will prove successful. The prognosis of relapses is very doubtful. There are some morphiomaniacs who cannot be induced to leave off taking morphia because they suffer from painful incurable diseases, or because morphia would have only to be replaced by other still more dangerous stimulants (alcohol, tobacco, &c.). The prognosis is always better in proportion to the length of time which can be given to treatment and for the patient's restoration to strength.

Forensic Aspect of the Subject.—In all judicial proceedings by morphiomaniacs (will, sale, purchase, &c.) it is a question of the responsibility of the person concerned, because intoxication by morphia can produce mental derangement. It is not sufficient to have proved morphiomania, but in every single case it must be proved that a mental derangement is present, and that therefore the person is not responsible for his actions. It is well known that morphiomaniacs forge prescriptions. Prescriptions are, from a legal point of view, deeds, and the forgery of deeds is punishable. Great caution is necessary as regards life insurance. Healthy people who have insured their lives and who afterwards become morphiomaniacs lose, like drunkards, their claims on the insurance company. Chemists and druggists who act contrary to the laws of those countries which forbid the sale of morphia to the public, are justly liable to punishment. Albrecht Erlenmeyer.

[*References.*—Die Morphiumsucht, von Albrecht Erlenmeyer, 1887. Morphinisme, par M. Ball. Les Morphinomanes, par Dr. H Guimbail, 1890.]

MORTALITY, RATE OF. (*See* Statistics.)

MOUSSE ÉCUMEUSE.—The French term for frothing at the mouth in epilepsy and hydrophobia.

MOVEMENTS AS SIGNS OF MENTAL ACTION.—All mental action is known to us only by its expression in movements. The movement of a part of the body is a physical fact; we may describe the part moving, and the time and quantity of the visible action, which are here called the attributes of the movement; the results of the movement, and its necessary antecedents, though not parts of the act itself, often help to determine the mental character of the act.

A single movement of an individual part of the body is less often considered as a sign of mental action than a series of movements of many parts. Hence we have to consider the modes of studying a single movement and series of movements, and their relations to their antecedents and sequents, as well as to surrounding objects.

We are here dealing with purely physiological action, no metaphysical considerations or concern with the facts of consciousness will disturb the line of observation and argument or enter into any definition or explanation given. From this point of view the study of mental action is simply a study of visible movements and the corresponding brain action; we are concerned with their accurate description, their causation and outcome. It is convenient to describe modes of movement as observed, then to infer the modes of brain action corresponding thereto; various mental states may be described in terms indicating movement and the brain action corresponding.

The greatest number of signs that we have to observe are movements of small parts of the body, parts of small mass and weight, such as the eyes, the mobile features of the face, the hands and fingers. We shall proceed to study a visible movement, then some series of movements and the corresponding action in nerve-centres.

A visible movement may follow some impression received through the eye or ear, something seen or some word heard; the action, if it follows immediately upon the stimulus, may be clearly produced by it. When there is the least amount of present brain stimulation the brain centres are the most free and ready for control through the senses. The boy who has been impressed before school by talking of a bird-nesting expedition is inattentive to his master's explanation of Euclid. When the movements seen have apparently no known circumstances immediately stimulating them they are sometimes said to be "spontaneous," and the occurrence of many such acts is said to indicate spontaneity in the subject. Examples of these uncontrolled movements are seen in the wandering eyes and fidgeting fingers which indicate some emotional states. The movements of the new-born infant which we have described under the term microkinesis are similarly "spontaneous."

The sequents of movements seen may also be observed, the results following the action are not parts of the physiological phenomenon but serve to give it a certain character; a muscular contraction, stimulated by a nerve-centre is always itself a physiological fact, the first outcome of the visible movement may be a mechanical act such as lifting a weight, or writing, &c. The sequents of movements may be very complex although the movement itself be a simple fact. We may observe the antecedents and the sequents of an action; noting the time and the quantity of each. If light be allowed suddenly to fall upon the eye the iris immediately contracts the pupil; if we speak to a child there may be a period of delay before he moves.

It seems impossible to give any definition distinguishing action of a purely mental kind from such as effects other purposes, but the general characters of some acts distinguishing them as intelligent will be given.

Certain characters of brain are essential to the manifestation of mental action, they are inferred from the attributes of visible movements and may be described as Spontaneity, Retentiveness, Delayed expression of impressions, Double action in nerve-centres, Controllability of nerve-centres by physical forces.

Spontaneity as a character of brain is specially characteristic of infancy and childhood. It is indicated in visible action by a large number of movements of different parts of the body apparently occurring without any present circumstances stimulating them; the child and the young animal are full of such movements, they are specially seen in small parts. Probably in all cases such movements, if not really stimulated by surrounding forces, are due to previous impressions received by the individual or inherited.

Separate brain centres appear to be capable of acting without any external stimulus; such mode of action is seen in many conditions of adult life, and it seems likely that in mental function this is the foundation of mental spontaneity and spontaneous thought.

Retentiveness as a property of brain is somewhat analogous to inertia as a physical property of inanimate objects. Retentiveness may be indicated by the recurrence of a movement, or a certain series of acts, following a certain impression by sight or sound; a similar sight being followed by similar action, or movements of the same parts in similar order upon different occasions. Retentiveness in nerve-centres tends to repetition of similar action under similar stimulation; as in the case of some common reflex-action, *e.g.*, knee-jerk. The common "automatic movements" of some low class idiots show the retentiveness of their unimpressionable brains. Frequent repetition of the same words and phrases shows great retentiveness and little aptitude for fresh mental action. The increasing vocabulary of the developing child is a sign of advancing power. A parrot is very retentive of the few words he has become capable of speaking.

Delayed expression of impressions is indicated by a relation between the time at which the impression is produced in the nerve-centre, and that of the visible action by which it is subsequently expressed. Retentiveness preserves the impression which may not be known to us till it is subsequently expressed. This delay in observing the visible effects of the impression may be prolonged, there may be no outward manifestation till some further impression is made, or the expression may come out, as it is said, spontaneously.

A child four years old quietly looks at some one putting a letter into a pillar-post; we cannot at the time see the impression produced upon the child's brain, but we guess that an impression has been produced because the child's head and eyes turned towards the pillar-post. We know that an impression has been made when next day, on the child finding a letter on the table, "he takes it and posts it behind the door."

Double Action in Nerve-Centres.—It seems that a nerve-centre, when affected by an impression, may undergo some local molecular change, and also send efferent currents to muscles, producing visible movements at the same time. When speaking to another man he replies—immediate outcome—his subsequent actions show that some impression was produced.

Double action as thus explained probably does not always occur, as in the case of simple reflex actions, and other unintelligent movements. When an impression has been produced in a nerve-centre, the time of observation must be prolonged to see if you may find any delayed expression. Delayed expression of impressions is very common in mental phenomena, the expression is always by movement. Memory is due to impression on nerve-centres; the expression of an impression may be often repeated.

When we study movements we study the outcome of efferent currents; in studying brain action expressing mind (psychosis) we mainly consider the local or molecular changes in the nerve-centres. The evidence of a permanent local impression is its expression when the subject is stimulated. Evidence of local impressions in the centres, as produced by the sound of a word, is seen when immediate action follows in the hearer, and later signs of memory of that word are found. The stimulus of the sound of the word may produce efferent currents from the centre leading to movements, and also a permanent impression in the centre itself, such expression of the impression must be by movements, as by speech.

Controllability of Movements by Physical Forces.—Observations on the antecedents of acts show that many may be controlled by physical forces acting upon the senses, such as light, sound and touch, or mechanical impact. When such forces immediately determine the action, it is clear that they must decide the combinations and series of movements in the parts of the body.

Compound Series of Acts.—In noting the relations of an observed series of movements involving, as to their antecedents, many parts of the body, it is very usual to see a long series of acts follow some slight stimulus, such as the sound of a word of command, or even a gesture in another person. This may be termed *a compound series of acts;* it does not necessarily terminate in a strong movement, but in an action which—as it is said—is well adapted to the circumstances; this is probably due to the nerve arrangements for such action having been previously adapted by similar circumstances. In all such cases of movement adapted to the surroundings it will be found that impressions had been received previous to the slight stimulus which started the compound action observed. The kind of action now referred to is thus in part an example of delayed expression of previous impressions upon the brain, and is a mode of action absent in the infant at birth, and in the early stages of infancy, the necessary arrangements among nerve-centres must be built up. As to the theory of adapted action, it appears that a stimulus acting upon one of the senses may be followed by nerve-currents passing from certain cells to other groups of cells, to be finally succeeded by movements well adapted to the circumstances which produced the primary stimulus. Spontaneous movements must commonly be controlled, or temporarily inhibited, in any attempt to produce a new line of action by any educational method.

The most obvious signs of mental action are special series of movements in the body which must be observed in their relations to surrounding objects, and actions in other persons.

The principal intrinsic character of a series of acts is the relation in time of the movement of the visible parts of the body. There are four great classes of movements: (1) Uniform series, (2) Augmenting series, (3) Diminishing series, (4) Action adapted by circumstances. *A uniform series of movements* is the repetition of the movement of the same parts in uniform degree, or quantity of displacement, and in uniform time; this is seen when the individual does the same things over and over again. Walking is a uniform series of acts, and is not considered as necessarily a sign of intelligence, for it is not necessarily much controlled by the senses. Some manipulative processes consist of purely repetitive action. Some of the "awkward habits" of children are the repetition of uniform series of movements, such as lateral movements of the head in rotation, grinning, shrugging the shoulders, movement of the head to one side with slight inclination and rotation to the same side, putting fingers in the mouth, such movements frequently occurring spontaneously, or on any and every stimulus. In commencing an educational system with a young child, the spontaneity may at first be more easily controlled to become a uniform action than one adapted to any useful purpose.

Augmenting Series of Movements, or Reinforcement of Action.—A series of movements may occur, sequential to some stimulus, in which the final movement is much stronger than would be expected from the force of the primary stimulus, each group of movements, as the series progresses, increasing in number and in force. It is the spreading of the area of movement, or number of parts moving as the action proceeds, that is here specially indicated, such augmenting series of movements being started by a very slight stimulus, the force expanded in such series being out of all proportion to the strength of the original stimulus. The sound of a sharp word to a child may be followed by depression of the angles of the mouth; alternate tonic contraction and relaxation of the orbicularis oculi, altered respiratory movements, causing screaming, flushing of the face, and finally clonic contractions of many parts from action spreading to all the motor areas of the brain.

It appears that a nerve-centre may be stimulated by an afferent impulse, and may then discharge its efferent impulse to more than one centre, so that the nerve-currents become reinforced or strengthened, as they proceed finally to the muscles which produce visible movement.

Such reinforcements occur at the earliest stages of existence, whereas "compound cerebral action" occurs only as a later development.

An augmenting area of action is often considered a sign of emotion or mental excitement. Visible action in the body may rapidly spread as the return of the natural spontaneous action of the nerve-centres; in this case respiration is less interfered with than in the morbid displays of augmenting action: this is well exemplified in the march of spasm in an epileptic fit. In the child let out from school the crowd of movements seen results from the resumption of natural brain action uncontrolled; when fatigue leads to an increasing area of fidgetiness the state may be a return to the more childish condition where spontaneity of movement is usual.

In observing augmenting action (cerebral reinforcement) it is necessary to note if the movement spreads from large parts to small parts, *e.g.*, shrugging of the shoulders, then lordosis with lateral bending of the spine, and later drooping of the head, then movements of the facial muscles, eyes, and fingers; in other cases movement spreads from small parts to larger ones. To set the teeth, double the fist and hit out from the shoulder is to use larger muscles than when the mouth quivers, and the eyes are turned away, with many words and crying. With an augmenting area of movement, the time of action is often quickened, as in conditions of mental excitement.

Diminishing Series of Movements.—Conversely, we may observe a diminishing series of movements, fewer and fewer parts being in visible action, indicating a corresponding limitation of cerebral activity. This may be a quelling of the storm of nerve-action, it may indicate a return to aptitude for mental activity or approaching somnolence, *i.e.*, subsidence of all action, or it may signify cerebral exhaustion. The order of subsidence should be observed.

It may be well to touch briefly upon some points which illustrate the advantages of studying mental phenomena by the methods here described.

(1) We may find certain new signs by which to define the intellectual condition of a subject, its evolution or its deviations from the normal.

*(2) We are enabled to note precisely certain signs indicating the evolution of

* See Author's Paper, *Journ. Ment. Sci.*, April 1889; and *Proceedings of Roy. Society*, June 21, 1888.

mental function from infancy upwards, and—as we think—the organisation of the spontaneous movements of the new-born infant (microkinesis) to become the signs of intelligence.

(3) Movements observed at different ages may be classified and grouped, so as to show the ratio of action due to spontaneity in relation to that due to surrounding conditions and the impressions which they produce.

(4) It may be shown that thought, as a physiological action, is probably some kind of molecular change among nerve-cells, while its outward manifestation is always by visible movement—as a directly reflex-movement, or as a delayed expression of some previous impression.

Voluntary and Mental Movements.—Movements studied as signs of mental action are often said to be voluntary, more or less voluntary in contrast to others described as automatic or spontaneous. Probably we cannot define a voluntary movement, but we may explain what conditions observed make us call it more or less voluntary. A movement following quickly upon a word of command may be considered voluntary.

Respiratory movements when occurring in a uniform series are not considered voluntary; when the action is specially modified, as in speaking or singing; when the action is controlled by the sound of music they are more voluntary. Respiratory movements in the infant are uniform, except when the child cries as an expression of pain or other mental phenomena; in the adult many forms of emotion are expressed by variation in respiratory action, as in fear or anger. The modified respiratory actions termed sighing, laughing, singing, &c., may be signs of mental states, because they indicate nerve states, modified by special circumstances or antecedents. We consider such signs as mental phenomena, not so much on account of these (attributes or) intrinsic characters as because of their relation to antecedents—the previous sight or sound. When no special antecedent of the act of sighing is known it is often said to be spontaneous, automatic, or involuntary. The voluntary character of a movement appears to be indicated partly by its relation to some antecedent impression, and in part by its sequence; useful acts are often considered to be voluntary, and these are such as produce some result. The voluntary character is also in part due to its control by some fresh impression in place of spontaneous action; it may also be a change from one series of acts to another. In other cases the voluntary character is admitted because the act is obviously an example of delayed expression of some previous impression. As examples of voluntary and intelligent action see the ready reply, the exact copy, the act appropriate to the circumstance.

A complex series of movements of many parts in succession—*i.e.*, a compound series of movements following some slight stimulus through eye or ear without reinforcement of action, and producing some result or impression, is usually intelligent and voluntary; the more distinctly we see the action controlled by circumstances without reinforcement, the more is it like an intelligent and voluntary action. We see a cat sitting on the doorstep of a house, a dog comes by, the cat simply moves behind the railings without any excess of movement or display of emotion; that is a voluntary and intelligent act, the outcome of experience or previous impressions.

Action adapted by circumstances is a high-class manifestation; such action usually ends in something being done, or something said, which produces an impression so that the outcome of action is not lost. Adapted action appears in the child late in its evolution, it is increased by training, and is more easily acquired when the ancestors have been similarly trained. A large amount of spontaneity and reinforcement is antithetical to action adapted to circumstances.

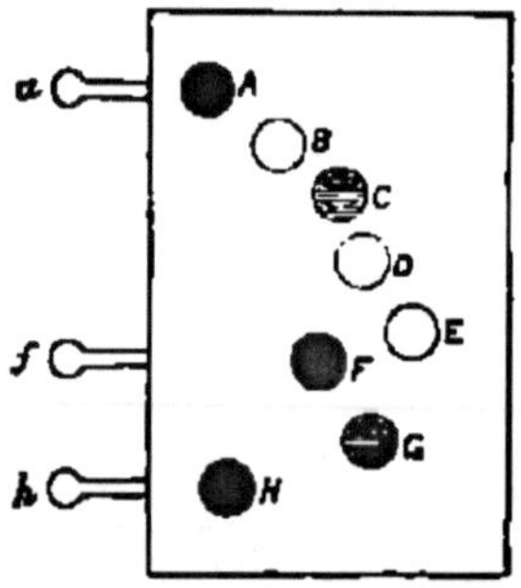

A mechanical diagram, representing a certain area of the brain. The circles represent brain centres. When a centre is represented as black, it is sending out force to muscles and producing visible movement in the body as expressed by elevation of signals at the side. The full action of A causes elevation of signal *a*, &c.; centres C G are supposed to be active, but not to be sending nerve-current to muscles; centres B D E are not acting.

Adapted action may begin with a slight stimulus, and may consist of many acts, the final act being such as is not usually produced directly by the primary stimulus.

The corresponding neural action we have termed compound cerebration. The primary stimulus forms one diatactic union, the currents from this form a secondary union, and so on—during the period of quelled spontaneity—and at last a fourth or fifth union, as the case may be, sends efferent currents to muscles producing a visible expression indicated by movement. The hypothesis of compound cerebration may be illustrated by a mechani-diagram represented on page 824.

An advantage of such modes of study as are here presented may be to enable us to apply to psychology the principles known as evolution, reversion, and antithesis.

If we describe certain mental states in terms of series of movements which indicate them, then when we see similar acts recur, we may say that reversion has taken place. In infancy we see series of movements of very small parts, not under control by the circumstance; in adult life (e.g., in chorea and conditions of mental irritability) we may see series of spontaneous movements of many small parts, not under control by the circumstance. This is a reason for speaking of such conditions as reversions to a lower—an antecedent, or more infantile—state. Such statements have at least the advantage of being intelligible, and are capable of criticism founded upon the observations of other men.

Again, if the attributes of action in the cellular elements of the brain be taken as the means of description, the processes of action in brain-cells may be compared with processes and conditions (of growth) in other living cellular organisms. Further, the physical forces controlling the attributes of cellular action in general may be studied as to their power to control action among the brain-cells.

Antithetical (or opposed) mental states are such as do not commonly co-exist, but are capable of replacing one another. The mental states termed kind and unkind, defiance and shame, joy and pain, may be called antithetical, as they do not commonly co-exist, the presence of the one mental state for the time precludes the other. The antithesis of the states joy and pain is expressed by the opposition of the signs which indicate these states. The antithesis of the mental states joy and pain, might be anticipated by the student of the physical expression of these states, for the two modes of facial action cannot co-exist. This illustrates one reason why the student of mental science should observe the expression of mental states as seen in visible action of the parts of the body. Hands cannot at the same time be both motionless and full of movement; now in the mental state called attention the hands are mostly still, in the fidgety child the fingers present numerous spontaneous movements; the physical signs are opposed to one another as are the mental states corresponding. Those emotions whose physical expressions are antithetical are the most unlikely to occur together, or if they do coincide momentarily there is a conflict seen in the body between the two physical states, as in an individual who, while suffering pain, still tries to look happy, and soon one or other condition gains the ascendency. Suppose a child has hurt his finger, but is trying hard not to cry, we shall see the muscles about the mouth quiver, until finally, the effect of the injury to the finger acting upon the nerve-centres becomes so strong that the angles of the mouth are depressed and the outbreak of sobbing follows. The opposite emotions, pain and self-restraint, or the conflicting nerve-currents acting upon the nerve-centres, result in one action predominating. This principle of antithesis is very useful in trying to gain knowledge as to the causation of mental states, and may serve to guide practice in education.

Spontaneous Movements and Spontaneous Thoughts.—The mass of spontaneous movements in the infant (microkinesis) has already been referred to, the corresponding brain action seems to be the spontaneous activity of many small nerve-centres, as a result of nutrition, with discharge of weak nerve-currents to the muscles of small parts of the body, *i.e.*, to those parts which in adult life are most concerned in expressing mental action. Later we see definite series of movements, and the expression of mental states. In our theory of the physical changes corresponding to mental action, it is supposed that intelligent acts depend upon the arrangement or "getting ready" (diatactic action) of certain groups of nerve-cells *before* the movement. It is this arrangement among the nerve-cells that seems to correspond to the mental act. Observation of movement in the infant seems to show that such unions for action occur very early, there may be arrangement among the cells not expressed by movement corresponding to initial mental acts. When the child is three years old, we still see much spontaneous movement, there is continuous chatter with the disconnected use of a few words and gesticulations. It seems probable that there may be many spontaneous arrangements occurring among the centres, corresponding to the visible movements. The microkinesis is in adult life replaced by co-ordinated or intelligent acts, but micropsychosis seems to continue. Spontaneous movements in the adult appear to be due to a reversion to the microkinesis of the infant, and often correspond to spontaneous, irregular uncontrolled "little thoughts." As rough analogy:—A child is fidgety (full of uncontrolled movements), and is inattentive (uncontrolled thoughts); nervous children have many spontaneous movements, and often have many strange, disconnected, imaginative, precocious thoughts; during sleep impressionability is lessened, and dreams are spontaneous. In adult life this spontaneous occurrence of many thoughts may or may not be accompanied by much spontaneous movement, there are wandering, unbidden, wild, ungoverned thoughts, a mass of thoughts, a cloud or rush of thoughts through the brain; such may occur in a man who is motionless, or in one who presents many movements.

This spontaneous thinking may result from fatigue, and unchecked it may lead to exhaustion; it is best controlled by things heard and seen.

Illustrations of Movement and Expression in the Face.*

Fig. 1.

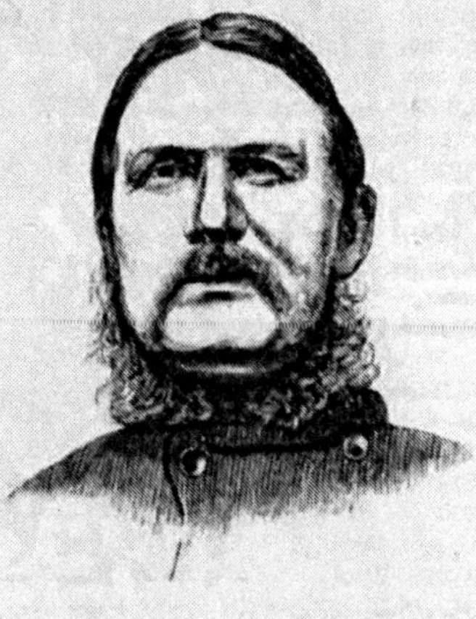

Thomas P., aged 52. Right hemiplegia, with cerebral facial palsy, right side. The face is asymmetrical, and the muscles in the right lower zone about the mouth act very indifferently. The naso-labial groove on this side is almost lost; this is well seen on comparing the two sides. No asymmetry is seen in the upper and middle facial zones.

Fig. 2.

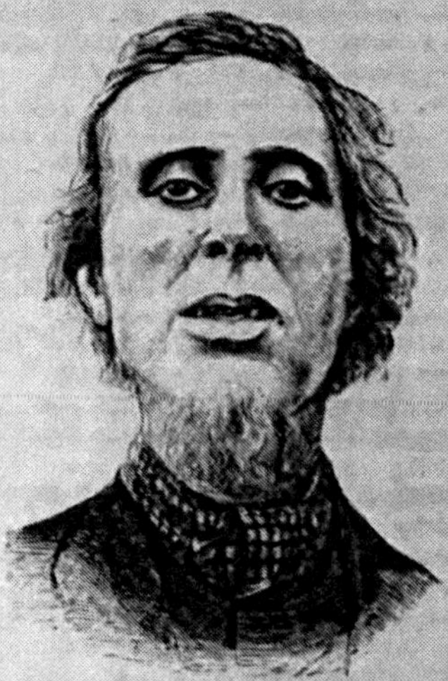

John H., aged 52. Left hemiplegia, with cerebral facial palsy, left side. The facial asymmetry is less marked than in Fig. 1. From the median line to the angle of the mouth is a longer distance on the right than on the left side. The hemiplegia is of long standing: there was much rigidity of the paralysed arm. There was well-marked valvular disease of the heart.

Fig. 3.

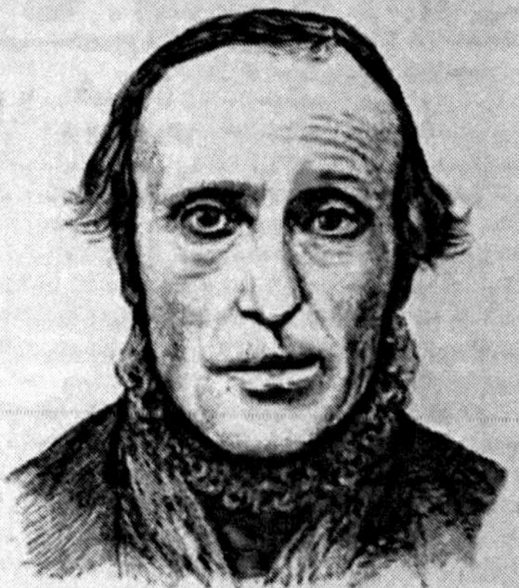

Bell's paralysis of the face, right side. Thomas C., aged 50. Seen November 1880. Four days previously he had suddenly found his face drawn to the left side; no other paralysis. The paralysis appeared due to the effect of cold; recovery was complete in three weeks. The symmetry in each zone of the face is striking. The orbicular muscle of the right eye is much weakened, as seen in the lower eyelid; the right eyebrow has fallen a little lower than on the left; the line of the eyebrow is nearer to the level of the pupil on the right than on the left, owing to the paralysis of the occipito-frontalis. The right cheek is flattened, the mouth and nose are drawn to the left.

* The engravings have been executed from photographs taken from life.

FIG. 4.

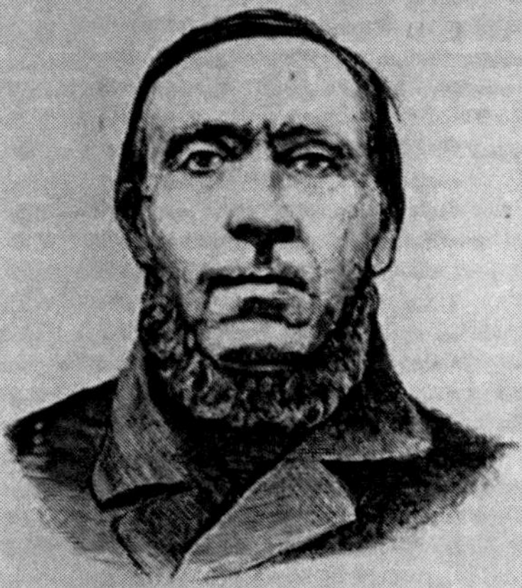

John Walker, aged 67. Seen April 1882. Paralysis agitans, in advanced stage. Face almost expressionless, with loss of all the fine adjustments of expression. He presents one dull monotony of facial expression. At the same time he can occasionally be made to grin, can show his teeth, elevate the eyebrows, or close the eyes, &c. The face is symmetrical in its passive condition and in its movements, and the condition is similar in all its zones. His voice is as monotonous as his face—one uniform low monotone. The right hand was the earliest limb affected; there is little tremor now, but, when held out, it presents the posture of the "writing hand" described by Charcot.

FIG. 5.

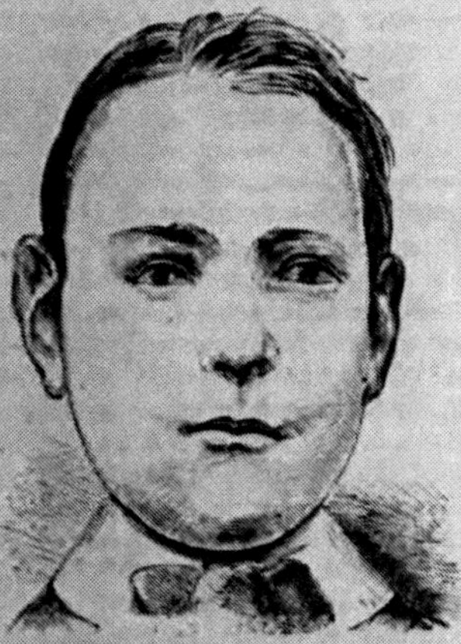

John B., aged 7 years. A high-class imbecile. Head well-shaped and of fair size; no paralysis. He has illusions, and has had maniacal attacks. His hands present much finger twitching, and they often assume the "nervous posture." Any excitation causes smiling; pain, pleasure, strong light, all cause the same expression.

FIG. 6.

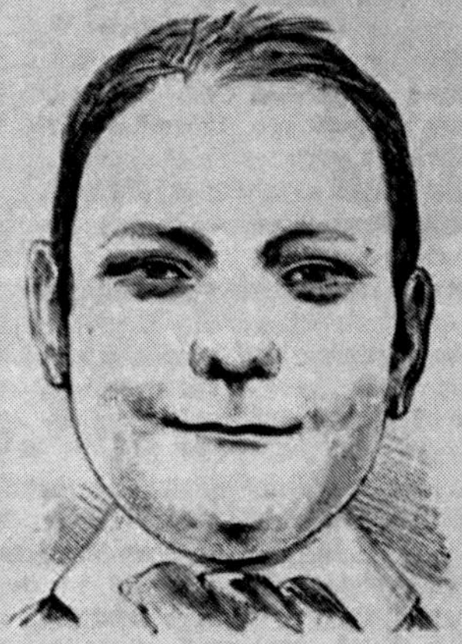

John B., smiling. The greatest change is in the lowest zone—*i.e.*, the zone that is most paralysed by brain-disease. This is the only active expression possible in the boy; it is symmetrical, and affects the upper zone the least, the lower zone the most. Exaggerated muscular action is common with brain defects.

FRANCIS WARNER.

MUSIC IN THE TREATMENT OF THE INSANE. (*See* TREATMENT.)

MUSICOMANIA, MUSOMANIA (*musica*; *μανία*, madness). A variety of insanity in which the passion for music has been fostered to such an extent as to derange the mental faculties.

MUSSITATIO (*mussitare*, to murmur). A condition in which the tongue and lips move as in the act of speaking, but without sounds being produced. An unfavourable sign in disease, indicating great mental debility.

MUTILATION, SELF. (*See* SELF-MUTILATION.)

MUTISM.—Dumbness from mental defect or disorder. In addition to the cases of Deaf-Dumbness (*q.v.*), mutism occurs in the course of various mental disorders, as Mental Stupor, Delusional Insanity, &c. As an instance of the latter, the following may be mentioned. The writer asked a patient in Bethlem Hospital, who had been mute for a long period, why he did not speak. He wrote down, "Because I have not been ordained." Subsequently, Dr. Rhys Williams took him to Archbishop Tait at the Palace. He had previously told the doctor that he could not go through any mimic form of ordination, but he spoke kindly to him. The patient was much gratified, spoke from that time, and was discharged not long after as recovered. A year or two afterwards he relapsed, and was re-admitted. (*See* DIAGNOSIS.)

THE EDITOR.

MUTITAS SURDORUM (*mutitas*, mutism; *surdorum*, of the deaf). Deaf-mutism, speechlessness from deafness, congenital or acquired. (Fr. *sourdsmuets.*)

MUTTERPLAGE, MUTTERSUCHT, MUTTERZUFALL.—German terms for hysteria.

MYODYNIA, HYSTERICAL (μῦς, a muscle; ὀδύνη, pain; hysteria). Hysterical muscle-pain. A term for what is regarded by some as ovarian tenderness, but which Briquet maintains is simply muscular.

MYSOPHOBIA (μύσος, an action of disgust; also filth; φόβος, fear of). Morbid dread or fear of filth, or of personal impurity or uncleanness.

MYXŒDEMA AND INSANITY.—Attention was first directed to what he called cretinoid degeneration in adults, by Sir William Gull, in a paper published in the *Clin. Soc. Trans*, vol. vii. 1873. This he showed to be marked by a change in the features, which become broad and flattened, the eyes appear unduly separated, the lips large and thick, and the folds of connective tissue about the eyes become loose and baggy, while under the jaws and about the neck the skin becomes thickened and lies in folds. The hair comes out, the hands become broad, the skin dry and harsh, not sweating; the temperature becomes sub-normal, the complexion generally is sallow, bearing, in some cases, a jaundiced aspect. But with the alteration in complexion there is almost always a bright patch of red, due to capillary congestion, over the malar bones. The disease occurs most frequently in women about forty to fifty years of age. The above description applies fully to myxœdema, which occurs more rarely in young patients, though we have met with it in both young men and women. There is some distinct relationship between this condition and the state of the thyroid gland (*q.v.*). A special name has been given by continental physicians to an allied state called by them cachexia strumapriva. Sir William Gull recognised the mental deterioration occurring in these cases. In his first report on the disease he says: "The mind which had previously been active and inquisitive assumed a gentle, placid indifference, corresponding to the muscular languor, yet the intellect was unimpaired." In a second case he describes the mind as generally placid and lazy, liable to being suddenly ruffled. There is certainly a degree of habitual and mental indifference, though this may under occasional circumstances be absent, since the intellect is unimpaired.

In 1880 we published notes on myxœdema with nervous symptoms in the *Journal of Mental Science*, and we shall refer later to these observations. In 1883 the committee of the *Clinical Society* of London appointed to investigate the whole subject of myxœdema published an exhaustive report on the disease, and this committee recognised the mental degeneration which is common in myxœdema. It reports that convulsions occur, though rarely, that of the intellectual changes, slowness in apprehension, thought and action, is the most constant, its absence being noted in only three cases. Abnormal persistence in thought and action is recorded in about one case in four. In a rather larger proportion there is more or less imperfection of mental processes, the defect being, as noted before, one of retardation or sluggishness. Writing is sometimes slow, sometimes imperfect; in the case of educated persons the handwriting is usually good, and the length of letters, in all respects well indited, is remarkable. Irritability is a marked feature, though in exceptional instances there is the reverse. In some cases placidity alternates with occasional outbursts of fretfulness and irritability. In a large proportion sleep is noted as good, but in many of these there is excessive somnolence, especially in the daytime. In about one-third of the cases wakefulness is recorded, and sleep is often disturbed by horrible dreams and sensations. It may be noted that drowsiness during the day is very common in myxœdema in both good and bad sleepers. Delusions and hallucinations occur in nearly half the cases, mainly where the disease is advanced. Insanity as a complication is noted in about the same proportion as delusion and hallucination. It takes the form of acute or chronic mania, dementia, or melancholia, with a marked predominance of suspicion and self-accusation; exalted ideas may occur. Memory is usually impaired from an early period, especially in respect of recent events. It is recorded as deficient in forty-six out of seventy-one cases. It may be mentioned that exophthalmos has been observed once or twice in the early periods of myxœdema; the special senses may be more or less affected especially in the later stages of the disease.

Myxœdema, though not common, is by no means exceptionally rare among the insane, and every large asylum has examples of the disease. It occurs chiefly in middle-aged women, and the disease, as a rule, has made considerable progress before any symptoms of insanity have become well marked. The symptoms divide themselves into two well-marked groups, those of disorder, and those of decay or weakness. A certain number of patients suffering from myxœdema become slowly self-conscious and distressed by the alteration in their appearance, so that, from simple exaggeration of self-consciousness they become suspicious and pass through a stage of watchfulness and expectancy into one of doubt, dread, timidity, and suspicion, till in fact they become fully developed examples of the delirium of suspicion or chronic mania. And as such they may have ideas of exaltation; thus, in one elderly patient in Bethlem, the idea that all sorts of things were being done which she did not understand led her to believe that these things were being done against her; with the increase of the disease, loss of hearing came on, and this caused still greater mental confusion and doubt. Instead of being actively dangerous or violent she slowly passed into a state of satisfaction with all the many attentions which she imagined were being paid to her, so that she became one of the queens of Bedlam.

In these cases it is pretty certain that all the mental symptoms have their origin in the impaired conduction of sensory impressions, so that as there are alterations in the structure of the skin and probably also in the structure of the conducting and receiving nervous organs, the ideas derived from these impressions differ materially from the ideas which were previously originated by similar healthy impressions. This leads to confusion, doubt, and either suspicion or dread; the loss proceeds further so that there is definite intellectual change as evidenced by defects of memory, will-power, and the like. In one group of cases, the chief cause of mental disorder is the idea that persons are noticing their physical peculiarities. Most of these in the end exhibit the same symptoms as those already described; the chief cause of trouble is the idea that being peculiar in aspect they are particularly noticed by people in the streets.

It is from this set of ideas that dread of going out arises. We have met with two such cases, and Dr. Wilks has recorded another; in the one the patient slowly, from being a good-looking young lady, became conspicuously broad-faced and ugly. Living as she did in a small country-town, the change in her face was remarked, and rude village boys used to jeer at her. Later, as the disfigurement became still more pronounced they followed her, calling out that she was "the pig-faced woman." Naturally this caused her a great deal of distress and worry, so that she avoided going out of doors as much as possible, and then took active steps to defend herself against real or assumed insults. Under these circumstances being violent and threatening she had to be sent to an asylum. In this case it is noteworthy that there was complete sexual perversion. In the asylum she steadily lost power and died of bronchitis with the onset of cold weather. And it is noteworthy that in all such cases the change of temperature is likely to produce serious and often fatal complications in the disease. It will be seen then that with myxœdema there may be a delirium of suspicion, developing out of the personal disfigurement and there may be, primarily or secondarily to the above, progressive mental weakness showing itself in chronic mania with suspicion, doubt, irritability and occasionally violence. The natural termination of these cases is in dementia which may become very pronounced and may be associated with loss of physical power, so that the patient is confined to bed; death generally depends upon some secondary cause. The pathology of the disease does not require special consideration here, but it is noteworthy that the mental symptoms may depend directly upon some alteration in the nervous tissues themselves. In some cases in which we have examined both brain and spinal cord we have been convinced that there were distinctly visible changes which would account, at all events, for progressive weakmindedness.

It is possible that in some cases the mental disorder really originates from the slowness and imperfection of the nervous conduction due to the changes in the peripheral nervous structures, while in some the defect lies in the changes which have taken place in the higher nervous structures.

Imperfect reception of messages leads to doubt and suspicion, while the progressive degeneration of the highest nervous elements leads to loss of control and later to loss of memory.

Myxœdema is not specially a nervous disease either by origin or alliance.

Mental symptoms may arise from changes in the peripheral or central nervous tissues, so that altered impressions, conductions, or ideations may arise, leading to various forms of mental loss or confusion.

The dulness produced and the alterations of aspect may be associated with suspicion of an insane type.

The general tendency of myxœdema is to produce mental weakness sooner or later.

GEO. H. SAVAGE.

[*References.*—Gull, On a Cretinoid State supervening in Adult Life in Women, Clin. Soc. Trans., vol. vii. 1873. Dr. Ord, On Myxœdema, Med. Chir. Trans., vol. lxi. 1878. Kocher (Berne), Langenbeck's Archiv f. Chirurgie, vol. xix. 1883. Dr. Savage, Journ. Ment. Sci., 1880. Dr. Felix Semon, Clin. Soc. Trans. 1883. Report of a Committee of the Clinical Society of London on Myxœdema, Clin. Soc. Trans., Supplement to vol. xxi. 1888.]

N

NAJAB UD DIN UNHAMMAD.—To this Arab physician, who flourished about the middle of the eighth century, we owe our knowledge of the symptoms and also the treatment of insanity as recognised by the Arab physicians. The title of his treatise was Asbab wa Ullamut. On this work a commentary was written in Arabic by Nafis bin Awaz in 1450, entitled Sharh ul Asbab wa Ullamut. It was translated in the seventeenth century into Persian by Muhammad Akbar under the name of Tibb i Akbari.

The various forms of mental disease are as follows:—

I.—**Souda a Tabee.**
- (1) *Souda.*
- (2) *Janoon.*

II.—**Murrae Souda.**

III.—**Malikholia a Maraki.**

IV.—**Diwangi.**
- (1) *Kutrib.*
- (2) *Mania.*
- (3) *Daul Kulb.*
- (4) *Sadar.*

V.—**Haziyan.**
- (1) *Mibda a illut dimagh.*
- (2) *Mibda a illut Marak.*
- (3) *Bukharat Had.*

VI.—**Raoonut.**

VII.—**Himak.**

VIII.—**Ishk.**
- (1) *Huram.*
- (2) *Pak.*

IX.—**Nisyan.**
- (1) *Zikr.*
- (2) *Fikr.*
- (3) *Takhil.*

Insanity is defined as "a state of agitation and distraction, with alteration and loss of reason, caused by weakness or disease affecting the brain."

It is not very clear to what types of insanity the preceding terms correspond.

I. **Souda a Tabee** appears to resemble dementia in most respects. The patient disregards clothing, cleanliness, and the calls of nature; the memory may be impaired, and there may be childish laughter. In some cases—and here the symptoms resemble melancholia—intense anxiety is manifested, and the patient suffers from the constant dread of approaching evil. With these symptoms are associated extraordinary movements of the hands and feet, leaping and beating the ground. When Souda becomes chronic it terminates in Janoon, in which the patient is restless, sleepless, taciturn, but at times roars like a wild beast. The prognosis was considered very unfavourable.

As to the treatment of Souda a Tabee the patient was bled and purged in the early stage, but nutritious food was given to him, baths were ordered, and milk was rubbed on the skin of the head and body. In fact, notwithstanding venesection and purgation, the patient was far better treated than in the good old days of the lancet in England. He had not only nutritious food, but his taste was consulted; he was allowed to have sweets, dry fruits, grapes, apples and water melons. Further, change of climate was recommended, and everything likely to cause irritation was to be avoided in order that the mind might enjoy complete rest. Nay, pleasure was to be afforded him by soft music, gardens planted by trees and fragrant shrubs—shady places to allow of protection from the heat. By this means it was intended to induce sound sleep, which was acknowledged to be a better remedy for mental disorder than medicines. Very remarkable is the following passage from an Arabian writer, Shaik la Ajub, unsurpassed by anything in the writings of Pinel, or in the principles of treatment enunciated at the York Retreat at the latter end of the eighteenth century:—"Be it known that of all remedies, to strengthen the heart and brain is the safest and most sure, by which means the mind and action are guided aright. Do nothing to frighten a patient, and let him select his own employment. Make the senses a special subject of treatment, and occasionally give stimulants. Rest and fresh air are required for the miserable men afflicted with insanity. They should be shown every possible kindness; in fact, they are to be treated by those under whose care they are placed as if they were their own offspring, so as to encourage them to place confidence in their caretakers, and communicate their feelings and sufferings to them. This will be at least a relief to those unfortunates, and a charity in the eyes of God."

Should the patient continue to be unduly excited or distracted, drugs were to be administered, some of a soothing nature, and others calculated to drive melancholy away. Actual prescriptions are given.

II. **Murrae Souda.**—In this form of mental disorder the patient is "morbidly anxious and "constantly full of doubts." Here we are confronted with the Grübelsucht of German alienists. In walking, his eyes rest on the ground, his head and face are thin, his pulse weak, sometimes fast and other times slow, his urine thin and clear. Among the earliest symptoms of ill-health is insomnia. As to treatment, blood-letting if necessary must not be large, or it would add to the debility. Before resorting to it the effect of certain prescriptions was to be tried. "Do nothing to agitate the brain, avoid violent purgatives, give nourishing drinks, also flesh and fish. The patient should live in a place where the temperature is mild, and be surrounded by many trees and roses."

III. **Malikholia a Maraki.**—The humoral pathology comes in here. From the limbs, the humours and the heat of the body pass to the brain. This heat (Marak) ascends, it destroys the soul and darkens intellect. The patient, if not relieved, loses all power of reasoning and action, and the disorder terminates in dementia. He is quarrelsome and dangerous, if the humour affected be bile; but if it be the saliva he will be quiet, and as if under the influence of liquor. The treatment must depend upon whether there are signs of inflammation or not; if the former, bleed and put the patient on a milk diet; if the latter, feed him up.

IV. **Diwangi.**—The sub-division (*Kutrib*) of this type derives its name from a small animal which is for ever on the move, and therefore serves to represent the extreme restlessness which is present in this disorder. As the same word signifies a jackal, it also indicates the howling which such patients sometimes indulge in. They are represented as suspicious, and hiding themselves during the day in woods and among tombs, only coming out during the night. Their expression is sad, they are acutely melancholy, sometimes they lacerate their bodies with thorns and stones. The treatment consisted in compelling the patient "to be constantly employed, it being of the utmost importance to get the patient to work." The patient might be bled at the outset. If the above treatment failed, water was to be constantly dashed on his head, and he was to be prevented from sitting in the dark. The prognosis was good. We next come in the second sub-division of Dīwāngī, to the familiar title of "Mania," the Arabic equivalent being "*Janoon Tabee,*" termed by one Arab writer Razuo, "*Janoon Haeeg.*" Those labouring under this malady smash and tear whatever they come across. In short, they are maniacs. Another sub-division (*Daub-Kulb*) resembles hydrophobia. The patient fawns like a dog. If he bites another person, the latter speedily dies with symptoms similar to those observed in men bitten by a mad dog. The fourth sub-division (*Sadar*) is described as mania associated with "swelling of the brain." We notice here the first reference to restraint. The hands and feet were to be tied, and this for three reasons:—That the patient's restlessness may be controlled; that his brain may have rest, and lastly that he may be prevented from killing himself and others.

V. **Haziyan** is a disorder of judgment involving the loss of the power of thought. It is unnecessary to detail its sub-divisions.

VI. **Raoonut,** and VII. **Himak.**—The symptoms under these forms appear to be very similar to the foregoing.

VIII. **Ishk.**—This word signifies a creeper which twines around a tree and gradually causes its death. Grief and weeping, love of solitude, concentration of the mind on a loved object, anxiety and silence characterise this form. The patients labouring under it must be amused and kept merry. Marriage is prescribed as the best remedy of all. The cause given is excessive venery.

IX. **Nisyan** is the loss of memory, the treament of which was unknown to Najab ud din Unhammad. Neither Mr. Stokes nor M. Loisette appears to have had his analogue in Arabia.

THE EDITOR.

[*Reference.*—Dr. J. G. Balfour, "An Arab physician on Insanity," Journ. of Ment. Sci. July 1876, from which Paper this article is derived.]

NANOCEPHALUS (*νάνος*, a dwarf; *κεφαλή*, head). A term meaning the possession of a diminutive head, the size of the rest of the body being normal. (Fr. *nanocéphale*; Ger. *Zwergkopf.*)

NARCË (*νάρκη*, stupor). An old term meaning diminished activity of the nervous system. Applied by Hippocrates to mental torpor. (Fr. *stupeur*; Ger. *Fühllosigkeit.*)

NARCOMA, NARCESIS (νάρκη). Narcosis (*q.v.*).

NARCODES (νάρκη; ὄδες, terminal). An adjective meaning "having stupor"; narcous. (Fr. *narceux*; Ger. *betäubt.*)

NARCOLEPSY (νάρκη; λαμβάνω, I take). Irresistible attacks of sleep, short in duration, but occurring at frequent intervals.

NARCOSIS (ναρκόω, I become torpid). A condition of insensibility produced by the action of certain drugs, poisons, and retained excretory products on the nervous system. (Fr. *narcose*; Ger. *Betäubung.*)

NARCOTICS (ναρκόω). Certain drugs and poisons which act on the nervous system, and in small doses promote sleep, but in large doses bring on complete insensibility and death. (Fr. *narcotiques.*) (*See* SEDATIVES.)

NARRENHAUS (Ger.). A madhouse.

NARRHEIT (Ger.). Lunacy, madness.

NASAL TUBE.—A soft india-rubber tube which is passed through the nose into the œsophagus, for the forcible feeding of those either unable or unwilling to take food naturally; it is also used for washing out the stomach in cases of poisoning and in certain gastric diseases. (*See* FEEDING.)

NATIVISTIC THEORY.—The theory that asserts that visual and other sensations give rise to perceptions of space, form, distance, &c., not through a mental interpretation as the result of experience, but through the agency of some innate power.

NATURAL.—A common term for an idiot.

NAUTOMANIA (ναύτης, a seaman; μανία, madness). Morbid fear of a ship. By some authors it has been applied to a form of insanity, said to be occasionally observed among seamen, characterised by a morbid dread of water, and a furious, destructive, and homicidal mania. (Fr. *nautomanie.*)

NECROMIMESIS (νεκρός, a corpse; μίμησις, imitation). The delusion in which a patient believes himself to be dead. (Mickle.)

NECROPHILISM (νεκρός; φιλέω, I love). A term used in two senses, either a morbid desire for eating dead bodies, or an insane impulse to violate a corpse. Those so affected are called necrophiles.

NECROPHOBIA (νεκρός; φοβέω, I fear). Either morbid fear at the sight of a dead body, or morbid fear of death. (Fr. *nécrophobie*; Ger. *Leichenscheu.*)

NEGATIONS, INSANITY OF (*Délire des Négations*).—The French term was introduced by Dr. Jules Cotard in 1882, to designate a state to which Griesinger made special reference in describing melancholia:—"A state of mental pain, becoming always more dominant and persistent, and increased by every impression, is the essential mental disorder in melancholia; and, so far as the patient himself is concerned, this mental pain consists in a profound feeling (Unwohlsein) of *ill-being*, of inability to do anything, of suppression of the physical powers, of depression and sadness, and of total abasement of self-consciousness. . . . The disposition assumes an entirely *negative* character (that of aversion)." *

The employment of the word in question by the Germans, as also by the French, includes the antithesis of that healthy condition of the mind which may be termed positive. It involves a repulsion, and may therefore be said to be a negation of mental health. It is not necessarily accompanied by verbal denials. The idea which those intend to convey who employ the term is expressed in Griesinger's words, "Die Stimmung nimmt einen durchaus negativen Charakter (des Verabscheuens) an." Without this explanation the reader would naturally expect a morbid mental condition similar to that of "insanity of doubt," and in truth one variety of the insanity of negations appears to the writer to be almost if not quite identical. From the above, however, it will be seen that Griesinger had in view one phase of melancholia. He would have included mania of persecution. It has been the object of M. Cotard to extricate it from this category, and he gives with great perspicuity the differential diagnoses between the two.

In the **insanity of negations** there is anxiety, groaning, præcordial distress; the patients are typical examples of anxious melancholia; others fall into mental stupor; some exhibit alternations of mental stupor and acute melancholia.

Hypochondriasis, especially *moral*, is observed at the onset. The patient accuses himself; he is incapable, unworthy, guilty, lost; should the police come to arrest him and conduct him to the scaffold, he only too richly deserves death for his crimes. Suicide and self-mutilation are frequent, homicide is rare. There are disorders of sensation, including anæsthesia. Hallucinations are often absent. When present they are simply confirmatory of delusions; hence there is no

* "Die Pathologie und Therapie der psychischen Krankheiten," 1861, pp. 227–8. See also Syd. Soc. transl., 1867, p. 223.

antagonism between the patient and voices that speak to him—no dialogue; when such patients speak to themselves it is in order to repeat in the form of litanies the same words or the same phrases addressed to real persons around them. Visual hallucinations are tolerably frequent. *Physical* hypochondriasis follows. Patients think they have no brain or stomach, &c. They may either deny that they are alive or that they will ever die. The personality is transformed; some speak of themselves in the third person. Patients deny everything, they have no parents, no family; everything is destroyed, there is no longer anything; they have no mind; God himself does not exist. There is a morbid desire to oppose everything. Food is *entirely* refused; such patients refuse because they are unworthy, because they cannot pay, because they have no stomach, &c. The course of this form is at first intermittent, then continuous.

On the other hand, the symptoms of **persecution mania** are as follow:—The patient does not as a rule present the usual *facies mélancolique*. Hypochondriasis, especially *physical*, is observed at the onset. The patient holds aloof from the external world and the harmful influences coming from various sources—especially from the midst of social life. He does not accuse himself: he rather boasts of his physical and moral force, and the excellent constitution which allows him to bear so many evils. Suicide is comparatively rare. Homicide is more frequent. Disorders of common sensation are very rare. Auditory hallucinations are constantly developing themselves as is well known. Visual hallucinations are very rare. Moral hypochondriasis is secondary. Patients declare that their persecutors attack the moral faculties, and that they are made idiotic. There is *délire des grandeurs*. The refusal to take food is *partial*. In consequence of the fear of being poisoned, patients eat voraciously such food as they believe not to be poisoned. The course of the disorder is remittent or continuous, with paroxysms.

The above presents in a lucid form the points of differential diagnosis between insanity of negation and that of delusions of persecution as sketched by M. Cotard. Examples are given. One is that of a lady who when asked, "How do you do, madame?" replied, "The person belonging to myself is not a dame, call me Mademoiselle, if you please."

"I do not know your name. Will you tell it me?"

"The person belonging to myself has no name; I desire that you do not write it."

"I still desire to know your name, or rather what you were formerly called?"

"I understand you. I was Catherine X——. It is needless to speak of what took place. The person belonging to myself has lost her name, She gave it away when she entered the Salpêtrière."

"How old are you?"

"The person belonging to myself has not an age."

"Are your parents still living?"

"The person belonging to myself is alone, has no parents and never had any."

"What have you done? and what has happened to you since you became the person of yourself?"

"The person belonging to me has remained in the Asylum of . Experiments, physical, metaphysical, have been and are still made upon it."

In attempting to trace the pathological evolution of those melancholiacs who accuse themselves, and of those patients who labour under the insanity of negation, M. Cotard sketches in the first instance the principal characters of the mental condition of the former. In the simplest form they are those which belong to the variety of melancholia known as "simple" or "without delusion," or, as some term it, moral hypochondriasis (J. Falret). Already such patients present a negative condition of mind. They mourn over their lost energy and feeling; they assert that they no longer feel affection for their friends or even their own children. Ideas of ruin arise and appear to be a *délire négatif* of the same nature. There is a veil interposed between the patient and his surroundings, which, as in cases of mental stupor, may become so opaque as to entirely mask the world of reality. There is, M. Cotard holds, only a difference of degree between the foregoing conditions of moral hypochondriasis, self-accusation, and the systematised delusion of negation. It is easy to understand the transition from a sense of the external world being changed and the denial of its existence. Even the state of mind which leads the patient to deny the possibility of his recovery, logically ends in an absolute disbelief in his environment and his own existence. While some patients believe in their immortality, asserting to the last moment that they shall not die, patients who pass into a state of delusional stupor, imagine that they are dead.

In classifying cases of insanity of negation, M. Cotard gives **three categories**, the **first** of which comprises what he calls the simple condition (*état de simplicité*), the **second**, those cases in which it is a symptom of general paralysis, and the

third, those in which, associated with persecution mania, it constitutes those complex forms of insanity which account for the confusion between melancholia and delusions of poverty, culpability, distrust, and of persecution.

As an example of the **first** category, the case of a lady is given, suicidal, hypochondriacal, and with delusions of guilt. During paroxysms of distress she asserted that all her organs were displaced, and that she was lost, that she had no longer a head, and that in short she was dead. After a time she denied having arms or legs, and in short believed that all parts of her body were metamorphosed. The disorder terminated in dementia.

Under the **second** division a case is given in which the patient expressed negative ideas of a very absurd character; he denied that there was any night, and refused to go to bed; he passed whole nights in his office, asserting that he could not retire to bed because it was still day. He refused to eat any more, and however abundant the food, he became infuriated and denied that there was anything on the table. He asserted that he was in a desert where no one lived, and from which he could not escape, because there were no more carriages or horses. Shown a horse, he said, "This is not a horse, it is nothing." He refused to have his clothes put on because the whole of his body was not greater than a hazel-nut. He would not eat because he had no mouth, or walk because he had no legs. He died from general paralysis.

The **third** class is illustrated by a patient who had severe attacks of hysteria, followed by melancholia, with ideas of guilt; mystical ideas, and paroxysms of wild excitement, and believed herself to be possessed. One delusion was that she had become a scorpion, and she displayed remarkable contortions in imitation of its movements. She imagined herself to be persecuted by people who could read her thoughts. She denied at last being any longer human.

We have thought it well to put the reader in possession of the views entertained by certain French alienists in regard to the *délire des négations*, but an English alienist finds it difficult to see the force of the various forms or divisions which are laid down by M. Cotard. That there is a mental condition to which the terms "negation" and "negative" as ordinarily understood might very properly be applied, cannot be doubted. An instance in which the term may be very properly used has been already given in this article (p. 833), for no statement, however elementary as regards its truth, could be made without the patient instantly denying it. If a man is asked his name, and he says he has none; or his age, and he denies being of any age; where he was born, and he replies that he never was born; who was his father, and he denies ever having parents; if he has headache or stomach-ache, and he responds that he has not either of these organs; or lastly, if a patient is shown the commonest flower there is, and he denies that it is that flower—well then, we admit that no better term can be found for such a mental condition than the one under consideration, but this is only a small part of the area covered by the cases which French alienists have in view. Moreover, we should be falling far short of Griesinger's "revulsion"—the negation of mental health. In truth, his description appears to us to be so comprehensive that it ceases to be distinctive.

THE EDITOR.

[*References.*—Leuret, Fragments psychologiques, Paris, 1831, pp. 121, *407 et suiv.*; Traitement moral de la Folie, Paris, 1840, pp. 274, 281. Esquirol, Des maladies mentales, chap. Démonomanie, Paris, 1838. Fodéré, Traité du Délire, t. i. p. 345. Morel, Etudes cliniques sur les maladies mentales, t. ii. pp. 37, 448. Macario, Annales médico-psychologiques, t. i. Baillarger, De l'état désigné sous le nom de stupidité, 1843; La théorie de l'automatisme (Ann. Méd.-Psych. 1855); Note sur le Délire hypochondriaque (Académie des Sciences, 1860). Archambault, Annales médico-psychologiques, 1852, t. iv. p. 146. Petit, Archives cliniques, p. 59. Michéa, Du Délire hypochondriaque, Ann. Méd.-Psych. 1864. Materne, Th. de Paris, 1869. Krafft-Ebing, Lehrbuch der Psychiatrie, obs. ii. et vii. M. Cotard, to whom we are indebted for the above references, has written an article in the Ann. Med.-Psych., 1880, entitled Du Délire hypochondriaque dans une forme grave de la mélancolie anxieuse. See also Archives de Neurologie, 1882; and his Etudes sur les Maladies Cérébrales et Mentales, 1891. Preface by Falret.]

NEGRO-CACHEXY. A form of pica or depraved appetite not uncommonly found in negroes when afflicted with some diseases; akin to the pica of chlorosis and pregnancy. Syn., Cachexia Africana.

NEGRO-LETHARGY. (*See* NELAVAN.)

NELAVAN.—The "African sleep disease." An endemic disease of negroes on the West Coast of Africa characterised by morbid somnolence, headache, and emaciation. It is usually fatal.

NERVE STORMS.—A name loosely given to paroxysmal attacks of emotional disturbance functional in character. It is also applied to certain diseases, such as epilepsy, migraine, paroxysmal vertigo, &c., some of whose characteristics are a regular succession of phenomena in each attack, an inverse relation between the severity and frequency of the attacks, and a culmination to a certain pitch of intensity followed by subsidence. It has been thought by some that the pathology of these diseases is best summed up by the term "nerve-storm" on the supposition that there is a gradual accumulation of nervous force which is suddenly discharged, with the result of producing the peculiar symptoms.

NERVOSISM. — The doctrine which maintains that all morbid phenomena are due to variation in nerve force.

NERVOUS DIATHESIS. (*See* DIATHESIS, INSANE.)

NEURÆMIA (*νεῦρον*, a nerve; *αἷμα*, blood). A term used for functional disease of the nervous system (Laycock).

NEURALGIA in its Relation to Mental Derangement. — It would be more correct to substitute for "neuralgia" the term "derangement of sensibility," for we are going to treat here not only of circumscribed affections of one or another nerve with the characteristic painful points of Valleix (*Valleix'sche Schmerzpunkte*), but likewise of hyperæsthesiæ, anæsthesiæ and paræsthesiæ, of central or peripheral origin, and of a circumscribed or diffuse nature, and of their connection with mental processes.

Symptoms. — Considered from this wider standpoint, the *anomalies of sensory nerves* form a frequent element in the clinical aspect of mental disorders, and also—as we are about to prove—an important factor in their production. Such anomalies are part of the acute as well as chronic forms; they sometimes precede the mental derangement and sometimes accompany it throughout its course; they sometimes are mere accidental, and sometimes, on the contrary, exciting causes, by constituting a basis for the mental disorder, or by causing the outbreak of an actual attack. Thus we may speak of (1) a **psycho-physical**, and (2) of a **pathogenic** function of neuralgia in its relation to mental derangement.

(1) Under **psycho-physical** function we understand the *psychical interpretation of neuralgia—i.e., the explanation of abnormal sensations by a deranged mind.* From the pathology of the nervous system we know those abnormal perceptions through which anæsthetic limbs are often considered to be foreign bodies, or the frequent delusions following the amputation of limbs in consequence of irradiation from the nerves of the stump. Such illusory interpretations take place in a still higher degree in mental derangement when all critical power is absent, or all perceptions are determined by one predominant fixed idea. Thus every "pressure" on any part of the body is explained by the melancholiac as a "warning of his guilty conscience," and by the paranoiac as a "point of attack on the part of his persecutors." In the so-called "maniacal rage" (*Zorn-manie*), a frequent form of mania in anæmic patients, the præcordial pain causes the patient to make violent attacks. In consequence of such interpretations of derangements of sensibility, neuralgia becomes the direct foundation, *i.e.*, the cause, of delusions or fixed ideas. The *quality* of the abnormal sensation most frequently decides the *subject-matter* of the delusions; painful sensations and those of pressure produce ideas of persecution and danger in melancholic and paranoiac patients; abnormal sensations in the viscera produce the idea of "strange animals in the stomach" or of "displaced viscera" in the hypochondrium; the ideas of "pregnancy" and of "rape" are caused by uterine disorder. Abnormal sensations in the male genital organs are explained as "attempts to castrate." On the other hand, abnormal sensations of the skin produce changes in the sense of bodily limitation: the patient feels smaller or larger, he even becomes the "universal spirit" or feels "wings growing, which carry him as if he were as light as a feather." Sometimes local hyperæsthesia and anæsthesia occur combined; a melancholiac feels a "hole" (anæsthesic portion of the skin) in his chest, through which the devil has fetched his *evil soul* (deep intercostal pains)." The "ogres" (*Wehrwolf*) in the epidemics of the Middle Ages must probably to a great extent be considered as abnormalities of cutaneous sensation in melancholiacs. In the same way the sensations of motor-inhibition in the persecution-mania of certain tabic patients become man-traps and snares which the supposed enemies of the patient have laid for him.

We find an analogy to these psycho-physical relations in *dreams*. Here also certain sensations (in the viscera, and muscles) produce a "dream of flying," or a "dream of falling;" and in certain individuals approaching internal disorder (indigestion, &c.) announces itself in certain ever-returning dreams. "Nightmares," also, with the sense of suffocation and of danger to life, belong to this category.

The connection of certain delusions with certain abnormalities of sensation is a clinical fact, not only of psychological but practical interest. For if the psychical quality of a delusion corresponds to the physiological *timbre* of a neuralgic sensation, we seem justified in concluding *from the subject-matter of the former, the quality and seat of the latter.* Experience confirms this in a great number of cases.

Thus the complaints of "depression and possession" of some melancholiacs or the localised "persecutions and attacks" of a certain group of paranoiacs are produced by local disorders of sensation or painful nerve-tracts. To this class we have to refer, especially, the frequent *præcordial sense* of weight in conditions of depression, which in a great number of cases corresponds to a neuralgic tract of intercostal nerves (*vide infra*). Thus certain qualities of the delusions become for the physician important *psychical indications* for the bodily *loci dolentes*, the subject-matter of the delusion becomes an important *mental auscultation*, so to say, a semeiotic indicator of the corresponding diseased nerve-tract. For both—the neuralgia and the delusion—form a whole: the physical irritation and its psychical equivalent.

Derangement of sensibility, clinically most different, may assume this psychophysical character and become the cause of *delusions*, examples of which have already been given. In addition to the latter, we have to mention diffuse and local hyperæsthesiæ and anæsthesiæ of central and spinal origin (in paralysis and other organic diseases of the brain) and local neuralgiæ of spinal or constitutional anæmic origin (paranoia, melancholia) as vaso-motor neuroses (especially in their primary stages). Clinically, the most frequent are intercostal neuralgiæ, especially in neuropathic women; after these, neuralgic affections of the nerves of the head, especially of the forehead and occiput. Both conditions frequently accompany melancholia, the former being the objective sign of the patients' guilty conscience or "heartache," which—a most significant fact—is localised in the posterior boundary of the axilla (sometimes even on the *right* side) and the latter causing the mental confusion which the patients complain of ("so that they are even unable to think of their relatives"). For, in a normal condition of mind our *thoughts* are accompanied by certain sensations on and in the head, and of slightly oscillating visual pictures. In addition to the tract of the intercostal nerves *irritation of the vagus* plays frequently a great part in melancholia which is indicated by alterations in the beats of the heart and by a sense of weight in the chest, by dryness of the throat and hoarseness. These sensations also indicate to the patient "the seat of the evil one in his breast," or point out to him that "part of the throat by cutting which he must commit suicide." The præcordial pressure or so-called *præcordial anxiety* consists of *affections* of the intercostal nerves, of the vagus and of the corresponding vaso-motor tracts—united or separately—and is felt by the patient according to its nervous origin as situated *externally* in the pit of the stomach, above the heart in the axillary line on the lower part of the sternum, or as an internal weight. Next in frequency to this group of derangements of sensibility follow the numerous *visceral neuralgiæ*, which occur especially in hypochondriac melancholia, and there produce the illusory sensation of an abnormal *situs viscerum* or delusions of all sorts of incurable disease, of the presence of foreign substances and of animals, of the absence of certain organs or their transformation into glass, metal, &c. Then follow the hyperæsthesiæ, anæsthesiæ and paræsthesiæ of the genital organs, which especially in paranoiac *women* produce delusions of pregnancy and of rape, in *men* the delusion of nocturnal castration, and of sexual assaults, and in *both sexes* under certain conditions the delusion of perverse sexual sensation and transformation. In many conditions doubtless cutaneous hyperæsthesiæ play a great part and cause the delusion of "burning" followed by constant reflex attempts to undress. In paralysis and hysterical insanity the abnormal cutaneous sensations in connection with abnormal muscular sensations produce the delusion of the change of cutaneous limitation, of becoming greater or smaller (macromania and micromania), of bodily deformity, of levitation and of the flying away of single limbs. The whole spinal cord even may be attacked by neuralgia as in the so-called spinal paranoia (of masturbatory or hereditary neuropathic origin); in this case all forms of perverse sensations occur, partly localised, partly diffuse, and produce "physical persecution-mania," a disease, in which every spot of the body in consequence of the altered sensibility seems to the morbid *ego* to be the points of attack of the persecutor.

The principal condition for such an interpretation of abnormal sensations is a morbid consciousness, because the delusion we have spoken of is only possible under the influence of a deranged state of the mind, and only so far as the critical faculty—*i.e.*, the normal association of ideas—has been injured. Thus, the subject matter of the delusion depends on the quality of the sensation *and* on the predominant condition of the mind; consequently, a central (psychical) *and* a peripheral (neuralgic) factor act together. From this it follows that, in the course of the mental derangement, the psychical results—*i.e.*, the subject-matter of the delusion—of those two factors undergoes changes; during convalescence from melancholia, when the consciousness becomes clearer, the former "guilty conscience" in the pit of the stomach becomes a natural "painful home-sickness," and gradually the painful nervous sensation is correctly interpreted.

(2) The pathogenetic function of neuralgia is connected with the psycho-physical factor, and still more closely with the physiological origin of the genuine affection. The connection of both has already been mentioned in the co-operation of the central and peripheral factors—the morbid consciousness and derangement of sensibility—spoken of above; but here it is essentially of a psychical nature and is the cause of the delusion as an elementary psychosis, and the latter is the psychical equivalent of the physical cause. From this differs the importance of neuralgia as a physio-pathological factor of the psychosis, in which case it is an essential factor in the production of the latter; not a single element of psychical importance only, but a *conditio sine quâ non* of physiological importance, and as such it forms *necessarily* part of the cerebral affection, because without its co-operation we should not find an *entity* of mental derangement.

In the latter interpretation it finds, as mentioned above, its analogue in the normal process of emotion, which also has physiologically a centro-peripheral origin. For in emotion (and especially in depressive emotion, which corresponds to the condition of depression) there is a central and, of necessity, a peripheral process (vaso-motor and sensory).

We daily experience, at the very moment of perception, that something refers to ourselves; we feel certain physical sensations, which, though changeable and different according to the individual, generally return with typical regularity. We remind the reader of the vaso-motor rush in the emotion of *shame*, the sensation of weight at the pit of the stomach, difficulty of breathing, dryness of the throat, palpitations and the feeling of intense coldness, &c., in the emotions of *fear*, *grief*, and *fright*. Anger even influences the vaso-motor action and inhibits breathing, whilst the rolling of the eyeballs, the mimicry, and lastly, the movements of defence or attack of the arms, indicate the spreading of the irritation from the oculo-motor nerve downwards over the spinal cord. And as the latter movements liberate the inhibition felt at first in the emotion of anger (the anger expending itself), so in grief and sorrow the flow of tears acts as a reflex, relieving the painful (irradiated) sensation of weight at the pit of the stomach. It is understood that, in the process just described, the *cerebral* conditions of the emotion—*i.e.*, the mental inhibition in the process of ideas and the altered relations—precede the fresh idea, which causes the emotion, but that the *ego feels* this disturbance and is *affected* by it, is produced by the accompanying physical sensations, which give the emotion its typical *timbre*. In this way it becomes clear how certain peripheral sensations resembling that *timbre* are able to suggest to the *ego* certain morbid emotions. Thus, a choreic patient is, in consequence of the emotions caused by his abnormal muscular movements, constantly in an angry temper; and in a patient suffering from depression, new attacks of anguish are continually caused by the præcordial weight. Those attacks are at first without any motive, but before long the *ego* interprets them in the manner indicated.

What is the **physio-pathological explanation** of the accompanying sensations? They consist of affections of the cranial nerves, so far as we are able to analyse—especially of the vagus and glosso-pharyngeal—of the spinal nerves of the thorax and abdomen, and of the vaso-motor nerves according to the particular affection. Certain affections, especially of the vagus and of the intercostal nerves, accompany the normal conditions of depression as well as decided melancholia, in which they produce distinct points of localised pain, generally over the lower part of the sternum, and in the epigastric region (præcordial anxiety, præcordial pain). Through their connection and their action simultaneously with the cerebral disorder, which produces the condition of melancholia, the sensory tracts just mentioned become *psychical* nerves in the strictest sense. It is possible, and seems to be confirmed by experience, that especially in grief and in analogous mental conditions first the vagus is affected (sensations in the pharynx, alteration in the voice, respiration, and the heart's beat), and that gradually, and in proportion to the strength of the emotion, the excitement spreads downward over the medulla oblongata and the spinal cord, and affects the intercostal nerves, thus causing the sense of weight on the chest, and especially the "heartache" (Herzweh) of which the patients complain, with the reciprocal influence on the patient's interpretations, mentioned above. According to the individual disposition, the vaso-motor system is also affected, probably in the brain (contraction of the cortical arteries with inhibition of mental function), and spreading downward over the thorax and abdomen (*cf.* "Die neuesten sphygmographischen Untersuchungen," von G. Burckhardt).

In normal depression the depressor nerve (according to Cl. Bernard) counteracts this increase of blood-pressure and cardiac pressure in consequence of the arterial tension, by causing relaxation of the capillaries and afterwards also dilatation of the contracted arteries. This self-regulation of the normal emotion is probably annihilated in conditions of morbid depression by the circumstance, that the sympathetic (vaso-contractor) is by some peripheral stimulation (intercostal neuralgia) kept in a condition of reflex irritation, which cannot be counteracted (Goltz).

To return to **clinical observations.** In the group of conditions of melancholia *the co-operation of the cerebral affection (inhibition of psychical function) with the peripheral irritation of a sensory nerve-tract* is an undoubted fact. There are two reasons for this: (1) We always find associated with the cerebral excitement—*i.e.*, the psychical paroxysms—the vasomotor symptoms; (2) the exacerbation of the latter is invariably followed by a psychical crisis—*i.e.*, an exacerbation of the mental condition. As soon as the patient feels his melancholia increasing, the *loci dolentes* on the chest, &c., become more distinct *with* or *without* the vasomotor conditions mentioned, and, *vice versâ*, as soon as the neuralgia is excited (by some physical condition, as menstruation, &c.), the anxiety returns or the pain and delusion increase. *The patient lives in a vicious circle of circumstances.* The occurrence of the so-called *raptus melancholicus*, especially, is frequently caused by "epileptoid" irradiation from a neuralgic zone. This pathogenesis belongs to the "neuralgic reflex-psychoses," of which we shall treat separately below. A group also of maniacal conditions belongs to this neuralgic circle, especially *mania furiosa*, which has nothing in common with *amenomania* (with *couleur de rose esprit* and graceful manner), but consists, on the contrary, of a sulky mood, acts of violent resistance, and assaults. Here also the angry temper and the painful inhibition of consciousness, with constant return of one and the same furious idea in the midst of an otherwise rapid flow of ideas, are accompanied physically by a peripheral neuralgia, the motor reflex discharges of which are represented by the acts of destruction, and the movements of defence and motiveless attack. The patient, when asked in a quiet condition where his anger is situated and what causes his rage, points to his chest or the pit of his stomach.

Of *paranoiac* conditions, the wide-spread so-called spinal persecution-mania is caused by various derangements of peripheral sensibility, and its course is, *among other circumstances*, essentially connected with the course of this diffuse spinal neurosis. We have spoken above about the relations of the latter to the formation of delusions, and have especially pointed out the importance of the *timbre* of the peripheral sensations, which is reflected in the subject-matter of the delusion (sexual neuralgia with obscene delusions, &c.). Here we must say more about the pathogenic element, which consists in the connection of the cerebral process with a sensory spinal neurosis, and especially about the further development of these cases of paranoia. In *one* group of cases we find the co-operation of the mental derangement (ideas of persecution) with physical paræsthesia, in such a manner that the ideas of persecution are completely made up of the interpretation of the paræsthesia: wherever the patient perceives a sensation, to that point the attack of the persecutor is directed; every pain is explained by the patient as a new sign of the action of his enemies or of the demons. This circle of ideas becomes gradually narrower, so that the change of the sensation into the delusion becomes more and more *direct*, without any intervention of reasoning or of *critique*. Thus, colicky pains in the stomach are at once interpreted as "operations on the abdomen," itching of the skin is *bonâ fide* explained as "bites of snakes which the persecutor has secretly placed in the bed of the patient." On the other hand, every thought of the persecutor is reflected in a peripheral paræsthesia or paralgia. In *another* group of cases we find a transference of the sensory irritation to the *motor system*: in the parts affected by neuralgia, temporary or permanent spasms and contractures (especially in the extremities) occur, a sort of *status attonitus*. In this form of development of the neuralgic psychosis consciousness generally sinks to a more or less profound stupor, though with a dream-like internal life, in which the altered muscular sensations are also interpreted as "persecution" (especially demoniacal). The patients lie down still and motionless, often spasmodically crying; they have to be fed, and object to being approached. The contractures of the limbs frequently cause swelling of the joints and local abscesses. During convalescence the patients state the exact localisation of the painful sensations which compelled them to hold their limbs contracted, and also their delusional perceptions—*e.g.*, that the evil one had been sitting on their chest and taken their breath (intercostal neuralgia with consequent tension of the muscles of the thorax); that he had made their limbs touched so that they were bewitched and unable to move (interpretation of neuralgia of the fifth nerve with consequent contractures of the muscles).

It does not escape our notice that the cases of paranoia which we have mentioned represent in their full development a sort of *cerebro-spinal reflex-mechanism*, in which ideas and emotions on the one hand, and the manifold physical abnormalities of sensation on the other, enter into *direct relation and reaction*, and in which, after the disappearance of the inhibitory function of the brain, the *ego* gradually becomes dissolved—dissociated—into individual mental acts without any connection. This is actually the psycho-physiological character of the secondary stages and of the termination of this group of spinal paranoia.

As an addition to the pathogenic notions of neuralgia we have to mention the *sensory-trophic reflex-action* of certain cases of *traumatic* neuralgia on the brain. We find peripheral lesions of the nerves of the head (fifth nerve or occipitalis major) giving rise sometimes to conditions of chronic depression or excitement with severe headache radiating from the cicatrised part, with congestions, numbness, vertigo, loss of memory, sometimes also with hallucinations and attacks of *mania furibunda*. The trophic derangements appearing with the psycho-neuralgic cerebral disorder on the affected side of the head are: falling off of the hair, local secretion of sweat, and sometimes itching exanthema. Thickening of the membrana tympani has also been observed. As a rule, pressure on the cicatrix is followed by an increase of the radiating headache and usually also by an outbreak of mania. The latter therefore seems to be a sort of *epileptoid equivalent* (in some cases actual convulsions are present during the attack), and the mental disorder an actual *reflex-psychosis*. By excision of the painful scar, and production of a new and painless one, a complete cure of the severe mental disorder has been sometimes effected (*vide infra*).

In the same neuralgic-reflex manner the attacks of mental derangement in prolapse of the uterus are probably brought about, which soon subside after the introduction of a pessary, but return after its removal. The relapses of mania often observed as a consequence of a painful whitlow cannot be explained otherwise than by the same pathogenesis. Vasomotor influences undoubtedly form here, as in all neuralgic psychoses, an important connecting link.

The **therapeutics** of these derangements of sensibility, especially of the neuralgiæ, must be founded on the consideration that the sensation of local pain or the paræsthesia proceed from some central or peripheral source (by irradiation), but it must be kept in mind that in the former case also the central irritation of the nerves does not persist as such, but spreads over a certain sensory tract, settles down in it, and thus causes, sooner or later, an *independent* neuralgia. The mental pain and the ideas of persecution in paranoia are, so to say, formed in the sensory nerves of the body. Thus, in the course of states of depression different intercostal neuralgiæ, with the characteristic points of pressure and the altered cutaneous sensibility, are differentiated from the (what is at first a vague) præcordial weight.

This relation must be kept in mind in treatment. As long as the cerebral affection predominates, and irradiation over a certain peripheral tract has not taken place (*i.e.*, as long as no definite neuralgia has been caused), ordinary therapeutics are sufficient, as applied in the commencement of conditions of depression. A methodical treatment with opium, together with the corresponding general treatment, will have a soothing effect on the brain, as well as on the peripheral tracts of irradiation. But as soon as the latter become marked out and prominent, local treatment has an excellent curative effect. In these cases, especially of melancholia with definite intercostal affections, the internal exhibition of opium may be changed for subcutaneous injections of morphia with methodically increasing doses at the neuralgic points, or in their neighbourhood. If the attacks are paroxysmal, especially in cases of periodical anxiety, it is important to *prevent* them by making the injection before the attack. In many cases this method of treatment has excellent results, assuming that, in addition to this, general treatment, somatic and mental, is applied. In slighter cases, in which the paroxysms are not so violent, and the anxiety or pain less severe, the local application of chloroform on cotton-wool, or the internal application of anodynes, especially of antipyrin, render valuable service, especially as this process may be repeated several times a day at the commencement—*i.e.*, before the increase of the pain. In more severe cases, daily galvanic treatment of the painful intercostal tract, according to circumstances, with simultaneous galvanisation of the spinal cord (descending current) has very good results. Massage has also been successful.

It must be understood that if the neuralgia is very distinct and persistent, we have to attempt to find the peripheral reflex origin. Disorders of the abdominal functions, and especially affections of the sexual organs, are often the first cause, in which case the treatment should be directed accordingly. Other indications belong to gynæcology, and the general treatment of anæmic conditions (iron, hydro-therapeutics) so frequently necessary, belongs to internal medicine. We must make it our principle to apply one sort of treatment after the other (often also combined) when one of them has failed, and always to proceed with *methodical persistence*. Medicinal treatment has as yet had most unsatisfactory results in the neuralgiæ and paræsthesiæ of spinal paranoia (the so-called physical persecution-mania); electric treatment can frequently not be applied on account of the specific delusion of the patient that he is under the influence of hostile electrical machines, but if applied is, according to our experience, of little use, and the good achieved is but temporary. But, if the spinal hyperæsthesia is caused by a peripheral irritation accessible to treatment, as affections of the genital organs (especially in women), a good influence may be exercised over the spinal reflex neuralgiæ by the treatment of the peripheral irritation.

The treatment of *reflex psychoses* in consequence of *traumatic neuralgiæ* has been much more successful, as in a certain number of cases a complete and lasting cure of the irradiated mental affection was effected by *operative removal* of the painful cicatrix (on the head).

HEINRICH SCHÜLE.

NEURÄMIE (*νεῦρον*, nerve). Neurasthenia (*q.v.*).

NEURAMOEBIMETER.—An instrument for the measurement of Reaction-time. (*See* PSYCHO-PHYSICAL METHODS.)

NEURASTHENIA (*νεῦρον*, the nerve; *ἀσθένεια*, weakness).—**Definition.**—By this term we denote a peculiar condition of the nervous system, deviating more or less from the normal state, and characterised by a loss of resistance, the latter in its turn producing an increased irritability and debility, so that the nervous system is in a condition which may vary from that of apparent health to severe and distinct nervous disease. Thus neurasthenia extends over the whole sphere lying between health and the more severe forms of nervous disorder, without however separating them distinctly; on the contrary, in the neurasthenic condition of the nervous system lie the roots of the symptoms of the nervous disease, and out of it, if not checked, the roots grow and form the disease. Neurasthenia therefore represents to a certain degree the starting-point of all the more severe nervous disorders, and the soil from which they grow. The phenomena, however, are in neurasthenia much less marked than in actual disorder, and are often but slightly indicated; at the same time they are invariably present.

If the conditions mentioned continue to develop, hysteria, epilepsy, locomotor ataxy, or general progressive paralysis appears; if they do not continue to develop, the individual in question remains *neurasthenic*, or, after a shorter or longer time, is restored to health, having had only a severe attack of neurasthenia. Compared with the other nervous disorders, neurasthenia has many peculiarities, or else it would not have been possible to separate the two groups. These peculiarities consist more in negative than in positive qualities, inasmuch as neurasthenia is distinguished from other more marked nervous disorders, less by the qualities it possesses than by those which it does not possess. There will be scarcely one neurasthenic patient in whom there are not a number of hypochondriacal symptoms; in a great number of neurasthenic patients we also find hysteroid and epileptoid, in others again tabiform and paralytiform symptoms; these symptoms, however, are not so well marked as to enable us to speak of hypochondriasis, hysteria, epilepsy, locomotor ataxy or general progressive paralysis. Although they may develop into these diseases, they do not yet represent them. It is the same with gastro-intestinal derangements, at a time when dysentery, cholera or typhoid fever is prevalent, or with slight catarrhal and rheumatic affections at the present day when influenza prevails over the globe. The slight affections mentioned are undoubtedly connected with the epidemics, but are the simulation only of the more severe forms. They are not as yet the cholera, dysentery or typhoid fever itself; the characteristic element is absent.

Nomenclature. — Neurasthenia has also been called *nervousness* or *irritable* weakness. About 1850, Hasse termed it *morbid irritability* and also *exaggerated sensibility*, but before him some English and French authors had at least partly described it: in the sixteenth century, Jean Fernel; in the seventeenth, Lepois, Thomas Willis and Sydenham; in the eighteenth century—especially towards the end—Robert Whytt, Raulin, Pomme, Tissot and Erasmus Darwin, and at the commencement of this century, F. W. Jaeger, Louyer-Villermain, and others. The terms *cachexia*, *diathèse nerveuse*, *marasme*, *état nerveux*, *affection vaporeuse*, *névropathie* and *vapeurs*, which afterwards became *marasmus nervosus*, *status nervosus*, neuropathic diathesis, neuropathic disposition or constitution, were formed at those periods. About 1840 Bouchut described it as *névrospasmie*, and Valleix as *névralgie générale qui simule des maladies graves des centres nerveux*; and not much later—about 1850—Sandras, Cérise and Gillebert d'Hercourt described it as *névropathie protéiforme*, *surexcitation nerveuse*, *état nerveux*, &c. From 1860, when Bouchut published his monograph: "*Du nervosisme et des maladies nerveuses*" it was often called by the awful name of *nervosismus*, and after 1868, when George M. Beard published his first treatise on the disease in question, it was termed *neurasthenia*, a name which undoubtedly is the best, because the most significant. Weakness in all its conditions and with all its consequences is the characteristic of neurasthenia, which no other international term has expressed so well.

From the time when Bouchut and Beard wrote, we may date a new era in the history of the disease in question. Each of them claims more than once that *he* was the first to shed light on this affection, and that up to his time there had been only confusion and want of clearness on the subject! They say that *nervosismus* or neurasthenia has mostly been confounded with hysterical and hypochondriacal conditions. They—and they only—had introduced a separation of these conditions. But if we are completely unprejudiced, we must confess that an absolute separation is impossible, and we actually find Bouchut and Beard describing symptoms as belonging to neurasthenia, which undoubtedly belong to hysteria and hypochondriasis, or even to mental disorders. Beard, indeed, maintains that neurasthenia is a modern and especially an American disease, scarcely known in Europe, and not at all in some European countries, as Germany, Russia, Italy and Spain.

Neurasthenia, however, is neither a modern nor an American disease only. It existed thousands of years ago in the old world, and already in Hippocrates we find descriptions of morbid conditions which must be referred to it. In addition to this we remind the reader of the descriptions in former times, mentioned above, in order to prove that these statements are quite erroneous.

In many other places we find also some very characteristic descriptions of the subject in question, which however appeared under a different name or as passing statements in other treatises, and therefore escaped the notice of many. We mention among others the article on "Spinal Irritation," by Brown (*Glasgow Medical Journal*, May 1828); a treatise on Neuralgic Diseases by Thomas Pridgin Teale, sen. (1829); remarks on Spinal Irritation by Parrish (1831); "Practical Observations on Diseases of the Heart, Lungs, &c., occasioned by Spinal Irritation," by John Marshall (1835); the remarks of Henle on the Erethism of the Nervous System in his *Pathologische Untersuchungen* (1840), and in his *Rationelle Pathologie* (1846–51); also on Spasmophilie or Convulsibilitaet as a special morbid condition, by Hirsch, in his *Beitraege zur Erkenntniss und Heilung der Spinalneurosen* (1843); the description of Cerebral Irritation by Griesinger in the *Neue Beitraege zur Physiologie und Pathologie*, in the *Archiv fuer physiolog. Heilkunde* (1844); the treatises on Spinal Irritation and Habitual Spinal Debility, by Wunderlich, in his *Handbuch der Pathologie und Therapie* (1854); and lastly, the remarks of Hasse, when speaking of Nervous Weakness in his *Krankheiten des Nervensystems* (1855).

The claims of Bouchut and Beard are therefore groundless, and the circumstance that the works of these two men were received with an enthusiasm which they did not deserve, is due to the fact, that the study of nervous diseases had been neglected for a long time. It is however a merit of Beard's, whose work is entirely in accordance with Bouchut's, to have invented the suitable term "neurasthenia," a fact which, considering the international importance of science, is of great value.

Symptoms. — The character of neurasthenia is weakness, loss of power of resistance, decrepitude. The nervous system is weak, partly in consequence of faulty development, in which it remained more or less behind, and partly in consequence of insufficient or inappropriate nutrition, which has produced a condition of more or less advanced atrophy or paratrophy; it may be compared to a not yet fully developed, or worn out, or diseased single nerve, because its functions have undergone the same changes. It reacts according to the law of stimulation of the fatigued nerve, just as in hypochondriasis, hysteria, epilepsy, and in mental derangement. It is not surprising, therefore, that neurasthenia has, according to the views of Bouchut and Beard, often been confounded with hysteria and hypochondriasis, and that in spite of this, Bouchut and Beard do the same, describing distinctly hysterical, hypochondriacal, epileptic, and epileptoid conditions as belonging to neurasthenia.

Whilst in the conditions mentioned the reaction may be that of profoundly fatigued or even degenerating nerve, in neurasthenia it is always that of slightly fatigued nerve. Neurasthenia is, from this point of view, we repeat, the commencement of all these more fully developed conditions; it is the soil in which they take root and from which they grow. Neurasthenia, occurs as mentioned above, in all possible degrees of intensity, and varies from the condition of perfect health to that of fully developed disease. It is therefore to a certain degree nothing more than a greater or less disposition to assume the symptoms of the diseases mentioned; it is what in neuropathology is called the neuropathic diathesis, as long as it keeps itself within certain limits; as soon as it steps over these limits it becomes actual disease or a symptom of disease with well-marked characters—hypochondriasis, hysteria, epilepsy or psychosis. On the other hand, it is clear that the commencement of the latter diseases necessarily coincides with the symptoms of neurasthenia, and that it is impossible to separate them clearly. It will always be at the discretion of the physician to consider symptoms as neurasthenic or as belonging to hypochondriasis, hysteria, epilepsy, or to mental derangement; this was the case with Bouchut and Beard in classing under neurasthenia, as new discoveries, symptoms which by others were regarded as belonging to more serious conditions.

The same holds good with regard to the relation of neurasthenia to the so-called organic diseases of the nervous system. Both Bouchut and Beard maintain that neurasthenia is distinguished from the latter in not being caused by organic changes. But is it possible to imagine an alteration in function without organic change? If we consider as organic changes those only which are obvious to the blindest observers, we shall frequently not find them even in cases in which during a whole lifetime abnormal phenomena presented themselves in a most striking manner. If, however, we keep in mind that there is no function without an organ, and that every function is but the product of the action of the latter, and must vary according to the nature of the organ, we cannot possibly doubt that there are organic changes in cases in which the functions are altered, however slightly, the more so if we have learned in our own researches to recognise those changes chemically and physically. From a large experience we shall derive the conviction that there can be no difference between the so-called functional and organic diseases, but that when the former develop and when disorders of function have existed for a longer or shorter time, they can have sprung only from organic changes.

The so-called functional diseases must therefore be always regarded as possibly serious; and this in proportion to the degree in which they are developed and the sufferings they cause. The history of many a case of encephalitis, myelitis, neuritis (neuralgia), locomotor ataxy, and of general progressive paralysis has unfortunately but too often proved this. Beard, who lays special stress on the difference between functional and organic disease and calls neurasthenia a purely functional disorder which causes much pain, is quite wrong in maintaining this distinction. All the affections mentioned are caused by profound organic changes, and their character does not develop except after a prodromic stage of many years; yet the symptoms were considered merely functional disorders, and under the circumstances naturally so. Their relation to the prodromic stage is the same as that of hypochondriasis, hysteria, epilepsy, and mental disorders to pure neurasthenia; they spring from it. Such is the case, also, with multiple sclerosis, with progressive bulbar paralysis, and with sclerotic *plaques* in the spinal cord, a sufficient reason for taking every case of neurasthenia very seriously, because we never know whether more serious disorders may not at last develop, or whether the neurasthenia is not already an indication of more severe troubles. Of course the longer neurasthenia has been present, and the graver the symptoms, the less favourable is the prognosis.

According to the law of stimulation of a fatigued or degenerating nerve, the nervous excitability as such is decreased, but nevertheless appears at first increased on account of the greater capacity of conduction in consequence of the decreased resistance; this exaggerated excitability still increases, at first rapidly, thereby producing painful and spasmodic symptoms, which are far from being proportionate to the stimulation, but afterwards the increased excitability decreases rapidly, so that strong stimulation only is able to produce any effect, until at last no effect at all can be produced. The increased excitability being produced by a decrease of the normal resistance, which naturally is followed by a decrease of nutrition and consequently by a condition of weakness, it is clear that the increased excitability which a degenerating nerve at first presents, cannot last long, and that soon decreased excitability, bluntness, paresis, or whatever we call fatigue and exhaustion, must take its place. Excitability, with a tendency to rapid fatigue or exhaustion, is therefore a characteristic of neurasthenia. Sensory nerves being normally more excitable than motor ones, it follows that, with a few exceptions, neurasthenia will present itself first in the sensory sphere in the form of hyperæsthesia, and afterwards also in the motor sphere of the nervous system, in the form of hyperkinetic, hypersecritic, and hypertrophic symptoms, which, however, often soon change into the opposite condition. As among the latter states the kinetic symptoms and the fatigue are the most conspicuous phenomena, *hyperæsthesia* and *muscular weakness* are considered the principal symptoms of neurasthenia.

Hyperæsthesia, with the corresponding hyperkinesia, spasmophilia or convulsibility, is the principal symptom of *spinal irritation* which we have mentioned above, and which was for some time thought to be caused by a greater or less excitability of the spinal cord due to hyperæmia or inflammation. This was, however, a mere hypothesis, to which, on the whole, little value was attached. It was an attempt at an explanation, but more stress was laid on the phenomena themselves. There was naturally a great difference of opinion about these phenomena and their importance, but many authors were of the same opinion, especially in this, that spinal irritation and its symptoms were closely related and formed the transition to hypochondriasis, melancholia, mania and dementia, and that—as Romberg especially points out—it would not be well, to attribute too much to spinal irritation, thereby taking away from hysteria and neuralgia, in order to gain material for a new interpretation, or rather misinterpretation. The enthusiastic advocates of neurasthenia as a condition of its own, widen, nowadays, its sphere at the cost of hysteria and of the more severe neurotic conditions—*e.g.*, *locomotor ataxy* and *general paralysis*; in this way many a patient has met an early fate, who by timely and appropriate treatment might have been saved. We therefore cannot too strongly emphasise that neurasthenia, although not yet a disease properly speaking, is often the *commencement* of a disease, and that all the more serious neurotic conditions, not the result of some sudden special accident, have their origin in neurasthenia. Neurasthenia, after having reached a certain degree, does not necessarily continue to develop; it may exist unchanged for years, thus representing the neurasthenia of most authors of our times; it may be relieved and its symptoms may be suppressed, but they may also at any time become aggravated and glide into one or the other nervous disease; it is impossible to say with certainty that the latter will not occur. If anybody believes that he has been able to assert this in a number of cases, we must say, to put it mildly, he deceives himself. Many reasons and arguments have been pressed upon us, but we have not found them sufficiently forcible to make us alter our opinion.

The characteristics of neurasthenia are, therefore, hyperæsthesia and muscular weakness, or, in other words, *increased excitability* with a *tendency to rapid fatigue, especially of the muscular system*. If, instead of the mere fatigue, spasms occur, and if in the muscular and vascular, and the corresponding processes in the glandular system, neurasthenia passes over into hysteria or epilepsy, the symptoms have now attained a certain height and periodicity, and have developed into paroxysms which by most authors are considered the proper and only criterion of either pronounced hysteria or epilepsy. In the same way, if more severe mental excitement follows on a sense of uneasiness, with or without oppression and anxiety, then we shall see hypochondriasis or melancholia develop according to the subjects with which the mind of the patient is occupied, or even the imperative ideas or false sensations which usher in some forms of insanity.

However this may be, hyperæsthesia, as the most widely spread phenomenon, especially attracts our attention, because it is completely of a subjective nature, and even in the most painstaking examination no objective foundation can be found, so that it is generally regarded as imagination, exaggeration, or a product of the craving to appear interesting, &c. It causes the patient, however, enough trouble and discomfort to make him lose his happiness for a considerable period of his life. This hyperæsthesia occurs most frequently in the muscular system and its belongings, especially the bones. This sphere is the most excitable, because offering the least resistance, and hence it is intelligible that it is so easily exhausted and so soon fails to perform its functions. All kinds of unpleasant sensations and even vivid pains in the muscles or limbs are therefore of usual occurrence in neurasthenic individuals. These pains appear mostly in the muscles of the back and in the spinal column, and are therefore regarded as pathognomonic of neurasthenia; as in former times they were attributed to spinal irritation. Beard, who objects to considering neurasthenia as the "spinal irritation" of former times, maintains therefore that it is only a symptom of neurasthenia, which, however, may obscure all other symptoms, and then actually represent the spinal irritation of our forefathers.

Next to pains in the back, which have been wrongly referred to the spinal cord, because pain cannot be anything else but a cerebral function, many other cerebral symptoms—symptoms of Griesinger's cerebral irritation—are regarded as characteristic of neurasthenia, and are therefore next to spinal irritation of pathognomonic importance in neurasthenia.

The symptoms of cerebral irritation are manifold. Strictly speaking, all subjective symptoms and conditions of altered, especially increased, excitability belong to them, and this includes pains in the back and in the joints, in short, spinal irritation. We comprise, however, among the symptoms those phenomena and conditions only which present themselves in the cranial nerves, especially in those of the higher senses, and particularly in the mind (in the strict sense)—the sphere of abstract imagination and its relations. The frequent occurrence of headache, especially of *migraine*, of a sensation of numbness and heaviness of the head, of pains in the eye, of photopsia and chromatopsia, of scotoma, of indistinctness of vision, of noises in the ear, of humming and buzzing, of bell-ringing, of sensitiveness to smell, and of subjective sensations of smell as well as of taste, and of idiosyncrasies (*e.g.*, pica), are important phenomena of cerebral irritation. In addition to all these, we have to mention, as equally important, instability of mental equilibrium, easy and rapid changes of temper, a sudden and apparently unaccountable sense of discomfort, dissatisfaction, depression and sadness, of oppression, anxiety, fear, and anger, a tendency to vertigo and absent-mindedness, more or less numerous antipathies and sympathies, certain *tics* and whims, the more or less frequent occurrence of imperative ideas, and, lastly, most troublesome insomnia or somnolence.

Of the conditions of mental oppression and anxiety some that are produced by certain external causes are remarkable. Of these, *hypsophobia* is a type. Under just the reverse conditions oppression may occur in some individuals as *batophobia* when they pass by a high wall and look up, or when they are in a deep and narrow valley. In others, again, the sense of anxiety is produced when they are about to cross a large open space as *agoraphobia*, or when they are compelled to stay in small closed rooms as *claustrophobia*, or, better, *cleistrophobia* or *domatophobia*.

According to the cause of this fear, many special conditions have been described, and Beard especially has taken great pains in particularising them. Thus, we find *monophobia*, fear as such; *anthropophobia*, the fear of being with others; *pathophobia*, the fear of becoming ill (otherwise comprised under hypochondriasis); *pantophobia*, fear of everything; *astrophobia*, fear of lightning; *rupophobia* (Verga), the fear of being dirty; *siderodromophobia*, the fear of going by train; *nyctophobia*, the fear of night; *phobophobia*, the fear of becoming afraid. Were we to carry this absurdity further, we might distinguish a much greater number of conditions of fear: *skopophobia* and *klopsophobia*, the fear of spies and thieves; *thanatophobia*, the fear of death; *necrophobia*, the fear of the dead and of phantasms; *triakaidekaphobia*, the fear of the number thirteen, &c., but what should we gain? The conditions in question are nothing but a kind of *idiosyncrasy* or *antipathy*, which in its turn is a kind of imperative idea. If very slight and temporary, it is a symptom of neurasthenia; but if more severe and permanent, it passes over into the gravest condition of mental disorder. This proves the connection between neurasthenia and mental disorder, and also that neurasthenia is frequently only the earliest and slightest indication of a psychosis.

Of pains in the muscles, which are said to be symptoms of neurasthenia, we have to mention peculiar and vague sensations of great fatigue, stiffness, heat and uneasiness, which occur principally in the legs and feet, and sometimes also in the upper extremities; they induce constant changing of the position of the limbs, so frequently met with in nervous and restless people, as the layman calls them. This uneasiness, mostly due to hyperæsthesia of the muscles, is considered a pathognomonic symptom of neurasthenic conditions.

Among the other conditions of hyperæsthesia, those of the skin must be mentioned as the most frequent; as dragging and tearing pains in the course of the various nerves, hyperalgia and hyperalgesia as well as hyperpselaphesia. Among the latter conditions we have specially to mention the feeble resistance to either a high or low temperature. Neurasthenic individuals will rarely bear a high temperature, and on the other hand they are very liable to catch cold; even a slight draught is troublesome and hurtful to them; such individuals are also very ticklish and complain of subjective sensations of heat, of paresthesia, pruritus, formication, &c.

In the visceral sphere we find as symptoms of hyperæsthesia, conditions of *cynorexia* and *polydipsia* as well as of *anorexia* and *adipsia*. Special stress is laid by Beard on adipsia as a neurasthenic symptom. He considers the adipsia or hypodipsia of the Americans to be partly a cause of frequent and well developed neurasthenia, especially as compared with the Germans, for whom the copious use of beer serves as a preventive. Another marked consequence of this hyperæsthesia is a certain liking for stimulants, as coffee, tea, alcoholic beverages and tobacco. Most nervous individuals like sweets and fat, and frequently also gelatinous substances, preferring gelatinous to ordinary meat; they possess little power to resist alcohol, and are affected and even intoxicated by small doses in a striking manner, especially if in a warm place. Some of them, however, are able, under special circumstances, as, *e.g.*, after cold, fatigue, &c., to take a great amount not only for the moment, but also without any evil effects afterwards. For these, alcohol may be the best medicine in all their slight complaints, among which we have mentioned frequent colds.

Neurasthenic individuals are in their youth, as a general rule, very susceptible to sexual feeling, and have a tendency to all kinds of improper practices. Like all sensations caused by hyperæsthesia, these are not permanent, and the sexual capacity is not proportionate to the susceptibility—the best gift which nature could provide for such individuals in order to keep them from excess and its evil consequences.

As oxyæsthesia or acroæsthesia is not distinct from hyperæsthesia or anæsthesia, but represents merely the commencement of the alteration of sensibility which terminates in these conditions, it is quite natural that hypæsthesic or anæsthesic conditions should be sometimes developed where hyperæsthesia is present. Only so long as this hypæsthesia or anæsthesia is slight and temporary, is it allowable to attribute it to neurasthenia, whilst if not so, it is due to hysteria or to other grave disorders of the nervous system. The slight and temporary hypæsthesia and anæsthesia in the region of the spinal cord are comprised in the term *neurasthenia spinalis* which is almost the same as the spinal irritation of old authors. The same symptoms arising from disease in the region of the brain, and especially of the part connected with psychical functions, are produced by *neurasthenia cerebralis*, which is on the whole the same as Griesinger's cerebral irritation. Similar conditions affecting the visual organ are called *neurasthenia retinæ*, *asthenopia* or *kopiopia*; affecting the digestive organs *neurasthenia gastrica;* affecting the sexual apparatus *neurasthenia sexualis*, *nervous impotency*, &c. Here we might create quite as many forms of neurasthenia as we have seen terms ending in *phobia*, without however doing anything more than creating new names for forms long known, without making matters any clearer. *Cui bono!*

Seeing that hyperæsthesia is, so to say, nothing but the commencement of anæsthesia, in the same way hyperkinesia is the commencement of hypokinesia or akinesia. We have already mentioned that a certain uneasiness and increased restlessness may be considered as pathognomonic of neurasthenic conditions. The rapid exhaustion of the muscle is due to the readiness to contract more or less violently, however slight the stimulation may be. Besides this hyperkinesia, there occur in neurasthenic individuals spasmodic movements, and even actual convulsions, which, if exceeding a certain degree and not being merely slight and temporary, belong, we maintain, to hysteria, chorea and other related conditions.

These spasms occur most frequently in the muscles of the face and eyes, as *malleatio*, *nictitatio*, twitching of the angles of the mouth and of the lips, as nystagmus, dilatation, contraction or inequality of the pupils, and extremely slow or rapid reaction of the pupils so as to be scarcely perceptible. In addition to this, all sorts of cramps present themselves, especially in the calves, the *levatores scapulæ* and in the muscles which produce erection and ejaculation. The tendon reflexes are often very much exaggerated. Further, the like spasmodic conditions occur also in the intestinal tract, and in the circulatory and respiratory apparatus, and produce—in a less marked degree however—all the symptoms, which we find more especially in hysterical patients—globus, flatulency, constipation, and diarrhœa, palpitation and a sense of oppression and anxiety, which latter especially are due to abnormal processes in the circulatory apparatus, particularly in the heart. To these abnormal conditions of the circulatory system is due the tendency to blush which is so often observed in neurasthenic individuals, and which Beard rightly counts among the most characteristic symptoms of neurasthenia. In addition to this there is a tendency to œdema, which appears especially in the face, and on the hands and feet, and cannot be ascribed to renal disease or more grave disorders of circulation; telangiectasis, hæmorrhoids and capillary aneurism also develop, which afterwards may become very troublesome and even fatal. To the abnormal conditions in the respiratory apparatus are due the almost irrepressible fits of yawning, so frequent in neurasthenic individuals, a troublesome singultus and cough for which the most careful examination is unable to find cause, and lastly, some forms of asthma, among which Beard reckons *hay fever*, some kinds of pollen producing the asthmatic paroxysms on a soil prepared by the neurasthenia.

The hypokinesia presents itself in the first instance in a certain languor and immobility. Neuropathic individuals, if they do not happen to be excited, are very easy in their manners, they like to have much rest, stay long in bed in the morning, and lounge in the daytime on a sofa or in a comfortable arm-chair. Actual paresis is rare, and if paralysis is present, it may almost always be attributed to other more serious disorders. Among the paretic conditions must be reckoned a certain relaxation of the muscles of the larynx, in consequence of which the voice sounds very hollow, some forms of strabismus—especially *strabismus internus*—slow reaction of the pupil, which sometimes is scarcely perceptible, and, lastly, decrease or even absence of the tendon reflexes.

In the secretory and trophic sphere the reaction is similar to that in the motor sphere. To the hyperkinesia correspond hyperecrisis and hypertrophy, which are indicated by increased diuresis and diaphoresis, salivation and steatosis, as well as by an increased nutrition and an increased production of heat. To the hyperkinesia correspond hypuresis, hyphidrosis, hyposialosis, hyposteatosis, a faulty nutrition, although perhaps tending to produce obesity, and a decreased production of heat. Neurasthenic patients, therefore, readily complain of a troublesome sense of heat or cold, and, in fact, they often have their heads very hot, or hot hands and feet, and *vice versâ*; they also frequently suffer from shivering and horripilatio, not only at a low temperature, but sometimes when the sun of July or August shines upon them, and have often a feverish attack; which occasionally, when accompanied by more severe nervous symptoms, may develop to such a height, that it seems to be the commencement of typhus, pneumonia or meningitis, but it mostly disappears again as suddenly as it came.

The secretion of *urine* is very changeable; in one and the same individual there may exist, other circumstances being equal, sometimes hyperuresis, and at other times hypuresis; sometimes more phosphates and carbonates, sometimes more urates are secreted. Generally the urine is rich with substances reducing salts of copper (*kreatinin*, Schwanert) and may be mistaken for *diabetes mellitus*, especially as a number of symptoms, such as a sense of weakness and actual debility, comparative impotency and an increased sense of thirst, seem to assist the latter diagnosis. Undoubtedly secretion of sugar occurs, which is sometimes more and sometimes less marked, and may cease for some time, thus representing a kind of intermittent melituria, sometimes observed to be precursory to an attack of actual diabetes mellitus, which often breaks out suddenly and unexpectedly after catching cold or after getting wet. According to Beard, oxalates are also abundant in the urine of neurasthenic patients; it often emits, when fresh, a most disagreeable odour caused by some very volatile substances, with a goat-like smell when concentrated and rich with urates, and not quite so strong, but nauseous when more dilute, and containing phosphates and carbonates. The smell, especially in the latter case soon disappears, and this may be the cause that it has not yet been sufficiently observed. Bouchut says that the urine of neurasthenic patients represents *diabetes insipidus* and is without smell. On the contrary, the smell is sometimes so strong as to cause vomiting.

The secretion of *sweat* is very much increased in neurasthenic individuals, especially on the extremities, so that perspiring, and in consequence, damp, cold hands and feet are of common occurrence.

But the reverse also, as we mentioned above, may be the case, and dryness of hands and feet as well as over the whole of the body may be observed. There are neurasthenic patients who have never perspired in their lives. Not rarely the sweat carries with it foreign substances—smelling, coloured or sticky—thus representing the products of parhidrosis, osmidrosis, and bromhidrosis.

Neurasthenia is said to occur frequently in well-fed or even robust individuals. Beard, however, when giving the differential diagnosis between neurasthenia and hysteria says: "Neurasthenia is always associated with physical debility. Hysteria, in the mental or physical form, occurs in those who are in perfect physical health," but in another place he says of a neurasthenic patient: "The man was tall, vigorous, full-faced, and physically and mentally capable of endurance" (pp. 104 and 30). In fact, therefore, he admits the statement made above, but his other view is the correct one. Nothing but a total misunderstanding of what good nutrition and a robust constitution are, could lead any one to assume that neurasthenia occurs in strong robust individuals.

The good nutrition, which has its source in the moderately increased excitement of the nervous system, is but apparent; it corresponds to the plethoric condition of former physicians, which for a long time is taken for health and strength, but when affected by some attack or other, proves to have not the slightest power of resistance. When the latter circumstance is the case, the good nutrition is the result of an increased or even decreased excitability of the nervous system and therefore undoubtedly indicates weakness or a kind of paralytic condition, which is the consequence of an exaggerated excitability. As hyperkinesia or hyperæsthesia is nothing but the commencement of akinesia and anæsthesia, in the same way hyperecorisia and hypertrophy are the commencement of hypeccrisia and aneccrisis, and of hypotrophy and atrophy. The premature involution which takes place in so many fresh and healthy individuals, and which has its symptoms in becoming grey or in loss of the hair, the loss of teeth, and of the sexual appetite, &c., is mainly due to this, while as the last cause must be regarded a chlorotic constitution, and hypoplasia of the blood corpuscles together with hypoplasia of the nervous system.

The symptoms of neurasthenia appear sometimes on only one side, and then in preference on the left. Beard calls this hemi-neurasthenia, but in reality it only appears because the usual condition is so much more strongly developed, that the left side is more excitable on account of its smaller power of resistance than the right. This is also the reason why anæsthesia, as well as hemianæsthesia is mostly left-sided, and why we also find hyperkinesia and hypokinesia as well as dysecorisis and dystrophy on the left side. If the secretion of sweat is abnormal, it occurs usually on the left side only. *Hemiatrophia faciei progressiva* is also usually left-sided. The hair frequently becomes sooner grey on the left than on the right side, and rarely *vice versâ*.

According to the different symptoms, which in different individuals come into the foreground, and of which we have treated above as useful for distinguishing different groups of neurasthenia, several forms have been described with reference to the *nervosismus*. Bouchut already mentions *nervosisme aigu* and *chronique*, meaning by the former the conditions of fever with all their accompanying and consequent symptoms, which so easily occur in nervous individuals, and by the latter the habitual condition of irritable weakness, which we have attempted to describe. According to the different symptoms of these conditions, he speaks of *nervosisme cérébral, spinal, cardiaque, laryngé, gastrique, utérin, séminal, cutané, spasmodique, paralytique,* and *douloureux;* of *nervosisme simple, hystérique,* and *hypochondrique;* corresponding to which modern authors have described quite as many forms of neurasthenia, like *neurasthenia cerebralis* or cerebrasthenia, *neurasthenia spinalis* or myelasthenia, *neurasthenia sexualis, gastrica,* &c., all of which are merely like the endless varieties of roses, carnations and hyacinths which we find in the price-list of nurserymen when compared with the original stock!

Neurasthenia being, partly at least, due to a faulty development of the nervous system, its form depends very much on the individual. It is essentially a congenital and mostly hereditary condition, and in cases where it appears to have been acquired its development was furthered by certain injurious influences.

Neurasthenia might be compared to chlorosis, the character of which is smallness, delicacy, and faulty development of the *vascular* system. The character of neurasthenia is smallness, delicacy, and faulty development of the *nervous* system. All chlorotic individuals are neurasthenic, and all neurasthenic individuals are chlorotic, although the chlorosis may be *rubra* and may be disguised by a healthy and robust appearance, as mentioned above.

Causes.—The development of neurasthenia is specially favoured by overwork, more particularly of a mental kind, by late hours, disappointment, grief and care, by unsatisfied ambition, exhaustion, long or severe illness, sexual excesses, frequent or profuse seminal losses, loss of blood during menstruation, confinement, lactation, &c.—that is to say, by circumstances which, on the one hand, bring about a direct wearing out of the nervous system and, on the other, injure the general nutrition by loss of blood and strength, thus also weakening the nerves. The latter influences often cause poverty of blood, olichæmia or hydræmia—Bouchut well calls it *hypoglobulie* (*i.e.*, chlorosis)—and this is the easier because the individuals in question are chloræmic, and therefore also comparatively olichæmic, to begin with. This olichæmia or hydræmia necessarily influences the nervous system. It explains also why the influences mentioned above are not dangerous when the special disposition—*i.e.*, neurasthenia, however slight—is absent, because then the nervous system and the blood-corpuscles are more highly developed, and are able to supply easily from their own strength and from the nourishment ingested the force which is used up in the wear and tear of life.

Inasmuch as neurasthenia is mainly congenital, and always associated with chlorosis, or at least with a chlorotic diathesis, it is natural that the female sex, being more sensitive, should be more subject to it. It occurs most frequently in middle life, from puberty down to the climacteric. It is rare in early age and in old age, perhaps because in the former the strength of the individual is not yet taxed, and in the latter it has ceased to be so, whilst in a full-grown individual non-fulfilment of the duties of life makes the insufficiency and weakness of the nervous system conspicuous.

Neurasthenia, being caused by or representing a constitutional anomaly, is chronic in its course, which, however, is not always uniform, but subject to many variations, the cause of which is not always clear. There is frequently a striking periodicity in its symptoms, as is mostly the case in nervous disorders caused by weakness, and is especially characteristic of those disorders which are congenital or transmitted by heredity.

Course.—It has been repeatedly mentioned before that under unfavourable circumstances graver nervous disorders may develop out of neurasthenia. It may also give rise to a number of other diseases representing their first symptom, when the disease itself cannot yet be recognised. Neurasthenia may for years precede cancer or cancerous formations and sarcoma. Gout also is often preceded by it, or rather people with a gouty diathesis are mostly neurasthenic. As such individuals have a great tendency to apoplexy (it is an open question whether or not the greater number of cases of apoplexy may not be associated with gouty conditions), neurasthenia also precedes or accompanies those morbid cerebral conditions which at last terminate in apoplexy. Thus, neurasthenia frequently appears to be only a symptom of other disorders, especially those of a constitutional character, out of which, in the seat of least resistance, certain local disorders develop. This is proved by the fact that neurasthenia is the consequence of faulty development of the vascular and nervous systems, thus representing a chloræmic and nervous constitution with faulty metabolism and a tendency to all kinds of disorders. The products of an abnormal metabolism, as an excess of urates, phosphates, and oxalates, and the strong aromatic substances found in the urine, sweat, and breath, and sometimes also ptomaines and leukomaines, serve to increase neurasthenia and to develop out of it still more serious disorders. The urates—*e.g.*, may produce gout, and in connection with it hysteria and mental disorder. The aromatic substances also may produce hysteria, hystero-epilepsy, and psychoses. If, in addition, the interstitial connective tissue is influenced in its growth, as—*e.g.*, by some dyscrasia like syphilis, alcoholism, or saturnism, so that it commences to proliferate and to become inflamed or even neoplastic, then we find the so-called organic changes of the nervous system, like myelitis, encephalitis, peri-encephalitis, and grey degeneration. The last-mentioned circumstances, however, being less frequently met with in women than in men, it follows that the latter serious disorders are much less frequently met with in women than in men.

On the other hand, even highly developed nervousness may be cured or so far improved that the individual is able to bear his condition or even that he feels quite well. Relapses, however, frequently occur as soon as the duties of life make themselves felt again or nutrition becomes deranged. It always takes a long time before the patient feels permanently well, and a strict *régime* is necessary in order to obtain this result.

Treatment.—It is easily seen that in neurasthenic conditions medicines do not do much good; they may be used as palliatives, but they will never cure the disorder. This holds good especially of the narcotics and anæsthetics, which often are used against insomnia and troublesome sensations. In addition to this there is always a danger lest the patient falls a victim to morphinism, cannabism, alcoholism, cocainism, coffeinism, &c.

Here we might mention that a perfectly healthy man rarely becomes a morphinist, cannabist, &c., but that such individuals are without exception neuropathic. In these cases cause and effect have often been confounded, and to the substances mentioned has been attributed what in reality was due to the constitution. However, we do not mean to say that those substances do not exercise any harmful influence, but the matter lies thus: in a neurasthenic individual a stimulant gives temporary relief, but leaves the neurasthenia as it is or even increases it, and afterwards the neurasthenia causes an irresistible desire for the stimulant which, while it gave relief, aggravated the disorder. Therefore the substances in question cannot be considered as the only causes of the disorders mentioned, but they form a secondary link in the vicious circle, which always in pathology plays such an important *rôle*, the primary link being the morbid constitution.

We might almost entirely dispense with the use of narcotics in the treatment of neurasthenia, especially if we want to effect something more than merely temporary improvement. We most highly recommend iron with small doses of quinine; the iron improves the condition of the blood, whilst quinine decreases the excitability of the nervous system, and it may be given in small doses of 1 to 2 gr. *per diem* for weeks without any injurious effects. It has been maintained that quinine weakens the stomach and impairs digestion, but this is probably only the case when the gastric secretion is not sufficiently acid.

After this, we recommend the nervine stimulants; as Valerian, assafœtida, and castoreum, remedies which have almost entirely gone out of use, but which, nevertheless are invaluable. Valerian, if constantly used, is an excellent remedy for the troublesome sensations, for some spasmodic conditions, and especially for insomnia. We consider tinctura assafœtidæ et castorei āā 20 to 25 min. in infusum valerianæ the most reliable remedy, giving relief in conditions of oppression and distress, and having no bad after-effects. We also recommend electricity in all its forms, as the condition of the patient requires it. General galvanisation, faradisation, and franklinisation often give results we scarcely expect.

Above all, however, we have to regulate nutrition and everything connected with it. Living in healthy surroundings is necessarily required. In vain the physician applies all his remedies if the patient lives in a place which is damp in winter and hot in summer, and which at all times is close and stuffy.

With regard to food, we recommend mixed food in moderate quantities; in some cases Mitchell-Playfair's treatment gives good results, in others vegetarianism. The latter seems to be useful when neurasthenia is a symptom of a gouty condition, the former when a symptom of hypoplasia. In cases in which neurasthenia is produced by gouty disorders—cases more frequent than usually supposed—alkaline waters must be freely used, whilst beer and wine, with the exception of light hock taken in moderate quantities, must be forbidden. The same holds good for corpulent neurasthenic patients, who, however, must never undergo an anti-fat treatment.

The patient must stay out as much as possible in the fresh air, in the woods, on the mountains, or at the seaside. For some patients, exercise, as walking, riding on horseback, and gymnastics, is beneficial, whilst others require rest in bed. The former seems to be required when there is a certain sluggish nutrition, the latter when there is an excess. In the same manner baths may be recommended; moderately cold if nutrition is to be increased, warm if it is to be decreased. Actually cold or hot baths ought not to be ordered. It is, however, evident that we may sometimes also recommend hot baths and vapour baths if the neurasthenia seems to require them. Massage has also been highly recommended, and with good reason. Carefully practised, we consider it suitable for cases of slow nutrition, whilst it may be harmful in cases of an opposite character.

Although medicines are unable to do much for neurasthenia, we cannot get on without them. In patients in whom nutrition is low, small doses of arsenic, taken for some weeks, are useful. The bromides have been recommended for conditions of troublesome excitement and insomnia. They are good, but if used for some length of time they produce derangement of nutrition, and make the patient drowsy. The same holds good of sulphonal, paraldehyde, chloral, and chloral-amide, which must be given only for a short time, and, if they are indispensable, must frequently be changed. We must keep in mind that in neurasthenics small doses have a greater effect than they have in non-neurasthenics, and that, therefore, intoxication is much more easily produced.

For the same reason, neurasthenic persons do not bear tobacco, coffee, tea, &c., so well as healthy individuals; sometimes they cannot bear it at all. According to the case, some foods and stimulants must be forbidden or given with extreme care.

Neurasthenic patients mostly suffer also from irregular digestion and costiveness. Both must be regulated, but if possible by mild means, as sour milk or butter-milk, whey, kefir, vegetables, fruit, and saline draughts; rarely, if ever, by drastic purgatives.

Lastly, we may mention the application of hypnotism and suggestion in the treatment of neurasthenia. Both have exercised, according to our experience, an undoubtedly beneficial influence on this disorder, but only for a short time. Afterwards the neurasthenic condition easily returns. Therefore we cannot, at least for the present, recommend the application of hypnotism and suggestion, with hope of permanent success. RUDOLF ARNDT.

NEURHYPNOLOGY. (*See* NEURO-HYPNOLOGY.)

NEUROBLACIA (*νεῦρον*, nerve; *βλακεία*, stupidity). A dulled state of nervine sensibility. (Fr. *névroblacie.*)

NEUROGAMIA (*νεῦρον*, a nerve; *γάμος*, marriage). A term given to "animal magnetism" because of the alleged nervous community of feeling between the magnetiser and the magnetised. (Fr. *névrogamie;* Ger. *Neurogamie.*)

NEUROHYPNOLOGY (*νεῦρον*, a nerve; *ὕπνος*, sleep; *λόγος*, speech). The name given by Braid to his theory of magnetic sleep. (*See* HYPNOTISM.)

NEUROHYPNOTISM (*νεῦρον*, a nerve; *ὕπνος*, sleep). A term for the state induced by hypnotic manipulations. (Fr. *neuro-hypnotisme.*)

NEUROMETADRASIS (*νεῦρον*, a nerve; *μετά*, with; *δρᾶσις*, efficacy). A term for animal magnetism, signifying the influence of one body upon another.

NEUROMIMESIS (*μιμέομαι*, I imitate). Mimicry of disease in nervous or hysterical persons. (Fr. *névromimosie.*)

NEUROPYRA (*νεῦρον*, a nerve; *πῦρ*, fire or fever). Nervous fever. (Fr. *fièvre nerveuse;* Ger. *Nervenfieber.*)

NEUROSES (*νεῦρον*, a nerve). Nervous diseases. A neurosis is usually described as a functional disorder of the nervous system—that is to say, a disorder such as migraine, which, so far as we know at present, is unattended with any constant organic lesion. (Fr. *névroses;* Ger. *Neurose.*)

NEUROSES, FUNCTIONAL, The Systematic Treatment of (so-called Weir Mitchell Treatment).—The treatment of functional neurosis has, until of late years, been the despair of physicians and a real "opprobium medicinæ." No one can contest this statement who will honestly reflect on his experience of such cases. Take a confirmed neurotic of many years standing, whose social position and means enable her to follow any advice she may have received, and consider what her probable history has been. Ever since her illness began she has been going from one health resort to another. She has tried Schwalbach, St. Moritz, and the Riviera; she has swallowed pints of drugs, iron, quinine, bromides, chloral, and anti-spasmodics; she has exhausted the virtues of hydropathic establishments; she is lucky if she has not also run the gauntlet of innumerable pessaries, and much uterine treatment; of late years almost certainly she has "tried a little massage," and most certainly it has failed to do good; and lastly she has had hosts of sympathetic friends, many nurses, and a whole phalanx of doctors. This is no exaggerated picture. It is a simple statement of what almost all well-to-do patients of this kind have gone through, and their last state is always worse than their first. To have systematised a scientific and rational means of dealing with such illnesses, which rarely, if ever, fails to effect a cure in well selected cases, or if not a cure, at least a great amelioration, is no slight achievement and, to my mind, constitutes one of the greatest gains to practical medicine of which the present generation can boast. This we owe to the sagacity and intimate knowledge of this form of disease possessed by Dr. Weir Mitchell, of Philadelphia, by whose name the method of systematic treatment, a brief description of which it is the object of this article to give, is now very generally known. His claim to originality with regard to it has been contested. All that need be said, in passing, on this point is, that while many have suggested and adopted individual portions of this treatment, such as the removal of unhealthy influences and the like, no one else has laid down a complete scheme by which a serious attack on the disease, on rational principles, is carried out, and to him alone this merit is due.

Before describing in detail the method to be adopted, it would be very desirable to study the forms of functional neurosis for which it is adapted; for success depends quite as much on the proper selection of cases, as on the intelligent and sufficient carrying out of the treatment itself. Nor is a word of warning on this point unnecessary. The remarkable results which have often followed the application of this method in proper cases has not unnaturally attracted a good deal of attention, and many have been tempted to try it without sufficient study of the subject, and they have used it in altogether unsuitable cases, with the natural result of failure and disappointment, which have cast discredit, and very unfairly, on the treatment itself. It will be advisable, therefore, to state briefly the kind of case in which alone it should be used, but this the limits of space will oblige us to do in the baldest and briefest way. To describe the course and symptoms of the functional neuroses concerned would require a volume in itself, a volume much needed, since we are satisfied that there is no department of medicine so little understood, and so much requiring study. We shall content ourselves with enumerating some of the more prominent classes of neuroses for which this treatment is adapted, without any attempt at classification, adding a few observations as to the cases in which it should not be tried, but in which, we are sorry to say, from want of sufficient caution, we have often seen it used.

(1) **Nervous Exhaustion or Neurasthenia.**—The form of disease in which it answers best is, in our experience, that species of general nervous breakdown which constitutes a very real and very important malady, the existence of which, however, has only been recognised of late years, and which we have not seen sufficiently recognised in any of our medical text-books. We are sadly in want of a name for it. By some it is called "nervous exhaustion," by others, "neurasthenia," and both these names have been objected to because of their associations, and not unreasonably. Yet no better ones have been proposed, and they seem to us to describe what we believe to be the real, essential nature of the illness better than any other designation we have seen suggested. It is often called "hysteria," a word associated with fanciful and imaginative illness, no doubt often complicating this condition, but, on the other hand, often entirely distinct from it. In our experience many of these cases occur in clever, emotional and excitable, but not fanciful, women, who would give all they possess to be well, and heartily long for good health if they only knew how to obtain it. A condition such as this, in such women, is as far removed as possible from the state that is known to us as "hysterical." In a large proportion of these cases the origin of the illness can be directly traced to some shock or over-strain affecting the nervous system. Amongst the most common of the former are the death of some near relative, money losses, disappointments in love affairs, and the like; of the latter, overwork in the modern system of high-class education in girls, whose physical health is unfitted for the efforts they are unwisely encouraged to make. The disease is not, as a rule, suddenly established, but is the gradual outcome of deteriorated health. No one symptom can be mentioned as distinctive, but the result is a state of continuous inability for any exertion, and a constant feeling of weariness and fatigue on the slightest effort, until at last all effort is given up, and the patient's life is practically passed on the sofa or invalid chair. The appetite gradually fails and little or no food is taken, and dyspepsia, with its train of evils, such as flatulence, constipation, and so on, is constant; emaciation, more or less marked, is very general, and sometimes it is excessive. On the other hand, there is a comparatively rare but well-marked type of this class of disease in which, while the muscles are wasted and flabby, there is an abnormal development of unwholesome subcutaneous fat, the whole appearance being of great obesity. We have observed in cases of this kind that the fat is deposited in masses in particular parts, such as near the joints or on the outside of the thighs, and that its distribution is irregular.

Marked evidence of mal-nutrition is to be found in the urine, which is generally pale in colour, containing abundance of phosphates, sometimes a trace of albumen, with an amount of urea always markedly below the average. Other indications of nervous disturbance besides those mentioned are frequently met with, but are too variable to be described; amongst the most common are severe headaches, sleeplessness, vaso-motor disturbance of many kinds, such as palpitations, irregularities of the pulse, flushings, cutaneous erythematous patches of a transient character. Emotional and mental phenomena are pretty sure to become developed in long-standing cases of this type, and although, as we have said, many cases are not "hysterical" in the ordinary acceptation of the word, unquestionably few protracted cases can escape some moral conditions which may fairly be so classed. There is generally some devoted and over-sympathetic mother or sister, husband or nurse, in the background, and eventually the constant watching of symptoms, the incessant trial of all sorts of cures and drugs, have produced a mental condition that is most unwholesome. The fact, however, must be insisted on that at the bottom of all this is a condition of real disease, and so far as our present knowledge goes, the author believes that this disease is in reality one of defective nerve-power, on which the other phenomena mentioned have become engrafted.

(2) **Hysteria.**—The second class of case may more properly be termed "hysterical," and it includes a vast number of neurotic conditions impossible to classify.

One of the most common, and one which most readily and certainly answers to treatment, is that form of neurosis which has been called "hysterical apepsia." Generally it begins with ordinary dyspeptic symptoms, leading to pain and discomfort after eating. To avoid this, one article of food after another is dropped, until at last scarcely any food at all is taken. It is quite astonishing to see how patients of this kind can exist on the almost starvation diet to which they have accustomed themselves. The emaciation in old-standing cases is so excessive that all the sub-cutaneous fat is absorbed, and the patient assumes a wizened and strange appearance, which is highly distinctive and most remarkable. One peculiar feature of these cases is very characteristic of the nervous origin of the disease, and that is a strange unrest, if it may be so described. The patient will not keep still. She takes long prostrating walks, and other forms of muscular exercise, for which her wasted body is quite unfit. It is only in the worst cases, when the strength has absolutely broken down, that patients of this class get bedridden and completely laid by.

Other types of neuroses are more or less distinctly mimetic, and are apt to be confounded with organic disease. These assume such protean and varied forms that any enumeration of them is impossible, and yet they are probably the most important of all, since in them the difficulties of diagnosis are often immense; and yet it is in these forms of nervous disease that accurate diagnosis is most important, for if the mistake is made of treating organic disease as functional, not only is failure certain, but real injury to the patient may follow. It is in cases more or less simulating disease of the central nervous system that such difficulties are most apt to occur. Such are, among others, various forms of paresis, often closely simulating sclerosis; hysterical paralysis; hysterical locomotor ataxy; various spasmodic and convulsive conditions, chorea, and the like. In some cases of this type accurate diagnosis may be said to be impossible; in all a most careful examination, and a full knowledge of the most advanced neurology is necessary. Moreover, in certain old-standing cases, originally purely functional, eventually certain obscure and little understood changes in the nerve centres may become established, which render complete cure impossible, although judicious treatment may effect great amelioration. Still it is in bad cases of this type that the most successful and brilliant cures are often effected. This class, moreover, includes simulated diseases of many other organs besides those of the central nervous system: thus we may have the most intense neurotic vomiting; or again cardiac affections, such as pseudo-angina, or palpitations; or some simulated chest disease, such as asthma, or spasmodic cough. None of these, however, present the same difficulties in diagnosis as those already alluded to, and all of them are amenable to treatment when properly conducted.

(3) **Narcosis.**—Another class of case, which may fairly be called neurotic, is according to the writer's experience, better treated in this than in any other way, and that is the acquired habit of taking narcotic drugs, such as chloral or morphia, or alcohol in excess. In a large proportion of the functional neuroses already alluded to the patients had insensibly fallen into the practice of consuming large quantities of narcotics, which had originally been prescribed for the relief of symptoms, but which had gradually been taken in increasing doses until the habit had been fully established. The comparative facility with which this pernicious custom was abandoned, when the patient was under treatment, as the nutrition improved, and health and strength were gained, was very striking. The author has since treated many cases in which the habit was not merely incidental to a functional neurosis, but in which it alone was the cause of ill health, and for the express purpose of breaking it off. The result has been nearly uniformly successful, and it has been obtained at the cost of far less physical and mental suffering than is possible under any other way of dealing with these unfortunate cases. This is doubtless due in part to the complete control which the isolation of such cases under a thoroughly competent nurse gives the practitioner, but largely also to the regular habits, the full occupation of the

patient's time, and above all to the rapid improvement of the nutrition under treatment, which enable the patient to resist the craving for narcotics or stimulants in a way which is quite impossible under any other conditions. In some of the author's cases the amount of narcotics taken for a lengthy period has been quite enormous, and yet the habit has been completely abandoned in a few weeks, with comparatively little suffering, and has not, as a rule, been again resumed.

(4) **Mental Disease.**—It is important to lay stress on the fact that there are certain forms of neurotic disease in which this systematic treatment should not be attempted. This is a point of real importance, for the striking success which has followed treatment in suitable cases has led, far too frequently of late, to its being heedlessly tried in cases in which it is practically certain to fail, and thus a really good thing comes to be discredited.

One form of nervous case in which this, like everything else, is sure to be unsuccessful, is that of the comfortable, well-feeding, well-nourished, and thoroughly selfish, nervous patient, to whom her illnesses are sources of enjoyment, and who has neither the wish nor the intention of being bettered. Cases of this kind are not rare, and the wise physician will leave them alone.

This treatment is often unfortunately tried in cases of real mental disease, especially in chronic melancholia. The relatives and friends of such patients are often, and very naturally, exceedingly desirous of shirking the real facts, and will do anything rather than admit that the patient is insane. The term "hysterical" is a very convenient cloak in cases of this kind for masking the truth, and strong pressure is often brought to bear on the medical man to treat cases on this assumption. No doubt there are some few cases in which the diagnosis is uncertain, and in which the treatment may do good. There are patients who, being predisposed to insanity, are, from defective nutrition, some temporary shock, and the like, walking along the edge of a precipice, as it were. On the one side is mental disease, on the other health. It is conceivable that, under the improved nutrition resulting from systematic treatment, the patient may be drawn away from the precipice along which she is walking, in the direction of health; on the other hand, however, it is quite as likely that the isolation, &c., may precipitate her over it, sooner than would otherwise have been the case. We have seen both results occur, and we know no class of case requiring more care in selection. If there is any decided symptom of insanity, such as marked religious delusions, suicidal impulses, and the like, then we hold the rule to be absolute that this treatment is positively contra-indicated. We have cases constantly brought to us for treatment under such conditions. More than once we have been persuaded to try treatment against our own better judgment, and we have never done so without regretting it. In one sense, most well-marked neurotic cases are closely allied to cases of mental disease. For example, it is quite common to meet with cases admirably adapted for systematic treatment, where the family history clearly shows an hereditary disposition to insanity. We have even seen cases quite cured by treatment, who subsequently became insane; and the more we see of such cases, the more convinced we are that the rule we have laid down should be strictly adhered to.

The rationale of systematic treatment is abundantly simple, and it is well that this should be thoroughly understood. There is nothing mysterious or complex about it; it is nothing more or less than a rapid means of putting the patient into good physical condition, of raising her health from the low level into which it has fallen to the highest level which is possible in the individual case. And, coincident with good physical health, we hope for the disappearance of the functional neurosis which in most cases is incompatible with perfect health. The rank weeds of neurotic disease will only grow and flourish in suitable soil—that is, in a state of depressed vitality; improve the soil, and the unhealthy growth will disappear. That this can be done through the chemist's shop, the health resort, or the injudicious tending of unwise friends, all experience shows is an impossibility; these, as a rule, only make the patient go from bad to worse. Get rid of all these, put the patient under thorough physical and moral training, such as systematic treatment enables us to do, and it is surprising how rapidly her whole being seems to alter, how the confirmed invalid may be changed into the strong and healthy woman, and how all her acquired neuroses vanish.

The chief elements of systematic treatment are:

(1) **Removal** of the patient from her usual surroundings, and putting her completely at rest, under the care of a suitable nurse.

(2) **Massage**, combined generally with the use of **electricity**, as a means of pro-

ducing tissue waste, and enabling the patient to consume large quantities of food.

(3) **Over-feeding**, as a means of rapidly increasing nutrition.

Each of these will require separate consideration.

(1) **Removal**.—Isolation is generally found to be the great obstacle on the part of the friends to the adoption of this treatment, and strong pressure is invariably brought to bear on the medical attendant to secure some modification of this most unpleasant necessity, a pressure to which unfortunately he too often yields, and thus ruins the success of his treatment. It is impossible to speak too emphatically on this point. Increasing experience convinces the author that any compromise in this respect will assuredly prove disastrous. No doubt the difficulty of securing it is often great. In London and other large cities there are an abundance of medical homes where it is easy enough to place patients, but in the country and in small towns these are not to be had. On this account the attempt is often made to isolate the patient in her own house, under the belief that she can thus be separated from her friends and relatives, a belief that will certainly mislead. Even if they can be persuaded really to remain away, which is almost impossible, their vicinity is known, there is an incessant passing of messages and notes, and a fret, which is entirely avoided if the absolute removal of the patient is secured. Still more fatal is the concession often made of the occasional visit of a relative or friend. The medical man will almost certainly be told that this plan of complete removal from the usual domestic surroundings is admirable for Mrs. Brown, Jones, or Robinson, but that this particular patient is so sensitive, so deeply attached to her mother or sisters, that it is an absolute impossibility in her case, and that they will readily submit to everything proposed but this, and that, therefore, they must be allowed to visit her as before. All that need be said on this point is, that if the medical man who proposes to carry out systematic treatment cannot resist pressure such as this, he is quite unfit to treat the case at all, and had much better not make the attempt.

When the writer first began to treat these cases he placed them in lodgings with a nurse. This he never does now, much preferring that they should be in a medical home. In the first place, they are there spared the trouble and worry of housekeeping, which is incompatible with perfect rest of body and mind, and, what is of more importance still, they are not placed absolutely at the mercy of the nurse, but are, in some degree, also under the supervision of the manager of the home, who can report on their general progress. This is a matter of great importance, since it places a check on the nurse, and enables the medical attendant to judge if she and the patient get on well together.

The selection of a suitable nurse is of primary consequence, and a good nurse for neurotic patients is a *rara avis* indeed. As a matter of fact, nine nurses out of ten, however large their experience and thorough their training, are quite unable to manage these cases properly. The majority err by supposing that they must rule the patients, and endeavour to do so by a harsh assumption of authority which is sure to fail in its object; or if they do not do this, they fall into the opposite error of being over-sympathetic and yielding. What is wanted is tact, kindness, common-sense, and firmness, a combination of qualities which, it is needless to say, is not easily found. One practical rule should be borne in mind, and that is, that when a case is not doing well, when the patient is fretting and dislikes her attendant, an immediate change should be made. The nurse is there for the good of the patient, not for her own advantage, and the fear of hurting her feelings should never stand in the way of the patient's welfare. It is always advisable that the nurse should be, if possible, a person of some culture and education. She is shut up for many weeks with the patient, whom she must be able to read to and otherwise amuse. To condemn a cultivated lady to a lengthy and intimate intercourse with a coarse, vulgar, and illiterate woman would not only be a positive cruelty, but would certainly defeat the object desired.

Combined with isolation, the patient is placed absolutely at rest in bed, and is practically kept there during the whole treatment. In some severe cases it is advisable that the rest should be so absolute that no physical exertion of any kind should be allowed, and the patient is not permitted to leave her bed to pass her evacuations, nor should she wash herself, nor use any other form of physical exertion. It will presently be seen how complete repose is associated with extreme tissue-waste produced by massage, a process so fatiguing that it could not possibly be borne, unless all voluntary effort both of body and mind is avoided. It is not until the fifth or sixth week of treatment, when the physical powers are resteered, that the patient is allowed to sit up for an hour or two, and shortly afterwards she may go out for a short walk or drive, until gradually healthy habits of life are resumed.

(2) **Massage.**—Combined with rest and isolation, a process of massage is commenced on the second or third day. Now, with regard to this it is necessary to make some observations. This is in itself a new therapeutic agent; it strikes the imagination, and, in spite of all that the writer and others have said about it, both the public and the profession have insisted on looking upon it as the main factor in this method of treatment, which is called by many "massage treatment," or some other term indicating that this is the essence of the cure. Accordingly, many who have not taken the trouble to study the matter have thought that if they only order their patients to undergo some amount of massage, all is done that is essentially necessary, and they believe that they are carrying out this treatment. The result is necessarily failure and disappointment, and a really good therapeutic agent is discredited and looked upon with suspicion. When the writer first began to treat cases in this way, there was no such thing as a masseuse to be had; now they exist by hundreds. Schools for massage have been established, whence numbers of perfectly useless operators are turned out after a short perfunctory training; every nursing institute professes to supply them; works on massage have been published, which render a perfectly simple matter obscure; and, in fact, the author believes he was quite justified in stating, as he has done elsewhere, that massage has become the prevailing medical folly of the day. Against such a state of things it is necessary to protest. In the view of the writer, massage, properly applied in suitable cases, is an invaluable remedy, which may perhaps best be called a mechanical tonic. It works all the muscles passively, without effort on the part of the patient, and thus enables her to consume the large amount of food which it is necessary to assimilate. In this there is nothing mysterious. It is simply a remedy, just as cod-liver oil or quinine are remedies, and a remedy of a strictly scientific and common-sense character. As to the details and method of applying it, the writer deems it quite unnecessary to say anything. A very short experience is necessary to enable the practitioner to judge whether it is being properly done or not. It is quite needless for him to be acquainted with the technique of the process. The simple rule is, that if in a week or ten days the patient is unable to assimilate with ease all the food that is given to her, then assuredly the massage is ineffective, and the operator should at once be changed. In the author's experience not one woman in a dozen who professes to be a "masseuse" is of any use at all. At first not more than a quarter of an hour to twenty minutes' massage is given twice daily; then the time is gradually increased, until an hour to an hour and a half is given, also twice in the day, and by the time this amount is reached the patient should be taking the full amount of food prescribed. During the process she is freely lubricated with oil, and when each rubbing is over she is left to lie in the blanket for an hour's absolute rest, the room being darkened, and complete repose enjoined. In very feeble and delicate patients it may be necessary to proceed more slowly, and then the full rubbing will not be reached for perhaps a week or ten days longer. At the end of the treatment, when the patient leaves her bed, the afternoon rubbing is omitted, and then by degrees the massage is stopped altogether.

Combined with the massage in most cases electricity is used as a subsidiary means of exercising the muscles. It is generally given by the masseuse for about twenty minutes to half an hour, twice daily. The interrupted current is used, and the rheophores, well wetted, are placed on the principal muscles of the upper and lower extremities, the back, thorax, and abdomen, at a distance of about four inches from each other, until the muscles are thoroughly contracted. It requires a good deal of skill and practice to use this so as not to pain the patient needlessly. The electricity is not commenced, as a rule, until the patient has been about a fortnight under treatment, and should she object to it strongly, or appear to suffer much pain, it should certainly be discontinued. It appears to be of very secondary importance to the massage, and the author very frequently treats cases without using it at all.

(3) **Feeding.**—The very essence of this method of cure is the dietary, the object of which is to improve the nutrition of the patient, and place her in a condition of perfect physical health. The other modes of treatment adopted are all subsidiary to this. It is quite surprising to witness the facility with which a patient who for years has been subsisting on an almost starvation diet, who has suffered from every possible form of dyspeptic derangement, and who has loathed the very name of food, can, in nine cases out of ten, be got, under rest and effective massage, to take, in a week or ten days, an amount of food which

is quite incredible to those who have not seen it, and not only to take it without repugnance, but perfectly to digest and assimilate it. It is well from the first for the nurse to feed the patient, and she commences by administering about three ounces of fresh milk every third hour. In a day or so this is increased to five, and then to ten ounces, at the same interval. By this time the patient is getting from a quarter to half an hour's massage twice daily, and then the administration of solid food is commenced. At first some breakfast is given, then a fish dinner, afterwards a finely divided chop; and so, by degrees, the full diet is arrived at. When a case is doing well, in about ten days the full amount of three hours' massage is given, and with it the full diet. A careful record should be kept by the nurse, in a book provided for the purpose, of all that the patient takes, and with it a journal of her general progress, such as her sleep, the action of the bowels, and the like. The following may be taken as a fair sample of the dietary consumed. Breakfast: a plate of porridge and a gill of cream, fish or bacon, toast, with cocoa, or café au lait; 11 A.M., a cup of beef-tea, with two teaspoonfuls of beef peptonoids; luncheon, 1.30 P.M., fish, cutlets, or joint, with a sweet, such as stewed fruit, or a milky pudding; 5 P.M., beef-tea and peptonoids, as at 11; dinner at 7, soup or fish, joint or poultry, and sweet. In addition, not less than 80 ounces of milk is given in twenty-four hours; 10 ounces—that is, a full tumbler—every third hour. It is not uncommon for this amount to be exceeded, and patients often take as much as 100 or 110 ounces. It is very rare to find any inconvenience follow this apparently enormous dietary. Every now and again a patient may become bilious, or may even vomit, when solid food should be stopped for twenty-four hours, after which it is resumed. As a rule, however, all this is taken easily; and it coincides with a rapid gain in flesh and strength. In an emaciated case a patient may at first gain 5 or 6lbs. in weight per week, afterwards 2½lbs. is a fair average gain. It is quite common to see cases which gain 15 to 30lbs. in the course of six weeks, and it is to be observed that this is not a gain of fat, but of good substantial flesh, the muscles previously wasted becoming firm and resistant, while the pallor of the skin disappears, and a good ruddy glow of health takes the place of the anæmic, sallow look of the patient. The change in the appearance of many of these cases at the end of a course of treatment must be seen to be believed. It is no exaggeration to say that they are often hardly recognisable as the same persons. Coincident with the gain in flesh and strength is often to be noticed a change for the better in all ways; the bowels, before so obstinately confined, act regularly and without drugs; sleep becomes good, sedatives being no longer required; and gradually the invalid habits of years are dropped. These results of course are not invariable. It is needless to say that practical difficulties are often met with, which can only be dealt with by experience and tact, but it is very rarely that they cannot be overcome; one may almost say never, provided only that the case has been well selected.

The best test of progress is the gain in weight, and therefore the patient should be weighed every fortnight. Unless at least 2lbs. per week is being gained the case cannot be considered to be doing well; and this is often largely exceeded.

In that type of neurotic disease, previously alluded to, in which the patient is abnormally fat, another form of management is required. It is no use commencing to massage and feed cases of this kind at once. Some means must first be adopted to clear the tissues of the unwholesome fats with which they are loaded. This is a tedious and a trying process, but the results are generally eminently satisfactory. For this purpose the patient is put to bed and completely at rest; and at first she is placed on a diet consisting of two quarts of skimmed milk daily, given in small quantities every two hours. After this amount has been taken for a day or two, it is gradually lessened until not more than a pint a day is consumed. Under absolute rest, and the absence of any muscular exertion, this apparently starvation diet does not cause any discomfort or inconvenience. Of course it is necessary to watch the patient closely to see that no ill effects follow. If there should be any appearance of undue weakness, some beef-tea or good soup should be temporarily substituted for the milk. After the amount of milk has been reduced to a minimum, the weight will gradually lessen at the rate of half a pound a day, and the fat with which the tissues are loaded will rapidly disappear. The length of time the patient may safely be treated in this way will, of course, vary according to circumstances; and it is essential that she should be weighed daily.

Probably from three to four weeks will be about the outside time that this process should be employed, and from fourteen to twenty pounds taken off the weight. When this has been done, pure milk may be substituted for skim milk, and the treatment conducted from this point precisely as in the case of an originally emaciated patient. The writer has now treated many fat, anæmic, neurotic patients in this way, and the results have been extremely satisfactory. He has never met with any serious trouble from it, nor has he found the patients rebel against what would seem to be a very trying *régime*. As a matter of fact, they are all without appetite to start with, and little complaint is made, nor does much discomfort appear to be experienced.

Nothing has been said as to the use of drugs. The writer generally prescribes some ferruginous tonic, such as Blaud's pills, or a mixture containing dialysed iron and arsenic; and some form of aperient is usually required at first, although the bowels almost invariably soon take on a healthy action, however constipated they may have previously been. As a matter of fact medicines are so entirely secondary in importance to improved nutrition, that they may very generally be dispensed with altogether.

Something must be said as to the moral management of these cases. It is obvious that a good deal must depend on the medical man's aptitude in dealing with the multiform peculiarities of patients of this class. Just as a nurse of great experience may be found quite unfit for managing patients of this type, so it is with doctors. The necessary combination of tact, knowledge of human nature, patience, and temper, are qualities not possessed by all, and not easily acquired. Difficulties are to be met, not by bullying, nor by weak yielding to the fancies of a sick person, but by firm kindness, and by showing that the practitioner has the superior will which intends to have its own way. If he cannot succeed in impressing this fact on his patient, and at the same time in securing her regard and esteem, it is to be feared that she may gain the upper hand, and the case may be a failure. How this is to be done it is not easy to teach in a short article. Perhaps it may be said of the doctor who is suited to cure such cases—that, like the poet, "nascitur non fit."

Finally, whenever it is practicable, after the treatment is concluded, the patient should be sent away with her nurse for an after-cure, in the way of travel by sea or land. It is of the utmost importance that the gain should be perpetuated, and if she returns at once to all her old habits and ways of life, the danger of relapse is naturally much increased.

W. S. Playfair.

NEUROSTHENIA (νεῦρον, a nerve; σθένος, strength). Great nervous power or excitement. (Fr. *névrosthénie*.)

NEUROTIC (νεῦρον, a nerve; ικος, terminal). Of or belonging to nerves. Used also as an adjective to describe a temperament characterised by hypersensibility to subjective and objective impressions. (Fr. *névrotique*.)

NEUROTIC INHERITANCE.—An inherited tendency to nervous diseases and to exalted nervous sensibility.

NEW SOUTH WALES, THE INSANE IN. (*See* Australia.)

NIGHTMARE.—A troubled dream with sense of oppression and great anxiety. (Fr. *cauchemar*; Ger. *Alpdrücken*, imp-pressure.)

NIGHT TERRORS.—An affection of children akin to nightmare. An hour or two after onset of sleep, the child affected suddenly screams out and wakes in a great fright, not at first recognising its surroundings or nurse. The child often has difficulty in getting to sleep again, the fright passing off gradually. As a rule there is no recurrence the same night, but there usually is on succeeding nights. (*See* Developmental Insanities.)

NOASTHENIA (νόος, mind; ἀσθένεια, debility). Mental debility. (Fr. *noasthénie*.)

NOCAR (νῶκαρ, drowsiness.) Heaviness, lethargy.

NOCARODES (νῶκαρ, drowsiness; ωδης, terminal). Lethargic.

NOCTAMBULATION (*nox*, night; *ambulo*, I walk). Literally night-walking, but from the association of night with sleep, sleep-walking. (Fr. *noctambulation*; Ger. *Nachtwandeln*.)

NOCTAMBULISMUS. Noctambulation (*q.v.*)

NOCTAMBULUS (*nox*, night; *ambulo*, I walk). One who walks during sleep.

NOCTISURGIUM (*nox*, night; *surgo*, I arise). Sleep-walking.

NOCTURNAL CRISES.—The name given to the nightly exacerbation of symptoms sometimes observed in the insane. There seems to be an exaggeration of, or alteration in, the nightly cyclic changes common to every individual, which in health produce sleep, but in the insane produce sometimes, increased violence and other symptoms. No doubt the altered surroundings of the patient at night, the seclusion and the quietude, account for much of the change in the patient's condition, but probably it is partly due, as already mentioned, to a perversion of a natural phenomenon common to every one. (*See* Bevan Lewis's "Mental Diseases.")

NOCTURNAL VERTIGO.—The sudden sensation of falling from a height sometimes experienced just after going to sleep. Akin to nightmare.

NOËMA (*νοέω*, I think). A thought. (Fr. *pensée*; Ger. *Gedanke*.)

NOËSIS (*νόησις*, thought). Reflection, thought.

NOMENCLATURE. (*See* CLASSIFICATION.)

NON COMPOS MENTIS.—A medico-legal term, meaning unsoundness of mind. Under this term, Coke included: (1) Idiota. (2) Acquired weakness. (3) A lunatic who has lucid intervals is non compos mentis so long as he has not his understanding. (4) One who deprives himself of his understanding, as the drunkard. Plural—Non compotes.

NON-RESTRAINT. (*See* TREATMENT.)

NOÖLOGIA (*νόος*, mind; *λόγος*, a discourse). Noölogy, the doctrine of mind. (Fr. *noölogie*; Ger. *Verstandeslehre*.)

NOÖSPHALES (*νόος*, mind; *σφάλλομαι*, I am deceived). An adjective applied to one disordered mentally. (Ger. *verrückt*.)

NOÖSTERESIS (*νόος*, mind; *στέρησις*, deprivation). Loss of intellect. Dementia. (Fr. *noöstérèse*; Ger. *Verstandesberaubung*.)

NORWAY, INSANE IN. (*See* SCANDINAVIA.)

NOSOMANIA (*νόσος*, malady; *μανία*, madness). A form of monomania, in which the patient suffers mentally from an imaginary bodily disease. Allied to hypochondriasis. (Fr. *nosomanie*.)

NOSOPHOBIA (*νόσος*, malady; *φόβος*, fear). A form of monomania in which, through fear of a malady from which the patient is not really suffering, he adopts most stringent precautions, and undergoes dieting and medical treatment quite unnecessarily. For example, some individuals diminish their food and become anæmic and dyspeptic through fear of apoplexy. (Fr. *nosophobie*.)

NOSTALGIA.—There is a kind of melancholia which ætiologically has been called nostalgic melancholia, or nostalgia. We do not intend to speak of this form of disease only; we shall consider nostalgia from a more general standpoint.

Definition.—Under nostalgia we must understand the abnormally exaggerated longing for his home of a man who lives away from it, whether it be that relatives or friends who were left behind, or the peculiarity of the home as regards landscape or climate, are the object of his longing. This longing often does not come into the circle of full consciousness. Nostalgia always represents a combination of psychical and bodily disturbances, and for this reason it must always be defined as disease, and may become the object of medical treatment.

We must be careful to find out whether the alteration in the patient's feelings is in a strict sense the primary cause. In that case we can effect the cure only by sending the patient back to his own home. But if in becoming accustomed to other surroundings, another sphere of activity, and a different climate and food, a fever with gastric disturbances comes on, which may be observed in most men who become acclimatised, and which is followed by a melancholy depression of nostalgic character, then a cure is possible without sending the patient home. We have to take care not to confound nostalgia with disappointment, and moroseness, produced by bad temper and discontent with the temporary position abroad. This point in the differential diagnosis is of great importance.

Conditions and Symptoms.—It is not every one who resides abroad that is attacked by nostalgia; there are no general rules for its occurrence in the different sexes, ages, and temperaments. Most people will probably never suffer from nostalgia, whilst many are attacked by it each time they leave home. Some nations who inhabit mountainous countries, as the Swiss, the inhabitants of the Tyrol and others, are said to have a great tendency to nostalgia, and this especially out of love for the landscape of their native country. The nostalgia of the rural population is peculiar, and their want of education is of great importance in considering it, as it is a predisposing cause. Nostalgia also occurs more frequently in young persons than in old. Epidemic nostalgia has been observed in soldiers, and prisoners of war, and in troops sent to distant colonies. Homer has sung about the nostalgia of Ulysses, and Goethe has created in his Mignon an immortal representation of home-sickness. In animals, also, phenomena are said to occur which are similar to nostalgia. Dogs, for example, refuse to take food in the house of a new master, begin to sicken, become weak and languid, and pine away.

Compulsory absence from home has great influence in causing nostalgia, as in the case of prisoners, or of servants who have undertaken to stay a certain time abroad, and are prohibited by their contract from returning when they wish; such persons are more liable to nostalgia than those who are at liberty to do what they like. The most important bodily symptoms of nostalgia are loss of appetite (which may increase to the refusal of food) disturbances of digestion, and emaciation. In this condition phthisis sometimes develops itself. Besides this, sleeplessness, congestion of the brain, and acceleration of pulse have been observed. Among the psychical disturbances, that alteration of the feelings which appears in the form of pure melancholia is of greatest importance, indicating mental distress with a desire to commit suicide. Frequently, and in cases of longer duration, we find also hallucinations and illusions.

It is an exceedingly important point, not yet sufficiently appreciated, to consider nostalgia from a *forensic* point of view, because it is an abnormal state of mind which suspends the free determination of will in an individual, and because it is apt to cause certain acts and crimes which bear the character of impulsive actions. Very frequently, nostalgia, especially if it originates from the pressure of unalterable and involuntary conditions, is the motive to incendiarism, infanticide, and suicide. Nostalgia may easily end in impulsive actions, if it assume a form of mental affection involving anger or rage against those persons who are thought to be the cause of suffering. The impulsive action then bears the character of an act of vengeance. We ourselves have observed a case where a servant attacked by home sickness, and repeatedly hindered by her mistress from leaving the service and returning home, threw a child of her mistress into the water and drowned it. It was an act of vengeance committed in an emotional condition, but under the influence of a deranged mind. Cases like this have to be very cautiously judged *in foro*, and the limit between genuine nostalgia and mere ill-will has especially to be strictly defined.

ALBRECHT ERLENMEYER.

NOSTOMANIA (*νοστέω*, I return; *μανία*, madness). The longing for home so morbidly intense that it has become a monomania. (Fr. and Ger. *nostomanie.*) (*See* NOSTALGIA.)

NOSTRASIA, NOSTRASSIA (*nostras*, of our country). Similar to nostalgia.

NOTENCEPHALUS (*νῶτος*, back; *ἐγκέφαλος*, brain). A deformity of the skull in which the brain protrudes behind and lies over the upper part of the neck. (Fr. *notencéphale.*)

NULLITY OF MARRIAGE. (*See* MARRIAGE, THE PLEA OF NULLITY OF, ON THE GROUNDS OF INSANITY.)

NURSING; or, TRAINING SCHOOLS FOR NURSES.—The history of nursing in hospitals holds a large place in that of modern hospital reform. The present era of scientific hospital construction had its forerunners in the little pavilion hospital at Plymouth, and in the advanced views advocated by M. Tenon in France, and Dr. Jones in America, more than a century ago.

One of the marvels of our time is the great reform in the nursing of the sick. It is marvellous also that so good a thing, and one so eagerly accepted, should have waited so long for the world to be shown its need. But it is a woman's work, and it waited for the woman and for the time when her inspiration and faith could have their way. The reform of Miss Florence Nightingale has placed in the hands of the physician a new order of instruments, intelligent and thinking, that teach their users, and that give a new embodiment to the spirit of humanity.

But the work of Miss Nightingale also had its forerunners, and they are found to have been at Kaiserswerth, where she went in 1849, to strengthen her inspiration by a year's training in nursing. Pastor Fliedner had there founded the first of the modern orders of nursing "sisterhoods" in the Protestant Church, and the antecedents of these organisations were those in the Roman Catholic Church. While the humane labours of Fliedner were going on, in the same Rhenish province, but a few miles distant, Dr. Maximilian Jacobi had already, in 1836, been eleven years at the head of the hospital at Siegburg for the insane of those provinces. He had developed there the ideas that we accept today, which no one could put in clearer terms, or with a more humane spirit, than he did—the needs of the unhappy sufferers from mental disease. When Samuel Tuke republished in England, in 1841, Jacobi's work on "Hospitals for the Insane," he presented in his own views a like humane conception of the need of intelligent and sympathetic personal attendance. We have only to examine the writings of Jacobi and Tuke to find that while these writers knew what they wanted, they missed the way of going to work to get it.

Pinel's reform in France included the claim for humane attendance, but he simplified the question, which has been difficult from the beginning, by employing *filles de service*, the patients who were completely cured of their former insanity or subject to the lucid interval of periodical mania. Esquirol adopted this plan and advocated a system of pensions for superannuation, but the French alienists in later years found no practical escape from the defects of the ordinary attendants. The religious orders did not prove satisfactory. They were approved by some and objected to by others. Lay societies of persons devoted to the care of the sick were advocated, and the formation of an institution which should furnish attendants for all the asylums of the country, but with no practical results. Pinel's teachings were early taken to Germany by his pupils, notably by Heinroth, and inspired the humane conception of the proper provisions for the insane in the dozen new asylums opened there in the first thirty years of the century.

Dr. Jacobi then evolved his noble views of the right of the insane to have kind and intelligent attendants. But Jacobi was not prompted alone by the French influence. The work of William Tuke, begun independently of and contemporaneously with Pinel's, had gradually developed a truer idea of humane attendance upon the insane, and attendants were trained at the York Retreat for other asylums. Such were the operative influences in Germany, when in 1825 Jacobi at Siegburg, and Fliedner at Kaiserswerth, commenced their work. The latter devoted his first years to prison reform, but not beginning till 1836, as before stated, the first deaconess's house and small hospital.

Tuke's reform progressed slowly in England, but being sustained at York, it found its expression at Lincoln and Hanwell by Charlesworth, Hill, and Conolly, who published his "Teachings for Attendants." The few American asylums of the first three decades were founded upon the humane teachings of Pinel and Tuke. In the notable fourth decade, and contemporary with Jacobi and Fliedner, equally advanced work was being done in America. Dr. Bell's "Directions for Attendants" was published, and a similar treatise by Dr. Woodward, before the publication of Conolly's book. Within the next ten years similar works were produced by Drs. Kirkbride, Curwen, and Ray.

Dr. Browne, at the Crichton Institution, Dumfries, in 1854, made the first attempt "to educate the attendants upon the insane" by a course of thirty lectures to his staff. He strove to get for his patients the ideal nurse, and in this, as in other matters, he anticipated many of the best ideas of the present day; but the leadership went over to the general hospitals when Florence Nightingale took into them the good things which she found in the sisterhood system, by which Fliedner put into practice the main ideas then adopted by all the leading alienists.

The important question of nursing and attendance for the insane continued to receive serious consideration. The Commissioners in Lunacy for England made it a special subject of comment and inquiry in their report for 1859. They declared "that the engaging of competent attendants of good character, and in some instances of superior education, cannot be too strongly insisted upon;" and they endeavoured "to impress upon all who are responsible for the care and treatment of the insane, the paramount duty of adopting means for securing the zealous service of competent attendants." But the Commissioners, twenty years later, referring to their former report, said—"Although the care and treatment of the insane have in most respects altered greatly for the better, improvement in the character and position of attendants has not been nearly so marked," and they were still convinced that "much of the evil arises from the insufficiency of wages."

A notable article on "Sisterhoods in Asylums," appeared in the *Journal of Mental Science* for April 1866. It advocated the employment of women for the care of the insane of both sexes, by having recourse to the religious orders, or something like them, in which there would be a survival of the better features of the old monastic system.

Dr. Clouston, in a paper read before the Medico-Psychological Association in 1876, lamented the unattainableness of the ideal asylum and asylum attendants. (See Insane, Attendants on, p. 694.)

During the ten years previous to 1880, the system of infirmary wards became more common. In those for men, married attendants and their wives were sometimes employed, and in a few instances there were single women; but there did not exist in any asylum in the world as recently as that date, an organised school for the training of nurses for the insane. Dr. Clouston's stirring words stated the position to which the alienists had come. It was still, as for many years, an attitude of knowing what was wanted, and asking how to get it. The asylum physicians were the first to recognise what was required, but they did not get at the principle which Florence Nightingale had discovered from the general hospital point of view. The principle was that the way to get good nurses was to give them knowledge and thus quicken their sympathy, and to attract intelligence to the service, by giving it a worthy field for its exercise. The alienists, from the asylum point of view, only made attempts that were not sufficiently organised—the scope of every plan of teaching was too limited and gave nothing that the attendant could use elsewhere; they never got beyond the idea of improving the attendants upon the patients immediately concerned. In the hospitals the nurses were fitted for a new profession. The hospital was made a school, and in the process of giving the training it received its reward in trained service. The motive influence of a wholesome self-interest was brought into play, and the nurse, like the physician, was asked for no more philanthropy than she could afford to give while gaining self-support in the world's work. The career of the asylum attendant was made to end only in the asylum; that of the hospital nurse only began in the hospital where she was anxious to learn her profession. The question of the inducement of better wages which troubled the asylums and the Lunacy Boards for so many years, was quickly disposed of in the new hospital schools, and became of minor importance. The inducement of the education offered was the potent factor in the reform because it opened the way to higher rewards. Wages became nominal for the major part of the work, which was done by pupils, and even an income has been derived from the giving of instruction. The compensation to the few qualified nurses retained in the hospitals could be made satisfactory, because they became practically part of the teaching staff. These are principles which underlie all practical nursing reform.

The next decade after 1880 witnessed the beginning of a change in the asylums that is destined to become as radical and beneficent as that which has taken place in the general hospital. In January 1884, Dr. Campbell Clark published in the *Journal of Mental Science* the first results of his practical experiments in training attendants in the Glasgow District Asylum. Upon its being opened in 1881, having many female patients with serious bodily diseases, he employed a matron especially trained to hospital work, and an attendant who had been trained in a London hospital. He advocated the hospital idea, and taking up the subject where Dr. Clouston left off, he urged the expediency and necessity of so training the attendants, that they would have something reliable and desirable as a permanent occupation, and he argued that "*by raising the value of the training to them better material will be attracted to the work.*" Here is touched the foundation principle; Dr. Clouston almost stated it in his proposition—and better than those who preceded him. In Dr. Clark's report for 1889, he speaks with rightful satisfaction of his new departure as having "become an organised system of our asylum work," and is able to say that many asylums in this country have given practical effect to the principle of specially training attendants and nurses with very good results. Dr. Clouston's plan, developed upon the reorganisation of the female hospital at Morningside in 1882, required that all new attendants should pass through it, and be taught the nursing of the sick with bodily ailments and acute mental diseases. It is significant that those so instructed were reluctant to leave the hospital because the duties were more interesting than in the ordinary wards.

In 1885 there was published the excellent "Handbook for the Instruction of Attendants on the Insane," prepared by a Committee of the Medico-Psychological Association.

The ultimate development of this important reform is stated at length in the *Journal of Mental Science* for October 1890. It consists of a report by the committee appointed by the Medico-Psychological Association of Great Britain and Ireland, to inquire into the question of systematic training of attendants in asylums for the insane. (*See* Insane, Attendants on, p. 692.)

In New South Wales effective work is reported by Dr. Norton Manning, the Inspector General. It was begun in 1885 by the official publication of a manual on the care and treatment of the insane for instruction of attendants and nurses.

The contemporary movement in America is equally interesting and instructive. The writer of this article being familiar with the work there, can best illustrate by reference to it, the variety of method in the organisation and conduct of training schools. The first effective American work in the general hospitals began in 1873. Under the stimulation of this the McLean Asylum employed a trained nurse, an unmarried woman, in the common wards for men as early as 1877. It was determined in 1879 to establish there a fully organised system of training nurses on the plan of the schools of the general hospitals, in one of which the superintendent of the asylum had just previously established such a school. The problem having thus been studied practically from the hospital point of view, the motive forces were recognised. The preparations were begun in 1880 and a number of hospital-trained nurses were employed, but with indifferent success, they having acquired a preference for "bodily" nursing. The practice of placing unmarried women as nurses in the common wards for men was made successful. General hospital methods were introduced with some practical class work, such as massage, &c.,

and special difficulties were overcome that seemed to stand in the way of accomplishing the purpose of giving instruction in general nursing. The asylum school was formally established in 1882 upon the appointment of a nurse with both asylum and hospital training as the head of it. Subsequently a more successful arrangement was gained by sending the supervisor, who had been long in the service, to a general hospital to learn the technique of school work. She was then promoted and became an excellent superintendent of nurses and also matron. Regular instruction was given in cooking for the sick, and later in physical exercise and medical gymnastics.

In a little over three years six nurses, who had been under training three or four years, were graduated as qualified in general bodily nursing as well as special nursing of the insane. The training of male nurses was begun in 1886 and the first five were graduated in 1888. In 1890 the product of the school reached an aggregate of 92 nurses, 70 women and 22 men. In July 1890 there remained in the service 22 graduate nurses, 12 women and 10 men. About 32 were engaged in private nursing, all but 4 being women, and others had married, gone to their homes or into other work. Three had taken responsible positions in other institutions as teachers and matrons. The plan of development of the McLean Asylum may be briefly stated as (*first*) the establishment of a complete organisation for teaching in the practical work and classes, exercises in text-books, &c., and (*secondly*) the final addition of personal instruction by the medical staff by means of didactic lectures and demonstrations. The first step required only some extra work from the superintendent of nurses and the supervisor, but they were carefully prepared for it long before the formal work began. The second step was easier and was complementary to the main organisation of the school system.

The McLean Asylum has not been alone in this labour in America. At the Buffalo Hospital, at the Willard Asylum, at the Kankakee Asylum, at Essex Asylum, at the Hampshire Asylum, at the Danvers Hospital, similar work has been undertaken.

But the results obtained at the McLean Asylum are typical of those gained in all the asylums under the new system. The trained nurses preferring to remain in asylum work may eventually constitute about one-third of the whole service as the substantial part of the nursing staff becomes more and more permanent. The other two-thirds include pupils of the first and second years. This system of classification leads the head nurses to regard the pupils as subjects for instruction and correction and to feel they have a share of responsibility in this respect and as to their own example. *The pupils learn the right way from the outset.* Minor faults are quickly brought to light. The current courses of instruction, besides the technical teachings, continually stimulate the acquirement of the qualifications most desirable in a nurse. In fact, the service largely disciplines itself. The employment of ward-maids to do the drudgery leaves the nurses more free for their legitimate duties and for companionship, which should be the rule.

There is now proof to demonstration that these asylum schools can effectively teach general nursing, both medical and surgical, particularly the former. This implies the hospitalisation of asylums, and is of immense importance in promoting the coming asylum reform. The plan of organisation most likely to give assured results is undoubtedly that of providing at the outset an adequate teaching staff of trained women and adopting a definite curriculum of study, the work of the medical officers being complimentary. This is the plan of the general hospitals. Another way is to begin with lectures. This plan may be pushed to success, but history shows how many failures these have been.

The greater part of the service should always be done by pupils. The life of the school depends on keeping its work of teaching active, not letting the service become clogged by too many lingering graduates. Eagerness to go into private nursing should be fostered in every way. The graduate should have the feeling of being possessed of the ability to undertake any general nursing. There is then the courage to seek it.

It is important that the asylum schools should press their products upon the public. They may take advantage of the demand created by the hospital schools. When their value is known the demand for the asylum-trained nurses will stimulate and benefit the schools that trained them. It should never be forgotten, moreover, that all this is but the means to a greater end. The duty of the asylums to promote the public good demands their best efforts to diffuse a general knowledge of the mental aspects of illness, of mental hygiene and the proper early care of the insane.

It will be long before the movement of nursing reform will pass the first stage in which the supply is creating the demand.

It is compulsive that every hospital and asylum must, for mere economy's sake, train its own nurses. No asylum can much longer hold aloof from this movement. Such is the breadth of the field in which the asylums are beginning to do this new work and thus better repay their cost, that while they are simply perfecting their own internal service, they are promoting most effectively preventive psychiatry. These ideas are not simply Utopian. They result from the observation of what has happened during the last eighteen years, while the writer was directly engaged in establishing training schools in the general hospital and in the asylum. He draws the following conclusions: *First*, The teaching should be systematic, definite in its aim, and comprehensive enough to give the nurse *knowledge* of her proper work. Then an enlightened interest is enlisted, repugnance is overcome, sympathy is quickened by knowing how to relieve suffering, and her motherliness does the rest. She knows the *wrong* of withholding sympathy and faithful care. *Secondly*, The plan of training should include the intention of making the pupil successful in private nursing. While the hospital and asylum exist primarily for the benefit of the patients, the school within them for its own sake should do thoroughly the work of a school. The interests of the asylum and the school are one. The better the nurse is qualified for all the manipulations of nursing, the better she is for the asylum in which she is taught. The value of the professional training is made so great to the nurse as to stimulate a cheerful doing in the best way of what is expected of her.

These are the lessons to be learnt from the history of nearly a century of gradual amelioration in the condition of the insane since Pinel and Tuke recognised the importance of humane personal attendance. It is to be hoped that a liberal interpretation will be put upon the maximum of requirements of the Medico-Psychological Association of Great Britain in regard to the training of attendants. The principle that history teaches is that general training in nursing for the nurse, and in general medicine for the physician, are alike essential as a proper basis for special practice in either case. The danger of keeping up the old barriers to the progress of reform lies in a limitation in the training of medical nursing when "all the manipulations" may be taught so easily. The characteristic of the American plan is that the attendant should be made a nurse, and that the nurse should be assured of such a recognition as will command employment in her calling. The main reliance is not to be upon "sufficiency of wages," or "religious vows to do good works," upon the taking of honest-hearted human nature as we find it, respecting its right to a wholesome self-interest, keeping to the conservation of values in the giving and taking of philanthropic personal service, imparting knowledge to the woman, and thereby revealing the way to the exercise of a natural motherliness, and having due regard for the duty of hospital and asylum to the public that supports them. These are the common sociological principles that underlie the whole matter.

E. Cowles.

[*References.*—Handbook for the Instruction of Attendants on the Insane, prepared by the sub-Committee of the Medico-Psychological Association of Great Britain and Ireland, appointed at a branch meeting held in Glasgow on the 21st of Feb. 1884: authors, A. C. Clark, C. M. Campbell, A. R. Turnbull, A. R. Urquhart, octavo, 64 pp.; London: Baillière and Co., 1885. Nursing Reform for the Insane, American Journal of Insanity, October 1887. Training Schools of the Future; Seventeenth Annual Report of the National Conference of Charities and Correction at Baltimore, 1890, by the writer of this article.]

NYCTEGERSIA (νύξ, night; ἔγερσις, a waking or rousing). Nocturnal excitement. A rousing in the night. (Fr. *nyctégersie*.)

NYCTEPLANCTOS, NYCTIPLANCTUS, NYCTIPOLOS, NYCTIPOLUS, NYCTIPORUS (νύξ, night; πλανάομαι, πολεύω, and πορεύομαι, I wander or march). Terms for one who walks during sleep. (Fr. *somnambule*; Ger. *Nachtwandler*.)

NYCTOBADIA, NYCTOBASIS (νύξ, night; βαίνω, I step). An old term for sleep-walking. (Fr. *nyctobase*.)

NYCTOBATESIS, NYCTOBATIA (νύξ, night; βατέω, I move). Sleep-walking.

NYCTOPHONIA (νύξ, night; φωνή, the voice). Term for the loss of voice during the day; an occasional symptom in hysteria. (Fr. *nyctophonie*; Ger. *Tagstimmlosigkeit*.)

NYMPHOMANIA. — **Definition.** — Under this term we understand a morbid condition peculiar to the female sex, the most prominent character of which consists in an irresistible impulse to satisfy the sexual appetite—the same pathological condition which in the male has received the name of satyriasis (*q.v.*). Some alienists have with Esquirol attempted to distinguish erotic insanity of purely cerebral origin from an irresistible impulse caused by morbid irritation of the reproductive organs. This thesis may be maintained as a theory, and cases may be quoted to support it. It would, however, be rash to affirm that it is always so, and the proof is difficult to establish. Nobody disputes that morbid love may be entirely intellectual or platonic, and may have as its object a living or dead person, a *souvenir*, a statue, or a picture, but in addition to this, there exists a violent, irresistible sexual appetite which must be satisfied, regardless of age or any other consideration. Of these two kinds of phenomena, the former is the consequence of a disorder in which the brain predominates over the sexual organs; the latter is the result of a reverse action of the sexual organs upon the brain, but with reciprocal re-action, without our being always able to determine, however, the starting-point with sufficient precision. Nymphomania must not be considered as a morbid entity, but rather as a form or variety of mental derangement connected with affections which may differ as regards their seat, nature, and development. We describe it as an impulse, even if the doctrine of pure impulsive monomania has disappeared from mental pathology. Its ætiology is the most interesting part of its history. The appetite in question is not the same in all women. There is also a difference betwen the sexes, and there are racial differences also. In some women it appears early, and remains to a very advanced age; in others it develops slowly, is dormant, and becomes prematurely extinct, so that such women never reach their full sexual development. Longitude and latitude have but a limited effect on this function, but a high temperature, together with stimulating food, intensifies it. Thus, the negro in his tent under the burning rays of the sun, and the Esquimaux, during the long winter nights in his over-heated hut, equally give themselves up to repulsive excesses in the midst of orgies which constitute their festivals; the civilised man obeys the same instincts when his imagination, excited by sensuous representations, and his stomach filled with exciting aliment, have aroused his animal passions. Temperature, food, surroundings, and example increase, therefore, the activity of this sense, and moderate excitement is too often followed by an irresistible morbid impulse. Education may diminish or augment the appetite, and hence impressions received in childhood, and especially at puberty, have a great influence on its development; the innate morbid germs or proclivities do not necessarily thrive, but may be easily fostered. On the one hand, a pathological predisposition, wisely restricted, may be even turned to the benefit and preservation of the species, whilst on the other hand, if not moderated, it terminates in the premature extinction of the individual, or in the degeneration of the race. The final result often depends upon accidental causes: the woman, as a child or an adult, very easily receives impressions from her environment; she unconsciously receives the motive of her actions from her reading, from pictures, statuary, plays, or daily scenes. When the neuropathic condition affects and dominates her, all the impressions appeal to her morbidly impressionable state, and she often becomes the slave of her instincts.

Nymphomania frequently appears in the course of various mental disorders, differing in seat and lesion: idiocy and its varieties, mania, circular insanity, hypochondriasis, hysteria, epilepsy, general paralysis, hypochondriacal insanity, and brain degeneration. Exceptionally, it persists during the whole duration of the principal disorder, but generally it is only a transitory phenomenon. Nymphomania is frequent at the commencement of different forms of insanity, but its duration is short; it is frequently observed during the first two stages of general paralysis, and seems to be directly connected with lesions of the brain and spinal cord. After the nerve-cells and fibres have become atrophied, sexual impotency ensues, and we no longer observe erotic insanity or sexual excitement. Nymphomania is observed as a temporary phenomenon in old women whose intellect has become deranged, and who later on are affected with cerebral softening and encephalitis around a localised lesion. In religious insanity of mystic form, erotic insanity amounting to an irresistible impulse is by no means rare; later it is succeeded by remorse which causes the patient most painful suffering.

The affections of the spinal cord, myelitis, incipient softening, and locomotor ataxia, cause the same sexual disorders (reflexly), which we have described as resulting from cerebral disease.

Causes.—Nymphomania may have as a cause disease of the genital apparatus: eruptions on the labia majora and minora, inflammation of the vagina, uterus, Fallopian tubes, and organic affections of the uterus and the commencement of the vagina. Women given to the use of opium, morphia, and haschisch may, in the same way as men, exhibit sexual excitement bordering on nymphomania—a condition in which their imagination dwells in consequence upon erotic ideas and images. Later on, when the intoxication has become chronic, the sexual appetite slowly diminishes and becomes extinct; the annihilation of the intellectual faculties, combined with general exhaustion, becomes complete.

Nymphomania presents various degrees of existence. At first it shows itself by simple excitement of the reproductive organs, which is brief, and upon which the will still exercises control; subsequently there is irresistible erotic impulse. The patient's expression is bright, the face turgid, the respiration quickened, the sexual organs are congested, and the gestures amatory. The appetite demands satisfaction without regard to age or person; the desire may even lead to murder if resistance is offered to the patient's desires. The duration and termination of such a disorder depends upon the primary cause; most frequently temporary, it becomes a permanent and predominant phenomenon in certain idiots and chronic lunatics, and causes general weakening with disorders of the bodily functions; diseases and traumatisms of the genital organs are the consequence; very exceptionally death is the direct result; if it occurs, it is in consequence of some accidental affection, for the enfeebled organism is more disposed to contract any malady.

Various intoxicants are apt to produce nymphomania: poisoning by cantharides was formerly supposed to have this effect, but subsequently it was denied; irritation of the genito-urinary apparatus is noticed after the absorption of cantharides, but it does not cause eroticism. This subject requires fresh investigation, as the observations reported by former observers can be interpreted in various ways. It is well known that fatal poisoning by cantharides causes painful turgescence of the generative organs without any sexual impulse. From the moment we are able to prove that nymphomania is accompanied by a mental disorder or is its immediate consequence, a nymphomaniac must be declared to be irresponsible from a legal point of view, if under such circumstances she obeys an irresistible morbid impulse. As a general rule, the man solicits and the woman complies, but it may be that she is the one to solicit. It would be unjust to attribute all the actions of libertinism in women to morbid proclivities; perverted immorality often accomplishes actions which the most vivid imagination would scarcely be able to conceive, and such actions fall within the reach of the law, if not caused by mental derangement. But insanity must be suspected and looked for, if a woman after a long life of propriety and modesty gives herself suddenly to debauchery, thus bringing scandal and contempt upon her family and herself. This sudden change of conduct frequently finds its explanation in commencing organic lesions or in an insanity as yet doubtful, but which will soon become obvious. General paralysis in its commencement often produces in women a condition of sexual excitement liable to become nymphomania; such excitement strikes the observer from its exaggeration, whilst the insanity remains obscure or passes by altogether unrecognised. Nurses and servants, to whom the care of children is confided, should be kept under strict surveillance by the parents, because it is not uncommon that under the influence of hysteria or of a morbid disposition they subject the children to manipulations which affect their health and compromise their existence. Many cases have been divulged, but how many happen of which we hear nothing! A habit of our times, which is far spread and most dangerous for our children, is, not to keep the dogs, which are now in almost every house, in the yard or in the stables, but to allow them to come into the house and even into the bed; their habit of introducing their tongues everywhere causes the child to contract habits against which it is unable to strive, whilst the parents are too much absorbed in their pursuits to notice what passes around them. For many years a whole literature of romance and plays has been occupied in the description of Lesbic love, to the great damage of young girls and neuropathic women; curiosity at first attracts and soon misleads them; the sensation experienced enslaves them, and then, aided by the use of morphia, ether, and cocaine, nymphomania establishes itself. The word has spread from the unfortunates to the women of the theatres, and from thence has taken possession of unoccupied women of all classes of society with unsatisfied desires.

Hypnotism is stated to have been used for the purpose of committing crimes on women, and this may be done under hypnotism as well as any other anæsthetic. It is useful to keep here in mind that simulation may always be expected in hysterical women, and that it is well to remember the possibility of its existence. We cannot, however, discuss these questions here, and it must therefore suffice merely to indicate them. A hypnotiser, who, by repeated manœuvres, has tried the disposition of his subject (a woman easy to hypnotise), might experience little resistance if he wished to excite her amativeness. His responsibility is exactly the same as that of an individual who abuses a weak imbecile or idiotic person.

Intercourse calms the natural want but

does not cure the morbid excitement. Marriage only results in introducing unhappiness into two families, and in addition to this a child resulting from the union will probably be a source of new pathological conditions. Hence abstention from marriage is the best advice to give both for the individual and for society.

The **treatment** must be directed to the principal disease which causes nymphomania. Anaphrodisiacs are useful, without, however, being very effective; bromide of camphor and of potassium, Sitz baths and sedative lavements, moderate exercise, regular work, life in the open air, and a good physical, moral and intellectual hygiene should be prescribed.

As regards surgical operations, clitoridectomy, nymphotomy, circumcision, and oöphorectomy, are useless, and some of them are even to be condemned. It is evident that the cause of nymphomania is a lesion or a disease of the cerebro-spinal axis. To revive here an old subject of debate would serve no useful purpose. It has been demonstrated in important discussions in medical societies, the authority of which is indisputable. Observations made on different sides, seem to confirm their conclusions.

GUSTAVE BOUCHEREAU.

[*References.*—Esquirol, Maladies mentales, tom. ii. Foville, Nouveau Dictionnaire de Médecine et de Chirurgie pratique, Jaccoud, tom. xiv. Guislain, Leçons Orales, tom. i. Morel, Études cliniques, tom. ii. Trélat, La Folie lucide.]

NYSTAGMUS (*νυσταγμός*, nodding of the head when sleepy). A constant involuntary movement of the eyeballs, generally horizontal, observed in some forms of disease of the nervous system. May occur in the insane, but is not pathognomonic. (Fr. *nystagme.*)

O

OAF (A.S. *ough*, an elf). A fool, or idiot, so called from the notion that all idiots are changelings left by the fairies in the place of the stolen ones (Brewer, "Phrase and Fable").

OBJECT CONSCIOUSNESS. — The consciousness of the presence of an object which is really at the time affecting the sensation of the observer. In this mental state, that which occupies consciousness is an object contemplated as something belonging to the *non-ego*. Objective science is the theory of the known.

OBLIVIO (*obliviscor*, I forget). A word used occasionally in psychological medicine for forgetfulness or lethargy. (Fr. *oublier;* Ger. *Vergessen.*)

OBNUBILATION (*ob*, towards; *nubilo*, I am cloudy). A cloudiness. The word is used to express such a state of mind as that immediately preceding syncope or death. The term is also applied to giddiness. (Fr. *obnubilation;* Ger. *Umwölkung.*)

OBSESSION.—In the occult sciences, "obsession" is the state of a person tormented by a demon, while "possession" indicates the permanent sojourn of the devil in the body. It is also used in the present day to mean the haunting of a person's mind by a dead person's spirit (Soc. for Psych. Research.) In psychological medicine it is synonymous with IMPERATIVE IDEAS (*q.v.*).

OBSESSION, AND IMPULSE IN GENERAL. — Obsession and impulse are two phenomena observed in normal conditions and forming a part of cerebral biology.

Every cerebral manifestation, either of the intellect or of the affections, which in spite of the efforts of the will, forces itself upon the mind, thus interrupting for a time, or in an intermittent manner, the regular course of association of ideas, is an obsession. Every action consciously accomplished, which cannot be inhibited by an effort of will, is due to an impulse.

Impulse bears the same relation to acts which obsession does to ideas. Obsession may exist alone; impulse is mostly the consequence of a series of obsessions. The two phenomena are connected with each other by means of the psychological process, which always connects actions with cerebral life; thought is transformed into act; the idea shows itself externally by a series of muscular actions. And like the idea or group of ideas originating them, this series of actions could not be inhibited by the will. In reality, these two physiological conditions are rare: we may even say, that without having a distinctly pathological character, they indicate generally a temporary derangement of the mind. One centre cannot work for a long time isolatedly in an individual who is otherwise sane, but suffers from impotency of will, without causing profound derangement in the regular operations of the intellect, the result of which will be a state of suffering, and consequently a pathological condition. In a normal individual, obsession and impulse are the consequence of a violent irritation of certain centres, transmitted by molecular vibrations, which continue for a variable length of time, gradually decreasing until the primordial excitation is exhausted. We remind the reader of the impulses of passion, of those which follow violent excitement of the mind, and strong or exaggerated affection, &c.; the violence of the emotional phenomenon is so great that the reaction comes on suddenly before the will has time to exercise its inhibitory influence; such are the impulses following a sudden outburst of anger and the impulsive actions caused by excessive love, &c.

What are the physiological conditions accompanying these phenomena? The regular succession of operations of the intellect is normally this: an idea arises which is logically connected with a series of associations of ideas, or with a sensation, or with an affection; the mind then comes into play, controls the idea, and the latter is transformed into an action, with intervention of the will. Let us suppose an idea to rise suddenly within the field of consciousness, without being apparently connected with the usual generating factors, and let us further suppose this idea to be the expression of an exaggerated irritation of the centres which originate it, and that its incessant repetition hinders the normal course of all former associations of ideas; volition will be paralysed and obsession is constituted.

Two elements are indispensable to obsession:

(1) A centre which suddenly and isolatedly enters into function, its action not being required by the mental needs of the moment.

(2) Temporary impotence of the will to remove this obsession.

Such is obsession in the first analysis. If now this obsession is transformed into an action, which by its suddenness interrupts the regular succession of the actions of life, or if an action or series of actions is suddenly accomplished, being caused only by exaggerated affection or sensation, and in consequence of its suddenness altogether escaping the control of the reason —the will being paralysed—an impulse is constituted.

To resume: loss of the equilibrium of mental operations, caused by the exaggerated function of a certain number of centres, and causing temporarily impotence of will —such are the causes of obsession and impulse.

It is true, will is neither annihilated nor inhibited, because it is not a simple faculty connected with a definite group of cells. Imagine a centre, irritation would cause it to enter into action, but its activity has degrees proportionate to the intensity of the irritation. In the normal condition of cerebral equilibrium, this irritation never exceeds a certain degree, which allows the faculty of will to exercise its inhibitory influence. If the primary irritation is exaggerated, the activity of the centre excited will also be exaggerated, and surpassing the normal limit, will continue for some time and escape the controlling action of the will; the normal equilibrium will be suspended for the time being. We see that in this case the will appears neither weakened nor paralysed, but, its energy being in the normal state, it is unable to strive efficiently. Let us now suppose this primary irritation to be still more exaggerated, and to be specially favoured by the susceptibility of the individual, then the activity of the centre will assume a still more lasting intensity, the phenomenon will be followed by other conditions which we are about to study, and the pathological condition in question is constituted. We then recognise between the physiological and pathological phenomena only a difference in degree, the cause of which lies in an innate cerebral defect.

Physiological obsession and impulse are incidents without importance in intellectual life. They appear as a temporary difficulty. The periodical return of the obsession is troublesome, but the will is not absolutely disarmed. On the other hand the patient easily directs his attention to another point. With regard to impulse, the will is completely annihilated, for it appears with such suddenness that the mind becomes aware of it only at the moment it is accomplished, and the will has not had time to intervene; but, like obsession, it is followed by only slight moral suffering. After the deed has been accomplished the mental condition is again quite normal.

What is psychologically necessary in order that physiological obsession and impulse should become morbid syndromes? Let us suppose that these two phenomena, instead of remaining isolated facts in the mental processes, assume considerable importance, and that their incessant *persistency* and *repetition* during a long time make the constant fatigue a condition *of actual suffering*. Let us also suppose that obsession and impulse instead of originating in an idea, sentiment, or a trifling sensation, spring from eccentricity, perverted affections and abnormal sensations, suicidal impulse, sexual perversion, &c., which represent so many pathological conditions of the cerebrum, what will happen? The consequence will be moral suffering and inexpressible anguish, increased tenfold by the absolute impotence in which the individuals know themselves to be to expel the obsession or to arrest the impulse by a free effort of will. The mind is wide awake and the patient is at first quite astonished with this kind of automatism of one part of himself. He tries to get rid of it, but the obsession becomes dominant, and from that time he is engaged in a continuous struggle in which he knows he will be defeated. Henceforth the normal course of operations of the intellect is interrupted, the obsession usurps the whole attention of the patient and makes him its powerless slave. The anguish is now complete and shows itself by physical symptoms (præcordial anxiety, tremor, &c.) which invariably are the consequence of every pathological obsession or impulse. When the impulse has followed the obsession the contest is suspended for a while, leaving the patient still deeply afflicted with his impotence, but in reality relieved from a great burden. The idea of having satisfied a temporary and dominant need gives the patient a sort of undefinable sense of well-being, whatever the nature of the impulse may be. But this remission is of short duration; the obsession comes back and must be again satisfied. The anxiety returns and the struggle recommences, leaving the patient once more in a state of helplessness; the will also succumbs. And so it goes on, subsides, and again returns, until the first cause of automatism disappears.

Such are pathological obsession and impulse. We see that they may be reduced to the same character as the physiological phenomena; we only have to add the accompanying moral suffering and anxiety. The impotency of the will as regards inhibition is always a principal, but not the most important symptom. Are obsession and impulse caused by a sort of temporary and morbid loss of energy of the will, or in other words, does there in reality exist a *disease of the will?* This does not seem probable. The truth is that the normal amount of voluntary energy is often increased in the struggle against the obsession. And that the will succumbs is not the consequence of temporary weakness, but because it strives against a power stronger than itself. It will be well, however, to add that in this loss of mental equilibrium which precedes the appearance of obsessions and impulses, diminution of power of resistance may actually exist and favour the defeat of the patient in his struggle, but this diminution of power is never the most important fact.

In short, *incessant recurrence* of obsession and impulse, to which the patient offers only *useless resistance; consciousness* of the phenomenon; energetic *struggle* to get rid of it; *moral anguish* in consequence of the sense of impotency; *relief* after the impulse has been satisfied; are, briefly, the psychological characters of pathological obsession and impulse.

We see, therefore, that these patients are completely conscious, even in the midst of the most fearful anguish, and when the impulse is on the point of being carried into effect. (*See* IMPERATIVE IDEAS.)

M. LEGRAIN.

OBSTUPESCENTIA (*obstupesco*, I grow or become stupefied). An old term for that state of stupefaction in which the patient remains perfectly quiescent with his eyes open as if astonished, and not moving or speaking. (Fr. *obstupescence*; Ger. *Bestürzung*.)

OCCUPATION. (*See* TREATMENT.)

OD FORCE.—Od is a suffix proposed by von Reichenbach for the peculiar force alleged to be produced on the nervous system by all magnetic agents. According as it is found in magnets, heat, light, &c., he called it magnetod, thermod, photod, &c. The influence of magnets on the body is not proved.

ODAXESMUS (ὀδαξάω, I bite). Term applied by Marshall Hall to the bitten tongue, cheek, or lip which is an important sign of an epileptic fit. (Fr. *odaxesme*).

ODOUR OF THE INSANE.—In common with other functions in the insane, the function of the skin is often disordered and its abnormal secretion leads to a smell of a disagreeable character. The skin is often dry and harsh at the same time. If perspiration be induced and baths afterwards given the smell can be greatly lessened. Much diversity of opinion exists as to whether there is an odour peculiar to the insane or not.

ODYL.—A so-called new "influence" said to be developed by magnets, heat, electricity, &c. The odylic force is alleged to give rise to luminous phenomena visible to certain sensitive persons, and to them only.

ODYNEPHOBIA (ὀδύνη, pain; φοβέω, I fear). A morbid dread of pain. (Fr. *odynéphobie*; Ger. *Schmerzscheu*.)

ŒCIOMANIA (οἶκος, a house; μανία, madness). A variety of moral insanity characterised by domestic perversity. No doubt many unstable natures are able to get on fairly well when away from home, but "œciomania" is one of the many examples of the needless multiplication of physiological terms.

ŒNOMANIA. (*See* OINOMANIA.)

ŒSOPHAGEAL TUBE. (*See* FEEDING (FORCIBLE) OF THE INSANE.)

ŒSTROMANIA (*οἶστρος*, a gadfly, also amorous desire; *μανία*, madness.) An old term for nymphomania (*q.v.*). (Fr. and Ger. *Œstromanie.*)

OHRBLUTGESCHWULST (Ger.). Hæmatoma auris (*q.v.*).

OIKEIOMANIA (*οἰκεῖος*, belonging to a family; *μανία*, madness). Œciomania (*q.v.*).

OIKOPHOBIA (*οἶκος*, home; *φόβος*, fear). A morbid and unreasoning dread of home.

OINOMANIA (*οἶνος*, wine; *μανία*, madness.) A term meaning a morbid craving for wine, and also madness produced by drink. It is used especially for that form of drunkenness in which there are long intervals of sobriety between isolated drinking bouts. (Fr. *oinomanie*; Ger. *Säuferwahnsinn.*)

OLD AGE AND ITS PSYCHOSES.

Senile Involution.—In many cases man preserves in old age a fair amount of mental and bodily power. Not unfrequently, indeed, old age seems to be the time of actual ripeness and perfection, on which a man like Jakob Grimm is in the happy position of being able to pronounce an enthusiastic eulogy. Usually, however, old age is that period of life in which mental and bodily power suffer loss in the form of increasing weakness. It would not be in accordance with facts to fix a certain year, or even years, at which old age commences. The transition is generally gradual, and the limit differs according to the individual. In one man we see the symptoms of old age appear between sixty and seventy, whilst in others they may appear ten years before that time, or still earlier. This however we may say, that in the female sex the period of general involution, which may be considered as the commencement of old age, begins at the end of the menopause, which, although there is no certain rule for all, nevertheless is finished in most cases about the fifty-fifth year.

As in the male, evolution mostly begins a little later than in the female, we may fix the time of the commencement of senile involution about the sixtieth year. Inasmuch as the transition is gradual, and the symptoms of old age only become pronounced later on, we assume, in accordance with most other authors, that senile involution definitely begins from sixty to sixty-five.

Pathology.— Senile involution commences mostly with slowly developing constitutional changes, as atheromatous degeneration of the walls of the vessels, changes in the blood (hydræmia), and increasing atrophy of all organs. The only exception is the heart, which in old age becomes greatly hypertrophied; in more advanced age, however, atrophy also takes place. These changes become externally manifested by symptoms of senile weakness, which develop gradually in mind and body, and which are termed "*habitus senilis.*"

Symptoms.—This pathological involution commences with headache, sense of pressure on the head, dizziness, sense of weakness and fatigue, subjective phenomena of vision and hearing, paræsthesia (which are manifold and vary much in the beginning), decrease of the functions of the senses, temporary vaso-motor and cardiac derangement accompanied by dyspnœa and asthmatic troubles, which appear often and severely, especially by night, disturbance of sleep, intercurrent states of somnolency during the day, and disturbance of digestion. There is often great sexual appetite, frequently in the form of perverted sensations and impulses; there is often also a craving for alcoholic stimulants.

The objective examination shows the symptoms of the "habitus senilis," slight emaciation or a tendency to corpulence in many cases, atheromatous arteries, irregular vaso-motor and cardiac action, tendency to venous stasis, emphysema of the lungs, and chronic bronchitis. Frequently the knee-jerk is lessened or entirely absent, and there is also lessened sensibility of the lower extremities.

In regard to the mind there is greater or less weakness, especially forgetfulness of recent events, apathy and indifference with weakness of will, a tendency to temporary hallucinatory states, absence of mind and sensory derangements. Moreover, there are other symptoms of mental excitement, as increased recollection of things long past, hypochondriacal depression with an inclination to cry, excitability often to the extent of fury, motor restlessness, especially by night, in connection with phantasms, illusions of visions and hallucinations, disturbance of consciousness and mental confusion. The patient sees fire, animals, and pictures, and hears noises; he believes that somebody is going to rob him; lastly, he has immoral ideas with sexual hallucinations and an intense apprehension.

All these bodily and mental symptoms of pathological involution may be temporary and come on in paroxysms; but they also may become permanently established. They must be regarded as so-called functional derangements, and they are probably closely connected with the derangements of circulation and nutrition of the central nerve-substance, caused by the morbid condition of the organs of circulation.

Idiopathic anæmia and hydræmia of the nerve-centres cause and accompany these derangements. In other cases cardiac disorders, derangements of the organs of digestion or of the bladder may be the cause of the derangements of circulation and nutrition of the central nervous system, which then are secondary symptoms. This, at least, is certain, that all these abnormal states may entirely disappear or appear as paroxysms, or as attacks which last rather longer, or even if chronic, they remain stationary. Also with regard to intensity and variety of the symptoms, they may range from slight disturbances to fully developed disease. We consider them identical with those conditions of transition between mental and nervous health and disease, which have been frequently observed in recent times as inherited or acquired neuropathic and psychopathic diathesis.

We draw attention to the great importance of these conditions in forensic medicine, because they frequently lead to crimes, or by weakening the patient's power of control cause damage to his own interests as well as to those of his family, and thereby entail prosecution by civil law. Sexual crimes of all kinds play a prominent part; theft, incendiarism and assaults have been observed. The examination of the mental condition frequently offers very great difficulties to the physician, especially as lucid intervals are frequent and often of long duration.

Actual mental derangement occurs in old age, but nothing certain is known about its frequency. It is highly probable that it is more frequent in the male sex than in the female. We have found 8 per cent. of all mental disorders to belong to old age (and of this number 10 per cent. were males and 6 per cent. females), whilst Schuele found for the whole 6.5 per cent.

In former times the mental disorders of old age were divided into functional and organic derangements. We think Fuerstner is right in adding to these two groups a third, which, of more uncertain character, lies midway between the functional and organic psychoses, and does not belong to either the one or the other group entirely. Our observations completely confirm this. We therefore have in old age:

(1) **Functional psychoses;**

(2) **Psychoses which are no longer functional, but do not wholly bear the stamp of organic psychoses;**

(3) **Organic psychoses.**

(1) **The functional psychoses** of old age are not rare, but certainly much rarer than the organic. If we were to reckon under this heading all mental derangements which occur in women after the cessation of the menses, their number would be still greater, but we are not allowed to do so, because all these psychoses do not belong to old age. We may speak of senile psychoses only when those constitutional changes occur in the organism which we call senile, and when the psychoses can with certainty be regarded as caused by them. According to this view, many cases during and after the cessation of the menses cannot be reckoned in this group, while, on the other hand, cases have to be included which, as regards the age of the patient, would not have been considered as psychoses of old age (cases of premature old age). Old age causes the senile psychoses; it creates those conditions of body and mind which lead to mental derangement; it acts predisposingly as heredity does for the earlier periods of life. But the mental disorders of this group have, with regard to ætiology and symptomatology, nothing characteristic; they are, on the whole, like the mental derangements of earlier life. There is, however, sometimes less intensity in the onset of the disorder; less force in the delusions, which are of a more limited number; and the psychopathic process is often less marked. This, however, is, according to our experience, not the rule, but the exception.

Taken in the order of frequency, the following forms are observed:

(*a*) *Hypochondriasis.*

(*b*) *Melancholia*, or still more frequently a mixture of both forms as hypochondriacal melancholia. We must here mention that hypochondriacal elements often accompany other forms of senile psychoses.

After hypochondriacal melancholia, the most frequent is the passive form, *melancholia passiva or simplex*. Pure dysthymia—constant depression, without delusions—frequently occurs. The excited form is, according to our experience, more frequent than the stuporous form.

Sometimes we have observed melancholia complicated with elements of paranoia.

(*c*) *Mania*, almost exclusively in the mild form of simple maniacal exaltation (*mania levis*). Acute mania with frenzy was observed by us in only a few cases.

(*d*) More rare than the forms mentioned

above is *paranoia*, but we have several times observed typical paranoia even at the age of eighty. They were mostly cases in which at first hallucinations came on and remained for some time with general clearness until at length delusionary ideas appeared. Subjective phenomena played therein a great part, and almost always introduced and accompanied the hallucinations. Hallucinations of vision were the most frequent, and organic and functional derangements of the peripheral sensory organs could always be found. Paranoia occurred in the acute and chronic form, the latter more frequently because many cases of originally acute paranoia became chronic. In the subject-matter of paranoia, the hypochondriacal element was predominant.

Sexual illusions are generally, and *kleptomania* is often, found. The latter may be considered as the affection most marked in old age, although it may be absent in some cases.

The symptoms of these forms have, however, nothing absolutely characteristic, neither has their course, which is in no way different from that of the other functional mental derangements. We lay stress upon this, the more because Fuerstner arrived at different conclusions, and found striking remissions and even intermissions.

In respect to the **prognosis**, the functional psychoses of old age terminate as frequently in recovery as those of earlier age. We have repeatedly observed this termination in patients who were between seventy-five and eighty. However, this course is very rare in paranoia.

As regards **treatment**, we are not in a position to give other indications besides those which are accepted in the treatment of mental disorders in general; only they will have to be modified according to the conditions of more advanced age. We some time ago pointed out in an article on this subject that in the mental derangements of the old great caution must be exercised, and that exact observation must be employed. Characteristics of old age are a great reticence and desire for seclusion; the former, however, is sometimes followed by loquacity. On the other hand, there is a certain mistrust and great irritability, qualities which lead the patients often to simulation and to sudden and unexpected actions of a violent character. Assaults on others and on themselves are not rare.

(2) With regard to cases of the **second group**, we find in them not only intellectual defects, as Fuerstner states, but also other central derangements, as they are found in organic diseases of the brain. The difference between the second and third group is that in the former the cases terminate favourably or, if not, they remain stationary. They give the impression of commencing senile dementia, but their further progress shows that this is not so. They frequently commence in an acute manner in so far as attacks of apoplexy and vertigo precede the actual outbreak, although already long before this, premonitory phenomena appear, similar to the symptoms described above.

The disease itself appears in the form of acute mania, melancholia, stupor, or mania. Its symptoms are much more variable than Fuerstner supposed. It is characteristic that all these forms are not pure but are accompanied by regular sensory disorders, which are at the beginning very severe, but later on are milder.

These patients are in a state of confusion and absent-mindedness; perception and apperception are faulty; there exists amnesia, and occasionally also aphasia. There are disturbances of the optic nerves, the facial and hypoglossal; sometimes there are actual paralytic attacks. After some weeks, or it may be months, the patients become mentally clearer, and the psychoses disappear, together with other cerebral derangements. Recovery may take place without any relapse; on the other hand, recovery is often very incomplete, and there remain conditions of weakness of the central nervous system, which sometimes influence the body most, sometimes the mind. It is clear that cases of this group are more severe than those of the former. We suppose with Fuerstner that there are disturbances of the circulation and nutrition of the central nervous organs in consequence of atheroma which make the disease more severe. We have here to point out the essential importance of the influence which the heart exercises when fatty, mostly in conjunction with dilatation, but also with valvular disease.

The **treatment** of these patients is extremely difficult. The severe stupor, the inability to localise his symptoms, the obstinate sitophobia, the frequently dangerous bodily weakness, the often exaggerated motor impulses, and persistent insomnia, interfere with the usual indications. One must be most cautious in the employment of remedies, on account of the great change in the heart and vessels, and the often critical bodily weakness. Everything has to be administered to the patients by force. We think the main point of the treatment to be sufficient nutrition, to carry out which we have to resort early to artificial feeding. This indicates the kind of food which ought to be given; it must be easily digestible, readily assimilated, nourishing, strengthening and stimulating—*e.g.*, broth, milk, eggs, peptones, extract of beef and similar food. In addition to this, give alcohol in a concentrated form as egg-flip or punch, sherry, old Bordeaux, &c.

Of hypnotics the least dangerous and most efficient seems to us to be sulphonal; we have learned to prefer this to any other. According to circumstances we may make use of opium or digitalis, as Fuerstner recommends.

(3) To the third group belong the distinctly **organic psychoses of old age**, the characteristic of which is the progressive nature of the disease. There is an increasing stupor and bodily weakening which have their anatomical foundation in increasing atrophy of the central nerve substance in the form of retrogressive metamorphosis. The process originates in the disease of the arterial system, especially of the cranial cavity and of the heart. We mention this, because often the arterial system in general is found relatively well preserved, whilst the carotids and the vertebral arteries are found to be much diseased. There are even cases, in which the great arteries of the brain appear to be healthy, whilst the small arteries and capillary vessels are diseased. The disorders caused thereby lead on the one hand directly to a chronic change, on the other hand, indirectly in a more acute manner (through softening which is partly multiple, partly metastatic) to disintegration and primary atrophy of the nerve substance. That hæmorrhage into the latter plays a great part is equally a consequence of arterial disease. The membranes of the brain also often partake of the disease. Internal, external and bilateral pachymeningitis, simple and hæmorrhagic, chronic leptomeningitis, and above all ependymitis are frequently found at the post-mortem examination. The whole is accompanied by an excess of fluid in the ventricles, corresponding to the wasting of the brain, &c. Senile dementia is mostly for some time preceded by senile marasmus of mind and body. These manifold symptoms are found as we have described them above, as the stage of transition between physiological and pathological old age. We have to add that sometimes this disease is observed without being preceded by any conspicuous premonitory symptoms.

The transition to the state of actual disease is mostly gradual, the sensory derangements becoming more permanent, and the symptoms of bodily and mental weakness more and more distinct. In rare cases only the transition is an acute one introduced by symptoms which may be violent in character. This takes place in the form of an acute mental derangement with the character of hallucinatory confusion, of mania, of stupor, or with apoplectiform symptoms, and also after epileptiform attacks. It is quite exceptional for the disease to commence in the form of general disorder with fever. Cases of the latter kind which begin acutely, pursue frequently an acute course. After some weeks or months they terminate fatally with symptoms of central irritation, and especially of increasing cerebral weakness and paralysis. These are cases which, in their symptoms, bear great similarity to those of galloping paralysis, which, however, distinguishes itself by more conspicuous central disorders. We find processes like that of pachymeningitis, with or without hæmorrhagic exudation, foci of softening — especially multiple — and hæmorrhage into the central nervous substance. In a few cases only there is acute atrophy with strongly developed effusion of fluid with severe ependymitis. These forms have been long known and have been described by Lobstein as "morbus climactericus," and by Virchow as "febrile atrophy in old men."

This transition is mostly gradual.

The symptoms of senile dementia depend upon whether the disease is diffuse or localised; they are also influenced by complications. Processes like pachymeningitis often, although not necessarily, modify the symptoms, which then are characterised by sleepiness, complete lethargy, flushing of the face, weakness of the lower extremities, staggering gait, and almost absolute sitophobia; in semi-lateral sclerosis by symptoms of conjugate deviation of the eyes, and temporary spasmodic motor disorders.

Another complication is a spinal one with symptoms like those of tabes. Although typical locomotor ataxy rarely occurs in old age, symptoms like tabes often occur (absence of the knee-jerk, hyperæsthesia, anæsthesia and weakness of the lower extremities, paresis of the sphincters, &c.).

According to our experience, general paralysis occurs in a few cases. But altogether, these symptoms are much rarer than those which arise from localised lesions. We must here add that we have to take great care not to connect all the symptoms of the latter with changes of a definite anatomical nature. We have often experienced this with regard to symptoms of aphasia, and also with regard to permanent symptoms of monoplegia and hemiplegia.

Senile dementia assumes the form of progressive central degenerations. Most characteristic of this are the profound sensory disorders, the continuous and common conditions of obliviousness and the prominent amnesic derangements, which often render old men completely incapable of setting themselves right.

The well-known pathological weakness of mind, tendency to sentimentality and emotion, are symptoms of senile degeneration, but not of complete senile dementia; they belong to the prodromic stage of the disease. Frequently, however, but not always, a chronic mental change may be observed, in which the patient believes that he lives again through periods long gone by, or thinks he is in surroundings and in situations of the past. We have often thought that the elements of this derangement bear the character of plasticity (*Plasticität*) and a certain degree of sensuality, and sometimes even take an hallucinatory character. They are more frequent and vivid by night than in the daytime. Aphasic disorders are frequently only temporary, but not always so. Vague illusionary ideas of hypochondriacal character and of sexual intercourse, theft, poisoning, persecution, &c., and sometimes also macromania occur, but are not stabile, and assume more of the character of insanity. Morbid excitability of temper may often be observed.

The most characteristic bodily symptoms are motor weakness, tremor, often to the extent of paralysis agitans, failure of the senses, caused by various anatomical changes in the external sense-organs, lowered temperature of the body, the changing states of somnolency and insomnia, the former of which appears in the day, the latter by night, and, in connection with all these, great weakness of the heart.

Duration.—There are forms which terminate fatally after a few weeks or months. The greater number of cases last some years; but cases of still longer duration are of not infrequent occurrence. We do not know any other termination of the disease but death, which comes on slowly, through gradual, general weakening, and marasmus, but more quickly in consequence of disease of the brain (as pachymeningitis, softening, or hæmorrhage), or frequently also in consequence of affections of the pulmonary organs. In the case of general marasmus, bed-sores often occur, and in connection with them general disorders, or affections of the bladder, with their consequences.

We have already pointed out the naked-eye pathological changes. They are different from those of general paralysis. The brain is generally lighter, softer, more atrophied, but sclerotic foci are not excluded, leptomeningitis is less marked and less diffuse; the dura mater is nearly always adherent to the cranium; ependymitis is very distinct; the spinal changes consist more in general atrophy than local disease; but we sometimes find grey degeneration of the posterior and lateral columns.

The microscopical results confirm this statement. The disease of the vessels of the brain is mostly general and much more intense, and therefore the disease of the nerve-tissue is much more extensive. Not only the convolutions of the cerebrum, and especially the ascending frontal and parietal, are affected, but all other parts of the brain, and the degeneration extends especially into the white substance. The degeneration and atrophy of the nerve-tissue are the same in all parts of the central nerve-substance. As in general paralysis, we find also here absence of tangential fibres (Exner) and atrophy of the nerve-cells of the third layer, but we also find the cells and fibres absent wherever we look for them. There are also more strongly developed peri-vascular and peri-cellular cavities, an enormous number of spider-cells, and in all parts of the tissue emigrated lymph-corpuscles and leucocytes, the latter often in foci in consequence of hæmorrhage. In other places the elements of decay are more prominent, as granular cells, stratified and pigmented cells, but also often elements without form, as characteristic of capillary foci of softening.

As we sometimes find in old men from sixty to seventy, symptoms of mental disease which we cannot distinguish from those of general paralysis, so with regard to anatomical examination, we sometimes find central changes which bear the characteristics of senile involution as well as of paralysis. This circumstance favours the belief in the occurrence of general paralysis in old age, or rather, as seems more probable, of a complication of both diseases. LUDWIG WILLE.

OLD MAID'S INSANITY.—A form of insanity so called by Dr. Clouston, and "Ovarian Insanity," by Dr. Skae. It is characterised by a morbid alteration in the normal state of affection of woman towards the other sex. The patients are as a rule unattractive old maids about from forty to forty-five, who have led very strict and virtuous lives. The lady becomes seized with an absurd and reasonless passion for some particular individual of the opposite sex, very often her clergyman. She believes him to be deeply in love with her or accuses him of seduction or other misdeed in connection with herself, and uses the merest trifles as proofs of her beliefs. Recovery is rare, the insanity often passing into some other form. There is no proof that the ovaries are affected (Clouston).

OLIGOMANIA (ὀλίγος, few; μανία, madness). A needless word used by some authors instead of the term monomania, on the ground that the latter is an insufficient term for any form of insanity, there always being more than one morbid phenomenon in an insane person. (Fr., *oligomanie.*)

OLIGOPSYCHIA (ὀλίγος, little; ψυχή, the soul, mind). Imbecility or fatuity. The term is quite unnecessary. (Fr. *oligopsychie;* Ger. *Geistesarmuth.*)

ONEIRODYNIA (ὄνειρος, a dream; ὀδύνη, pain). A painful dream. The term includes both incubus and somnambulism.

ONEIROLOGY (ὄνειρος, a dream; λόγος, a discourse). The doctrine or theory of dreams. (Fr. *oneirologie;* Ger. *Traumtheorie.*) (*See* DREAMING.)

ONEIRONOSOS, ONEIRONOSUS (ὄνειρος, a dream; νόσος, disease). Morbid dreaming, uneasiness while dreaming. (Fr. *oneironose.*)

ONOMATOMANIA (ὄνομα, a name). The irresistible impulse to repeat a particular word, or the morbid dread of a particular word. (*See* IMPERATIVE IDEAS.)

OÖARIE. Hysteria (Fr.) (*q.v.*).

OÖPHORECTOMY. (*See* OVARIOTOMY.)

OÖPHORIA (*oophorum*, ovary). A name given to hysteria from its supposed connection with affection of the ovaries.

OÖPHORO-EPILEPSY.—Epilepsy depending on ovarian disease.

OÖPHOROMANIA.—Insanity resulting from ovarian disease.

OPEN DOOR SYSTEM. — Allowing the doors in an asylum to be unlocked.

OPIOPHIL (*opium;* and φιλέω, I love). A lover of opium. There is an opiophil club in Paris. Akin to morphinomania (*q.v.*).

OPISTHOTONUS, HYSTERICAL. (*See* HYSTERIA.)

OPIUM. (*See* SEDATIVES.)

OPIUM CRAVE.—The intense craving for opium and morphia leading to moral and other insanity. (Ger. *Opiumsucht.*) (*See* MORPHIOMANIA.)

OPSOMANIA (ὄψον, aliment; μανία, madness). Either a craving for some particular aliment to the extent of insanity, or a morbid craving for dainties. (Fr. *opsomanie.*)

OPSOPHAGIE.—Morbid daintiness as to food.

OPTICAL DELUSION.—The popular term for a visual hallucination or illusion.

OPTIMISM. (*See* EXALTATION.)

ORCHESTROMANIA (ὀρχηστήρ, a dancer; μανία, madness). Chorea, St. Vitus's dance.

ORGANIC DEMENTIA.—Dementia accompanying and resulting from gross brain lesions such as hæmorrhage, tumours, &c. Distinct from general paralysis. (*See* DEMENTIA.)

ORGANIC MELANCHOLIA.—Melancholia accompanied by gross brain lesion and causally connected with the lesion (Clouston).

ORTHOPHRENIA, ORTHOPHRENISMUS (ὀρθός, right; φρήν, the mind). Right-mindedness. A term also used for the cure of a disordered mind. (Fr. *Orthophrénie.*)

ORTHOPHRENICUS.—Of or belonging to orthophrenia, the cure of a diseased mind.

OSTEOMALACIA. (*See* BONE DEGENERATION IN THE INSANE.)

OSTEOPOROSIS. (*See* BONE DEGENERATION IN THE INSANE.)

OTHÆMATOMA. — A synonym of Hæmatoma Auris (*q.v.*). The appearance of the commoner forms of sanguineous

FIG. 1.

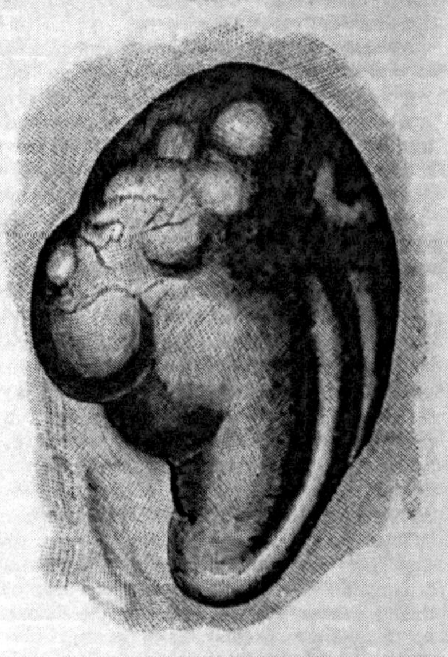

1. Othæmatoma in the acute or *primary* stage. Tumour of extraordinary size occupying the

entire cavity of the auricle, and obliterating its ridges and hollows. Surface uneven, and in parts of a plum colour. *Result*, slow absorption, with extreme contraction, and finally the almost complete distortion of the auricle, and obliteration of its several component parts. Case of E. H., affected with active melancholia (taken from life).

FIG. 2.

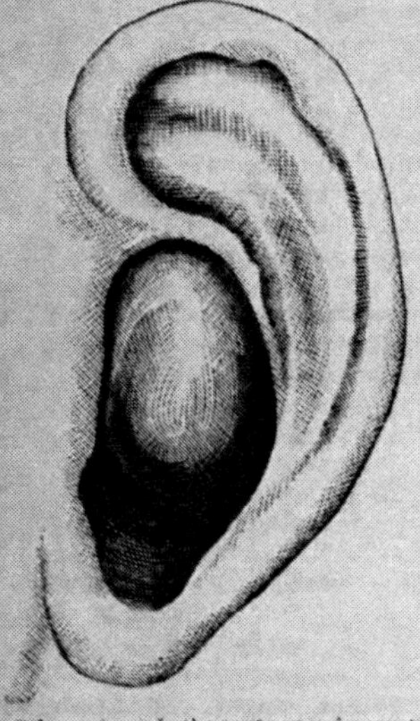

2. Othæmatoma in the acute or *primary* stage. Tumour of moderate size filling up the cavity of the concha; full and rounded above where it is bounded by the ridge of the antihelix, being lost below in the lobule. *Result*, disappearance with but little subsequent deformity. Case of C. H., affected with recurrent paroxysmal mania (taken from life).

FIG. 3.

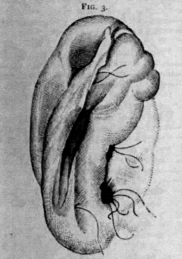

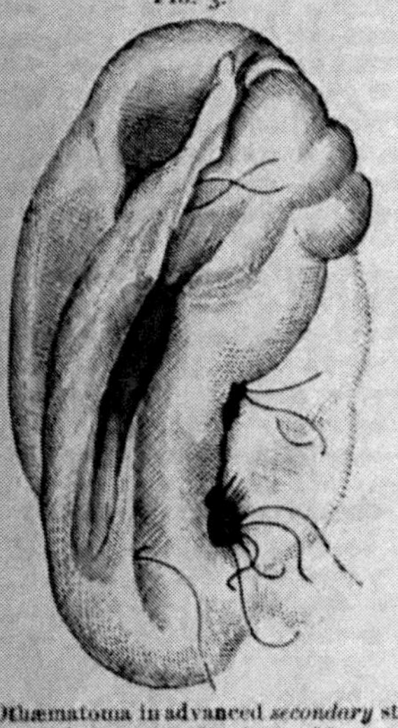

3. Othæmatoma in advanced *secondary* stage. Helix folded over antihelix, fossa of latter completely obliterated, the upper portion of the auricle was transformed into an irregularly tuberculated misshapen mass; on section a triangular portion of bone had become developed in the centre, surrounded with cartilage and connective tissue. Affection of very long standing. Case of J. M., affected with chronic dementia (taken after death).

sub-perichondrial effusion of the auricle in the recent state, or of the puckering or shrunken condition of the ear in the secondary stage of this affection, is so familiar as to need no special illustration, but the rarer varieties, such as (1) involvement of the whole of the anterior auricular surface, and (2) implication of only the concha and external auditory meatus are here figured. The first illustration shows the limitation of the effusion to the cartilaginous portions of the auricle, and the freedom from implication of the lobule and the outermost portion of the helix. The third shows the secondary stage after effusion and absorption. The wood-cuts are inserted by kind permission of Dr. Macnaughten Jones from his work on the ear. Dr. Ringrose Atkins (Waterford) drew them from cases under his care.

J. F. G. PIETERSEN.

OVARIAN INSANITY.—A name for old maid's insanity (*q.v.*).

OVARIOTOMY and OÖPHORECTOMY in relation to INSANITY and EPILEPSY.—The subjective and objective signs revealed by the ordinary methods of clinical observation teach us much, but how infinitely more precise our knowledge becomes when the opportunity is afforded of studying the condition of the economy when these organs are taken away. Of course we know that removing the organs of reproduction entails sterility; but this is not all. What is the effect upon the organism as a whole, or upon the nervous system in particular? One factor in the question is the immediate influence of the operation itself. Severe injuries, starvation, shock of great catastrophes, sunstroke, have been followed by insanity; surgical operations other than those with which we are now concerned are occasionally followed by insanity. The shock of labour may be enough to overturn the nervous equilibrium. Temporary delirium, hallucinations, violence to self or child, in some cases passing into mania, are evidence of this. No doubt there are other factors; simple shock can hardly be.

Knowing this, we have inquired whether abdominal surgery, involving the removal of the ovaries and uterus, is especially causative of insanity. If it be shown that insanity follows these operations in a sensibly larger proportion than it does other operations, then a reasonable presumption arises that it is the deprivation of the uterus and ovaries and not the mere surgical operation which leads to the insanity. The facts actually acquired strongly support this proposition. A point to bear in mind is, that the effect of shock is likely to be immediate, whilst privation of the uterus and ovaries may not be felt until after a considerable lapse of time.

This proposition established, do we not see in it a proof that these organs exercise a motor and governing power over the nervous centres? We have long been familiar with the effect of castration upon the male economy. The eunuch retains the voice of the boy; the essentially virile attributes are not developed. Does history record an undoubted example of a great discovery or a great invention made by a eunuch? It would be interesting to learn the relative prevalence of insanity amongst entire and castrated Orientals. The application of this to our argument is obvious. To unsex a woman is surely to maim or affect injuriously the integrity of her nervous system. Observations of the effect of castrating and spaying animals might throw some light upon this question. Appeal may be made to the experience of veterinary surgeons to help. M. Barthélémy (*Journ. de Méd Vétérinaire*) says that œstrum or rut can occur in pigs after complete removal of the ovaries. We have no opportunity of making anything approaching to an exhaustive summary of cases, but the following facts are instructive:—Sir Spencer Wells writes (June 1890) to the writer: "Twice during convalescence after ovariotomy I have seen maniacal attacks, but both patients were of lunatic families. . . . . In some cases where double oöphorectomy has been performed without, as I think, sufficient reason, I have seen patients almost melancholic at their mutilated condition and sterility." Dr. Savage, of Birmingham, informs us (July 1890) that he has removed the appendages on both sides in 483 cases. Of these, twenty-six died after the operation; three aged respectively 25, 25, and 30, became insane and recovered; one, aged 38, committed suicide six months after the operation. Dr. Thomas Keith writes (May 1890):—"So far as my limited experience goes, I would say that the removal of the ovaries for disease has not been in any case followed by any disturbance in the mental conditions, nor have I seen any change after the removal of the ovaries for checking the growth of bleeding fibroids; but after hysterectomy and removal of both ovaries, the effect has been decided, and I cannot consider the results accidental. Of sixty-four hysterectomies (supra-vaginal or complete removal of entire uterus), there have been six cases of insanity—three acute, and three chronic cases. In one of the acute cases, the patient, a hospital nurse, had been in Morningside Asylum with an attack of acute mania. Two of the acute cases died after operation, the other four are alive, but none of them well."

Lawson Tait, referring to Keith's statement cited above, says:—"I have operated upon a very much larger number of cases of hysterectomy, and I know of no case of insanity in my practice. Instances of insanity occur after all surgical proceedings, even the most trivial, and even after the administration of an anæsthetic." On the other hand, Tait states that "there are three cases of insanity of the most pronounced type completely cured by the relief of the sufferings incurred by the hæmorrhagic myoma. Besides this, there are a number of cases of striking eccentricities and ill temper, clearly due to the sufferings which have been equally relieved."

One lesson to be deduced from this apparent conflict of experience is, that the question demands earnest and extended inquiry. One difficulty in the way is that the subsequent history of the subjects of operation can hardly be complete.

We will offer this one reflection. It seems more rational to look for freedom from mental disease in those women who have undergone a successful operation for the cure of an ovarian or uterine disease. Such diseases we know are apt to entail nervous disorders, and we have seen that the nervous disorders, when complicating disease of the sexual organs, are frequently cured when the diseased organs are removed. But another inquiry should also be instituted as to the influence of removal of the healthy organs on the nervous system.

As to the question, are we justified in operating on a lunatic who cannot give a responsible assent? In a case which came under our notice, the indication to remove the ovaries was to our judgment decisive. We were supported by the assent of her guardian, of an eminent hospital physician, and of a distinguished alienist, but we declined to undertake the responsibility without the sanction of the Commissioners in Lunacy. The patient continued insane. Sir Spencer Wells, in a case somewhat different, being consulted as to the legality of ovariotomy upon a lunatic, asked Sir William Harcourt, then Home Secretary, who said, "If she is incapable of judging for herself, treat her as if she was an infant!" So the operation was done; the patient recovered and married. Surely this dictum is good sense as well as good law.

Does epilepsy, often so intimately associated with menstruation, justify removal of the ovaries? Lawson Tait ("Diseases of the Ovaries," p. 328) has removed the ovaries—Battey's operation—in five cases under this indication. All recovered from the operation, but the results as regards cure were not so satisfactory as to encourage him to pursue the practice. We believe that the cases are quite exceptional in which it can be advantageous in epilepsy.*

ROBERT BARNES.

OXALURIA AND INSANITY.—It has been noticed that the continued presence in the urine of oxalates has often been associated with symptoms of nervous depression, dyspepsia, hypochondriasis and even melancholia. These affections have been said to be dependent on as well as associated with the presence of oxalates. It must however be owned that oxalates are frequently found in the urine of persons in excellent health, and it seems as likely that the oxaluria is dependent on the deranged digestion, want of assimilation and nervous depression, as that the latter are dependent on the former. (*See* URINE.)

OXYÆSTHESIA (ὀξύς, sharp, acute; αἴσθησις, sensation). Abnormally acute power of sensation, such as occurs in certain forms of hysteria.

OXYGEUSIA (ὀξύς, sharp, acute; γεῦσις, taste). Excessive acuteness of taste.

P

PACHYMENINGITIS INTERNA HÆMORRHAGICA. — **Arachnoid Cysts. Arachnoid Hæmatoma. Hæmatoma of the Dura Mater** (παχύς, thick; μῆνιγξ, membrane).

I. Cerebral.—The conditions variously described under one or other of the above names, although not unknown under other circumstances, are nevertheless met with in overwhelming preponderance in association with the various forms of mental disease. Hence it follows that it is chiefly in asylum practice that they come under notice. Among the insane inmates of asylums, indeed, the condition is far from uncommon; nevertheless, in spite of the opportunities thus afforded for the study of the affection, much difference of opinion has existed as to its pathology, which perhaps even now can hardly be said to be thoroughly elucidated.

Since the morbid appearances met with vary greatly in different cases, it will be convenient to single out two or three of the leading types of the affection for brief description.

In what may perhaps be styled the simplest form, the inner surface of the dura mater is found to be covered to a greater or less extent with a thin, delicate, gelatinous film or pellicle, which is almost always more or less coherent, so that whatever be its degree of tenuity, it can generally be detached, to a certain extent at any rate, as a distinct membrane; the film may be colourless and translucent, or have a slightly yellowish tint, or may present a reddish hue over a large portion of its area, and it is, in any case, very generally spotted or blotched with black, rust-coloured or ochreous dots or patches. On raising the film with forceps from the inner surface of the dura mater, to which it is loosely adherent, the epithelial surface of this latter membrane is seen to present its usual smooth, shining character, and to be, to all appearance, unaltered.

The most common situation for such a membranous film is the convexity of the hemispheres, and if occurring to but a small extent it may be confined to the parietal region of one or both sides; frequently, however, it extends down towards the base, and occupies a portion of the middle and occipital fossæ, one or both; or it may reach into the middle fossa on one side and the occipital on the other. When spread over a more extended area the membrane is usually thicker than that above noted, as will be shortly described. It tapers off gradually, so that its boundaries are not clearly defined. At other times the membrane, although still preserving a soft, filmy character, has a more decided hæmorrhagic appearance than is indicated in the above description; indeed,

* See Paper read before the Brit. Gynæcolog. Soc., by Dr. Barnes, "On the Correlations of the Sexual Functions and Mental Disorders of Women," Oct. 8, 1890, and the discussion which followed, in which Drs. Savage, Wilks, Hack Tuke, Mercier, Bantock, R. T. Smith, Heywood Smith, Hugh Fenton, Percy Smith, Macnaughten Jones, Lankford (U.S.A.), took part.

one of the most common forms under which this condition occurs, is that of a thin, reddish, or reddish-black pellicle, spread over the inner surface of the dura mater and loosely attached thereto, which both to the naked eye and to the microscope has much the appearance of recent blood clot. Frequently, however, the morbid phenomena met with are much more pronounced than those above described. It is not uncommonly the case that large, soft, reddish, reddish-black, chocolate-brown, or buff-coloured membranes are found lining the whole, or a large portion, of the inner surface of the dura mater, occupying not only the convexity, but spreading also over the fossæ, and varying in thickness from 1 to 3 mm. or more; they are still but loosely attached to the inner surface of the dura mater, from which they can be readily peeled off. It is usually the case, under such circumstances, that a considerable quantity of reddish serum is found in the sub-dural space, and the surface of the cerebral convolutions may present in places a flattened appearance as if they had been subjected to pressure, and here and there they may be tinged with a rusty red or ochre hue, as if from imbibition of blood-colouring matter. The surfaces of these soft membranes are frequently paler and more fibrinous-looking than the central parts, so that on section the membrane shows a dark centre bounded by paler lines, and sometimes they consist of two distinct laminæ, the space between which is occupied with broken-down or variously altered blood, or serum. When this is the case, the whole presents something of the appearance of a cyst, hence one of the names under which this condition has been described. Like the thin filmy pellicles, these larger membranes taper off gradually at their extremities.

Under other circumstances the membrane is found to have acquired a firmer consistence and a paler tint, and to present much more the appearance of a layer of fibrin; these characters may prevail throughout its whole extent, but more commonly, perhaps, portions of the lamina are pale and fibrinous-looking, whilst in other portions the signs of recent hæmorrhage predominate. The union with the dura mater is somewhat more intimate than in the cases hitherto noted, but the membrane can still be readily stripped from the surface to which it is attached.

But at times, although somewhat rarely, the whole of the inner surface of the dura mater is found to be lined with a firm fibrinous membrane varying from 2 to 4 mm., or more, in thickness; this membrane is not homogeneous, but consists of several distinct layers of fibrin, which are more or less separable from each other; the adhesion to the dura mater is much more intimate than in any of the cases hitherto described, the whole, in fact, appearing to form one laminated membrane; the adhesions, which are, for the most part, vascular in nature, can however always be broken down without difficulty. The entire surface of the dura mater may be thus coated, including all the fossæ at the base of the skull, with the exception of that beneath the tentorium cerebelli, in which position it is rarely met with; the membrane is, however, seldom or never equally thick throughout; almost invariably it is thickest over the convexity, and gradually tails off in the fossæ, being generally thinnest over the orbital plates.

Although the leading types of the affection have been described separately, it must not be supposed that any hard-and-fast line can be drawn between them. Contrasted as they are in their extremes, as instanced in the delicate gelatinous films, and the thick laminated fibrinous membranes, they nevertheless graduate into one another by an almost perfect gradation of transitional forms; not only so, but it is common to find the different forms mixed up in the same case; thus, a portion of the dura mater may be lined with a *fibrinous* lamina of greater or less thickness, and on the surface of this latter lamina may be found a distinctly *hæmorrhagic* membrane of obviously much more recent origin.

A word or two as to the microscopical appearances. In the case of the thin hæmorrhagic membranes first described, we find a meshwork of fibrin in which are entangled red and white corpuscles, the whole having much the character presented by a layer of blood-clot. But as the membrane becomes thicker and more fibrinous we find the appearances change. Bands of imperfectly formed fibrous tissue now make their appearance, running parallel to one another, and to the surface of the membrane, and containing long oval nuclei; between the bands may be seen in places collections of red blood-globules without definite boundary wall, whilst delicate newly formed capillary vessels are numerous. Whilst in the case of the firm fibrinous membranes the fibrous bands have become closer, the nuclei more distinct and the capillary vessels less numerous, collections of red blood-globules are no longer met with, but little heaps of hæmatoidin granules are frequent.

But although the above are the chief types of what has been described as *pachymeningitis*, an incorrect idea would be obtained of the affection did we not include other cases which, though not usually grouped under this term, nevertheless appear to the writer to have a most important bearing on the question of pathology.

Allusion is made to the presence of fluid blood in the sub-dural space, or of this combined with recent blood-clot lying upon the surface of the arachnoid or dura mater, but not forming a continuous membrane. Such cases occur more frequently than is supposed. Thus, out of 54 cases observed by the writer in which blood or membrane or both combined were found in the sub-dural space, no less than 8—about one-seventh of the whole—presented fluid blood or recent clot without the presence of any trace of membrane on the inner surface of the dura mater.

Before, however, discussing the pathology of the affection, it will be convenient to consider certain facts bearing on its ætiology.

The writer has elsewhere given* an analysis of 42 cases of this disease, which had come under personal observation in Rainhill Asylum, and to these, 12 others can now be added, raising the total to 54.

These 54 cases occurred in a series of 637 unselected post-mortem examinations of insane patients, which gives a percentage of 8.47 cases of hæmatoma, on the whole series of autopsies.

In the 54 cases, the age of the youngest patient was thirty, that of the oldest eighty-five, the average age of the whole being 51.61, the average age of the asylum population from which the cases were drawn being about 43.33. Taking the cases according to the decades at which they occurred, we get the following result:—

	Cases.
From 30 to 40 years	11
" 40 " 50 "	13
" 50 " 60 "	18
" 60 " 70 "	6
" 70 " 80 "	3
" 80 " 90 "	3
Total . .	54

Hence it appears clear that hæmatoma or pachymeningitis is an affection of advancing years, the decade between fifty and sixty seeming to be the one most obnoxious to the disease. Of the 637 autopsies, in 330 the patients were males, and in 307 females; whereas of the 54 cases of hæmatoma 31 were males, and 23 females. This gives a percentage of 9.39 on the total number of male cases examined, and of 7.49 on the total number of females. These figures indicate, therefore, that hæmatoma is more common in males than in females, a result which is in accordance with the usual opinion.

The greater preponderance of male cases becomes more pronounced if we take examples of general paralysis only. Thus, out of 126 cases of this disease in males, hæmatoma was met with in 23—a percentage of 18.25; whereas out of 49 female cases, 6 occurred—a percentage of 12.24.

Coming now to the form of mental disorder, we find that the 54 cases of hæmatoma can be classified as follows:—

	Cases.
General paralysis	29
Melancholia, acute	3
" chronic	2
Mental stupor	1
Mania with epilepsy	1
Chronic mania	4
" " with dementia . .	2
Senile mania	1
Dementia, secondary . . .	5
" senile	6
Total . .	54

Hence it appears that hæmatoma is somewhat more common in general paralysis than in all other forms of insanity put together. This great preponderance of cases of general paralysis is also shown by the statistics of Sir James Crichton Browne, who found * that, out of a series of 59 cases of all forms of insanity in which hæmatoma was met with, 29 were examples of general paralysis.

It is further apparent from the above statement that it is chiefly in cases of chronic insanity that this affection comes under notice, for in only 3 out of the 54 cases had the mental disease been of less than three months' duration, and in the vast majority it had been reckoned rather by years than by months.

Although it is not unusual for the affection to be unilateral, it is more common to find both sides of the brain involved. Of the 54 cases, 20 were entirely unilateral, and 34 bilateral. In many of these latter cases, however, the disease was more marked on one side than the other, and in 7 of them the difference was pronounced. When one side only is involved, the disease does not appear to have a marked preference for either; thus, of the above 20 unilateral cases, in 10 the right side was affected, and in 10 the left. Sir James Crichton Browne, however, thinks

* "On Hæmorrhages and False Membranes within the Cerebral Sub-dural Space occurring in the Insane," *Journal of Mental Science*, Jan. 1888.

* *Journal of Psychological Medicine*, Oct. 1875.

that the left side is the one most prone to be attacked.

Although it is chiefly among those recognised as insane that the affection is met with, it also occurs in the subjects of chronic alcoholism, a neurosis which is indeed closely allied to insanity, and which connotes a similar brain degeneration. Apart from these conditions, and excluding traumatic cases, the affection appears to be extremely rare.

What is the **pathology** of the conditions above described under the name *pachymeningitis* or *hæmatoma of dura mater?*

Two opposing theories have been formulated with reference to it. The one describes the phenomena met with in terms of inflammation, and, whilst recognising the hæmorrhagic element, regards this as secondary to a primary inflammatory change; the other ignores the agency of inflammation, looking upon this at the most as secondary and trivial, and attributes the appearances presented to the organisation more or less partial or complete of a primary hæmorrhagic effusion.

According to the inflammatory theory, the thin gelatinous film which is met with on the inner surface of the dura mater is the result of an inflammatory exudation from the vessels of the dura mater itself. This film becomes permeated with delicate thin walled capillaries, and gradually becomes organised. Other similar films are developed upon this in slow succession, until at length a laminated membrane is formed. To account for the hæmorrhagic element it is supposed that the delicate newly formed vessels which ramify through the membrane frequently become ruptured, and pour out their contents in greater or less amount; and that the presence of recent clot, or of pigment granules and other forms of altered blood, may thus be explained. This interpretation of the phenomena was especially advocated by Virchow, and it is to the authority of that great name that we are indebted for the predominance of the inflammatory theory. The opposite view, according to which the primary mischief is a hæmorrhagic effusion, was insisted on by Prescott Hewett * and others before Virchow's researches on the subject; Huguenin † has since then revived this view, and more recently the present writer,‡ as the result of an entirely independent investigation, has come to the same conclusion.

It is reasonable to suppose that, if the affection were a primary inflammation of the dura mater, evidence of this would be afforded by the condition of the dura mater itself. This, however, is far from being the case. As previously stated, when the membrane is stripped from the dura mater to which it is loosely attached, the epithelial surface of this latter membrane is seen to be smooth and shining. There is no capillary injection or other evidence of inflammatory mischief; nor, indeed, in the earlier stages at least, is there any increase of thickness. It is true that, in association with the thick laminated fibrinous membranes, it is not uncommon to find the dura mater slightly thicker than normal, and, on stripping the false membrane from it, a certain roughness may be left, due to the separation of the vascular adhesions. These changes are, however, very slight, and, occurring as they do late in the progress of the case, are much more readily explicable on the idea that they are occasioned by the irritation set up by the clot, than that they are marks of a primary inflammatory process. It is reasonable to suppose that, if the latter supposition were correct, the signs of inflammation would be abundantly manifest, and not either altogether absent, or trivial and equivocal. As is well known, a thrombus in a vein sets up irritation in the walls of the vessel with effusion of leucocytes, and it is through the agency of these migratory cells that the clot becomes adherent to the vessel, and subsequently undergoes organisation. Now, the inner surface of the dura mater may be compared to the inner wall of a vein within which coagulation has occurred, and the fibrinous membranes found beneath the dura mater may be looked upon as clots, which have undergone partial organisation through the agency of the leucocytes which have migrated from the vessels of the dura mater, in response to the irritation set up by these clots.

The structure of the membrane itself supports this view. The reddish or reddish-black membranes have much the appearance both to the naked eye and to the microscope of recent clot, whilst the pale laminated membranes closely resemble the fibrinous thrombi met with in veins when the coagulation has been of some standing, or the layers of fibrin occurring in the sac of an aneurism.

The laminated membranes are doubtless at times caused by successive hæmorrhages; but a single large hæmorrhage appears quite capable of producing a laminated appearance owing to the changes which take place in the clot.

In an organising membrane also rupture

* "Medico-Chirurgical Transactions," 1845.

† Ziemssen's "Cyclopædia."

‡ *Loc. cit.*

of newly formed vessels undoubtedly at these occurs, producing fresh hæmorrhages, but these appear to be always small in amount.

On the theory that the membrane is formed from the blood, and not the blood from the membrane, it is reasonable to suppose that the hæmorrhagic effusion would occasionally occur to a sufficient extent to prove fatal before there was time for a membrane to become developed. As a matter of fact, as indicated above, such cases are by no means rare.

If it be argued that these cases are not to be included in the same category as those in which a sub-dural membrane is present, it may be replied that the two classes of cases occur under just the same sets of conditions, and there is a very gradual transition from one to the other.

The rarity with which the affection occurs in the cerebellar fossæ is also worth noting. Whilst it is quite common to meet with a hæmorrhagic membrane on the upper surface of the tentorium cerebelli, it is very rare to meet with one beneath it. On the inflammatory theory such a condition of things is quite inexplicable, but the mechanical obstacle which the tentorium must present to the gravitation of blood into the cerebellar fossæ, supplies us at once with the interpretation of the exemption of this region.

The period of life at which this affection occurs is also significant. As shown in the statistics previously quoted, subdural hæmatoma is distinctly a disease of advancing years, and the connection between age and arterial degeneration and tendency to hæmorrhage scarcely requires emphasising.

The affection is indeed relatively common in very aged dements where the conditions are as little favourable to inflammatory action as can well be imagined.

The inflammatory theory is rejected then in favour of that which ascribes all the phenomena met with to the simple effusion of blood into the arachnoid cavity, in greater or less quantity, and it may be more or less frequently repeated. But we have yet to inquire into the source of these hæmorrhagic effusions, and into the reasons for their occurrence. With reference to the origin of the hæmorrhage, there can be but little doubt that it comes in the majority of cases from the vessels of the pia mater, which occupy the summits of the gyri; in these regions the pia mater and arachnoid have in many cases of insanity an intimate union, whilst in most cases of general paralysis they are so glued together as practically to constitute one membrane, so that if a vessel were to rupture, it would tend to pour its contents direct into the arachnoid cavity, and not diffuse them into the sub-arachnoid space.

Sometimes, however, as the writer has observed, the blood first diffuses itself to a small extent beneath the arachnoid, and afterwards bursts into the sub-dural space.

As regards the reasons for such rupture, the writer has previously expressed his opinion that a solution of the problem is to be found in two of the conditions, which singly or combined occur in most cases of insanity—viz., wasting of the hemispheres, and general or localised congestion of the meninges, assisted as these conditions undoubtedly are in many cases by actual degeneration of vessel walls. Since the writer published this view, he has found that Sir James Crichton Browne had expressed a similar opinion, and that Huguenin, in laying stress on the brain-wasting which occurs in the class of cases in which hæmatoma is met with, appears to have had the same idea in mind. It is clear, indeed, that the atrophy of the convolutions must tend to remove a good deal of support from the vessels of the pia mater occupying the summits of the gyri, and thus create a tendency to congestion and rupture, and if we analyse the conditions under which the so-called pachymeningitis occurs, we find that brain-wasting is the one feature that is common to all cases alike. It is not asserted that hæmatoma never occurs without cerebral atrophy, although the writer has not met with such cases, but the two conditions are at any rate associated in such an overwhelming majority of cases that the connection can hardly be accidental. This it is which explains the comparative frequency of the disease among the insane, especially where the mental affection has been of some standing, and the rarity with which it occurs outside asylums.

If along with loss of support from atrophy of convolutions, there is attendant congestion of meninges, either local or general (which again may itself be partly occasioned by loss of support), it is clear that the conditions favourable to rupture are enhanced. As a matter of fact, the vessels of the pia mater which occupy the summits of the gyri are subject in many cases of insanity to repeated and violent attacks of congestion, such attacks being especially frequent and intense in general paralysis. Thus, it is not uncommon in cases of this disease to find patches of extreme congestion of the pia mater so extreme as almost to resemble an ecchymosis. Such a condition is of course highly favourable to actual rupture, and if combined with this there is weakness of vessel walls from degeneration, we have another powerful factor in favour of hæmorrhage.

Hitherto no mention has been made of the symptoms which the affection occasions, and, as a matter of fact, in the majority of cases, any symptoms that may be produced pass unrecognised.

This circumstance of itself points to the compensatory nature of the affection; for making every allowance for the fact that the disease is usually met with in demented persons in whom symptoms of all kinds are masked, there can be little doubt that even in such cases an inflammatory process would make itself known more frequently than is found to be the case in the affection before us.

On the supposition, however, that the blood as a rule does little or nothing more than fill up the space left by the wasting brain, we find a ready explanation of the comparative rarity of symptoms. As a matter of fact, indeed, the affection is usually discovered after death in cases in which during life there had been no suspicion of its presence.

But this absence of symptoms does not always occur. Occasionally, as indeed one might expect would happen at times, the effused blood does not stop short with filling up the vacuum left by the wasting brain, but spreading further compresses the surface of the brain, acts as an irritant, and declares itself by such signs as convulsions, paralysis, &c. Thus, in one case, a female general paralytic, aged forty-four, fell down one morning in a fit, and for some twelve hours after this she lay completely comatose with all her limbs perfectly paralysed, and flaccid, stertorous breathing, abolition of reflexes, and lowered temperature. Death occurred nine months after this attack, and a thick fibrinous membrane was found coating the whole of the inner aspect of the dura mater.

In another case, that of a female aged fifty-eight, who had melancholia with delusions of persecution, the patient one evening was found comatose, with complete paralysis of left side. After death, which occurred in 34 hours, a recent clot, mostly black in colour, was found in the sub-dural space, covering the frontal, parietal and temporo-sphenoidal lobes on the right side only, and weighing altogether 92 grammes.

In a third case, a female senile dement, aged seventy-one, was seized with convulsions, bilateral, but more marked on right side than on left, with conjugate deviation of head and eyes to right. Death occurred in the course of twelve hours, and at the autopsy recent clot was found, loosely attached to the dura mater, spread over both hemispheres, but being distinctly more pronounced on the left side than the right.

In a fourth case in which a female general paralytic, aged twenty-eight, died seven days after being seized with severe left-sided convulsions succeeded by paralysis, followed three days later with signs of irritative contracture of right arm, there were found at the autopsy two hæmorrhagic membranes, already commencing to organise, a small one on the left and a larger one on the right; the latter occupied the whole of the convexity and dipped down into the fossæ; it was about 3 mm. in thickness, attached loosely to the dura mater, and its surfaces were already becoming fibrinous.

If these last cases, instead of proving rapidly fatal, had been prolonged for a few weeks or months, the inference is that a fibrinous membrane would have been found, as in the first case.

In two or three other cases observed by the writer when the hæmorrhage was less in amount, and death did not occur for a few days, an irregular elevation of temperature was noted, also occasional vomiting, and a tendency to frequent restless movements of the upper extremities. Drowsiness, or a deepening of the usual hebetude, and headache, were likewise at times observed. Even, however, when the hæmorrhage has been sufficient to produce localised paralysis, it is often a matter of extreme difficulty to determine whether the effusion has taken place within the substance, or upon the surface, of the brain.

Huguenin mentions as very important gradually appearing symptoms of superficial lesions of both hemispheres, facial paralysis, hemiparesis on the same side, and then symptoms of irritation or paralysis on the opposite side.

The writer thinks also that *cæteris paribus*, the coma is not so profound when the effusion takes place upon the surface of the brain, as when it occurs within its substance.

It will be observed that the diagnosis, unsatisfactory as it is, rests upon the recognition of the initial hæmorrhage, and the symptoms of irritation set up the clots, and that the formation of membrane does not declare itself by symptoms.

The question of treatment may be dismissed in a few words. Having regard to the secondary nature of the affection, and to the fact that it is comparatively seldom recognised during life, treatment is for the most part alike uncalled for, and of no avail. Where, however, a copious hæmorrhage produces recognisable symptoms, the indications for medical treatment are the same as those for cerebral hæmorrhage generally, with the exception, perhaps, that local measures, such as ice to the head, are likely here to be more efficacious. When the symptoms are obviously those of brain compression, surgical interference may at times be resorted to with a successful result. The *rôle* of the trephine in this affection is, however, a very limited one, and its frequent use would be likely to have a deleterious, rather than a beneficial effect.

2. **Spinal.**—Under this head it is not proposed to deal with the affection commonly known as pachymeningitis of the cord, descriptions of which may be found in all works on neurology. Allusion is rather made to the presence of hæmorrhagic and fibrinous membranes within the spinal canal, which appear to be analogous to those already described within the cranium. This affection is far less frequent in the spinal canal than in the cranium. Mickle* alludes to the occasional occurrence of old durhæmatomata within the spinal canal, and also traces of spinal hæmorrhagic pachymeningitis, as well as softish dark clot from recent spinal meningeal hæmorrhage in general paralysis; and Savage has also seen pachymeningitic membranes, and recent spinal hæmorrhage under similar circumstances. In all these cases the membrane or blood was found within the sac of the dura mater between it and the surface of the cord.

In all cases observed by the writer, however, the membrane was situated on the outer aspect of the dura mater, between it and the walls of the spinal canal. In three such cases† there was a fibrinous-looking membrane from 2 to 4 mm. thick, occupying the cervical or dorsal region of the cord lying upon the outer surface of the dura mater on its posterior aspect, and being loosely attached to this, and to the posterior aspect of the spinal canal; the membranes were for the most part pale in colour and soft in consistence; in one case the membrane extended along some of the nerves proceeding from the cord.

Dr. Percy Smith has described an exactly similar case, and Dr. Clouston alludes to two others. All these cases occurred in general paralytics.

It may be taken for granted, therefore, that although hæmorrhagic effusions may be found within the spinal arachnoid cavity in general paralysis, there are also, though somewhat rarely, met with in this disease, fibrinous membranes lying upon the *external* aspect of the dura mater between it and the spinal canal, and occupying usually the cervical and dorsal regions of the cord. The balance of evidence seems to be in favour of these membranes being of hæmorrhagic origin, and comparable to the somewhat similar membranes so commonly met with beneath the cranial dura mater in this disease. It is doubtful how far they produce symptoms. In one of the writer's cases a diagnosis was made during life by the presence of symptoms of irritation of spinal nerves—viz., retraction of the head and rigidity of the extremities; but here the effusion had extended along some of the spinal nerves, to the irritation of which the symptoms were doubtless attributable. (*See* PATHOLOGY.) JOSEPH WIGLESWORTH.

* "General Paralysis of the Insane," 2nd ed.

† *British Medical Journal*, Sept. 21, 1880.

PACK, THE WET.—A form of treatment in some varieties of insanity. (*See* BATHS.)

PALATE IN IDIOTS.—In genetous idiocy the shape of the hard palate is often very characteristic. It is high, very arched and narrowed from side to side, so that the molar teeth are closely approximated. This kind of palate is sometimes met with in healthy individuals, but if it is present in a young subject who is showing signs of mental incompetency, it is useful in indicating that the mental affection is probably congenital. (*See* IDIOCY.)

PÂMOISON (Fr.). Hysterical swooning.

PAMPHOBIA. (*See* PANOPHOBIA.)

PAMPLEGIA. General paralysis.

PANOPHOBIA, PANPHOBIA (derivation disputed; either, πᾶς, all; φόβος, fear; or from the legend in Herodotus, which relates that Pan assisted the Athenians at Marathon by striking causeless terror among the enemy, who therefore fled panic-stricken; and φόβος, fear). A variety of hypochondriasis characterised by groundless alarm. Indefinable fear. Morbid apprehension. (Fr. and Ger. *pantophobie*.)

PANTAPHOBIA (πᾶς, all; α, priv.; φόβος, fear). Absolute fearlessness.

PANTOPHOBIA. (*See* PANOPHOBIA.)

PARABULIA (παρά, beside; βουλή, will or purpose). Disordered mind or purpose; perverted will. (Fr. *parabulie*.)

PARACHOLIA. (*See* POLYCHOLIA.)

PARACOPE (παρακόπτω, I strike falsely). Literally, coining, but used by Hippocrates for delirium, especially for the slight delirium accompanying fevers. Used also for insanity. (Fr. *paracope.*)

PARACOPTIC. Insane; pertaining to insanity.

PARACOUSIA (παρακούω, I hear imperfectly). False sensations of hearing. Auditory illusions. (Fr. *paracousie;* Ger. *Falschhören.*)

PARACROUSIS, PARACRUSIS (παρακρούω, I strike aside). Literally, striking a false note. A term used similarly to paracope; applied to madness by Hippocrates. (Fr. *paracruse.*)

PARACUSIS IMAGINARIA. The hearing of imaginary sounds, not existing outside the body. (Fr. *paracouse imaginaire.*)

PARÆSTHESIA (παρά, beyond; αἴσθησις, sensation). Perverted sensation occurring in the form of "tingling" or "pricking" sensations, when a part of the body is touched or injured. A symptom in various forms of mental disease. Also applied to perverted emotional states (emotional parsæthesia). (Fr. *paræsthésie.*)

PARAGEUSIS (παρά, beyond; γεῦσις, taste). A term for morbid taste. (Fr. *parageusie.*)

PARAGRAPHIA (παραγράφω, I write improperly). The making of mistakes in writing, such as using one word for another, or omitting the end of a word; a manifestation of cerebral disorder.—**P. literalis,** form in which the patient cannot write even letters, but only signs.—**P. verbalis,** form in which the patient is able to write letters or syllables, but not complete words.

PARAHYPNOSIS (παρά; ὕπνος, sleep). Abnormal sleep as in hypnotism or somnambulism.

PARALALIA (παραλαλέω, I talk at random). A permanent or temporary alteration in oral expression characterised by the retention of the power of thought, and of formation and combination of ideas, and yet at the same time by the impossibility of finding the right words to express those ideas, or of co-ordinating those words which can still be articulated. (Fr. *paralalie.*)

PARALDEHYDE. (See SEDATIVES.)

PARALEREMA (παρά, beyond; λήρημα, foolish talk). Delirium.

PARALERESIS (παρά, beyond; λήρησις, dotage). A term for slight delirium, as from fever. (Fr. *paralérème;* Ger. *Irrereden.*)

PARALEROS, PARALERUS (παράληρος, talking foolishly). Delirious. (Fr. *délirant;* Ger. *Irreredend.*)

PARALEXIA (παρά; λέξις, a word). Difficulty in reading, though the person may be able to write readily from dictation; a form of aphasia with word blindness.

PARALGESIA (παρά, beyond; ἄλγος, pain). The abolition of pain. Anæsthesia.

PARALLAGE, PARALLAGMA.
PARALLAXIS (παραλλάσσω, I pervert or change). The terms really apply to the overlapping of bones, but have been applied to mental aberration.

PARALOGIA (παρά, beyond; λόγος, speech). A slight degree of madness or delirium. (Fr. *paralogia.*)

PARALYSIE CÉRÉBRALE, PARALYSIE GÉNÉRALE (Fr.). Terms for general paralysis of the insane.

PARALYSIE DES ALIÉNÉS (Fr.).
PARALYSE DER IRREN (Ger.) General paralysis (*q.v.*).

PARALYSIS AGITANS, Insanity associated with.—The mental disorders to which paralysis agitans may give rise have not as yet attracted much attention. This is not surprising, when we consider that the history of this affection is but of recent date, and that all its peculiarities have not yet been fully recognised. In 1817 Parkinson first described this disease, which has sometimes been named after him, Parkinson's disease, but in spite of most careful investigations, the anatomical lesions connected with the affection have not yet been elucidated.

In order to study the psychical consequences of paralysis agitans, we must discriminate between three groups of mental abnormality.

(1) Those patients belong to the first who present nothing but a change of temper and character; they become impressionable and excessively irritable, are troubled and excited about trivial matters, are unable to bear contradiction, and fly into a rage at the slightest provocation. They insist on having incessant and undivided attention shown them, while they are restless, distrustful, and suspicious; they will not allow any one to speak near them in a subdued voice, and imagine that people try to hide themselves from them; some of them are ashamed of themselves by reason of their affliction and the inconvenience that results therefrom; they become taciturn, and indulge in emotional weeping on the slightest occasion; this disposition is reflected in their features, which, in many cases, partake of an expression of intense grief. Lastly, they become indifferent and apathetic, lose their inclination for work, and no longer derive any pleasure from matters formerly interesting to them. None of the symptoms mentioned, properly speaking, appertain to insanity, but the transformation brought about by them may well be con-

sidered as a first stage of mental aberration. Although we may meet with similar modifications in many other nervous diseases, we have to recognise that grief and irritability are two tendencies common to paralysis agitans.

(2) Patients of the second group are those who present weakening of the intellectual faculties, which may vary from simple blunting of the mind to complete dementia. Authors have paid special attention to this form of insanity in paralysis agitans, and most of them describe it. The disorder manifests itself in a weakened intellect, memory becomes unreliable, thought is slow and difficult, and those who come into contact with the patient note that he no longer possesses his ordinary mental lucidity. The symptoms become aggravated, and mental decrepitude ensues long before the advent of old age. These mental conditions are nearly always reflected in the features of the patient and give him a peculiar aspect, which may be considered as pathognomonic of the affection; the face is immobile and mask-like in its changelessness of expression, the eyes at the same time are fixed, and, as Ball aptly remarks, the expression simulates certain cases of stupor with melancholia; in the latter, however, the intellect, although much disordered, persists, whilst here, on the contrary, it fails, and the patients are in a condition of actual dementia which, as the malady proceeds, becomes aggravated and is at last quite incurable.

(3) The third group comprises those who present symptoms of insanity properly speaking. The knowledge of this third group is of recent date, and is to be reckoned only from the time when Ball drew attention to it by his paper read before the Section of Mental Medicine at the International Congress in London in 1881. Before that time only two or three isolated observations, of which, however, little notice had been taken, had been published. Since then, Ball has resumed his inquiries into the subject, while opportunities have likewise been afforded us of investigating this psychosis.

Positive observations leave no doubt that paralysis agitans may bring about mental disorder; in fact, none of the usual causes of insanity can be found in these cases, and notably one prominent factor is wanting — viz., hereditary influence. There is no reason to dispute the assumption that paralysis agitans may effect this mental disturbance, because we have parallel instances in chorea, epilepsy, and other neuroses, in which lesions of the nerve-centres have not been discovered, but which may equally be the causes of mental disorder.

The symptoms of insanity in paralysis agitans are variable. The most common is a morbid exaggeration of the sentiments or the grief in which the patients have been steeped since the commencement of the malady, into a melancholia proper, which may either be simple, or consist of a more or less profound depression complicated and accompanied by hallucinations and insane ideas. The hallucinations may affect either hearing or sight. The patient believes he hears threatening, insulting or mocking voices. The hallucinations of sight are very prominent; he may see himself surrounded by enemies, and he may hear them at the same time; another patient sees his bed surrounded by individuals who threaten him; while another imagines his room to be full of robbers, and sees them groping and feeling about the walls; or he sees his wife surrounded by suspicious-looking persons who wish to annoy her. These hallucinations may occur by day as well as by night. There are, however, some to whom they occur only at night, and who, with the approach of day, cease to be troubled by such sensory disorders.

The insane conceptions, if hallucinations are present, are in conformity with the latter, and partake of the character of ideas of persecution. The patients believe themselves besieged by enemies, of whom they see traces everywhere; they imagine that they are about to be robbed, or that people are endeavouring to injure them in some other way. Under the influence of these ideas they become still more irritable and distrustful; they carry weapons in order to defend themselves, and, as may readily be understood, may become dangerous to those about them. It is, however, necessary to bear in mind that the ideas of persecution observed in such cases are not those of true persecution mania, especially because they do not develop in the same manner; and, in addition to this, the frequency of visual hallucinations proves that we have here a morbid condition quite different from persecution-mania, in which hallucinations of sight are very rare.

Besides hallucinations and insane conceptions we have to mention disorders of sensibility, which may be connected with either of these two forms of mental aberration. One patient believes himself consumed by an internal fire; another feels pricks and cuts on his skin; a third believes that he has more than two legs, and has the sensation of having one in front and one behind. Some patients have an impression that their legs gradually grow longer until they reach an obstruction at some distance from them. These disorders are undoubtedly connected with the cutaneous hyperæsthesia sometimes met with in the course of paralysis agitans.

One of the most serious and common symptoms of melancholic depression in paralysis agitans is the tendency to suicide which is found in the majority of those labouring under this affection, and is due either to hallucinations, insane conceptions, or to the restlessness and weakness induced by the disease itself.

The symptoms of insanity which we have here enumerated are those most commonly met with in paralysis agitans; they are always, therefore, of a depressive type, bordering in some cases on simple melancholia, but most frequently constituting a melancholia accompanied by multiple hallucinations, or suicidal impulses. There are few exceptions to this rule. Patients are sometimes to be met with who are continually or intermittently the subjects of excitement. There are also some who, without being actually excited, present animated accessions of a gay, self-satisfied character, which, by their alternation with depression, recall the symptoms of circular insanity.

A remarkable peculiarity of the insanity connected with paralysis agitans is that sometimes its paroxysms and intermissions coincide with the exaggeration and diminution of the tremor. According to Ball, this coincidence is almost the rule. He says: "The disorders of the intellect in paralysis agitans are not permanent, but appear to become exaggerated with the aggravation of the sensory symptoms, and they seem to disappear when the tremor decreases or ceases entirely." Our observations, however, point to the fact that in some well-determined cases intellectual disorder is developed in a manner absolutely independent of the motor and sensory disorders.

The usual tendency of the insanity—whatever its form may be—is to lead rapidly to dementia, and therefore the patients of the third group are easily confounded with those of the second.

Is insanity frequent in the course of paralysis agitans? If we are to judge merely from the small number of observations recorded it would appear that it is not. Ball, however, thinks this to be a mistake, and he maintains that paralysis agitans is more frequently accompanied by mental disorders than is generally supposed. The reason why we do not see it is because the patients in some way hide their mental symptoms, because their physical disorder overshadows their mental obliquity, or because they advance towards dementia rapidly, and the weakening of their mental faculties prevents the symptoms of insanity from becoming obvious. With regard to insanity, properly speaking, we have, according to the opinion expressed by Bucknill and Rayner at the Congress in London in 1881, to limit ourselves, until further investigations have been made, to the assertion that it is sometimes met with in the course of this neurosis. We have, however, at the same time to admit that there are but few such patients who could not in various degrees be classified under one of the first two groups which we have enumerated.

It remains for us to study the pathogenic relation between paralysis agitans and insanity; of the relation itself there can be no doubt as we have already indicated, but the fact remains that in the observations published, insanity did not develop for some time after the commencement of the tremor; there is an interval ranging up to eight years between the two; beyond this statement, however, everything is hypothetical. If it were proved, as Ball avers, that the fluctuations of insanity are intimately connected with the variations in intensity of the tremor, it would undoubtedly be necessary for these two phenomena to be attributable to one and the same case. On the other hand, we know almost nothing about the pathological anatomy of paralysis agitans, so that we are unable to refer the symptoms of insanity to gross cerebral lesions. As, however, science in its progress has established the fact that every form of insanity is due to an organic or functional change of the nervous centres, we may be permitted to assume that insanity in paralysis agitans obeys the same law, and that if mental disorders occur in this neurosis it is because some modifications have been brought about in the brain which are apt to alter and pervert the normal mental operations.

The prognosis and the treatment of insanity in paralysis agitans are the same as those indicated for the disease which causes it.

V. Parant.

[*References.*—B. Ball. De l'insanité dans la paralysie agitante, Encéphale, 1882. V. Parant. La paralysie agitante examinée comme cause de la Folie, Annales médico-psychologiques, 1883. Ringrose Atkins. A Case of Paralysis Agitans in which Insanity occurred, Journ. Ment. Sci., Jan. 1882. Proceedings of the International Congress of London, Journ. Ment. Sci., Oct. 1881.]

PARALYSIS, ASCENDING.—Term applied to cases of general paralysis which commence with tabetic symptoms. (*See* Locomotor Ataxy.)

PARALYSIS, GALOPPIRENDE (Ger.) Term applied to the form of general paralysis which runs a rapid fatal course, and is characterised by extreme mental and nervous excitement with sudden collapse. It is a subdivision of the *agitirte Form* of general paralysis (Kraepelin).

PARALYTIC IDIOCY, OR IMBECILITY. (*See* IDIOCY and IMBECILITY.)

PARALYTIC INSANITY. Term applied to general paralysis, but it should be restricted to insanity following ordinary paralysis.

PARAMIMIA (*παρά*; *μιμέομαι*, I imitate). Disordered expression; use of tone or gesture not in accord with the words employed.

PARAMNESIA (*παρά*, beyond; *μνῆσις*, memory). An affection of the faculty of expression caused by a loss of memory of the signification of words heard and seen. (Fr. *paramnésie*.) (*See* MEMORY, DISORDERS OF.)

PARANEURISMUS (*παρά*, beyond; *νεῦρον*, a nerve). A term for a nervous affection. (Fr. *paraneurisme*.)

PARANŒA. (*See* PARANOIA.)

PARANOIA (*παρά*, beyond, the opposite of; *νοέω*, I understand).—The use of this word has become very frequent in Germany and in the United States, but it has not obtained favour in Great Britain. It was the term employed by Dr. von Gudden in regard to the mental malady under which Leopold II. of Bavaria laboured. The Greek etymology does not render us any assistance in the endeavour to comprehend the particular class of case to which it is applied. It is regarded as **synonymous** with that very favourite word of the German alienists, *Verrücktheit*, in respect of which there has been so much difference of opinion, and so much change since the time of Griesinger to the present day, that a lamentable amount of confusion and obscurity has been introduced into the nomenclature of this form of mental alienation.

Definition. — A condition of which chronic and systematised delusion is the essential sign. English alienists have considered "delusional insanity" a sufficiently distinctive term. As Koch says, "without delusion, no *Verrücktheit*"; and he adds "it is always primary." He adopts the view that there is no secondary form, and that therefore it is needless to speak of "primary" and "secondary" in relation to this mental affection. On the contrary, Griesinger held that emotional disturbance was the first link in the chain, that, in short, it was the basis of *Verrücktheit*. We are not prepared to admit that this alienist was wrong, and to say with Koch and the majority of German alienists that delusions do not develop out of the moral soil. Heredity is so common in this form of insanity that it is usually assumed that it springs out of a mental constitution which is by nature abnormal and unstable. At the same time, there is not originally a state of weakmindedness. Mental instability is usually present from the earliest period of life; the development of insanity may not occur until the patient has attained his majority, or later in life. The prevalent use of the word no doubt implies a constitutional tendency to mental disorder of a delusional type. Long before he is recognised as an actual lunatic he is styled "a crank." Hallucinations may be and frequently are mixed up with delusions, but they are not essential to paranoia. Delusions of persecution are extremely common, and lead to the commission of homicidal acts.

Drs. Amadei and Tonnini have made an elaborate classification of systematised insanity or paranoia.*

It consists of two great classes—degenerative and psycho-neurotic paranoia. In the former it is congenital, being due to insane inheritance. Subdivisions of this class are (1) cases in which there is a very early and sudden outburst of abnormal symptoms, (2) cases in which there is a gradual development of mental disorder. From both conditions may arise ideas of persecution, ambition, morbid religious views, and eroticism, these states being accompanied by hallucinations, or not. And the same holds good of that form in which the symptoms appear gradually.

Psycho-neurotic paranoia comprises cases in which there is no hereditary degeneration. It develops slowly, as in ordinary mania and melancholia. It terminates in either recovery, or more frequently in dementia. Its course is more rapid, and it is more intense in character than degenerative paranoia. This group, like the first, is subdivided, the genera being primary and secondary.

The primary division is the most frequent, and may be acute or chronic. The secondary cases follow an attack of melancholia or succeed to one of mania. Further, there may be the persecution and other manias above mentioned, and these may run their course with or without hallucinations.

Course.—It is essentially chronic. The tendency is to an increase of the congenital mental degeneration, but it may last for years without passing into profound dementia. Time tends to weaken the inten-

* "Archivio Italiano per le Malatie Nervose," &c. (Anno xxi.).

sity of the delusions, and therefore renders the patient less and less dangerous to society. As Krafft-Ebing forcibly expresses it, "the delusion of the *Verrückten* remains a dead mass of ideas which cannot undergo any modification. It becomes more and more a mere phrase." This alienist is one who holds that the disorder is the outcome of melancholia or mania, much more commonly of the former.

Paranoia occurring in two sisters has been reported by Dr. Peterson.* They differed but slightly from other persons when they were young. Only trifling eccentricities and some excess of self-consciousness were observed. Ideas of persecution and suspicion developed so gradually that their friends did not recognise them until actual insanity declared itself. When Dr. Peterson first saw them they wore veils, the removal of which revealed the fact that their faces were patched all over with small square pieces of cloth covering sores. An eruption of acne had been made much worse by picking and by their wearing wet cloths all night in order to prevent poisonous vapours entering their lungs, as also by the cloths being torn from the bleeding surface. These patients had hallucinations of hearing, taste, and markedly of smell. Moreover, they had illusions of sight and cutaneous sensibility. Their mother laboured also under paranoia with delusions of a religious character, and one of the sisters was conceived when her mother was insane.

The same physician has published an autobiographical sketch of a religious paranoiac who was a patient for more than seven years in the Hudson River State Hospital for the Insane, having been thirty years of age when he was admitted. As regards heredity, his great-uncle was a paranoiac, living on a farm in intimate companionship with the patient until the latter was twenty-three; his father was exceedingly eccentric, and Dr. Peterson suspects was himself something of a paranoiac; his wife was his first cousin. She said that her son had always been despondent, and since the age of twenty had done very little on account of his bad health. A year before his admission he shot himself in the head, and subsequently fancied that people influenced him by magnetism. He laboured under auditory hallucinations all the time he was in the asylum; and in the early period of his residence he manifested suspicions of persecution. After seven years' confinement delusions of grandeur developed. He rarely lost his self-control, and was allowed a great deal of freedom. His autobiography covered 400 manuscript pages. "He had unusual talents and aptitudes, and we find him studying, in the original, many of the classic Latin authors; while among his favourite companions were the works of Boethius, Lucretius, Josephus, and the Bible. His literary style and modes of thought are in themselves an evidence of more than ordinary attainments in rhetoric, philosophy, and logic."

A very elaborate history of a male paranoiac in the Bloomingdale Asylum, in New York, has been given by Dr. Noyes.* It is, in fact, a study of the evolution of systematised delusions of grandeur. He possessed much artistic skill. As a child marked peculiarities of manner and dress were observed. It was difficult to him to concentrate his attention on books, although he learnt readily. Among his peculiarities of conduct it may be mentioned that on his return from a half-hour's smoke out of doors after each meal, he had one method of procedure from which he never varied. "He first washed his hands in the bath; then going to the dining-room, he filled a glass with water from the cooler, and holding this extended in his right hand, he would balance himself on one heel and suddenly whirl about, always to the right, and then drink the water." At one time he was an art student in Paris, where he was regarded as exceedingly bright, but so wanting in application that he was styled the "unfinished artist." Naturally, repeated attempts were made when he was in the asylum to induce him to execute works of art continuously, but his constant excuse was, "the Spirit does not move me." In view of the remarkable sketches which are reproduced by Dr. Noyes, we must acknowledge with him, that "the grace, beauty, and poetic conception shown in these sketches and drawings, and also in the quotations, are such that it must cause the most profound regret that such talent and originality should have been hampered in their growth by a faulty physical development, and that an incurable mental disease should have clouded such a brilliant intellect" (*op. cit.* p. 375).

Prognosis. — Very unfavourable. If decided improvement takes place it is very likely to be followed by relapse. Delusional insanity, the outcome of an attack of mania or melancholia, may run a more favourable course, inasmuch as

* *Alienist and Neurologist*, Jan. 1890, St. Louis.

* *The American Journal of Psychology*, vol. ii. 1889.

[illegible] original mental constitution may have been sound. From the point of view taken by those who deny secondary [illegible], the prognosis must always be [illegible] unfavourable, if not hopeless. (See VERRÜCKTHEIT.) THE EDITOR.

PARAPATHIA (*παρά*; *πάθος*, an affection). Moral insanity.

PARAPHASIA (*παρά*; *φάσις*, a speech). A term for using one word when another is intended, or for mispronunciation of words, due to cerebral disorder.

PARAPHIA (*παρά*, beyond; *ἁφή*, a touching). A morbid sense of touch. (Fr. *paraphie*.)

PARAPHORA (*παραφέρω*, I move in a wrong direction). A going aside, generally applied to the mind, and to mental derangement or distraction. It has been applied to the unsteadiness of intoxication. (Fr. *paraphora*.)

PARAPHRASIA (*παρά*; *φράσις*, speech, expression). Incoherent speech.

PARAPHRENESIS (*παρά*, beyond; *φρήν*, the mind). A term for amentia, delirium, or any mental derangement. (Fr. *paraphrénésie*.)

PARAPHRENIA (*παρά*, beyond; *φρήν*, the mind). Paraphrenitis. (Fr. *paraphrénie*.)

PARAPHRENITIS (*παρά*, beyond; *φρενῖτις*, inflammation of the brain). A term for mental derangement, but also used for inflammation of the diaphragm.

PARAPHROSYNE, PARAPHRONESIS (*παράφρων*, out of one's mind). Derangement or wandering of mind. Used by Hippocrates in the same sense as he used paracope and paracrousis. (Fr. *paraphrosyne*.)

PARAPHROSYNE CALENTURA (*παρά*, beyond; *φρήν*, the mind; *caleo*, I am hot). The name given by Sauvage to a mental disease formerly observed in sailors in the tropics. The characteristic symptom said to exist was a delusion that the sea was green fields, the result being that the men attempted to throw themselves into it. Le Roy, of Méricourt, has demonstrated that the descriptions of this malady show it to be a delirium produced by insolatio or residence in a hot climate, aggravated by excessive fatigue. (Fr. *paraphrosyne calenture*.)

PARAPLECTICUS, PARAPLECTUS (*παράπληκτος*, struck on the side). Stricken on one side; paralysed; frenzy-stricken. Also used by the Greek poets for one who is brain-struck or crazy; *cf.* Soph. "Ajax," 229. (Fr. *paraplectique*.)

PARAPLEGIA, HYSTERICAL. (*See* HYSTERIA.)

PARAPSIS (*παρά*, beyond; *ἅπτω*, I touch). A morbid sense of touch.

PARARTHRIA (*παρά*; *ἀρθρόω*, I articulate). Any disorder of difficulty in articulation of speech.

PARATERESIOMANIA (*παρατήρησις*, an observing; *μανία*, madness). A rage for observing. (Fr. *paratérésiomanie*.)

PARATHYMIA (*παρά*, beyond; *θυμός*, the mind). An overstraining of the mind. (Fr. and Ger. *parathymie*.)

PARENTS.—Where a parent or other guardian, whose consent is necessary to a marriage, is insane, application may be made to any division of the High Court of Justice, and the marriage may be declared to be proper. This declaration is equivalent for all purposes to a consent (4 Geo. IV. c. 76, s. 17; *Ex parte Reibey*, 7 Jur. 589). A. WOOD RENTON.

PAREPITHYMIA (*παρά*, beyond; *πιθυμία*, a longing). Morbidly depraved longings and desires. (Fr. *parépithymie*.)

PARERETHISIS, PARERETHISMUS (*παρά*; *ἐρεθίζω*, I raise to anger). Abnormal excitement. An irritated condition of a part. (Fr. *paréréthèse*.)

PARESIS (*πάρεσις*, weakness, want of strength). Partial paralysis.

PARESTHESIS, PARESTHESIA (*παρά*, beyond; *αἴσθησις*, sensibility). Perverted sensibility.

PARETIC. Pertaining to or affected with paralysis. **P. DEMENTIA.** General paralysis (*q.v.*).

PARLIAMENT (Law of) in Relation to Insanity.—Idiots and lunatics (except during lucid intervals) are disqualified for being chosen members of Parliament (1 Whitlock's "Notes on the King's Writ," 461); and the *permanent* mental incapacity in a member, returned while of sound mind, has from a very early period in our law been regarded as a ground on which his seat might be vacated. In the 28th year of his reign, Edward I. issued writs directing the sheriffs to summon those members who had been elected for the Parliament holden in the preceding Easter, and in all cases where the person so elected should be prevented by death or infirmity from attending to elect others in their room. It is stated in Brooke's Abridgment (tit. Parl. s. 7) that similar writs were issued in the 38th year of the reign of Henry VIII. without making any distinction between illness curable and incurable. But it must be recollected that at those periods the session of Parliament was usually of so limited a duration that it might reasonably be presumed that any severe illness, however short, would incapacitate a member from attending. In subsequent cases* the House appears uniformly to

* In the "Journal of the House of Commons," vol. i. Feb. 14, 1609, there is the following entry :—

have inquired into the nature of the alleged malady and to have granted or refused a new writ according as there seemed to be a permanent or temporary incapacity in the member previously returned.*

The present practice is regulated by the Lunacy (Vacation of Seats) Act, 1886.† The provisions of this statute may be summarised as follows: If a member of the House of Commons is henceforth committed into or detained in any asylum as a lunatic, the fact must be certified forthwith to the Speaker, by the Court, judge, or magistrate, upon whose order, and by every medical practitioner, upon whose certificate, such committal or detention has taken place, and by every superintendent or other person having the principal charge of the asylum aforesaid.‡ Any two members of the House of Commons may certify to the Speaker that they are credibly informed of such committal and detention. The Speaker is required to transmit the certificate or certificates aforesaid, to the Commissioners in Lunacy in England or Scotland, or to the Inspectors of Lunatic Asylums in Ireland according as the place in which the member is detained is situated in England, Scotland or Ireland. It is the duty of the department, to which such certificates are transmitted, to examine the alleged lunatic and report to the Speaker whether he is of unsound mind. If the report is to the effect that the member is of unsound mind, a second examination and report by the same department are required by the Speaker at the expiration of six months from the date of the first, if the House of Commons be then sitting, and if not, then as soon as may be after the next sitting thereof. If the Lunacy Department reports that the member is still of unsound mind, the Speaker lays both reports on the table of the House of Commons; the seat is thereupon vacant and a new writ is issued by the clerk of the Crown.

An idiot cannot vote at a parliamentary election. A lunatic during a lucid interval can do so. The returning officer must satisfy himself that a lucid interval exists at the time of voting. It seems that the test of competency in such a case is the capacity of the voter to distinguish between the candidates, and generally to understand the nature and consequences of his act. A. Wood Renton.

"Hassard, 69, incurable—bed-rid—a new writ." See also in 162 Hansard, 3rd ser. 1941—a complaint that Mr. A. Steuart, a certified lunatic patient, had voted in a division, May 13, 1861.

* 66 "Commons Jour.," 226, 265, appendix 687 (1811). Mr. Alcock's case; Shelford's "Lunacy," 490-1.

† 49 Vict. c. 16.

‡ A medical practitioner or superintendent failing to comply with this requirement is liable to a penalty not exceeding £100.

PAROENIA (*παρά*, from; *οἶνος*, wine). In medical jurisprudence, an act committed while under the influence of wine.

PARONIRIA (*παρά*, near; *ὄνειρος*, a dream). Disturbance of sleep by disagreeable dreams. (Fr. *paronirie*; Ger. *die krankhaften Träume*.)

PARONIRIA AMBULANS (*ambulo*, I walk about). A synonym of somnambulism.

PARONOIA. Paranoia.

PAROPHOBIA (*πάρος*, intens.; *φόβος*, fear). A synonym of hydrophobia.

PAROPSIS (*παρά*, beyond; *ὄψις*, vision). False seeing, illusion, or hallucination of vision. (Fr. *paropsie*; Ger. *Falschsehen*.)

PARORASIS (*παρά*, beyond; *ὁράω*, I see). An old term for weak or disordered vision. It has been also used for hallucination of sight. (Fr. *parorase*; Ger. *Falschsehen*.)

PAROSMIA, PAROSPHRESIS (*παρά*, beyond; *ὀσμή*, a smell). Morbid sense of smell. (Fr. *parosphrèse*.)

PAROXYSMAL INSANITY.—Sudden mental attacks characterised by strong emotional distress or excitement passing off in a short time. (*See* Epilepsy and Insanity; Insanity, Paroxysmal.)

PARTIAL MORAL MANIA. (*See* Kleptomania, Pyromania, &c.).

PARTNERSHIP (Law of) in Relation to Insanity.—The lunacy of a partner does not *ipso facto* dissolve the firm; but the *permanent* lunacy of an active partner is a ground for the *judicial* dissolution of a partnership at the instance either of the sane partner or partners, or of the proper representative of the lunatic partner himself.

Dissolution at the Instance of a sane Partner.—In the leading case of *Jones* v. *Noy*, 1833 (2 M. & K. 125), the principle and the conditions upon which such a dissolution will be allowed were very clearly explained. Two persons had agreed to become partners as solicitors for a period of twelve years. One of them became lunatic before the expiry of the stipulated period, and subsequently died in a lunatic asylum. The other carried on the business for some time and then sold it. The representative of the deceased lunatic was held to be entitled to a share of the profits up to the time of sale. The judgment of Sir John Leach, M.R. in this case is at once so short and so instructive that it deserves quotation *in extenso*.

"It is clear upon principle that the complete incapacity of a party to an agreement to perform that which was a condition of the agreement is a ground for determining the contract. The insanity of a partner is a ground for the dissolution of the partnership because it is immediate incapacity; but it may not in the result prove to be a ground of dissolution, for the partner may recover from his malady. When a partner, therefore, is affected with insanity, the continuing partner may, if he think fit, make it a ground of dissolution, but in that case we consider with Lord Kenyon that in order to make it a ground of dissolution, he must obtain a decree of the Court. If he does not apply to the Court for a decree of dissolution, it is to be considered that he is willing to wait to see whether the incapacity of his partner may not prove merely temporary. If he carry on the partnership business in the expectation that his partner may recover from his insanity, so long as he continues the business with that expectation or hope, there can be no dissolution."

All the distinctive doctrines of English law upon the subject are logically implied in these sentences: (1) Lunacy is merely a ground of dissolution (*cf. Anon.*, 1855, 2 K. & J. 441; *Helmore* v. *Smith*, 1887, 35 Ch. D. at p. 442; (2) the lunacy which will justify a dissolution must be permanent (*Jones* v. *Lloyd*, 1874, L. R. 18 Eq. 265); (3) it must also be existing when application for the interference of the Court is made (*Anon.*, *ubi sup.*);* and (4) it must be of such a nature as to render the partner *incompetent to conduct the business of the partnership according to the articles*. In *Anon.* (*ubi sup.*) a motion for an interim injunction to restrain a partner who six months previously, being temporarily of unsound mind, had attempted to commit suicide, from interfering in the partnership affairs, was refused, the evidence not showing that, at the time of the motion, he was incompetent to conduct the partnership business.

All causes or matters for the dissolution of partnerships or the taking of partnership accounts are assigned to the Chancery Division (Jud. Act, 1873, s. 34 (3)).†

* If the lunatic is not so found by inquisition, the Court will, if necessary, direct an inquiry into the nature and extent of his malady.

† The Lunacy Act, 1890, provides (s. 119) that, "where a person being a member of a partnership becomes lunatic, the judge may by order dissolve the partnership;" and the Partnership Act, 1890, enables (s. 35 (a)) the Court to decree a dissolution "when a partner is found lunatic by inquisition, or in Scotland by cognition, or is shown, to the satisfaction of the Court, to be of permanently unsound mind, in either of which cases the application may be made as well on behalf of that partner by his committee or next friend, or person having title to intervene, as by any other partner."

Dissolution at the Instance of the Representative of a Lunatic Partner.—"A dissolution," says Sir F. Pollock ("Partnership," p. 91), "may be sought and obtained on behalf of the lunatic partner himself, and this may be done either by his committee in lunacy under the Lunacy Regulation Act, or where he has not been found lunatic by inquisition by an action brought in his name in the Chancery Division by another person as his next friend. In the latter case the Court may, if it thinks fit, direct an application to be made in lunacy before finally disposing of the cause."

Date from which a Judicial Dissolution takes Effect.—(1) The articles may authorise a dissolution, and the partnership be dissolved under the articles. Here the judicial dissolution takes effect from the date of the actual dissolution, and not from the date of the decree. (2) The partnership may be at will. Here the date of dissolution is the time fixed in the notice to dissolve. (3) In all other cases the dissolution will be from the date of the judicial decree.

When the Court dissolves a partnership on the ground of insanity it directs the costs to be paid out of the partnership assets. A power under the articles to dissolve a partnership upon any ground may be exercised by one partner notwithstanding the lunacy of the other. Thus in *Robertson* v. *Locke*, 1846 (15 Sim. 235), by articles of partnership between A. and B., the partnership was to be dissolved upon either party giving the other a six months' notice. A. gave the required notice. It was held effectual notwithstanding the insanity of B. at the time.

A. Wood Renton.

PASSIO CADIVIA. A synonym of epilepsy.

PASSIO HYSTERICA. A term for hysteria (*q.v.*).

PATENTEES (INSANE).—Insanity creates no disability which will prevent any person from applying for and obtaining letters patent for an invention. The Patents Act 1883, sec. 99, expressly provides for such cases in the following terms: "If any person is by reason of . . . . lunacy . . . . incapable of making any declaration or doing any thing required or permitted by this Act, or by any rules made under the authority of this Act, then the . . . . committee if any of such incapable person, or if there be none, any person appointed by any Court or Judge possessing jurisdiction in respect of the property of incapable persons, upon the petition of any person on behalf of such incapable person, or of any other person interested in the making such declaration or doing such thing, may make such declaration or a declaration as nearly corresponding thereto as circumstances permit, and do such thing in the name and on behalf of such incapable person, and all acts done by such substitute shall for the purposes of the Act be as effectual as if done by the person for whom he is substituted."

This section applies not only to patents but to trade-marks and designs.

A. Wood Renton.

PATHEMA (πάθος, a suffering or passion). A term for suffering. Disease of body or mind. (Fr. *pathème*; Ger. *Ein Leiden.*)

PATHEMATOLOGY (πάθος, passion; λόγος, a discourse). The doctrine of passion or affection of the mind; or merely pathology. (Fr. *pathématologie.*)

PATHETISM (πάθος, feeling). A term for animal magnetism, hypnotism, or any doctrine of mental influences.

PATHOCRATIA, PATHOCRATORIA (πάθος, passion; κρατέω, I am strong). Self-restraint. The holding of the passions under control. (Fr. *pathocratie.*)

PATHOCTONUS (πάθος, passion; κτείνω, I kill). The killing of the passions; that is, self-restraint. (Fr. *pathoctone.*)

PATHOLOGY.—Insanity is not a disease: it is a symptom of many diseased conditions of the brain, the term disease being for the moment employed in its widest sense, and being held to comprise not only well-marked morbid changes, but also imperfect development and malformation of the organ and its envelopes. Insanity may therefore be defined as *a symptom of various morbid conditions of the brain, the results of defective formation or altered nutrition of its substance; induced by local or general morbid processes, and characterised especially by non-development, obliteration, or perversion of one or more of its psychical functions.* This definition obviously covers a large number of abnormal mental conditions which conventionality does not include under the term "insanity." Comà, delirium, and intoxication (amongst others) are not regarded as insanities; an arbitrary line is drawn between them and so-called mental disease. But it is a line which cannot be acknowledged by the scientific observer; it is one drawn solely for social and legal purposes, and demanding no attention in an article which deals with the causes of morbid mental manifestations, irrespective of the duration, degree, or social consequences of the abnormal conditions. To the pathologist and physiologist the patient under coma and delirium, and the drunkard under alcoholism, are as much insane as the maniac or melancholiac. The two sets of conditions are, or may be, linked together by causation, anatomical relations, symptomatology, natural history and results, and to exclude their relative consideration would only tend to narrow the field of inquiry, and would divest the observer of the power of employing argument based on analogy. Griesinger asserted the position correctly when he said, "diseases of the nervous system form one inseparable whole, of which the so-called mental diseases form only a certain moderate proportion."

The results of experiments and observation bearing on the region of the brain specially affected by insanity, are best expressed in the words of Ferrier: "We have many grounds for believing that the frontal lobes, the cortical centres for the head and ocular movements, with their associated sensory centres, form the substrata of those psychical processes which lie at the foundation of the higher intellectual operations. It would, however, be absurd to speak of a special seat of intelligence or intellect in the brain. Intelligence or will has no local habitation distinct from the sensory and motor substrata of the cortex generally. There are centres for special forms of sensation and ideation, and centres for special motor activities and acquisitions, in response to, and in association with, the activity of sensory centres; and these, in their respective cohesions, actions, and interactions, form the substrata of mental operations in all their aspects and all their range." *

The *ganglionic cells* of the *cortex* are the organs through whose instrumentality all cerebral action is manifested, and on the implication of their healthy condition morbid phenomena depend. The object of this article is to indicate the various morbid influences which may act on these organs, their methods of action, the causes of solutions of the continuity of their connections, and to seek for explanation of the resultant mental conditions by deductions drawn from direct and comparative pathological and physiological argument.

The *remote causes* of nervous disease accompanied by insanity are dealt with under Heredity, Statistics, &c.

The influence of nationality, civilisation, education, and occupation, can rarely be brought to bear on the circumstances of a particular case, whilst that of sex and

* "The Functions of the Brain," 1886.

age fall to be considered in the body of this article. In regard to heredity, it may be remarked that through whatever channel a tendency to nervous degeneration may have been introduced into the constitution of a family, or of an individual, it may make itself felt in two directions: either in arrest of development of the bones of the skull, or of the brain itself, and consequent idiocy or imbecility; or by the development of the nervous diathesis. The former are conditions fixed by the pathological circumstances under which their subjects are born (constituting a true congenital insanity), and are effectually marked off from the results of the nervous diathesis. They present themselves in two forms: first, a liability to break down under circumstances which would not affect persons of originally stable constitution; and second, in irregular and abnormally defective nervous action. Thus, hereditary predisposition may act as a factor common to all classes of insanity, whatever their immediate causes may be; or it may be an independent factor in itself. The nervous diathesis affects actually or potentially the whole nervous system, and it is by no means certain that it will appear in the same form in the descendant as it did in the parent; hence, if we take a family stock in which the nervous diathesis is strongly developed, we may find in the first instance individuals in no way affected by it; in some it may result in outbreaks of insanity, in others of uncontrollable drinking, in others of epilepsy, in others of violent neuralgias, while in some we may have varieties of unstable, passionate, and eccentric tempers which never break down into actual disease at all. Once established there is no possibility of predicting in what direction it will act.

An important preliminary question to determine in pathology is, do morbid processes going on in the brain or its membranes act under conditions materially different from those occurring in other regions? It has been generally asserted that they do act under a special condition in consequence of the assumption that the cranium is a "practically closed sac," which assumption has actually taken the position of an axiom. The cranium is not by any means a closed sac. The dura mater, which is practically its periosteum, and the pia mater, have numerous and extensive conduits, the sectional area of which is considerable, to the extra-skeletal lymphatic system, passing through each foramen at the base of the skull and in the vertebral column. The immense activity of the contained organ, and its constant changes of size, demand free exit of the products of waste and unused material, and for the fluctuation of the normal cerebro-spinal fluid. The patency of these conduits may under certain conditions of disease, mainly increase of blood-pressure, be compromised to a considerable extent; still they are never completely closed, and an interchange of fluid constantly goes on between the interior and exterior of the cranium.

Were the cranium a "practically closed sac" pressure would be diffused equally all through its contents, which we know is not the case in brain abscess or apoplectic clots; and local tension can even exist, limited by the resistance of connective and other tissue, as in other regions of the body. Were the axiom alluded to correct, the rigid skull would be as much a cause of death under diseased conditions, as it is a protector of the delicate organ it contains against the ordinary accidents of life. But the brain is liable to suffer under pathological conditions from a circumstance which does not affect many other important organs; it can obtain no vicarious aid, it cannot delegate any of its functions to other systems, it must do its own work, and rid itself of its own products of waste and disease.

When we analyse the list of *immediate* causes assigned as the producers of insanity in cases, as they present themselves, we find them to be divisible into nine great classes. It may be admitted that in a certain proportion accuracy of statement cannot be guaranteed; but, allowing for error, there is adequate warrant for ranging immediate causes under the following heads:—

(1) Over-excitation of the higher brain function.
(2) Idiopathic morbid processes.
(3) Adventitious products.
(4) Traumatism.
(5) Secondary effects of other neuroses.
(6) Concurrent effects of disease of the general system.
(7) Toxic agents.
(8) Concurrent effects of evolutional and involutional conditions.
(9) Heredity.

Over-excitation of the Brain is universally acknowledged as an inducer of insanity without the intervention of any other morbid factor. Over excitations, whether produced by such emotions as joy, sorrow, fright, anxiety, or by unduly prolonged intellectual action, are generally spoken of as "moral" causes, and in many works on insanity are placed in strong contradistinction to "physical" causes, the psychical influence of the former being apparently held to be sufficient to account for the subsequent phenomena irrespective of their action on the tissues of the brain. Very generally a psychical continuity is suggested, and we very rarely find any attempt made to connect the action of the cause with its effects in disease on the cortical constituents. But due consideration of the facts of anatomy and physiology ought to demonstrate that no distinction exists between "moral" and "physical" causes; that, in effect, the former are as much physical as traumatism and alcoholic poisoning.

There is sufficient evidence founded on direct observation to prove that when the psychical functions of the cortex are exercised hyperæmia of the active region is an immediate consequence. The observations of Mosso (*Ueber den Kreislauf des Blutes im Menschlichen Gehirn*) cannot be called in question. We have observed, in two cases, distinct hyperæmic bulging of the cortex through openings in the skull during mental action, and amongst others, Dr. G. Gibson, of Edinburgh, has recorded the tracings taken in a similar case. In the latter case, and in those that came under our own observation, the bulging was steadily maintained whilst mental action continued. In degree it depended on the intensity of the action, and steadily increased according to the length of time the action persisted, until a certain maximum point was gained. With the withdrawal of stimulus the bulging gradually disappeared. The deduction to be drawn from this phenomenon is aptly put by Crichton Browne:—"The blood-vessels were clearly made for the brain, and not the brain for the blood-vessels; and the amount of blood supply to the brain and its several parts is determined, not by vascular domination, but by the functional activity of the nervous tissues." It is of importance to consider by what circulatory and nervous apparatus this functional hyperæmia is induced.

The vessels directly involved are those which supply the cortex of the superior, frontal, and superior-lateral aspects of the brain; whilst the central or ganglionic vessels influence the nutrition of the organ through the nutrition they afford the vaso-motor centres. The relative supply of blood to the cortex and to the white matter is as five to one, the supply to the central ganglia being intermediate. Reference to BRAIN AND MEMBRANES will show that the regions above mentioned are supplied with blood by the three cerebral arteries, which are the terminal branches of the internal carotid. These vessels are at the extreme limit of the circulatory apparatus; they are furthest away from the heart, and the effect of gravity tells more upon them than on the vessels of any other part of the body. Further, those running directly perpendicularly (the main branches of the middle cerebral) must feel the effects of variation of pressure more than any other of the cerebral arteries. The effects of gravity come into play even more definitely and effectively in connection with the venous system after the blood has reached the sinuses, when its weight determines its course into the large veins passing through the base, and almost directly to the heart. Under ordinary circumstances, notwithstanding certain mechanical obstruction to the venous flow in the pia mater, the current of blood through the brain is very free; it is evident that this is necessary, and that anything that interferes with this free circulation must exert a most injurious effect on the nutrition of the cerebral tissues.

The vaso-motor influences are of two kinds, vaso-constrictor and vaso-dilator. The centres of vaso-motor action consist of numerous ganglionic cells in the floor of the medulla oblongata, lying in groups on each side in the upward continuation of the lateral columns after they have given off their fibres to the decussating pyramids (Ludwig, Dittmar). The results of stimulation and paralysis of this centre are mentioned in BRAIN, PHYSIOLOGY OF; but for the sake of convenience it may be stated here that reflex stimulation (*e.g.*, from the cortex) is followed by contraction of the arteries, increase of arterial blood pressure, distension of the systemic veins and of the right heart: whilst, on the other hand, paralysis causes relaxation of the arteries, with resultant lowered blood pressure. This centre is, under ordinary circumstances, in a state of moderate tonic excitement; but there is experimental evidence that, although there is no reason to believe in the existence of a cerebral vaso-constrictor centre, alterations in blood pressure may be produced reflexly, by stimulation of the cerebral cortex acting on the medullary centre. The course of the fibres connected with this centre is circuitous. According to Gaskell and Foster, those going to the head, after passing down the cord, leave by the anterior roots of the dorsal nerves below the second pair, run along the mixed nerve trunk, pass along the visceral branch, the white ramus communicans to the chain of sympathetic ganglia, through the annulus of Vieussens to the lower spinal ganglia, and thence to the cervical sympathetic. After passing through the sympathetic ganglia they are fine unmedullated fibrils.

Gaskell says (*Journal of Physiology*, vol. vii.):—"The presence of special vaso-dilator nerves for the blood-vessels of every part of the body is an article of faith accepted by almost all physiologists of the present day. Owing, however, to the fact that in most instances such nerves are found mixed up with the vaso-motor nerves, the evidence upon which their existence is based is in the majority of instances indirect rather than direct. Fortunately, we possess among the vaso-inhibitory nerves a few examples, the separate existence of which is beyond dispute. In these cases these nerves run separately from the vaso-motor, so that an examination of their structure and distribution may fairly be expected to give indications of general laws, if such exist, which may afterwards be tested in the case of the other vaso-inhibitory nerves. The nerves in question are *par excellence* the inhibitory nerves of the heart, the vaso-dilators contained in the chorda tympani and small petrosal nerves, and the nervi erigentes."

The distribution of these dilator nerves differs materially from that of the vaso-constrictors, as they pursue a more or less direct course to their destination. Thus, the vaso-dilator fibres for the sub-maxillary gland run in the chorda tympani, and may be traced back to the facial; the ramus tympanicus of the glosso-pharyngeal nerve contains similar fibres for the parotid gland, and it appears probable that the trigeminal nerve contains vaso-dilator fibres for the eye and nose, and possibly for other parts (Foster). The centre in each case appears to be in the central nervous system not far from the centre of the ordinary motor fibres which they accompany (Foster). Considering the close analogy between the active functional congestion of the cortex and of various glands, it may fairly be assumed that these and other nerves as they pass to their ultimate areas of distribution send off vaso-dilator fibres to the membranes and the convolutions. There are, moreover, certain characteristics of the vaso-dilator system, which afford support to the assumption of their extensive distribution to the brain. As stated by Foster, their action is less complicated than that of the vaso-constrictors, as they appear to have no tonic influence; stimulation, as in the salivary gland, here producing reflex dilatation of the glandular vessels by active extension of the muscular fibre; and "the effects of the activity of vaso-dilator fibres appear to be essentially local in character. When any set of them comes into action, the vascular area which they govern is dilated, and the vascular areas so governed are relatively so small that changes in them produce little or no effect on the vascular system in general." Further, under ordinary circumstances their influence is of shorter duration than that of the constrictor fibres. But there may be cited here an interesting experimental result as possibly bearing on future remarks. Foster states: "When a nerve [he instances the sciatic] after section commences to degenerate, the constrictor fibres lose their irritability earlier than the dilator fibres, so that at a certain stage a stimulus, such as the interrupted current, while it fails to affect the constrictor fibres, readily throws into action the dilator fibres. The latter, indeed, in contrast to ordinary motor nerves, retain their irritability after section of the nerve for very many days."

That the products of metabolism have considerable effect on the capillaries of a region called into activity may be almost accepted as a postulate, and Roy and Sherrington have advanced a theory that such products alone cause variations of the calibre of the cerebral vessels.* Their opinion is based on the absence of anatomical proof of the existence of cerebral vaso-motor or vaso-dilator nerves; and in the effects of the injection of filtrates prepared from brains showing acid reaction. The injection of such filtrates is followed rapidly by hyperæmia. They conclude that "the chemical products of cerebral metabolism contained in the lymph which bathes the walls of the arterioles of the brain can cause variations of the calibre of the cerebral vessels: that in this reaction the brain possesses an intrinsic mechanism by which its vascular supply can be varied locally in correspondence with local variations of functional activity." The observations of Langendorf and Gescheidlen† are conclusive as to the alkaline reaction of normal brain tissue, and the rapid production of acidity under abnormal conditions; but the additional deduction we feel inclined to draw from these observations and the ingenious experiments of Roy and Sherrington is, that acid lymph may so increase the irritability of the muscular wall of the vessels as to render it all the more susceptible to nervous vaso-dilator or vaso-constrictor influence. As will be shown later, we also believe that

* *Journal of Physiology*, vol. xi.

† *Biolog. Centralblatt*, 1886.

the products of disease exercise a very marked influence in the maintenance of congestion.

In the present state of knowledge of the subject it is impossible to come to a definite conclusion as to the mechanism of cortical functional hyperæmia. The views of most physiologists seem to be in favour of the inhibitory theory. But *à priori* the theory of stimulation for a definite hyperæmia necessary for a special functional activity is supported by the analogy of the vaso-dilator nervous influence on the blood supply of muscles and of certain glands. When, as we have seen, the cortex of a man's brain bulges through a hole in his skull on the application of mental stimulus, the resemblance to the turgescence of the salivary glands on stimulation of the chorda tympani and small petrosal nerves is highly suggestive. We have also the results of stimulation of the nervi erigentes, and the phenomena of angioneuroses of the head and face afford a degree of support. Our belief is that both sets of nerves may exercise influence—that stimulation of the vaso-dilator system is the immediate producer of functional hyperæmia, that subsequently inhibition of the vaso-motor system of nerves assists its maintenance; and that the products of metabolism, especially under diseased conditions also exercise a powerful influence. However impossible it may be at the present moment to demonstrate the actual mechanism, or unravel its mode of action, there can be little doubt that we have a vaso-constrictor centre in the medulla, and vaso-dilator centres (probably in the cerebrum), which under ordinary circumstances control the supply to the cortex, and which are controlled by the cortex itself through the action of intercurrent nerves. No organ of the body has such sudden and frequent calls for rapid change of blood supply to definite areas, and, even were we in total ignorance of the existence of vessel-controlling nerves acting upon it, there is such an array of accessory facts as to warrant the assumption of their presence.

Functional hyperæmia is in every respect a condition of health; one necessary for the provision of temporary nutriment during temporary activity, ceasing with the withdrawal of stimulus, when the calibre of the vessels is reduced to its original dimensions through the constricting nervous influence. The vascular supply of the brain is so arranged as to favour the rapid production of hyperæmia. Moxon pointed out that the greater veins of the pia enter the superior longitudinal sinus at such an angle that as the blood enters the sinus it is directed against the general backward running current, so that unless the blood in the sinus is much diminished in quantity there is always retardation of the venous flow from the pial vessels, and maintenance of a mild mechanical congestion. As B. Lewis observes, this maintains the patency of the vessels both of pia and cortex so long as the heart works with ordinary vigour; and marked phenomena result from either diminution or increase of arterial or venous pressure. At the base (as the same author points out) "a sustained pressure of no inconsiderable degree" is maintained on the vessels of the pons by the combined streams of the two vertebrals being poured into the basilar artery, the sectional area of the former being but slightly greater than that of the latter single artery; this sustained pressure may not be entirely expended on the vessels of the pons, but may extend to the arteries given off from the circle of Willis, thus supplementing the supply of the internal carotids. Undoubtedly under such conditions arterial vaso-constrictor action must be in force, and any interference with it by morbid processes must produce specially definite results. The combined action of these influences favours a full and constant—it might be said an over-full—blood supply, as is shown by the slight bulging of the dura mater into a trephine hole, and by the hernia cerebri in fracture of the skull: although in the latter condition the protrusion may be extreme in consequence of paralysis of the vaso-motor system produced by traumatic shock. The increase of bulk of the convolutions due to functional hyperæmia is, under conditions of health, provided for by the displacement of cerebro-spinal fluid into the elaborate system of lymph spaces existing in the pia, the sub-dural space and the dura mater—into which two latter spaces, and into the longitudinal sinus, it is conducted by the Pacchionian villi—and into the cisterns at the base, between the dorsal surface of the medulla and the posterior part of the cerebellum, in the inter-peduncular space, in front of the optic chiasma, between the under surface of the cerebellar hemispheres and the lateral portions of the medulla, on both sides of the transverse fissure, and at the lower ends of the Sylvian fissures. All these spaces and cisterns are in direct communication with the ventricles, and with the great spaces in the spinal column. The fluid reaches the extra-skeletal lymphatics by peri-vascular and peri-neural conduits passing out through every foramen of the skull and vertebral column. The amount of this fluid produced daily has not been estimated, but surgical results show that it must be considerable.

We have said that so long as functional hyperæmia is merely sufficient to supply the temporary extra demand for the nutrition of the cells during functional activity, and for the making up of the loss of energy, there is a return of the normal circulation as soon as the extra demand ceases, and the cell has got rid of its extra excretory products. But the demands on the local circulation may be so great and may be so long continued that, as in other organs and other parts of the body, the physiological line may be passed, and pathological conditions may be induced, not confined to the vessels themselves, but extending to the tissues they supply. On account of the basal position of the openings of the skull it is evident that even slight pathological alterations (either at the vertex or the base, but especially at the vertex), if they interfere with the removal of lymph fluid, must implicate the maintenance of the perfect vascular unity of the cerebrum; and that any long-continued angio-neurotic changes extending beyond the limits of normality, must have considerable effect on the tissues of the brain.

If the nutrition of the cells is unduly interfered with for any long continued period, there ensues a series of changes not only in the cerebral cells, but also in the vaso-motor and vaso-dilator control systems, which may be temporary, or permanent according to circumstances. The circulatory apparatus has been adjusted to meet the increased demand, but the cells, being stimulated beyond the health limit, a condition of unstable equilibrium between nutrition and function is reached —they receive the increased blood supply and a certain amount of nutrition, and consequently, instead of the normal discharge of energy, irregularity of discharge is produced by the prolonged maintenance of over-vascularity. The continuous excitation demands a greater supply of nutriment, and in consequence a gradually increasing strain is laid on the vaso-control system, till at length one of two events occurs; either a diseased balance between nutrition and function is reached, or the balance is completely destroyed.

In the first case discharges take place at a lower level of cell nutrition and function; in the second, vascular changes become so advanced that what must be regarded as a series of sub-inflammatory processes ensues. To take a parallel example from the field of general pathology; the over-exercise of function of the special cells of the kidney, whether induced by excess of blood, by effete substances, or by the presence of poisonous agents, is the immediate cause of parenchymatous nephritis; and we have the first symptoms of the disease associated with cell changes, followed by vaso-motor disturbances, which, in their turn, re-act on the cells and the tissues of the organ through histological alteration of the vascular and lymphatic apparatus. It may be objected that the parallel does not exist in the case of excess of blood acting on the cells; but it must be remembered that the excess of blood, especially of blood loaded with effete matter, is only an irritant, and the producer of the permanent hyperæmia which is the first efficient factor in the production of histological changes.

The implication or alteration of the relation of nutrition to function constitutes the preliminary or primary factor in the production of the prodromal symptoms of idiopathic insanity; the arteries of the cortex are dilated, and send an abnormal amount of blood inwards, and as a result there is increased and sustained pressure in the veins. This condition may persist for considerable periods of time before definite mania or melancholia is developed, unnoticed by any but those immediately surrounding the patient, and its symptoms of restlessness, irritability and bodily decadence, are even by them often disregarded or misconstrued. If early recognised, appropriate treatment very generally prevents degradation of tissue, and procures recovery; but if the condition is neglected the sequence of events, common to all tissues under similar circumstances of irritation, ensues. A sub-inflammatory stage is reached, evidenced by deposits of leucocytes much greater than normal between the adventitia and the muscular coat, and by various degrees of proliferation of the fixed connective-tissue cells of the vessel. Both leucocytes and fixed cells break down, and a *débris* is formed, which, along with masses of blood pigment, occupies the peri-vascular space in large quantities, and can be found distributed along the whole course of a cortical vessel to its ultimate ramifications, although it can be most readily demonstrated at the bifurcations. This material has been found in quantities so large as to interfere with the patency of the lymphatic sheath, and to procure its distension by the obstruction of exudation fluid. Implication of the lymphatic circulation is one of the most important, if not the most important, of the pathological factors in the production of insanity. It may act in two ways; first, by submitting, through diminished drainage, the cells to the action of waste products, and secondly, by affecting the conductivity of vaso-motor fibres. It must be remembered that each cell is surrounded by a capsule connected by the the "spur-like" process of Obersteiner with the hyaline sheath, forming the main lymphatic apparatus of the individual cell. This process is a very fine tubule, and necessarily is easily occluded. Not only does the occurrence of exudates in the hyaline sheath dam back the flow from the capsule, but the deposits of leucocytes, epithelial cells and masses of pigment, may actually occlude the openings of Obersteiner's processes. Under these circumstances the cell lies bathed in a poisonous fluid, the reaction of which is acid, and therefore opposed to its healthy alkaline constitution. Degradation is a necessary consequence, shown first by granularity of the protoplasmic body, and subsequently by changes of the cell presently to be described. This granularity does not at first exceed the "cloudy swelling" of all active cells; it only becomes morbid when persistent and exaggerated. But exudation fluid may also affect the exercise of the function of the vaso-constrictor fibres. Possibly a certain amount of pressure may be caused, and it is well known that pressure at first tends to stimulate, and, if continued, to paralyse the action of these nerves. In their case also the acid exudate acts in a similar manner, procuring intensification of function, followed by exhaustion from extreme stimulation. In whatever manner exudates act on the vaso-constrictors it is certain to be finally in the direction of reduction of inhibitory function and consequent dilatation. When the pia mater becomes infiltrated, as it often does in severe cases, there can be little doubt that pressure acts strongly on the branches of this system running between its layers. Wherever a vaso-constrictor nerve is involved in an inflammatory mass we have the same condition as where it is actually cut, and this alone would be sufficient to account for the obstinate congestion of the brain causing delirium or death, not only in cases of idiopathic insanity, but also in many other head affections.

We can only speak from the experience derived from the examination of four cases of idiopathic insanity, which proved fatal within two months of the development of mania and melancholia, as to the period at which the products of inflammation show themselves and exercise any marked influence. In two cases, one symptomatised by mania, the other by melancholia, deposits of leucocytes, pigment, and nuclei of endothelium were found in considerable quantities, here and there in aggregated masses, in vessels taken from the superior convolutions; the proliferation of fixed cell nuclei was marked. In two others, one of mania (death having resulted from exhaustion) and one of excited melancholia (the subject of which committed suicide), stasis of a very well-marked character was found; the lumen of many cortical vessels of all sizes was occupied by blood corpuscles, the peri-vascular lymphatics were much distended and blocked by *débris*, and wide spaces between the sheath and the brain substance were seen in the maniacal case. There can be little doubt that these morbid products are deposited much earlier in the history of a case than two months, but in the absence of data it is impossible to assign any definite period for their appearance. It is highly improbable that such intensity of diseased action occurs, save in extreme cases, but in the first two instances adduced, the pathological products were not much more strongly marked than those presented in subjects of older standing insanity of a milder type. In such we have constantly found the products described, and have noted the evidence of extensive exudation. It is not often that the observer is fortunate enough to get the cellular capsule and its process in absolute relation to the lymphatic sheath; but in three instances we have procured evidence of their continuity, and noted the distension of the whole apparatus, the cell lying in a clear open space in connection with a wide canal. This can be easily demonstrated, as regards the capsule alone, in chronic cases. If, as B. Lewis asserts (and we entirely agree with him), each cell is surrounded by a looped capillary, and if the vessel becomes implicated to the extent of stasis, or even short of it, it is not difficult to understand how degeneration of cell protoplasm is hastened by two sets of action; toxic from within, and deprivation of nutriment from without.

But further morbid instrumentality is at work. We have direct evidence that during sleep the cortex of the superior convolutions is anæmic; according to Mosso's experiments (*loc. cit.*) and observations, the supply to the cortex is much diminished, the vessels—both arteries and veins—being contracted, and the brain is smaller. Insomnia is one of the earliest symptoms of incipient insanity, and continues during its acute period; sleep is not obtained in its natural degree till convalescence, or terminative dementia, is reached. It cannot be doubted that this insomnia is due to hyperæmia. In those rare cases of insanity, in which there is no interference with the periodicity or intensity of sleep, the fact of its presence ought to influence diagnosis. Sleep is the condition necessary for the recuperation of cell-tissue; in its absence the downward tendency to degeneration must necessarily be assisted.

The question which now naturally presents itself is, how can we reconcile the dependence of three such apparently widely divergent morbid mental symptoms as mania, melancholia, and dementia, on one common pathological condition. The following clinical observations support the position as to the unity of pathological causal conditions:—

(a) During the prodromal period the symptoms of excitement and melancholia frequently alternate.

(b) In many acute cases mania and melancholia co-exist—*i.e.*, it is impossible to say whether they are cases of maniacal melancholia or of melancholic mania.

(c) As many cases run their course towards recovery the symptoms are consecutively melancholia, mania and dementia.

(d) In *folie circulaire* the same sequence of symptoms occurs time after time.

(e) In general paralysis of the insane, the inflammatory nature of which is beyond doubt, a certain proportion of cases is characterised by exaltation of feeling, another by depression, and a third by obfuscation, from beginning to end; whilst in certain others we may have all varieties and degrees of symptoms presenting themselves.

(f) The effect of the administration of certain poisons, especially alcohol, is a sequence of psychical phenomena of much the same character.

These observations point, not to a difference in kind of primary causation, but to variation of symptoms in accordance with the progress and nature of pathological processes, which vary principally in accordance with the constitution of the tissues of the individual. It must be borne in mind that the deposits of inflammatory products and congestion are not identical or constant in the individuals of a series of subjects, because the individuals and their tissues are not constant quantities. We have thus a constant condition of irritation acting on inconstant subjects. We know that the pathological results of over-taxation of brain function are accompanied by morbid excitement of action of the organ; but we are apt to forget that although mania is accompanied by exaltation, and melancholia by depression of feeling (speaking of each in the mass), they are both manifestations of excitement of feeling. Given this common psychological condition of excitement of feeling we must seek for an explanation of the varieties of its phenomena either in some quality or quantity of its exciting cause, in some peculiarity of its pathological products, or in some idiosyncrasy of the affected individual. We derive no material assistance from psychological considerations, for there is no necessary connection between depressing emotions and melancholia on the one hand, or between stimulating emotions and mania on the other. Intense grief produces mania as often as melancholia, and the insanity of the man of saturnine disposition is as often as not characterised by mania. The peculiarity of the exciting cause appears to be, not its psychological characteristics, but its intensity and rapidity of incidence; the latter depending not only on the former, but also on the stability or instability of tissue. According as excitement of feeling is rapidly produced so the more likely is mania to be the symptom, especially when it acts on an extremely irritable but unstable protoplasm. It is not only to the constitution of the cortical cells and their network to which we may look for evidence of instability and irritability, but also to the ganglia which govern the vaso-motor systems of nerves. Inherent weakness of these centres may play an even more important *rôle* in the production of insanity than instability of the peripheral ganglia, more especially in the rapidity of its production. That melancholia often supervenes on depressing emotions, gradual in their incidence and action, does not imply a psychological nexus; but, that as their irritating influence is slowly applied to cells of diminished vitality and nutritive power, so the results of the irritation are slowly produced; and, as in the case of every organ of the body, we have variety of degree of symptoms in conformity with the rapidity of the progress of pathological events. In extreme cases of recent excitement, maniacal or melancholic, we have found stasis and the products of inflammation: in chronic cases the same appearances are presented, although in a less degree, whatever the symptom may have been: and if we have any right to connect post-mortem demonstration with the indications of disease during life the inference is unavoidable that considerable variety of clinical phenomena may be dependent on a common cause acting on differently constituted tissues.

Evidence of inflammatory action is constantly met with in the encephale of the insane, and is frequently alluded to by writers on the changes observed, without, however, any definite reference to it in connection with the natural history of the various diseases causing insanity, with the occasional exception of general paralysis and traumatism. But setting aside all cases of these two conditions and chronic alcoholism, estimating them as together forming one-third of the insanities, in the remaining 70 per cent. we find evidences of inflammatory action having been at work at some period or other in about one-half. In the other half, where such evidence is not seen, the insanity has been dependent on anæmia or other causes presently to be spoken of.

The marks of inflammatory action are met with in the (*a*) **Skull**, (*b*) **Membranes**, (*c*) **Blood-vessels**, (*d*) **Neuroglia**, (*e*) **Cells**.

(*a*) There can be little doubt that inflammation plays an important part in producing thickening of the **skull**, and increased density and rarefaction of its diploë; and that these changes are the result of irritations common to the bone, the membranes, and, in many instances, the cortex itself. The dura mater is the periosteum of the calvaria, and is supplied by the same vessels and lymphatics, and the two must always inevitably suffer from common causes of irritation. The thickenings of the inner table, causing a nodose appearance, often correspond to adhesions with the membrane. The frequency of the coincidence of a thickened vitreous lamina and a rarefied diploë are strongly suggestive of the change being a compensatory one, a view held by Rokitansky and others; but the strong probability is that such thickening is, to say the least, marked by previous or contemporaneous inflammatory action.

(*b*) **Membranes**.—B. Lewis states that his records show that in 20 per cent. of those dying insane the dura mater was found adherent to the skull. In our own experience the proportion is much greater, for in 300 autopsies we noted 109 cases in which this condition existed. This is all the more curious as in Scottish asylums the proportion of general paralytics and epileptics is less than in England. Adhesion may be complete over the whole dome, so complete indeed as to necessitate section of the dura before the calvaria can be removed. This is rare; the adhesions are generally local and are most frequently over the frontal lobes, at the sagittal suture and under the parietal eminences. They are evidences of "bygone inflammatory change" (Lewis), which, judging from the frequency of frontal or vertical headache in the prodromal period of idiopathic insanity, must be of early incidence. It is of importance to emphasise the early occurrence of this pain as bearing on the inflammatory theory. As Duret points out, inflammatory conditions of the bone or of the dura mater are accompanied by pain set up by the compression of the branches of the fifth, twelfth, and sympathetic nerves, produced by exudates. Given such testimony as to the conditions of the envelopes it is the natural inference that the brain elements which are primarily affected must be under the agency of similar conditions. Marked thickening of the dura is not common, but wherever the membrane is adherent to the bone a certain increase of its thickness can be found. The microscopic characters are irregular dilatation, tortuosity, and thickening of the vessels. Adhesions between the dura and arachno-pia are rare. When found, there is invariably accumulation of subdural fluid producing flattening of the subjacent convolutions. Granularity of the epithelium of the external surface of the arachno-pia is occasionally but rarely met with.

Pachymeningitis has been discussed in a separate article (*q.v.*). Whilst agreeing that in certain cases the *modus operandi* is as there stated, it is necessary to mention that German authorities lay great stress on the production of this condition by inflammatory processes. In Ziegler's "Pathologische Anatomie," Band ii. 1890, par. 129, p. 373, his views are thus stated:—

"*Pathological Anatomy of the Dura Mater.*—The dura mater is a membrane closely adherent to the bone within the cranial cavity and forms its inner periosteum. It is accordingly subject to all those changes that affect the periosteum of other bones; but as the sheath of the central nervous system certain special changes occur in it which require consideration.

"This membrane is very frequently the seat of an inflammatory process known as chronic internal pachymeningitis, which evidently appears in consequence of various injuries whose precise nature is not exactly understood. The inflammation is most frequently "hæmatogenous" and appears either independently or associated with inflammation of the pia mater and subarachnoid tissue; it may also accompany inflammation of the adjoining bones. It appears either unilaterally and in circumscribed areas, bilaterally and in scattered areas, or generally diffused over the entire cranial cavity.

"So far as is known, the outset of the inflammation is characterised anatomially by the formation of exceedingly thin deposits on the inner surface of the dura, which consist essentially of thin, granular, thready, or, at times even more homogeneous, fibrin with scanty round cells.

"After some time the membranes become pervaded by active (*lebensfähige*) cells, and interpenetrated by vessels growing as offshoots from the dura. From this germ tissue is afterwards formed a delicate fibrous tissue which lines the interior surface of the dura in the form of a membranous, transparent deposit, abounding in wide, thin-walled vessels filled with blood.

"The newly formed vessels of the membrane are particularly prone to bleed, the very slightest circulatory disturbances apparently sufficing to cause hæmorrhages through diapedesis and rupture. Consequently pachymeningitic membranes nearly always contain recent hæmorrhagic areas or pigmented deposits proceeding from older hæmorrhages, a peculiarity which has led to the process being described as hæmorrhagic pachymeningitis. The hæmorrhages are usually small, but may, however, attain such very considerable dimensions as partly to separate the already formed membranes from the dura and thus to form hæmatomata enclosed in a membranous sac which compress the brain more or less. If the new membranes (the blood-cysts or hæmatomata) give way, blood finds its way into the sub-dural space.

"When once the inflammation has set in it seems very rarely to be recovered from. The extravasated matters are indeed re-absorbed, but, where discharges are great, the process is both slow and imperfect, while, at the same time, the presence of the extravasated and disintegrated blood keeps up an irritation tending to fresh inflammation. Hence the inflammation continues, fresh exudations and fresh membranes are formed, which assume more and more a tough scar-like or callous character and contain more or less pigment, fibrinous residue, disintegrated blood and lime. Sometimes after absorption of a larger extravasation a local collection of liquid appears between the dura and the neo-membrane; this is known as hygroma of the dura mater or partial pachymeningitic hydrocephalus.

"In older, tougher membranes less rich in cells and more fibrous, a portion of the vessels usually atrophies, but a cure is not attained through this obliteration. Other parts remain highly vascular and fresh hæmorrhages maintain the inflammatory condition.

"Pachymeningitic membranes do not usually form any adhesions in their immediate neighbourhood; it may, however, happen that more or less firm connections are formed between them and the arachnoid, in consequence of which blood-vessels from the false membranes pass into the soft meninges.

"In addition to pachymeningitis interna chronica, there is also an external form, in which the inflammatory processes are confined essentially to the outer surfaces of the dura, and are associated with thickening of the latter membrane and with resorption and new formation of the bone substance. Moreover, the dura is very frequently inflamed through injuries and through inflammatory processes in the contiguous parts. When for example the skull is injured by a stab or blow, in consequence of which various inflammatory processes have been set up, the dura may also be involved sympathetically. In the same way inflammation of the middle ear, of the petrous bone or even of the orbital cavity may extend to the dura. When once suppuration sets in, the dura appears of a yellowish white or grayish-yellow colour. If previous hæmorrhages have occurred, the shade of colour may be dirty gray or grayish-green and brown."

In the pia mater in which the arteries ramify before their passage into the brain, and in which the veins are contained on their exit, the results of frequent and pathological congestions are extremely well marked to the naked eye; and, as might be expected from the intimate relation of the cortical pia to the exterior and interior of the brain substance, pathological processes in the one are usually associated with similar or allied morbid conditions in the other. Milky opacity is the most prominent departure from the normal condition; it is by no means confined to the brains of the insane, and may be often noted in the post-mortem rooms of general hospitals. It appears first as an opalescent streak on either side of the larger veins, and is doubtless due to occasional pathological congestion, superadded to the normal mechanical obstruction induced by the peculiar anatomical relations of the vessels to the longitudinal sinus. But the condition is never so well marked as in the insane, in whom the cloudy opacity is found involving the whole of the superior surface of the brain, and sometimes, although rarely, implicating its inferior aspect. In such cases the arachno-pia is often much thickened and separated from the visceral pia by the fluid, the trabeculæ being stretched, and its lymphatic spaces immensely dilated.

This condition, according to our own records, has been noted in 58 per cent. of those dying insane. Occasionally we find great tortuosity of the vessels, especially of the veins; lately we examined a case in which certain vessels were twisted three times on themselves like a coil of rope. The patient died from hæmorrhage into the sac of the pia mater, thin clots and fluid blood occupying the greater part of the cavity. Adhesion of the visceral pia to the brain substance has been noted by us as occurring in 37 per cent. of our dissections. The morbid connection between the membrane and the cortex is of two kinds, (a) the thickened sheath of the vessels, and (b) a fine reticulum produced by increase of the connective-tissue corpuscles of the external layer of grey matter. These are undoubtedly indications of inflammatory action, but not the only ones. We have said that such adhesions are found in 37 per cent. of insane persons, but they probably would be found in a larger proportion were it not that in many instances they have been obliterated (at least in the case of the reticulum) by the floating up of the membrane by fluid finding its way to the surface from below. In many cases we find the visceral pia separated from the surface of the cortex by a considerable open space, the membrane being attached by the hyaline sheaths only. A space in this position has been described by His as the "epicerebral lymph space," and the under surface of the visceral pia has been stated to be lined by endothelium. This lining we have failed to demonstrate, and the existence of such a lymphatic space is difficult to realise, as no provision has been suggested by which the fluid could reach the main currents. The only means of communication would be by stomata, and their existence has never been demonstrated. In connection with these adhesions B. Lewis says, when speaking of the subject generally, without definite reference to general paralysis or other inflammatory conditions, "*In earlier stages* [the italics are our own] the appearance is suggestive of inflammatory implication in the distinctly pinkish appearance of the cortex, sometimes diffused, sometimes limited to the areas of recent adhesions; the pia is thickened, tumid, and the seat of nuclear proliferation, its vessels deeply engorged, and the superjacent arachnoid also thickened, opaque, and œdematous. The distended vessels are coarse and tortuous, their sheaths thickened by multiplication of their cells and the traversing of their structure by wandering leucocytes"—a very picture of inflammatory action.

(c) Exactly the same state of matters exists around the vessels. We have already indicated the appearance presented by vessels during the earlier and later stages of congestion. If a vessel is carefully removed from the brain matter, laid on a slide, and gently washed with a camel's hair brush and water, it will often be found full of blood, sometimes so firmly packed as to defy all attempts to remove it. In such, and in bloodless vessels, especially at bifurcations, deposits of blood pigment and the other *débris* above alluded to, are found in large quantities, and the nuclei of the sheath are seen increased in number and size. In hardened sections the lumen, both of the vessel and lymphatic sheath, are seen fully occupied, the former by blood, the latter by leucocytes and fatty-looking *débris*. We repeat: the whole position points to the action of subinflammatory processes, the effects of which present themselves to the naked eye more prominently over the vertex and immediately surrounding parts, leaving the base and inferior lateral regions of the brain unaffected. The condition of the arachno-pia affords a very fair index of that of the subjacent convolutions; it is in fact (in addition to the lymphatic function) the connective-tissue capsule of the brain, and its intimate relations with the neuroglia that involve, almost necessarily, a liability of the two kinds of connective tissues to be affected by similar pathological processes.

(*d* and *e*) **Neuroglia and Connective-tissue Cells.**—The clinical fact that a very large proportion of idiopathic cases (70 per cent.) recover indicates that resolution can be procured by appropriate treatment, and that the channels becoming again nearly normal, the various functions of the organ can be again healthily exercised. The theory has been advanced by B. Lewis that the connective-tissue corpuscles exercise an important influence in the removal of effete products. In Brain, Anatomy of, it will be found stated that these bodies are of two kinds, one considerably larger than the other. The larger, called after their discoverer, Deiter's cells, are branched, and it is held that they are connected with the hyaline sheath by a process which may be canalicular, but which has not as yet been proved to be so. It is difficult to demonstrate these Deiter's, or spider, cells in healthy subjects; but in morbid conditions they are frequently met with, and can easily be made evident, especially in frozen sections stained with aniline black. In health neither the larger nor the smaller cells take up staining agents readily, and it is therefore inferred that their ready colouring in sections taken from diseased subjects indicates some molecular change in their protoplasm. It is undoubtedly true that it is impossible to obtain a demonstration so perfect in health as in disease. B. Lewis holds that these Deiter's cells are the "lymph connective" elements of the brain, that they are "scavenger" cells, and that they take a very active share in the processes of disease affecting the nervous centres. In his own words :—

"The delicate system of lymph connective elements permeating in the normal state the whole of the cerebral mass of white and grey substance takes a more active share in the pathogenesis of mental decadence than any other, and the more the question is investigated the greater importance, we feel convinced, will be attached to these elements in the processes of disease as affecting the nervous centres. Their physiological indications are clear; they are *scavengers of the brain*, and the evidence obtainable renders it now incontrovertible that they are liable to excessive and rapid development under certain morbid conditions affecting cerebral nutrition and repair in the normal condition of healthy cerebration. . . . . Whatever leads to increased waste of cerebral neurine; whenever structure disintegration is slowly proceeding either in nerve cell or fibre; whenever accumulation of *débris* occurs from disease of the vascular tracts; then we invariably note an augmented activity registered in these scavenger elements of the brain. That their activity is in direct ratio to the functional activity of the essential neurine tissue we think there can be no doubt, nor that with each accession of the nerve-tide they are stimulated to increased activity in the removal of the products of waste and the plasma effused from the vessels. In healthy states, however, they assume the hypertrophied form, the deep staining, the coarse fibrillation, the rapid multiplication, and the evidence of obvious intra-cellular digestion, which are readily observed in pathological states."*

The hypertrophied processes being distributed between the nerve elements and surrounding the vascular walls replace the delicate neuroglia, and as the cells undergo further alteration they produce a fully formed felt-like material. Hamilton, Zeigler, and B. Lewis agree that this material is liable to contract and seriously interfere with the permeability of the vessels. The last insists that these changes belong to the latter stages of disease, so that they are always associated with very rapid and advanced pathological processes or with chronic conditions. He believes that this condition is due to the irritation of certain specific poisons, but that it is also, in part at any rate, brought about wherever "a large accumulation of degenerated material has to be carried off from the cortex, or where effete material as the result of some obstruction to the normal transit of lymph from the brain has accumulated; in such positions we are likely to meet with this development of fibre cells."

Although we agree in the main with the above, we cannot help thinking that too much importance is attached to the function of these so-called scavenger cells on the one hand, and too little on the other; and that we must guard ourselves against the theory that there is associated with them in the brain, a pathological process different from that which occurs in other organs. There can be no doubt that the connective-tissue cells play an important phagocyte *rôle* in all parts of the body both in health and disease. It is equally certain that where there is material to be removed we find an increased development of connective-tissue cells. The greater the amount of effete material to be removed the more rapid is the development of these cells, and the more embryonic is the character they assume. It is during the embryonic stage that they appear to be specially active as scavengers, and it is only in the later stages when the protoplasm is losing its phagocyte activity that the reticular material is most fully developed, and we feel inclined to regard the large "scavenger cells" of B. Lewis as cells that have passed through a more active phagocyte stage than that in which they are when they assume the forms and appearances he so vividly describes. Still in this condition their phagocyte function is not, in all probability, entirely lost, and the substitution of the reticulum of processes serves to implicate the association system of ganglionic cell poles. The relation of these cells to the lymph spaces of the brain is indicative of the part they have to play in the absorption of neurine material and in the digestion or transformation of foreign matter and waste products. A parallel example of phagocyte function is afforded by the connective tissues of the lung, where the cells lining the lymphatic spaces and those free cells that are budded off from the fixed cells, have been shown to take up foreign particles of carbon or blood pigment, pass them on from point to point, and eventually get rid of them into the general stream; or, if the mass be large, they

* "A Text-Book of Mental Diseases."

attempt to surround it, so that it may be temporarily, or even permanently, cut off from the general lymphatic system. Wherever this takes place there is proliferation of the cells, and an alteration of the whole connective tissue arrangement. This proliferation may be the most permanent feature in the disease-processes, whilst in other cases it appears to play only a secondary part. To instance the lung again: during the early stages of a catarrhal pneumonia there may be a marked increase in the number of epithelial cells lining the air vesicles of certain lobules, but this is accompanied by comparatively slight connective tissue change or proliferation. After a time, however, if the process becomes chronic, we find that there is an absorption of irritant material formed from the mass of degenerating epithelial cells in the lymphatics, and as a result there is a marked proliferation of the connective-tissue cells. Here the proliferation is evidently quite secondary to the processes that have been going on in the air vesicles. But in certain other cases of pneumonia (as also in specific disease affecting the brain and in chronic alcoholism), there is apparently an almost primary increase in the amount of connective tissue, the irritant appearing to pass directly from the blood-vessels into the lymphatics, there setting up connective tissue proliferation. Whenever this is the case there is of course interference with the nutrition of the epithelial cells, in consequence of which there may be either proliferation and degeneration or degeneration only. We are inclined to apply this analogy to the connective tissue changes in the brain, and to assign very different degrees of importance in various forms of insanity to them, and to the action of the scavenger cells. In the forms of insanity in which a new formation of connective tissue takes place there will necessarily be a greater tendency to the removal of partially devitalised nerve tissue which, once removed, can so far as we know at present never be completely replaced; and nerve cells and processes which, if left to themselves, might have regained under proper nutrition a portion, if not the whole, of their former activity, will be removed by the over-active connective-tissue cells, by which they are as a matter of fact replaced. Although we make this general statement it must be borne in mind that without the removal of degenerated cells and effete products there can be no possibility of a return to health, so that the scavenger cells doubtless play a double *rôle*—reparative and destructive. Except in the most acute cases of idiopathic, and probably other forms of, insanity, their proliferation is not a marked feature in the early stage. In that stage we have increase of endothelium and *débris* occupying the lymphatic sheaths. With reduction of congestion this morbid material is removed; but if it is not got rid of by flushing we find, as in the case of chronic catarrhal pneumonia, well marked increase of these connective-tissue cells in the neighbourhood of vessels. This must be regarded as an effort of nature to remove the effete material collected in the ganglionic cell capsule. In cases of rapid recovery reduction of inflammation may be assumed; when recovery is protracted the slower process of elimination by phagocytes is at work; in the case of chronic terminative dementia the scavenger cells have failed, and in the abortive effort have so proliferated that they cause destruction of nerve fibre, of the lateral processes of the nerve cells, and finally of a considerable number of the cells themselves. We can only deduce from clinical observations the length of time taken by this destructive process. In the case of acute idiopathic mania, symptoms of recovery show themselves in from one to six months; if no improvement shows itself during the next six months, and a tendency to dementia is manifested, the case is all but hopeless, and we may infer that cell degradation has taken place to such an extent as to preclude the possibility of repair, and that certain other morbid products have been thrown out as a result of degeneration of fibre.

Lately we have obtained evidence of leucocytes taking on phagocyte action. In a case, the subject of which died of intercurrent disease, within nine months of the appearance of insanity, accompanied by obscure motor symptoms, the large cells of the motor area were found undergoing degeneration, and had evidently been attacked by leucocytes. They were clearly distinguishable from the scavenger cells of Lewis; when observed under high powers (×2000) the character of the nucleus was observable, and, moreover, no appearance of processes existed. The substance of the cells was in many instances invaded by one, two, or three such bodies, and were also surrounded by large numbers of the small nuclei of neuroglia. Throughout the whole specimen connective-tissue proliferation was extreme, especially on the vessels; but Deiter's cells were not to be found.

The first and most frequent evidence of over-action in idiopathic insanity is an excessive deposit of pigment in the large cells of the fifth layer. Pigment is found in these cells even in healthy subjects. We lately examined the brains of twelve adult subjects taken casually from the pathological department of the Edinburgh Infirmary, and in every instance an amount of pigment (variable indeed) was found, which, however, was specially well marked in those cases in which delirium had been a feature; in no instance were the cells changed in shape or size. We have examined the brains of six cases, terminating fatally in from two to ten months from the incidence of insanity from exhaustion, or some intercurrent disease, with the special object of observing the condition of these cells. In all there was great pigmentation, beginning at the base and extending to the apex. It was impossible to say whether this was preceded or accompanied by increase of size, an appearance produced as if by distension, the angles being obliterated and the sharp outlines destroyed. The pigment seemed to creep round the nucleus, occasionally displacing it. In all cases the nucleus itself was the last part to be affected by any degenerative change, and the first evidence of its implication seemed to be a white translucent spot, as if the nucleolus had disappeared and a transparent material had been substituted. The basal poles in the earlier cases presented a broader appearance, and, like the whole cell, readily took on pigment; but in no case did the staining agent affect these processes for more than three millimetres from the body, at which distance the pole first became less colourable, and then refused to receive any stain. In the later cases neither cells nor poles took on the staining reagent to such an extent as in the earlier ones; the lateral or protoplasmic processes could not be traced, and the cells presented the appearance of possessing a distinct cell wall. In the ten months case many cells had broken down, leaving nothing but the nuclei, and in certain instances these had been destroyed, the original body being represented by a mass of coloured granules, rounded, or diffused over a space three or four times that which had been originally occupied. As was pointed out by Howden, pigmentation is always associated with hæmatoidin deposits round the vessels. The cells of the outer layers do not seem to suffer so severely from this process, only faint tingeing of a much finer yellow material being observable at their bases, and this but rarely. In the two cases of longest standing many cells were noticed undergoing a granular degeneration unassociated with pigmentation. These also had changed shape, the nuclei were displaced, and the lateral poles lost, although the apical processes could be traced for considerable distances. In cases of chronic terminative dementia, this is invariably to be noticed. In some instances we have found immensely "inflated" or swollen non-granulated cells in the motor area, almost uncolourable by carmine or logwood. Meynert speaks of this condition as "œdematous." Here it is often very difficult to demonstrate any cellular elements; those in the three outer layers are withered and collapsed-looking, showing as mere streaks slightly more coloured than the surrounding tissue. Often they will not take on carmine at all, but hæmatoxylin usually is absorbed slightly. The larger cells, again, in such cases are often highly granular, and present little or no pigmentation: they may be reduced to fatty-looking masses, irregular in outline, the nuclei having even disappeared. Both in connection with pigmentary and granular degeneration resulting from idiopathic mania, vacuolation is occasionally met with, but not nearly to the extent to which it is observable in other forms of insanity.

We have said that the condition of the pia mater affords a fair index of the condition of the immediately subjacent tissues. Membranes covering the convolutions which are believed to contain identical centres—those of the frontal lobes, are as a rule much less deeply affected by diseased action than those of the superior, and superior lateral aspects. This is mainly due to anatomical arrangements already described, and the presence of mental symptoms must be largely referable to imperfect drainage of the region of intellectual action. It is impossible to say how far the almost invariable implication of the large cells of the motor area is productive of hebetude and other motor symptoms so constant in the insane.

The loss of the protoplasmic lateral or associative processes of the cells must be regarded as a most important feature, probably even more important than the destruction of individual cells. If we accept the theory of ideational centres, the cutting off of one from another must form the basis on which to found a system of morbid psychology. In this connection we cannot do better than quote the words of B. Lewis:—

"The interdependence of the structural elements of the cortex, due to its terminal system of arteries, is of primary importance to us in correctly appreciating the morbid appearances presented in insanity. Another factor, however, must be invariably considered with respect to all morbid lesions of the cortex, and that is the sympathy betwixt *distant* territories which are functionally associated in their activities, and structurally linked together by 'association' fibres. The former condition—the interdependence of parts in terminal systems—was the direct outcome of elaborate differentiation; the latter condition of sympathy betwixt distant territories is established by an equally elaborate structural integration."

Atrophy of the brain, general or local, is a sequence of inflammatory action. General atrophy is rare; it is usually confined to the superior or lateral convolutions, and may be induced by pressure from exuded fluid, or by phagocyte action. In the former case inflammatory exudates are poured into the cavity of the pia (subarachnoid space) more rapidly than they can be carried off by the natural channels, they flood the sub-dural space, and produce pressure of no inconsiderable degree. In dealing with intra-cranial fluid in connection with insanity it seems to have been assumed by most authors that all such accumulations are "compensatory;" by which is meant, passive accumulations of fluid. We find inflammation credited with the production of many lesions, but its influence in the production of exudate fluid is studiously ignored. Still in fatal cases of recent acute insanity we find large accumulations, which had they occurred in the subject, say, of basal meningitis, would be regarded as a direct result of the condition. We have no direct evidence of this during life so far as idiopathic insanity is concerned, but we have most undoubtedly observed a marked bulging of the dura mater in two early cases of general paralysis, a condition distinctly due to inflammatory action. As we shall have to consider the subject of fluid pressure in the production of atrophy *in extenso* when speaking of general paralysis, it is, to save repetition, relegated to that section.

Shrinking of the brain may be caused by contraction of sclerosed regions and pathological phagocyte action. In this case, of course, compensatory fluid is called for and provided; as also in the case of local atrophy. Local atrophy is generally produced by plugging or serious congestive interference with the patency of the terminal arteries of the convolutions. One of the most important of Duret's observations is that these vessels are strictly terminal and do not anastomose with those of immediately adjacent regions. If this assertion be correct, when such an artery is plugged atrophy, confined to the area which it supplied, is a necessary consequence. The frequency of atrophy, general and local, in the insane is remarkable. The statistics of B. Lewis, referring to insanity in the mass show that out of 1565 fatal cases, it was present in 1055 (or 67.4 per cent.) "that the wasting was general throughout the hemisphere in 574 cases, although 261 also showed a special implication of certain areas, and that in 481 other cases partial or localised atrophy was observed." The occurrence of local atrophies occurred in the following sequence of frequency—the fronto-parietal segment, postero-parietal lobule, the central gyri, the separate frontal gyri and Sylvian boundary, the temporo-sphenoidal, the occipital and angular gyri.

The most important of the degenerative changes shown by the microscope are *miliary sclerosis* and *colloid bodies*. The former was first described by Drs. Batty Tuke and Rutherford,* and their observations were confirmed by Dr. Kesteven.† Many attempts have been made to prove that these appearances are produced by hardening agents and spirit; but this theory is shown to be utterly unsubstantial by the fact that miliary sclerosis is easily demonstrable in fresh frozen sections. Were it artificial it would be found in all brains hardened in spirit, which is not asserted by Savage and others who have tried to discredit it; that it is found in the spinal cords of animals is what might be expected, when we consider how liable they are to spinal injuries and to inflammation of the cord in early life. Spirit was never used by us in our hardening methods; we have since tried various methods of hardening, and also of cutting in a fresh condition and always with the same result. But the question has been set at rest by B. Lewis, who shows that miliary sclerosis can be traced in sections prepared both by hardening and in the fresh state. This we had observed ourselves previous to the publication of Lewis's important work. The original description of miliary sclerosis still holds good: "as a rule the spots are unilocular, occasionally bilocular, and in rare instances multilocular; but whatever their condition in this respect is, they possess the same internal characteristics. A thin section prepared in chromic acid, viewed by the naked eye, shows a number of opaque spots irregularly distributed over the surface of the white matter; they are best seen in a tinted section, as they are not colourable by carmine. When magnified under a low power, they have a somewhat luminous pearly lustre, and when magnified 250 and 800 diameters

* *Edin. Med. Journ.*, 1868.

† *Brit. and For. Medico-Chir. Review*, 1868.

fusing, they are seen to consist of molecular material, with a stroma of exceedingly delicate, colourless fibrils. They possess a well-defined outline, and the neighbouring nerve fibres and blood-vessels are pushed aside and curve round them. In well-advanced cases the plasm seems denser at the circumference of the spots than at their centres, and a degree of absorption of the contiguous nerve fibres is evident; this solution of continuity is only noticeable at the point where the lateral expansion is greatest. The spots are generally colourless, but in some instances they are of a yellowish-green tint, which may be attributable to chromic acid. They vary much in size; multilocular spots are $\frac{1}{10}$ of an inch to $\frac{1}{100}$ of an inch in diameter, the unilocular from over $\frac{1}{100}$ to $\frac{1}{500}$ of an inch. As many as eleven locules have been observed in one patch, separated one from the other by fine trabeculæ of nervous tissue."

These spots are very rarely found in the grey matter, and then only at its edge; in the white matter they may be seen with the naked eye, studding the white matter in considerable numbers. B. Lewis states that the condition is, at a certain stage, invariably associated with an increase of Deiter's cells, and that the peri-vascular nuclei frequently exhibit proliferation and granular hæmatoidin, in the vascular sheaths, in sections in which miliary sclerosis exists. We have found it in the superior convolutions, the pons, medulla, cerebellum, and cord. B. Lewis has figured with great accuracy its appearance in longitudinal sections of the spinal cord: "The morbid product is then seen to be aggregated in oval or elongated elliptic patches measuring 139μ to 186μ in length, by 40μ to 70μ in breadth . . . . and its appearance at once suggests to the mind the forcible extravasation at numerous points of a coagulable material which has driven the textural elements asunder before it." We are entirely at one with this author as to the nature of this product, having changed our opinion on the subject after having examined his preparations. These patches undoubtedly consist of altered myelin exuded in droplets from the medullated tubes and coalescing more or less completely, the axis-cylinder being forced aside along with the neighbouring tissues, or undergoing solution of continuity. Miliary sclerosis is "not a primary sclerotic change," but is an accident occurring in the course of sub-acute inflammatory action (Lewis). The term miliary sclerosis does not express the nature of the condition except so far as certain of its results or accompaniments are concerned; but it has been so long in use as to make it difficult to suggest a change in nomenclature.

Colloid degeneration is a condition allied to miliary sclerosis. Hamilton from a series of experiments on the spinal cord of animals came to the conclusion that colloid bodies were developed from the axis cylinder as the result of inflammation. He describes them as occasionally showing concentric rings, undergoing fissiparous division, and producing "depôts" of similar round translucent bodies of smaller size: in a later stage developing nuclei, becoming transparent and granular, presenting the appearance of "mother cells," with small cells in their interior, which are set free as pus-corpuscles. This description can only apply to these bodies under the condition of acute inflammation. Woodhead described a similar condition as due to a more chronic inflammation of the cord in a case of locomotor ataxia.* We have never seen this form of degeneration in the human brain except as round or oval translucent bodies, a little larger or smaller than a blood corpuscle. In the pons, medulla, and cord certainly they are found somewhat larger; and we have met with them much smaller in the brains of birds undergoing irritation—*e.g.* in pigeons we have seen them 3μ in diameter. They stain with hæmatoxylin; osmic acid renders them black; but they do not readily take up carmine, and are unaffected by aniline blue-black. They are, without doubt, produced like miliary sclerotic spots, by change occurring in the hyaline sheath. It is possible the axis-cylinder may assist, but the changes in that organ noticed in connection with colloid degeneration are usually the result of affections of the sheath. In fact the axis-cylinder may often be traced through a tumour or ampullation consisting of swollen hyaline. Colloid bodies are found in groups in the white matter, sometimes near vessels, or in lines following the course of fibres of the part. In old-standing cases of senile dementia we have found them (small in size) immediately below the visceral pia, and below the epithelium of the ventricles. Dr. A. Miles, of Edinburgh, has lately found them in great numbers and of large size in the brains of persons dying after traumatic injury to the head. He examined specimens by both the fresh freezing and hardening methods; and found them in a boy who died fourteen hours after an accident, and in another case which died in two hundred and fifty-six hours. They were distributed

* *Journ. Anat. and Phys.*, vol. xvi. p. 364.

all through the white matter of the convolutions near the seat of injury, in the most superficial layer of the grey matter, and in the lymphatic system. In the white matter they appeared as small round droplets, 7μ in size, gradually increasing in size as they approached the cortex, and most numerous in the vicinity of punctiform hæmorrhages. They were largest (30μ to 50μ) on the free surface of the brain below the visceral pia, suggesting that several droplets had coalesced after finding their way outwards by the space between the hyaline sheaths and the brain substance. When seen in the meshes of the pia mater they were always near lacerations of the visceral pia: "when in relation to the intra-cortical vessels, they were found in the peri-vascular lymph space of His."* It is evident that colloid bodies can be produced by inflammatory processes, and by direct injury to the head, causing, so to speak, a bruised condition of the nerve fibre. But it is probable that in those suffering from chronic insanity they are secondary lesions, the result of impaired nutrition of fibre consequent on cell degeneration. It is also more than probable that their composition is identical with miliary sclerosis, and that the more highly organised appearance of the latter is due to a slower process of production, and a greater accumulation of material.

The examination of nerve fibre requires to be conducted with special precautions on account of the rapidity with which post-mortem changes occur in it. Even in winter, and when subjects have been removed to a mortuary, the temperature of which is not greater than that of the atmosphere, the examination should not be delayed for a longer period than twenty-four hours; under any circumstances it is better to keep the head surrounded by ice till the autopsy can be conducted. The myelin sheath is the structure first implicated, although it appears to resist the action of inflammatory processes for a long period. The degeneration is first marked by a tendency to ampullation under very moderate pressure on the cover-glass; later on the myelin breaks down and forms masses of a fatty nature, colloid bodies and points of "miliary sclerosis." The axis cylinder may be traced for a considerable distance denuded of its medulla. Although we have sought very carefully for changes in the axial cylinder, such as those described by Ranvier, we have failed to detect them in the brains of the insane: this is probably due to the rapid obliteration of the axial cylinder after destruction of the sheath has taken place. The small slightly refractile bodies often seen in recent specimens are apparently the detritus of degenerated myelin.

* *Brain*, July 1890.

The pathological appearances presented in *general paralysis* have occupied the attention of many observers; and lesions of the various constituents of the encephale have been described with considerable accuracy. But it remained for Bevan Lewis to collate these observations with his own, eliminate error, and put the whole together in consecutive form: adding to existing knowledge the most accurate and minute descriptions of diseased tissues; advancing and demonstrating their *modus operandi* in producing the naked eye appearances, and co-relating, as far as possible, the clinical phenomena with the results of pathological research. His account of the morbid anatomy of the disease must be accepted as the most perfect which has as yet been produced, and we therefore give a summary of it, interpolating remarks where his conclusions seem open to doubt.

Three well marked stages in the morbid implication of the cortex are to be observed: (1) A stage of inflammatory change in the tunica adventitia with excessive nuclear proliferation, profound changes in the vascular channels, and trophic changes induced in the tissues around; (2) a stage of extraordinary development of the lymph connective tissue of the brain, with a parallel degeneration and disappearance of nerve elements, the axis cylinders of which are denuded; (3) a stage of general fibrillation with shrinking and extreme atrophy of the parts involved.

(1) Stage of inflammatory engorgement. Lesions are first noticed in the vessels of the pia, and the lymphatic sheath is where inflammatory change originates. Although in early cases slight cloudiness of the arachno-pia may be noted, and there may be greater difficulty than in health in removing the visceral pia, there is no general adhesion to the brain substance. In our own experience we have, in two very early cases, both dying from lung affections within six months of the definite symptoms of general paralysis, and in two others who died within nine months, observed a much greater degree of adhesion than B. Lewis mentions, and feel inclined to the opinion that the disease may either first affect the visceral pia and extend to the hyaline sheath, or that the two portions may be synchronously affected. But it may be admitted that in most cases the proliferation of the cells of the adventitia is better marked than in those of the outer layer of grey matter. Still, in the four

[illegible] alluded to the difference in amount was slight. The amount of proliferation may be enormous, so much so as to conceal the vessel; it is a genuine inflammatory process, accompanied by the usual signs of inflammation, transudation of fluid, diapedesis, and collection of hæmatoidin crystals, especially at the bifurcations of vessels. From the cells of the pia processes are sent downwards even to the deepest layers of the cortex. As the disease advances the soft membranes become more and more gravely implicated.

"The nuclear proliferation around the vessels of the pia, their distension and engorgement (from paralysis of the vital contractility of the muscular coat) lead to a very free exudation into the meshes of the pia. The connective trabeculæ lying between the intima pia and arachnoid (arachno-pia) . . . . become saturated with a fluid exudate, present a swollen and gelatiniform aspect to the naked eye, streaked with opaque lines, or assume a patchy, or a general and uniformly diffused opalescence. . . . . Into this space exude the cellular and fluid products of the inflammatory sheath. This tendency to the accumulation of exudate in the subarachnoid (pial) lymph-tissues receives a marked increment at a later stage of the disease; for when atrophic changes occur in the cortex as the result of impaired nutrition and degeneration of nerve elements, a great compensatory serosity of this lesion is established, and the membranes become fairly water-logged. The atrophy, which is the result of a genuine sclerotic change in the cortex, is necessarily more marked in the sulci than over the summits of the gyri, the area of cortical surface involved in the one case being far greater than in the other, and, in consequence thereof, the gyri become *narrower* and *attenuated*, the thinning of the cortical layers being the most marked feature."*

Whilst fully agreeing with this author as to the compensatory nature of the fluid at a later stage of the disease, when shrinking has taken place consequent on the contraction by the sclerosed condition of the glia cells, we have pretty definite data for holding that in the early inflammatory stage the fluid is, as he states, a true exudate, and is being poured out in such quantities that it cannot be removed by the normal channels,† and so acts by pressure on the convolutions in the production of general atrophy of the superior gyri. The question is one of great importance in its bearings on treatment. Dr. B. Tuke, in three, and Dr. Claye Shaw‡ in two, cases caused the parietal bones to be trephined, on the presumption that exudates cause pressure on the convolutions. If such is not the case, and if the fluid is purely compensatory, of course such an operation is not justifiable. But in the case so treated definite evidence was afforded that positive pressure did exist, as on removal of the disc of bone the dura mater bulged freely into the hole, and after the operation in each case, marked remission of symptoms took place, and in three instances the progress of the disease was distinctly stayed. In two of Dr. Tuke's cases where the arachno-pia was laid bare the naked-eye evidence of inflammation was most evident and definite; no doubt could exist for a moment, but that the pia as a whole was in a state of actual inflammation, more evident however on one side than the other. Negative pressure could not have produced bulging, and the demonstration of positive pressure is complete. One of our first cases died of pneumonia eight months after the operation. The dura mater had not been opened. On post-mortem examination a large accumulation of fluid in the sub-dural and pia-matral spaces was found in the left side on which the bulging took place; on the other side, where no protrusion had occurred, the amount of fluid was slight. On the left side corresponding to the accumulation of fluid, the whole subjacent area of the convolutions was atrophied; on the right side no marked change in the bulk of the gyri presented itself. The localisation of the effusion was probably due to inflammatory thickening and adhesion of the two layers of pia, forming a closed sac, and occluding the lymphatic channels. Into this sac the fluid was being constantly poured, and the only means of escape was by the Pacchionian villi into the sub-dural space and the longitudinal sinus. The pressure caused by rapid infiltration and slow absorption gradually caused atrophy of the subjacent convolutions. From these definite observations we are of opinion that Bevan Lewis has overlooked the important fact that intracranial fluid, especially at the earlier stages of this and other diseases, is a producer of pressure, and is often not compensatory. He proves to demonstration the presence of inflammatory action, but excludes from the process one of its first and most important products.

Epileptic Insanity.—The whole subject of epilepsy having been fully considered in a special article, it is only necessary to refer to the morbid appearances presented in the brains of the epileptic insane. An

* Bevan Lewis, *loc. cit.*, pp. 497–8.

† *Brit. Med. Journ.*, 4 Jan. 1890. ‡ *Ib.* 6 Nov. 1889.

amount of interest connected with the subject generally surrounds the observations of B. Lewis. Founding certain physiological deductions on the fact that he has noticed a diseased condition of the cells of the second layer, and of the large ganglionic cells of the motor tract, he infers that the former possess inhibitory powers over the latter. The change in the cells of the second layer is peculiar, inasmuch as the nucleus is the first part affected: "the centre of the nucleus is occupied by an extremely bright, highly refractile, spherical body—obviously of a fatty nature." In stained specimens this spot shows as a "bright spherical bead," standing out all the more strongly on account of the deep tint taken on by the body of the cell.

Vacuolation takes place as the disease advances, caused by the "bursting out from the cell of the globular bead of fatty substance. . . . . This extreme degree of change may occupy the whole of the second layer of the cortex, but in certain cases it has been found to affect every layer down to the spindle-series of the cells." Although the cell protoplasm becomes eventually affected, it resists for a long time the action of the nuclear disease; in the long run, however, the whole cell disappears, or is reduced to *débris*. The large ganglionic cells suffer in the earlier stages in the manner we described in the fourth edition of Bucknill and Tuke's "Manual"; they are abnormally large and distinct, stain much more deeply than in healthy subjects, become distended in appearance, and lose their natural contour. According to Lewis, they lose their special processes.

Still following B. Lewis's statements, there is no associated vascular change, and spider-cells are not present. On the assumption that the cells of the second layer possess inhibitory power over the motor cells he finds in their affection, and in the destruction of all means of communication with the ganglionic cells, an explanation of the convulsive phenomena of epilepsy. Were these statements applicable to all cases, the pathology of epilepsy would have had considerable light thrown upon it. It may be admitted that in a certain class of epileptics Lewis's observations may hold good: but it is certainly not applicable to all, inasmuch as the appearances described do not present themselves in every case of brain disease symptomatosed by epilepsy. We have seen the appearances spoken of, although never to such a marked degree as Lewis describes; but we have also examined many cases by the same methods, in which the lesions differed entirely or in part. Besides the condition of the ganglionic cells already spoken of, we have noted in them the brightly refracting nucleus, which has been absent in the superior layers, and the apical, along with the other poles have, in common with the cell, presented an appearance suggestive of the term hypertrophy, the apical poles being traceable for long distances. At the same time vascular changes have been well marked; the vessels have been thickened, and the lumen of the channel in the cerebral matter has been distinctly dilated. It may be suggested that this was the result of hardening agents causing retraction of the tissues, but all our specimens, morbid and healthy alike, were treated in exactly the same manner; the wide open spaces around the vessels were particularly well-marked in the case of epileptics. And, again, we have never procured more typical specimens of spider-cells than around the vessels in epileptic brains, in which the connective tissue generally was markedly affected. There can be no doubt that during attacks of the *grand mal* great cerebral congestion exists. This has been duly considered elsewhere. But the effects of constantly recurring extreme congestion tell on the whole economy of the cells, and in the case of a certain proportion of epileptics, insanity of a pretty definite character results from the implication of these cells. It is frequently of an impulsive, "explosive" type, and suggests an interesting correlation with the muscular phenomena of the affection.

Another change met with, and frequently described as associated with the epileptic condition, is the formation of granulations on the floor of the ventricles. This is usually associated with proliferative or other changes of the cells of the ependyma, or with proliferation or increased new formation of the subjacent connective tissue. Along with this there is usually evidence of congestion of the blood-vessels in this region. The simplest form, and the one most frequently met with, is a simple throwing into folds of the ependymal covering—really a further extension of the choroid fringe. A second form consists of a kind of granulation tissue, in which the young connective tissue first projects the ependymal cells before it into the cavity of the ventricle, and then breaks through, leaving a solution of continuity of the cellular layer.

In the third form, in which the granulations are not nearly so large, there appears to be simple swelling, accompanied by vacuolation, of the ependymal cells. There is some diversity of opinion as to whether these granulations are really the cause of any clinical symptoms; but the strong probability is that they interfere with the free movement of the upper part of the brain over the base, and that the friction generated by the rubbing together of the two surfaces, or even by the passage of fluid through the ventricular cavity in cases of sudden movement, may cause considerable irritation and excitation of the areas covered by these granulations. They will certainly impede the free movements of fluid, and also of the brain, so necessary to keep up compensatory changes in connection with alterations in the blood supply of the various parts of the cerebral cortex; they will thus interfere, not only with the nutrition, but also with the actual function of the nervous tissues.

In the *acute maniacal delirium* which occasionally presents itself during the course of acute infective fevers two factors have to be taken into consideration: first, the specific poison which appears to act directly on the nerve cells, giving rise to stimulation and impaired nutrition, and consequent granular degeneration; and, secondly, the high temperature, during the persistence of which metabolic, or, to speak more accurately, catabolic, processes go on more rapidly. In such cases we have always clinical evidence of a more or less well-marked affection of both sensory and motor cells. In very acute cases there is, accompanying the changes in nerve elements, extraordinary proliferation of connective tissue cells around the vessels, and migration of leucocytes, a condition commonly associated with the presence of micro-organisms, and well marked in cases of acute exudative meningitis. The insanity following fever is more frequently of an anæmic type.

The insanity of *sunstroke* is a toxic condition allied to that just spoken of. It is the result of catabolic changes produced by high temperature. In certain instances it may be caused by carbonic acid poisoning.

There is strong reason for believing that in *puerperal insanity* a considerable proportion of cases is due to toxic influences. It must be remembered that, although a woman may become insane during the puerperal period, her case need not be referable primarily to childbirth. Mental symptoms may be, in point of fact, idiopathic—*i.e.*, the result of so-called moral causes—the effect of which culminating at the birth of her child show themselves some three weeks or a month later by an attack of simple mania or melancholia. But the violent delirous mania which is apt to develop within fifteen days after delivery has all the aspect of being due to toxic influence. Its sudden inception, delirious character, rapid development, inflammatory complications, and tendency to death are eminently suggestive of septic origin. Such cases rarely present themselves later than a fortnight after childbirth (the period during which septic changes go on in the uterus), and more frequently within ten days. Absorption from the uterine surface of disorganised material and blood, acting on a system which has been already subjected to considerable drain, exercises its influence on the most highly organised cells, and acute violent mania, temporary in character but followed by prolonged brain weakness, is the result.

It is of importance to note, from an ætiological point of view, the *absence* of insanity as an accompaniment or sequela of certain complaints which *à priori* might be supposed to be prolific causes, but, to which morbid mental symptoms can in fact, be rarely referred. Insanity is never the pathological consequence of diseases of individual organs, but is occasionally more or less closely associated or connected with those forms of disease which result from diathesis or cachexia, such as tuberculosis, rheumatism, gout, and syphilis. There are many diseases painful in character and very depressing to the nervous system, such as calculus, fistula, cancer of the rectum and uterus, stricture, with its often miserable complications, and many others which suggest themselves, which might be presupposed to be probable fertile causes of insanity, but which, in point of fact, are not inimical to brain health. They may be so indirectly, inasmuch as they prevent sleep; but even in this wise their effect is very slight. Nor does there appear sufficient evidence to warrant the connection of diseases of the heart, liver, or kidneys with insanity. It has been sought to show that certain forms of heart disease are associated occasionally with simple or hypochondriacal melancholia, and others with mania. These observations, however, are not supported by extended clinical observation. Nor do we think that diseases of the liver or kidneys have any real connection with the induction of insanity; except, perhaps, that in Bright's disease a temporary mania is rarely met with, probably the first indication of uræmic poisoning. The direct production of insanity or delirium of short duration has been observed, but it is very doubtful whether prolonged mania or melancholia can be clearly shown to be associated with such diseases except as producers of over-excitation of the brain.

Much stress has been laid on diseases of the *uterus* and *ovaries*, and more especially on tumours of those organs, as the primary factors in the production of insanity. Skae laid down as special forms, utero- and ovario-mania, and Hergt has described the various morbid conditions of the female organs found on post-mortem examination, and has connected them with mental symptoms. But authors on gynæcology make no mention of insanity as a sequela of uterine disease, except in so far the mental depression which in many women follows on the knowledge that they are affected by serious, perhaps fatal, disease, and the pain and anxiety inseparable therefrom, may produce sleeplessness and consequent melancholy; and there is no proof of such tumours exercising an extensive influence on causation by peripheral irritation. The fallacy that such connection exists has, in the great majority of instances, probably arisen from the observation often made in asylums that insanity arising from whatever cause is conditioned by the presence of uterine growths, and that delusions of a sexual character may arise from the sensations thereby produced. For all practical purposes peripheral irritation may be dismissed from the list of producers of insanity. Did it so act the records of surgical hospitals would surely produce endless examples of its morbid action on brain health. We are aware that there are reported cases of mania being produced by such slight causes as a splinter of wood in the hand or foot: in all such we are convinced more important underlying factors have been overlooked. It is an interesting but unexplained fact that insanity occasionally follows on extirpation of the ovaries; and that in all the insanities resulting from morbid conditions of the female generative organs, delusions of mistaken identity are commonly met with.

It cannot be said that any strong pathological evidence has been advanced to connect such *diathetic conditions* as tuberculosis, gout, and rheumatism with the production of insanity. The strongest case has been made out in favour of tuberculosis; there is a probability that its accompaniment, anæmia, may exercise a certain influence. There is apparently no toxic agent at work in such cases. But on the whole we are inclined to think that insanity is more conditioned than induced by the tubercular state. In the same way gout and rheumatism undoubtedly exercise an influence on the progress of a case. The connective tissues, predisposed by the diatheses to morbid changes no doubt now and then increase, probably in the immediate neighbourhood of blood-vessels, and, by the consequent affection of motor areas, choreic movements are induced. These may also be induced by similar affection of the cord. But a true gouty or rheumatic insanity—*i.e.*, an insanity arising out of structural changes produced primarily in the nervous centres by the action of the several poisons is extremely doubtful. Did such cases exist it might be expected that motor symptoms would be the first to occur, whereas in all the reported cases the choreic movements presented themselves after the mental symptoms were more or less confirmed. The rheumatic, and especially the gouty, poison attacks regions undergoing degeneration or weakened by disease, and, given vessels in a sub-inflammatory condition, the strong probability is that these toxic agents will fasten on their connective tissue, and complicate the condition and its symptoms.

Excluding the consideration of depression, *contre coup*, and laceration, as results of *traumatic injury* of the skull, the lesions produced are the diffused clots in the pia-mater (sub-arachnoid space), and under the visceral pia, and bruise of the substance of the convolutions. This bruise affects the small vessels and the myelin sheath of the nerve fibre. In the case of the former, small rounded clots are seen in section in the grey, and extending for some distance into the white matter. We have already drawn attention to the results of injury in the myelin sheath. In the attempt of the tissues to remove the morbid materials produced by traumatism, the connective tissue becomes increased in quantity, and the consequence is a local sclerosis, extending probably for some distance from the area of injury. Cases of "general paralysis" as a consequence of local injury are not uncommon, and are induced by this pathological process.

Toxic Insanity.—In considering the various insanities associated with toxic conditions, there may be taken as types three different forms of poisoning, and under one of these three headings may be approximately arranged the various forms of insanity which are looked upon as toxic. (1) In the first place, the toxic group associated with *alcoholic* poisoning, may be divided into (*a*) those acute conditions in which alcohol appears to act directly on the nerve cells, along with which may be associated such forms as chloroform and ether poisoning; (*b*) the condition brought about by chronic alcoholism, where in consequence of frequent acute poisonings the cells gradually undergo a process of degeneration, associated with which are marked lesions in the blood vascular and connective tissue systems. (2) In the second group may be placed those acute maniacal conditions in which poisons developed *within the body* appear to act first in stimulating and then in depressing the nerve cells; such conditions as are found in the delirium of fevers and septic poisonings. And (3) we may arrange in a third group those forms of insanity, comparatively chronic in character, which result from poisons which continue to be developed in the system after their first introduction; of this group *syphilis* is probably the most typical. A more minute subdivision might undoubtedly be made, but most of the characteristic forms of toxic insanity may be brought under one or other of these headings.

The alcoholic or etherial poisoning, of which acute alcoholism may be taken as the type, induces acute symptoms through two channels: first, by acting directly on vaso-motor cells, the motor cells of the fifth layer, and the presumably inhibitory cells of the second layer; and secondly, by acting through altered vascular supply, through the vaso-motor cells. It has been experimentally shown by Binz, that after the exhibition of chloroform, ether or alcohol, there is distinct alteration in the appearance of the larger cells in the brain, characterised by a parenchymatous or cloudy, granular swelling of their protoplasm. There is in fact marked evidence of increased activity of their protoplasm, but, so far as has been noted, there is little or no change in the appearance of the nucleus. There is thus evidence of increased activity and of increased functional discharge of and from the brain cells. If, however, this condition is maintained for any length of time, it is found that not only is the protoplasm affected, but slight alterations take place, even in the nucleus. Along with this change in the cells of the cortex there appears to be sometimes, in the earliest stages, increased vascularity of the cerebral tissues, a condition which must be associated with the increased functional activity of the cells; this is invariably accompanied by a greater functional activity of the lymph-vascular system—in which we find an increase of nuclei—and a greater prominence of the endothelial plates lining the lymph spaces, changes that must be associated with the increased quantity of the effete matter that has to be carried away from the more active cells. This condition of stimulation and exaltation appears to be so intense that the cells are rapidly exhausted, and a condition of stupor supervenes, a condition which allows of the ready excretion of the poison, of a rebuilding up of the cell substances, and of a comparatively rapid return to the normal condition of the vaso-motor system. In acute alcoholism we have in fact a temporary mania, with increased motor discharge, diminished inhibition, rapid running down, and a temporary degeneration of the nerve cells, accompanied by abnormal blood supply and production of waste materials, for the removal of which there is increased activity of the blood and lymph-vascular systems. By an easy transition we pass from acute to chronic alcoholic insanity, in which essentially the same structures are affected, but in different degrees, and giving rise to different symptoms. In chronic alcoholic insanity the convulsive element very frequently predominates, and in many respects the pathology is similar to that of epilepsy. The blood-vessels are found to have invariably undergone very marked changes. In the smaller vessels these conditions are evidenced in the one case by marked proliferation of the nuclei, leading to great increase in their number, by which the lines of the vessels are very distinctly marked out in the cortical substance (Lewis). In other cases the cells are distinctly fatty, they do not take on the staining reagents, and have a peculiar granular appearance. Bevan Lewis points out that in addition to these changes there is a very great increase in the number of "scavenger" cells in the outer layer of the cortex, where the connective tissue is intimately associated with the vessels of the pia mater, and a similar increase along the line of blood-vessels running towards the deeper layers; this being accompanied by other evidences of inflammatory change, such as the characteristic amyloid bodies in the lymph spaces and proliferation of the connective tissue nuclei.

The pathological changes enumerated by Bevan Lewis are as follows:—(1) Vessels in cortex large and tortuous; coats in advanced stages of atheromatous and fatty degeneration. (2) Nuclei in adventitia proliferating, or protoplasm of cells fatty. (3) In superficial layer of cortex and along line to blood-vessels scavenger cells numerous. (4) Amyloid bodies in *epicerebral* spaces. (5) Numerous lymphoid elements in peri-vascular and peri-cellular paces. (6) Lesions in second and third layers are only seen after implication of the motor cells of fifth layer. These and the layer of spindle cells immediately beneath the deepest cortical layers then become degenerated and fatty. Invasion here appears to be from the medulla and the central gyri.

The changes in the vessels are nuclear proliferation, atheroma, and aneurysmal dilatation, the latter of which eventually gives rise to the cribriform condition. The motor cells are swollen and rounded, stain deeply, become granularly pigmented, and the apical process degenerates. This, according to Lewis, accounts for the interference with the inhibitory action of the cells of the second layer in chronic alcoholism. The cell wall is thickened, which shows that it is losing its functional activity. There is a considerable quantity of pigment deposited between the shrinking protoplasm and this cell wall. The processes of the cells are stunted and are covered with nuclei, and the protoplasm is granular or vacuolated. In the lowest layer "scavenger" cells and nuclei cover the spindle cells, which are very much altered and degenerated, and are practically being devoured by these proliferating cells. The medullary sheath of the nerve processes gradually disappears, or is so altered by the invading connective tissue that the axis cylinder, which is frequently fusiform as in other cases of inflammation of the nerve fibres, can be perfectly well stained with the aniline colour when it becomes a prominent feature in the cortex. These are to be demonstrated with great difficulty in a normal brain, but in senile decay of the cortex they are even more evident than in alcoholics. In the white matter the blood-vessels are found much dilated and aneurysmal; they are atheromatous, and are undergoing fatty degeneration of the intima; and proliferation of the cells of the adventitia, small collections of extravasated blood, hæmatoidin crystals, and sometimes fat embolisms, are observable. Along with these changes in the brain somewhat similar changes go on concurrently in the cord. There is apparent thickening of the muscular coat of the vessels, but this is due to an increase of fibrous tissue and not to any true increase of muscular fibre. Along the lines of the larger vessels are patches of sclerosis which are not in any way due to ascending or descending degenerative changes; but are rather the result of a process which is usually met with in other organs in which there is chronic endarteritis, and one almost invariably found in chronic alcoholics.

It is a noteworthy fact that in the cord, as in the brain, the membranes, with their free vascular reticula, are especially affected; and at those points where the pia mater is most closely associated with the cord and with the cortex—*i.e.*, along the lines of the columns of Goll, and in the motor area of the brain—the connective tissue and vascular changes are always most marked. It will be observed that we have here two processes, both of which must be associated with the presence of irritative material, which, first causing stimulation of the protoplasm, eventually leads to marked interference with nutrition, inducing development of the more stable, but less highly developed, tissues, which is followed by further degeneration of the more highly endowed cells. Thus we find that in this condition we have both fatty degeneration and sclerosis going on simultaneously; the one resulting from impaired nutrition of the pre-existing cells, the other being due to increase of the cells of the lymph connective tissue system, which cells are called upon to perform a gradually increasing amount of work in the removal of effete products.

In different individuals these processes go on at different rates, and consequently different pathological appearances are presented and different clinical symptoms may be the result; but in all cases the difference is one of degree rather than of kind. Lewis contends then that certain cases of chronic alcoholism are very similar to cases of general paralysis, not only in their clinical history but in the fact that the membranes of the brain often present, in the two sets of cases, similar appearances, "both as regards naked-eye aspects and distribution of lesion." He then goes on to say, however, that in alcoholism "the morbid change is centred in the (atheromatous) change of the inner coat," whilst "in general paralysis the morbid change is concentrated in the adventitial sheath, and is a far more acute irritative process in the loose external tunic of the vessel, which explains the more rapid implication of the nervous structures lying immediately around by direct extension," and he explains on the ground of this difference in the site of the original change "the slow yet progressive impairment of nutrition of the nerve centres," and the "steady enfeeblement of the mental faculties akin to the advancing imbecility of senile atrophy, in which similar changes of the vessels" are found. In general paralysis, on the other hand, "the early implication and rapid spread of morbid activity along the adventitial tunic of the vessels" induce the more acute changes "in the nerve cells of the cortex." When in chronic alcoholism the adventitia is also affected, especially in the peripheral zone of the cortex, not only the nerve fibres of this region but the deeper ganglionic cells are affected and symptoms similar to those of general paralysis are the result of similar pathological changes. Lewis states that "extensive atrophy of these large elements of the cortex is coincident only with the most advanced forms of alcoholic dementia; the earlier stage of vascular impairment and the growth of young scavenger cells in the peripheral zone, ere the cells themselves are involved, being apparently associated with the maniacal excitement and early delusional perversions of alcoholism. . . . . Whilst the cortical lesions of general paralysis indicate an invasion from without inwards, affecting the sensory elements and apical (? sensory) poles of the motor-cells; alcoholism induces in addition thereto, extensive vascular changes from within outwards, implicating the medulla of the gyri and affecting a destructive degeneration of the medullated fibres."

These points, insisted on by Lewis, are of very considerable interest in connection with ætiology of the alcoholic condition and of general paralysis. We have in alcoholism the condition of an etherial poisoning rapidly making its way to the blood, giving rise to irritation of the intima. The effect of this poison on the extremely active connective-tissue cells, with which it comes into contact, is not marked, and such of the alcohol as is not directly and rapidly excreted is rapidly broken down, so that the effects on the lymphatics, except in the later stages of the poisoning when nutrition and activity of the cells is very greatly impaired, is not a very marked factor in the process; but when that impairment of activity and nutrition does come on the changes in the lymph connective tissue go on rapidly, and we have the conditions associated with general paralysis.

In Lewis's statement, although he does not use it, we have a strong argument in favour of the occasional syphilitic origin of general paralysis. It is a well-known fact that the poison of syphilis circulating through the body, attacks, not only the intima of the vessels, but also the adventitia, and the lymph connective system; in point of fact the poison, comparatively stable, passes from the vessels into the lymph spaces, disturbs the functional action of the various cells, interfering with their nutrition, giving rise to abnormal stimulation, and bringing about the conditions met with in general paralysis.

Stating the matter briefly *alcohol* acts on the blood-vessels and on the nerve cells in the first instance, and only later affects the lymph connective tissue; whilst the syphilitic poison acts almost from the first on the whole three, and so gives rise to marked tissue changes, and clinical consequences; the congeries of symptoms of which are summed up under the term general paralysis.

Lewis here makes an exceedingly laudable attempt to associate symptoms with ætiology and pathology, and he sums up thus:—

"The constitutional state engendered in chronic alcoholic insanity is identical with what forms the basis of chronic Bright's disease; and as in this affection we have a multiplicity of local expressions of the morbid lesions, so, here, we find the tendency is towards a concentration in the nervous centres; atrophic states of brain, or of spinal cord, or of both combined, are thus induced by predominance of (*a*) simple fatty degeneration of their nutritive vessels and tissues; (*b*) from fatty degeneration associated with interstitial sclerosis; (*c*) from diffuse sclerous, interstitial change; (*d*) from peri-arteritis and hypertrophy of the tunica muscularis.

"In the peri-arteritis, occasionally engendered in chronic alcoholics of a certain age, we probably see the boundary line overstepped betwixt simple alcoholic insanity and general paralysis of the insane; and we have resulting therefrom, in a more acute spread of the cortical lesion, what might be regarded as general paralysis accidentally evolved out of chronic alcoholism, or, as some would less correctly state the case, general paralysis caused by alcohol. Alcohol has its own *rôle* to play, and a most extensive one it is; but, the tissue changes engendered thereby are always as highly characteristic as are the morbid sequences of general paralysis, and we must seek to dissever from the latter disease our notions of alcohol playing the part of a direct ætiological factor, in the sense of originating the primal tissue changes by which the disease is characterised."

Following out the analogy of the kidney it may be pointed out that even the changes in the brain in acute alcoholic mania may be likened to acute changes in the kidney also due to alcoholic poisoning. We have cloudy swelling of the functionally active or secreting cells of that organ; they become swollen, their protoplasm is even more granular than normal; the vessels are dilated. One of three things may happen in either case; first, excretion of the alcohol, and the cells, if allowed to rest, return to the normal condition; secondly, in consequence of chill, or the results of any extra exertion being thrown on the kidney during this stage of exhaustion, acute inflammatory changes are set

We append a scheme for practical use in post-mortem examinations as employed by Dr. Barrett, Pathologist, Royal Infirmary, Edinburgh :

Name
Sex **Age**
Case Book : vol. page **Pathological Record : vol. page**
Died
Autopsy date time Weather

EXTERNAL EXAMINATION.

Height **Circumference at Shoulder**
Pupils **„ of Head**
P. M. Rigidity
P. M. Lividity
State of Nutrition
External Markings
External Injuries and Evidences of Disease

INSPECTION OF CAVITIES.

Cavity of Abdomen
Fluid
Cavity of Right Pleura
Left Pleura
Fluid Right **Fluid Left**
Cavity of Pericardium
Fluid
Cavity of Skull—Dura mater reflected
Fluid

WEIGHTS OF ORGANS.

Encephalon (including Cerebrum, Cerebellum, Pons, Medulla, and ½in. of Cord, and Fluid) **Fluid (measure)**
„ (weight)
Cerebellum
Pons and Medulla and ½in. of Cord
Liver Spleen Right Kidney Left Kidney Right Lung Left Lung Heart
Other Organs

SPINAL CORD

Membranes ***Vessels***
(a) Cervical
(b) Dorsal—Upper
Do. Lower
(c) Lumbar
Section above Lateral Ventricles **at level of Lateral Ventricles** **Basal**
1. Grey Matter *(a) Colour*
(b) Consistence
(c) Atrophied
(d) Layers visible
2. White Matter *(a) Colour*
(b) Consistence
3. Vessels and Peri-vascular Spaces
Lateral Ventricles *dilated* *contain* **oz.** *clear turbid fluid*
Membrane *thickened*
Granulations *absent*
Vessels and Choroid Plexuses
Third Ventricle
Fifth Ventricle
***Basal Ganglia*—(a) Colour**
(b) Consistence
(c) Vessels and Peri-vascular Spaces
***Cerebellum*—Arrangement of Lobes, &c.**
Pia and Arachnoid
Section—1. Grey matter, with Corpus Dentatum
2. White matter
Vessels and Peri-vascular Spaces

Pons and Medulla. **External Alterations in shape**
Section—1. Consistence
2. Colour of grey matter
3. Ditto of white matter
4. Softenings
5. Hæmorrhages
Fourth Ventricle: 1. Membrane
2. Granulations *absent*
3. Choroid Plexus
Pituitary Body and Infundibulum
Pineal Gland
Microscopical Examination, **Results of—**

MORBID ANATOMY OF ORGANS.

HEAD.

Scalp
Skull-Cap: **Capacity** **weight** **sp. gr.**
Outer table
Diploë
Inner table

ENCEPHALON.

Dura Mater: **1. Adhesions (*a*) to Bone**
(*b*) to Pia Mater
2. Thickenings
Sinuses
Veins from Pia
Arachno-Pia:* **1. Milky**
2. (*a*) Adherent to Dura
(*b*) Separated from Brain by Fluid { **i. Anterior** / **ii. Vertex** / **iii. Posterior** / **iv. Basal** }
3. Fibrous Bands to Dura
4. Pachymeningitis **Extent** **Position of**
5. Hæmorrhages
Pia **(*a*) Adherent to Brain matter**
Blood-vessels
External Configuration **of Brain as a whole *as regards complexity of convolutions, shape, &c.***

CEREBRUM.

Convolutions, superficial atrophy, &c.
1. Frontal—Right
Left
2. Parietal—Right
Left
3. Temporo-sphenoidal—Right
Left
4. Occipital—Right
Left
Sulci ***wide*** ***compressed***

SYMPATHETIC GANGLIA AND NERVES.

THORAX.

Left Lung ***Right Lung***
Heart. **Cavities: Size and shape**
Contents
Valves— **Cone Diameter.**
Pulmonary ***competent***
Aortic ***competent***
Tricuspid
Mitral
Muscle
Vessels
Blood
Mediastinum

ABDOMEN.

Liver ***Right Kidney***
Gall-Bladder ***Left Kidney***
Spleen ***Stomach and Intestine***

*** The terminology here differs from that of Dr. Barrett.**

up, there is breaking down and desquamation of the epithelium, dilation of the blood-vessels, proliferation of the connective tissue, and partial or complete stoppage of the functional activity of the organ, corresponding to similar conditions in the brain; thirdly, there may be a continuation of the irritation, impairment of the nutritional and functional activity of the epithelial cells—here also corresponding to the similar conditions already described in the brain—increase in the amount of connective tissue, preceded, however, by proliferation of the endothelium of the intima of the vessel, fatty degeneration of the endothelial cells, atheroma of the larger branches, and a thickening of the muscular coat by an increase of fibrous tissue; a condition similar to that met with in the vessels of the cord in chronic alcoholic insanity. Exactly similar stages may be observed in the brain.

From what has already been said the effect of syphilitic poisoning in the production of cerebral disease and mental symptoms must be very marked, and it is a remarkable fact that nowhere in his admirable work on mental diseases does Bevan Lewis refer to syphilis as an ætiological factor, though in his chapter on general paralysis he gives a most excellent description of the pathological processes set up by this disease without association of cause and effect. In the brain and cord, as in other organs, the manifestations of the action of syphilitic poison are exceedingly varied. The congenital idiocy associated with this disease must be looked upon as the result of an increase in the amount of connective tissue, similar to that met with in congenital syphilitic cirrhosis of the liver and lung of children, in which we find a marked increase in the connective tissue around the liver cells, or lung alveoli, in connection with the lymph channels and with the vessels themselves. In the liver this may be so extensive as to cause atrophy of the parenchymatous cells. They are cut off into small groups and their connection with bile-ducts is interfered with. Similarly, in the brain, we have a diffuse sclerosis; the communicating network of the nerve cells is interfered with, and the cells themselves are atrophied or degenerated in structure and function. The presence of the syphilitic condition may be manifested in acquired syphilis by slightly impaired nutrition of the cells, by increased irritability of the motor cells and by impaired activity of inhibitory cells. More gross lesions are the gummata, which are sometimes met with as the result of localised inflammation set up by the syphilitic poison, in which case we have the symptoms of cerebral tumour associated with those of the more marked or modified forms of the general syphilitic condition. Gummata may also be met with in cases of acquired syphilis, where the symptoms are much the same as those already described; except that instead of a condition of imbecility or idiocy, or congenital irritability and want of inhibition, there is a gradual retrocession from the normal mental activity through the various stages of degeneration to a more or less marked condition of dementia.

J. Batty Tuke.

German Sims Woodhead.

PATHOMANIA (πάθος, passion; μανία, madness). Mania without delirium. Another name for moral insanity. (Fr. *pathomanie.*)

PATHOPATRIDALGIA (πάθος, passion; πατρίς, fatherland; ἄλγος, pain). Nostalgia. (Fr. *pathopatridalgie;* Ger. *Heimweh.*)

PATHOPHOBIA (πάθος, suffering; φόβος, fear). Another term for hypochondriasis. Morbid fear of disease.

PAVITATION (*pavor*, fear). A term for fright or fear, with trembling. (Fr. *pavitation.*)

PAVOR NOCTURNUS (*pavor*, fear; *nocturnus*, at night). A term for the night terrors of children. (*See* Developmental Insanities.)

PEDICULOPHOBIA (*pediculus*, a louse; φόβος, fear). Morbid dread of phthiriasis.

PELLACIA. Pica (*q.v.*). (Fr. *allotriophagie;* Ger. *die krankhafte Begierde.*)

PELLAGRA (*pellis*, the skin; ἄγρα, a seizure—an affection of the skin; but more likely derived from the Italian, *pel agra*, "sore skin.") **Syn.** Maïdismus, Psycho-neurosis maïdica, Mal della Rosa, Mal rosso, Mal del Sole, Mal del Padrone, Cattivo male, Mul della Vipera.—**Def.** A disease of comparatively recent origin, induced by the toxic action of diseased or damaged maize, the chief characteristics of which are morbid conditions of the skin and of the mucous membrane of the digestive tract, with symptoms referable to the cerebro-spinal system.

History and Distribution.—The earliest account of this malady as an endemic affection came from Spain in the beginning of the eighteenth century (in the Asturian district of Oviedo in 1735), while it appeared in Italy in the vicinity of Sesto Calende (on Lago Maggiore) just prior to 1750, where it was first scientifically investigated in 1771. It invaded Lombardy and Venetia, spread over Æmilia, and in the last decade of the eighteenth century extended over Piedmont and Liguria and later on over Central Italy. In the beginning of the present century it first appeared in the south-west of France (in 1829), in Roumania (in 1846), and in Corfu (in 1856); it has never disappeared from the regions in which it has implanted itself, and a noteworthy fact remains that the number of cases has increased in the earliest seats of the disease. Its present distribution embraces the districts of Europe situated within a zone extending from 42° to 46° N., and comprising the north of Spain, its especial haunt (the provinces of Asturia, Aragonia, Burgos, Guadalagara, Navarra, Galicia, Zaragoza, Cuenca, Granada, Frabelos and Zamora being those in which the disease mainly occurs), the south-west of France (in the departments Girondes, Landes, Hautes Pyrénées, Basses Pyrénées, Haute Garonne and Aude), Italy (the provinces of Venetia, Lombardy, Æmilia, more recently in Piedmont and Liguria), Roumania and Corfu. In Italy about ten per cent. of all cases are insane, and the deaths vary from 2.5 per cent. of all the inmates in the district asylums, to 5 per cent. in the city ones. The disease attacks males and females indiscriminately, and no age is exempt, while those who most readily succumb are the aged and infirm; the extent and ravages of the disease vary in persons living under the same nutritive and hygienic conditions.

Ætiology.—The evidence that the appearance of pellagra was coincident with the first general cultivation of maize in large quantities, that its area of distribution is and has been confined to rural districts inside which maize forms the exclusive or principal food, and where the grain does not grow to perfection, coupled with the fact that such imperfect and diseased maize is at certain seasons the staple food-stuff of the populace, help us to conclude what the source and character of the actual material disease agent are. In those districts, moreover, where mixed food is taken—*e.g.*, along the sea-coast of affected areas where fish is eaten, or where rice or potatoes are substituted for maize, the people remain exempt. With the recurrence of bad seasons and the consumption of damaged maize, the disease increases in extent and severity, and the deduction to be made from these facts is that pellagra is due to certain toxic substances developed in the course of the decomposition of Indian corn, and possibly, under the influence of epiphytes on the corn. The consumption of good well-cultivated maize never causes pellagra, a fact that militates against the opinion adopted by some observers, that the disease is due to the low nutritive value of a maize diet. The maize cut before it is ripe, gathered in rainy seasons, stored away damp, sown from affected seed or what is known as quarantine seed (*zea mais præcox*), all contribute to the engendering of some toxic development in the grain which forms the true pellagra-poison. In Corfu the maize consumed is chiefly imported from Roumania, an infected district, and in all the areas in which pellagra prevails it is usually the poorest classes, the small tenant-farmers and labourers, who suffer. The nature of the pellagra-poison is still an open question. Balardini attributed the symptoms to the development of a parasitic mould on musty maize (named by him "verderame"), while Lombroso conjectures it to be due to the occurrence of a fatty oil and an extractive substance, the products of decomposition or of bacterial action, which are never found in sound maize. An indirect heredity, the transmission of a congenital feebleness to the offspring thus increasing its susceptibility, has been noticed. The affection is not contagious.

Symptoms.—The phenomena, as well as the periodical recurrence of this affection, occur in most cases in the beginning of spring, and the earlier symptoms point to lesions of the gastro-intestinal tract and the cutaneous structures, while the more advanced symptoms evince the implication of the cerebral and cerebro-spinal system.

From observations personally made, the disease presents the following characteristic signs:—a premonitory feeling of lassitude and disinclination for exertion, with occipital headache, vertigo, tinnitus aurium, and a sense of pain in the gastric region with burning pain in the back and extremities, usher in the attack; these are succeeded by furring of the tongue, marked anorexia, and occasional diarrhœa; coincident with these symptoms an exanthem appears, at first limited to those parts of the body exposed to the sun's rays, the skin becomes red and swollen, desquamating after some weeks in large flakes, there being a sense of burning tension about the affected parts. At the height of the attack the tendon reflexes are much exaggerated, there is great mental depression, thinking is an effort, and the patient is irritable, excitable and obtuse. After lasting three or four months the symptoms decline, the skin where affected remains dark-coloured, rough and dry, and all the objective and subjective phenomena disappear. The next spring it recurs with increased severity, and at perhaps the third attack the symptoms become serious. An increase in the general feebleness, so great that the patient cannot walk, paræsthesia of the trunk and extremities, acute headache, ptosis, mydriasis, diplopia, hemeralopia, amblyopia and other visual defects occur; the exanthem now implicates larger areas, the skin thickens and cracks, diarrhœa becomes frequent, the tongue is thickened and red, the gums bleed readily. The muscular weakness attacks preferably the lower extremities, and occasionally a paretic affection of the extensors ensues, by reason of which the flexors come into excessive action, and phenomena of motor excitation, such as increased resistance against passive movement, spasms, cramps, tonic and clonic convulsions ("pellagrous attacks") and, rarely, well-marked epileptic seizures, are to be observed. Atrophy of certain muscle groups with paralysis, a paretic, at times spastic, gait, and idiomuscular and fibrillar contractions on mechanical stimulation are additional phenomena. In the tense or paretic muscles faradisation shows decreased excitability, sensory abnormalities are not constant, but hyperæsthesia to cold and hypalgesia are occasionally found. The muscular sense is not affected. Vision is impaired as stated above, and Lombroso describes retinal implication in 80 per cent. of the cases he investigated—cloudiness of the retina, atrophy of the arteries, dilatation of the veins, and marked atrophy of the papilla. In 66 per cent. of the cases examined the patellar tendon reflexes were highly exaggerated, and all the tendon reflexes were in a state of hyper-excitability, but variations in the intensity of the knee-jerk phenomenon up to total absence of response were in a few cases noted (without, however, any concurrent tabetic signs). The vaso-motor derangements are a general contraction of the cutaneous vessels with pallor, coldness of the skin and in the later stages œdema due to vaso-paralytic dilatation of the veins and capillaries. The trophic affections are the above-mentioned erythematous eruption; the skin after the exanthem fades, becoming dark brown, smooth, dry, thin, and non-elastic; the subcutaneous cellular tissue disappears and white cicatricial striæ develop, or it becomes infiltrated, bluish, and ichthyotic. The nails too crack and peel off. Emaciation, anæmia, and general cachexia ensue, paralysis of the bladder supervenes, the patient is bedridden, diarrhœa becomes incessant, and death occurs owing to cardiac failure and general weakness. Occasionally phthisis or septicæmia from bedsores puts an end to the patient's sufferings, while the not infrequent supervention of "typhus pellagrosus" (an acute and intense exaggeration of all and especially the mental symptoms to a delirious stage, with more or less hyper-pyrexia which otherwise is absent in pellagra) terminates the malady.

Mental Symptoms.—These which are rarely absent in the more advanced cases bear chiefly the character of melancholia. The milder signs of mental implication—the mere retardation of ideas, the disinclination for thought or activity, and simple mental depression, occur in the earlier stages of the affection and in slight cases. The later developments of the disease are associated with a profound melancholia with a sense of painful apprehension, pauphobia, micro-maniacal symptoms, self-accusation, delusions of persecution, demonomania, hypochondriacal delusionary ideas, refusal of food, and a tendency to suicidal impulses. The retardation of the flow of ideas becomes more marked until a likeness to stuporous melancholia ensues, the patient being apathetic, resistful and suspicious. Consciousness is rarely impaired. Occasional instances of homicidal, more frequently suicidal, impulse occur. The mental, like the physical, symptoms, run through a steady course; if showing improvement, recurring at repeated intervals, until a permanent insanity is induced. Secondary dementia, owing no doubt to the periodicity of the disease, is a rare sequela of the mental affection. Maniacal symptoms are still rarer, and when such occur, gay excitement, an acceleration in the flow of ideas, with general mental exaltation and increased motor impulses, mark the disease. *Folie circulaire* has also in a few instances been observed, but actual paranoia, in its typical form, is rare, and sensory hallucinations are seldom met with. Imperative ideas, movements, positions, &c., are frequent, and the combination of the spinal symptoms with euphoria often renders the diagnosis between pellagrous insanity and general paralysis difficult.

Prognosis. — Pellagra may run its course with intermissions through a period extending over ten, fifteen or more years, without reaching even then its highest degree of development. Recovery can only be expected if the patient has gone through no more than one or two slight attacks, and is immediately placed in more favourable hygienic conditions. If the disease is already far advanced the prognosis is unfavourable, the most hopeful of these cases exhibiting permanent nervous lesions—*e.g.*, chronic insanity and motor paresis; suicide occurs among a fairly large percentage, the inclination being towards death by drowning; death ensues in other cases from marasmus or from the complications of this affection, especially tuberculosis. Or the advent of typhus pellagrosus or severe intestinal affection may bring the patient to his end.

Diagnosis.—In cases where the subjective symptoms are especially prominent, the diagnosis has to be made from neurasthenia and hysteria; here the ætiology and history of the case, the periodicity of the affection, its exacerbations in the spring, with the tendon reflex abnormalities, will help to distinguish between the affections. The exanthem may be absent ("pellagra sine pellagrâ"), but when present, and with the other symptoms in abeyance, the distinction must be drawn between it and pure solar erythema. The condition of the tongue and intestinal tract will in such instances frequently assist in the diagnosis. In all cases where the spinal symptoms primarily attract our attention, the coincident mental disorder, the erythematous eruption, and the gastro-intestinal lesions will be of great value in determining between pellagra and a pure neurosis. The spinal symptoms are not, moreover, progressive, but with frequent changes of intensity remain stable for years, so that even in long-standing cases complete paralysis or contractions are not developed. Where the mental symptoms stand out prominently, the other associated affections will help us in the differential diagnosis. A special difficulty may arise when the mental condition corresponds to that of general paralysis of the insane, if at the same time the tendon reflexes are increased, or lessened, or entirely absent (pseudo-paralysis pellagrosa); in such cases, the absence of motor speech derangements is an important distinctive sign—*i.e.*, if the speech derangements are not a symptom of the transition of the disease into general paralysis, an event which undoubtedly sometimes occurs. The predominance of the gastro-intestinal symptoms, with abeyance of other pellagrous signs, sometimes occurs. Here a careful inquiry into the history of the case will frequently clear up any doubts which might be felt as to their origin. The diagnosis between typhus pellagrosus and other febrile affections, notably typhus, enteric fever, pneumonia, &c., may be made by noting the irregular course of the fever, the negative results of examination of the suspected organs and urine, the absence of any specific exanthem unlike that of pellagra, and the positive gastro-intestinal symptoms.

Pathology.—Putting on one side appearances incidental to the general constitutional disturbance, and those due to intercurrent disease, &c., found in pellagra—*e.g.*, general nutritional derangements which are not constantly present, such as wasting of the adipose and muscular tissues, fragilitas ossium, degeneration of the cardiac muscular tissue, fatty degeneration and atrophy with a slight degree of sclerosis of the liver, spleen, and kidneys, we have to consider the more constant post-mortem results obtained in pellagrous patients. These are: (1) Changes in the intestinal tract—attenuation of the intestinal wall in consequence of atrophy of the muscular coat, with occasional hyperæmia and ulceration of the lower parts of the canal; (2) Abnormal pigmentary deposit, such as is usually met with only in senility, is commonly found, especially in the ganglionic cells, the muscles of the heart, the hepatic cells and in the spleen; (3) Changes in the nervous system; these are by far the most important and constant post-mortem signs. The hyperæmic and anæmic conditions, or the œdema of the central nervous system, though frequently present, are by no means the characteristic changes, neither are those inflammatory conditions such as pachymeningitis and cerebral and spinal lepto-meningitis, or the obliteration of the spinal canal by granulations, or ossific arachnitis, at all peculiar to this malady, they being common to many chronic nervous affections; the most noteworthy and constant lesion, and one that may be taken as peculiar to this disorder, is an affection of the spinal cord and especially of its lateral columns. The brain when examined furnishes generally negative results, apart from the occasionally found pigmentary deposits in the cortical cells, and in the adventitia of the smaller vessels, with fatty degeneration or calcification of the intima; atrophy of the cerebrum and its cortex has been found in cases of long-standing mental derangement. The cord lesion, though mainly one of the lateral columns, frequently implicates also the posterior columns; in the former the pyramidal tracts are generally affected with partial involvement of the anterior columns; in the latter the postero-lateral columns are generally left free. The lesion of the lateral columns is shown most prominently in the dorsal region of the cord, while that of the posterior columns is limited to, or rather most distinctly marked in, the cervical and dorsal regions.

Microscopically, the affection seems to be a primary degeneration of the nerve-fibres, with secondary proliferation of the neuroglia, the walls of the vessels not being necessarily implicated; sometimes granular cells, and more frequently amylaceous corpuscles, are met with in the degenerated areas. Degeneration of the anterior root-fibres along the anterior cornua has also been demonstrated, while there is to be found in addition a more or less considerable degree of pigment-atrophy of the ganglion cells in the anterior cornua, with sclerosis of the matrix and atrophy of the nerve-roots. Besides the excessive pigmentary deposit found in the peripheral ganglia, both spinal and sympathetic, there are no characteristic microscopical evidences in other parts of the nervous system. "Typhus pellagrosus" furnishes us with definite post-mortem results—chronic gastro-enteritis with formation of ulcers and swelling of the mesenteric glands, and well-marked changes in the central nervous system, associated with secondary affection of the kidneys, lungs, pleura, &c., being the main features on examination. It is to be noted that the spleen is usually involved in the general visceral atrophy, and is never enlarged. Majochi has found micrococci in cases of typhus pellagrosus both in the blood during life and post-mortem in the intestines, liver, spleen, and other viscera which he regards as characteristic; but successful cultivation of these has not yet been carried out.

Pellagra may therefore be regarded as a disease occasioned by the action of some toxic substance, bearing in its clinical aspect a close resemblance to another affection of similar origin—ergotism. A like mental derangement is found in each, and the lesions which occur in both are certain degenerative changes in definite portions of the spinal cord, the posterior column, being especially implicated in ergotism, while the lateral, or both lateral and posterior columns, are affected in pellagra. It may be regarded as taking, so far as its spinal symptoms go, a position midway between ergotism and another disease, similarly induced by toxic influence, lathyrism (a condition produced by the use of the seeds of lathyrus cicera, a species of vetch, as food, the symptoms being hyperæsthesiæ, convulsive movements and paraplegia), in which the actual cord lesions have not, however, been demonstrated. The exanthem, though undoubtedly in part the result of solar influence, owes its origin in the first place to the poison, as it is only to be observed during the spring months when the disease is at its height, and in the later stages implicates cutaneous areas to which the sun has had no access. The intermissions and exacerbations at definite periods have been explained by the fact that maize forms in the affected districts the only food during the winter, and it is at its close that the symptoms first begin to assert themselves; while it is during the winter too that the specific poison, whether bacterial or chemical, has the best chance of developing in the grain. Other causes, however, of which we as yet know nothing, also come into play in determining this periodicity, as during the treatment of patients so affected, and when maize in any form has been withheld for years, the vernal recurrence is never entirely absent. Belmondo's view that typhus pellagrosus is due to the sudden impregnation of the blood by the toxic influence, which has either been taken in large quantities or acts cumulatively, is certainly tenable.

Treatment.—The first and most natural step in treatment is the prohibition of maize in any shape or form as food, or if this be impossible, the use of only such grain as is ripe to perfection, is well dried and stored, and which is the result of the sowing of a good quality. The encouragement of cultivation of unaffected maize, of other cereals, potatoes, &c., as well as the improvement in the hygienic and social condition of the rural population which has of late been the especial care of the State in Italy, have furnished extremely good results. When once the disease has broken out in a district, it is curable if taken in hand early, but a vigorous crusade against the affection has hitherto been frustrated by the action of the peasantry themselves, who conceal the fact of an outbreak, regarding it as a "mal de miseria," but the erection of special institutions where sufferers can be received, and in which for a trifling cost they can be provided with good food and find healthful occupation, has lately served in some measure to remedy this condition of things. With regard to medical treatment there is little to add; the various affections must be treated symptomatically as they arise, there being no known drug which can act as a specific.

F. TUCZEK.

[*References.*—Art. Pellagra in the Encyclopedia Medica Italiana. Salveraglio, Bibliografia della Pellagra, 1887. Belmondo, Le alterazioni anatomiche del midollo spinale nella Pellagra e loro rapporto coi fatti clinici, 1890. Tuczek, Ueber die nervoesen Stoerungen bei der Pellagra, 1888. Tonnini, Disturbi spinali nei pazzi pellagrosi. For other and less recent works see Hirsch, Handbuch der historisch-geographischen Pathologie, 1883.]

PERCEPTION (*percipio*, I take up wholly). Perception is a mental process; it is the result of a very complex activity of the mind, involving the synthesis of a number of sense-data. The sensations are merely modes of our being affected by external stimuli, but perception is purely psychical. Perception has been divided by Wundt into simple perception and apperception, the former being the simple knowledge that we are somehow mentally affected, the latter being the mental state after discerning attention has been given by the observer to the sense data. (*See* PHILOSOPHY OF MIND, p. 27.)

PERCEPTIVE FACULTIES.—In phrenology—term for the faculties recognising the existence and physical properties of external objects; form, size, order, eventuality, language, &c. (Spurzheim.)

PERIALGES (περί, very; ἄλγος, pain). Very painful, sad, or melancholy. (Fr. *périalge*.)

PERIBLEPSIS (περί, around; βλέπω, I stare). The wild look in those who are delirious. (Fr. *périblepsie*; Ger. *Umhersehen*.)

PERICHAREIA (περιχαρής, glad in excess). Sudden or vehement joy. The opposite of ecplexia, or stupor.

PERICHONDRITIS AURICULÆ. (*See* HÆMATOMA AURIS.)

PERIMENINGITIS. (*See* PACHYMENINGITIS.)

PERIODICITY IN MENTAL DISEASES.—Periodicity is more marked in mental depression than in exaltation, and rarely occurs in hallucinations and in delusional insanity. In depression, the duration of the disorder is frequently about a year. In exaltation the disorder may continue from four to six months or more (Kraepelin). Periodicity and circular insanity must not be confounded, although the latter may be periodical. The reader will find a valuable chapter on the subject in Clouston's "Clinical Lectures on Mental Diseases."

PERIPHERAL NEURITIS.—Paralysis, usually more or less generalised over the upper and lower extremities, and dependent upon peripheral neuritis, is a frequent result of chronic alcoholism.

Symptoms.—(1) *Motor*. It commonly happens that the patient, when first seen, is unable to stand; it may be that the power of flexing the thighs upon the pelvis is fairly preserved, and sometimes the knees can be flexed, although with greater difficulty. But the feet will usually be found "dropped," that is, they lie flaccidly in a position of over-extension, and the patient is unable, when requested, to dorsal-flex them. The knee-jerks are absent. The muscles of the legs, especially those on the anterior surface below the knee, are probably atrophied, and are found to yield no response to induced currents of electricity, but to contract slowly to galvanic currents of moderate strength. The arms are thin, and the thenar and hypothenar eminences may be atrophied. There is more or less "wrist-drop," so that the patient presents the appearance of one suffering from lead palsy. The extensor muscles in the forearm as well as the intrinsic muscles of the hand may exhibit, like those of the lower extremities, signs of degenerative reaction to electrical currents.

On the (2) *sensory* side we may expect to hear of pains, which are often of lightning character, coming and going in sudden darts, like stabs of a knife or the boring of a gimlet, and quite recalling those characteristic of tabes dorsalis. These are usually most pronounced in the lower extremities. It is commonly observed that much tenderness of the muscles is complained of when these are grasped by the hand. The patient will sometimes describe a sensation of aching in the muscles, and very commonly a feeling of "numbness," "deadness," or "pins and needles," which is referred especially to the hands and feet. More or less cutaneous anæsthesia is found in the extremities, especially in the feet and hands. As a general rule the functions of the bladder are not disordered, and there is no tendency to bed sores.

In females affected with alcoholic paralysis the writer has observed that the catamenia are almost always suppressed, and often for many months during the illness.

Although in the majority of instances it is the extremities which are most seriously affected, yet in some cases the facial muscles, the external muscles of the eyeballs, the respiratory muscles, and those subserving deglutition may be more or less involved. Exceptionally there may be no pains, and but little or no disturbance of cutaneous sensibility, indicating the probability that in some rare cases the efferent fibres only are involved. There is often a considerable amount of œdema of the feet and legs, and the hands may look puffy and sodden. In some cases it is chiefly a tottering gait which is noticeable. This often precedes the paralytic state, which may sometimes arrive quite suddenly.

(3) *Mental*.—There is considerable diversity in the amount and kind of mental disturbance in cases of alcoholic neuritis, and it does not necessarily happen that

the most marked paralysis goes with the most serious mental disorder. There is usually in severe cases, a remarkable loss of memory. Patients who may perhaps have been confined to bed for many weeks will describe the long walk that they have taken, and the various things they have done that very day, and this with an air of such *vraisemblance* that it is difficult to disbelieve their story. There is very often a condition of complacent indifference to their state, and apparent incapability of grasping the fact that they are helpless. There is usually no anxiety for the future, though the circumstances may signify utter ruin. This is the more frequent condition, but now and then the symptoms are those of delirium tremens with hallucinations of sight and hearing, with sleeplessness and depression.

Course of the Disease.—Patients who are cut off from further supplies of alcohol, who have not advanced too far, and who are well nursed and cared for generally recover. There is gradual remission in the pains and sensory disturbances with a slow return of power in the affected extremities. In severe cases, months, and sometimes years, are required for recovery. The paralysis, at first flaccid, becomes marked by troublesome contractures as the muscles which are least affected overpull those most seriously involved. In fatal cases the termination may be by increasing exhaustion, pneumonia, or more suddenly by cardiac failure.

Morbid Anatomy.—The spinal cord is usually found free from change. The peripheral nerves, unaltered in appearance to the eye, are found on microscopic examination to be the seat of marked changes which are most pronounced towards the distal extremities. The changes in the nerve-fibres consist in segmentation of the myelin, with multiplication of nerve-corpuscles, and disappearance of many axis cylinders. With these there is often proliferation of the nuclei of the endoneurium, and the walls of the minute vessels are stuffed with cells, affording evidence of interstitial neuritis. The changes are usually most marked in the lower portions of the sciatic nerve and distal ends of the median, ulnar and radial nerves; they are also often apparent in the intercostal nerves, the vagus, phrenic, and it may be in the oculomotors.

Imperfect striation and a tendency to fatty change may be noted in the affected muscles.

Diagnosis.—The absence of knee-jerk, ataxic gait, and lightning pains cause a strong *primâ facie* resemblance to tabes dorsalis, in the course of which disease, too, mental disorder may sometimes supervene. In cases of peripheral neuritis, however, the pupils retain their power of contracting to light. Examination of the affected extremities by electrical currents reveals a wide-spread loss of faradic excitability which is no part of the symptoms of tabes dorsalis. In this latter disease there may occasionally be a narrowly localised change of this kind from peripheral neuritis, but this is rare. The kind of mental disturbance, too, differs much from that which may occasionally occur in the course of tabes dorsalis, where it is apt to be characterised by the features of general paralysis. There is also the history of chronic alcoholism, which cannot fail to be evoked by inquiry.

From anterior polio-myelitis the disease is differentiated by the presence of marked sensory disturbance, and from this as well as from other acute affections of the spinal cord by the presence of mental disorder.

Treatment.—Rest in bed, abstinence from alcohol, nutritious food, are the chief requisites. Salicylate of soda in doses of twenty grains, or antipyrin in doses of from ten to twenty grains, three times a day, if not contra-indicated, may be given to relieve the pains. When the acute symptoms have subsided the galvanic current should be applied in order to keep up the nutrition of the muscles, as well as massage with active and passive movements, especial care being taken to overcome the tendency of the feet to become rigidly contractured in a position of over-extension. This treatment will require a long time and patience, which will usually bring about a satisfactory recovery without the necessity of dividing tendons.

T. Buzzard.

PERKINISM, PERKINS' TRACTORS.—Dr. E. Perkins of Norwich, Connecticut, U.S.A., introduced a novelty into therapeutics, which has been called Perkinism, after him. He treated some diseases by drawing two metallic rods (of different metal) which he called "tractors," over the surface of the affected part. He obtained a fair amount of success, due no doubt to the influence of the mind upon the body, and possibly to the determination of afflux of blood to the part by mechanical action. The same effects were produced by wooden tractors.*

PERNOCTATION (*per*, through; *nox*, night). A term for insomnia or night-

* *Cf.* "Illustrations of the Influence of the Mind upon the Body in Health and Disease," vol. ii. p. 250.

wakefulness. (Fr. *pernoctation:* Ger. *Nachtwachen.*)

PERSECUTION, IDEAS OF. (*See* PERSECUTION, MANIA OF.)

PERSECUTION, MANIA OF.—Syn. Delusion of suspicion; Monomania of suspicion; Monomania of persecution; Délire des persécutions; Folie des persécutions.

Definition.—Monomania of suspicion is a mental disorder of chronic form, which is essentially characterised by hallucinations, by general sensory derangement and by insane ideas, in consequence of which the patient considers all his morbid sensations as the result of persecutions, of which he believes himself to be the victim.

History.—The first treatise on the delusion of suspicion was published in 1852 by Lasègue, who proposed to group under this term a number of symptoms, all of which possessed a striking resemblance. According to him they were all peculiar to a morbid type which in itself was so distinct as to allow of its being detached from other conditions of mental alienation. In this he was not mistaken; numerous works which followed his discovery, and the almost unanimous assent with which the name he gave to it was adopted, show the importance of the step taken.

We do not mean to say that before Lasègue persecution mania had never been observed. At all times there have been persons labouring under this disorder, and in reading the observations of ancient authors, we shall soon find that persecution-mania of former times, although different in form, was the same in principle. In the works of Pinel, Esquirol and others, many symptoms are described, which, when examined, will not be found less significant than those mentioned above.

The classifications, however, established by these masters of psychical medicine, placed those symptoms under the category of lypemania, and the influence of these men was so great, that even at a time when the type indicated by Lasègue was almost universally admitted as a special morbid condition, alienists continued to describe it as one of the varieties of lypemania, a fact of which we may easily convince ourselves by referring to the works of Bucknill and Tuke, of Marcé, Foville, Dagonet, and others.

In his first essay on persecution-mania, Lasègue treats principally of the course of the disorder when it has assumed its characteristic form. He has himself contributed to the study of other peculiarities of the derangement in question, and was also assisted in his work by other observers, and it seems as if there is not much left to be done in the study of this subject.

One of the most important complementary works is certainly that of Foville, in which he shows that persecution-mania is intimately related to insanity of ambition, and that the latter frequently follows the former.

The last and most complete work has been recently published by Ritti in the *Dictionnaire encyclopédique des Sciences médicales.* Every one who intends to thoroughly study this subject must certainly refer to the article mentioned.

General Description of the Disorder.—In giving a clinical description of persecution-mania, we shall treat separately of the period of incubation, and then pass on to the development of the disorder as such.

According to Falret and Ritti, the development comprises the following four periods:—

(1) Period of insane interpretation.
(2) Period of visual hallucinations, the disorder being established.
(3) Period of general sensory derangement.
(4) Stereotyped state; or, mania of ambition.

This classification has undoubtedly the great advantage of dividing all the various phenomena observed in the course of the disorder. There are, however, two objections to it. First, it may happen that the hallucinations of vision develop almost at the same time as the hallucinations of the other senses, and with various disorders of general sensibility. And secondly, at the period when it becomes stereotyped, the ambition may be absent; as a matter of fact, it is frequently so, and therefore we are not justified in counting the insanity of ambition among the characteristic symptoms.

Under these circumstances it appears to us to be more rational, in spite of the high authority of Falret and Ritti, to describe in persecution-mania three principal periods:

(1) Period of insane interpretation.
(2) Period of sensory disorders.
(3) Period of stereotyped or systematised insanity.

Period of Incubation.—The period of incubation of persecution-mania is almost always long; it takes place slowly and gradually, and mostly without the knowledge of the patient and his friends. There are individuals who, from their childhood seem to be predisposed to become victims of this form of mental disease. From the earliest times they have had a tendency to seek solitude; they are taciturn and distrustful, and always believe that people mock at or ridicule them.

Others begin by being hypochondriacs. Morel was one of the first to describe hypochondriasis as a phenomenon precursory to persecution-mania; he says that a tendency to melancholia contains the germ of this disorder. And it is easy to understand this if we consider the facility with which hypochondriacs retire into themselves, analyse the slightest impressions, and believe that being ill they ought to be constantly an object of the care of others. When this care, however, is not practised according to their wish, they become uneasy, angry, and distrustful. They begin to imagine that nobody cares for their more or less imaginary sufferings, and that they are neglected by every one. Thus disposed they are only too ready to plunge into persecution-mania.

Morel was wrong in giving hypochondriasis as the necessary prelude to persecution-mania. There are certainly patients who suffer from this disorder, but who have never been, strictly speaking, hypochondriacs. It would be more exact to say that almost all patients labouring under monomania of suspicion, have during the period of incubation, passed through a period of moral depression, which made them receptive of their morbid impressions. In addition to this, hypochondriasis and a tendency to melancholia may be observed at the commencement of almost all forms of mental disorders, even of simple acute mania, and under these circumstances there is no reason why we should represent hypochondriasis as a premonitory symptom peculiar to persecution-mania.

We have to add that, as Lasègue has stated, the disease commences sometimes at the first onset in a sort of cerebral attack, which consists in a kind of vertigo or giddiness, which may be more or less prolonged, and of which the patient is able to state not only the time, but sometimes even the exact date of commencement, and after that date the insane ideas begin to appear quite suddenly.

Period of Insane Interpretation.—This period consists essentially in the fact that the patient interprets everything that happens in a bad sense and as intended to do himself harm. Although in reality the disorder is already in full activity, nevertheless his insane ideas are but rudimentary and vague, and do not attach themselves to anything special. He suspects everything and is constantly on his guard, and the slightest incidents acquire in his eyes an extraordinary importance. He imagines that everybody looks at him and talks about him. If he sees several persons speaking to each other, he believes that he is the object of their conversation, and that they are certainly speaking ill of him. The slightest movement made in front of him by any unknown passer-by appears to him as an insult. If somebody spits on the floor, it is in detestation of himself. He believes all the words he hears to refer to himself, and they acquire in his eyes a significance in connection with his predominant ideas. If one speaks to him, every word seems to have a double meaning. He suspects everybody and everything, even tokens of affection or esteem. He mistrusts his parents and friends as well as strangers. He believes that everybody deceives and abuses him, and this idea gains ground in him because he fancies that people exchange among each other mysterious signs referring to himself. Even when he is alone in his house, he is not safe from the universal ill-will; he imagines that people listen and spy at his door and that he is kept under a secret surveillance. When he happens to go out, he has a feeling that he is followed by persons whom somebody has paid to watch his footsteps. Even the way in which the things around him have been arranged gains in his eyes a special significance. A casement or a door which is half open, linen clothes hanging out of a window, or a curtain newly hung, means for him something important, and only adds to the signs of hostility shown him from all sides.

At this stage, however, the patient does not give himself entirely up to his insane ideas; he reflects and says to himself that he imagines all the things and that they are absurd; he is ashamed of it. He also tries to conceal his suspicions; he often succeeds in it so well that nobody around him knows about his infatuation. There are a great number of cases who pass through this period, and even through the greater part of the following one, without having shown the slightest external sign of mental disorder. The mistrust, however, which is one of the elements of their malady, prevents them from showing confidence to any one, fearing lest this trust itself might turn against them; consequently they are extremely reserved.

But whatever the patient may do, and in spite of the unconscious resistance he offers, the disease, stronger than he is, follows its course. At first, the insane interpretations have been vague, indefinite and confused. The patient imagines that *somebody* is about to do him harm, but he does not know who, nor why, nor how. *Somebody* is the expression he uses, and *somebody* he complains of. Soon he goes one step further and commences to attribute to a body of men the animosity of which he is the object, to secret societies, to the freemasons, to the Government, or to the police. The number of his enemies is legion, but an organised legion which marches in a body against him. One more step, and his suspicion turns against this or that individual, who becomes his persecutor. In many cases he shows great ill-will towards this pretended persecutor, on whom he wishes to take vengeance. It is, however, necessary to add that the last step mentioned takes place in the following period.

At this point, the patient who labours under persecution-mania has not any hallucinations strictly speaking, his senses, however, begin already to be disordered. Occasionally he believes that he hears a vague noise, a murmur or a whisper. Natural noises, as the rattling of a cart, steps on the staircase, or the opening or shutting of a door, become sounds for him which are connected with his prepossession. One of our patients was unable to go to the railway station because the whistling of the engines appeared to him to be signals given to his enemies; he imagined that the whistling said, "There he is; there he is;" and he ran back to his house.

From this point it is one step only to the period of actual hallucinations, which soon appear at the same time with a variety of troubles of general or special sensibility.

Period of Sensory Disorders.—This is the period when persecution-mania is at its height, and when that factor appears which is essential to, and characteristic of, this form of mental disorder, viz., hallucinations.

Of all hallucinations the principal one is that of hearing; it is of such importance that most authors following Lasègue, consider it as the only one essential to persecution-mania. There are, however, a few cases in which other forms of hallucination are met with. In any case, the auditory hallucinations are almost always the first to appear.

We have mentioned above that at first hallucinations consist of simple noises, and, to use a term which Ball applied to them, are elementary; afterwards they become more defined, and the patient begins to hear voices, which, however, are still at some distance and confused so that the patient does not easily understand the words; in addition to being distant, they are also uttered in a deep voice. Rapidly they seem to be nearer, and become more distinct. At first the patient hears only isolated words which are abusive, insulting and obscene; the patient hears himself called murderer, assassin, drunkard, or similar epithets. Then the isolated words become framed into more or less lengthy sentences, which are all of the same character, and in which accusation, insults and threats always predominate.

These auditory hallucinations are heard by day and night, but they are generally most intense at the beginning of the night. Most patients hear them with both ears, but some also, as Régis has proved, hear them on only one side. They may come from all directions, through the ceiling or the walls, and through the chimney, or out of cupboards and wardrobes; sometimes they come from underneath the ground, and are then heard not only with the ears but by means of a transmission of the vibrations by the whole system. This is analogous to the fact observed in deaf-mute individuals, who perceive the sounds of music with their stomach.

At the moment, the patient believes that he hears clearly and well-articulated words; he also believes he recognises the voice of a certain person whom he considers as the originator of all the persecutions of which he himself is the victim; the voice of this individual, who is the cause of all misfortune, harasses the patient incessantly. Thus he recognises a physician, a priest, or even his father or mother, and consequently directs against these his hatred and desire for vengeance.

Hallucinations of sight are very rare in persecution-mania. Lasègue was of opinion that patients presenting them do not belong to the classical type, and most authors agree with this view. According to him, the patients are incapable of generating visual hallucinations. They are indignant if considered capable of having visions. Some declare that they have often tried to get their persecutor face to face, but that they have not succeeded, because he has run away or has hidden himself without any possibility of tracing him.

Hallucinations of smell and taste are frequent, although much less so than those of hearing, and they soon impress their mark upon the character of persecution-mania. The patient smells foul, nauseating, and intolerable smells, which he attributes to vapours or chemical agents placed in his neighbourhood. Some believe that they are surrounded by an atmosphere of sulphur. One of our patients who had studied chemistry distinctly smelt the whole series of odours which he had studied in the laboratory, carbonate of sulphur, the vapours of arsenic and chlorine, and many other smells.

If under the influence of hallucinations of taste, the patient finds an unpleasant smell in everything which he takes into his mouth; all food appears to him bitter or bad. It is only one step to the idea that people try to poison him, and most patients arrive at this conclusion.

Hallucinations of general sensibility in persecution-mania are extremely numerous and of remarkable variety; they may affect all parts of the body and cause the patient great physical suffering. The skin is tormented by all kinds of pain; the patient feels itching, he has a sense of heat or of burning, and he has *bizarre* impressions, which he attributes at once to mysterious agencies, to electricity, chemistry, magnetism, or to hypnotism; he feels that somebody strikes or pinches or pricks him with needles. The same sensations are perceived in the internal organs, and many patients believe that somebody is twisting their intestines about. The most painful impressions, however, are experienced in the genital organs. Female patients imagine that they are being outraged, and some arrive at the conclusion that they are pregnant. Male patients imagine that they are being emasculated, and that they are being subjected to masturbation; some also believe that their genital organs are penetrated by the mysterious agencies we have spoken of above.

Before finishing the subject of hallucinations, we should like to mention a peculiar transformation due to auditory hallucinations; some patients greatly troubled by the voices which they believe that they hear, identify these voices so completely with their own thoughts that they finally believe that they are no longer masters even of their own ideas. They are actually possessed by what Baillarger describes as psychical hallucinations. The patient believes that people read his own mind, that somebody steals his ideas, and that the voices which he hears immediately transform his ideas into words.

Ball reports a case where the patient, an old sufferer from persecution-mania, said one day: "Somebody steals my ideas before I have had time to conceive them." Under the influence of this idea, some patients when questioned as to what they feel, do not answer at all, but look at their questioner in such a manner as to indicate that they do not want to be made dupes by his pretended ignorance, or they will even say, "What is the good of telling you, you know it quite as well as I do." Such a condition is most serious, as indicating an advanced stage of the disorder, and not leaving any doubt that the derangement has become chronic. After this it may also happen that the patient feeling that his ideas escape him, and are known to every one when he would rather conceal them, imagines that he has in himself two separate individuals. He experiences an actual doubling of his personality, and in addition to this he is quite prepared for other modifications which may occur at a later period.

Period of Stereotyped Insanity.—Foville has used a very expressive term to describe the condition of the patient at this stage; he says that it is a kind of crystallisation. And, as a matter of fact, when this point is reached, persecution-mania is definitely established; if it undergoes any more modifications, it is only to eliminate elements of secondary importance, and not to acquire fresh ones; the ideas of persecution peculiar to the various individuals, the hallucinations and the sensory disorders have reached the stage of complete development. The patients do not add anything more; they are, so to say, crystallised in their insanity. Such patients we may see living for a great number of years, and find them at the end of this time in the very same condition as at the commencement; they have exactly the same hallucinations, and they are persecuted by exactly the same persons. They repeat constantly the same words and phrases, and their actions are also the same as before.

It may, however, happen that at this point rather insane ideas are formed, thus giving the disease a new appearance. Although there is an intimate connection between the former and the latter, these ideas do not change the nature of persecution-mania and do not alter its proper character. As Lasègue and Falret aptly remark, there is simply juxtaposition of the ideas, and no transformation of the disease. To a certain extent, the position of this class of patients is analogous to that of melancholiacs, whose mental troubles Cotard has described under the name of insanity of negation. (*See* NEGATIONS, INSANITY OF.)

These fresh insane ideas are ideas of ambition, of haughtiness, and of superiority. The patient who presents this symptom, attributes to himself every high quality, grand titles, great riches, and power and superiority over all who are around him. He believes himself to be a duke, prince, marquess, king or emperor; some go still further and regard themselves as saints or as God. They are millionaires, and are possessed of boundless wealth. They make the most marvellous discoveries, and imagine they have the power to perform miracles; nothing is impossible for them.

Insanity of grandeur, so far as it is connected with persecution-mania, has been admirably described by Foville, whose works on this subject are of the greatest importance.

It is an interesting question to elucidate how persecution-mania develops out of insanity of ambition.

One element of this transformation is undoubtedly the doubling of the personality spoken of at the end of the preceding period. The patient says to himself—consciously or not: "There are in myself ideas in which I recognise myself, and others in which I do not recognise myself; there are therefore in me two individuals, one who is myself, and the other who is not myself." And pursuing this train of ideas the patient forgets more or less completely his real personality, and attributes to himself an imaginary one.

Let us now consider how the ideas of ambition are formed. The patient returns into his own personality, and considering on the one hand his social position, artisan, labourer, or whatever he may be, and on the other hand the persecutions, of which he believes himself to be a victim, and the power which he attributes to his persecutors, he questions himself whether he is really a person of so little importance as he appears to himself. He says to himself that he must be a person of distinction, because people take so much trouble to torment him and to persecute him in so many ways. He imagines that he has been changed in the nursery, that he is evidently the descendant of princes, kings, or emperors, and that those whom he has hitherto regarded as his parents, are not his parents at all. Then he begins to say, and to believe, as we have indicated just now, that he is a grand personage, and sometimes he raises himself even to the ranks of divinity.

This mode of production of ambitious ideas has been called by Foville "transformation by logical deduction;" the logic in these ideas is evident in spite of their absurdity. We have however to add, that in other cases insanity of grandeur appears spontaneously and almost suddenly; the patient may present himself quite unexpectedly with all the attributes of the new position which he gives himself. This may be induced by one word which the patient happens to hear, and which appears to him to be revelation, or it may be caused by auditory hallucinations, and in the latter case the reasons for this transformation cannot be understood, because these new ideas are self-suggested.

Arrived at this stage, the patient has gone through all the phases of persecution-mania. We have described the symptoms peculiar to each period, but this will not yet be sufficient to give a perfect idea of the malady. Therefore, we proceed to occupy ourselves with peculiarities which, although varying in different individuals, are nevertheless identical, and are valuable additional characteristics of this form of insanity; these peculiarities refer to the actions of patients labouring under this disorder.

Actions of Patients in Persecution-mania.—It is evident that in consequence of his malady, the patient never passively yields to the attacks of which he believes himself to be the victim. All either try to escape the persecutor, or to take vengeance upon him. We must keep in mind that although the patient's intellect has undergone changes, the wheel-work is nevertheless intact, and that he reacts to certain impressions in almost the same manner as healthy individuals.

As Régis aptly remarks, the first thing they do is to complain; they immediately apply to the authorities asking them to put a stop to the persecutions, the origin and cause of which they are unable to discover. In this manner police-officers, magistrates, ministers, and even sovereigns are constantly assailed with their applications.

Just as their insanity is still vague and consists in insane interpretations only, in the same manner their suspicions and accusations are also vague. The patient will say: "I have enemies, but I do not know them, I try to discover them, but I fail to do so; I most certainly have enemies who want to do me harm, but I am ignorant who they are."

The more the insanity becomes definite the more precise also become the accusations; then the patient begins to direct his accusations against his doctor, against a certain friend, or even against his father or mother. Foville remarks that such individuals are sometimes actually happy, if they can address themselves to men who, understanding their mental condition, take the necessary steps to have them admitted and cared for in an asylum.

On the other hand, people often do not recognise that they are insane, and listening to their complaints try to quiet them and afterwards leave them to themselves, thus exposing them to the dreadful consequences of their insanity. And, as a matter of fact, they then abandon their complaint, and, taking to more effective measures, they become aggressive. Their attacks are mostly absolutely spontaneous and unexpected. The patient will rush up to any one who happens to pass by in the street, and who he believes has spoken of him, or has looked at him with contempt, and attack him with his fist or stick. In many other cases, however, the attacks are premeditated, and are directed against the person by whom the patient imagines himself to be constantly tormented.

Lastly come the more serious attacks, namely, murderous assaults. The patient generally does not reach this stage all at once, but passes through a long period of hesitation. His ideas however drive him on, and seeing no other way out of such a deplorable situation, he commits some frightful deed. Some become homicides in the hope that they will have peace after their persecutors are dead; others, because they hope to be given over into the hands of justice, and that on the day of the trial they will be able to denounce their persecutors, to cleanse themselves from all imputations they believe to be made against them, and to have their innocence publicly proclaimed. In the same manner, patients with ideas of grandeur wish to obtain acknowledgment of the rights to which they believe themselves entitled.

The number of assaults committed by individuals labouring under persecution-mania is extremely great; if we were to count those which have been published under different titles since the days of Pinel and Esquirol, we might fill volumes.

It follows from what we have said, that in most cases the patients who commit homicidal attacks, have definite motives and act with reflection and determination, but we must also keep in mind that in certain cases the patient executes his plans in the paroxysms of the disease, so that it seems as if such patients could only be impelled by a morbid influence or impulse. We have to mention a fact to which Blanche has properly drawn attention. He has shown that patients before they act, pass from time to time through a condition of exaltation. Habitually calm they become at times excited without any other cause than a cerebral modification, of which they are not conscious, and in one of these moments of excitement they commit the deed. Generally speaking, we may say that the motives which drive the patient to murder, are as numerous as the ideas which, according to the mind of the patient, form the foundation of persecution-mania.

Frequently it is not characterised by violence, but the patient addresses writings of all kinds—letters and petitions—to those whom he believes to have power to protect him. The patient generally writes at great length, and we must remark, that frequently his writings give a better account of his condition than his words and conversation. There are few alienists who have not met with patients whose letters alone revealed the mental disorder. Such patients have sufficient power over themselves to control their conversation, and knowing that their words would be considered unreasonable, take good care not to say anything that might compromise them; they are not so suspicious when writing, and thus soon expose their insane ideas. Usually the letters of the patient, especially when he is in an asylum, are denunciations, couched in precise and categorical terms, against the physician and the management. These denunciations are sometimes so plausible, that we must carefully investigate the character of the individual who wrote them, and not receive them in earnest.

Having regard to the actions which we have mentioned above, the patient may often become himself an actual persecutor to others.

Individuals labouring under persecution-mania are not always aggressive, and there are many cases in which the patient, instead of trying to avenge himself, endeavours to avoid the evils planned against him; this is done in various ways, according to the insane ideas which predominate in the patient, and according to his character.

The most troublesome insane conception from which a patient can possibly suffer, is certainly the fear of being poisoned; this fear causes him first of all to examine all his food minutely, then instead of taking his meals with his family, or continuing to go to his usual restaurant, he constantly changes without however trusting the food placed before him. Then he begins to buy his provisions himself, and does so by enveloping himself in mystery; every day he goes to a different shop, and preferably to one where he thinks he is unknown, but at last he finds everywhere signs of poison, and distrusting even himself ceases to eat altogether. If this happens with a patient in an asylum, the only remedy is to resort to artificial feeding.

Again, the patient may try to escape persecution by flight. Foville has described this condition under the name of migratory insanity (he calls these patients *aliénés migrateurs*). The patient commences by changing his lodgings or his house; then he changes from one quarter to another, and later to another town. At last, when this migratory insanity is fully developed, he changes to another country, soon, however, removing again, in order to seek in the most distant countries the rest which he cannot find anywhere.

It would seem natural that suicide should be common in cases of persecution-mania, but that is not the case. Suicides are rare. Some authors, especially Régis, go so far as to deny that there are any, and attributes this tendency to melancholiacs alone.

Course of Persecution-mania.—Although the progress of insanity in persecution-mania is very regular, there is nevertheless a great irregularity in the duration of each period. Generally, as we have pointed out before, the period of incubation is very long. There are individuals, who, from early childhood, have shown themselves predisposed to this mania, but who arrive at middle life before succumbing to the disease. It is generally impossible to assign a definite period to the actual commencement of the malady. The period of insane interpretation is also sometimes very long, but in the greater number of cases, it is comparatively the shortest period. We must not, however, think that there is always a well-marked division between each of these two periods; the characteristic symptoms of one period always extend into the succeeding one. The separation is most distinct between the period of insane interpretation and that in which the sensory disorders appear. A great number of patients present almost unexpectedly hallucinations, and acquire in a short time all their sensory disturbances to which they become victims. There are numerous cases in which persecution mania does not develop beyond the period of sensory disorders, but the greater number arrive at least at the stage of systematisation. After this time, some plunge into dementia; their ideation becomes weak, the impressions become confused, and the insane phenomena lose their acuteness. Others remain for an indefinite time in the same condition; their disorder does not undergo any more modification, and in spite of the disease they may retain a pretty normal mental activity, which under certain conditions may deceive us.

Many patients have intermittent attacks of agitation which border on maniacal excitement; they then become very aggressive, and abusive, talk with great animation, and are very angry, so that at such times it would not be prudent to approach them. This agitation may last for several hours or even days, and may return with almost regular periodicity. One of our patients becomes thus excited every day for two hours after dinner. In female patients an exacerbation takes place at the time of menstruation.

Some patients have actual remissions, during which they cease to suffer from hallucinations of persecution, being, however, thoroughly convinced that their previous experience was quite real. These remissions are rare, and we must be careful not to be deceived by appearances and regard as remission what frequently is nothing but simulation.

This is the place to consider a very interesting question lately raised at the medico-psychological society of Paris. Magnan and his pupils maintain that persecution-mania ought no longer to be considered as a morbid entity, but rather as a symptom of a more complex condition, to which at first they gave the name of chronic insanity, but which on account of the many objections made to this term, they now call by the name proposed by Cullerre, of "progressive systematised insanity." The new morbid condition thus called, is said to be characterised by a progressive and systematic evolution, and by the succession of four distinct periods which invariably appear in the same order.

In the *first* period, called that of *incubation*, the patient is uneasy and absorbed in himself; in short, he is in a kind of hypochondriacal condition, and after a shorter or longer period of hesitation, arrives at the stage of insane interpretation.

The *second* period is marked by organised persecution-mania, when the morbid ideas incessantly nourished by sensory disorders, establish themselves, and become coördinated and systematised.

The *third* period is characterised by the occurrence of ideas of grandeur, which indicate the ultimate systematisation of the disorder.

The *fourth* and terminal period consists in an incurable decay of the mental faculties.

It cannot be disputed that this classification corresponds to a great number of cases accurately observed, and that it has a right to be quoted in science; the mistake, however, made by those who introduced it, is, that they generalised its application too much. They maintain, in the first place, that the progressive systematised insanity is invariable in its evolution; but how will their classification include patients whose disorder comes to a standstill after the period of sensory disorders? They also assert that persecution-mania always terminates in insanity of grandeur. There are, however, plenty of patients who suffer from persecution-mania only, and live in this condition for an indefinite number of years, and who may fall victims to dementia, without having ever had any ambitious ideas.

Lastly, with regard to the dementia which characterises the last period, it is quite as often absent as insanity of grandeur. The authors in question have generalised all these latter facts because it suited their scheme, and in order to justify their manner of observation, they were compelled to create a new variety of dementia. In the present case, dementia is, according to their opinion, less the annihilation of the intellectual faculties than the disintegration of an insane structure which up to that point had been of remarkable fixity and solidity; but even this granted, one must admit that it often appears long before the period assigned to it in progressive systematised insanity. As a matter of fact, we see patients who, as soon as their insanity is organised, begin to separate its elements and abandon some of their insane conceptions. From this it follows that if we consider all the facts with impartiality, we must admit that we may under the name of progressive systematised delirium class all the symptoms which in former times were considered as cases of persecution-mania with megalomania, but also that there are other symptoms almost as numerous, in which persecution-mania preserves its individuality and autonomy, and that it certainly is in itself characteristic enough to preserve, as the type discovered by Lasègue, the special place occupied by it hitherto.

Prognosis.—The prognosis is almost always unfavourable. If there are cases cured, they are certainly not numerous, and we for our part have not yet met with one. In this respect we must not allow ourselves to be deceived by appearances and attribute cures to persecution-mania, which concern other morbid conditions in which ideas of persecution may be met with.

The duration of the disease is always long, and the patient may live to an advanced age, provided that other complications do not shorten his days.

Diagnosis.—When persecution-mania is fully established, it is generally easy to recognise. The great number of hallucinations, especially of those of hearing, and their influence on the life and actions of the patient, are excellent diagnostic means. The greatest difficulty with regard to persecution-mania is simulation, to which a certain number of patients have a great tendency. This simulation may in some cases embarrass even the most experienced alienist; still more so those who have no practice in the treatment of mental disorders. Magistrates are frequently deceived when they have to deal with lunatics of this class. There are, indeed, patients who are remarkably clever in concealing their insanity, wholly or partially. They know that their ideas are considered to be devoid of reason and take every care not to allow them to be noticed. Some succeed marvellously, and defy the most minute examinations. Clouston reports the case of a patient who believed himself in constant danger of being poisoned, and who was possessed by a hundred morbid suspicions, but who for a great number of years did not confess his troubles except to one person. To all others he pretended to be free from any anxiety; he was pleasant and behaved as if he was not at all troubled. Marandon de Montyel has recently published an astonishing account of a patient who for almost two years was of irreproachable behaviour; he was considered cured, and by a decision of the Court, he was allowed to leave the asylum in which he had been confined. The very same night he killed his mother whom he accused of all the persecutions of which he believed himself to be the victim. The next morning he gave himself up to the police after having posted a letter to the magistrate thanking him for having facilitated the accomplishment of an act, which put a stop to all the misery with which he had been afflicted for so many years. In this same letter he confessed to have simulated.

If one has time to observe the patient, it is not difficult with a little experience to make a correct diagnosis. Certain words which always return in the same form, the gesticulations — sometimes rather *bizarre*—and the way of acting in connection with his fixed ideas are significant indications, and in addition to this, patients who seem to be healthy in mind, so far as their words and conversation are concerned, are not afraid to confide their insane ideas to paper. Once on the track of the disorder, it only remains to ask the

put a few questions, or to throw into the conversation a few leading insinuations.

The insanity of grandeur, which appears in the third period, cannot be confounded with general paralysis if we remember that paralytics are generally incoherent and confused, and they exhibit a satisfaction with themselves which is in inverse ratio to the mistrust and the reserve shown by patients suffering from persecution-mania.

We often meet with ideas of persecution and hallucinations in alcoholism. The specific symptoms, however, of the latter disorder, enable us to avoid mistakes, and, in addition to this, there is another fundamental difference, in so far as that in persecution-mania the hallucinations are mostly auditory, whilst in alcoholism they are mostly visual. Lastly, alcoholism is of short duration, whilst persecution-mania may last for an indefinite period. One individual may suffer at one and the same time from delusion of suspicion and alcoholic insanity—that is to say, a patient suffering from the former disorder may also fall a victim to alcoholic intoxication.

Patients suffering from delusion of suspicion cannot be confounded with melancholiacs, if we keep in mind the condition of depression of the latter, and also their anxiety and distress.

Speaking generally, we must not confound persecution-mania with ideas of persecution met with in a great number of morbid conditions. These latter ideas taken isolatedly are incoördinate, and are not necessarily founded on hallucinations. Among the conditions in which they are present, we mention specially organic affections, locomotor ataxy, sclerosis *en plaques* and paralysis agitans. There is often in hysteria a marked tendency to make accusations and complaints, but it is rarely accompanied by auditory hallucinations, and the patients are not subject to general sensory disorders. In *folie raisonnante*, or in moral insanity, the patients often complain of being persecuted, and more frequently still they become in their turn terrible persecutors, but their disorder has no analogy at all with true persecution-mania.

We have specially to mention the ideas of persecution which mark the commencement of senile dementia. Old people, timorous and distrustful under the influence of old age, begin to exaggerate this tendency when senile dementia supervenes; they believe that some one wants to do them injury, to rob and ruin, or even to kill them; they accuse their dearest and most devoted friends and relatives of ill-will. They also believe that they are neglected and looked upon with contempt. Under these circumstances they have an aversion to every one, and intercourse with them becomes most difficult. Although this condition is extremely similar to persecution-mania, it differs from it because it is not based on hallucinations; it is nothing but the product of a cerebral alteration, and the progressive and rapid intellectual weakening will soon reveal the true nature of the disorder.

Ætiology.—The conditions under which persecution-mania develops, and the causes which produce it, are of a very complicated nature. Ritti has in his excellent description of persecution-mania made some statistical researches, which it will suffice for us to review.

Persecution-mania is a mental disorder of frequent occurrence, and cases seem to become more and more numerous. In this respect it bears some analogy to general paralysis.

The statistical returns of several asylums show that there are a greater number of female than male patients, namely, in the proportion of five to three.

Speaking generally, ideas of persecution-mania make their appearance in individuals before they reach an advanced age. The greater number of patients in asylums, whose disorder is at the stage of full development, are from thirty to fifty years old.

Persecution-mania attacks individuals of every profession and of every class of society. It seems, however, that the greater number of cases belong to the wealthy class.

With regard to the influence of heredity, we may state that some authors, especially Krafft-Ebing, consider it an important factor. According to these authors, we find among the ancestors of most of the patients in question various morbid conditions, either well-developed insanity, or more frequently an eccentric character and behaviour, or symptoms of hysteria, hypochondriasis or alcoholism.

The investigations of Christian and Ritti at Charenton do not attribute to hereditary degeneration such a marked influence as the authors just mentioned. There were among 134 patients admitted at Charenton in seven years suffering from persecution-mania not more than 36—about 26 per cent. among whose ancestors traces of mental disorders could be found.

Contrary to the general opinion, moral causes play only an unimportant part in the production of this form of insanity. It is so, however, with all other forms of insanity. Moral causes, to which some importance has been attributed in the cases which concern us here, are, principally: prolonged grief, loss of fortune, jealousy, excessive religious exercises, every kind of anxiety, vicious education, &c.

It is necessary to add that these various moral influences have a powerful effect on the physical constitution of the individual; they weaken nutrition, debilitate the organism, and prepare the soil for all kinds of morbid conditions; moreover, the more we study mental disease, the more we become convinced that physical causes are among the most important factors in producing insanity, and applying this to the disorder with which we are now occupied, we have good reason to say that moral causes are connected with the production of mental disorder, but only indirectly.

Ritti divides the physical causes of persecution-mania into three classes: (1) causes which act on the brain and nervous system (meningitis in childhood, infantile convulsions, cranial traumatism, apoplectic attacks, complications of various diseases, &c.); (2) causes which have their origin in the reproductive organs or in sexual life (faulty formation of the organs in question, seminal losses, onanism, and the various forms of venereal disease, &c.); (3) general causes of physical debility (privation, misery, and insufficient nutrition, anæmia, chlorosis and related conditions).

Treatment.—The indications for treatment are to arrest the development of the disorder or to mitigate its effects.

Those which refer to the former are almost all of doubtful efficacy. Distractions do no good because the patient does not feel interested in them. Travelling has sometimes done good, but frequently it is more harmful than useful. As a matter of fact, the patient carrying with him all his insane ideas and hallucinations, is the more irritated, because he finds them everywhere, and instead of becoming better, his condition becomes still worse. Hydrotherapeutics have yielded many good results, but a tonic *régime* according to the wants of the organism is the best of all.

In most cases it is necessary to place the patient in an asylum; first, because he is dangerous to public order and security; and secondly, because methodical and effective treatment can only be properly applied there.

We must add that the symptomatic indications are numerous, and that according to the case we have to allay insomnia, excitement, and various disorders of the alimentary canal. Lastly, in cases where the patient is afraid of being poisoned we have to resort to artificial feeding.

Forensic Medicine.—From a medico-legal point of view, cases of persecution-mania afford matter for consideration of the greatest importance. We cannot go deeply into it here, and must limit ourselves to stating the elementary principles.

In almost all patients there is at certain times a perfect contradiction between their reasonable manner and the gravity of their condition. Their attitude is habitually that of healthy people, although an experienced eye is not easily deceived and soon discovers the anomalies. For inexperienced people, however, the anomalies pass unnoticed. The same holds good of the conversation, which may be neither incoherent nor improbable, because the account of the persecutions is so plausible that it may appear as by no means impossible. Then, putting aside the external symptoms, there are many internal manifestations, which might pass as signs of a healthy mind. The patient is fully conscious of his doings and sayings; most of his actions are fully considered and premeditated, and even if reprehensible they are accomplished with real discernment of good and evil. Nevertheless, in spite of all this apparent reasonableness, an individual suffering from persecution-mania is a lunatic in the strictest sense of the word. Constantly beset by hallucinations, and governed by the disorder, he acts only under the influence of morbid ideas which do not allow him one moment's personal liberty. To maintain that under these circumstances he can be declared responsible would be to misunderstand the essentials of psychiatry, to pretend that one individual can be insane and sane at the same time, and that although he has no longer his *liberum arbitrium*, he is in the same position as if he had got it. Therefore, if an individual labouring under delusion of suspicion commits a criminal act, he must be exonerated from responsibility, and ought not to be sent to prison, but an asylum.

The criminal actions committed by this class of patients are numerous, and vary according to the predominating tendency in every individual: calumnies, libels, assaults on any class of society, and lastly attempts at homicide. We might indefinitely extend the nomenclature, but whatever the actions are, we are able to find in all of them, contrary to appearance, the influence of insanity.

Therefore, generally speaking, individuals attacked by persecution-mania are from the commencement of their malady not responsible for their actions.

From the same standpoint, they must be considered incapable of having the not dispoal of their person and property. It sometimes happens that a patient makes a will depriving his whole family and relatives of their due, and giving all he possesses to strangers, and sometimes even to persons of whom he has no knowledge. He does this to be revenged for the persecutions of which he believes himself the victim; and full of spite against his natural heirs he will disinherit them, rejoicing beforehand in the idea of having returned evil for evil.

With patients suffering from this mental affection, attempts made by designing persons to inveigle them into leaving their property to them are likely to be successful; but, in law, such bequests would be annulled.

We have already mentioned that, as a rule, it is necessary to confine this class of patients in an asylum, on account of the treatment as well as the danger to public order and personal safety. Once confined in an asylum, the patient commences to make accusations; not believing that he is insane he complains of being made a victim of arbitrary sequestration; he writes letter after letter to the administration and the authorities, demanding his release, and claiming damages against those who have caused his confinement. It is necessary that the authorities should be instructed about the dangers which may arise if release is granted under such circumstances. Cases are very numerous in which patients have been set at liberty because the magistrates did not appreciate their condition, and soon after they committed the most frightful crimes.

In conclusion, we may say that by their apparently reasonable accusations and complaints, patients have frequently been the cause of making the public believe that the sequestrations have been arbitrary, whilst impartial investigation by competent authorities has not hitherto been able to find one single case of the kind.

VICTOR PARANT.

[*References.* — Baillarger, Des hallucinations, Paris, 1846. Ball, Leçons sur les maladies mentales, Paris, 1880. Blanche, Des homicides commis par les aliénés, Paris, 1878. Bucknill and Hack Tuke, Psychological Medicine, London, 1879. Christian, Etude sur la mélancolie, Paris, 1876. Clouston, Mental Diseases, London, 1883. Cullerre, Traité pratique des maladies mentales, Paris, 1889. Esquirol, Des maladies mentales, Paris, 1838. Falret, De l'évolution du délire des persécutions: Annales médico-psychologiques, 1881. Foville, Ach., Lypémanie, dans le nouveau dict. de méd. et chirurg. vol. xxi.; Etude clinique de la folie avec prédominance du délire des grandeurs, Paris, 1871; Les aliénés voyageurs ou migrateurs, Annales médico-psychologiques, 1875. Lasègue, Du délire des persécutions, Archives générales de médecine, 1852. Legrand du Saulle, Le délire des persécutions, Paris, 1871. Magnan, Formes et marche du délire chronique, Leçons faites à Ste. Anne, 1883. Marandon de Montyel, De la dissimulation en aliénation mentale, Annales d'hygiène publique et de médecine légale, 1889. Morel, Traité des maladies mentales, Paris, 1859. Parant, Rapport médico-légal sur l'état mental du sieur A., meurtrier du Dr. Marchant, délire des persécutions, Annales médico-psychologiques, 1881; La paralysie agitante examinée comme cause de la folie, Annales médico-psychologiques, 1883; La Raison dans la folie, Paris, 1888. Pinel, Traité médico-philosophique de l'aliénation mentale, Paris, 1809. Régis, Manuel de médecine mentale, Paris, 1885. Ritti, Délire de persécution, Dictionnaire encyclopédique des sciences médicales, Paris. Rougier, Essai sur la lypémanie et le délire des persécutions chez les tabétiques, Lyon, 1881.]

PERSONAL EQUATION. The special reaction time of each individual. (*See* REACTION TIME.)

PERSONALITY, DISORDERS OF. (*See* DOUBLE CONSCIOUSNESS.)

PERTURBATION (*perturbo*, I disturb). Excessive restlessness, especially of the mind.

PERTURBATIONES ANIMI. Disturbances of mind.

PERVERSION. — Alteration for the worse in instincts, feelings, habits, appetite, or any other previous characteristic of the patient, is a constant accompaniment of insanity. Perversion of some of these attributes is, however, an essential sign of moral insanity.

PERVIGILIUM (*pervigilo*, I watch through). Disinclination or inability to sleep. Night watching. (Fr. *vigilance;* Ger. *die krankhafte Schlaflosigkeit.*)

PESSIMISM.—The making the worst of everything, a common mental condition in hypochondriasis and melancholia.

PETIT MAL. (*See* EPILEPSY.)

PEUR DES ESPACES. Agoraphobia. (*See* IMPERATIVE IDEAS.)

PHAGOMANIA (φαγεῖν, to eat; μανία, madness). A term for a paroxysmal and uncontrollable craving for food leading to thefts.

PHANTASIA (φαντασία, a making visible). An imaginary representation; phantasy. (Fr. *phantasie.*)

PHANTASM, PHANTASMA (φαντάζω, I make appear). A hallucination or illusion (*q.v.*). The term has been largely applied to so-called apparitions. The authors of "Phantasms of the Living" have excluded the alleged apparitions of the dead, and restricted their inquiries to the apparitions of persons still living, although on the brink of physical dissolution. Auditory, tactile or even purely ideational and emotional impressions in addition to visual phenomena, are "included under the term *phantasm;* a word which, though etymologically a mere variant of *phantom*, has been less often used, and has not become so closely identified with visual impressions alone" (*op. cit.* vol. i. p. xxxv). (Fr. *phantasme;* Ger. *Luftgebild.*)

PHANTASMAGORIA (φάντασμα, a phantom; ἄγω, I lead along). Term for the raising or recalling of spirits of the dead as formerly supposed to be practised. Patients sometimes say they see "phantasmagoria," meaning ghosts or spirits of the dead. (Fr. and Ger. *phantasmagorie.*)

PHANTASMATOMORIA (φάντασμα, an image; μωρία, folly). Silliness or childishness, with absurd fancies. (Fr. *phantasmatomorie.*)

PHANTASMOPHRENOSIS (φάντασμα, an image; φρένωσις, instruction). Schultz used this term for dreamy fancies while in a waking state. (Fr. *phantasmaphrénose.*)

PHANTASMOSCOPIA (φάντασμα, an image; σκοπέω, I see). A seeing of spectres, ghosts, or spirits. (Fr. *phantasmoscopie;* Ger. *Gespenstersehen.*)

PHANTASTON, PHANTASTUM (φανταστός, conceiving visions). Term for a mental conception or idea.

PHANTOM TUMOURS.—In hysterical women there occasionally occurs a rounded prominence of the abdomen which is thought by them to be due to the presence of a tumour or to pregnancy. It is uniformly smooth, resonant, soft, and movable from side to side. No pain, tenderness, or pressure symptoms are present, and the tumour disappears entirely under the influence of an anæsthetic, returning gradually as the patient regains consciousness. The cause is unknown, but the condition has been said (Roberts) to be probably due to paralysis of the intestines, a consequence of disordered nervous influence. The treatment is that for hysteria (*q.v.*); galvanism may be tried, and the bowels should be kept well open.

PHANTOMA (φαντάζω, I make visible). A ghostly appearance. A phantom.

PHARMACOMANIA (φάρμακον, a drug; μανία, madness). A mania for taking medicines. Applicable to morbid craving for drugs. (Fr. *pharmacomanie;* Ger. *Arzneiwuth.*)

PHARYNGEAL ANÆSTHESIA.—A symptom in hysteria. Anæsthesia of the pharynx is so uncommon, except in hysteria, that it is a useful aid in the diagnosis of that disease. (*See* HYSTERIA.)

PHILŒNIA (φιλέω, I love; οἶνος, wine). Addiction to wine or drink. (Fr. *philœnie;* Ger. *Weinliebe.*)

PHILOMIMESIA (φιλέω, I love; μίμησις, imitation). A love of mimicry, not uncommonly seen among the insane. (Fr. *philomimésie;* Ger. *Nachahmungssucht.*)

PHILOMIMETIC.—Of or belonging to philomimesia (*q.v.*).

PHILOPATRIDALGIA (φιλέω, I love; πατρίς, fatherland; ἄλγος, pain). Morbid home-sickness. (*See* NOSTALGIA.)

PHILOPATRIDOMANIA (φιλέω, I love; πατρίς, one's country; μανία, madness). A craving for home so intensified that it has become insanity. It occurs in young soldiers and sailors on foreign service. (*See* NOSTALGIA.)

PHLEBOTOMANIA (φλέψ, a vein; τέμνω, I cut; μανία, madness). An excessive belief in and rage for phlebotomy. (Fr. *phlebotomanie;* Ger. *Aderlasswuth.*)

PHLEDONIA (φλεδονεία, idle talk). Delirium. (Fr. *délire;* Ger. *Wahnsinn.*)

PHLEGMATIC TEMPERAMENT. (*See* TEMPERAMENT.)

PHOBIA (φόβος, fear). A termination literally meaning "fear of." The compound word so formed often has its meaning much extended, as for example, hydrophobia: in other cases, such as agoraphobia or photophobia, the literal meaning is the one usually understood.

PHORODIPSIA (φόβος, fear; δίψα, thirst). A synonym of hydrophobia.

PHOSPHATURIA AND INSANITY.—It has been observed, that in connection with excess of phosphates in the urine, hypochondriasis, irritability, depression of spirits, and even melancholia, have occurred. It is, however, doubtful what relation these symptoms bear to the phosphaturia; it seems possible that the latter is as likely to be the effect as the cause of the symptoms. (*See* URINE OF THE INSANE.)

PHOTOMANIA (φῶς, light; μανία, madness). The inability in some of the insane to bear the presence of light without increase of symptom. (Fr. *photomanie.*)

PHOTOPSIA (φῶς, light; ὄψις, sight). A subjective sensation or appearance of light. (Fr. *photopsie.*)

PHRENALGIA (φρήν, mind; ἄλγος, pain). A term for melancholia.

PHRENES (φρήν, the mind). Ancient term for the præcordium and also for the diaphragm, each of which has at some time been considered to be the seat of the mind.

PHRENESIS (φρήν, the mind). (*See* PHRENITIS.)

PHRENETIC. Frenzied, wildly delirious. (Fr. *phrénétique;* Ger. *phrenetisch.*)

PHRENICA. Mental diseases.

PHRENICULA, PHRENITICULA (φρήν, the mind). These terms have been used for "brain fever," and for acute hydrocephalus. (Fr. *phrénicule;* Ger. *Hirnfieber.*)

PHRENITIS (φρήν, the mind). Literally inflammation of the mind; it has been used for inflammation of the brain and its membranes, and for inflammation of the diaphragm.

PHRENOBLABES (φρήν, the mind; βλάπτω, I damage). Damaged or impaired understanding. (Fr. *phrénoblabe;* Ger. *am Verstande beschädigt.*)

PHRENOBLABIA.—A lesion of the intellect. (*See* PHRENOBLABES.)

PHRENOLEPSIA EROTEMATICA (φρήν, the mind; λῆψις, a seizing; ἐρωτηματικός, pertaining to interrogation). Doubting insanity (*q.v.*).

PHRENOLOGY (φρήν, the mind; λόγος, a discourse). The study of the faculties of the human mind in connection with the so-called "organs" in the brain associated with those faculties. These "organs" are studied through the impressions they are supposed to make on the shape of the cranium. Gall's hypothesis. (Fr. *phrénologie.*)

PHRENO-MAGNETISM.—Same as phreno-mesmerism.

PHRENO-MESMERISM.—A compound term applied to the supposed discovery that the manipulations practised in mesmerism, being directed to any particular phrenological development of the brain could call into action the corresponding faculty, sentiment or propensity.

PHRENONARCOSIS (φρήν, mind; νάρκωσις, a benumbing). A benumbing of the intellect; a dulling of the senses. (Fr. *phrénonarcose;* Ger. *Phrenonarkose.*)

PHRENOPATHIA (φρήν, the mind; πάθος, disease). Disease of the mind. (Fr. *phrénopathie;* Ger. *Gemüthskrankheit.*)

PHRENOPLEGIA (φρήν, the mind; πληγή, a blow). A sudden failing or upsetting of the mind; fatuity. (Fr. *phrénoplegie;* Ger. *Seelenlähmung.*)

PHRENORTHOSIS (φρήν, the mind; ὀρθός, right). Rightmindedness.

PHRENSY (φρήν, the mind). The same as phrenitis. Inflammation of the brain and its membranes, and the accompanying delirium.

PHRICASMUS (φρικασμός, a shuddering). Shivering from mental emotion.

PHRONEMOPHOBIA (φρόνημα, thought; φοβέω, I fear). A dread or hatred of thought. (Fr. *phronémophobie;* Ger. *Denkscheu.*)

PHRONTIS (φροντίζω, I think). Thought, reflection, anxiety. (Fr. *adémonie;* Ger. *Sorge.*)

PHTHISICA SPES.—The phthisical hope. It is a characteristic of patients suffering from tuberculous diseases (to which the term "phthisis" is usually applied) that they are to the last hopeful of cure and convinced they are getting on well. (*See* PHTHISICAL INSANITY.)

PHTHISICAL INSANITY.—It is now commonly admitted, as the result of the observations of many keen observers of the psychological condition of patients suffering from certain bodily diseases, that the emotional and even the intellectual state of such patients seems to be affected differently according to the seat and nature of the disease present. There is, in fact, a psychology of many diseases and of the great organs of the body. Many of the symptoms are apt to be obscure till looked for. A certain subtilty of mind as well as a trained observation are required to see them. Not every physician of great general diagnostic skill in cardiac disease will observe that the patient is morbidly fearful in mind, or will ascertain that this mental condition appeared coincidentally with the first symptoms of the heart troubles, or even preceded their detectable signs. No doubt the glaring anomaly of a calm hopefulness of recovery in the minds of multitudes of patients on the point of death from consumption could not fail to attract attention. The *spes phthisica* was an early generalisation in medical psychology. To estimate the precise mental and emotional condition of their patients would imply a double series of mental acts on the part of the physicians in attendance for bodily diseases, that cannot fairly be expected of many of them. And we must keep in mind that the observation of mental symptoms is not yet generally taught or insisted on in our medical curriculum. Yet the importance of the patient's subjective condition is very great in regard to the effect of treatment on the objective symptoms of many diseases. Why do change of scene, pleasant society, travel, and suitable occupation often "cure" certain diseases? Unquestionably, in many cases, they do so through the change they produce on the patient's mental condition, and the subsequent nutritional improvements. When medical psychology is taught as a part of the course of study of every medical student, we believe the science will advance far more rapidly than it has hitherto done in some directions, for we shall have a hundred observers of mental symptoms where now we have only one. Not only are we deficient in an exact knowledge of the psychology of bodily disease, but we have too few facts as to the precise mental symptoms present in the deliriums of the different febrile disorders, and as to the exact differences between the febrile delirium of childhood, of adult life, and of old age. Such additions to our psychological knowledge can only be made by the general practitioners of medicine, after being trained to observe mental symptoms, as a part of the examination of their patients.

Recent physiological and clinical investigation more and more tends to set up the brain as the great inhibitor and stimulator of all nutrition, the master of the functions of all other organs and tissues. It influences strongly both the blood formation and the blood supply. We lately had a case in which, when the excessive brain energising of a five years' elevated stage of *folie circulaire* suddenly ceased, and the low stage of the disease began, one effect was that the blood lost half its red corpuscles, and otherwise altered greatly in quality in a fortnight. This seemed to us to be a direct trophic effect of an alteration in the brain state. On the other hand, we are coming more practically to recognise that the condition of the nutrition of all the tissues and organs affects the brain directly through the changes they produce in the blood, and reflexly through their afferent nerves. We are not surprised when an attack of indigestion causes irritability and depression of mind, or when impaired metabolism results in lassitude, or when badly working kidneys produce sleeplessness with hallucinations of the senses. The recognition of the action and reaction of peripheral organs and brain are now parts of our ordinary medical state of mind. This clearly implies an intense reactiveness of the highest of the brain functions, that of mind, to all abnormalities of function and nutrition throughout the body, for the mental centre is necessarily the highest and the most universally related of all the nerve centres. We know these physiological and pathological facts, but we do not always apply them and endeavour to extend them in our daily work as physicians.

From the time of Hippocrates a special connection has been assumed to exist between sluggish action of the liver and melancholia, and modern physiology has enabled us partially to realise the reason of this. But to the lungs and their diseases was attached no special mental symptom. Two facts only had attracted attention half a century ago. One was the great frequency of phthisis pulmonalis among the insane in asylums. This had been noted by various observers in this country, France, and Germany. The second fact was later in being noticed. It was, as expressed by McKinnon in 1845: "The scrofulous and insane constitutions are nearly allied," and by Van der Kolk: "Lung phthisis especially appears to me to stand very frequently in close connection with insanity."

In 1862–63 * we made a careful examination into the connection of phthisis pulmonalis and tuberculosis generally with mental diseases, both statistically and clinically, with the result that ever since it has been generally admitted that there are important relationships between the two diseases. The first of these relationships is the much greater frequency of phthisis pulmonalis as a cause of death among the insane than among the sane of the same age. Whether the assigned causes of death among the insane are taken, or the frequency of tubercular deposit in their lungs, as found post mortem, the fact is equally proved that the insane are more prone to consumption than the sane. In the older institutions, where the hygienic conditions were bad, the number of deaths from phthisis was often from 25 to 30 per cent. of the whole number who died. And when the post-mortem records of those institutions were examined, from 30 to 60 per cent. showed signs of tubercular deposit to a greater or less extent. The sanitary conditions of the modern hospitals for the insane are, however, much better than they were fifty years ago; the diet of the patients is far better, and the clothing and warmth needed by those suffering from insanity are also far better attended to, so that the recent statistics of the prevalence of phthisis are far more favourable than they used to be. In the Royal Edinburgh Asylum for the Insane, from 1842 to 1863, the percentage of deaths from phthisis on the whole number of deaths was 29, while for the ten years from 1879 to 1888 it was only 13.6 per cent.

The true test of the prevalence of phthisis among the insane is got by comparing the proportion of those who die from this cause in asylums with the same proportion in the general population at the same ages, that is, in those over twenty years of age. According to Dr. James,† the very highest rate of mortality from phthisis at any age occurs in women from twenty-five to thirty—viz., 0.40 per cent. of those living at that age. Now, in the Royal Edinburgh Asylum in the ten years 1879–1888, when the phthisis mortality had been reduced to a rate below the average of similar institutions, it amounted to 1.19 per cent. of the average population of the asylum, the average numbers being 9.7 deaths a year from phthisis,

* *Journal of Mental Science*, April 1863.

† "Pulmonary Phthisis," by Alex. James, M.D.

and the average population 818.18. A low tubercular mortality in an asylum is therefore three times the highest rate to be found at any age in the general population. This mode of ascertaining the prevalence of any disease is now admitted by all statisticians to be the true one, and not the percentage of deaths from any disease out of the whole number of deaths. Much misconception as to the prevalence of phthisis among the insane has arisen from an ignorance of the proper mode of estimating it. It is to this ignorance alone that statements about phthisis not being more prevalent in good asylums than in the general population are due.

In many respects the insane in well-conducted asylums are now far better off than many great classes of our working population. Their diet, their amusements, their clothing, are all regulated on medical principles, and they are not exposed to cold unduly in winter and spring.

The fact that, under the most favourable conditions of life and treatment that we can at present devise for the insane in the best asylums, three of them die of pulmonary phthisis to one person in the general population at the same age, is one full of interest and significance to the student of brain function. When it was discovered that vascular disease was found in an enormous proportion of all the cases of a certain kind of kidney disease, an important light was considered to have been thrown on both classes of disease, leading to very practical results in regard to our conceptions of blood supply, vascular tension, and processes of excretion. So this fact of the combination of two such apparently dissimilar diseases as insanity and consumption should have attracted more attention than it has done to the pathological character of both diseases. It is certain that writers on phthisis have not referred to it as its importance demands. If the bacillar theory of phthisis is true, the general conditions within the body and outside it that produce a suitable nidus for the development of the tubercle bacillus must always be of the highest consequence. And here we have something that increases the fertility of the soil threefold for the bacilli. We know that almost everything that depresses the nutrition tends towards phthisis if long continued. We know also that insanity has in most cases trophic symptoms. The nutrition of the tissues is commonly depressed, this going along with the mental phenomena as an essential part of the morbid process. No such trophic symptom could be of more importance than this general reduction of the bodies of the insane to that state in which they form fertile seed-beds for the tubercle bacillus. The resistiveness of the healthy body against this the most destructive of all the enemies of longevity is evidently reduced enormously by the mental disease. We have for many years preached the "gospel of fatness" in the treatment of insanity. No better proof exists of the grounds on which this "gospel" is based than the fact that thereby we also fight against consumption, the twin sister and the common sequel of insanity. The frequency of phthisis in chronic insanity is the strongest proof that mental disease has marked trophic symptoms. The frequent association of the depraved nutrition known as scrofula with idiocy and congenital imbecility has long been known. Ireland says:* "perhaps two-thirds or even more are of the scrofulous constitution." Idiots and congenital imbeciles are very often of the strumous diathesis, having weak circulation, a low temperature, a pale complexion, bad and badly set teeth, the glandular and mucous structures being especially liable to disease. The likeness of idiocy and secondary dementia to each other trophically is in many ways marked, and therefore it is not matter of surprise that so many patients suffering from both states fall into consumption and die. Ireland says that "fully two-thirds of all idiots die of phthisis. It may be asked, is idiocy itself not another though a rarer manifestation of this diathesis?"

The hereditary relationship of insanity and phthisis was observed by Van der Kolk,† who says: "It is remarkable when in the very same family some of the children suffer from mania or melancholia, and the brothers and sisters who have remained free from these diseases die of phthisis." This we have observed so many times that we cannot regard it as a mere accident. Our experience and conclusions on this point are precisely those of Van der Kolk, and Guislain ‡ says: "Pulmonary tuberculosis appears to me to be in direct relationship with insanity; it is frequently seen in the descendants of the insane and in their progenitors." Dr. James quotes Thompson as showing that as to heredity the two diseases are similar in the following respects—viz.: (1) Transmission is from either parent; (2) The disease may appear in the child

* "Idiocy and Imbecility," by W. W. Ireland, M.D.

† "Mental Diseases," by J. L. C. Schroeder Van der Kolk. Translated by Rudall.

‡ "Leçons orales sur les Phrenopathies," Guislain, 2nd ed. by Ingels.

before it is developed in the parent; (3) The disease may be transmitted by the parent without development; (4) Atavism is a frequent and important characteristic. He might have added that the age at which the two diseases are most commonly developed is somewhat the same. They both appear first to any marked extent at adolescence, they attack full maturity and middle life freely, and they both tend to decline in old age. The tendency to insanity is strongest in the male sex from thirty to thirty-five, while consumption attacks its victims in that sex in greatest numbers from twenty-five to thirty-five. In the female sex insanity is later in reaching its acme, being at the age of from fifty to fifty-five, while consumption plays greatest havoc in that sex from twenty-five to forty.* In our investigations we found that a hereditary predisposition to insanity was 7½ per cent. more common in those patients who had died of consumption than among the inmates of the asylum generally. This seems to indicate that a strong neurotic heredity not only produces insanity, but that, after having thus tended to mental death, such a heredity leads also to bodily death by consumption. We have not been able to get statistics showing the hereditary relationships of the two diseases, but we constantly meet with families where both diseases exist. We lately had two insane patients, brother and sister, whose mother had been insane, and in whose father's family consumption had been prevalent, and who had had two sane sisters die of phthisis. Few practitioners but have met with many similar cases. It is our impression that a simple phthisical heredity is not so dangerous in leading to insanity, as an heredity to insanity is in leading to phthisis. Where both diseases have appeared in the ancestry, we believe that the risk to the descendants from both diseases is greater than the same amount of hereditary taint of phthisis or insanity singly would have produced. For example, if we have a couple marrying, the husband's mother having been insane, and the wife's father phthisical, we believe that the children would run a greater risk of both phthisis and insanity than if those grandparents had been both consumptive or both insane.

The most important questions to the psychiatric physician in regard to the relationship of insanity and phthisis are: Which is first commonly seen as an actuality in the cases where both are ultimately combined? Is the relationship of the primary disease to the secondary causal? Does the one influence the symptoms and course of the other? And, if so, how? Is there any form of phthisis that can be called that of insanity? Is there any form of insanity that can be called phthisical? If so, what are the special symptoms of the insanity? and of the phthisis so tinctured?

It is certain we cannot as yet answer all these queries satisfactorily. But the statistical and clinical observations we made in 1863, as well as our subsequent experience, do enable us to answer some of them. There can be no doubt that taking all the cases of insanity that fall into phthisis, in the majority of them the mental disease appeared first. We found that of 282 insane patients, who died tubercular, about one-third only died within two years after the insanity had first appeared. As the average duration of pulmonary consumption in the cases in whom it was the cause of death was found by Ancell to be about eighteen months, it is clear that in two-thirds of the cases at least, the mental symptoms preceded the pulmonary. But then in some of the cases the phthisis preceded the insanity, and we found that 66 out of the 282, or 23½ per cent., died within a year after becoming insane. This proportion of cases in which the two diseases had arisen so very nearly together is far too large to be accidental. The predisposing cause of both we ascertained in many of the individual cases, to be a heredity to both insanity and phthisis.

All recent investigation points to the fact that every severe disturbance of brain function of whatever kind is accompanied by lowering or disturbance of its trophic energising, and that such trophic lowering means sooner or later functional or structural change in the peripheral organs and tissues of the body. The fact that, out of the three-fourths of the cases in which the insanity preceded the phthisis by more than a year, 7.5 per cent. were cases of secondary dementia, shows clearly that it is the trophically lowest and terminal variety of insanity, the true "mental death," that leads most to consumption.

The next question as to whether the one disease influences the other, apart from causation, and how this influence takes effect, can chiefly be determined by clinical observation. First, as to how the insanity influences the phthisis. The most common effect is this, that the subjective and many of the objective symptoms of the disease are abolished. The disease is frequently rendered latent, in

* James on "Phthisis," and the 30th Report (for 1888) of the Commissioners in Lunacy for Scotland.

[illegible] as regards cough, pain, conscious [illegible], and discomfort. It is this effect, being a very striking one, that has given rise, even among careful observers, to the idea that an acute attack of insanity benefits the phthisis. Guislain even thought that there was an "antagonism" sometimes between the two, and Griesinger says that "even the nutrition slightly improves in certain cases on the outbreak of the mental disease." Our experience is that the facts that seem to point in this direction are fallacies. If we take the three tests of careful physical examination of the patient's lungs, his evening temperature, and his body weight, we have never known any phthisical case really improve on the outbreak of insanity. No doubt, if the mental attack is one of maniacal exaltation, the patient will entirely cease to complain of any symptom of his chest disease; he will say he is cured, he will take exercise, and run and leap, he will no doubt eat more food, but he will lose in weight, and his lungs will not heal. That there may be a tendency to a temporary arrest of the morbid process in the lungs, we are not prepared absolutely to deny. Nature often seems unable to carry on two active pathological processes in different organs simultaneously in their full activity.

It is certain that the tubercular deposition is often very localised at first in the lungs of the insane, that it is lobular, and that it is at first often very difficult of detection by auscultation. The absence of wearing cough, of pain, of any subjective sense of illness must save the patient from the exhaustion which those symptoms cause. In addition to the signs that can be got by examination of the chest, we trust for the early detection of the disease in many cases also to the facial expression of the patients, to their losing weight, to their diminished appetite, to observing little clearings of the throat as a baby does, and to small rises of the evening temperature.

We do not think there is any special variety of phthisis that prevails among the insane. The "fibroid" variety is certainly rare. Though many insane patients live for many years after they have become phthisical, yet we believe the duration of the disease from its commencement till the death of the patient is much less on the average among the demented class when it is distinctly secondary to the insanity than among the sane. Such patients go down very fast at the last. We have seen many of them walking out and uncomplainingly at work in the garden one week and die the next without any acute inflammatory attack at the end.

The low innervation of the lungs in such cases is seen in an extreme degree when gangrene of the lungs takes place at the last, though this is more common in the cases of melancholia with refusal of food, where the phthisis is not a sequel to the insanity, but almost contemporaneous with it in first appearance.

As to the effect of phthisis on the mental disease we have more evidence. Griesinger said in 1845:* "It has not been proved that the insanity which is accompanied by or developed from tuberculosis presents any peculiar character." In this opinion he was, we are convinced, quite wrong, acute clinical observer though he was.

The observations of some of the older authors were more correct. They had distinct inklings of the true facts of the case. When Laycock ascribed to this insanity "a certain capriciousness, a whimsical fluctuation between extremes," and when Neumann noted "self-absorption, great irritability and morosity, and tendency to swear," when Morel† directed the attention of physicians in charge of phthisical patients to the "nervous states complicated with depression, morosity, and eccentricities of character" they were likely to meet with, it is clear that many of the clinical facts of "phthisical insanity" had been observed before it was segregated as a distinct form of mental disease, or got a name.

Many years' careful study of this subject, from a clinical point of view, have led us to the conclusion that there are two entirely distinct ways in which the mental disturbances stand related to phthisis. The one is where the insanity has arisen at first quite independently of any phthisical cause or relationship, and run an ordinary course usually into dementia or chronic melancholia, and then after many years the patients fall into phthisis and die of it.

In such cases physiological and pathological considerations relating to the general solidarity of brain function, and the way in which the trophic energising tends to become lowered with the lowering of the rest of the brain functions, especially with the mental—all point to the insanity as a direct causative influence. One fact is very suggestive—in dementia we found the average temperature to be lower than in any other form of insanity—viz., 96.98,‡ and most of the

* *Op. cit.* p. 193.

† "Traité des Maladies Mentales," Morel.

‡ *Journal of Mental Science*, 1868, "Observations on the Temperature of the Body in the Insane."

chronic cases of insanity who die of phthisis are, as we have seen, laments. In this class of cases the phthisis, when it comes on, has commonly the following effect. In the early stage the patients are more demented, more sluggish, have less inclination for food, and tend to become more dirty in habits, and less inclined or able to employ themselves. In fact the mental symptoms of their dementia become aggravated. Then when the temperature begins to rise, such patients will often waken up somewhat. They will become more talkative, even more reasonable, much more irritable, more suspicious, and in a few cases just before death, will seem to become intelligent and sane. All this more active mental energising seems to be due to the higher temperature of the brain, and to the effects of more blood circulating through it. We have no doubt that it was these mental symptoms—simulating improvement as they do—that led some of the older authors to attribute a really curative effect on the insanity to the lung disease in some cases. The amount of intelligence that some patients, apparently for years "demented," will thus exhibit under the influence of the elevated temperature of phthisis, would suggest that there had been no great cell atrophy and no extensive degenerative changes in the cells of the cortex, but rather a trophic lowering and an asthenic energising, which had caused the mental symptoms of the dementia. It may be the dementia in such cases is more allied to stupor than true secondary dementia.

Another suggestive fact is that in asylums cases of epilepsy with insanity die of phthisis in a proportion greater than most other forms of insanity. Van der Kolk attributed this to the direct influence of the pneumogastric nerve whose centres are in the medulla, and which he believed to be specially affected in epilepsy, the pathological seat of which he placed there. We think a far more reasonable hypothesis as to the cause of the frequency of phthisis in old epileptics and congenital epileptics is that the disease causes a deep form of dementia, in which the general trophic condition is lowered, and that after each fit we have congestion of the lungs from impeded respiration, one effect of this being that the lungs become a more ready seat of the tubercle bacillus. The most complete forms of secondary dementia that exist are those occurring in the cases of adolescent insanity that do not recover, and in epileptic insanity. Both yield phthisis in the highest degree.

The other way in which the two diseases are related is much the more interesting, and by far the most important. It is where they arise either simultaneously, or within a year or two or three of each other, when there is usually a heredity to phthisis or to innutrition as well as to insanity, or to some of the graver neuroses, and when, above all, there is a series of mental symptoms present that constitutes, in our opinion, a distinct clinical form of insanity, to which we gave the name of "Phthisical Insanity" in 1863. In such cases the ætiology of the mental disease, and its clinical characters, its duration, and its termination, are all connected with the accompanying phthisis or the tubercular diathesis of the patient. The best of the most recent authors on mental diseases, Spitzka in America, Ball in France, Krafft-Ebing in Germany, and Maudsley, Blandford, Bucknill and Tuke, and Savage in this country, all recognise phthisical insanity as a true clinical variety of the disease. Ball, after quoting our general description of the disease, says "that description is without doubt exact in a great number of cases."* Savage sums up his chapter on the subject in these words: "Phthisis in the insane is associated with certain groups of symptoms characterised by suspicion and refusal of food on the one hand, and with masking of the phthisical symptoms on the other."†

Before describing the special features of this form of insanity, it is necessary to say that there is a certain general likeness of some of the symptoms in every kind of insanity that is accompanied or caused by an anæmic brain. We all know that where we have, for instance, an attack of simple melancholia resulting from slow starvation, the first symptom is usually morbid suspicion. So with another essentially anæmic insanity, that of over-lactation. Now, as we shall see, morbid suspicions form one of the marked symptoms of phthisical insanity. But in that disease we have something far more than that one symptom. We have a group of symptoms, mental and bodily, in a certain sequence, and the whole case standing out clinically as following a certain course. No descriptive picture of any disease can, however, apply to all the cases. Nature does not so uniform herself. We therefore cannot differ from Ball when he says that our clinical picture of a typical case does not absolutely cover the whole ground. Our sub-

* "Leçons sur les Maladies Mentales," par B. Ball.

† "Insanity," by George H. Savage, M.D.

sequent clinical experience of twenty-six years, tends strongly to confirm our original conclusion in 1863 that phthisical insanity differs from the ordinary anæmic or diathetic insanity. It does not arise in asylums from their hygienic defects. It arises commonly from a combined heredity towards insanity and phthisis, or when heredity insanity arises in a subject whose trophic energy is low. It is met with, not in the cases where long-continued insanity or the bad conditions of life in asylums could have produced it, but in the newly occurring cases. It is capable of diagnosis at once, or within the first year commonly.

The general characters of phthisical insanity are such as might be expected to be found in persons of weak vitality. If classified from the mental symptoms alone, some of the cases would be called mania, of the asthenic mildly delusional type, more of them monomania of suspicion or unseen agency, and some of them melancholia, also of the mildly delusional kind. A few of them have an element of mental stupor, and the wrongly named acute dementia. It is a remarkable fact that most cases of monomania of suspicion sooner or later die of phthisis. The symptoms of a morbid mental suspicion run through nearly all the cases of phthisical insanity. Sometimes, but not commonly, they have an acute stage at first, but this is short and not very intense. Most frequently the disease begins by a gradual alteration of disposition, conduct, and feeling in the direction of morbid suspicion, of irritability, of moroseness, and of unsociability. The social instincts and the keen enjoyments that arise therefrom are lessened in intensity or gone. There is often a morbid fickleness of purpose, a want of buoyancy and enjoyment of life, a depression of spirits, and sometimes senseless, and to the patient himself causeless, and unaccountable dislikes. Sometimes there is a lassitude and utter incapacity for exertion. There is in young women a waywardness and perversion of feeling that simulates hysterics. Often in bad cases there are delusions as to the food being poisoned. With these symptoms of lowered brain vitality and force, there are in some of the cases fitful gleams of high spirits, of happiness, and spurts of unsustained energy. Both the low unsocial and the high energetic phases are apt to be accompanied by an intellectual condition, characterised by want of sustained reasoning, by a changeable volitional state, and by a lack of common sense in the conduct of life.

The early bodily symptoms are commonly a loss of weight, a diminished appetite, a pigmented dirty-looking skin, indigestion, often perverted taste in regard to food, which no doubt suggests the delusions of poisoning. There is sleeplessness, incapacity for continued muscular exertion of all sorts. The temperature is low, the extremities especially cold. Commonly there are no pulmonary symptoms detectable at this early stage.

The next stage is one of actual maniacal excitement or melancholic depression, or openly expressed insane suspicion, or some act of mild violence. If the patient is melancholic, the symptom specially noticed by Savage—viz., refusal of food—is very common. Sometimes, on the contrary, if maniacal, the extra muscular exertion improves the appetite, and makes the patient look better. In this stage asylum treatment becomes necessary, and the phthisical insane are especially apt to resent this and to denounce their friends for having placed them in asylums. But up to this time many of the cases are curable, and proper treatment, of the hygienic, dietetic and open-air kind, is frequently followed by at least temporary recovery. If our studies and conclusions in regard to phthisical insanity have done nothing else, they have made us give patients in the state we have described the benefit of much milk, many eggs, cod-liver oil and maltine, the hypophosphites, quinine, extra warm clothing, an extra amount of fresh air, the airiest bedrooms, hospital treatment generally, and all the mental and moral influences that can be brought to bear on him for the diversion of his mind from his suspicions into healthy channels, our own mind being hopeful of cure from our experience of other cases. If chest symptoms have actually appeared, the usual local treatment is required in addition. The result of such treatment at this early stage is that over 30 per cent. of the cases may recover at least for a time: and this percentage is an increasing one, as such cases are diagnosed early. Both the morbid mental condition and the phthisis are in some cases recovered from, the patient gains weight, becomes cheerful and sociable again, and gets rid of his suspicions.

But in the cases who do not recover, all the symptoms we have described persist, except that the initial maniacal excitement or melancholic refusal of food passes off, and the patient has a period of months or years during which he is a typical phthisical mental case. He makes no friends in the asylum, he is moody, discontented, suspicious, commonly, though not always, idle, with a capricious appetite. He has slight spurts of maniacal excitement, or sometimes periods of stupor. His brain behaves like a lamp ill-supplied with oil, giving a fitful light. If you examine the chest during this time, you find either no active lung symptoms at all, or only evidence of slight and non-progressive lesions.

In the cases where this state lasts for several years, the patient, when the disease has not assumed the form of monomania of suspicion, gets partially demented, but is not so enfeebled in mind as he looks. The state of utter mindlessness seen in typical secondary dementia following adolescent insanity does not commonly supervene. The patients can be roused into wonderful exhibitions of intelligence for short periods. The adolescent cases are most apt to exhibit the deepest dementia: the cases over thirty commonly tend to monomania of suspicion.

In the majority of the cases of phthisical insanity we have distinct physical signs of phthisis within two years after the mental symptoms have appeared. There can be no doubt that in by far the majority of the cases the insanity precedes the detectable signs of lung disease. But that the "pre-tubercular stage of phthisis" is as real a part of the disease in some cases as the tubercular, few physicians of experience can doubt. The trophic failure that leads to the formation of the right nidus, without which the tubercle bacillus would be perfectly harmless, must be held to be as important a stage in the disease as the local lung destruction. In a few cases five years elapsed between our diagnosis of "phthisical insanity" and the appearance of the symptoms of tuberculisation. In about 5 per cent. of those who died of consumption in the Royal Edinburgh Asylum, the lung affection distinctly preceded the mental symptoms, for it was diagnosed on admission. In a few of those cases the insanity consisted of a transitory delirium that soon passed off.

We know no better proof that the mental symptoms in insanity may be influenced by lung tuberculosis than the fact which we ascertained statistically, that general paralysis, so commonly characterised by morbid exaltation, delusions of grandeur, ambitious delirium, happy facility, and an exaggerated sense of *bien être*, is apt to be attended by melancholic symptoms, morbid fears, and refusal of food, when its subjects also suffer from pulmonary consumption. We found that in most of the 27 general paralytics, whose lungs were found tubercular out of 92 in all, the mental symptoms had begun by depression, or had been those of depression throughout. The few suicidal general paralytics were nearly all tubercular. We have repeatedly been led to suspect lung disease in our general paralytic patients, when we found them beginning to be melancholic, or stuporous, and to refuse food, and we have often had our suspicions confirmed by an examination of their lungs, and by finding phthisis, bronchitis, or pneumonia.

In order to rest this connection of insanity and phthisis on a statistical basis, so far as this is possible, we have gone carefully through the case-books of the Royal Edinburgh Asylum for the past fourteen years—1874 to 1888 inclusive. There have been 1031 deaths in that time, of which 140 were from phthisis. This is a percentage of 13.6, or one in seven deaths. During these fourteen years, out of the 4891 admissions, 134 were diagnosed within the first twelve months of residence as being cases of "phthisical insanity" in the case-books. This is a proportion of 2.7 per cent., or one in every thirty-seven patients. It was by no means those 134 phthisically insane patients, however, who furnished the majority of the 140 who died of phthisis. They only furnished 30 of the 140, or about 21.5 per cent. of the mortality for that disease. Of the 134 phthisically insane, there have, up to this time, died 22.4 per cent. of phthisis. But 49 of the 134 have been removed from the asylum, some of them in the last stages of phthisis to die at home, or by transfer to other asylums, so that it would be a more correct statement to say that of those diagnosed as phthisically insane, and whose cases could be followed up to this time, 35.3 per cent. have died of phthisis.

One of the most interesting facts revealed by these statistics is this, that out of the 134 there have been 44 recoveries from their mental disease, and some of them also from these lung symptoms, or a percentage of 33. We certainly did not anticipate in 1862 that such a proportion of recoveries was possible in this clinical variety of insanity. In fact, one of our conclusions from our then data was that it was very incurable. But we had not then had a very long clinical experience, and our conclusions on the whole subject had largely to be formed from the descriptions of the mental condition of those patients who had died of phthisis, as we found them in the asylum case-books, for phthisical insanity had not been known or thought of till then. The hygienic state of the older asylums, too, was not so good as it is now. Nor was the dietary, or clothing, or exercise in the fresh air at all as they are at present. The fact that we now think we can diagnose phthisical insanity in its early stage before the actual lung disease has appeared, or while it is incipient, makes us take energetic therapeutic means to combat the disease by special treatment, medical, dietetic, and general. We find the percentage of recoveries is rising under such means of treatment, though the numbers we diagnose as labouring under the disease are about the same from year to year. A percentage of 33 of recoveries is a very low one for recent uncomplicated cases of insanity. Excluding all cases of organic brain disease, senile insanity, and cases over twelve months insane, the recovery rate has been at least 70 per cent. The cases diagnosed as phthisical insanity recover, therefore, in less than half the proportion of recent insanity uncomplicated with brain disease.

But we do not for a moment say that in some of the 44 who recovered, or of the 49 who were removed from the asylum unrecovered, or of the 11 yet in the asylum, or of those who died of other diseases, we did not make a mistake in diagnosis, calling cases "phthisical insanity" which were really not so. It cannot yet be claimed that it is so entirely distinct that it is not liable to be confounded with insanity (non-phthisical) accompanied by anæmia or caused by syphilis or alcohol, or with ordinary idiopathic hereditary delusional insanity.

We found that, statistically, morbid suspicion was the most frequent mental symptom in all those who died tubercular. It existed in 43 per cent. of 282 who died of phthisis. A suicidal tendency we find to be more common among the tubercular than among the ordinary inmates of the asylum, having been present in 21 per cent. of them. Melancholia and monomania of suspicion existed in undue proportion among those who afterwards became phthisical. The very deeply melancholic cases that had refused food and had to be fed, died of phthisis more frequently than almost any other class, some of them having been phthisical before the onset of the insanity, and in some the lung disease was secondary. It was in such cases that gangrene of the lung was sometimes associated with phthisis. Hallucinations of the senses existed in 20 per cent. of the cases, the order of frequency being of hearing, of sight, and of smell. In our 1063 cases the ordinary symptoms of lung disease were latent in about 30 per cent. of those whose lungs were found tubercular after death, but this proportion is not so great now since we make a more careful physical examination of our patients on admission, weigh them at regular intervals, and use the thermometer in every case night and morning after admission. It is one of the many important uses of the thermometer among the insane, that its valuable indications do not depend in any way on dulled reflexes or sensibility, or want of attention, or lack of power on the patient's part to tell of subjective symptoms. Latency is most seen in general paralysis. It is surprising how slight is the apparent effect of even advanced phthisis on some of the insane. They go about, do work, take food, make no complaint, and even look fairly well with advanced tubercular deposition—large cavities and enormous disorganisation in their lungs. Sudden terminations are not uncommon. A man who had only been failing in strength and appetite for a few weeks and in whom the physical signs of phthisis had been discovered, sat down to dinner as usual, took his food, and died suddenly of syncope immediately afterwards. His lungs were found riddled with tubercular cavities. Though tubercular ulceration of the intestines is very common in the phthisical insane, yet diarrhœa is not so common or so troublesome as in ordinary phthisical patients.

We shall only cite two typical examples of the disease, showing its clinical features. The first is one occurring at adolescence, and was more acute and rapid in its course than the average case.

H. S., aged 20, a map-colourer, of ordinary education, cheerful disposition, steady and industrious habits. She had been subject to "fainting fits," but otherwise had been in good health. She had been engaged to be married to a respectable young man, but shortly before the commencement of her illness—or rather, perhaps, at the commencement of her illness—she began to entertain fears that he was not a Christian, and she came to the conclusion that in those circumstances it was her duty to postpone her marriage. She then became melancholy, took a gloomy view of everything, and proposed going as a missionary to the Indians. She then began to fancy her food was poisoned, became irritable and dangerous to her relations when in a passion. She was sleepless, and her appetite was diminished, and she was sent to the asylum.

On admission, she was excited, her eyes were very bright, her countenance animated and expressive; she talked freely; she did not express much surprise or astonishment at finding herself in an asylum. She evidently, though apparently pretty rational, did not appreciate her position. She had dark hair, beautiful dark eyes, and delicate, refined features. Phthisical symptoms and physical signs were well marked.

At first she became very melancholy at her catamenial periods, but under the influences of fresh air, good food, and quiet, she became apparently well, and was removed from the asylum. Her phthisical symptoms abated also. But in a very short time she was brought back to the asylum with all her symptoms aggravated. She was more suspicious, and more incoherent when excited. She was very listless and weak, suffered from cough, night sweats, expectoration, and pain, when free from excitement. But when she became excited she got out of bed, dressed herself, walked about the ward, never coughed, never spat, talked almost constantly, imagined herself a person of importance, or hinted her suspicions in a vague way to those about her. Her pulse was quicker when excited, however, than when free from excitement. Those attacks came on irregularly till, in six months, she died. Her appetite was better during her excitement, but she did not sleep then. When free from excitement she sometimes was quite rational but listless, and was so before she died. Both lungs were completely disorganised.

The following is a good example of the disease developing in a man of middle life. E. M., aged 37. Admitted to asylum March 1886, and died December 1888 of phthisis pulmonalis. He was of a quiet, reserved, and somewhat suspicious disposition. His habits were steady and hard-working. He was a "rubber worker," a healthy trade, at all events as regards tubercular complaints.

Heredity—a half sister (same mother) who was insane and recovered, and more insanity than this is supposed to be in his mother's family. For two years before admission to asylum he had exhibited morbid suspicions and jealousy of his wife, and was generally suspicious about trifles. His general suspicions became gradually organised into delusions that his food was poisoned, and that his wife introduced men into the house at night. He would put his food into the fire, and would go out and dine off a crust. He fancied bloodhounds were sent after him. He would not take off his clothes at night, and behaved altogether strangely. Next he began to have hallucinations of hearing, and imagined his life was in danger. He fancied his child, ten months old, was "reading his thoughts," and in consequence sharpened a razor to murder it. He got more and more unsocial too. For ten months before admission he had been quite insane.

About the time his morbid suspicions first arose two years ago his chest "got weak," and he was advised to take cod-liver oil, which he did at times, always carrying the bottle in his pocket in case any poison should be put into it.

On admission he was suppressedly excited and somewhat exalted instead of being depressed as formerly. He had some difficulty in restraining his desire to smash things. He was quite coherent, and his memory good. He complained of paræsthesia such as a peculiar "creepy" sensation up one side of head, with an oppression at the top. His right apex was consolidated, and in the left apex there were moist sounds. T. 98.4, weight 8 stone, pulse 117, weak.

He was placed in our hospital ward, put on extra milk and eggs, malt liquors, hypophosphates and cod-liver oil.

His being placed here seemed to have the effect at first of strengthening his inhibitory power, so that his conduct and speech for two months were almost those of a sane man. He was unsocial, and admitted he heard voices, but seemed to agree with one when he was told they were "in his head" and not real. His bodily health improved a little, and he put on a few pounds more of flesh. But he had cough, expectoration, and hæmoptysis. He got apparently so well that we let him go home on pass. But it turned out that we were wrong in doing so, for he said afterwards, that when out he was tempted to throw himself into the canal.

Then his old suspicions returned. He would trust no one. He would ask day by day to get home, and could not see that he could not work to support his family. He would not read or talk with any one. Kindnesses to himself and to his wife were not appreciated. He became gradually more irritable and more delusional, fancying his wife and family were here. He was very suspicious of the medical officers, fancying they kept him here for some occult purpose which he could not state. He wanted to be sent from one ward to another on account of his suspicions of the attendants, but was never contented in any place. After a year and a half he was more insane, and showed some signs of mental enfeeblement tinctured with suspicions. His lungs gradually got worse. He had several severe attacks of hæmoptysis, and he died very anæmic and exhausted. His mental state did not improve before death. He had no hectic, and his temperature did not rise very much.

His brain after death was found to have a small spot of limited softening on the tip of the left occipital lobe, there were four bony spicules projecting into the dura mater from inner table of skull-caps; over first frontal convolution. The brain substance was otherwise normal in appearance. There were cavities, purulent infiltrations, and tubercular depositions in both lungs. The liver, kidneys, and pancreas were waxy.

Pathology.—Strictly speaking, phthisical insanity cannot as yet be definitely connected with any pathological change demonstrable after death in the brain. Deposition of tubercle in the organ is very rare indeed in the insane. We found it in only eight cases out of 282 who were tubercular. But there was one morbid appearance in so many of the cases, that one cannot but connect it in some way with the mental symptoms during life. This was a general and great anæmia of the grey matter of the convolutions with more or less of atrophy, with a great pallor of the white substance, and a distinct tendency to loss of consistence in most parts, and limited areas of congestion. The loss of consistence was especially marked in the fornix and its neighbourhood, being sometimes diffluent at that part. Louis noticed this softening of the fornix in many of his cases of phthisis who *were not* insane, and he associates the lesion with the tuberculosis. The specific gravity of the grey matter Skae found to be considerably below the mean in those who had died of phthisis.

The whole condition of the brain gives the impression of an ill-nourished organ. As yet we know nothing for certain of the direct influence on the mental functions of the brain of the myriads of specific bacilli that must circulate in the blood in the various infective diseases, or of the poisons which the bacteria either create, or in which they find a nidus, but we do know that the delirium is different as in different fevers, being low and "muttering" in one, fierce and noisy in another, gently chattering in another; this difference in character not being accounted for by differences of temperature. We know, too, that most men may take a catarrh, and have a temperature of 104°, without much risk of "wandering" at night, while few patients go through an attack of typhoid without more or less delirium, or mental confusion, though the temperature may never rise much above 100°. So in phthisis pulmonalis we have the unknown effect of the tubercle bacillus and its ptomaines circulating in the brain to account for the spes phthisica, or the suspiciousness, or the moroseness exhibited by various phthisical patients.

Many acute observers, Dr. Maudsley amongst them, think that there is not only a phthisical insanity, but a morbid psychology of phthisis in many cases apart from technical insanity, and apart from the *spes phthisica*. Persons of a strongly tubercular diathesis and with a consumption heredity, have been observed in too many cases to be a mere coincidence to exhibit an irregular mental brilliancy without balance, a fancifulness, a causeless changing from hope to despondency, an incapacity for continued mental exertion, a causeless suspiciousness at times, that we cannot but connect with the influence of weak respiratory organs on the brain. And if careful inquiry is made of those who have been their constant attendants during their last illness, and have observed the mental condition of two or three consumptive relatives, they will often tell you of the whimsical notions, the mental unrest, the vivid fancies, almost amounting to delusions, that they have noticed. It stands to physiological reason, that, as consumption is often essentially a disease of innutrition, the brain cortex should suffer like the rest of the body, at all events in some cases. T. S. Clouston.

PHTHISIOPHOBIE (Fr.). A morbid dread of phthisis.

PHYGANTHROPIA (φυγή, flight; ἄνθρωπος, a man). Misanthropia.

PHYSIOGNOMY OF THE INSANE.—The article on the Expression of the Face (p. 482), by Dr. Warner, and the description of the facial expression and gestures in melancholia, &c., under the head of various forms of idiocy and insanity will afford the reader a large amount of information. In this connection should be also read the article by Dr. Crochley Clapham, on the size and shape of the head (p. 574).

The reader of Lavater's "Physiognomy" finds him advising those who would study this art to begin with the insane. It has been pointed out, however, by Dr. Bucknill,* that "to commence the study of physiognomy in a lunatic asylum, would be not less impracticable than to study physiology in the first instance by means of pathology. It would have been as irrational to expect that the functions of the lungs could be discovered by the inspection of a piece of hepatised pulmonary tissue, as that the signs of natural expression could be determined solely by the observation of that which is strange

* "Manual of Psychological Medicine," 4th edit. p. 420.

and unnatural. It would seem, that in all the departments of investigation, it is right to commence with the study of that which is most normal, simple, and regular; and from thence to proceed with inquiries respecting that which is unusual and irregular." Hence it is justly affirmed "that no one can become proficient in the recognition of the facial expression of the various forms of insanity, who has not acquired a considerable amount of physiognomical tact by his intercourse with the sane portion of mankind." In this study, the reader will find in addition to the great work of the founder of the science, two treatises of the utmost value — Pierre Gratiolet's remarkable publication "De la Physionomie et des Mouvements d'Expression," and Charles Darwin's "Expression of the Emotions." The much earlier work of Sir Charles Bell, "The Anatomy and Philosophy of Expression as connected with the Fine Arts," must be studied. Sir Alexander Morison published in the year 1826 a work which contained several striking illustrations of the insane. Recently, Dr. Byron Bramwell has in his "Atlas of Clinical Medicine," reproduced some of these, and given others which are beautifully executed.

Portraits of patients labouring under various forms of mental defect and disorder will be found in the Frontispiece (Plate I.) viz.:—

Fig. 1.—Acute mania; female patient in the St. Hans Hospital near Copenhagen, photographed by Dr. Pontoppidan.

Fig. 2.—Chronic mania, with exalted ideas; believes herself to be Princess Beatrice. Photograph of a female patient taken by Dr. Walter P. Turner, at that time Assistant Medical Officer, Kent County Asylum (Chartham).

Fig. 3.—Acute melancholia; male patient, Bethlem Hospital. Never speaks.

Fig. 4.—Mental stupor. (Melancholia cum stupore.) Bethlem Hospital.

Fig. 5.—General paralysis. Dementia. Bethlem Hospital. Figs. 3, 4, and 5 were under Dr. Savage's care.

Fig. 6.—Idiocy. Photographed by Dr. Walter P. Turner.

Fig. 7.—Sporadic cretinism. Case reported to the International Medical Congress, 1881, by the writer. The patient, a male, had a girlish appearance, and, it will hardly be credited, was 39 years of age when photographed.

In the plate which accompanies this article (Pl. II.) the physiognomical expressions are of the most marked character, and illustrate cases of erotomania; delusional insanity (megalomania); apathetic dementia with asymmetry of the forehead, under certain emotional conditions; melancholia with similar asymmetry of the forehead; acute melancholia, with facial asymmetry under emotion; and secondary dementia with asymmetry of the forehead.

Fig. 1, Pl. II.—The patient whose physiognomy is here represented, laboured for many years under the fixed delusion that she was a queen. Her expression and bearing were to the last degree characteristic of exaltation and a sense of her royal dignity. Her dress was studded in front with silver coin to mark her exalted rank. When photographed by the writer, she was delighted with this mark of attention, and exclaimed, "Now photograph my back!"

Fig. 2, Pl. II.—Represents the face of a patient formerly in the Norfolk County Asylum under the care of Dr. Hills. She developed a large head and moustache. Her case was one of sexual perversion. It is referred to at page 129 of this work.

Dr. John Turner (Essex County Asylum) has photographed the faces of a number of patients in the asylum in which asymmetry of the facial muscles is strikingly shown. He observes, "It is a significant fact that the muscles of the upper part of the face display asymmetrical action much more frequently than do the muscles of the lower part—viz., in the proportion of 3.7 to 1." He adds that he has been impressed, while observing the faces of the female insane, by "the frequency with which the muscles of expression of the lower part of the face are called into play under emotional states which would in the sane result in expression more confined to the muscles of the upper parts, or to paraphrase Warner's remarks, their expressions are more animal-like, less mental. . . . To take the occipito-frontalis, it is the largest and most powerful muscle of the upper part of the face, and although described in the books of anatomy as one muscle, or at most of a right and left half, yet we must further subdivide it into at least an inner and outer division for each side, each of these divisions being capable of contracting by themselves, and frequently doing so. It is important also to note that the inner or median division of the muscle is more concerned in the production of the physical signs of the higher (more idealised) forms of expression, whilst the outer halves when they contract alone, produce no definite form of expression, but give to the face an inane aspect frequently seen in dements. Asymmetry of action is more frequently seen in this muscle (alone or in combination with the corrugator supercilii) than in any other of the muscles of expression." And Dr. Turner thinks that "by carefully studying the symptoms of paralysis of movements, together with the pathological appearances of the brain in suitable cases, we shall ultimately be enabled to identify the site or sites in the cortex, whose integrity is necessary for the proper accomplishment of those physical changes which accompany these emotions, and which are eventually expressed at the periphery in the form of muscle contraction."

Ch. Féré in "Les signes physiques des Hallucinations" endeavours to show that "with the various hallucinations there may be special expressions which may become organically fixed and may thus serve as aids to diagnosis," and that in some cases there are special wrinkles formed about the eyes, the mouth, and nose, in direct relation with the habit of mind induced by chronic hallucination. In at least one case he found that when the hallucinations were on only one side, the wrinkles were also one-sided. Referring to these statements Dr. Turner observes: "It seems to me highly likely that these one-sided wrinkles to which Féré refers have no other relation to the one-sided hallucinations than exists in the fact that whilst disorder of some of the higher centres in one half the brain may produce hallucinations of the senses, it also produces paralysis of certain movements accompanying certain emotional states."*

We are indebted to Dr. Turner for photographs representing the facial characteristics of four patients in the Essex County Asylum, asymmetry being common to all.

Fig. 3, Pl. II.—F.M.L., aged 21, her insanity on admission two years ago was of two years' duration. She was then maniacal for a week or so, but quieted down, and ever since has been in an apathetic condition, gradually drifting into dementia, sitting huddled up with her head bent down, speaking in a whisper and never spontaneously; only moving when urged—fond of chewing bits of paper. With the increase of degenerative brain-changes, asymmetrical conditions appeared first in the face and then in the trunk. These began by slight elevation of the left eyebrow, which was more arched than the right. The elevation became more and more marked, when present, but at no time was it a fixed condition, being only assumed with certain emotional states.

The pupils, which on admission were equal, became unequal, the right being slightly the larger, and now when standing up she droops over on the right side. The asymmetery is described in a note made recently as follows:—She keeps elevating her left eyebrow, which is angular, causing well-marked furrows on the left side of the brow. When she frowns and brings into play the internal portions of the occipito-frontalis and the corrugators, although there is very considerable furrowing of the outer half of the left side of the brow, the right outer half is quite smooth.

Since the foregoing was written she has died of phthisis. There was adhesion of the meninges to the incus on both sides, but very much more on the left, which was decidedly softer than the right, being almost diffluent. Over the pre-frontal lobes, the meninges were thickened in patches, the ventricles were dilated and full of fluid. Lungs extensively infiltrated with tubercle, the left being more disorganised than the right.

Fig. 4.—Annie T., aged 32, admitted in good health and suffering from acutely melancholic symptoms which had appeared within a few weeks of admission. She was restless, resistive, and troublesome; her face wore a mingled expression of perplexity, misery, and fear. She exhibited a most extreme condition of asymmetry, called forth when she was startled, or by a reference to some topic displeasing to her. Sometimes the occipito-frontalis on the right half of her forehead contracts, but when it does so it is as part of a symmetrical associated action in the *voluntary* elevation of both brows. The asymmetry appears to be due to the non-action of the right half of the occipito-frontalis, whilst at the same time the left half and both corrugators are acting. The paralysis of the occipito-frontalis on the right side allows the unantagonised corrugator of the same side to pull down the skin on this side more forcibly, it being in

* It will no doubt be objected to the importance attached to facial asymmetry, that a great many sane people present the same physiognomical signs. On this point Dr. Turner observes: "We must not expect asymmetry of expression to be peculiar to insanity, inequality in the size of the pupils occurs comparatively frequently in others than the inmates of asylums, and I have met with many and marked instances of asymmetry in the lines produced by the contraction of the muscles of expression; but although I have no tabulated results as to these cases, I am certain that they are more frequently to be met with in nervous, excitable people, in whom an unstable condition of the higher nervous centres exists. I have seen good instances in those who come to visit their insane relations here [Brentwood]; in hysterical girls, religious fanatics, and rarely, if ever, in robust, healthy individuals" (*Journ. Ment. Sci.*, Jan. 1892).

a more or less flaccid state; the result of this is to produce the furrows running upwards from the inner end from the right eyebrow, and across the middle line where they coalesce with the transverse furrows formed by the action of the left occipito-frontalis. This woman, after a little while, lost most of her active symptoms, became silent and mulish, her face grew fat and expressionless; she developed two forms of asymmetry, one caused by contraction of the outer half of the right occipito-frontalis, and both corrugators; this expression was easily evoked if her attention was drawn to unexpected sounds on her right side; but when so startled from the left, her forehead sometimes assumed the expression here figured. This latter condition was now more difficult to evoke, and much more rarely seen than the former.

Fig. 5.—Female patient who had delusion that her child was dead. Whenever reference was made to the subject her face assumed the expression seen in the figure. At times she complained of great pain on pressure of the abdomen. Her left leg was swollen, œdematous and painful, and if the abdomen was pressed or her leg touched, her face assumed exactly the same expression as that caused by allusion to her child. It began by elevation and retraction of the left nostril and left half of the upper lip, causing a deep naso-labial fold to appear on this side; it then gradually spread to the other muscles.

Fig. 6.—Face of female patient showing strong contraction mainly of the outer half of the right occipito-frontalis; neither corrugator is acting. She is in a state of secondary dementia, her insanity being of very many years standing. She is intensely silly, gives and makes foolish and irrelevant answers when spoken to; she can only be usefully employed in carrying articles, and for this simple duty requires considerable personal supervision. If left to herself she will sit unoccupied all day with her right eyebrow elevated more than an inch. This condition gives a stupid look to her face, it assimilates to no recognised form of expression, is not intensified with any emotional states; indeed, if her attention is attracted in any way it generally disappears.

Dr. Turner observes: "That the highest nerve-centres represent movements and not muscles is brought forcibly to our minds in observing these asymmetrical appearances. In any of these cases when the muscles on one side show evidence of weakness when contracting under the influence of certain emotions, or perhaps are incapable of contracting at all, it is only necessary to ask the patient to *voluntarily* frown or elevate the brows as the case may be, to see that all evidence of one-sided weakness disappears altogether; both sides will now contract with equal force." *

To complete this brief sketch of the more notable physiognomical indications of mental disease we must mention the marked changes which occur in the face of a patient suffering from myxœdema. Fig. 7 is from a photograph of the Case referred to in the article on this form of insanity (p. 829, l. 17). The illustration is, we can testify, an excellent representation of the features of the original—a patient under Dr. Savage at Bethlem Hospital, to whom we are indebted for the engraving.

FIG. 7. THE EDITOR.

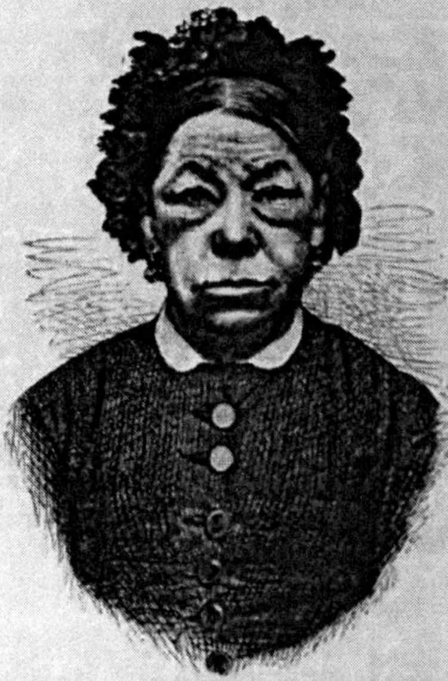

[*References.*—Duchenne (de Boulogne), Mécanisme de la physionomie humaine ou analyse électro-physiologique de l'expression des passions, avec Atlas composé de soixante-quatorze pl. photographiées représentant cent quarante-quatre figures. Dagonet, Maladies mentales, avec huit planches en photoglyptie, représentant trente-trois types d'aliénés, 1876. S. Schack, La physionomie chez l'homme et chez les animaux, 1887. Mantegazza, Physiognomy and Expression, Havelock Ellis's Contemporary Science Series (N.D.).]

PHYSIOLOGICAL PSYCHOLOGY. (*See* MENTAL PHYSIOLOGY.)

PHYSIOLOGICAL TIME.—A name for reaction-time (*q.v.*). The astronomers

* The reader is referred to Dr. Turner's able articles in the *Journal of Mental Science*, Jan. and April, 1892, entitled "Asymmetrical conditions met with in the Faces of the Insane, with some Remarks on the Dissolution of Expression," in which Dr. Turner explains the mechanism of asymmetry.

long ago discovered that impressions on the sense of sight were much more quickly apperceived when they were expected; the interval elapsing between the external stimulus and its apperception was by them called Physiological Time.

PHYSOSTIGMA. (*See* SEDATIVES.)

PICA (the magpie, either from its varied colour or because it was supposed to subsist on mud and earth). A term for depraved appetite with regard to the quality of the food. It is seen commonly in insanity, pregnancy and hysteria, and less commonly in chlorosis. (Fr. *pica*; Ger. *Elster*.)

PIQUEUR. — Term corresponding to the English "Jack the Ripper."

PLAGIOCEPHALIC IDIOCY. (*See* IDIOCY, FORMS OF; IDIOCY, PLAGIOCEPHALIC.)

PLANOMANIA (πλανάομαι, I wander; *μανία*, madness). A morbid tendency to wander away from home and to throw off the restraints of society.

PLATZANGST. Agoraphobia (*q.v.*).

PLEA OF INSANITY. (*See* CRIMINAL CASES, PLEA OF INSANITY IN.)

PLEAD (Capacity of Insane to).— Before a person is actually placed upon his trial, there are some preliminary steps which have to be taken. In the first place, the indictment goes before the grand jury, which, however, has no power to take into consideration the question of the mental condition of the accused, but which is required to say whether it finds a true bill or not, irrespectively of any question of sanity or insanity. In the event of a true bill being found by the grand jury, the accused is then arraigned, and is called upon to plead: and then may arise the question whether he is in a fit state of mind to be placed upon his trial; for as Blackstone* says, "If a man in his sound memory commits a capital offence, and, before arraignment for it he becomes mad, he ought not to be arraigned for it; because he is not able to plead to it with that advice and caution that he ought."

So, too, the Act of 1800,† enacts in the second section, that "if any person indicted for any offence shall be insane, and shall, upon arraignment, be found so to be by a jury lawfully impannelled for that purpose, so that such person cannot be tried upon such indictment, or if upon the trial of any person so indicted such person shall appear to the jury charged with such indictment to be insane, it shall be lawful for the Court . . . . to direct such finding to be recorded, &c."

* "Commentaries of the Laws of England," by Sir William Blackstone, Knt., book iv. ch. ii.

† 39 & 40 Geo. III., c. 94.

But here the question at once arises as to the degree of unsoundness of mind which has to be proved before it can be said that a person cannot be tried; and in order to endeavour to arrive at an answer to that question it may be well to consider a few recent cases, which, for the sake of convenience may be grouped as follows:—

(1) **Simple unopposed cases.**

(2) Cases in which counsel for the defence submits that the accused is **unfit to plead**; whilst counsel for the prosecution maintains **the contrary.**

(3) Cases in which counsel for the prosecution submits that the **accused is insane**, whilst the **accused himself** objects to this, and **insists on pleading.**

(4) Cases in which the **accused is mute** on arraignment.

(1) As an instance of a simple unopposed case the following may be taken. At the Spring Assizes for the County of Cambridge, held in February 1890, before Mr. Justice Denman, Walter Lawrence,* a labourer, aged 36, was charged with the murder of his son, on the 18th of February, 1890. The prisoner, on being arraigned, made no plea, and the learned judge asked whether any one suggested anything as to the man's state of mind, and said that before any evidence could be taken, there must be some suggestion, however informal, to the effect that the prisoner was not capable of taking his trial. The foreman of the grand jury then intimated to his lordship that one of the witnesses (Mr. Kidd) who had given evidence before the grand jury, had stated that he had attended the prisoner for an affection of the brain. The jury was then sworn to try the question whether the accused was capable of taking his trial. The report then goes on to say that his lordship explained to the jury that a man was supposed to be sane until the contrary had been proved. But when it was suggested that his state of mind was such that he was incapable of answering such a question, for instance, as whether he wished to employ counsel, or to object to any juryman, then it was not a case which would be put on trial. It was suggested that there was a doubt about this man's state of mind, and it would be the duty of the jury, after hearing evidence, to say whether they found him capable of being tried or not. Evidence was then given by Mr. Kidd that he had had the prisoner under his care for epilepsy and general cerebral disturbance. He thought the man was incapable of knowing what was taking place, and that

* The *Cambridge Chronicle*, Feb. 28, 1890.

his mental condition put it out of his power to plead; and for this opinion the witness stated his reasons in detail. Witness, being further questioned by his lordship, said, from what he knew of the prisoner, and what he saw of his behaviour that day, he did not think he was capable of distinguishing between a plea of guilty and one of not guilty. Dr. Rogers, the medical superintendent of the Cambridge County Asylum, said that he had had the accused under his charge at the asylum, and had formed a judgment as to his state of mind, and thought it was such that he could not do any of the things his lordship had suggested. Witness thought it would not be fair to try the accused, inasmuch as he would not be able to protect himself in such simple matters as had been mentioned. His lordship remarked that that evidence was conclusive, and he thought the jury would find the accused insane. The jury agreed upon this decision, and his lordship ordered Lawrence to be detained during Her Majesty's pleasure.

In another unopposed case, Nathaniel Curragh, aged 53, was arraigned at the Central Criminal Court, before Mr. Justice Wills, in July 1889, charged with the wilful murder of Charles Thomas Goran, the chief of a troupe of bicyclists, known as the Letine troupe, by stabbing him, at the door of the Canterbury Music Hall.

Mr. Mead, who prosecuted for the Treasury, said that he was informed that the prisoner was undoubtedly insane, and on account of his mental condition quite incompetent to plead to, or understand the nature of, the offence with which he was charged. Dr. Charlton Bastian, who had examined the prisoner upon instructions from the Treasury, was then called, and was examined at length, and gave the opinion that the prisoner was undoubtedly insane, and that he was quite incapable of appreciating the position in which he stood or of pleading to the charge. The jury, upon this, at once returned a verdict that the prisoner was insane and unable to plead, and he was ordered to be detained during Her Majesty's pleasure. In this case the initiative was taken by the counsel for the prosecution; but sometimes, as in the following instance, the initiative is taken by counsel for the defence, no objection being made by the prosecution.

At the Kent Assizes,* held in February 1888, before Mr. Justice Mathew, A. W. Richardson, aged 34, was charged with the wilful murder of Charles Pillow, at Ramsgate, on January 1. Mr. Dering appeared to prosecute; Mr. Murphy, Q.C., and Mr. Poland being for the defence. Mr. Murphy contended that the prisoner was not in a fit state of mind to plead, and a jury was sworn to decide that point. Dr. C. E. Hoar, the medical officer of the Maidstone prison, and Dr. G. H. Savage gave evidence to the effect that the prisoner was insane, and not in a fit state to plead. The jury thereupon decided in accordance with the medical evidence; and the usual order was made for the detention of the prisoner during Her Majesty's pleasure.

With respect to the foregoing cases, it will be seen that Lawrence was stated to be incapable of "knowing what was taking place," or of "distinguishing between a plea of guilty and one of not guilty," or of "answering such a question, for instance, as whether he wished to employ counsel, or to object to any juryman"; and, therefore, in his case, no doubt could be felt, by any one, that he was not capable of taking a rational part in the trial.

In the case of Curragh, the report states that counsel for the prosecution opened the case by telling the jury that he was informed that the prisoner was "undoubtedly insane," and that, on account of his mental condition, he was "quite incompetent to understand the nature of the offence with which he was charged"; and this statement was confirmed by the medical witness called by the prosecution, who expressed the opinion "that the prisoner was undoubtedly insane, and that he was quite incapable of appreciating the position in which he stood, or of pleading to the charge."

In the case of Richardson, the medical witnesses gave evidence to the effect that "the prisoner was insane, and not in a fit state to plead"; and it does not appear that any objection was made to receiving the evidence in that form.

It is unnecessary to multiply examples of unopposed cases; but the following may be given for the purpose of illustrating the effect of delusions as bearing upon the question of capacity to plead. The report is taken from the *Carlisle Express* of January 14, 1882.

William Jones, aged 43, a doctor of medicine, was arraigned at the Carlisle Assizes, before Mr. Baron Pollock, on a charge of having committed criminal assaults on four girls under the age of twelve years, whom he had decoyed into his house by promising to give them Christmas cards. He was labouring under the delusion that he had invented some wonderful medicines, which he called his Alpha and Omega medicines; and Dr. Clouston gave evidence to the effect that the accused

* The *Kent Messenger*, Feb. 18, 1888.

believed that it had been revealed to him that the offspring of a virgin was to transmit his theories, as to his medicines, to posterity; and that, underlying these delusions, there was a condition of morbid exaltation and mental enfeeblement. Mr. Baron Pollock, in charging the jury, said "If the balance of a man's mind was disturbed by some hallucination, or if he believed there was a special and Divine interposition in his favour, for the benefit of the world, by which a male child should be born to him, and that the office of that child in the world should be something special, one could hardly imagine anything that could be more dangerous." His lordship laid stress on the evidence of Dr. Clouston, who said that in spite of the prisoner's position the dominant idea in his mind was the delusion as to his medicines and the benefit they were destined to do to the world.

The jury returned a verdict that the accused was "not capable of defending the case against him," and his lordship made his customary order for detention during Her Majesty's pleasure.

Although this man was unquestionably insane, and was incapable on that account of pleading to the charge "with that advice and caution that he ought," or of "taking a rational part in the trial," yet it could scarcely be said that his mental derangement was such as to render him incapable of knowing when he was in prison, or when he was going to take his trial, or what was taking place in Court.

One more case may be cited for the sake of the terms in which the same learned judge directed the jury.

Thomas Mills, aged 57, was charged at the Ipswich Assizes in May 1884, before Mr. Baron Pollock, with the murder of his wife. He had beaten her to death, with a stake, and then he gave himself up to the police, and said he did not know why he had done it. When about to be arraigned, evidence was given by Dr. Eager, the medical superintendent of the Suffolk County Asylum, to the effect that the prisoner was insane and unfit to plead. Upon this, the learned judge directed the jury that "there was a law that no man could be tried except he was present at his trial; and present, not only in body, but also in mind, in such wise that he could take a rational part in the trial, understand the evidence against him, and do his best to defend himself against such a charge."

The jury returned a verdict to the effect that the prisoner was insane and unfit to plead .

In this case, again, it will be seen that a prisoner may be quite aware of the nature of the act that he has committed, may give himself up to the police for it, and may know quite well when he is in prison and when he is being tried, and yet may be held to be unable, by reason of his mental condition, to "take a rational part in his trial, understand the evidence against him, and do his best to defend himself against such a charge."

(2) Leaving for the present the unopposed cases, and coming to those in which the point, whether the accused is in a fit mental condition to take his trial, is closely contested, the following may be taken as useful examples:—

The first of these is reported in the *Leeds Mercury* of the 17th of February 1888.

William Taylor was indicted at the Yorkshire Winter Assizes, held at Leeds, in February 1888, before Mr. Justice Day, for the wilful murder of his daughter, and also of a police superintendent, at Otley, on the 24th of November, 1887.

The prosecution was conducted by Mr. Hardy and Mr. C. M. Atkinson; and the prisoner was defended by Mr. Waddy, Q.C., and Mr. Kershaw.

Mr. Waddy said that, acting on the advice of several eminent medical witnesses, he would ask his lordship to enable him to put an issue, in the first instance, as to the power of the prisoner to plead. He was prepared with evidence to show that at the present moment the man was insane. The jury having been sworn to decide this issue, Dr. Clifford Allbutt was called, and stated that he had examined the prisoner on the previous Saturday, and also on that (Thursday) morning before the sitting of the Court.

Mr. Waddy then put this question: "And on Saturday was he sane or insane?" But Mr. Hardy, for the prosecution, objected to that question, and his lordship sustained the objection, observing that the condition of the man's mind was a matter for the decision of the jury. Upon Mr. Waddy urging that he was entitled to ask the witness, as an expert, what his opinion was, his lordship said, Certainly not. That was a matter on which he was perfectly clear. Experts were not to be asked their opinion on subjects which it was the function of the jury to decide. He was not laying this ruling down with reference to that particular case, or with reference especially to questions of sanity. He laid it down in all cases in which scientific or expert witnesses could be called to give evidence as to their opinion. Mr. Waddy then said that he proposed to put witnesses into the box for the purpose of showing, from the prisoner's past history, his present state of mind; but his lordship deprecated that course, and said that it might be possible that the prisoner had spent his whole existence in a lunatic asylum, and properly; but the question before them now was whether he was at present a sane man and able to distinguish between a plea of guilty and one of not guilty. He was not going to shut out the evidence, but if proceeded with he considered it would represent so much wasted time. Mr. Waddy then suggested that he might ask Dr. Allbutt whether, from the investigation he had made, he thought the prisoner was, or was not, capable of understanding his position; but his lordship ruled that that was not a proper question at all; and went on to say that it was not for doctors to give verdicts. The witness could describe the prisoner's conversation and his manner, and the jury would decide as to his sanity. He could not allow their functions to be delegated to professional witnesses. Mr. Waddy then asked Dr. Allbutt to simply describe the course of his interviews with the prisoner. In reply, Dr. Allbutt said that when the prisoner was brought to the room, on the Saturday morning, he had the manner and aspect suggestive of an epileptic, looking confused and puzzled. He was vacantly smiling. Witness put a number of questions to him, and among other answers the prisoner gave was that he was born into this world with four endowments, which were health, strength, prosperity, and knowledge, and that these were given him by God. He also said there were two Gods, and that one of them had forced those qualities against him in a manner which he could not adequately explain. He appeared to be weak-minded, confused, and incoherent. Witness thought that, shortly, these were the facts observed at the interview. Counsel for the defence then asked: Had you any conversation with the accused with regard to the facts of the crime alleged against him? To which Dr. Allbutt replied, I had. I asked him, in the first instance, concerning the alleged shooting of his child. He told me that he remembered nothing, and was not prepared to admit that the event had ever happened. Concerning the evidence of the police superintendent, he said that he had no remembrance until one day, while in gaol, he saw an account of the affair in a newspaper. He then thought it must be true, and at that moment he was convinced he had done it. He added that he had a more or less distinct recollection of some one breaking into his house, and of his shooting at the intruder. In answer to further questions, witness went on to say that there was no sign of hypocrisy about the prisoner; that one might, at first, have a suspicion of malingering, but such suspicion was removed by the freedom with which the prisoner spoke. As a result of his interview he came to a certain conviction in his own mind. During the interview he had had with the prisoner that morning he seemed more excited, and his faculties, no doubt, were briaker. In reply to a further question whether, as a matter of medical science, where there is long-continued epilepsy, it affects the mind, witness said, it may, and often does, have that effect.

In cross-examination the witness said it was quite possible that the prisoner might have assumed his peculiar manner, but he did not believe that, in this case, there was any pretence. At that moment the prisoner certainly knew that he was on his trial, and probably he knew that he was being tried for murder. His insanity was more pronounced at one time than at another, and witness's impression was that he had gradually been becoming more lucid, up to the present time. In re-examination, witness said he thought the prisoner was then unfit to give adequate instructions to his solicitor, and that he did not fully appreciate his position and danger. His moods were very variable, sometimes indifferent and sometimes distressed.

Mr. Gladstone, solicitor, then deposed that he had had several interviews with the prisoner, but had been unable to extract any information with respect to his trial. Dr. Ritchie then deposed that he had known the prisoner for more than twenty years, and had attended him for epileptic fits. On the day of the crime he had been called to the prisoner. He would not believe that he had murdered his child and the police superintendent. He said a black cloud came over him, and in that cloud was the Lord Almighty, and whatever he commanded him to do he was bound to do it. He added that his wife had put some stuff in his tea for the purpose of poisoning him, and that she was also trying to poison the infant. Witness had seen the prisoner again that morning, and concurred with the evidence of Dr. Allbutt. In cross-examination, witness said that when he examined the prisoner on the day of the crime he was not then in a fit either of epilepsy or of *petit mal*. From what he had known of him for the last twenty years he thought his mind had now entirely given way. In reply to his lordship, witness said he had not tried to engage the prisoner in general conversation, but, with the exception of a reference to his wife, he had confined the conversation to the subject of his delusions. The Rev. Mr. Brooks gave evidence that he had visited the prisoner in prison about a dozen times and that he had found him subject to delusions the whole time. Prisoner said God had told him he could not kill, and, therefore, it was impossible. Dr. Wright, consulting physician to the West Riding Asylum at Wakefield, agreed with the account given by Dr. Ritchie and Dr. Allbutt as to the prisoner's manner; and he believed there was no feigning or exaggeration on the part of the prisoner. This concluded the evidence in support of the contention that the prisoner was unfit to plead; and then Dr. Clark, the medical officer of Wakefield Prison, Dr. Bevan Lewis the medical superintendent of the West Riding Asylum, and Mr. Edwards, the medical officer of Armley Gaol, were called by the prosecution for the purpose of proving the contrary, namely, that the prisoner was in a fit state of mind to be called upon to plead. Dr. Clark said that whilst prisoner was in the gaol at Wakefield he had enjoyed good health, had slept well, and had exhibited no symptoms that would lead to the supposition that he was insane; and that he answered all questions rationally and intelligently.

By his lordship: "Prisoner knew he was in gaol and that he was about to take his trial."

Dr. Bevan Lewis, in his evidence, stated that he had examined the prisoner on two occasions at Wakefield, and had not observed in him any appearance of insanity. He had conversed with the prisoner on general subjects, and the man talked rationally.

Mr. Edwards agreed, generally, with the two previous witnesses, but he admitted, in cross-examination, that the prisoner had spoken to him of the four endowments, health, strength, knowledge, and prosperity, mentioned by Dr. Allbutt, and that he had lately been incoherent in his manner. The prisoner had asked witness several times if he thought a man in his sane mind could commit such a crime as that with which he was charged. In reply to his lordship, Mr. Edwards said that at Armley Gaol the prisoner had been associated with two other prisoners; and, by the direction of the learned judge, these men were sent for, and one of them deposed that the prisoner did not seem to remember anything about the crime with which he was charged, but that he had said that he thought he should be confined in an asylum, as the result of the trial. Counsel having addressed the jury, for the prosecution, and for the defence, his lordship pointed out what he considered a very singular remark of the prisoner's, with respect to the asylum, which he did not think would be made by an insane man. And then, after a few minutes' consultation, the foreman announced that the jury were unanimously of opinion that the prisoner was sane.

The prisoner was then indicted for the wilful murder of the superintendent of police, and when called to plead, said, "I know nothing about it." The trial then proceeded, and occupied the remainder of that day, as well as the greater portion of the following day; with the ultimate result that the jury found a verdict to the effect that the prisoner was guilty of the murder, but that he was of unsound mind when he committed the act; upon which the usual order was made for his detention as a criminal lunatic.

The fact that the medical witnesses were divided in opinion in the foregoing case may possibly have formed one of the reasons which led the jury to say, by their verdict, on the first day, that, in their opinion, the prisoner was sane, so as to be fit to take his trial; but it would be by no means right to conclude that this was the only reason; as will appear from a consideration of the following case, in which, although the medical officer of the gaol, in which the prisoner had been confined whilst awaiting trial, regarded him as being unfit to plead by reason of his mental condition, and although he was supported in this opinion by the medical superintendent of the County Asylum, who had examined the prisoner upon instructions from the Home Secretary, nevertheless, it was decided otherwise, and the case was tried out; with, however, the ultimate result, in this case also, that the prisoner was declared by the verdict of the jury to have been "insane at the time he committed the act." The case is fully reported in the *Norfolk News* of November 19, 1887: Arthur Edward Gilbert Cooper, aged 34, clerk in holy orders, was indicted for feloniously, wilfully, and of his malice aforethought, killing and murdering the Rev. William Farley, at Cretingham, on October 2, 1887. The case was tried before Mr. Justice Field, now Lord Field, on November 15, 1887, at Norwich. In his charge to the grand jury, on a previous day, his lordship had referred to the case in the following terms: "It is a very sad case. It is one in which a clergyman, the rector of the parish of Cretingham, came by his death undoubtedly, upon the evidence, by the acts of the prisoner, who was his curate. There is no doubt whatever upon the facts. The only question which will arise, when it comes here, will be as to the prisoner's state of mind when he did what it is clear he did. That is a matter with which you need not have to do. It will, of course, be carefully inquired into in the Court below."

On the day when the prisoner was arraigned, he was about being called upon to plead to the indictment, when Mr. Murphy, Q.C., counsel for the prisoner, said that, before the prisoner was called upon to plead, he had certain information before him to which he deemed it imperative upon him to direct the attention of the Court, in order that an inquiry might first be made as to whether or not the prisoner was in a fit state to plead or to conduct his defence.

His lordship: "You deny prisoner's competence to plead?"

Mr. Murphy: "I do."

The jury was then sworn to try whether "the prisoner is of sound mind and understanding, so as to be capable of taking his trial on the charge whereof he stands indicted."

Mr. Murphy then said that it had come to his knowledge that Dr. Eager, a medical man of eminence, instructed by the Home Office, had inquired into the condition of the prisoner during the past month, and that the surgeon of the gaol, under whose charge the prisoner had been, had also formed an opinion on the subject, to which, in justice to the prisoner, an appeal ought to be made before he was put on his trial. The law presumed that all men were responsible for their actions until the contrary had been proved. Still, the law was merciful, for it neither made a man responsible for an act committed when insane, nor did it call upon him to take his trial when, through his state of mind, he would be unable to instruct his advisers to take the necessary steps to present his defence in a proper way. He, therefore, intended to call medical gentlemen who had that morning seen the prisoner, to give their opinion as to the prisoner's condition.

His lordship intimated that the sole question upon which evidence would have to be given was the *present* state of mind of the prisoner.

Mr. George Hetherington, the medical officer of the Ipswich Gaol, was called, and said, "I have had the prisoner under my charge from October 6 until within the last week, when he was removed to Norwich for trial."

His lordship: "Under charge is a general expression. What did he do?"

Mr. Dering (counsel for prisoner): "Was he especially put under your charge?"

Witness: "Yes."

His lordship: "What did you do with him?"

Witness: "My attention was called to him, particularly, because of the nature of his offence. I attended him daily during the time he was in Ipswich prison."

Mr. Dering: "What opinion did you form as to his state of mind?"

His lordship: "We must get at the facts. We can only now inquire as to his *present* state of mind."

Witness: "I examined him this morning. I asked him several questions."

His lordship: "What did you say?"

Witness: "I said, 'Can you recollect what happened that Saturday night?' My conversation was part of that carried on by Dr. Eager, who commenced it."

Dr. Eager was then called into the witness-box. He said: "I am the resident physician and superintendent of the Suffolk County Asylum. I first saw the prisoner on November 1 at Ipswich Gaol, in the Governor's room."

Mr. Murphy: "By whose instruction did you see him?"

Witness: "By the Home Secretary's. I conversed with him about an hour. I next saw him this morning, in the cell at the back of the Court. I spoke to him this morning for two or three minutes."

Mr. Murphy: "What occurred between you and him this morning? I may have to ask you what took place on November 1."

His lordship, interposing: "I think the first course you mention is the proper one. We are trying whether the prisoner is *now* in such a state of mind that he is fit to plead."

Mr. Murphy: "What occurred this morning?"

Witness: "I said, 'Good morning, Cooper.' He said, 'Good morning.' I said, 'How are you this morning?' He hesitated a good deal, and said, 'Pretty well.' I said, 'Have you felt any of the sensations of which you spoke to me when I was at Ipswich?' He said, 'I do not know that I have.'"

His lordship: "Did you say anything more to him?"

Witness: "I don't know that I said anything more. Oh yes, I said, 'Do you know the day of the month?' He replied, 'I do; it is November 15.' I said, 'Do you know the day of the week?' He said, 'It is Tuesday.' I cannot recollect that I said anything else to him."

Mr. Murphy: "Now tell me what occurred on November 1. Have you any notes you made at the time?"

Witness: "No, not here."

His lordship: "After this, do you think it necessary to go on?"

Mr. Murphy: "Oh yes; the impression formed at the previous examination, made on November 1, may be confirmed, in a few minutes, later on, by a look as well as by a question."

Witness: "I was with him for an hour on November 1."

His lordship intimated that he should leave the question to the jury upon facts, not upon opinions, so that it was important to have facts.

Witness: "I sent a report to the Home Office."

Mr. Mayd (counsel for the prosecution): "That report gives no details of any conversation."

His lordship: "In the second paragraph of your report, dated November 2, you say, 'He is now hopelessly insane, and irresponsible for the action.' Will you tell us what are the facts upon which you founded that opinion—that he was hopelessly insane?"

Witness: "From his appearance, which was very vacant. His manner was hesitating and doubtful."

Mr. Murphy: "Was he serious, or otherwise, in his conversation?"

Witness: "He was mostly serious."

Mr. Murphy: "Was he laughing?"

Witness: "At one time he stood up, his expression became fixed, his eyes half closed, and he seemed to be looking into space. He was perfectly unaware, apparently, that I was in the room until I called his attention to myself."

Mr. Murphy: "How did you call his attention?"

Witness: "I said, 'What are you doing?' He suddenly came to himself, jerked his head up, and laughed in a very foolish way."

Mr. Murphy: "Can you tell us any other facts upon which you founded this judgment?"

Witness: "He said, 'I feel that I am influenced by people I cannot see.' I think he volunteered that. I said, 'When do you feel that sensation?' He replied, 'More especially at night. I do not feel alone at night when I awake, but feel that I am surrounded by things in the air. I felt dazed when I got out of bed; I did not know what I was going to do.' During the conversation he said, 'I did not distinctly understand what happened until a few days ago.'"

His lordship: "All this is what we may have to hear by-and-by."

Mr. Murphy: "The issue we are to try is one upon which the prisoner can only have assistance from the people about him in gaol. From his manner and appearance did you form any judgment as to prisoner's condition to-day?"

Witness: "Yes."

His lordship: "What was his appearance this morning?"

Witness: "He was in the same condition."

His lordship: "Did you form any opinion that he is not in a condition fit to understand why he is here to-day, and to follow the evidence, and able from his state of mind to instruct learned counsel?"

Witness: "I think he is able to form a judgment as to why he is here; but I do not think he is able to form any judgment as to instructing his counsel."

"From mental disease, do you mean?"

"Yes."

"From what did you draw that inference?"

"From my own experience and knowledge."

"What are the facts which enabled you to form the opinion that he is not able to do so?"

"I think his mind naturally——"

"I know you think. What are the facts upon which you arrived at that opinion?"

"His hesitating manner; his apparent inability to answer simple questions."

His lordship: "The only question you asked this morning was, how he was."

Mr. Murphy: "Is it consistent with your experience that a man suffering from unsoundness of mind should be able to answer ordinary questions, and conduct himself like a reasonable man?"

Witness: "Quite so."

Mr. Mayd: "Is the prisoner able to understand the difference between a plea of guilty and one of not guilty?"

Witness: "I believe he is."

The foregoing evidence has been given *in extenso* for the purpose of showing more vividly the kind of questions that are likely to be put to a witness in a case of this sort; but considerations of space render it necessary to condense what follows.

Mr. Hetherington was recalled, and, in reply to questions, said: "I believe that, from the condition of his mind, the prisoner is unable to plead. I form that opinion from what I have seen of him in the gaol, and from what I saw of him this morning."

This witness was then examined and cross-examined at length as to his reasons for that opinion; and, ultimately, counsel for the prosecution put these questions:

"In your opinion, is the prisoner able to understand the difference between a plea of guilty and one of not guilty?" To which witness replied, "Yes." And then, "From what you have seen, do you think he is able to give instructions, for his defence, to his counsel?" to which witness replied, "No."

His lordship then, after counsel had addressed the jury, pointed out that the question at issue was whether the prisoner was in a fit state of mind to take his trial. "The law of England," said his lordship, "had not come to the position that a man was not to take his trial merely upon the opinion of some other person, however eminent he might be. The jury had to say whether or not *they* were of opinion that the prisoner was at that moment of such a sound mind as to plead and take his trial."

The jury, after very brief deliberation, found a verdict "that prisoner was able to understand, to plead, and to take his trial."

The clerk of assize then read over the indictment to the prisoner, and asked him if he were guilty or not guilty; to which the prisoner replied, "Not guilty, wilfully."

A fresh jury was then sworn to try the case, and ultimately, after a lengthened trial, the report goes on to say that "the jury consulted for about two minutes, and then returned a verdict that prisoner was insane at the time he committed the act."

His lordship: "You find that he was guilty of killing, but that he was insane so as not to be responsible, according to law, for his actions at the time the act was committed."

The foreman: "We do, my lord."

His lordship: "The prisoner will be detained during Her Majesty's pleasure."

The whole of the evidence which led the jury to this verdict is instructive, but a brief summary will suffice.

Counsel for the prosecution opened the case by stating that in 1878 the prisoner had been under the care of Dr. Harrington Tuke; that he was subsequently sent to Northumberland House Asylum, and afterwards to St. Luke's, where he was treated as a lunatic until September 1882, when he obtained leave of absence, and was ultimately discharged as relieved, but not cured. Since then he had assisted friends in clerical duty.

The evidence showed that he had officiated as Mr. Farley's curate for about a year, when, shortly after midnight on October 2, he rapped at Mr. Farley's bedroom door, and, upon obtaining admission, he walked up to the bed in which Mr. Farley was lying, and cut his throat with a razor, and then left the room.

Mrs. Farley, in giving evidence, stated that neither she nor her husband knew that the prisoner had been in an asylum, but they had noticed that he was very strange.

The parish clerk stated, in his evidence, that in a conversation which he had had with the prisoner directly after the occurrence, he had asked him, "Did you think about it before?" to which prisoner replied, "Yesterday."

Evidence as to the insanity of the prisoner was given by Mr. G. Jones, who was called to the deceased, and who afterwards saw the prisoner; by Dr. Wright, of Northumberland House; by Dr. Mickley, medical superintendent of St. Luke's; by Dr. Wood, physician to St. Luke's; by Dr. Harrington Tuke; and by an uncle of the prisoner, who stated that insanity was hereditary in the family.

In this case, the accused had been an inmate of different asylums for some years, and had then been discharged, not recovered, but only relieved; and, after being apparently at large for some four or five years, he killed his vicar in the manner that has been described. For this offence he was, six weeks afterwards, placed upon his trial; with the result that the jury found, without any hesitation, and without leaving the box, that, at the time he committed the act, he was insane so as not to be responsible. But, on the other hand, when he was arraigned, he was declared by the jury to be competent to plead and to take his trial. The jury had been sworn to try "whether the prisoner is of sound mind and understanding so as to be capable of taking his trial," but, according to the report given by the *Norfolk News*, they would appear to have avoided saying in so many words that he was "of sound mind and understanding," and to have limited themselves to saying "that prisoner was able to understand, to plead, and to take his trial." Both the medical witnesses who were examined at the preliminary inquiry said that, in their opinion, the prisoner was able to understand the difference between a plea of guilty and one of not guilty, and also, that he was capable of knowing that he was on his trial; but they both concurred in saying that, in their opinion, he was not competent to give adequate instructions for his defence to his counsel. If, then, the jury, in saying that the prisoner was able to understand, intended only to say that he was able to understand the difference between a plea of guilty and one of not guilty, they said, on this point, no more than was said by the medical witnesses, and indeed, with reference to this point, the fact that the prisoner, when called upon to plead, replied, "Not guilty wilfully," showed that the opinion as to his ability to understand this difference was well grounded, whilst that he knew the nature of the charge preferred against him may be inferred from the observation made by him to one of the medical witnesses to the effect that he "did not distinctly understand what had happened until a few days ago," implying thereby, that, at the time when he said this, he did understand what had happened. To say, however, that a person is able to understand the difference between a plea of guilty and one of not guilty is, of course, by no means equivalent to saying that such person is of sound mind generally, and yet, supposing for the sake merely of illustration, that the capacity to understand this difference were held to constitute the test of fitness to plead, a person who possessed this capacity might, no doubt, in the purely technical aspect of the case, be looked upon as being of "sound mind and understanding" so far as, but no farther than, that particular matter is concerned.

This use of the formula "sound mind and understanding" is, however, somewhat puzzling to those who are not accustomed to it, and indeed, the necessity for its retention is not very manifest, for if it is the case that the law says that a person is to be called upon to take his trial, although not of sound mind, provided that he is able to understand the difference between a plea of guilty and one of not guilty, or provided that he comes up to a certain standard of coherence, then it would appear that the only question for the jury, at that stage of the inquiry, would be whether the accused did or did not come up to such standard, and it would not appear to be necessary to require the jury, at that stage, to prejudge the wider question of whether the prisoner was or was not of sound mind.

Possibly an argument, in support of the view that persons may be called upon to plead although insane, might be deduced from the wording of the Act of 1883, the 46 & 47 Vict. ch. 38, the first section of which is to the effect that the Act may be cited as the "Trial of Lunatics Act." This might be held to indicate that the Act contemplated that lunatics might be placed upon their trial; but here again a question might arise as to whether this could only be done during a lucid interval, and a further question would be as to what constituted a lucid interval.

The question that was raised in this case, as to whether the prisoner was able to give adequate instructions to his counsel, does not appear to have been definitely answered, unless we may assume that it was answered by the jury saying that he was "able to take his trial." There was no dispute in this case as to the facts; and, indeed, the learned judge had, as we have seen, stated, on a previous day in his charge to the grand jury, that the only question was as to the state of the prisoner's mind; and, in a case of this kind, where it is the object of counsel to prove the insanity of his client, it is evident that counsel must rely far more on the instructions which he receives from others than on those which he receives from the client himself

It must not, however, be overlooked that one risk which is incurred by calling upon a prisoner, whose sanity is in doubt, to plead, even when there is no dispute as to the facts of the offence with which he is charged, is, that he may plead guilty; and if he does that, and if he persists in that plea, after having been declared fit to plead, the further inquiry into his mental condition by the Court would appear to be barred.

In that case it apparently becomes necessary to pass sentence, and then to leave the matter in the hands of the Home Secretary.*

The problem, therefore, in those cases where the facts are admitted, and where the only question is as to the mental condition of the accused, appears to be how to obtain a full and complete investigation into all the circumstances, without incurring such risk as may be involved in calling upon an insane person to plead.

(3) Cases occasionally arise in which, whilst the prosecution submits that the accused is insane, the accused himself objects. A case of this description was tried at the Central Criminal Court in February 1887, before Mr. Baron Pollock. Isaac Jacob Mauerberger, aged 36, a journalist, was charged with sending a threatening letter to Lord Rothschild. Mr. Poland, who appeared for the prosecution, stated that he had received a report from the medical officer of Holloway Gaol to the effect that the prisoner was not in a fit state of mind to plead, and a jury was thereupon impannelled to try that issue.

Mr. Gilbert, the medical officer of Hol-

* See the case of Swatman, p. 961.

loway Gaol, said that in his judgment the prisoner was insane, and not possessed of sufficient understanding to enable him to comprehend the charge or to defend himself. His lordship inquired what form this insanity took, and witness replied that the prisoner was subject to many delusions. Dr. Blandford having given similar evidence, the prisoner said he should cross-examine the medical men minutely as to the grounds upon which they based their opinions. He should prove that he had never been insane, but, on the contrary, was of perfectly sound mind. The jury, however, intimated that they were perfectly satisfied. Mr. Baron Pollock then, after referring to the medical evidence, said he need not tell the jury that according to the law of every civilised country a man could not be tried unless he could understand and appreciate the forms of trial. According to the statute law of this country a man could not be called on to plead unless he was of sound mind. If his intellect was such that he could not understand what was going on in a court of justice, it was the duty of the jury to say whether or not he was of sufficiently sound mind to take his trial. The jury then returned their verdict that the prisoner was not of sufficiently sound mind to take his trial; and the usual order was thereupon made for his detention during Her Majesty's pleasure.

It sometimes happens, however, that in cases where the accused himself objects to being thought unfit to plead by reason of unsoundness of mind, he is successful in maintaining this objection. John Ambrose Douglas was indicted at Maidstone* in July 1885, before Mr. Justice Hawkins, on a charge of shooting, with intent to murder. The accused was defended by Mr. Warburton, who said he apprehended the question would be whether the prisoner was in a fit state of mind to plead; whereupon prisoner exclaimed, "That is all nonsense, there is no better man in the country, and I shall not allow that there is anything wrong with my mind, it is as right as ever it was, and I will not be defended by a liar. I knew perfectly well what I was about." His lordship then asked: "Do you perfectly understand what the nature of the case against you is?" To which the prisoner replied, "Yes, what I am accused of is, I believe, firing, with intent to murder, and I say I did not intend to murder. I fired at him because the man is a thief, and stole my wife's horse"—and much more to the same effect. After further discussion, the case was adjourned to the following day, when it was tried out, with the result that the jury found that the prisoner was guilty of the act, but that he was not, at the time, responsible for his actions—the prisoner exclaiming upon hearing the verdict: "I can't agree with you." The usual order for his detention during Her Majesty's pleasure was then made.

* The *Maidstone and Kent County Standard*, July 17, 1885.

In this case it was at the prisoner's own request and insistence that he was placed upon his trial, although it is very doubtful whether it could be said that he was capable of taking a rational part in the trial, and certainly he was not of sound mind.

The following is a case in which the accused at first pleaded guilty, notwithstanding that there was ground for believing him to be insane. At the Carmarthen Assizes,* held in February 1888, before Mr. Justice Stephen, Henry Jones was arraigned and charged with the murder of his daughter.

The clerk of arraigns then said, "What say you Henry Jones, are you guilty or not guilty?"

Prisoner (weeping): "Guilty, my lord."

The judge: "Prisoner, if you take my advice you will say you are not guilty. You must recollect what you are charged with. Do you mean to say that you knew all about what you were going to do, and that you meant to kill your child?"

Prisoner: "Oh no, my lord, but I did it.

His lordship: "Then you are not guilty you say. He says he did not mean it."

The trial then proceeded, and resulted in a verdict to the effect that the prisoner was insane at the time he committed the act.

Here again is a case, reported in the *Hertfordshire Standard* of the 4th of August, 1888, in which a different course was pursued. Henry Cullum, aged 24, was indicted before Mr. Baron Pollock for the murder of Emily Bignall at Shenley in the month of March. Mr. Forrest Fulton appeared for the defence. The prisoner, on arraignment, pleaded guilty. Mr. Fulton then said that he was instructed to produce certain evidence as to the state of the prisoner's mind, but he had intimated to the solicitor by whom he was instructed that he did not think it right to interfere with the plea that the prisoner had thought fit to make. Mr. Wedderburn, counsel for the prosecution, said there were some medical reports which the judge might like to see. His lordship having had the reports handed up, said: "I think it will be best for me to take the usual course; yet, certainly, any documents

* The *Welshman*, Carmarthen, March 2, 1888.

sent in will be forwarded by me to the Home Office. It would be better to leave it unfettered, for the Home Office to deal with the matter of the state of the prisoner's mind." Mr. Forrest Fulton explained that the reason he had taken the course he had, with regard to the defence, was because it was extremely difficult to ask a jury to come to the conclusion that at the time of the commission of the crime the prisoner did not know the difference between right and wrong. Having regard to the family history of the man it would be for the authorities to consider his state of mind. His lordship then said: "I think the course you have adopted Mr. Fulton is the right one, I think it is better to leave it unfettered in the hands of the Home Office."

Sentence of death was then passed in the usual form. This sentence, however, was not carried out, but the prisoner was subsequently removed to the asylum for criminal lunatics at Broadmoor.

The reason assigned by prisoner's counsel in this case for not interfering with the plea of guilty has been already referred to in considering the answers of the judges to the questions put to them by the House of Lords after the trial of Macnaghten, in 1843.*

It does not appear that any one questioned the fitness of the prisoner to plead to the indictment, although it was evidently regarded as probable that the criminal lunatic asylum would be his ultimate destination. The case was, doubtless, a difficult one; but if difficult cases are thus deliberately left in the hands of the Home Office, this appears to almost amount to an admission that in dealing with questions involving the relation of madness to crime the ordinary rules of procedure of a criminal court are not precisely applicable.

Supposing that a Court of Criminal Appeal had been in existence, it may be asked, what would the result have been in this case? Supposing that the prisoner had again pleaded guilty, would the sentence of death have then been confirmed, without any possibility of intervention on the part of the Home Office?

Many questions of this description will present themselves for consideration whenever the proposal for the establishment of a Court of Criminal Appeal begins to take definite shape.

The following is a somewhat different case. Elizabeth Swatman was tried for wilful murder at the Ipswich Assizes on April 1, 1876. She had killed another woman, who lived in an adjoining cottage, by striking her on the head with a shovel. No one was near at the time, and there was no evidence either that there had, or had not, been a quarrel. At first, the perpetrator of the act was not discovered, but the next day the prisoner accused herself. She said she had often thought of killing the old woman, her neighbour, and at last she did it. At her trial she persisted in saying that she "hit the old woman," and this statement was taken as a plea of guilty, and she was sentenced to death. The learned judge then reported the case to the Home Office, with an expression of opinion that a further medical examination was desirable. This examination resulted in her being sent to Broadmoor. She was, if one may be allowed the phrase, very mad indeed—demented and incoherent—and she died in the month of September following, from disease of the brain. She was undefended, until counsel was assigned to her at the time of the trial; and it does not appear to have occurred to any one to suggest, before she was arraigned, that she was unfit to plead; and then, after she had been called on to plead, and had persisted in saying that she had "hit," and that she "had killed the old woman," it was decided that it would not have been right to go back to the consideration of the question of whether or not the prisoner ought to have been called upon to plead. The learned judge immediately made the necessary representation to the Home Office, with the result that we have seen; but here, again, it may be asked, what course would have been taken to set the matter right if there had been no Home Office to which to appeal?

(4) With respect to those cases in which the accused is mute on arraignment, it is not intended, in this place, to treat of deaf mutes generally, but only of cases in which the accused is mute by reason of mental disease or defect, either alleged or suspected.

Taylor, in his work on the principles and practice of medical jurisprudence, mentions (page 589, vol. ii., third edition) the case of Yaquierdo, who was tried at the Herts Summer Assizes in 1854, and gives the following account:—"The prisoner, who was charged with wilful murder, was found by the jury to be wilfully mute. The man refused to plead, although it was obvious that he was well aware of the nature of the proceedings. No counsel could be assigned to him, as this could not be done without the prisoner's consent. He was convicted." But to render the account of this case complete, it must be added that the prisoner, after conviction

* *See* CRIMINAL RESPONSIBILITY, p. 310 *et seq.*

and sentence, was found to be unquestionably insane, and was removed to the criminal wing of Bethlem Hospital, from whence he was transferred, ten years later, to Broadmoor.

A case in which the prisoner was mute on arraignment recently came before Mr. Justice Charles at the Stafford Summer Assizes, in 1888. Ernest Harper, 23 years of age, was charged with the murder of his brother. The prisoner when called upon to plead made no reply, and the learned judge then said that he should follow the course pursued by Baron Alderson in *Reg.* v. *Goode*, and should ask the jury to say, 1st, whether the prisoner is mute of malice; 2nd, whether he is able to plead; and 3rd, whether he is sane or not.

The jury having found that the prisoner was incapable of pleading, the learned judge said: "You find he is mute, not of malice, not on purpose, but of the visitation of God?" To which the foreman replied: "Quite so."

It may be noted, with reference to this case, that during the course of the inquiry as to the capacity of the prisoner to plead, Dr. Spence gave evidence to the effect that in May the prisoner had said that he was guilty, and that a voice inside him told him to do what he had done; from which it appears that, although the prisoner was mute when he was arraigned, he was not always mute, but had conversed on the subject of his offence whilst awaiting trial.

As a complement to the foregoing case, we may take another, which was tried at the Yorkshire Summer Assizes, and which is fully reported in the *Leeds Mercury* of August 5, 1890. Samuel Harrison, aged 30, a slipper-maker, was indicted, before Mr. Justice Charles, for the wilful murder of his wife, at Leeds, on the 9th of May. The report states that the prisoner, when placed in the dock, was unkempt and slovenly, and made no answer to the charge, but remained silent when addressed by his lordship, keeping his eyes downcast, and apparently being unconscious of what was going on. A jury was then impannelled to inquire "whether the prisoner stood mute by the act of God or out of malice." Addressing the jury, his lordship said the question upon which he wanted the help of the jury was, "Why did the prisoner stand mute? was he doing it on purpose, in which case he was standing mute out of malice; or was he doing it because his state was such that he did not know what was going forward, in which case he was mute by the visitation of God? Was he doing it on purpose, or, to use an ordinary expression, was he shamming?"

Mr. John Edwards, the medical officer at Armley Gaol, stated that he had had the prisoner under his observation since May 10; that, at that time, he was quite capable of understanding what was said to him; but that, about May 20, he began to change, and, when asked a question, replied that he "could not think on," and, at other times, that he "could not remember;" that the prisoner altered so suddenly, without there being anything to account for it, that he put it down that his manner was assumed. About a fortnight ago there was another change: he became quite dumb. His opinion was that the prisoner's attitude was assumed. In cross-examination, witness said that he believed it was after the prisoner had been visited by the Rabbi that he changed his demeanour. He was of opinion that the prisoner was quite conscious of what was going on in court. Dr. Bevan Lewis, the medical director of the Wakefield Asylum, stated that on July 19 he examined the prisoner, and came to the conclusion that he was assuming insanity. On that occasion he answered questions intelligibly as to an occurrence with his fellow-prisoners on June 30. He had examined him again and found his condition changed; but he was still of opinion that his state was assumed.

A temporary attendant at the gaol said he had had charge of the prisoner at night since June 16. At first he was communicative, but after the Rabbi had visited him he changed and ceased to talk.

His lordship, in putting the matter to the jury, said he saw nothing in the evidence to lead to the belief that the prisoner was mute by the visitation of God.

The jury immediately found that the prisoner was "mute out of malice."

His lordship then directed a plea of not guilty to be entered on behalf of the prisoner; and the trial then proceeded, and ultimately the jury found the prisoner guilty, and he was sentenced to death in the usual form:—the report stating that when the prisoner was asked if had anything to say why sentence of death should not be passed upon him, he made no answer, and gave no indication of consciousness of what was taking place.

A paragraph, however, appeared in the *Times* of August 19, to the effect that the Home Secretary had recommended Her Majesty to respite the sentence; the paragraph going on to say, "Harrison has been found to be insane, and he will, this week, be removed to the criminal lunatic asylum at Broadmoor."

Before leaving this branch of the subject it must not be overlooked that cases occasionally arise in which, whatever may be the mental condition of the accused, his counsel may desire to obtain a verdict on the facts; and, with that view, no question of ability to plead is raised when the accused is arraigned. A case of this description, in which Samuel George Milner was charged with manslaughter before Mr. Justice Mathew, is reported in the *Times* for July 30, 1890.

If we now turn to the statistical side of this matter, we find that the total number of persons admitted into the criminal lunatic asylum at Broadmoor, who had been arraigned in court, from the time at which the asylum was opened down to the end of 1888, was 1737, and that this total was made up as follows:—

Found insane on arraignment . .	265
Acquitted on the ground of insanity, or found insane in the terms of the Trial of Lunatics Act, 1883 . .	579
Reprieved on the ground of insanity .	29
Found to be insane whilst undergoing sentences of penal servitude . .	817
Found to be insane whilst undergoing shorter terms of imprisonment . .	47
Total . .	1737

That is to say, there were 1737 persons who were arraigned in court and were charged with criminal offences, and who ultimately were sent to the asylum for criminal lunatics, but, of these 1737 persons, only 265, or rather less than 16 per cent., were found insane on arraignment; leaving more than 84 per cent. who were found insane at later stages, whilst in custody.

This represents the general result for the whole period; but there are two useful subdivisions that may be made. First, the records show that the question as to the fitness of a prisoner to plead is much more closely examined into in grave than in slighter offences; and, secondly, they show also that, in cases of all kinds, the proportion of prisoners found insane on arraignment has been greater in recent than it was in former years.

To illustrate the latter point we may compare the period down to the end of 1882 with the six years from 1882 to 1888; whilst to illustrate the former point we may take the cases of murder and compare them with all the others.

We find then that, of the total of 1737 persons above referred to, 1395 were admitted up to the end of 1882, and 342 during the following six years. We find, further, that of the 1395, there were 193 who had been found insane on arraignment; whilst of the 342, there were 72 who had been so found. It will be seen from these figures that the proportion, found insane on arraignment, before 1882 was a little less than 14 per cent.; whilst for the six years from 1882 to 1888 the proportion rose to 21 per cent.

Next, with respect to those cases in which the offence was murder, we find that, during the whole period, the number of persons who had been arraigned and charged in court with that crime and who ultimately were sent to the asylum for criminal lunatics was 444, and that this total was made up as follows:—

Found insane on arraignment . .	109
Acquitted on the ground of insanity, or found insane in terms of the Trial of Lunatics Act, 1883	286
Reprieved on the ground of insanity .	29
Sentence commuted to penal servitude and afterwards found to be insane .	20
	444

And from these figures it appears that, of the total number of persons arraigned for murder who ultimately became inmates of the asylum for criminal lunatics, somewhat less than 25 per cent. were found insane on arraignment, leaving 75 per cent. who were considered sufficiently sane to be tried.

If we now go on to subdivide these cases with reference to the periods during which they occurred, the figures are as follows:—

Cases of Murder only.	Up to the end of 1882.		From 1882 to the end of 1888.
Found insane on arraignment	79	...	30
Acquitted on the ground of insanity, or found insane in the terms of the Trial of Lunatics Act, 1883 . .	228	...	58
Reprieved on the ground of insanity	18	...	11
Commuted to penal servitude and afterwards found to be insane	16	...	4
Totals .	341	...	103

These figures show a proportion of about 23 per cent. for the former period, and a proportion of about 29 per cent. for the six years from 1882 to 1888; and this increase in the proportion found insane on arraignment, of persons accused of murder, although not so great as the increase (from 14 to 21 per cent.) in the general total above mentioned, is yet sufficiently great to afford ground for surmising that the question of the precise degree of mental unsoundness that is sufficient to render a person, in the words of the statute, "insane so that he cannot be tried," has, probably, not yet reached a final settlement. On close examination, it might, indeed, be found to be as difficult to lay down hard-and-fast rules, which would satisfactorily meet every case in which the ability of an accused person to plead is in question, as it would be to frame an entirely satisfactory definition of the precise degree of insanity that renders a person not responsible according to law for his acts; and we know what the mature opinion of Lord Blackburn is upon this latter point.*

In Russell "On Crimes" (vol. i. p. 114), the test of capacity and fitness to plead to an indictment is stated in the following terms:—"Whether he (the accused) is of sufficient intellect to comprehend the course of the proceedings on the trial, so as to be able to make a proper defence." But here, again, it is evident that the term "proper" is by no means an exact or precise one.

The general rule of law may be said to be that every one is presumed to be sane until the contrary has been proved; and, in the application of this rule, it would appear that every one is presumed, in law, to be sane, with respect to any particular matter, until the contrary has been proved with respect to that very matter; and with regard to the manner in which, from the legal point of view, a person may be both sane and insane at the same time, Sir John Nichol has observed: "If it be meant by this that the law of England never deems a person both sane and insane at one and the same time upon one and the same subject, the assertion is a mere truism. But .... if it be meant that the law of England never deems a party both sane and insane at different times upon the same subject, and both sane and insane at the same time upon different subjects, there can scarcely be a position more adverse to the current of legal authority."

Looking at the matter in this light, it is quite clear that an accused person may be insane, and may be well known to be insane, and yet may declared to be sane so far as his ability and fitness to plead are concerned; and, this being so, it is not a matter for surprise that the proportion of insane persons who are found insane on arraignment is not large.

But there is another mode in which the subject might be approached. We have seen that out of a total of 1737 persons who, after having been arraigned in court, ultimately reached the asylum for criminal lunatics, only 265 (equivalent to less than 16 per cent.), were found insane on arraignment; leaving 1472 persons (equivalent to more than 84 per cent.) who passed through various further stages of trial, of sentence, or of imprisonment, before they reached their ultimate destination; and it is quite conceivable that, in the course of time, it may come to be thought that, with respect to a considerable proportion of such persons, if a decision were arrived at as to their mental condition at an *earlier stage*, and if action were taken upon such decision, it might be much to the advantage, not only of the accused themselves, but also that of the public at large.

W. Orange.

* *See* Criminal Responsibility.

PLEONECTICA ATHYMIA (πλεονέκτης, greedy; ἀ, priv.; θυμός, mind). A form of insanity characterised by greediness and desire for gain. Over-bearing arrogance. (Fr. *pléonexie*; Ger. *Mehrhabenwollen*.)

PLEONEXIA (πλεονεξία, greediness). Greediness, selfishness or arrogance regarded as mental disease. (Fr. *pléonexie*.)

PLETHYSMOGRAPH and BALANCE.—The plethysmograph was devised by Prof. Angelo Mosso, of Turin, for the purpose of studying the circulation by measuring the varying volume of the arm or foot, or even a single finger (Fig. 1).

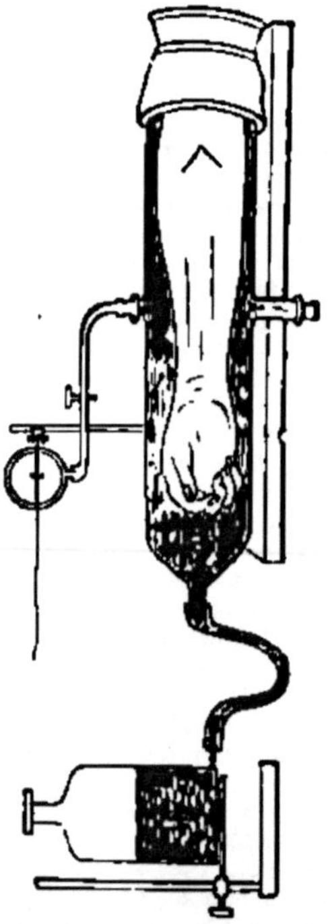

Fig. 1.

It consists of a glass cylinder (G), freely suspended, open at one end, and terminating at the other in a small tube. There are two openings on the side of the cylinder, serving to fill it with water, and to allow of the passage of electrodes when it is desired to study the influence of electrical irritation. These openings are hermetically closed, and into one is inserted a thermometer to measure the temperature of the water in the cylinder. The hand, forearm, and elbow are introduced into the cylinder, and a caoutchouc ring closes the cavity of the cylinder, slightly compressing the arm near the elbow. The ring must be sufficiently thick to prevent oscillations under the influences of slight increases of pressure. The tube at the farther extremity of the cylinder communicates with an open vessel (F), which is graduated, or contains a float, which may be put in connection with a lever to record the variations in level on a smoked cylinder. As the blood in the arm (and, therefore, the volume of the arm) increases, water is driven into the graduated vessel, or raises the float; as the blood in the arm decreases, water is drawn from the graduated vessel. Mosso found that mental exertion, or emotion, produced a diminution in the volume of the arm. This result is not, however, uniformly obtained, nor must it be supposed that the change of volume, when obtained, enables us to calculate the vascular changes in the brain; we have also to consider the probable changes in the lungs, connected with the concomitant variations in respiratory rhythm pointed out by Mosso.

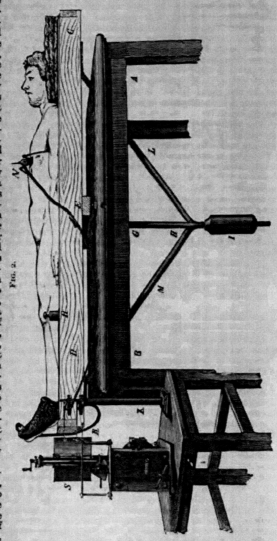

Fig. 2.

Another very ingenious instrument, devised by Mosso, like the plethysmograph, to demonstrate changes in the vascular system, is the Balance. This is a kind of delicately adjusted see-saw, on which the subject lies at full length (Fig. 2). It consists of a wooden case (*D C*) placed, as a balance, on a transverse bar of steel (*E*). This rests on a table (*B A*), pierced by three openings, one, in the middle, giving passage to an iron bar (*G H*), a metre in length, ending in an iron cylinder (*I*), weighing 25 kilos. The other two openings give passage to similar iron bars (*L H M*) fixed obliquely to the first. The centre of gravity being thus placed very low, the balance does not oscillate with too great facility. It is necessary that the subject should lie on the balance for at least an hour before the experiments begin, in order that the circulation may be adjusted to the horizontal position, and the excess of blood removed from the lower extremities. Mosso also applies two instruments, constructed on principles similar to the plethysmograph, to the hand and thumb, to aid in controlling the experiments. It is found that with every inspiration the balance sinks at the feet, and at the same time the lower extremities increase in volume; this movement is apparently due, not to visceral movement, but to increase of abdominal pressure interfering with the return of blood from the lower extremities. Mosso finds that during severe intellectual efforts the balance sinks at the head. During sleep it sinks at the feet, but if the subject is disturbed without being awakened, it sinks slightly at the head.

The plethysmograph is described or referred to in all works on general physiology, and it has led to the construction of various instruments on the same principle, such as Roy's oncometer. The balance has not come into general use, although, as Mosso points out, for the demonstration of psychic influences on the circulation it is much superior to the plethysmograph. A full description of it by Mosso will be found in the *Archives Italiennes de Biologie*, tome v. fasc. i. (1884)

[The figure of the balance is inserted by the kindness of Prof. Mosso, and that of the plethysmograph by the courtesy of Prof. Stirling and Messrs. Griffin.]

HAVELOCK ELLIS.

PLUMBISM AND INSANITY. (*See* LEAD POISONING.)

PLUTOMANIA (πλοῦτος, wealth; μανία, madness). Insane belief in the possession of large property—a kind of megalomania.

PNIGALION, PNIGALIUM (πνίγω, I suffocate). An old term for incubus or nightmare, because of the sense of suffocation in that affection. (Fr. *éphialte.*)

PODAGROUS INSANITY. (*See* GOUT AND INSANITY.)

POISONS OF THE MIND.—Definition. Limits of the Subject.—The study of the whole of the mental poisons embraces all substances, whatever may be their origin and nature, which are capable of exercising a morbid action on the intellectual processes, either by disordering them or by suspending them completely for a moment or longer. Speaking of poisons which act specially upon the brain, and of the influence which shows itself mainly or almost exclusively by cerebral disorders, we shall mention all the intoxications the symptomatology of which includes intellectual disturbances, whether the latter be prominent or latent. Strictly speaking, the former alone ought to be called *psychical poisons;* but on the one hand there is scarcely any poison—even among those which are commonly called by this name—which limits its action absolutely to the brain, and on the other hand, there are many injurious substances which, although injuring this organ in an indirect manner only, nevertheless disturb its functions occasionally. It is for this reason, and in order to be more complete, that we have extended our studies to all intoxicants which affect *primarily* the intellectual sphere, reserving, however, special attention for all toxic substances the action of which on the brain is predominant. It is necessary to understand the term "primarily"; as a matter of fact, there is no substance which introduced accidentally into the circulation, does not affect in some way the cerebral functions; all functions are connected one with the other, and in certain intoxications, which are not altogether psychical, we observe *secondary* (*deuteropathic*) intellectual disturbances, which may be the consequence of circulatory or thermic disorders, or of the disturbance of some other mechanism connected with the initial action of the poison. These, however, are not poisons of the mind, a term which must be definitely reserved for substances which act primarily, to a greater or less extent, on the cerebral cells.

As we have said, almost all substances introduced into the organism modify the cerebral processes, and the reason of this lies evidently in the delicacy of the organisation of the nervous system, which, like every complicated mechanism, is extremely vulnerable; the brain, as the terminus of all sensations, and as the regulator of even the most minute cellular functions, has to bear the brunt of all attacks, even the slightest, directed against the vital equilibrium, and has also to react in order to re-establish this equilibrium. In every intoxication, in addition to the cerebral reaction due to the effect of the poison itself, there are other reactions requiring as many reflexes for the defence of the body, and closely connected with the impressions, which the sensorium receives, of modifications of nutrition, or of changes which take place in other organs under the influence of the poison. These reactions are the symptoms common to every intoxication and are not specially important.

The cerebral reactions which take place under the more direct influence of the toxic substance are of two kinds: they are either diffuse, general and undefined, and are expressed by vague symptoms which indicate a lesion of the organ as a whole; or they are clear, well defined and localised, and are expressed by symptoms which indicate that the poison affects one special centre to the exclusion of all others (visual hallucinations, psychomotor derangement, disorders of ideation, &c.).

In addition to the disorders of the brain, we meet at almost every step with spinal derangement. The cerebrum and cord are the two great organs formed by a conglomeration of the same delicate elements; they react in the same manner, and it is therefore not surprising to see that in a great number of cases a spinal poison also affects the brain, and *vice versâ*. Chloroform, carbon monoxide, alcohol, &c., are principally psychical poisons, but at the same time entail cord disturbances. On the other hand, nux vomica and arnica, which are principally poisons of the latter class, nevertheless occasionally produce intellectual troubles.

Under which Class of Poisons ought we to include those of the Mind?—The two classifications generally accepted in France, are those of Rabuteau and of Tardieu, and even in these, it is clear that the poisons in question cannot form a separate class; the classifications are merely symptomatological, based on the preponderance of a special group of symptoms in the intoxication. Rabuteau has taken into his class of neurotics a group of cerebro-spinal poisons, under which he comprises the psychical poisons proper (chloroform, ether, opium, &c.). In Tardieu's classification, the latter have been subdivided into three classes: (*a*) stupefying poisons (tobacco); (*b*) narcotic poisons (opium), and (*c*) neurasthenic poisons (quinine). These classifications, although without solid basis, are the two most satisfactory. It is, however, clear that intellectual disorders may form part of the syndromes met with in all classes of toxic substances. Among the hæmatic poisons Rabuteau counts alcohol; among the *neuro-muscular* poisons, he gives the poisonous classes of nightshades; among the *muscular* poisons he includes lead; and, lastly, among the *irritant* or *corrosive* poisons, he enumerates ammonia and bromine. Each one of these poisons may have an influence on the mind, and as a matter of fact, some of them, like alcohol and the poisonous nightshade, produce such distinct and special disorders of the intellect, that it would be logical to class them under the "poisons of the mind." The same remark holds good with regard to the classification of Tardieu.

Psychical poisons, therefore, do not allow of being classified, and it could not be otherwise, because the symptoms of mental intoxication are sometimes predominant, but quite as often accessory, and these do not offer any safe basis for classification. With regard to the question of classifying psychical poisons among themselves, we shall see that the nosography is extremely deficient in documents about an extremely great number of poisons which affect the mind. Although many of them have been thoroughly investigated, many others are scarcely known.

General Symptomatology.—In spite of the dissimilarity of the substances which are capable of producing cerebral intoxication, there are, nevertheless, certain clinical characteristics common to all. We might even say, that there are no intellectual disorders more pathognomonic of one poison than of another. The artificial insanity produced by toxic substances is nothing but the reaction of the cerebrum, which is arrested in its full and regular function, and the coming into play of cellular elements, under the influence of an external and abnormal excitation, which is different from the usual stimulation. This excitation, naturally, may affect one part of the brain more than another; hence the apparent difference in the symptoms, which also may vary in different individuals although they are under the influence of the same poison. The toxic substance certainly does not add any new element to those which the normal brain possesses, and herein lies the great difference between the superadded insanity and the insanity which the brain produces itself—*i.e.*, between toxic derangement and psychosis. All, or nearly all, slight intoxications, be the poison animal, vegetable, or mineral, may be briefly characterised thus: excitation of the organ of thought, intoxication, and incoherence in ideas and actions; in toxic derangement there is only a functional disturbance and a *quantitative* modification of psychical expression while, in organic derangement (psychosis or encephalopathy), there is a *qualitative* ideational alteration.

The special symptoms are of infinite variety, although at bottom they are nothing but the expression of one and the same disorder, and this variation of the special phenomena depends on two factors—viz., on the localisation of the toxic effects in a special cell-group, and on the individual reaction. Nervous and predisposed individuals are evidently more easily affected than normal subjects. Alcohol, morphia and cocaine do not produce the same effects on all individuals, male or female, under all latitudes. Among all the poisons which we shall enumerate later on, a great number produce cerebral effects but rarely, in consequence of certain dispositions of the individual. Among the labourers who have to handle carbon disulphide or aniline, some only present mental disorders. The individual factor, therefore, with its idiosyncrasies plays here, as everywhere else, a very important part. In addition to this, there are other factors, the degree of education, habits and social condition, the course of ideas, fulness or emptiness of the stomach, the season, locality, &c., which serve to modify the symptoms of cerebral intoxication. The hallucinations of the western people under the influence of haschisch are not identical with the voluptuous dreams of the orientals. Lastly, we must take into consideration the dose absorbed, and the mode of preparation of the poison.

Generally speaking, the symptoms of cerebral intoxication may be divided into **three types:**

(1) Certain poisons produce a *general* disturbance of the intellect, a disorder of all the faculties, so that there is no longer any elective localisation of the intoxication in one faculty over another. If there is insanity, it is an incoherent insanity, absurd and without consistency, as in drunkenness or mania; there are neither fixed ideas nor any organised or hallucinatory derangement. If there are hallucinations (and this is frequently the case, because the cortical cells are uniformly over-excited) they do not influence the course of the ideas; they modify ideation at the moment they appear, but the phenomenon is transitory (derangement in pyrexia, &c.).

(2) Other poisons, without causing such intense disorder, nevertheless disturb the *ensemble* of the faculties, but *to a less degree*. To use a comparison, we might say that the former group is to the latter what alcoholic insanity is to simple drunkenness. General disturbance—although slight—of the intellect, in one word, intoxication, is the characteristic of this group. Save the intensity of the processes, the only difference separating the two groups is the partial or even complete persistency of consciousness (camphor, musk, betel, &c.).

(3) Other poisons, although producing temporary intoxication, seem to limit their action to one of the intellectual spheres, or to one cerebral department—either to ideation—or to voluntary movements or loss of sense of space (haschisch)—or to sentiments (instinctive impulse, erotic passions, &c.), or to sensory centres (hallucinations of various senses, belladonna, &c.). The conceptions also vary according to the predominance of the excitement in one psychical department, eroticism in some, and incessant restlessness, hyper-ideation, ambitious or mystic ideas, &c., in others.

We shall now group the various symptoms observed in cerebral intoxication, analyse them, and then extract from them some general truths.

Intoxication.—Intoxication is a symptom common to all forms of cerebral poisoning, and it is the first phenomenon observed after the absorption of the toxic substance, whether the latter be of an exciting or depressing nature. On account of the characteristic differences, authors have described intoxication by alcohol, quinine, chloral, ergot, atropine, iodine, &c. The study of these intoxications shows that they are all accompanied by the same cerebral disturbances and therefore may be embraced in the same description.

Intoxication has various degrees: sometimes very slight (*Physalis alkekengi*) or very profound, even making an individual semi-comatose (aniline); under other circumstances the patients deserve the epithet dead-drunk (alcohol, opium). The most typical intoxication which might serve as a standard for others to be compared with is alcoholic drunkenness. Certain poisons, like camphor, produce an intoxication very similar to it.

The intellectual troubles are: great excitement with exaltation (the ideas follow each other rapidly and are not logically connected, and imagination is more productive), volubility and incoherency, embarrassment of speech, difficulty of articulation (atropine), and sometimes actual aphasia (iodoform). In a case of poisoning with the honey of lecheguana (A. de St. Hilaire) total amnesia was observed with regard to the French language; when wishing to speak French the patient could express himself in Portuguese only. In addition to these phenomena, there is considerable neuro-muscular excitement; gesticulation is frequent and disordered, and the patient commits all kinds of eccentric actions. In certain cases (haschisch) we observe an exuberant sentimentality which is much more marked than in any other case. This last poison, as well as ether, produces also a singular stimulation of the memory: events long past recur with a clearness which they had lost. In certain cases (cignë) the intoxication produces an actual darkening of the intellect.

In the majority of cases, unless there is a special predisposition to the contrary, the intoxication induced causes a certain enjoyment. It is gay, pleasant and playful to the extreme under the influence of guarana, haschisch and maté, or it may manifest itself in hilarity, or even in insuppressible outbreaks of laughter (haschisch, codeine, laughing gas, opium, lecheguana). It may also produce a feeling of profound voluptuousness (haschisch), a kind of ecstasy, and an indescribable sense of well-being (datura, laughing gas, opium).

Lastly, we may observe at the same time a kind of sub-delirious condition (datura, Indian hemp). In haschisch intoxication we frequently meet with an exaggeration of the personality with ideas of self-satisfaction and ambition. Sometimes most singular illusions are observed. Individuals under the influence of haschisch make gross mistakes with regard to time, and completely lose their knowledge of locality. Opium-eaters have no longer an exact knowledge of place or time.

The attitude of the patients reflects the course of their ideas, and varies according to whether the poison acts upon the general sensibility or on the vaso-motor system. They are pale and depressed, and their eyes are sad and dull (kawa); or the face is animated, and the expression bright and lively; again, the patient may have a wandering look (lecheguana); or, lastly, he may lie down and be prostrated (iodoform).

The general phenomena are: cephalalgia, vertigo, giddiness, heaviness of the head, sense of compression in the region of the temples, tinnitus aurium, vomiting, tremor, reeling and uncertain gait, sense of weakness in the lower extremities (pelletierine) and numbness of the limbs (kawa). In poisoning with aniline we observe actual automatic movements, and in that with datura or laughing gas the patient has an irresistible desire to move.

Consciousness is generally soon obscured although there are cases in which it may persist (benzene, chloroform, lecheguana); we then have conscious intoxication with exact perception and comprehension of the outer world. In some cases (laughing gas) the patient loses all relation to the external world, although his knowledge of it is preserved. In poisoning with carbon monoxide the intellect remains intact till nearly the approach of death.

Intoxication appears rapidly after the absorption of the poison. It may last a very short time, and terminate in a condition of more or less profound sleep. Exceptionally, the intoxication by chloral may appear after the narcosis; there is at first slight excitement of short duration, then deep sleep, and the intoxication appears on the patient waking up.

Intoxication is followed by recovery, although it may leave behind various cerebral troubles, which we shall describe later on.

Other Elementary Troubles of the Intellect.—The clinical picture is not always so simple, and the intoxication is not the *only* symptom to be observed. We have isolated it because it is so typical, but, on the other hand, it may have complications, and it may also be absent. The individual reactions to one and the same poison are of an infinite variety, and the dose absorbed, as well as all the accompanying symptoms, must be taken into account. Absorbed in great quantity the poison produces intoxication, or it may prostrate the patient and even kill him; it also may be taken in a dose insufficient to produce intoxication, but repeatedly, and in this case the intoxication is from the commencement chronic (certain forms of alcoholism, poisoning in certain professions, aniline, carbon disulphide, &c.). It is easy, therefore, to see that intoxication which is *par excellence* an acute phenomenon, may be absent, and we shall now analyse the intellectual disorders which may take its place, may complicate it, or may follow after the intoxication has disappeared. We shall first study the **general intellectual phenomena** and then the **insane conditions.**

The simple intellectual troubles produced by the various poisons are of two kinds: (1) condition of *excitement*, and (2) condition of *depression*. We have seen that both conditions may belong to the history of one and the same toxic substance, the latter following the former; there are, however, substances which may cause principally excitement, and others which more specially cause depression.

(1) *Condition of Excitement.*—The poisons which produce general excitement of the brain are very numerous, among them, betel, coffee, aromatic stimulants, mint, snake-root, benzene, &c. Some even produce actual erethism of the nervous system, as coffee, maté, and tea. Others stimulate particularly the intellect and produce exaltation, *e.g.*, Indian hemp, hydrocyanic acid, datura, hyoscyamin, iodoform, ginger, turpentine, lecheguana and opium; at the same time the poison may possess great power of motor excitation (anamirta).

It is easy to conceive the consequences of these various conditions of excitement. The most common one is *insomnia* (atropine, cocaine, copaiba, coffee, and guarana). This insomnia is connected with a sense of very great resistance to fatigue in larger doses; maté soothes and stimulates to work; tea keeps awake, coffee takes away fatigue, mint gives new strength and tone to the nervous system.

The character undergoes a profound change, and becomes irritable and *bizarre* (kawa, turpentine, carbon disulphide). In nervous subjects, especially in women, this irritability borders on insanity (turpentine). Some patients are very impressionable (nux vomica); others are restless, excited, and feel uneasy (iodine).

As regards ideation, the stimulus may make the course of ideas more rapid, but they are superficial (coffee); sometimes they may be incoherent or they may even be boisterous; the incoherence is due to a want of uniformity in the stimulation of the various faculties; the patient also may become unable to generalise and to reason (chloroform).

The imagination presents an almost delirious vivacity (haschisch and opium), and the passions become stronger (chloroform). The personality may become transformed, and the patient may have actual illusions; sometimes a sense of well-being and of quiet happiness is experienced (maté), and sometimes the patient believes himself to be much lighter than usual, and he seems to fly from the ground (camphor).

As to movements, there is generally an excessive impulse to be in motion.

(2) *Condition of Depression.*—There are various degrees of general depression, from simple tranquillity (maratia-moogho), with affection of the mental powers (bromides), to complete torpor (aniline, laurocerasus, iodine, quinine). Some patients suffer from extreme languor (lauro-rosatus). The most conspicuous effect of the depressing poisons is *narcosis*, which has various degrees, from a tendency to sleep (datura, hyoscyamin, turpentine), drowsiness (mushrooms), somnolency (urea), and slight narcosis (duboisia, thebane), to actual sleep, with apparent annihilation of all cerebral life (chloroform, haschisch, opium, lecheguana, mandragora). The characters of sleep are of an infinite variety. It may be absolutely irresistible, or only an actual craving for sleep (chloroform, bromides). It may be profound and quiet (chloroform), and heavy and fatiguing (haschisch, opium), agitated (benzene), and full of dreams (chloral), or of nightmare (kawa, haschisch). In former times, some country-people, imbued with ideas of witchcraft, would rub into the skin liniments of belladonna or stramonium, thus securing a sleep full of all the illusions of the witches' sabbath, or lycanthropy. The sleep may last many hours, and may be followed by either absolute amnesia, or by a fairly clear recollection of the dream.

Should no narcosis be produced, the depression may be diminished, or reduction of mental acumen and moral energy (carbon disulphide), enfeeblement of volition, to the point of suppression (duboisia) great fatigue after slight exertion (santonin), moroseness, sense of discouragement and annihilation (hydrocotyle), of atonishment and indifference, with dulness and immobility (haschisch).

The depression may be accompanied by a certain degree of well-being (coca), and by a sensation reminding us of the lassitude of the *siesta* in hot countries (kawa), of ecstasies and of enjoyment. In other cases, there is a happy satisfaction, similar to that of an idiot, with incoherency of speech (bromides).

The two conditions we have just mentioned do not exclude each other; we have already seen that the condition of narcosis or depression in many cases follows the initial excitement (Indian hemp, opium, tobacco, and kawa). Occasionally, we may observe alternations of torpor, somnolency and agitation (carbon disulphide). In other cases, agitation follows the depression, as in the case of datura, which, after having produced sleep, causes agitation, with obstinate insomnia.

After the various intoxications, the memory often undergoes singular alterations; sometimes comparatively intact with regard to events before or during the disorder, it may completely disappear (iodine, chloroform, œnanthe). Cases have even been observed of retrograde amnesia (carbon monoxide, datura, benzene).

Insane Conditions.—In addition to the intoxication and general disturbance of the mind just described, the mental poisons produce also mental disorder, which we term *insane conditions* (*états délirants*). These conditions are so intimately connected with the former, that it is difficult to separate them, except for the purpose of description. The individual variations are here very numerous, the same poison producing different effects in two individuals, thus proving again that the individual reaction is everything. The other symptomatic differences depend on the more special action of a poison on one special function, as is the case with the poisonous kinds of nightshade, which create, as Lasègue says, such a desire to wander, that the patient can never be kept quiet.

We shall describe several types of disorder, and at the same time, we shall class into groups those poisons which have similar effects.

(1) *Maniacal, or incoherent type*, which is the most frequent. The derangement is absolutely general. To this class belong—*e.g.*, all febrile disorders and those caused by auto-intoxication.

(2) *Alcoholic type* (maniacal condition of a depressive, painful and frightful form). The poisons of this class are numerous—alcohol, carbon disulphide, datura, absinthe, tea, mandragora, atropine, &c. (*See* ALCOHOLISM.)

(3) *Maniacal type of expansive form*—ambitious, mystic and erotic ideas, ideas of self-satisfaction and of exaggeration of personality (benzene, laughing gas, haschisch, cantharides).

(4) *Melancholic type* (kawa, lecheguana, and iodoform). Not well defined and always temporary.

(5) *Mixed forms.* Depression may alternate with excitement.

(6) *Vesanic conditions*—*i.e.*, attacks of insanity, which although excited by poisons, do not derive their special colour or character from the drug, but arise in persons strongly predisposed to insanity.

The elements which constitute the derangement are:

(1) *Disorders of ideation:* false and strange conceptions; gay, sad, ambitious and erotic ideas, and those of persecution. They are generally isolated and incoherent, and are very frequently caused by sensory disorders. It is noteworthy that the derangement is most intense during the night. Lastly, the individual reactions are in close relation to the course of these ideas (anger, stupor, hilarity, &c.).

(2) *Sensory illusions.*

(3) *Hallucinations* of all the senses, especially of vision.

(4) *Consciousness* is obscured or annihilated.

Other Pathological Phenomena which accompany the Intoxication.—In order to complete the general history of mental intoxications, we have to mention the disorders other than psychical, produced by the poisons which affect the mind. These are of great importance as aiding the diagnosis, if the latter is left doubtful when the mental symptoms alone are taken into consideration.

There are, first, some general, more or less severe, symptoms, caused by the impression which the nervous system experiences—*fainting, tendency to syncope* (camphor (?)), *lypothymia, profound syncope* (muscarine, cantharides, camphor, ciguë, œnanthe, quinine, and turpentine); *prostration* (cherry-laurel and iodides), *stupor* (mushrooms, atropine, Indian hemp (haschisch), hydrocyanic acid, datura, duboisia), and, lastly, *coma*, which is very frequent, and may terminate fatally; it is very distinct in alcoholic and lead intoxications, and as a terminal symptom of epileptiform attacks (V. Bertin, art. "Coma," in "Dictionnaire Encyclopédique"). The hypasthenic, stupefying, narcotic and neurasthenic poisons are characteristic in producing coma. In the *hypasthenic* class, coma is somewhat rare; "the functional depression here affects more the *ensemble* of the vital powers than the brain-centres" (arsenic, corrosive sublimate, tartrate of antimony, bromide of potassium, and phosphorus—in the last case the coma may follow the mental derangement — somnolency, derangement, coma, and death). In the class of *stupefying* poisons the coma is more profound (alcohol, lead, belladonna, hyoscyamus, datura, tobacco, and chloroform). The *narcotics* produce narcosis, which may pass over into coma. Lastly, in the class of *neurasthenic* poisons, the coma is the consequence of a loss of nervous energy (nux vomica, cantharides, and hydrocyanic acid). In febrile and septic diseases coma is frequent (intermittent fever, Planer and Frerichs), as also in the auto-intoxications (uræmia).

Motor Disorders.—Motility may be exaggerated, diminished, abolished, or perverted, and the disorders may be localised in various manners. Exaggeration of motility may present itself in simple *stimulation* of muscular contractility (coffee), increasing to the production of involuntary movements (carbon disulphide), in *contractures* (creasote and iodoform), in *cramps* (carbon disulphide and alcohol), and in *convulsions*, which are of great importance and very frequent. They may be *general* (argas, atropine, creasote, digitalis, duboisia, ergot, jusquiame, lauro-cerasus, lead, quinine, &c.) (due to a special action of the poisons or to individual reaction; they may be a precursory symptom of death, or are characteristic of the acute phase of the intoxication), or they may be *localised*—face, limbs, jaw (œnanthe); diaphragm (hiccough in digitalism); posterior cervical region (aniline and copaiba); neck, abdomen, pharynx (copaiba); or opisthotonos and trismus (œnanthe, santonin, and turpentine); they remind the observer of convulsions in hydrophobia (cantharidism).

The *diminution of muscular energy* presents various degrees, from simple muscular weakening (creasote, jusquiame, lauro-cerasus and all narcotic and stupefying poisons) to diminution of mobility (bromides), and even to its complete abolition. Paralysis is extremely frequent in the course of intoxications; either *general* in acute cases (chloroform, laughing gas, cantharides, chloral, atropine, jusquiame, belladonna and turpentine), or *local* (temporary or permanent) in chronic cases (alcoholism, lead-poisoning); hemiplegia and alternating paralysis (iodine); and paralysis of the extremities (lead); the most common form is paraplegia of the lower limbs (alcohol, carbon disulphide and chloral). In the presence of paraplegia we have always to consider the possibility of intoxication. In chronic cases we may observe generalised paralysis due to muscular changes (degeneration, sclerosis and trophic disorders).

Sensory Disorders.—These form, together with mental and motor disorders, the three great parts of the symptomatology of intoxications.

As regards *general sensibility* we find *pseudæsthesia*, a *general* and *local anæsthesia; hemianæsthesia* and *analgesia;* and lastly, *general* and *local hyperæsthesia*.

On the part of *special sensibility* we observe *augmentation* and *diminution* of sensory acuteness. With regard to vision we meet with hyperæsthesia of the optic nerve, photopsia, dyschromatopsia, diplopia, diminution of visual acuteness, disordered vision, amblyopia, amaurosis, temporary or permanent, blindness, and contraction or dilatation of the pupils. With regard to hearing we observe tinnitus aurium, paracousia, augmentation or diminution of auditory acuteness, and deafness. On the part of taste and smell there may be exaggeration or abolition of both. On the part of genital sensibility poisons may have an aphrodisiac effect, or they may be anaphrodisiac.

The disorders of sensibility, however, are not truly pathognomonic. Generally speaking, sensibility may be exaggerated or diminished, and it is easy to see that many poisons may produce both effects, according to the idiosyncrasies and doses, and according to whether the intoxication is acute or chronic.

Course, Duration, and Termination of Mental Intoxication.—We shall consider the development of the symptoms separately in acute poisoning (therapeutic, suicidal, criminal, &c.) and in chronic intoxications (voluntary, professional, &c.). In the former case we observe nothing but a pathological storm accidental in the life of the patient, and to this category belong the greater number of cases of poisoning (chloroform, quinine, cantharides, digitalis, mushrooms, &c.).

Many poisons produce nothing but insignificant and temporary troubles which disappear without leaving any trace behind; their effect is limited to a slight excitement or depression of the faculties, to a short intoxication, or to a more or less profound narcosis. Afterwards, perfect order is re-established. Other poisons cause more serious symptoms: confusion, stupor, convulsions, coma and even death. The duration varies according to the individual disposition and the dose absorbed, but generally speaking, the acute stage—if recovery should follow—does not last more than a few days or weeks. If death should slowly supervene it is due to exhaustion of the nervous system or to organic disorder. Recovery may be slow and may be accompanied by fatigue, malaise, intellectual inability, and by symptoms of neurasthenia, and in some cases the brain may be incurably affected, as—*e.g.*, poisoning by carbon monoxide is sometimes followed by persistent retrograde amnesia (Rouillard, Briand) and occasionally by so-called acute dementia (Bouchereau, Raffegeau). Lastly, we indicate as a possible consequence insanity itself in predisposed individuals.

In chronic intoxications, which comprise the great social intoxications, the course of the symptoms depends necessarily on the habits of the patient, including of course the influence of individual reaction. It is useful to distinguish between voluntary and involuntary intoxication, as the course of each is rather different.

In the former case, the chronic period does not generally establish itself from the first. At the commencement we observe acute symptoms which here more than anywhere else deserve the name of intoxication (morphia, cocaine, alcohol, haschisch, opium, kawa). These acute phenomena may reproduce themselves a number of times, without however preventing chronicity from establishing itself: they are nothing but epiphenomena which appear again and again in the course of this period; the two essential kinds of symptoms, however, are the *irresistible appetite* for the poison, with periodical return of the acute and subacute symptoms, and the *progressive decay* of the mental faculties. The acute symptoms correspond to the temporary saturation of the body with the poison, while the chronic symptoms are the expression of organic lesions, gradually developed under the toxic influence. Thus regarded it is easy to see that while both kinds of symptoms may coincide, the former are necessarily transitory.

The character common to all these varieties of poisoning at the chronic period, and which is at the same time the cause and effect of this chronicity, is the impulsive craving of the brain for the return of the sensations experienced. Once intoxicated, the patient glides down a dangerous slope, because deprivation of the stimulant produces cerebral symptoms of all kinds, which temporarily disappear again on a new dose being taken. At the same time the dose has to be increased progressively on account of the singular adjustment of the cerebral cells to these substances. If not by force withdrawn from the morbid influence, the patient falls a victim after a variable length of time, which counts by years, under particular cerebral symptoms, which are the same in all cases, and indicate definite organic lesions of the brain.

The professional intoxications (aniline, carbon disulphide, lead, mercury, and turpentine) have, strictly speaking, no acute phase. The disease is chronic from its commencement; the saturation takes place slowly and may for a long time produce only insignificant symptoms, but it also may terminate in the same lesions as the former class, a fact which depends on the individual resistance. The course is slow and insidious, although sometimes interrupted by the appearance of subacute phenomena as an expression of temporary over-saturation; but generally the cerebral symptoms are the work of time, brought about more by organic lesions which have slowly been formed under the poisonous influence than by a direct action of the intoxicant.

This terminal period of all chronic cerebral poisoning deserves special mention. It is essentially and uniformly characterised by a progressive weakening of the mental faculties, which may pass over into complete dementia (alcohol and lead). This weakening manifests itself by a condition of stupidity and moral degradation, and by disorders of ideation and of memory (opium, haschisch, alcohol, lead and betel); the patients are quiet and inactive, and nothing but automata, leading a material life. It is a singular fact, that the appetite for the poison outlives the intellectual decay. Le Roy de Méricourt says with regard to maté-drinkers, they know three things only: to take maté, to sleep, and to eat—and we might say the same of all inveterate inebriates. Physical decay soon produces marasmus and cachexia, and the patient dies from exhaustion or in consequence of some organic complication, which easily establishes itself on such a soil.

Many victims of mental poisons die before having reached the stage of complete dementia, if the poison is energetic enough to disorganise rapidly not only the mind but also the other functions. This is the case in morphinism and cocainism. If dementia supervenes, it shows all the symptoms of organic dementia, and may be complicated by motor and sensory disorders, especially by paralysis, as we have pointed out above.

To sum up, the life of chronic cases may be divided into two periods: a period of cerebral over-exertion—cerebral usury—and a period of cerebral annihilation, if the patient has not exceptional power of resistance or if death does not intervene; but however great the resistance is, the patient will always become an inferior creature in consequence of the poison; he may be brilliant in consequence of the stimulation of his brain, but the reaction afterwards brings him below the cerebral average. In addition to this, the cerebral energy wants reviving by a fresh toxic dose, and this is followed by another fall; thus the vicious circle is formed in which the patient finds his end.

General Characters of Mental Intoxication.—The following is the *ensemble* of the characters deduced from the study of poisons of the mind:

(1) Toxic insanity is artificial and not organic; heredity and mental conditions modify the symptomatic aspect of the intoxication.

(2) Most mental poisons produce a special acute phenomenon, a simple pathological manifestation, which has received the name of intoxication.

(3) The intellectual disorders produced by this class of poisons are *general*, and affect the whole of the cerebral manifestations, although there is a special localisation for certain poisons, which, however, does not diminish the clinical value of the general disorder; these disorders are of two kinds—excitement and depression; the former is the more common and is generally followed by the latter.

(4) In addition to intoxication, these poisons cause two kinds of mental disorder, some consist in simple disturbance of the normal mental processes, consciousness however being intact; others are constituted by deviation and perversion of the same processes and by loss of consciousness; the latter constitute *toxic insanity*.

(5) *Toxic insanity* is *secondary* insanity. It is *general*, all the departments of the mind taking equal part in it; sometimes the derangement is predominant in certain centres. It is *incoherent* and *proteus-like;* there is no clearly systematic insanity and no logical intellectual disorder; the

conceptions are rapid, diffuse, ill connected and without consistency; there is no tendency to systematisation, and it reminds the observer more of mania than of vesania. It is *polymorphous:* all forms of insanity may be observed not only in two different intoxications but even in the course of one and the same intoxication—sadness, ambition, mysticism, eroticism, and ideas of persecution. It is *hallucinatory:* the hallucinations play a predominant part, affecting all the senses, with preference, however, for *vision;* they are very mobile and fugitive, and impress upon the insane ideas the character of incoherency and instability. Lastly it is *temporary:* nothing but a momentary, acute effervescence, terminating with the elimination of the poison.

(6) Although the insane ideas may assume almost any form, they are in the majority of cases *painful;* the hallucinations, especially the visual ones, are *frightful.* The clinical picture frequently shows the character of *alcoholic insanity,* which is a perfect type of all toxic derangement. When the ideas are gay, and the conceptions happy, the condition will be more a sub-delirious state—a dream—than actual insane disorder.

(7) Prolonged abuse of mental poisons produces definite anatomical lesions, which manifest themselves in a progressive weakening of all the faculties, passing over into *dementia.*

(8) Toxic insanity is almost always complicated with extra-cerebral pathological disorders, indicating that the whole organism takes part in the morbid process. These disorders are spinal (sensory and motor), but all the other functions are liable to be disturbed, frequently in even a predominant manner, showing that the mental disorders are not essential, and that toxic insanity is, strictly speaking, only a symptom—a syndrome—of a general malady.

(9) Lastly, we mention the capital importance of *individual reaction,* which modifies profoundly the clinical picture of one and the same intoxication, and diminishes the clinical value of toxic insanity as a morbid entity, making it only a modification varying according to personal idiosyncrasies.

M. Legrain.

POLYCHOLIA (πολύς, much; χολή, bile.) Excess of bile in connection with mental disorder. Paracholia signifies any abnormality in the secretion of bile, and in accordance with the doctrine of the ancients is closely connected with insanity.

POLYDIPSIA (πολύς, much; δίψα, thirst). Excessive thirst. (Fr. *polydipsie.*)

POLYOPIA, POLYOPSIS (πολύς, many; ὤψ, the eye). Multiplication of images. Sometimes a symptom in hysteria (Charcot). (Fr. *polyopie;* Ger. *Vielsehen.*)

POLYPARÉSIE (Fr.). A term for general paralysis.

POLYPATHIA (πολύς, many; πάθος, disease). The existence of a multiplicity of diseases, mental and bodily. (Fr. and Ger. *polypathie.*)

POLYPHAGIA (πολύς; φαγεῖν, to eat). A synonym of Bulimia (*q.v.*).

POLYPHRASIA (πολύς; φράσις, a saying). A synonym of Logorrhœa (*q.v.*).

POLYPOSIA (πολύς, much; πόσις, a drinking). A term for a passion for drinking. (Fr. *polyposie;* Ger. *Trinksucht.*)

PORENCEPHALUS, PORENCEPHALY (πόρος, a pore; ἐγκέφαλος, brain). A form of brain found in some congenital idiots and fœtus. A large portion of the convolutions and centrum is wanting, so that the ventricle can be seen through the aperture. The commissural fibres being destroyed, idiocy is the result.

POSSESSION.—In olden times anyone suffering from epilepsy or other strange neurotic affection was supposed to be possessed with a devil. The idea is still extant in such phrases as "he behaves like a man possessed." (*See* Obsession.)

POST-APOPLECTIC INSANITY.—**Definition.**—As the term apoplexy has been applied to morbid conditions differing considerably from each other, it is necessary to explain the sense in which it will be here used. Some authorities restrict its application to cases in which there is sudden, nearly or quite complete, and prolonged deprivation of consciousness, with entire, or very considerable, loss of sensation and power of motion, but only when due to sanguineous effusion in or upon the brain. Others, who approve of this definition of symptoms, do not limit the causation to rupture of blood-vessels. But there are many more who employ it with a wider signification, though one which is fully consistent with the origin of the word (ἀπό, from, and πλήσσω, I strike). They describe as apoplectic not only cases presenting the profound symptoms mentioned, but also others in which the chief result of the seizure is a mono- or hemiplegia of sudden development and intra-cranial origin, even though the impairment of consciousness may have been only slight and of short duration. The degree in which consciousness is involved varies greatly, both in depth and duration in different cases; it is, therefore, not a sufficient ground of distinction. In describing the mental disorders following apoplexy, the word will be used in the most comprehensive of these senses. It will not, however, include cases of injury, which occasionally give rise to conditions and symptoms almost identical with those of disease; nor toxic states from self-generated poisons, as in Bright's disease, in which apoplectiform attacks, followed by mental disorder, occasionally occur.

Ætiology. — Effusions of blood from rupture of a blood-vessel, and damage to the brain from embolism or thrombosis are the leading causes of apoplexy and the after disorders of the mind. Obviously, the results, both psychical and somatic, will largely depend on the position and severity of the lesion. A small effusion of blood in the white matter of the occipital or pre-frontal lobe may produce slight and, for the most part, transitory symptoms; a similar effusion in the substance of the pons Varolii will probably cause death in a few minutes. The mental functions may be in complete abeyance, either from the pressure of a clot of blood or from the deprivation of a large area of the brain of its blood supply by the obstruction of a considerable vessel. But unless the plugged vessel is large, consciousness is usually little if at all impaired; or if lost directly after the attack, as happens in exceptional cases, it is quickly restored.

It is especially the artery of the Sylvian fissure, or one or other of its branches, which is most liable to rupture or plugging; though either lesion may occur in any of the other vessels of the brain. Should the patient recover from the primary effects of the seizure, he is exposed to fresh danger during the period of reaction. Then there may be congestion or even inflammation of the cerebral tissue, which may implicate the membranes in varying degree. If this happen there may probably be more definite mental symptoms, as will be explained.

The state of previous nutrition of the brain will exert an important modifying effect on the result. Should the blood-vessels have long been atheromatous, as is common in advancing life, the cerebral tissue may have become defective in constitution, even though no very definite impairment of function, mental, sensory, or motor, may have been obvious. Its resistive power will be weak, so that an effusion of blood or obstruction in a vessel may lead to disturbance in a much wider area than in a brain whose structure was previously healthy.

The influence of heredity is probably in some respects similar to that of senility. Where there is a disposition to mental disease, the substance of the brain, in its intimate composition and arrangement, does not attain the normal standard of development; it more readily gives way to strain or shock; in many cases it does not seem fitted to wear for an average number of years; and, it may be, at a period of life corresponding to that at which the morbid tendency showed itself in the parent, or other ancestor from whom it is derived, that its nutrition becomes more distinctly impaired. Should an apoplectic seizure occur in one so constituted, even though it does not cause important local changes, the disturbing influence which it exercises on the brain, as a whole, may be sufficient to overthrow the weak cerebro-mental stability, and insanity arises.

An abnormal state of the circulation sometimes distinctly influences the mental condition; in some very markedly. The heart's action may have become weak and irregular through the position or extent of the cerebral lesion, or both, especially if it be so situated as to act on the medulla oblongata; or its feebleness and irregularity may be dependent on disease of the heart itself. In such states mere position of the patient will occasionally modify the mental functions. One so affected may be confused and talk incoherently when erect or trying to walk, but comparatively clear and collected in the recumbent posture. The physician now and again sees similar psychical changes in the use of cardiac tonics. Thus, mental confusion and hallucinations will disappear at least for a time under the action of digitalis in steadying and strengthening the circulation through the brain, thereby removing states of congestion due to permanent lesions. This the writer has noticed in sub-acute softening of the brain consequent on a slight apoplectic seizure. It need scarcely be said that the tendency to disorder of the mind will also be increased should the blood itself be in an unhealthy state, charged, for example, with excrementitious matter which the kidneys have failed to remove.

Mere constipation has a bearing on the question. In ordinary cases of insanity, maniacal excitement or melancholic depression is usually intensified by confinement of the bowels, and marked relief to the symptoms often follows the action of a purgative. So in the psychical disturbance of apoplexy—particularly that which is due to occasional general congestive attacks of the brain in some cases of subacute softening—excitement and hallucinations may for a time pass away partially, or entirely when the bowels are freely moved. There is a derivant and depletory effect on the cerebral vessels by the discharge from the intestinal mucous membrane.

The influence of age is shown by its determining some forms of apoplectic seizure rather than others. Thus embolism from valvular disease of the heart, and thrombosis during and after severe attacks of the exanthemata, in post-partum states, and in syphilitic changes in the walls of the blood-vessels, are incident to the earlier decades, and are rare after middle life. The character of the psychical disorder, as will be afterwards explained, is frequently modified by the particular cause in operation.

How far the position of the lesion may determine the form and degree of the mental defects is a subject of great interest and importance. The opinion has been expressed by Bastian and others that tumours and disease, implicating the cortex of the occipital lobes generally, are more apt to be associated with marked disorders of the mind than when they involve any other part of the surface of the brain; and Hughlings Jackson, while concurring in this view, further holds that the derangement is more marked when the morbid condition is of the right rather than of the left side. It is also maintained by Ferrier and other observers that the power of intelligent attention suffers most in damage from any cause to the præ-frontal lobes. However, Bastian himself admits that the cases are not rare in which disease of the occipital lobe gives rise to only slight mental change, and that others occur where bilateral lesions confined to the præ-frontal lobes are attended with considerable weakness of intellect. Upon the whole, it does not appear that our present knowledge warrants any definite conclusions on this point, unless so far as the psychical defect partakes of one or other of the forms of aphasia. These aphasic complications are very important, and will afterwards receive special consideration.

Forms of Mental Disorder.—The mental defects that follow an apoplectic seizure range from a degree scarcely, if at all, appreciable, which may be very brief, to profound and lasting impairment of the faculties of the mind. Some of them occur within a short time after the attack; others, though directly related to it, do not assume their distinct and definite form till a later period. They will be described as primary and secondary.

(1) **Primary Disorder of the Mind.**—In most cases where a patient does not succumb immediately or within a few days to an apoplectic seizure, he gradually emerges first from the coma and then from the remaining stupor, which are usually present when the cause has been cerebral hæmorrhage, and may or may not be present when it has been plugging of one of the main arteries of the brain. The improvement is often slow, and some weeks may elapse before an estimate can be made of the amount of probable permanent damage to the mind; but though slow, the improvement as a rule is steady and uninterrupted, at least up to a certain point. Cases, however, occasionally occur in which after the patient has partially recovered consciousness and the power of speech, if it has been lost, in which he passes into a state of delirious excitement, talking incoherently, and tossing about in bed, so far as the paralysis permits, should any be present. The mental disorder is due to the inflammatory action around the lesion, and to the wider vascular and nervous disturbance to which it gives rise. It is accompanied by a quick pulse and an elevated temperature, which may reach 105° to 108° F., when a fatal termination may be expected. In other patients the acute mental and physical symptoms gradually subside after two or three days, and they pass into a chronic state of more or less mental enfeeblement.

(2) **Secondary Mental Disorders.**—They may be broadly divided into two classes—namely, the various states of mental weakness which do not amount in degree and kind to a condition which in a legal sense might be properly designated insanity; and the disorders which may be so regarded. These will be considered in the above order.

(*a*) **Mental Defects.**—This group includes the psychical weaknesses which follow apoplectic attacks. They differ from the class already noticed in not being dependent on acute action at the seat of lesion, or in the brain generally. They represent the stable, and to a large extent permanent injury to the nervous structures connected with mental action. In some cases the mind as a whole suffers pretty uniformly; in others, certain powers are markedly affected, while the remainder are less, if at all, involved. A general idea may be formed of the proportion in which the leading faculties are weakened by the following study of fifty cases. They were inmates of the infirm wards of a workhouse, and were all hemiplegic. The primary seizure had occurred at least a month before examination, and in several there had been an interval of some years. Twenty-six were men and twenty-four were women. The ages ranged from twenty-five to seventy-two. Care was taken to exclude cases complicated with senile mental changes. No attempt was made to differentiate between those apparently due to effusion of blood and others more probably the result of thrombosis or embolism. Indeed, though there is in a large proportion of patients usually slight but distinct alterations in the mental condition, which suggest the *nature* of the impending attack, before an apoplectic seizure due to thrombosis, after its occurrence the psychical defects do not appreciably differ from those consequent on the rupture of a blood-vessel.

Beginning with *apprehension*, it was found to be fairly quick and clear in 38 cases and dull in 12. This, however, is only applicable to simple remarks and questions which do not require sustained attention. *Memory* was regarded as correct in 19 and impaired in 31. In the latter section impressions produced since the seizure, more particularly, were faint and evanescent. In a few it was slowly improving, apparently *pari passu* with the other symptoms, physical and mental. *Judgment* was obviously affected in 28 cases, and was apparently sound in 22. The tests applied did not go beyond simple subjects, and it is probable that in many of those in whom it had apparently escaped injury it was really somewhat weakened. The *emotional powers* were normal in only 8 cases; they were more or less implicated in 42. The impairment was slight in 5 cases, moderate in 22, and very marked in 15. There was an undue disposition to weep from trifling causes in 20, to laugh in 6, both to laugh and weep in 15. Where the tendency was to weep, even a sympathetic tone of voice accompanying a remark which was not in itself calculated to excite feeling, would in some patients induce a paroxysm of sobbing. One woman would go off into a fit of laughter on a slight smile or shake of the head. Several who suffered from emotional weakness were also very irritable.

It is to be observed that the analysis of these cases probably conveys too unfavourable an idea of the degree in which the mind suffers in apoplexy. They were all of a severe kind and, as mentioned, were accompanied by one-sided palsy. In slighter attacks there are occasionally no apparent after mental effects; but when carefully examined it will be found that the cases which are absolutely free from permanent enfeeblement of mental power are by no means common.

With the lapse of months, or more generally years, a considerable proportion of weak-minded and paralytic patients become slowly feebler in mind and body; they cease to be able to move about and are bedridden; they lose control of the bladder and bowels, and if care be not taken bed-sores form, when death soon closes the scene. A still larger number have a second or third shock, in which they may die, or, if they survive, their condition becomes worse and the end is hastened. The old, it need scarcely be said, are most disposed to rapid degeneration and repeated seizures. The younger patients may recover to a large extent the power both of mind and body; and the recovery will or will not be enduring according to the nature of the cause or causes in operation.

(*b*) **Forms of Insanity.**—It is not uncommon for an apoplectic seizure to be followed by such unsoundness of mind as would warrant confinement in a lunatic asylum. Any of the leading forms of insanity, classified according to the symptoms, may occur. The maniacal disorders are the most common, but they are usually associated with more or less of dementia. Noisy excitement and incoherence, hallucinations and illusions, destructiveness and filthy habits, may all be features of the mania. Generally the paroxysm does not last longer than two or three weeks, but in some cases it is much more protracted. Sometimes it assumes the recurrent form; there may be an interval of a fortnight or so during which the patient is calm and nearly rational, but afterwards the mania returns as before. Melancholic depression may occupy the interval, and the condition approximates to that of circular insanity. Some patients are fairly reasonable in their conduct and what they say during the day, but talk nonsense and are noisy at night. Occasionally melancholia is the form, and is maintained throughout the entire attack, with or without a distinct suicidal disposition. The mental disorder, whether mania or melancholia, may follow quite a slight apoplectic seizure within a few days of its occurrence; or the patient may have emerged from the coma and stupor, and have been apparently rational for a time before the symptoms of derangement make their appearance.

In some cases there is a more gradual development of mental unsoundness corresponding to a comparatively slow increase of softening due to thrombosis and the amount of the associated cerebral disturbance. The following case illustrates this variety. An acute man of business had a slight apoplectic attack, inducing spasms and ultimately paralysis of the left side. His mind was not appreciably affected till about three weeks after the onset. Within another month psychical disturbance, beginning with mistakes in the days of the week and in identifying people, had developed into a mild mania. He saw imaginary forms and even threw articles at them. He talked confusedly and occasionally displayed considerable irritability with emotional weakness. This condition subsided to a large extent after about a fortnight, though it occasionally recurred in less degree till his death about two months afterwards.

Persistent delusional insanity may be the form of derangement. Thus, a woman about forty years of age, who had been long insane and paralytic on the left side of the body, was in the habit of bitterly denouncing the officials of the asylum for being privy to tortures by electricity which she declared were inflicted on her.

A progressive dementia with emotional weakness, and in some cases, occasional periods of excitement, is a common condition after apoplectic seizures of considerable severity. The majority of such cases among the poor gravitate into the infirm wards of the workhouse; some are certified as insane and spend their remaining days in asylums. There is little or no difference between the two classes, except that the latter are occasionally more noisy and troublesome than the former. The wreck of mind is much the same in them both.

Apoplexy in the Insane.—There is often considerable mental change in an insane person after an attack of apoplexy. Troublesome and demonstrative monomaniacs not unfrequently become quieter and more manageable. There is no improvement, however, but rather the contrary; they have sunk to a lower mental level. But there are instances where a mild dement changes into a noisy, destructive lunatic. Here, too, the psychical state has altered for the worse.

The Relations of Aphasia to Insanity.—One of the most serious consequences of an apoplectic attack is the occurrence of the condition which bears the name of aphasia (*ἀ*, neg.; *φάσις*, speech). In describing its relations to mental disease, a brief account of its various forms will be given at the outset, so that the manner and degree in which the mind is involved may be more clearly shown. The term will be used in its most general acceptation to include all varieties of partial or complete loss of language or power of expression, when these are of cortical origin or at least due to lesions situated on a higher plane than the centres immediately related to the muscles by whose action thought is communicated to others, whether by vocal sounds or otherwise. Many of these defects differ materially from each other, but they may be all grouped in three divisions, namely—

(1) **Motor aphasia**; (2) **Sensory aphasia**; (3) **Mixed forms.**

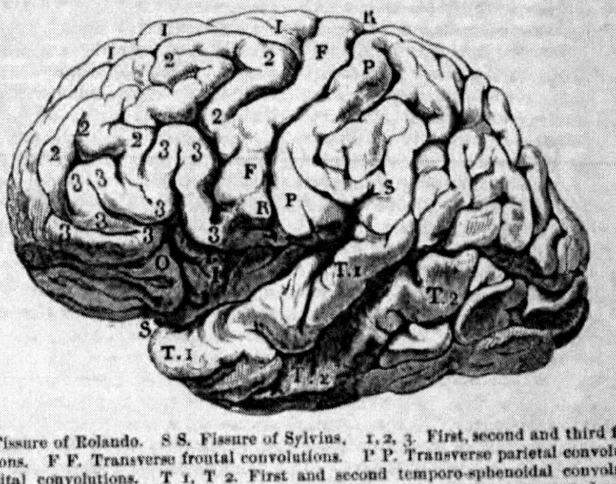

R R. Fissure of Rolando. S S. Fissure of Sylvius. 1, 2, 3. First, second and third frontal convolutions. F F. Transverse frontal convolutions. P P. Transverse parietal convolutions. O O. Orbital convolutions. T 1, T 2. First and second temporo-sphenoidal convolutions. I. Island of Reil (the superior and inferior marginal convolutions are represented as being drawn asunder so as to expose it).

We are indebted to Dr. Bateman for the use of this block, to which a special interest attaches, as it was sent to him by his friend, the late Prof. Broca, to illustrate the work on Aphasia, to which the Academy of Medicine has awarded the Alvarenza Prize for the year 1891.

(1) **Motor Aphasia.**—In uncomplicated cases of this kind the patients can understand what is said to them, they can read and comprehend written or printed words and also the language of signs. They are, however, unable to communicate their thoughts to others by speech, and in most cases also by writing. But the majority make use of a most expressive pantomime to convey their meaning. It is probable that in these cases the highest centres for the co-ordination of the nervous incitations for words spoken or written, or the channels for the transmission of these incitations to the lower centres directly connected with the nerves for the muscles involved, are specially if not alone implicated. The lesion is therefore motor in its nature; and there seems at first sight no sufficient reason why the mental powers should be distinctly impaired. The patient's organs for the reception of the impressions which give rise to language are not damaged, and those parts of the cortex on which previous impressions coming through the sensory nerves, particularly those of hearing and sight, were registered, are probably nearly in their normal condition.

The writer is of opinion that in thinking, words in most cases are revived in the sensory area of the convolutions. But he also holds that in their reproduction they are ordinarily accompanied by faint motor intuitions, which, in rare cases, especially in people who *speak* their thoughts, apart from conversation, may be so distinct as to be sufficient instruments for reasoning, independent of auditory revivals. In accordance with this view words in the motor aphasic may revive in consciousness much as before, though probably bereft of their non-essential motor accompaniment, and so far as verbal reproductions are concerned, there is no apparent impediment to the exercise of thought. That such patients really have the use of words will appear from a consideration of such acts as evince a process of reasoning in their execution. For thought *in the sense of reasoning* cannot be carried out without words, or, as in the case of trained deaf-mutes, without conscious motor intuitions of finger-language. This is the opinion of most metaphysicians, so far as words are concerned (Hegel, Mill, Schelling, Dugald Stewart, Condillac, Warburton, &c.). So eminent a philologist as Max Müller is very decided on the point; he says, "thought in one sense of the word—*i.e.*, in the sense of reasoning, is impossible without language." Assuming the soundness of this conclusion, it is only necessary to consider carefully the acts of patients suffering from this form of aphasia to enable us to determine if they have the use of words. It requires very little observation to satisfy the observer that their ordinary conduct is reasonable and in all respects correct. Indeed, cases are on record where the patients have succeeded in conveying instructions to others by gestures for the conduction of important business. This almost certainly indicates reasoning. But caution is here necessary. Accustomed acts even of a complicated kind cannot be taken as absolutely sure evidence of distinct reasoning on the part of the actor. The skilled musician plays intricate music while his mind is otherwise occupied. The chronic lunatic does excellent work at tailoring or shoemaking, or takes part in games, which he had learned and practised when of sound mind, even though his speech is now incoherent, and his replies to simple questions are irrelevant. So, many occupations, perhaps difficult to learn, when once their details have become thoroughly familiar require but little exercise of thought. The accustomed circumstances or combination of circumstances at once suggest wonted conclusions, and action, semi-automatic, follows in due course. The slight thinking necessary may perhaps not be more in many cases than can be carried out without the use of words.

A better way to ascertain the presence or absence of words in the minds of motor aphasics, and at the same time the condition of their reasoning powers, is to ask them to show by act or gesture what would be their course of procedure in certain circumstances, infrequent in their experience, and, as far as possible, out of the ordinary beaten path. Thus, the writer has asked a female patient to show what she would do if the nurse's arm were bleeding. She thought for a little, then went up to the nurse and began to wrap a piece of cloth round the arm, meanwhile, making signs that the bleeding would be stopped by that means. To another patient he said, "Show me what you would do if that bed were on fire." She went to the end of the ward, lifted a basin of water off the table, brought it to the bedside and indicated very clearly that she would pour the contents on the burning clothing. By questions and requests of this kind, varying, however, in different cases according to the social position, education, and other points, a very fair idea may be formed of the condition of the reasoning faculty and moral powers. The general faculty of memory has been proved to be good by asking patients, after the lapse of a number of weeks, to repeat what they did at the previous examination, no reference having been made to the subject in the interval: they have done the same things, after a little reflection, without the questions being put to them anew.

The conclusion which careful consideration, based on an inquiry conducted in this way, warrants, is that attention, perception, and memory are frequently not appreciably impaired, and moreover that the moral faculty and reasoning power are retained in some cases very fully. As a corollary to the preservation of the power of sustained thinking, words are not lost to the mind; the patients, though speechless, are not wordless.

It is improbable, however, that in any case the capacity for continuous thought is in no respect impaired. No doubt, as stated, the disability is motor, but motor intuitions, though quite unexpressed, arise in consciousness while thought is proceeding, and it is difficult to conceive that the mechanism for their production should be destroyed without the power of thinking also suffering to some extent. The defect will be greatest in those who have been in the habit of faintly or more distinctly articulating while reading or thinking, in order to make the subject-matter of their thoughts easier for their comprehension.

Cases of uncomplicated motor aphasia, though not rare, are far from being common. It is much more usual to find it associated with the sensory form; and in this combination it will again come before us. There still remain for consideration, from a mental point of view, two important varieties belonging to the first group, to which attention will now be directed.

(a) *Aphemia* (ἀ, neg.; φημί, I speak).—As already mentioned, most motor aphasics are unable to express their ideas either by speaking or writing. There are some, however, but not many, who, though unable to speak, except perhaps a few words or phrases, which they often do not use intelligently, have no difficulty in communicating with others by writing. A patient of the writer's, a man about twenty-three years of age, was in the habit of carrying a small slate with him on which he wrote his remarks in conversation. It was clear that he had a free if not a full use of words, though he had almost entirely lost the power of articulate speech. His general conduct was correct, and produced the impression that he was of fair intelligence and unimpaired moral sense. There are all degrees of this defect, ranging from a slight inability to express the last part of a long sentence, to absolute incapacity to utter a single word. The remarks already made on the state of the mental faculties in ordinary motor aphasia and the method of determining it are equally applicable to this variety of the disease.

(b) *Agraphia* (ἀ, neg.; γράφω, to write).—The existence of complete, uncomplicated agraphia without some other defect in the expression of language is doubtful, though one or two cases are on record where there was a near approach to it. But it is not by any means uncommon to meet with patients whose power of expression by writing has suffered to a much greater extent than by vocal speech, independent altogether of the paralysis of the arm. As patients in this condition retain to a large extent the power of speech, there is no difficulty in ascertaining the state of their minds. Any psychical defect which may be present is related to the accompanying loss of language, even though that may be slight, rather than to the inability to communicate by writing.

(2) **Sensory Aphasia.**—In a well-marked case of this form of aphasia, the patient can comprehend only very imperfectly, if at all, any remark that may be made to him. If asked to do some simple act, such as to hold up his hand, he fails to do so, unless the request be accompanied by a suggestive gesture, when he may perhaps comply, but without intelligence. He can in general mechanically repeat words emphatically spoken in his hearing, and there may be no hesitation in their expression; but a minute afterwards he cannot tell what he was asked to say. This is the condition to which the term "amnesia" has been applied.

It is clear that in this state the mind is much more deeply involved than in uncomplicated motor aphasia. The two great channels, hearing and sight, for the transmission of impressions from without that add to knowledge and give rise to thought, are still open, but the receiving mechanism—the part of the cortex of the brain in connection with these senses—is no longer perfect, and has perhaps been seriously damaged. New impressions can, therefore, be only imperfectly received, and perhaps not at all.

It may be here remarked, parenthetically, that the fact of an association between the auditory and optic nerves, and definite areas of the cortex, at least in their most distinctly psychical relations, if not established, is rendered highly probable by the results of post-mortem examinations. These have shown that where words are not apprehended, the lesion involves the upper temporo-sphenoidal convolution, and that a corresponding failure to recognise visual impressions points to a morbid change in the occipito-angular region. In a case under the writer's observation, where the symptoms corresponded closely to the description above given, more especially in the absence of intelligent apprehension of what the patient either saw or heard, complete destruction of the greater part of the parietal lobe, most of the upper temporo-sphenoidal convolution, and the back part of the frontal lobe, was found after death.

But it might be expected that the registration of previous impressions would be in the same district of the brain, and that damage to it would prevent or interfere with their revival in consciousness, as well as with the perception of those that are new. This seems really to happen in a large proportion of the sufferers. Sensory aphasics, though they may probably perform simple habitual acts as of old, give no indications by signs or in any other way of silent thought, at least, such thought as implies reasoning. No other result could be anticipated. The area of the surface of the brain, where, as stated, there is good reason to believe, that impressions from the two chief senses are received and recorded, has suffered damage or, as in the case referred to, been destroyed. We have seen that the revival of these impressions, more particularly those of spoken language, is necessary for sustained thought; consequently, a lesion of that part of the cortex must interfere with or prevent a reproduction of auditory or visual symbols in consciousness. Continuous thought or reasoning is therefore not possible to one in this condition.

The severe form of sensory aphasia, to which the foregoing remarks are applicable, is by no means uncommon, though it is not often seen in an extreme degree. The patient has generally the use of a number of words which, however, are uttered in a haphazard or recurring way, with, as a rule, little or no bearing on the observation that may have been made to him. If the lesion has been less severe, some meaning may be picked out of the disjointed expressions. The function of the more purely motor mechanism not being appreciably injured, words, as mentioned, may be repeated correctly, or nearly so, immediately after they are spoken to the patient; but there is no reason to think they are more than automatic utterances that do not enter into consciousness.

The degree to which the mind suffers appears to correspond very much with the extent of the actual loss of language, especially words. Should that be small, the patient's intelligence may be little impaired, but, if great, thought may be in abeyance. The patient may still respond to and be conscious of impressions that come to him from any of the other senses, such as touch or the muscular sense, but these, though they may give rise to *concepts*, are not by themselves sufficient to maintain continuous thought.

Just as in motor aphasia, there are partial defects, one channel of expression being free while the other is blocked, so in the sensory form either of the two main areas in the cortex for the reception of impressions may alone be affected. Thus there is a word-deafness and a word-blindness.

(*a*) *Word-deafness.*—In the complete and isolated development of this condition the patient hears the sound of any one's voice, and may even recognise the words, but fails to understand the meaning of what is said, however simple the remark. At the same time his perception of what he sees or feels, or of other sense-impressions, is normal. He can also converse, and his command of language may not be greatly impaired. He has no difficulty in the expression of words.

It is not a common condition, apart from other defects. There are all degrees of the affection. In illustration of a minor one, the case of a gentleman may be mentioned, who spoke to the writer about an inability he had in understanding the meaning of words. He was a highly intelligent, energetic man of business, about fifty-five years of age. "I hear quite well," he remarked, "all that is said, but the words sound strange; I cannot understand them as formerly." He spoke with fluency and gave a clear account of his condition, besides conversing on other subjects without hesitation. His disorder was almost entirely subjective, for there was scarcely any flaw to be detected in his power of apprehension during the interview.

This case may be regarded as the slightest of its kind. Many patients, besides being unable to understand clearly what is said, as in that instance, are unable to recall words, especially names and nouns generally. In them the power of reviving old impressions of articulate sounds as well as that of receiving those that are new is impaired.

The state of the mind in word-deafness has already been referred to when considering sensory aphasia generally. It is only necessary to add that the degree of mental defect will be modified by the extent to which the individual when in health was dependent for his knowledge on visual rather than on auditory impressions, and also on the amount of help he derived from silent articulations in thinking. There are persons whose perceptions of objects they see are exceptionally vivid, some of whom have the remarkable power of being able to project their visual percepts into space, and avow to have scenes and objects before them as clearly as when they saw them in reality, though that may have been many years before. The writer had an experience under the influence of medicine, which he may mention in illustration. He had taken a good deal of opium to relieve pain, and while under the action of the drug, which lasted for about three days after its administration was stopped, he was annoyed by the almost constant presence on the wall of the room of varying figures and landscapes, most of the latter being very beautiful. Some were American scenes, and were reproduced nearly in the form he had seen them thirteen years previously; others he failed to recognise. It is evident that if any one whose optical impressions in health are unusually clear and definite should suffer from word-deafness, involving the power of recollection, his visual mental revivals may furnish him with subjects of thought in greater degree than the average of people. His mind will be so much the richer for their possession, and from their distinctness they may be more readily called into consciousness in the absence of auditory percepts: they will thus help to compensate for the lack of the latter.

So, too, those who, in reading, either faintly articulate or distinctly pronounce what they read, and also such individuals as are much given to "thinking aloud," will probably suffer less mentally than others, for they may have the use of motor intuitions representing words, revived in motor areas, by means of which sustained thought may be possible to them. Their condition in fact approximates to that of the trained deaf-mute who, as previously stated, thinks by means of motor symbols derived from the movements of the fingers, internally reproduced.

(*b*) *Word-blindness.*—In a typical case of this variety the patient understands what is said to to him and can express his ideas correctly by speech. He may even be able to communicate his thoughts by writing. But though vision is perfect he cannot understand the meaning of words that he sees, whether they be written or printed. He may even fail to recognise individual letters. It is often part of a more general disorder, which has been named mind-blindness; but it occurs occasionally, though not often, in an isolated form. There is no difficulty in determining the condition of the patient's mind, as he has considerable, if not the full, use of language, and can converse much as before his illness. There may be clear mental loss should the lesion interfere with the power of reviving in the mind general visual images, as the ability to think on subjects into which they enter must necessarily suffer materially. But more particularly, the injury to the mind will be much greater if the patient have acquired the habit of thinking to a large extent by the revived visual impressions of words either printed or written, rather than by revived auditory impressions. This will happen to recluses or, generally, those who converse little or do not hear much spoken speech, and store their minds with knowledge derived from books. Their loss will be much more serious than that of the unlettered patient whose knowledge has been acquired through the sense of hearing. (*See* MIND BLINDNESS.)

(3) **Mixed Forms.**—Motor and sensory aphasia may be variously combined. In a large proportion, probably the majority of aphasics, there is, during the early period of their illness, almost complete loss of language, and also of the power of expressing what little remains. This holds true of cases which ultimately resolve themselves into simple motor aphasia; for a time the function of the sensory areas is also in abeyance, even though they may be free from organic lesion. This, however, is only a part of the shock which the brain generally, and especially its most complex part, has received, through the damage to an important section of it.

There are other cases in which the sufferer has the command of a very considerable amount of language and can freely express it, but the words are so utterly disconnected that the name *gibberish* aphasia has been applied to the condition. In one recorded case of this kind, the patient is stated to have understood spoken and written remarks and to have been able to write his thoughts correctly, seldom making a mistake. His mental powers, as a whole, were considered to have escaped injury, notwithstanding the jargon of his speech. It may be supposed that the association-fibres between the sensory and motor regions, rather than these parts themselves, are the special seat of lesion in this state.

Summary of the Mental Condition.—In simple uncomplicated motor aphasia, affecting both speech and writing, there is evidence of fair intelligence and no indication of marked defect in judgment. Care, however, requires to be exercised in judging these cases, lest too favourable an estimate be formed of the mental powers by the performance of familiar acts, which, having become largely automatic, do not evince the exercise of fresh thought. Indeed, in the great majority of these cases, careful examination and inquiry will show that the patient does not possess as much mental vigour and decision of character as he had previous to his illness. It is also to be noted that in proportion to the degree that motor intuitions enter into thought, varying much as they do in different persons, so will the lesion in this form of the disorder exert a corresponding disturbing influence on the reasoning faculty.

The interference with mental action in pure cases of aphemia or agraphia (if it occur) ought to be even less than is usual in complete motor aphasia, as only one of the channels for the expression of language is blocked, instead of both. This, as shown in the account of the former of these conditions, appears to be so, as aphemics manifest both intelligence and force of character.

In complete sensory aphasia there is profound affection of the mind. In almost all cases reasoning is not practicable owing to the obliteration of auditory and visual percepts, though a degree of thought may be possible to some patients by the exercise of the motor intuitions of speech or of writing. In the majority, however, the lesion is incomplete, and one sense is usually involved more than the other. Should it be that of hearing which is specially implicated, the mind generally suffers much more than where the visual sense is chiefly affected.

In word-blindness and word-deafness, if the defect be limited to the reception of new impressions, and the faculty of recollection be retained in full or little diminished vigour, the reasoning power and judgment may not be appreciably affected. This will be evident from the patient's conversation, the capacity for which is retained. However, cases in which the defect is so restricted are exceedingly rare. There is generally also some impairment of the memory of words, and then the mental power is more or less enfeebled.

These are briefly the mental conditions in the leading forms of aphasia. It will be observed that the most important defects, consist in partial or complete loss of the reasoning faculty, and that this corresponds closely with the extent of the loss of words, whether associated with the sense of hearing or of sight, but particularly the former. Judgment is weakened, not disordered. There are no illusions, hallucinations, or delusions. Should any of these be present, the case is not one of simple aphasia. There may be aphasia with insanity; but this is not common, unless as an incident in the course of mental disease. Reference will afterwards be made to this combination. The moral powers are not disordered or weakened, except in so far as they may be affected by the enfeeblement of the intellect. As a rule, there is no excitement of feeling, nor is there depression, at least not more than might be expected in one who appreciates the serious character of the disease from which he suffers. In some cases there is emotional weakness, but it is not so marked as in cases of hemiplegia, either left or right, especially the former, which are not associated with aphasia.

Civil Responsibility in Aphasia.—From the foregoing account of the diverse mental states in the various forms of aphasia, it will be inferred that the responsibility of patients for their acts must vary greatly. The motor aphasic, retaining reasoning power almost entirely, is an accountable agent, whereas the sensory aphasic, if the disorder be complete, and involve both auditory and visual cortical areas, cannot reason, and is therefore irresponsible. It is very different with the minor defects, word-deafness and word-blindness. In some cases of the former, such as in that of the writer's already referred to, it would be difficult to show ground for the reduction of the person's responsibility for a criminal act. And yet one might well hesitate to maintain that a derangement involving a part of the brain intimately connected with the revival of word-symbols, the very instruments of thought, even though the abnormality were scarcely noticeable by the observer, would have no disturbing influence on the reasoning faculty.

The uncertainty respecting the mental condition in slight forms of the disorder is greater in recent cases than in those of long standing. In the latter, active physical disease may have ceased for years, a small healed lesion exists, but exerts no disturbing influence on the neighbouring healthy tissues, which have accommodated themselves to the loss. There is some but no great defect in language, and apart from it normal psychical processes are not interrupted. On the other hand, should the disorder be of recent origin, its perturbing effect will probably extend much more widely than the area of definite morbid change of structure, and consequently the general mental equilibrium may be markedly upset for a time.

How the degree of mental deficiency may be best ascertained is obviously a matter of great importance. The apparently intelligent aspect of countenance and gestures are apt to mislead in many cases. The patient may seem to understand what is said, when a little observation will probably show that his comprehension has been very imperfect. Some idea of the person's mental condition will of course be formed by a study of his conduct. But, as explained, a better estimate may be made of the state of the reasoning powers and moral faculties by subjecting him to the test of a carefully considered series of orders and requests. In further illustration of the method of determining the condition of the sense of right and wrong, it may be stated that one of the patients referred to was asked what she would do if the nurse were to steal her shawl. She smiled, seized the nurse by the arm, and shook her fist very significantly. After this manner it may be practicable to find out the patient's views of dishonesty generally, and also his opinion of attacks on the person of others—subjects in connection with which the question of responsibility is most likely to arise.

The doctrine of modified responsibility with mitigated punishment is very applicable to aphasics. In regard to it they stand on similar ground to some of the insane. Fortunately several medico-legal trials of late years have shown that its soundness is becoming gradually recognised both by judges and the general public in certain cases of mental defect due to insanity, either congenital or acquired. Probably the risk in motor-aphasia may more generally be to hold the accused, when guilty of criminal acts less responsible than they actually are. A prisoner at the bar, speechless or only able to ejaculate yes or no, or an oath or two under emotion, would be very apt to impress the jury and court with the idea that his reasoning power was much weaker than a careful study of his condition would show. At the same time it is doubtful if in any case of that kind, however slight, the sufferer should be considered fully responsible for his acts; though on the other hand there are very many who should not be allowed to escape without punishment for their crimes.

Aphasia in the Insane.—A considerable number of the insane are more or less aphasic. The defect in language or speech or both, occurs in the congenital as well as the acquired forms of mental disease. There are profoundly dementated patients who seem absolutely to have lost all language, except perhaps a few words which they repeat in a parrot-like way, and with scarcely so much intelligence as that animal sometimes shows. In low types of idiocy a very similar condition exists. The unfortunate youths, though neither deaf nor dumb in the ordinary sense, notwithstanding all efforts at tuition, attain maturity without having acquired language of any kind, their only vocal expression being inarticulate cries; or in less severe cases they may have learned a few simple words.

The sensory defect is probably much in excess of the motor in most of these cases. Both the innate and post-natal forms are, however, only part of a wider and probably deeper morbid condition of the cortex of both hemispheres, in connection with which the general mental deficiency dwarfs and overshadows the aphasic element of its constitution. ALEX. ROBERTSON.

POST-CONNUBIAL INSANITY.—The mental excitement of marriage culminating in sexual excitation, often excessive, is liable to act as an exciting cause of insanity in an individual predisposed to mental affection. Sometimes an epileptic fit occurs. (*See* MARRIAGE AND INSANITY, ASSOCIATION BETWEEN.)

POST-EPILEPTIC AUTOMATISM (*post*, after; epilepsy (*q.v.*); *αὐτόματος*, acting spontaneously).—This is a name given to a series of phenomena occurring in certain individuals immediately after an epileptic seizure, and more commonly after those forms known and described as *petit mal*. It consists of involuntary motor performances which may range from extremely simple and objectless movements to advanced complex and apparently purposive acts; from interjectional speech utterances to connected sentences; from mild emotional displays to outbursts of ungovernable fury and passion. The degree of the epileptic seizure appears to bear some relationship to the range and complexity of the actions, as they are more intense after slight fits and *vice versâ*, but this rule is by no means constant. The wild and aimless clutching at persons and objects, sometimes observed in the immediate post-epileptic state, the frequent involuntary change of position from the supine to the prone, a serious automatic movement in which the patient may become suffocated, the purposeless gesticulations, the uncalled-for laughter or weeping, the efforts, in some cases violent, made by the patient to unclothe himself, to bite and scratch, to get up, to walk to and fro, to repeat some set word or phrase, these and kindred phenomena are easily to be recognised as indications of the milder less complex condition of post-epileptic automatism. The motor automatism may, as it were, assume an explosive character, taking the form of convulsive hysterical attacks immediately after a true epileptic seizure, either of the *grand* or *petit mal* type; this is commonly found in young women or men afflicted with epilepsy, whose mental instability is of a hysteric type, but by whom hysterical manifestations are ordinarily not obtruded, the fit being succeeded by a violent spasmodic convulsion accompanied or followed by unconscious acts, such as stamping, clapping the hands, acts of indecency, aggressiveness, &c. The more deliberate complex post-epileptic involuntary acts are of an extremely interesting nature, both from a clinical as well as from a medico-legal point of view. A patient will, after a *petit mal* attack, sometimes so extremely slight in degree as hardly to be perceptible, proceed either to acts foreign to his usual habit (*e.g.*, he will pilfer or secrete articles of little value to himself, will attack a bystander, destroy property, shout, sing, gesticulate, commit indecencies, &c.), or to quiet rational systematic actions which to an ordinary observer appear premeditated, voluntary, and responsible (*e.g.*, he will engage himself in his ordinary occupations, will indulge in a long walk, or even unclothe himself and jump into the water, &c.). Crimes of a serious nature, such as murder, arson, &c., have undoubtedly been committed by patients while in this condition. The period of duration of these motor phenomena is very variable, extending from a few seconds to, in rare cases, some hours; in the less complex forms the automatic acts are constantly repeated after each fit, but the more highly developed actions do not appear to recur so consistently. It is not easy to distinguish these motor phenomena from the motor automatism of larvated epilepsy, but in the former, the seizure, however slight, can, as a rule, be recognised to be an antecedent phenomenon, though the patient himself may subsequently be unconscious of having had a fit. Undoubtedly, the condition may be feigned by educated persons, but in such the complex acts will usually be found to be too purposive in character, a motive can usually be discovered to underlie the deed, and they will, on close questioning, betray their consciousness of the act itself. The automatism has been attributed by Hughlings Jackson and others to a temporary loss of controlling power of the highest over the next grade of nerve centres, so that the loss of inhibitory control over the motor centres results in the independent action of the latter. The condition being correlated to epilepsy and due thereto shares in its general treatment. (*See* EPILEPSIES AND INSANITIES, EPILEPSY AND INSANITY.)

J. F. G. PIETERSEN.

POST - EPILEPTIC INSANITY. (*See* EPILEPSY AND INSANITY.)

POST-FEBRILE INSANITY.—The name given by Dr. Skae to the insanity which sometimes occurs during exhaustion following fevers.

The occurrence of insanity as a sequel or complication of acute disease has been observed by many writers, among whom may be mentioned Westphal, Foville, Delasiauve, Christian, Webber, Sée, Cormack, Jaccoud, Sydenham, Graves, Burrows, Hermann, Baillarger, Thore, Griesinger, Greenfield, Tuke, Savage, Clouston, Mickle and others. Mental disorder may occur during any part of an acute febrile disease. It may appear:

(1) **As the earliest symptoms;**

(2) **During a later stage; or,**

(3) **More commonly toward the termination or period of convalescence.**

Dr. Bristowe has recorded a case of acute mania occurring as the earliest symptom of typhoid fever, and Dr. Murchison has noted three similar cases (Greenfield). Thore has given an account of an outbreak of acute mania preceding pneumonia, and Dr. Greenfield the occurrence of melancholia followed by general excitement, with hallucinations of sight and hearing, appearing and subsiding *pari passu* with an attack of pneumonia. The symptomatic delirium or febrile delirium is often difficult to distinguish from true insanity, and almost any of the affective states of mental disorder may be completely simulated in febrile delirium. According to Greenfield, "the intensity of the fever alone forms no criterion, from the more frequent association of delirium with prostration, and certain other conditions of the system;" this difficulty however, is somewhat lessened as the period of commencing recovery or convalescence is reached.

Nasse* has classified the mental affections originating in fever according as they are (1) the immediate result of the fever itself; or (2) as they constitute a prolongation of the delirium when the fever has subsided; or (3) as they arise during convalescence. With regard to the first two conditions we are in want of

* Bucknill and Tuke, "Manual of Psychological Medicine," p. 371.

data; the relation of high temperature to delirium is unknown.* Here we have chiefly to do with the consideration of the third group, which includes by far the greater number of cases of true vesania. The forms of acute disease commonly followed by insanity are the specific infectious fevers (Greenfield), intermittent fevers and long agues, especially if they be quartan, and this forms *sui generis* a peculiar form of mania (Sydenham),† erysipelas (Baillarger, Boyle), acute pyrexia of phlogoses (Voisin), articular rheumatism (Jaccoud, Contesse), acute angina, diphtheria, erythema nodosum, miliary roseola, purpura, febrile urticaria, guttural herpes, and others (Gubler).‡ Of the forms of acute disease enteric fevers, pneumonia, and rheumatism are nearly on an equality as causes.

At present we are not in a position to say whether the forms of insanity bear any definite relation to the nature of the febrile disease; nor do we know the relative frequency of the forms of mental disorder after any particular class of diseases. According to Thore,§ the commonest form of insanity consists in the sudden onset of acute maniacal delirium, characterised by great agitation with hallucinations of sight and hearing, its duration varying from fifteen hours to three or four days, and the termination often occurring as abruptly as the onset. This form occurs chiefly after rapid acute diseases, such as pneumonia and tonsillitis, and much more rarely after typhoid fever (Greenfield). A table of the relative frequency of the various forms of insanity has been compiled by Christian, and quoted by Greenfield. Christian found, that out of 114 cases, 4 had isolated insane ideas, 15 hallucinations, 34 mania or maniacal agitation, 8 ambitious delusions (*délire ambitieux*), 16 sadness or melancholia, 27 stupidity, and 10 intellectual weakness or dementia.

Considered *serialim*, after typhoid the cerebral condition may be one of torpor mingled with agitation and hallucinations.* This condition may be transitory, or may pass from melancholia into mania and chronic dementia.† In many of the more chronic cases, especially those which arise early, there is often great moral perversion with extreme irritability of temper,‡ sometimes there is weakened memory or general apathy and failure to form clear conceptions as to the objective significance of things. In one case at present in Bethlem there is complete failure to grasp the environment, together with some confusion and anergia. Delasiauve§ has described ambitious monomania as occurring temporarily during the period of decline of mild typhoid fever in a female aged twenty-three. Similar cases have been related by Christian‖ and Simon. A case of *délire ambitieux* in a male aged twenty-one during convalescence has also been described by Liouville.¶ A form of insanity has been described by many writers, in which there are many physical symptoms closely resembling those of general paralysis. These symptoms may be affections of the speech, or ataxy of movement. The speech is slow with deliberate drawing; the syllables are articulated in a monotonous tone, and with a nasal twang.** The affections of the motor system may further be evidenced by muscular weakness, with or without tremors or tremblings of lips, facial muscles, or even limbs.†† Westphal has described also a peculiar trembling of the head when unsupported, in a case in which there were no lip tremors, and in which sensation was unaffected. The pathology of this condition is little known. In chronic cases which have died in asylums, anæmia of the brain, or atrophy of the cortical substance, opacity of the pia mater, and excess of the sub-arachnoid fluid, have been found. Jaccoud ascribes the paraplegia following typhoid to congestion of the cord.

After typhus the character of the mental disturbance is not unlike that following typhoid. Greenfield is of opinion that there is more frequently some moral perversion than mania with distinct delusions or hallucinations. This observation is not confirmed by others. Thore says the most frequent sequents are, dementia, general maniacal delirium, continuous

* McDowall has reported a case of typhoid fever with physical and mental symptoms of "typical" general paralysis whilst the fever lasted, *Journal of Mental Science*, July 1881, p. 279. Dr. Savage has also seen a case of high temperature in a youth aged twenty-one, affected with ulcerated sore throat and a diffuse syphilitic rash, in which there were, in addition, mental symptoms such as restlessness, excitability, change of disposition and refusal of food. This case was of interest on account of the concomitance of the mental symptoms and the high temperature.

† See MALARIA.

‡ *Archives Gén. de Méd.*, 1860, t. i. pp. 257, 402, 534, 693; t. ii. pp. 137, 718; 1861, t. i. p. 301. Mickle, "General Paralysis," 2nd ed. p. 240.

§ *Annales Méd.-Psych.*, April and Oct. 1856.

* Delasiauve, *Annales Méd.-Psych.*, July 1849.

† Griesinger, "Mental Pathology" (Syd. Soc. trans.); also *Arch. d. Heilk.*, 1860.

‡ Greenfield, *St. Thos.'s Hosp. Reports.*

§ *Ann. Méd. Psych.*, 1850, p. 148.

‖ *Archives Gén. de Méd.*, 1873, t. ii. pp. 257, 421.

¶ *Ann. Méd. Psych.*, 1879, t. i. p. 428.

** Westphal, *Arch. f. Psych. u. Nervenkrank.* 1872, iii. 2.

†† Christian, *Arch. Gén. de Méd.*, Sept. and Oct. 1873.

or intermittent, and of varying duration, with or without hallucinations of the senses, or partial insanity, monomania, or ambitious monomania. The onset of acute transitory mania may occur during the early stages of convalescence, and this is believed by some to be due to some sudden change in the cerebral circulation. Weber calls this the "delirium of collapse," and states that with the symptoms of prostration the pulse is feeble, rapid, and irregular; further, that this condition is common at the period of crisis and may be due to sudden anæmia of the brain from heart failure. Westphal (*Arch. für Psych. u. Nerv.*, Band iii.) and Foville (*Ann. Méd.-Psych.*, January 1873) observed intellectual weakness in relation to variola and typhus, and such symptoms as change in physiognomy, slow clumsy movements, movements by fits and starts, trembling of the limbs, partial or general ataxy of limbs, stiff gait, disorders of speech, impaired deglutition, and in one case loss of the power of sneezing, whilst mentally there was some alteration with excitability. Westphal noted the scanned, nasal and monotonous speech in which the letters and syllables were not displaced, but separated by intervals and uttered jerkily, or with visible efforts, yet, as after typhoid, without co-existing tremblings of the lips and face

Foville, on the other hand, noted the occurrence not only of marked twitchings of the muscles of the face, but also a tendency to convulsive projection of saliva or the return of fluids by the nose during the act of deglutition. The pathology of these conditions is vague. The frequent substitution of convulsions for rigors in children is said to indicate the early implication of the nervous centres, and, according to Greenfield, the acute transitory mania may be the analogue of these convulsions affecting the psychical, instead of the motor, centres. In the early stage of typhus there is said to be an increase of the watery constituents of the white matter in the brain (Buhl). There may be no appreciable organic lesions, the symptoms depending chiefly upon cerebral anæmia, resulting from debility (Trousseau).* The atony, exhaustion, and anæmia of the brain may be furthered by moral shock or debility of the blood (Sydenham), the nutritive defect producing atrophy, serous exudations, &c. The hebetude due to wasting of the nervous matter and nerve tubules (Behier) may also occur after typhus or any of the more severe fevers.

* Clinical Lectures (Syd. Soc. trans.), vol. ii. p. 429.

After the delirium of **smallpox** melancholia with refusal of food and insomnia has been noted by Berti*, and is quoted in the *London Medical Record*, vol. i. p. 135.

Baillarger† has recorded a case of *délire ambitieux* of fifteen days' duration following **scarlatina.**

The most frequent form of insanity after eruptive fevers is said to be maniacal delirium, often with hallucinations. In children the exanthematous diseases play an important part in the ætiology of deafness, and secondarily in the causation of idiocy and imbecility.

Cholera may be followed by transient delirium, paroxysms of mania, or melancholia; but the form does not appear at all definite (Greenfield). In all febrile conditions, insanity arising early and due to toxic conditions of the blood, congestion of the internal organs (including the brain) may occur. These altered vascular conditions may be active or passive, general or partial, chronic or acute. Trousseau‡ would explain the cases of paralysis at the onset of acute disease as arising in one of these ways. Greenfield attributes the mental symptoms in some cases to direct excitation from peripheral irritation, as the influence of pain, organic disease, &c., producing central exhaustion or irritability; or due to reflex irritation, or peripheral irritation acting in a reflex manner, either on the vessels or the nervous tissue itself. Other conditions, such as sub-acute inflammation of the cortical substance or membrane of the brain, capillary embolism, or thrombosis (as in the melanæmia following ague), (Griesinger) have been cited as probable causes. Undoubtedly many of the forms of insanity may be regarded as instances of metastasis. Griesinger has noted instances of insanity alternating with articular rheumatism; Sebastian, with ague; the author, with thrombosis of the cerebral sinuses§ and many others.

Acute **Rheumatic Affections** are not uncommonly followed by mental disturbance. The development of the insanity mostly coincides with the fall of the temperature, cessation of joint affections, and subsidence of the symptoms. Trousseau, Clouston and Griesinger have recorded instances of mania with chorea following rheumatism. The form of the insanity following rheumatic fever is, as a rule, one of depression. In some cases there may be agitation with sensory disturbance, refusal of food, and a tendency to delirium,

* *Giorn Veneto delle Sc. Med.*, Jan. 1873.
† *Ann. Méd.-Psych.*, Jan. 1879, p. 79.
‡ Clinical Lectures (Syd. Soc. trans.).
§ *Brain*, 1886.

but the majority suffer from melancholia with or without hypochondriasis, or there may be some delusions present which gradually pass off or take the character of ideas of persecution. The more severe forms of insanity, such as dementia, paralytic insanity, and general paralysis have been observed but rarely. Affections of the special senses are not uncommon. Jaccoud, Contesse, and Voisin have recorded instances of articular rheumatism leading to general paralysis.

Pneumonia is sometimes followed by insanity, and the tendency to mental disturbance is not proportionate to the severity of the disease. Dr. Webber states that the onset of acute maniacal delirium usually occurs suddenly towards the period of crisis, or early in convalescence, and manifests itself first early in the morning or after waking from sleep. Many of the more chronic forms have no premonitory symptoms, or there may be loss of sleep and want of mental rest.

Any form of insanity may occur at any age associated with **rheumatic affections**. Transitory mania in a child does not generally appear so serious as in an adult (Greenfield). The male sex appears to be mostly affected, and the liability to affection is increased by heredity, previous mental strain, or intemperance.

In addition to the ordinary symptoms of exhaustion following an attack of pneumonia there may be local or general hyperæsthesia, loss of electro-contractility of muscles, and of reflex excitability, paralysis of special nerves or of systems of nerves, various forms of spasm and convulsions, ataxy of movement, hemiplegia or paraplegia. Griesinger has also described a transient form of hemiplegia, and Mickle quotes general paralysis as occurring, but does not give examples.

Other febrile conditions, such as **erysipelas** and **diphtheria** are apt to be followed by various paralyses or insanity. Erysipelas of the face and scalp was assigned by Baillarger as the cause of general paralysis in two cases. Boyle and Voisin have also each observed a similar case.

It is impossible to enter here upon the consideration of the various *paralyses* which follow febrile affections. General paralysis is said to follow typhus, cholera, typhoid, dysentery, diphtheria, pneumonia, articular rheumatism, erysipelas, &c. Localised and diffused paralysis may also follow pneumonia, erysipelas, cholera, dysentery, typhoid, typhus, and the exanthematous fevers, acute angina, diphtheria, erythema nodosum, miliary roseola, purpura, febrile urticaria, guttural herpes, and other disorders. According to Mickle* the diffuse form may be distinguished from general paralysis by the more frequent and obvious preceding anæsthesia, analgesia, numbness, pricking and arthritic pains, and by the circumstance that it often begins in the *velum palati*, almost always undergoes recovery in the space of a few weeks, and is rarely accompanied by intellectual trouble, and he further states that "should the paralysis be diphtheritic (and even in some other cases) it is apt to extend from the *velum palati* to the pharynx, thence to the lower limbs, then sight and hearing become affected, then the upper limbs, and finally the trunk and respiratory muscles, while the premonitory signs mentioned above are often present."†

The diagnosis of these conditions is often attended with extreme difficulty, and it is only late in the course of the disease that its true nature can be ascertained.

The treatment must depend upon the nature of the case. Lowering treatment is seldom efficacious, and not unfrequently the administration of drugs, such as opium, may possibly have had much to do with the excitement. THEO. B. HYSLOP.

POST-MORTEM APPEARANCES. (*See* PATHOLOGY.)

POST-PUERPERAL INSANITY. (*See* PUERPERAL INSANITY.)

POSTURES AND MUSCULAR BALANCE OF THE BODY AS INDICATIONS OF MENTAL STATES.—All writers on expression of the emotions and other mental states agree in ascribing some importance to the postures or attitudes of the body. The artist, in expressing emotion and character, has for centuries depicted on canvas the balance of the body, as well as indications of its movements, its form and proportions. The records of antique art, in the form of ancient statuary, engravings on gems, and the drawings on vases, are valuable indications that human expression centuries ago was much the same as in our day.

A posture of the parts of the body concerns us as a sign of the brain state, it is a result of the last movement, and its change is a movement. The posture indicates a balance of muscular action, and is usually temporary in character. This balance of visible parts corresponds

* "General Paralysis," 2nd edit. p. 241.

† See also Webber, *Trans. Amer. Neur. Assoc.*, vol. ii. For fuller information relating to these various paralyses the reader is referred to the works of Sée, *L'Union Medicale*, Nov. 8, 1886, p. 257; Westphal, *Archiv für Psych. und Nerv.*, Bd. iii. p. 376; Foville, *Ann. Méd. Psych.*, Jan. 1873, pp. 12, 40; Cormack, *Brit. Med. Journ.*, vol. ii. 1874; Jaccoud, *Leçons de Clin. Méd.*, 1886; Whipham and Myers, *Clin. Soc.*, March 12, 1886.

to a condition of nerve-centres in equilibrio, or a given ratio in the amount of force they respectively discharge. In studying postures we observe the outcome of certain ratios of nerve action.

Postures, like movements, may be either "spontaneous," or due to some present stimulation of nerve-centres through the senses; it is the former class that most directly indicates the average balance or condition of the brain. Spontaneous postures, in parts of the body that are free, may be described as indications of emotional and mental states; visible parts must be mechanically free in order that they may be balanced by the governance of the brain, the hand must not be in the pocket, or the back resting against a support; the nerve-centres should also be free, not strongly controlled by impressions from the surroundings at the time of observation.

When about to observe the spontaneous postures assumed in the arms, or upper extremities of a patient, we ask him to stand up and say, "Put out your hands with the palms down, spreading the fingers," speaking in a quiet tone, and not showing our own hands; it is then possible to notice the balance of the body, the head and the spine, the arms and the hands, as well as the movements of these parts. This action in the patient is convenient, leaving the arms and hands free, and ready for observation and description.

There are **four principal postures of the head**—(1) **flexion**, (2) **extension**, (3) **rotation** to one or other side in a horizontal plane, the head remaining erect, but the face being turned to the right or left, (4) **inclination** to one or other side, lowering that ear so that the two do not remain on the same level—inclination is said to be towards that side on which the ear is lowest. The posture may be compound, the head may be flexed, inclined and rotated to the right, or it may be extended and inclined to the left, &c. The head when held erect is in a symmetrical posture, so also when it is flexed or extended; to produce such balance both sides of the brain must act equally and at the same time. If the head be rotated to the right, this indicates more force sent from the left half of the brain than from the right; asymmetry of posture means unequal action of parts of the brain.

The typical hand posture (Fig. 1) seen in health and strength, is **the straight extended hand.** The fingers are straight with the palm of the hand, and on a level with the forearm and shoulder, the palm of the hand or metacarpus is straight and not arched transversely, or contracted as in the feeble hand. All parts are in the same horizontal plane.

The **second** typical posture (Fig. 2) is but a slight deviation from the first, the thumb with its metacarpal bone being drooped, all other parts being in the same plane as before.

The hand in rest (Fig. 3) is the natural posture when it is not being energised by the brain. There is slight flexion of the wrist and fingers, and slight arching of the palm of the hand.

The energetic hand (Fig. 4) is a posture produced under moderately strong brain stimulation. The wrist is extended, the fingers and thumb being moderately flexed. The four typical postures that have been given are normal, as signs of certain healthy brain states.

The nervous hand (Fig. 5) is due to an abnormal brain state, an ill-balanced condition of the brain centres. The wrist is flexed, the metacarpus slightly contracted, the thumb somewhat separated from the other digits, the fingers and the thumb are bent backwards at the knuckle-joints. This posture is in direct antithesis to the energetic hand, the wrist and knuckle-joints being in exactly opposite positions in the two attitudes.

The feeble hand (Fig. 6) presents general flexion, this is seen in the wrist, thumb and fingers, the palm of the hand being considerably contracted, thus approximating the thumb and little finger. It probably represents the least possible amount of force coming from the nerve-centres to the muscles of the limb; muscular tone is here lower than in the hand at rest.

The Convulsive Hand (Fig. 7).—The closed fist, or the clenched hand has the fingers strongly drawn over the thumb which is pressed upon the palm of the hand. The palm is contracted or drawn together.

To complete the types, the hand **in fright** (Fig. 8) will be described, but we do not think it is often seen in real life. The wrist is extended as well as all the fingers, this posture thus differs from the energetic hand only in the character of extension of the fingers.

While observing the hand posture look also for any finger movement. If the two arms be held out we may see a posture of weakness on one side only, more usually on the left side, or the characteristic posture may be more strongly marked on one side. Thus we frequently see the nervous-hand posture strongly marked on the left side, and less distinct on the right, thus indicating a different balance of the action

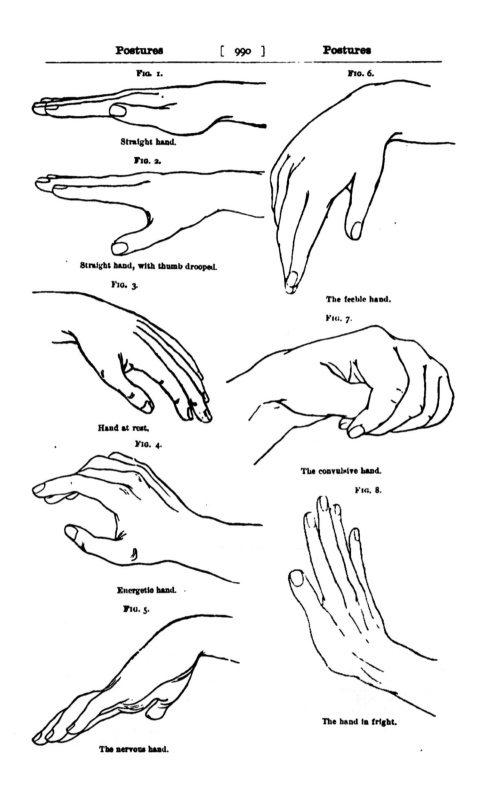

FIG. 1.

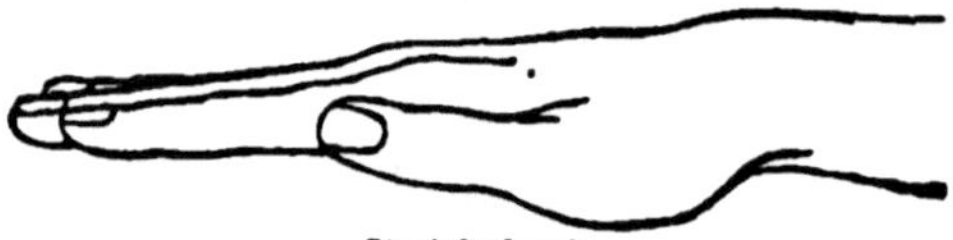

Straight hand.

FIG. 2.

Straight hand, with thumb drooped.

FIG. 3.

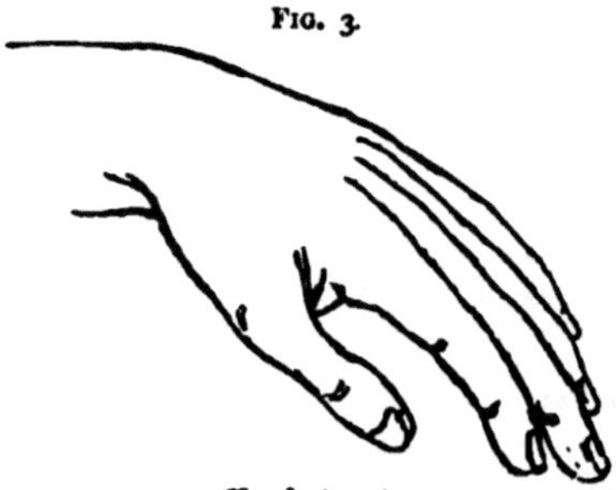

Hand at rest.

FIG. 4.

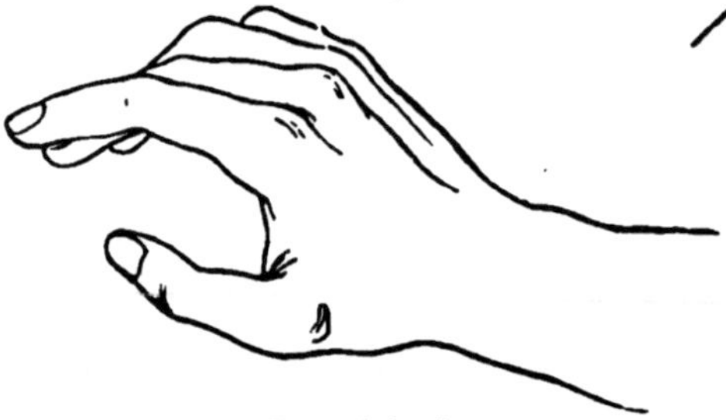

Energetic hand.

FIG. 5.

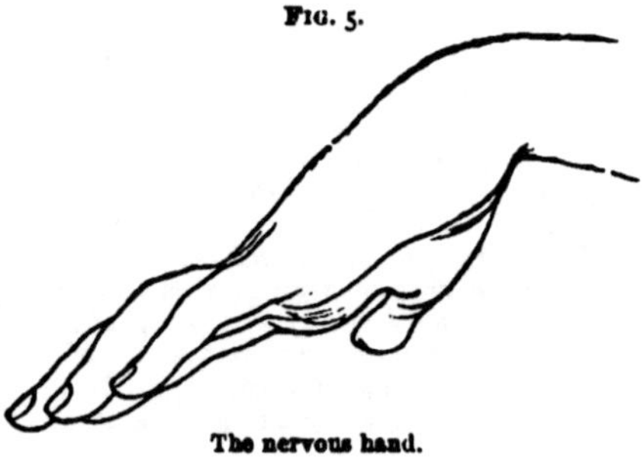

The nervous hand.

FIG. 6.

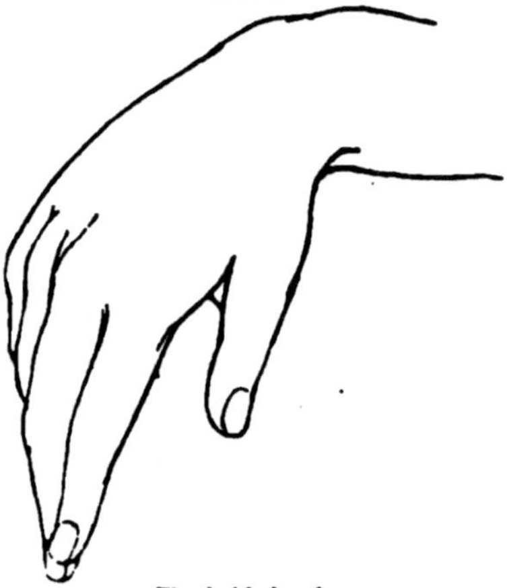

The feeble hand.

FIG. 7.

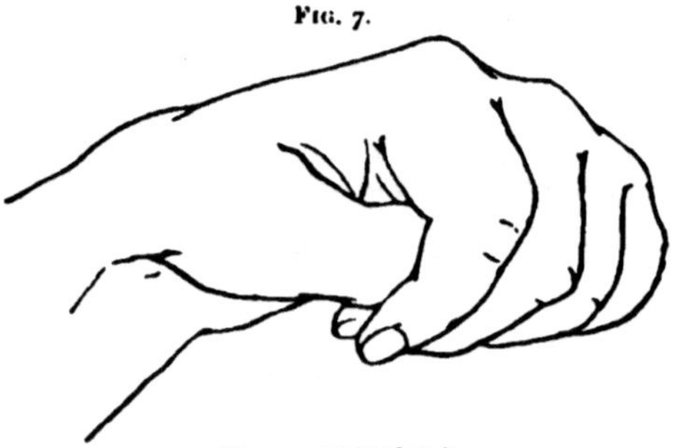

The convulsive hand.

FIG. 8.

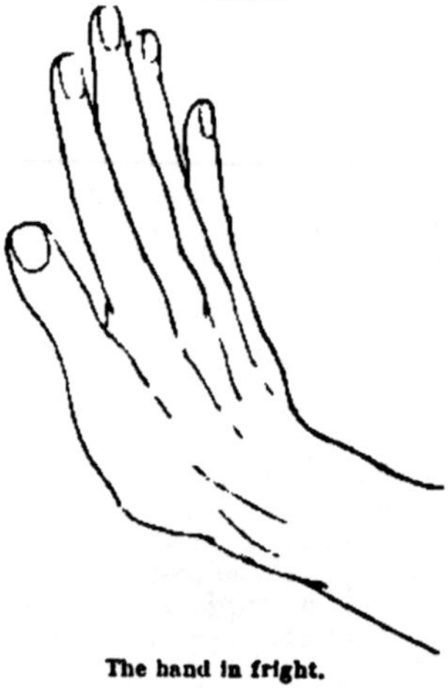

The hand in fright.

in the corresponding nerve-centres on the two sides.

The spine may be too much rounded, or it may be asymmetrical with slight temporary lateral curvature; this, as well as lordosis, is frequently found when the other balances are of the feeble type, and the hands asymmetrical.

Certain spontaneous postures and muscular balances are antithetical, and it may be shown that the mental states corresponding are likewise opposed to one another. The "nervous hand posture" and the "energetic hand" are anatomical opposites; in the former the wrist is flexed, the knuckles being over-extended; in the latter the wrist is extended, the knuckle-joints being flexed. The first posture is seen in weak and excitable children with other signs of feebleness, the energetic hand is commonly seen in strong and eager children. The antithesis of the mental states, joy and pain, is expressed by the opposition of the signs which indicate these conditions; this will be obvious to the student of physical expression, for the two modes of facial action cannot co-exist.

In speaking thus briefly of certain physical signs observable in man, it is found impossible to dissociate those that indicate general brain states from those **indicative of mental conditions.**

Following the method of describing only the physical signs seen, we shall never say that a feeling or emotion produces a certain balance or posture of the body, but that a certain brain state produces the postures, and these are the signs of its condition — certain subjective mental states may be constant accompaniments. Postures are more easy of description than movements, but their significance is far less indicative than the mobile signs.

Abnormal Postures. — A few words must be said about abnormal postures due to conditions of the nerve-system. We refer to such as are sometimes seen, often as a temporary matter, and differ from those previously described.

In the hand, *squaring of the fingers* with extension at the knuckle-joints, the internodes being flexed at a right angle, has been seen in cases of athetosis, hysteria, and a few cases of chorea, which proved to be very intractable. In other cases, flexion of the index and ring fingers, the other digits being extended is an unusual posture sometimes seen.

Among other indications of abnormal neural balance, we may mention as signs of feebleness, contraction of the metacarpus, *lordosis*, and a head flexed and slightly inclined and rotated to one side.

Over-extension of the head with arching of the spine is well known as an accompaniment of cerebral irritation; the same balance in less degree may be seen in mental excitement.

The coincidence of certain postures is a fair indication of the neural balance. In 143 cases presenting "nervous hand," we found coincident lordosis in 46 cases. In 54 cases presenting "weak hand posture," lordosis was seen in 13 cases. Other examples might be given. The balance on the two sides should be compared; it is usually to the disadvantage of the left if nerve force is weakened. In making observations, conditions of movements should always be noted together with the postures seen.

Conditions of muscular balance in the face and eyes are given in the article Expression.

A few examples of the artistic use of postures as indicating expression of nerve-states may be given from the antique.

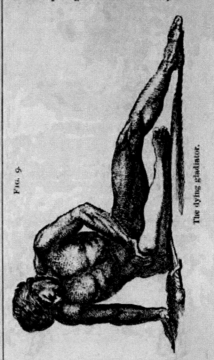

Fig. 9.

The dying gladiator.

Sir Charles Bell draws attention to this statue (Fig. 9) as representing postures of the body resulting from the urgent dyspnœa of a man in mortal agony. Here the limbs are not free to express the finer nerve-states.

Fig. 10.

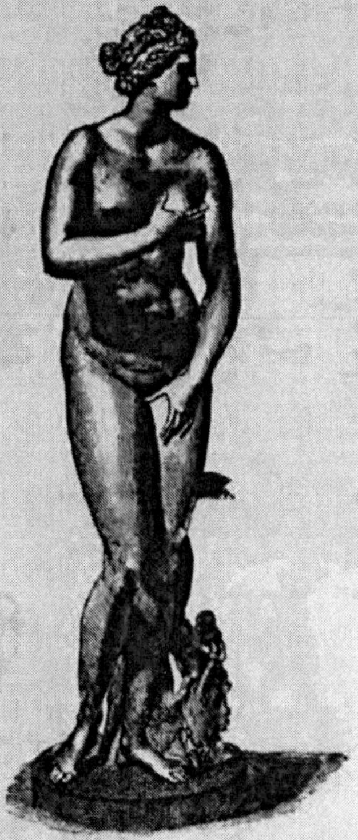

Venus de Medici.

It was this statue (Fig. 10) in the Pitti Gallery of Florence that taught me how to describe the balance termed "the nervous hand;" each hand is here thus balanced. The same may be seen in antique bronze statuettes.

Fig. 11.

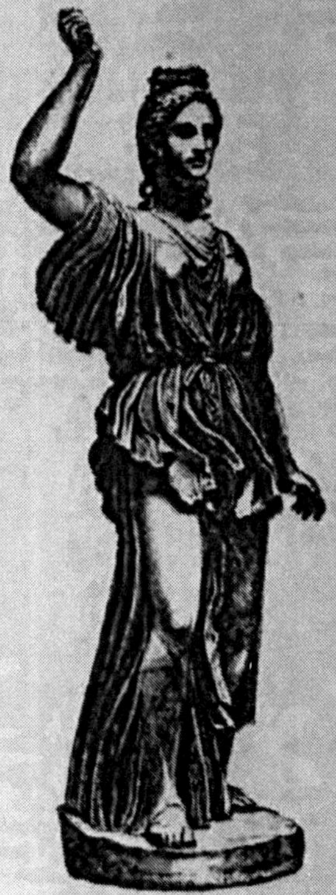

Diana. (British Museum.)

This is a strong figure (Fig. 11): the right hand held a spear, the left is free and balanced in "the energetic posture."

Fig. 12.

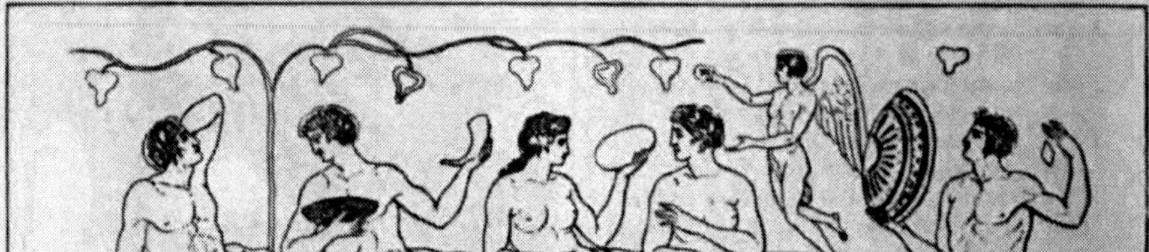

A feast of the gods. (From an antique vase.)

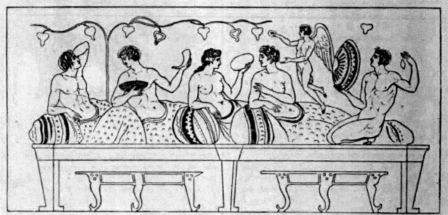

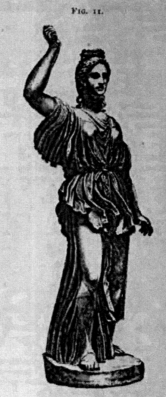

All hands among those at the feast (Fig. 12) present some feature of "the nervous hand" in over-extension of the knuckle-joints. The Genius, who is not a partaker of the feast, presents the energetic hand.

Fig. 13.

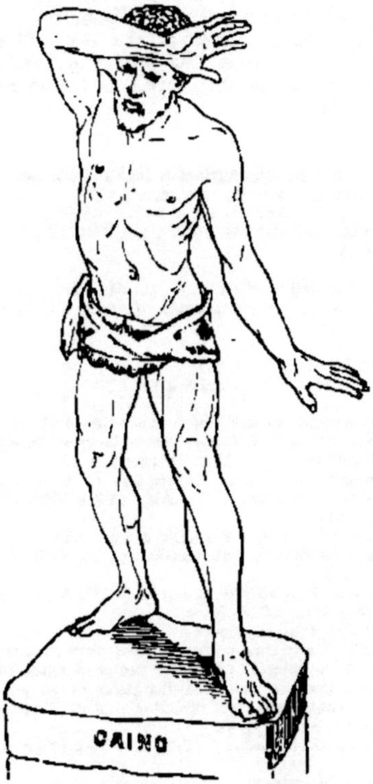

Cain. (Pitti Gallery, Florence.)

The whole figure (Fig. 13) expresses horror, or mental fear. Each hand is free and balanced in the posture of "the hand in fright." Francis Warner.

POTASSIUM BROMIDE. (*See* Sedatives.)

POTHOPATRIDALGIA (πόθος, a longing; πατρίς, one's country; ἄλγος, pain). A morbid home-sickness, seen sometimes in young soldiers and others in foreign countries. (Fr. *pothopatridalgie*: Ger. *Heimweh*.)

POTOMANIA (πότος, drink; μανία, madness). Drink-madness. Delirium tremens. (Fr. *potomanie*; Ger. *Trinksucht*.)

POTOPARANOIA, POTOTROMANIA. (*See* Pototromoparanoia.)

POTOTROMOPARANOIA (πότος, drink; τρόμος, trembling; παράνοια, madness or folly). Delirium tremens, or madness from drink. (Fr. *pototromoparanée*; Ger. *Zitterwahnsinn der Trinker*.)

POWER OF ATTORNEY (*See* Agency and Partnership).—(**1**) A power of attorney not given for valuable consideration, *and* not expressed in the power to be irrevocable, is, as between the donor and donee, *ipso facto*, revoked by the lunacy of the donor. Third persons dealing with the donee, without notice of the lunacy of the donor, are (probably) protected (Conveyancing Act, 1881, s. 47 (1), *Drew* v. *Nunn*, 1879, 4 Q. B. D. 661). (**2**) A power of attorney given for valuable consideration *and* expressed in the power to be irrevocable is irrevocable *in favour of a purchaser*, notwithstanding the supervening lunacy or unsoundness of mind of the donor (Conveyancing Act, 1882, s. 8). (**3**) A power of attorney, *whether given for valuable consideration or not*, if expressed in the instrument creating it to be irrevocable for a fixed time not exceeding one year from the date of the instrument is, *in favour of a purchaser*, irrevocable for that time, notwithstanding the supervening lunacy or unsoundness of mind of the donor (Conveyancing Act, 1882, s. 9). The last two provisions apply *only* to powers of attorney executed after December 31, 1882. (4) The capacity to grant a power of attorney would probably be determined in the same way as the capacity to appoint an agent in any other way. A. Wood Renton.

PRECOCITY.—It has been noticed that precocious children are as a rule connected with families some of whose members are insane. The mental defects of some members of a family seem to be made up for by the extraordinary mental acquirements of others of the family. Precocious children are more liable to insanity than others.

PREDISPOSITION. (*See* Heredity.)

PRE-EPILEPTIC INSANITY.—Morbid mental states frequently occur before as well as after an epileptic fit. Delusions may be present, hallucinations manifest themselves, or there may be a dreamy confused state of mind.

PREOCCUPATION.—A common symptom in some forms of insanity, especially in melancholia. The patients do not answer when spoken to, nor do they seem to hear anything, being so much wrapped up in their own thoughts.

PRESCRIPTION, and LIMITATION OF ACTIONS.—These subjects may conveniently be considered together. The terms prescription and limitation may with sufficient accuracy for the present purpose be defined as follows:—"Prescription" is the undisturbed and continuous enjoyment of a legal right for a period fixed by law, on the expiry of which all attempts to overthrow it are barred.* The time within which such attempts must be made is the period of "limitation." The doctrines of prescription and limitation rest upon the presumption of law, that a person who knowingly fails to enforce a legal right, which he alleges to be infringed, acquiesces in the infringement.† Now, if a person is prevented by mental disease from knowing that his rights are being invaded, clearly he cannot be said to acquiesce in such invasion. It would seem, therefore, *à priori*, that lunacy should suspend the operation of the law of limitation. Such, however, is the importance which the law assigns to the doctrines of prescription and limitation that lunacy has only received a very partial and half-hearted recognition as a ground of disability.

The present state of the law will be apprehended from the following table,‡ in which the leading forms of action are noticed :—

Account (action of)	Period of limitation runs against a lunatic from time of his recovery. (21 Jac. I., c. 16, s. 7.)
Admiralty (suits for seamen's wages)	Same rule. (4 & 5 Anne, c. 16, s. 18.)
Advowsons (recovery of)	Lunacy no bar to limitation. (*Cf.* 3 & 4 Will. IV., c. 27, ss. 30-33.)
Assault, battery, wounding, or false imprisonment	Same rule as in action of account. (21 Jac. I., c. 16, s. 7.)
Awards (actions upon)	Time runs from recovery of lunatic. (3 & 4 Will. IV., c. 42, s. 4.)
Bills of Exchange (including cheques and promissory notes)	Ditto. (21 Jac. I., c. 16, s. 7.)
Bonds	Ditto. (3 & 4 Will. IV., c. 42, s. 4.)
Common (rights of) and other profits *à prendre*, claims to	Same rule; except in cases where the right or claim is declared by the Prescription Act to be absolute and indefeasible.§ (2 & 3 Will. IV., c. 71, s. 7.)
Constables (actions against)	Lunacy no bar to limitation. (*Cf.* 24 Geo. II., c. 44, s. 8.)
Copyhold fine (action for)	Time runs from recovery of lunatic. (3 & 4 Will. IV., c. 42, s. 4.)
Copyright (action for infringement of)	Lunacy no bar to. (*Cf.* 5 & 6 Vict., c. 45, s. 26.)
Covenants (actions upon)	Time runs from recovery of lunatic. (3 & 4 Will. IV., c. 42, s. 4.)
Debt (actions of)	Ditto. (21 Jac. I., c. 16, s. 7; 3 & 4 Will. IV., c. 42, s. 4.)
Deed (action upon)	Ditto. (3 & 4 Will. IV., c. 42, s. 4.)
Detinue (action of)	Ditto. (21 Jac. I., c. 16, s. 7.)
Distress for rent charge	May be made at any time within 6 years from recovery or death of lunatic, whichever happens first, but utmost allowance for such disability is 30 years from accrual of the right of action. (Real Property Limitation Act, 1874, ss. 3 and 5.)
Distress for other rents	Lunacy no bar to limitation. (*Cf.* 3 & 4 Will. IV., c. 27, s. 42.)
Divorce	See article on MARRIAGE.
Dower (arrears of) action for	Lunacy no bar to limitation. (*Cf.* 3 & 4 Will. IV., c. 27, s. 41.)
Ejectment	Same rule as Distress for rent-charge (*q.v.*).
Justices of the Peace (actions against)	Lunacy no bar to limitation. (*Cf.* 11 & 12 Vict., c. 44, s. 8.)
Land (action for recovery of)	Same rule as Distress for rent-charge (*q.v.*).
Legacies (suits for)	Lunacy not a *statutory* bar to limitation. (*Cf.* 3 & 4 Will. IV., c. 27, s. 40; and Real Property Limitation Act, 1874, s. 8.)

* Prescription has no place in English law except in respect to easements and rights of common.

† "Vigilantibus non dormientibus jura subveniunt." But the doctrines of prescription and limitation are based upon public policy as well as upon equity. "Interest reipublicae ut sit finis litium." "If time," said Lord Plunket, "destroys the evidence of title, the laws have wisely and humanely made length of possession a substitute for that which has been destroyed. He comes with his scythe in one hand to mow down the muniments of our rights; but in his other hand the law-giver has placed an hour-glass, by which he metes out incessantly those portions of duration which render needless the evidence that he has swept away." Cited by Best, "Evidence," p. 31, note (*k*).

‡ Only lunacy existing *when the right of action accrued* will suspend the operation of the law of limitation.

§ The cases here referred to are—1. Where the right, profit, or benefit has been actually taken and enjoyed for the full period of 60 years. 2. Where any way, easement, or water-course, or the use of any water has been enjoyed for the full period of 40 years. 3. Where the use of light has been enjoyed for the full period of 20 years; unless in any of those cases it shall appear that the same was enjoyed by some consent or agreement expressly given or made for that purpose by deed or writing. The statutory periods of limitation are given in a convenient tabular form in Wharton's "Law Lexicon."

Libel (action of)	Time runs from recovery of lunatic. (21 Jac. I., c. 16, s. 7.)
"Merchant's accounts"	Lunacy no bar to limitation. (*Cf.* 19 & 20 Vict., c. 97, s. 9.)
Mortgage (redemption of)	Lunacy no bar to limitation. (*Cf.* 1 Vict. c. 28, s. 1; and *Kinsman* v. *Rouse*, 1801, 17 Ch. D., at p. 107.)
Mortgage (foreclosure of)	Same rule as Distress for rent-charge (*q.v.*).
Mortgage (money secured by), recovery of .	Period of limitation runs from accrual of right of action to some person capable at the time of giving a valid discharge. (Real Property Limitation Act, 1874, s. 8.)
Rent (by lease or deed), action for . .	Time runs from recovery of lunatic. (3 & 4 Will. IV., c. 42, s. 4.)
Rent (not secured by lease or deed) . .	Lunacy no statutory bar to limitation. (*Cf.* 3 & 4 Will. IV., c. 27, s. 42.)
Seduction (action for)	Time runs from recovery of lunatic. (21 Jac. I., c. 16, s. 7.)
Slander (action of)	Ditto.

The right of a person to recover land of which he has been deprived by fraud accrues at the time when such fraud might with reasonable diligence have been discovered (3 and 4 Will. IV. c. 27, s. 26). Nothing short of *absolute lunacy* will be recognised by the Court as disqualifying a person for the detection of "fraud" within the meaning of the section (*Manby* v. *Bewicke*, 1857, 3 K. & J. 342).

A. Wood Renton.

PRESENTATIONS OF SENSE.—Presentations of sense are those complex objects of consciousness which result from an act of mental synthesis of several simultaneous sensations. The elements of presentations of sense are therefore sensations, which are merely modes of our being affected, mere psychical states. The transference of these psychical states to definite presentations of sense is a mental achievement resulting from a long process of development. The characteristic of a presentation of sense is that it has space-forms, which the sensations composing it have not. For the formation of sense presentations the following are necessary: (*a*) A synthetic activity of mind; (*b*) A difference in the quality of the sensations, so that a graded series can be formed (spatial series); (*c*) Local signs; (*d*) Localisation and eccentric projection; and (*e*) As a rule, more than one organ of sensation (Ladd).

PRESUMPTIONS (LEGAL) RELATING TO INSANITY.—Legal presumptions are inferences or positions established by law for the regulation of judicial procedure,* and are of two kinds (1) conclusive or irrebuttable, called by the civilians **præsumptiones juris et de jure**, and (2) rebuttable, or **præsumptiones juris tantum.**

(1) In the law of insanity there are only two rules that seem to have belonged to the former class—viz., that idiocy is incurable, and that a lunatic upon the other hand is always capable of recovering his understanding.* With regard to these rules it must however be pointed out that the old legal incidents of idiocy are now of little importance, and that the presumption in favour of the recovery of a lunatic may now be rebutted.†

(2) The **præsumptiones juris tantum** relating to insanity are very numerous. The following are the most important:

(*a*) A person deaf and dumb from his birth is presumed to be an idiot.‡ But this presumption may be rebutted. Thus, in *Dickinson* v. *Blisset* (1 Dick. 268) a lady born deaf and dumb, having attained the age of twenty-one years, applied to the Court of Chancery for possession of her real estate, and to have an assignment of her chattel estate, and Lord Hardwicke having put questions to her in writing, to which she gave sensible answers in writing, granted the application.

(*b*) Every person who has attained the usual age of discretion is presumed to be of sound mind until the contrary is proved, and this holds as well in civil as in criminal cases.

This presumption of law rests upon the fact that sanity is the normal condition

* The *raison d'être* of such presumptions is admirably explained by Best: "Evidence," ss. 42, 43, 304 *et seq.*

* *Cf.* the Statute de Prærogativa Regis, 17 Edw. II., c. 10, as to lunatics; 17 Edw. II., c. 9, as to idiots. See also article on Idiocy, and *Fitzgerald's case*, 1805, 2 Sch. & Lef. 438, per Lord Redesdale, and *Ex parte Whitbread*, 3 Mod. 44, 2 Mer. 99.

† *Cf. Ex parte Whitbread*, 2 Mer. 99. *Re Blair*, 1 Myl. & Cr. 300, and *Re Frost*, 39 L. J. Ch. 808.

‡ See article Deaf-Dumbness. The opinion of Lord Coke was that a person born deaf, dumb, *and* blind, is included within the legal definition of any idiot as wanting those senses which furnish the human mind with ideas. But it was decided in *Elyot's case* (Carter 53), that a person deprived of only one or two senses, and who can convey his meaning by writing or signs, is not incapacitated. The *ratio decidendi* in this case—viz., the capacity to understand communications—clearly covers the case of a deaf and blind mute who is now capable of being instructed.

of human beings and upon the jealousy with which our law protects personal belief.*

(*c*) Mental derangement, once proved, or admitted, to have existed at any particular period, is presumed to have continued; and consequently the party who alleges a lucid interval or recovery must establish his allegation.†

The *onus probandi* may shift more than once during the progress of a trial. Thus, suppose the validity of a marriage to be in dispute. Here we start with the general presumption in favour of sanity, which the party impeaching the marriage must displace, if he can. Evidence that the person, whose competency to marry is in question, had, at or about the critical period, been found lunatic by inquisition, would throw the burden of proof upon the person supporting the marriage, who might again, partially at least, rebut the presumption of insanity arising from the inquisition by showing that the alleged lunatic had obtained liberty to traverse. (*Cf. Elliot* v. *Ince*, 1857, 26 L. J. N. S. Ch. at p. 824.)‡

(*d*) Unexplained delay in impeaching deeds, instruments or contracts on the ground of incapacity, will raise a presumption in favour of their validity.

This rule rests upon a clear principle of public policy. "*If property*," said Lord Chancellor Eldon in *Towart* v. *Sellars* (1819, 5 Dow. Parl. Cas. at p. 236), "*has been disposed of twenty or thirty years before, formally and with the concurrence and assistance of individuals of good character, and if that disposition is not quarrelled with as speedily as may be, and only challenged when the parties best acquainted with the whole circumstances of the transaction are dead and gone*, it is dangerous to set aside that disposition at the distance of twenty or thirty years upon a ground so fallible as human memory and testimony as to the state of the person making that disposition at other moments without at all applying to the moment when he executes the deed." The latter part of this judgment refers to the special circumstances of the case, but the clauses in italics explain and clearly justify the presumption above stated.

Thus, in support of an action (*Towart* v. *Sellars*, *ubi sup.*) brought in [illegible] to reduce certain deeds executed between 1782 and 1799, upon the ground of the insanity of the grantor, parol evidence was given that he was quite deranged from 1781 till his death in 1804; but this evidence applied to his insanity generally, and not at the particular moments when the deeds were executed, and it was encountered by positive evidence relating to those periods. The House of Lords, reversing the decision of the Court of Session in Scotland, held that the deeds were valid.

Still more emphatic effect was given to the same presumption in *Price* v. *Berrington* (1850, 3 Mac. & G. pp. 486, 495). In that case Lord Chancellor Truro dismissed a bill, filed to set aside a deed of conveyance twenty-seven years after its execution, although it appeared that the grantor had been found lunatic not only by inquisition, but upon an issue directed in the particular matter.

(*e*) "Where the persons who have prepared deeds and are the attesting witnesses to their execution are dead, when process is commenced for setting such deeds aside, it will be assumed in the absence of evidence to the contrary that they would have sworn that the party was of sane mind when the deeds were executed, although it be attempted to disprove the sanity of the grantor by general parol evidence of incompetency at other times" (per Lord Eldon, C., in *Towart* v. *Sellars*, *ubi sup.* at p. 245, and Shelford's Lunacy, p. 54).

A. Wood Renton.

PREVENTION OF INSANITY (PROPHYLAXIS).—To prevent insanity in persons predisposed, and to ward off subsequent attacks from those whose minds have already been disordered, are amongst the most important duties of medical practitioners. The first form the large class who have inherited a tendency to the malady from parents or forefathers, and are liable to transmit it in turn to their offspring. Those who are able to observe such individuals from their birth, and advise concerning their bringing up, their schooling, and entry into the world, may do much to save them from the hereditary scourge, whereas specialists will not come into contact with them till the evil has revealed itself. But the task is a difficult one. Every effort will be made to conceal or explain away the family taint. Any occurrence of the kind will be minimised, will be ascribed to natural causes, as bodily illness, old age, or brain disease, or, failing these, will be denied

* *Testamentary* capacity, however, must, in the interest of the persons entitled under the Statutes of Descent and Distribution, be proved affirmatively by the executor who propounds a will. See article Testamentary Capacity in Mental Disease.

† See *A. G.* v. *Parnther*, per Lord Thurlow, 3 Bro. C. C. 433.

‡ As to the meaning of "lucid interval," see article Testamentary Capacity. See also article on Evidence.

altogether without the slightest hesitation. The family medical attendant, however, if he is acquainted with the life-history of more than one generation, will for himself gain sufficient insight into the constitution and temperament of the members to guide him in his advice concerning the rearing and training of the younger branches, and denial of the family peculiarities and weaknesses will not be practised towards him, because he is too conversant with the facts.

It has often been urged, and cannot be too strongly insisted on, that a nervous inheritance may be derived, not only from parents or grandparents in whom actual insanity has developed, but from those who have suffered from epilepsy, dipsomania, hysteria, hypochondriasis, or neuralgia. A combination of two of these in the parents, or of one of them with phthisis or gout may lead to insanity in various members of a family, and to phthisis or neuralgia in others. It is evident, however, that children will be born under various conditions, and some will be far more liable to nervous disorder than others born of the same parents. For some may be born before the mother has shown any symptoms of the disease, others may be children of one who has been insane during her pregnancy, or has had repeated attacks of mania. In the case of others conception may have taken place after the father has shown undoubted symptoms of general paralysis. This is not an infrequent occurrence. Some may be born of a mother who becomes insane after every childbirth, and only recovers to a very partial extent by the time another is born. Such children stand in a different class from those whose parents have never been insane, but inherit a taint from their own progenitors, which shows itself, it may be, in brothers, sisters, or other collateral branches. Children born before insanity has shown itself in a parent are in a better position than those born after, and those born of parents in whom the disease has appeared at a very early age, are more likely to inherit it than the children of parents in whom it appeared later in life, especially if, in the case of the latter, there was an adequate and assignable cause. Those whose parents are cousins are liable to hereditary disease. If any, as insanity, exists in the family, it will most likely be intensified by the relationship, and the offspring are likely to be not only insane, but stunted and weakly in other respects, and very possibly idiots. In this they but follow the laws of in-breeding, which apply equally to man and animals.

If a medical man has under his observation and care a child born of a father or mother who has already shown signs of insanity, or is "nervous," epileptic, hysterical, hypochondriacal, or unstable in any way, what is he to observe and what precautions are to be taken? From the earliest age he may note symptoms enough to put him on his guard. The infant may sleep badly, may be cross, or over-excitable, or have infantile convulsions. If the mother is the affected person, it will be better for her not to suckle it, as a nervous, excitable woman, prone, it may be, to varying mental moods, is not likely to be a good nurse, and it is of the first importance that a nervous child should be thoroughly well nourished either by a good wet-nurse or hand-feeding. Bad sleeping is a point not to be overlooked, and judicious management and regular hours and habits may do much to remedy the evil. The child should be taught to sleep by day as well as by night till a very considerable age is attained.

When a few years have passed, other signs may show the nervous inheritance The child may suffer from "night-horrors," may be afraid of being alone or in the dark, or its temper may be fractious and capricious, or violent and passionate. Everything here will depend on the judgment and prudence of those who have charge of it. Many a child is frightened and rendered nervous and timid for life by tales told by foolish servants and nurses, of ghosts, spectres, and robbers, or is terrified into obedience by threats based on such fictions. The sensitive and imaginative brain carries such romances to bed with it, and wakes from its too vivid dreams in an agony of panic. Another evil, it is to be feared, comes occasionally from nurses, who, in order to make such children sleep, teach them habits of self-abuse. And while they are thus exposed to risks from servants, they may receive no less harm from parents, who will spoil them at one moment and indulge them with improper food and drink, while at another they behave towards them with intemperate fury and frighten them by noise and passion. It is above all important that the bodily health of these children should be regulated with discretion, that they should have abundance of plain wholesome food and no alcohol, live and play much in the open air, and be encouraged at an early age in such pastimes as riding, swimming, and other suitable pursuits. A love of and consideration for animals should be promoted, and the fellowship of other boys and girls should be cultivated, so that selfishness and egoism may be as far as possible repressed. The time soon arrives when education has to be considered. A certain proportion of these children are sharp and precocious, and learn their lessons with ease; others are backward and dull and hate their books. The choice of a school, especially a preparatory school, is of the greatest importance. When a precociously clever boy enters a preparatory school he will be hailed as a promising candidate for one of the scholarships for which boys of twelve or thirteen compete at most of our public schools. The competition for these scholarships is very severe, great numbers of boys entering for a few vacancies. Consequently, a large proportion are doomed at this early age to all the evil consequences of mental disappointment and sense of failure after years of brain work with all its dangers. Truly, modern education, with all its boasted advance, has here invented an ill for its children of which our grandfathers knew nothing. No less care must be bestowed upon the backward children. Where the brain development is slow and learning acquired with difficulty, great patience must be exercised by teachers. Such children may learn some subjects easily, but have no aptitude for mastering others. They must not be put in a class with a dozen or twenty others, and made to conform to a common standard, and punished according to rule if all their lessons are not learned uniformly well. Masters and mistresses are apt to mistake inability for idleness, and to unduly press and punish the backward, assuming that because one subject is well learned, it is mere idleness that prevents all being equally well done. They have not sufficient discrimination to see who are idle and who backward, and, no doubt, it is often a difficult matter to decide, and requires great judgment and patience.

The choice of a school for children calls for no less care. Are girls to go to school at all? Much will depend on the character of their home life, and the judicious or injudicious management of their parents. School may be the salvation of some girls by taking them away from uncomfortable homes, or foolish spoiling and petting, subjecting them to the rules and discipline and public opinion of a number, instead of the self-indulgence of home life and the caprices of an hysterical, violent, and indiscreet mother. The marvellous effects produced in some boys by the broad views and higher tone of a large public school cannot but be paralleled to some extent in the case of girls, and as a rule the larger the school the better will be the result. Where a boy or girl goes to school, it is above all things necessary that the bodily health should be carefully watched. Clothing should be adequate and dormitories properly ventilated. The food should be good and sufficiently tempting to be eaten, and outdoor play and exercise should be enforced.

Much controversy has lately arisen as to the propriety of making boys join in games in the playground, and not allowing them to "loaf" in their studies, or get into mischief in a town. Whatever may be said as to the propriety or impropriety of this compulsory play as a general rule, there are, beyond question, many of these peculiar and nervous children who would never play unless compelled, but would spend their time in solitary amusements, or get to the public house if opportunity offered. The writer has met within asylum walls in after-life more than one whom he recollects at school as loafing and idling in this manner, not stupid or neglecting his school work, but avoiding the playground and school games, taking no exercise, often dirty in dress, and remarkable for some peculiarity of habit or appearance.

There is a matter of great importance in a boy's school-life which cannot be passed over without notice. It is the subject of masturbation. It is a habit learned in a very large number of cases at an early age, and taught by one schoolfellow to another at a time when neither is old enough to know that it is likely to grow into a habit, or to be productive of evil; though they may be conscious that it is a practice which must be concealed as indecent and unclean. It is not wise to allow a boy to take the chance of contracting such a habit, often one most ineradicable, without his having the slightest idea that it is hurtful to health. It is almost certain that he will hear of it in school, and it is far better that he should be warned by a father, guardian, elder brother, or the family doctor, that he must on no account indulge in this vice than that he should take his chance of refraining therefrom. With girls it is different. Their chance of being taught the practice is far less, especially if they are educated at home, and this is a very strong argument in favour of home education. If they are to go to school, the greatest care must be taken in the selection of one where such things do not exist. It has been said that girls may find out the habit for themselves, and this is true, though probably not common. But no one would bring it to the knowledge of girls in general, because here and there one has made the discovery. Such knowledge would in truth be a dangerous thing. The time of puberty and of the first appearance of the catamenia is one fraught with considerable peril to these nervous and sensitive girls, and they should be carefully watched throughout it. It is a time when all extremes must be avoided. They should not be allowed to over-fatigue themselves with tennis, long walks, or rides. They should not be exposed to great heat or cold, or anything which will check the menstrual flow or render it too profuse. They should not overtax the brain with lessons or competitive examinations, and a strict watch must be kept upon their sleeping, as an inability to sleep in young people of such an age is often a warning and forerunner of coming mischief, and if a girl sleeps alone it may easily be overlooked. This period of life is one of greater peril to girls than to boys, to whom it makes comparatively little difference, and who break down at the time of adolescence rather than that of puberty. A boy of twelve develops slowly and gradually, and he is not a fully perfected man till he is twenty-five. But a girl of seventeen or eighteen is far nearer to a fully developed woman if we compare her with one of twelve, and as her time of development is crowded, so to speak, into a narrower space, so is it fraught with greater peril to her.

Dangerous as is the period of puberty to boys and girls, especially the latter, that of adolescence, between the ages of eighteen and twenty-five is far more so, and more break down and become insane at the latter than at the former epoch. In this time the lives of a great number of both sexes are virtually chosen and entered upon. Young men go from school to college, make choice of a profession and commence life. Many of the women do the same, they choose an occupation or calling; they also fall in love and marry. Some men do this too, but not so many. Few at any rate of those who have to earn a livelihood are able to marry at so early an age. It is a time, moreover, when a girl's religious feelings are apt to be highly excited, and she is especially liable to hysteria and hysterical emotion in connection with such subjects. From all this it will be seen that when we have to deal with a neurotic girl or young man inheriting insanity, it will be of the utmost importance that the career chosen should be one fitted to the mental constitution, and that everything about them should be equally studied and regulated with the view of constantly warding off the threatened evil.

Looking at the history of so many of these predisposed persons, and at the part which drink plays in filling our asylums, it surely is not too much to advise that all such should totally abstain from alcoholic liquors. The young are not likely to indulge to excess in other stimulants, as opium, haschish or snuff, but a liking for wine or spirits may be cultivated at an early age, and the liking may grow into a craving, and how hard this is to resist and overcome every medical man knows full well. To abstain in the first instance is not nearly so difficult. Girls at the present time are in great numbers accustomed to avoid beer and wine. They in no way suffer from the deprivation; on the contrary, with exercise and plenty of food they have grown and attained a stature and muscular development which is very striking. With young men it is not so common, yet a considerable number abstain, and, if the habit is commenced at an early age, the difficulty vanishes. In fact it is certain that apart from the question of drinking to excess, many of these neurotic persons suffer from various kinds of nervous dyspepsia which are aggravated by alcohol, and cannot be cured unless it is abandoned. If left to themselves, they will probably fly to brandy to relieve dyspeptic pain and spasm, and instead of curing will increase their sufferings, and so drift into the practice of constant stimulation. It is also important in the choice of a calling that none should be chosen which entails a constant tasting of wine or spirits, or the entertaining or drinking with others as is the practice in some walks of life. It is equally important that the feeding as well as the drinking of the predisposed should be carefully watched. Stimulants in the shape of alcohol they need not, but abundance of plain wholesome food they require, and many break down from want of it. It constantly happens that from hypochondriacal notions about dyspepsia, from fancies of various kinds as to what is or is not wholesome, or what agrees or disagrees with them, or a fear on the part of girls of getting fat, a small and inadequate amount of food is taken, and certain important items are frequently omitted. One cannot take bread, another milk, another potatoes or vegetables. So the diet list is reduced till little remains, and that innutritious or indigestible. If this occurs in men who are at the same time hard worked in brain, a break down is most likely to follow sooner or later, and it is often most difficult to induce them to take the food which is necessary for recovery. Another class think it carnal and sensual to indulge the appetite and eat their fill, and endless evil comes to many who fast during Lent and other such seasons, and mortify the flesh according to the doctrines of the ultra-ritualistic party. The whole of the religious training of the predisposed requires the most careful handling, a difficult matter, as they are for the most part averse to consult those best able to advise them, and seek the excitement of the followers of extreme views from revivalists and the Salvation Army to the Roman Catholic Church. Young people of both sexes should not spend an undue time in reading religious books or writing long accounts of their spiritual state. Their religion should be practical and not introspective, and they should not be allowed to remain an abnormally long time on their knees and thus expose themselves to cold. On the other hand, there are not a few who fancy themselves philosophers, and read Herbert Spencer's works, or worry their brains by reasonings which they cannot follow, parading their studies for the sake of effect or for the annoyance of those about them.

The time has now arrived when the young man has to choose the profession or occupation in which life is to be passed, and this choice has to be made by many young women as well. It is a momentous question, and one often decided, not by the individuals themselves, but by parents or guardians, or force of circumstances. Where a free choice can be made, what should influence the selection of a calling? Of the learned professions the Church is the least eligible; it appeals strongly to the emotional part of the mental constitution, the part which in neurotic people is apt to be easily and strongly aroused and least under control. Religious doubts and difficulties concerning creeds will probably arise in these excitable minds, questions as to whether a clergyman having doubts should retain his benefice or resign it, and in so doing reduce himself and his family to poverty. Fear may arise in a vacillating and doubting mind as to whether the duties of the parish are properly discharged, and on the slightest depression overwhelming religious remorse may ensue. And this profession once adopted cannot be thrown up or changed for another, so that it is by no means a desirable vocation for those whom we are considering. For the last reason law and medicine are preferable. The study of them, especially the latter, has great and practical interest for one who likes it, an interest which cannot flag, as new discoveries in science and new methods of alleviating disease are made and published. There may be a certain amount of anxiety in both professions, business may be slack and fees scarce, but in the calling of a solicitor or general medical practitioner there is usually a livelihood to be earned, and a certain amount of routine and unexciting work to be done without much worry. A clerkship in a Government office, where hours are short, responsibility small, and holidays long, is the place of all others for the "nervous" man. In the old time such posts were obtained without much difficulty, but now that a competitive examination is a necessary preliminary, the case is altered, and the work and disappointment which may follow failure make such less desirable. Still our neurotic people are not devoid of brains, and steady work for a time may gain this prize, to be held without detriment for many years with the consolation of a pension at the end. The army is unfavourable, as it may necessitate a long residence in an unwholesome tropical climate; the emolument is small, there is no great interest in the work during a large portion of the time, and desultory and idle habits often lead to drinking. Life in our colonies or in North or South America, tempts many young men, and it is a good calling for those who wish to work under others, and are fond of a hard out-door life; but it may entail much solitude and privation, and the vicissitudes of seasons and prices may cause great care and anxiety, if a man is farming land of his own. There is one piece of advice valuable to all. Besides his work or profession let every one have a pursuit, taste, or hobby, call it what we will, to which he may turn, and with which he may distract his thoughts and recreate his mind, tired and sick of work and worry. The want of this has caused many a one to break down, and many by it have been saved from mental ruin.

Besides choosing a profession, young people have another serious question to ask themselves: Shall they marry, and if so, whom? A vast number will answer for themselves without asking advice from others, even their own parents, but here and there the medical adviser of the family may be consulted. Unfortunately this is generally done when the engagement is made and marriage impending, and adverse advice, if given, is rarely heeded. But if we note the number of young men and women who break down during the time they are engaged, immediately after marriage, or in the honeymoon, it is certain that it is all fraught with danger to those predisposed to insanity by constitution and inheritance. That all persons who have insanity in their family should abstain from matrimony is more than can be expected. Not only do these marry, but they are specially prone to make ill-judged selections. There seems a tendency among these neurotic folk to choose for their partners people of a like nervous temperament, and from a shyness which is characteristic and constitutional, they often choose cousins whom they have long known in preference to strangers, whom they know not and are too shy to approach. It need not be said that the danger is increased if cousins from two families where insanity exists intermarry and have children. This, however, happens but too frequently, and parents do not oppose such unions, because they prefer to ignore the whole risk; they hope for the best, and invent excuses for the cases that have occurred, as drink, sunstroke, falls on the head, and the like, or deny that the malady has ever existed at all. If a member of such a family is to marry, it is important that he or she should be in good health and marry a person who is also in good health, and has a good family history. If a girl is delicate and neurotic she should not marry a very poor man, and have the additional anxiety of poverty and the constant and daily obligation to pinch and save for the sake of husband and children. The continual anxiety of small economies and the necessity of meeting small debts, may break down one who in more affluent circumstances might have gone unscathed. Another fertile source of insanity is a numerous family, one child following another in rapid succession. Many delicate women having no break or respite, succumb to this strain, even those in whom insanity may not be markedly hereditary. The nervous system has no rest or chance of recuperation, and mental or lung disease, or both, is the result. There is an idea prevalent amongst many that nervous or hysterical young men and women should marry as soon as possible, and that marriage is a sovereign cure for this state. Now it is probable that many men predisposed to insanity may benefit greatly by marriage if they are so fortunate as to meet with a suitable wife. Henceforth they lead a regular life, keep earlier hours, have a confidante to share their troubles, who also cares for their meals and domestic comforts, and nurses and guards them. On the other hand, if marriage does not benefit them, and they prove unfitted for it, it is a condition which the unfortunate wife cannot free herself from. An irritable man will quarrel more with his wife and behave worse to her than to any other being, and there is besides the risk that the offspring may be an idiot, epileptic or neurotic in some shape or way. The benefit to be derived from marriage by a predisposed woman is far less, and the danger far greater. There is marriage with all its trying surroundings in which so many break down. Then follow pregnancy and parturition, to recur, it may be, frequently. If there is immunity on the first or second occasions, later on insanity may be developed. One thing is certain, that women who have already had attacks of insanity should abstain from marriage, and the concealment of such a history from an intended husband and his friends is a most serious and reprehensible step.

The next question for consideration is this: What should be done when a man or woman who has not been previously insane, is threatened with symptoms of a mental disorder? In many cases the treatment is obvious. An exciting cause, if we are sure it is the cause, must at once, if possible, be removed. Overwork must cease, overworry may not be so easy to deal with, but the attempt must be made, and a long journey to a foreign land may by the mere effect of distance reduce it to a trifling amount. The effect of a fright or shock may subside, and the shock be unlikely to recur ere time comes to our aid. Over-excitement about religious matters must be stopped, and undue devotion and early services strictly forbidden. Drinking must be checked, and sexual excess, and excesses of all kinds. Betrothals must be broken off or suspended if it is plain that they are producing a state of mind which renders marriage an impossibility. In short, when we see that there is an exciting cause it must be removed, but it may happen that no definite or tangible cause can be ascertained. The individual is leading his or her ordinary life, yet there is a deviation from the normal state, there is depression or excitement, unfounded fear, suspicion or irritation with disturbance of health, and in the majority of cases want of sleep. The failure of sleep is a symptom of the highest importance, and one constantly disregarded both by the patient and his relatives. Yet by remedying this, more probably can be done towards warding off insanity than by any other treatment. Again and again it happens that a week's good sleep procured by sulphonal, paraldehyde, chloral or the like, will dissipate the fears and suspicions, allay the excitement and irritability, and bring the sufferer back to his sane mind. The most foolish prejudice exists against the production of sleep by such medicines, and there is often a difficulty in getting the patient to take them. It is objected that a habit of using such drugs will be set up, as if such a habit could be contracted in a week or two. Certain it is that if the sleeplessness goes on unchecked, the threatened insanity will rapidly develop, and will have to be dealt with in a more serious way. The next most potent weapon with which to avert the disorder is change of scene. It is wonderful how removal from the environment in which the symptoms have arisen, and the people amongst whom the patient has been living, working and complaining, will change the ideas and substitute others in place of the morbid. The removal will have to be of longer or shorter duration according to the time the mental disturbance has existed and its depth, but it is unwise to bring a man back to his old surroundings immediately on his showing signs of convalescence. The companion or companions must be carefully chosen. Friends are better than relatives, strangers than friends, for strangers bring fresh views and ideas, and are less able to talk about the troubles of the past. Anything like a delusion should be discussed as little as possible, for delusions grow and are consolidated, not dispersed, by discussion.

To prevent a recurrence in those who have already had an attack of insanity, the same precautions to a great extent must be observed. The previous illness will furnish valuable information, and a question may arise as to what was the real cause, and how it can be prevented from being the source of a second. The exciting cause, for instance, may be parturition. The patient may have made a perfect recovery, but there will be a risk of recurrence when the next child is born. Is she then to abstain from any risk of pregnancy? Much here must necessarily be left to the discretion of husband and wife, but beyond a doubt the risk must be pointed out, especially if insanity or symptoms approaching it have followed more than one confinement. With regard to other causes, it may be necessary that a man should even give up his profession or vocation, if his mental health does not admit of his continuing it. A soldier may have to give up the army; a civilian may be compelled to leave India, if it is plain that his brain cannot stand a tropical climate. In all this the physician can only advise. He may be able to avert the early symptoms by procuring sleep, or ordering rest or change of scene, but he may have great difficulty in persuading the patient or friends to forego that which is the chief danger, for the predisposed are self-opinionated and obstinate in no small degree. Great will be the difficulty in persuading those whose insanity depends upon drink to abstain altogether from alcohol. Yet there is no safety in any half measures, especially for women. Their only hope is in total abstinence; if they take a little, they will certainly want more, till excess is reached. And only by the closest vigilance and supervision can total abstinence be enforced. Insanity in spite of every care will return in those who by constitution are prone to break down periodically. The best that a physician can do is to bring the patient under treatment as soon as symptoms indicate the approach, and to try and shorten the attack by prompt and early measures.

Can anything be done to prevent the alternation of mania and melancholia, to which has been given the name of *folie circulaire*; or the periodical recurrence of the same form, mania or melancholia? Where the alternation or recurrence is once firmly established, the prognosis is most unfavourable, do what we will. Change of scene and constant moving from place to place may be of some use, if the case admits of it. Medicines avail little. As the attacks come round, each must be treated according to the symptoms, but they pass away to return with greater or less regularity perhaps through a long life. G. FIELDING BLANDFORD.

PRIMÄRE VERRÜCKTHEIT. (*See* PARANOIA, and VERRÜCKTHEIT.)

PRIMOGENITURE. — It has been stated that the first-born, especially if a boy, runs a greater risk of being an idiot than a later child. According to some, the right of primogeniture rests on the danger the eldest son runs at birth.

PRIVATE ASYLUMS (*See* GREAT BRITAIN, INSANITY IN).—It would be impossible in the space at our command to give a history of the legislation affecting the licensed houses of Great Britain and Ireland. They have formed the object of attack from the public, and the occasion of a vast number of legislative enactments during the greater part of this century. All that we propose to do in the present article is, to give some of the most important regulations now in force (53 Vict. c. 5, s. 207, 1890) in regard to them.

If the commissioners, in the case of a house within their immediate jurisdiction, or in the case of a house licensed by justices, are of opinion that a house has been well conducted by the licensees, the commissioners or justices may, upon the expiration of the licence, renew it for that house to the former licensees, or any one or more of them, or to their successors in business.

If at any time it is shown to the satisfaction of the commissioners or justices, as the case may be, that it would be to the advantage of the patients that another house should be substituted, they may grant a licence subject to the same conditions as may have existed in respect of the first-mentioned house.

In the case of joint licensees or proprietors desiring to carry on business apart, the commissioners or justices may grant to each licensee renewed licences for such number of patients (not exceeding in the aggregate the number allowed by the joint licence) as such joint licensees agree upon, or as the commissioners or justices determine.

Where the licensee of a house is a medical man in the employment of the proprietor of such house as his manager, the licence shall be transferable or renewable to him so long as he continues manager of the house or to his successor.

The most important section of all the sections of the recent Lunacy Act (respecting private asylums) is that which enacts: "Save as in this section provided, no new licence shall be granted to any person for a house for the reception of lunatics, and no house in respect of which there is, at passing of this act, an existing licence, shall be licensed for a greater number of lunatics than the number authorised by the existing licence."

It may be added, that a medical visitor to a private asylum shall be entitled to such remuneration as the justices may approve (Lunacy Act, 1890, 53 Vict. c. 5, s. 177, sub-s. 12). Medical visitors are not appointed to visit licensed houses within the Metropolitan area, but only those licensed by county justices (s. 177, sub-s. 1). THE EDITOR.

PROCEDURE, in laying Evidence before Jury, when the ACCUSED is ALLEGED to be INSANE.—The mode of procedure at the present time, with regard to the manner in which evidence as to the sanity or insanity of an accused person is laid before the jury, may be gathered from the following extract from Hansard's Parliamentary Reports, 3rd series, vol. 286, p. 40, giving a report of the proceedings in the House of Commons on March 17, 1884. In reply to a question asked by Mr. Mellor, the Attorney-General (Sir Henry James) said: "Perhaps it will be the better course for me, in answer to the question of my honourable friend, to state what directions I have given to the Director of Public Prosecutions. I lately received a communication from the Home Office to the effect that, in some recent cases, great inconvenience, if not injustice, had resulted from no responsible person being in charge of cases when the life of the accused was at stake. I was also informed that the Home Office had found great difficulty in dealing with cases of alleged insanity, in consequence of the facts not being brought before the jury, and being only suggested after the trial. It seemed to me, therefore, advisable to take steps to insure that all evidence bearing on the case, whether tending to prove the guilt or innocence of the prisoner, should be placed before the jury; and, with that object, I have requested that whenever an accused person is brought before justices on a capital charge, the magistrate's clerk shall communicate with the Solicitor of the Treasury, and that that officer shall take charge of the prosecution, unless he finds that some competent private person or local body has the conduct of it; but, in the absence of such proper conduct, it will be the duty of the Treasury Solicitor, acting as Director of Public Prosecutions, to see that the evidence in every capital case be fully brought before the jury. I have also requested that, in those cases where insanity in the accused is alleged, full inquiry shall be made, and, in the absence of his, or his friends', ability to produce witnesses, the Treasury Solicitor shall secure their attendance."

With reference to the foregoing statement of the Attorney-General, a few words of explanation as to the terms Public Prosecutor, and Treasury Solicitor, may be not altogether superfluous. A Public Prosecutor, in England, is a comparatively recent institution, dating only from the year 1879. In that year an Act, entitled the "Prosecution of Offences Act," was passed (42 & 43 Vict. c. 22), by which Act provision was made for the appointment of an officer to be called the Director of Public Prosecutions, whose duty it should be, "under the superintendence of the Attorney-General, to institute, undertake, or carry on such criminal proceedings, whether in the Court for Crown Cases Reserved, before sessions of Oyer and Terminer or of the peace, before magistrates or otherwise, and to give such advice and assistance to chief officers of police, clerks to justices, and other persons, whether officers or not, concerned in any criminal proceeding respecting the conduct of that proceeding, as may be for the time being prescribed by regulations under this Act, or may be directed in a special case by the Attorney-General."

In 1884, however, it was found expedient to amend the Act of 1879; and on August 14, 1884, an amending Act was passed (47 & 48 Vict. c. 58), by which all appointments made in pursuance of the Act of 1879 were revoked, and it was provided, amongst other things, that "the person for the time holding the office of Solicitor for the affairs of Her Majesty's Treasury, shall be Director of Public Prosecutions, and perform the duties and have the powers of such Director."

It will be observed that the date, at which Sir Henry James made the statement above quoted, was March 1884, and at that date the Solicitor of the Treasury was acting for the Director of Public Prosecutions, whilst, by the Act which was passed in the month of August of that year, he became actually the Director, and has so continued to be from that time. To say, therefore, that a prosecution is being conducted by the Director of Public Prosecutions is now the same as to say that it is being conducted by the Treasury Solicitor, and the latter term is the one which is the more commonly used.

Sir Henry James referred more particularly in his statement to capital cases, but, as has been seen from the extract setting forth the duties of the Director of Public Prosecutions, the prosecutions undertaken by that officer are by no means limited to capital cases; and the instructions with respect to "those cases where insanity in the accused is alleged" would appear to be interpreted as applying to any prosecutions undertaken by him. And thus, in the case of Richard Coolidge Duncan, who was tried at Carnarvon, in July 1891, on a charge of feloniously wounding his wife, the prosecution was undertaken by the Treasury Solicitor, and, in conformity with the usual practice, the medical superintendent of the neighbouring county lunatic asylum was applied to, and was asked to examine the accused and to give evidence at the trial. This was accordingly done, and a report of the trial may be found in the papers for July 14, 1891.

The general results of the working of the Prosecution of Offences Acts may be seen by reference to the annual reports laid before Parliament, the latest of which was ordered by the House of Commons to be printed on March 12, 1891 (No. 139).

In carrying out the instructions of the Attorney-General to the effect that, in those cases where insanity in the accused is alleged, "full inquiry shall be made," the general practice of the Treasury Solicitor is to apply to medical men of experience and repute, one of whom is usually the medical superintendent of the lunatic asylum for the county in which the accused is in custody, and to request them to examine the accused with a view to giving evidence at the trial, and in the meantime to draw up a report as to the mental condition of the accused, for the information of counsel; and then, if the gentlemen applied to are willing to comply with this request, they are afforded every facility for obtaining the fullest possible information as to the antecedents of the accused. It is the usual practice of the Treasury Solicitor to appoint a local solicitor as his agent in the assize town where the case is to be tried, and that solicitor will always take whatever trouble may be necessary to obtain full information as to the antecedents of the accused. The depositions taken before the magistrate or before the coroner afford the necessary information as to the offence with which the accused is charged, and every reasonable facility is given for the purpose of securing a satisfactory personal examination of the accused. Everything, indeed, is done to endeavour to give full effect to the instructions of the Attorney-General that "full inquiry shall be made," and that the evidence shall be "fully brought before the jury." One of the gravest objections that may be urged against a plan of this kind was very clearly pointed out by Dr. Bucknill, in a lecture* delivered by him at the London Institution, in February 1884. Dr. Bucknill observed: "The greatest objection to an examination forerunning the trial is that it would be almost impossible to prevent it from eliciting confession of the deed, which would often be embarrassing and contrary to the spirit of our law, although in France, as you may know, confession is encouraged or provoked. A solicitor for the defence would decide whether this danger existed or not, and would have a mental examination instituted or not, as he thought best for his client. An official examination, forerunning the trial, which had the misfortune to elicit a confession fatal to the prisoner would, I think, be condemned by English opinion. I do not know what legal right the prosecution or the executive has to order the examination of a prisoner committed for trial."

The difference between the English and the French modes of criminal procedure, to which Dr. Bucknill very rightly draws

* See *British Medical Journal*, March 15 and 22, 1884.

attention in the foregoing extract, forms the subject of a very instructive chapter in Sir James Fitzjames Stephen's "History of the Criminal Law of England," and that chapter will well repay perusal on the part of those who are interested in this matter.

Mr. Wood Renton, in an article contributed to the *Medico-Legal Journal*, of New York, for June 1891, puts the point very tersely in the following extract: "Criminal jurisprudence on the Continent is inquisitorial. Criminal jurisprudence in England and most English-speaking countries (Scotland excepted) is litigious."

Although, however, these two terms "inquisitorial" and "litigious" serve admirably to accentuate the essential distinction between the criminal jurisprudence of the Continent and that of England, it would be scarcely right to assume that, at the present time, the criminal jurisprudence of England is litigious and litigious only.

As the institution of a Public Prosecutor, whose business it is, not so much to obtain a conviction as to see that justice is done, is only, as already stated, of comparatively recent date, there has been scarcely yet time for the realisation of the full effect of the appointment of this officer. Then, again, the statement of the Attorney-General, that it appeared to him "advisable to take steps to insure that all evidence bearing on the case, whether tending to prove the guilt or *innocence* of the prisoner should be brought before the jury," is a strong indication that the attitude of the prosecution is by no means a purely litigious attitude; whilst the instruction, that in the absence of the ability of the accused to produce witnesses, "the Treasury Solicitor shall secure their attendance," affords further strong evidence in the same direction.

But, if it is, happily, no longer possible to say that, in England, criminal proceedings are purely litigious in their character, neither is there any desire that the "full inquiry," directed by the Attorney-General, should run the risk of defeating its object by becoming inquisitorial; nor is there any wish or intention to interfere with the perfect liberty of the accused to present his defence in whatever way may seem best to him and to his advisers.

And when the accused, or when his friends, on his behalf, are taking their own steps for the defence, and are employing legal aid, the risk, referred to by Dr. Bucknill, of eliciting "a confession fatal to the prisoner" would be guarded against by the medical examiner placing himself in communication with the solicitor for the accused. In other cases, where the accused is undefended, the medical examiner will be able to judge, from the documents in the case, as to the degree of risk on this point, and will proceed with due caution. If he finds ground for serious doubt as to the extent to which he would be legally justified in pushing his examination of the accused, his prudent course will be to lay a statement of his doubts before the Treasury Solicitor, who will advise him in the matter.

If more than one medical man is engaged in the examination, it is well that their report should, if possible, be a joint report. Sir James Fitzjames Stephen observes upon this point:* "If medical men laid down for themselves a positive rule that they would not give evidence unless, before doing so, they met in consultation the medical men to be called on the other side, and exchanged their views fully, so that the medical witnesses on the one side might know what was to be said by the medical witnesses on the other, they would be able to give a full and impartial account of the case which would not provoke cross-examination."

In any case, what is wished for, from the medical examiners, is a full and impartial report, for the information and guidance of the Court. It is very desirable therefore, in the first place, to ascertain accurately all the facts, and then to point out what are the medical inferences which may legitimately be drawn from those facts; carefully distinguishing between fact and inference. It is, perhaps, unnecessary to hint that a report loses much of its weight if there is any evident want of care in the manner of stating facts. A statement like the following naturally provokes suspicion: "The accused has no recollection of the occurrence." The question at once arises in the mind of any one reading a statement of this sort whether what is meant is that the accused is so fatuous as not to remember, from one moment to another, anything that he does, or that occurs around him, or whether it only means that the accused *says* that he has no recollection of the occurrence. And then, in the latter case, the further question naturally arises whether the accused says this spontaneously, or whether he says it in answer to a leading question.

It is, however, by no means right to suggest to an insane man that he has no recollection of acts committed by him. Excepting in those cases where either violent delirium or absolute dementia

* "History of the Criminal Law of England." By Sir James Fitzjames Stephen. Vol. i. p. 576.

is present, there is ordinarily very fair recollection; and to suggest the contrary is only to place the accused in a false position. There is perhaps only one more hint of importance to add. It is, that there need be no undue haste in coming to a conclusion, in cases of doubt or genuine difficulty. If, in spite of every endeavour to clear up doubtful points, the medical examiner still feels unable to arrive at a decision, his right course is to inform the Treasury Solicitor, and at the same time to state whether, in his opinion, a longer period of observation would serve to elucidate the matter. A trial can be postponed when there is good and sufficient reason for so doing.

When the case ultimately comes into Court, the medical examiner must not forget that he appears there as a witness: an independent witness whose sole object is to assist the Court to the best of his ability: but still, a witness, who is expected to answer the questions put to him in a plain and straightforward manner. The conduct of the case rests with counsel, subject to the direction of the presiding judge; but it may be remembered that the two points that will arise with reference to the mental condition of the accused are, first,* as to his capacity to plead to the indictment; or, secondly,† as to his criminal responsibility, or, in other words his liability to legal punishment.

W. Orange.

PROCESSIFS (Fr.). Persons labouring under what the French call *délire de la chicane* (Cullerre). (*See* Persecution, Mania of.)

PROGNOSIS.—Insanity is a disease requiring for its cure, even under the most favourable conditions, a period not of days but of weeks or months. Its nature in the majority of cases necessitates removal from home—from home surroundings and relatives. The treatment therefore becomes a costly matter, and the friends of a patient will anxiously inquire for the physician's prognosis, and ask first whether the sufferer is likely to die, then, whether he will recover; thirdly, at what time recovery is likely to take place; and fourthly, what is the danger of a recurrence of the disorder.

Before examining the varieties of insanity it may be well to consider generally the principles on which our prognosis is to be formed.

The **first** question will be as to the time during which the mental symptoms have been noticed, and the manner of their oncoming. If they have commenced recently, have developed rapidly, and are acute in character, the prognosis will be favourable. But if, on the other hand, the commencement is uncertain, and they have gradually and insidiously shown themselves so that the friends cannot fix the beginning, but think the patient has been changed during the last year or two, then will the prognosis be gloomy, especially if the bodily health be but little disturbed.

In the **second** place, the age of the patient must be taken into consideration. The young recover in larger proportion than the old, especially females. At Bethlem Hospital there were admitted in sixteen years 933 patients of both sexes below the age of twenty-five. Of these 595 recovered, being a percentage of 63.7. In the same number of years there were admitted 1872 patients between the age of twenty-five and forty, of whom 968 recovered, a percentage of 51.7, while of the whole number admitted the percentage of recoveries was only 50.4. Those under the age of twenty-five have a comparative immunity from the dire disease, general paralysis, which destroys so many between the age of twenty-five and fifty; and this may account for some of the difference, though not all, because at Bethlem general paralytic patients are not, or were not, admitted as at other asylums. From an acute attack of insanity, if it be the first, the young generally recover, unless it be complicated by some other disease, as epilepsy or phthisis. If it is a second attack, recovery is more doubtful, and so in each recurrence the prognosis becomes less and less favourable, especially if the intervals are shorter and recovery less complete.

In the **third** place, the insanity of the young is largely due to hereditary transmission. How is the prognosis affected by this? It is a popular idea that a patient will not recover if the malady is inherited. It is clear that boys or girls under twenty cannot have brought about their insanity by the cares and worry of life, by anxieties about money, or excess in drinking. They have become insane because they have derived from their fathers and mothers an unstable neurotic constitution prone to disturbance even from a very slight cause. But the figures given above show that recoveries take place in large proportion, so that the prognosis amongst the young is favourable. It may be that being so unstable by nature, they are often thrown off their balance by something which is but a slight and passing cause, and the equilibrium so easily disturbed is easily regained, and they recover, probably to be again upset

* *See* Plead.

† *See* Criminal Responsibility.

by something equally trivial. Much may be gained by a knowledge of the family history, for families in which insanity exists vary greatly in their average standard of health, and a member of one may be more likely to recover than a member of another more degenerate race. We see families in which, it is true, insanity has attacked certain members, yet the others are healthy and strong, mentally and bodily, and able to hold their own in the struggle for existence. In another, though there may have been less actual insanity, yet the general average is of a low character, and neurotic disorders of every kind abound—fits in childhood or at puberty, partial imbecility, early habits of drinking, the moral insanity of the young, excessive masturbation, sleep-walking and the like. If one of these has an attack of mania under the age of twenty-five, he either does not recover, but drifts at once into dementia, or he recovers partially, so as to be able to leave the asylum, whither he returns in the course of a year or two, and remains a chronic patient to the end of his life, swelling the ranks of the young demented people of whom we see so large a number in all our asylums.

In the fourth place, something may be learned by examining the cause of the insanity. In many cases the friends of a patient will plead ignorance of the cause, especially when it is family taint, but in some there may be an undoubted, exciting cause, without which the disorder would probably not have occurred. This may be the loss of a near relative or friend, a serious reverse of fortune, or a sudden shock, fright or accident; or it may be physical illness, a bout of drinking, or great fatigue, overwork or exhaustion, as that produced by over-lactation. Wherever there is a well-defined and appreciable cause, and the insanity follows at no great distance of time, the prognosis is good; so, too, the prognosis is better if the condition of the patient is markedly feeble, and his strength diminished, than if his health is excellent, his weight normal, and his sleep but little broken. By judicious medical treatment health may return, both bodily and mental, but the prognosis will be most unfavourable if we detect any symptom that points to organic brain change. In examining patients between the ages of twenty-five and fifty-five, particularly if they be males, the doubt will always arise as to whether we have before us a case of general paralysis of the insane. The onset of this fatal disease is so variable that the ordinary symptoms of exaltation may be wanting, nay, the disorder may present all the appearance of melancholia, or there may be excitement and exaltation without the physical symptoms of general paralysis. In many cases the prognosis must be very guarded, but where any physical symptoms are present, and where there is any history of fits, however slight, even faintings, or any ataxy or optic neuritis, the chance of recovery is small, though improvement may take place. The prognosis also is bad if we detect evidence of syphilitic brain disease, of tumour or sclerosis, or if the insanity is complicated by epilepsy.

The prognosis is bad in all cases marked by **periodicity**. This may vary from alternate days, on one of which the patient is very insane, melancholic, or maniacal, while on the next he is comparatively sane, up to periodical attacks recurring with tolerable regularity every two or or three months, or two or three years. In some cases the recurring attack is always of the same character and runs the same course, presenting the same delusions and lasting the same time. In others an attack of mania is followed after a longer or shorter interval by an attack of melancholia, and this again by mania, the regular recurrence constituting what the French have termed *folie circulaire*.

From this general view of the prognosis of insanity we may pass to the various forms of the disorder, and first to **mania**, or mental excitement, which ranges from slight but abnormal hilarity or irascibility to the most furious delirium. The latter is often called acute mania, but a better name is **acute delirious mania**, a grave form often fatal to life, to be distinguished from acute mania without delirium, which may exist for a considerable length of time without any danger to life.

If we are called to a case of acute delirious mania with sleeplessness, incessant singing or shouting, restless violence and incoherent raving, what must be observed in order to arrive at an accurate prognosis? The history is of importance: a patient is more likely to recover in the first than in subsequent attacks, his chance diminishing with each successive invasion. Young people, especially women, almost invariably recover from the first attack—recover both in mind and body. Later, they may die in the acute stage, or, recovering to a certain extent, drift into a state of chronic insanity. When repeated attacks occur, with no long interval of time, this result is greatly to be feared, especially when there is a history of marked hereditary taint. Besides the age of the sufferer and the question of previous attacks, the cause of the acute delirium must be investigated. It may be the delirium of drink to which the foregoing observations equally apply. In young and strong individuals, and in first or second attacks, the prognosis is favourable, while it is most gloomy in the old, or in men broken in health, who have had many such attacks already. The complications of serious bodily organic disease, tuberculosis, heart or kidney disease, may lead us to a grave prognosis, while, on the other hand, the delirium which supervenes not unfrequently in the course or during the decline of febrile disorders, as pleurisy, measles, scarlatina, or small-pox, usually passes away in a brief time and recovery follows.

Turning to the patient, the prognosis will be regulated by several important observations. It is more favourable in women than in men, and in persons whose previous health has been strong and sound. The mode and means of treatment will have much weight in pronouncing a prognosis. There must be suitable rooms, airy yet safe, with the windows carefully guarded, so as to obviate the necessity of perpetual holding or mechanical restraint. Many a patient, concerning whom a most favourable prognosis might have been pronounced, has been sacrificed to the prejudices of relations, who have refused the advantages of a good asylum, or grudged the expense of proper apartments and attendants. During the acute stage the prognosis will be affected (1) by the amount of sleep procured. Formerly, many patients died from the exhaustion caused by want of sleep, but in these days there are so many drugs available that by one or other sleep to some extent can generally be produced. (2) The quantity of food taken is an important consideration. The prognosis is favourable if it can be administered in sufficient quantity, and without a violent and exhausting struggle. For this an adequate staff of attendants will be required. (3) A very high temperature is not usually met with in acute delirium; where it occurs it is of very unfavourable import. (4) So also is a very rapid pulse. In times of great muscular movement and excitement, the pulse may become very quick, but in the intervals of comparative quiet fall again considerably. If it remains rapid throughout, the symptom is a grave one. (5) The tongue may afford us valuable information. Under very great excitement and sleeplessness it frequently keeps clean and moist, and this is a good sign. If, on the contrary, it becomes dry and furred, and this state gets worse, and the lips and teeth are covered with sordes, and assume a typhoid appearance, the prognosis is most unfavourable. Here inquiry should be made as to whether opium or its preparations have been administered, as the dryness may be due to a large extent to such medicines. If all things are favourable for treatment, if the patient's health has previously been good and attacks few, we may give a favourable prognosis, both as regards the danger to life and the recovery from the mental disorder. But if attacks recur with short intervals and with increasing violence, death will probably ensue, or at any rate there will be no mental recovery, and permanent insanity or dementia will supervene.

There are patients whose disorder is more fitly termed acute mania—mania without delirium. There is here no immediate danger to life, so in our prognosis this question need not detain us. The sufferers are violent, noisy, often dirty in habits; they sleep but little, but are quite conscious, and know perfectly what they are doing. They may have many delusions, or, on the other hand, the mania will vent itself in outrageous conduct without delusions; they are constantly destructive, mischievous and abusive. On what can we found a prognosis in these cases? (1) The first question is, how long has the attack lasted? If it is recent and proceeds from a definite cause, there is hope, and recovery takes place even after a year or two of such violence. (2) The character of the mania may assist us. If it is mere noisy turbulent violence, without delusions, or with perpetually changing delusions, the prognosis is better than if there are strongly fixed delusions or hallucinations. Hallucinations of sight and hearing, especially the latter, are always grave symptoms, and though they do frequently pass away as the acute stage subsides, yet they are always to be regarded as formidable, and the prognosis must be guarded in such cases. (3) We must examine the physique and age of the patient. The young and strong may have repeated attacks of mania, and recover on each occasion. It is the form of insanity which chiefly affects the young. If the patient is elderly, the prognosis is bad, especially if at the outset he is debilitated by some bodily disease, or the effects of some former wound or accident. He has not the strength necessary to combat the mental excitement, and being further reduced by the latter and by want of sleep, he will gradually sink and die.

Under the general term of mania are comprised various cases of insanity marked not by depression but by excitement, though this excitement differs much, ranging from suspicion and fear, almost amounting to melancholia, up to delusions of grandeur and exaltation of ideas with squandering of money, which may raise the suspicion of general paralysis. The prognosis in these cases appears to vary according as they are removed from the melancholic pole and approach the paralytic. The pathological condition of the former is more favourable to recovery than that of the latter. When we find a patient presenting most of the mental symptoms of general paralysis with exaltation of ideas and maniacal conduct in accordance therewith, we may be sure that his pathological condition is not far removed from that of the graver malady, and if speedy amendment does not take place under treatment, this condition may become chronic, and the brain will remain permanently damaged. Such are to be found in every asylum. They fancy themselves dukes or kings, millionaires, inventors. They are the class who invent fantastic dresses, and decorate themselves with trumpery and tinsel, or fill their pockets with stones and call them diamonds. They never recover.

Passing to the varieties of **melancholia** or mental depression, we meet with one which, like acute delirious mania, is dangerous to life, and may indeed be fitly termed **acute delirious melancholia.** We see not the dull gloom or stupor of ordinary melancholia, but frenzied and panic-stricken violence, the patient resisting everything and everybody, trying to escape from imaginary enemies by door or window, thinking he is going to be burned by fire in the house or the fires of hell, intensely suicidal, refusing all food, trying to strip of all clothing, resisting, in fact, everything that those about him wish him to do. Here, so far as prognosis is concerned, almost the converse of all that was said with regard to acute delirious mania holds true, and the prognosis is most unfavourable. The sufferers are not the young and strong, but the old and debilitated in health. As they will take no food, and much is required, there is a constant and exhausting struggle to administer it. There is a struggle, too, to dress them, and they will not lie down or remain in bed unless fastened, so that their failing strength becomes more and more exhausted, and the feeble power of life does not derive adequate nutriment and new nerve-force from the food that is given. Sleep, moreover, is entirely absent. The melancholia of such patients is often the outcome of bodily disease, of phthisis, pleurisy, or heart or kidney disease, the latter being frequently masked by the acute mental symptoms. A very short period of treatment will materially assist our prognosis. If it be properly carried out, we ought, in a few days to notice an improvement, the frenzy will be less, the patient more inclined to sit or lie down, food will be taken with less resistance and the aspect will improve. If there is no improvement in a short time, death from exhaustion quickly follows, and in fact the mental condition often appears to be one stage in the process of dying. If the patient does not die but the acute state passes away, then we have to deal with a case of ordinary melancholia, and there is no reason why recovery should not take place. For this nervous depression is a pathological condition, yet one which does not greatly affect the organic life and structure of the brain. It is the expression of a defect of nerve force, an insufficient genesis, whereby the individual's whole nervous energy is lessened, and so there are produced dull and gloomy feelings which in turn give rise to dull and gloomy ideas. Something of the same kind constantly occurs in persons who are not insane, but are overworked or overworried and get no sleep or rest. Melancholia then is the smallest departure from the normal state, and the one most likely to pass away. Many, indeed, suffer periodically from low spirits often for a considerable time, months or even years, yet when the fit passes away, they are as they were before it. The brain does not appear to suffer any permanent damage from the insufficient supply of nerve energy, and so it is that melancholia may last even for many years, and then the patient recovers and returns to perfect health, good spirits and sanity. It follows that the prognosis in melancholia is good; especially so is it in cases of so-called **simple melancholia** marked by depression only, and inability to follow an occupation or take pleasure in anything, yet without delusions of any kind. Hundreds of these patients recover without coming to an asylum or even to a doctor. Such attacks return again and again, often with regular periodicity, passing away with but little treatment. As the depression deepens, delusions of many kinds appear, or a strong suicidal tendency, but even here the prognosis, though graver, is not necessarily hopeless, and most of the lamentable suicides recorded in the newspapers are committed by persons who might have been cured if placed under proper treatment.

The conditions unfavourable to recovery from melancholia are chiefly those which indicate an enfeebled state of the bodily health. For this reason hypochondriacal melancholia is unfavourable; and those persons are less likely to recover whose symptoms are of a hypochondriacal nature, having delusions that the bowels never act, that their inside is gone, and delusions about various parts of the body, impotence and the like: moreover, the class of melancholiacs who, having been hypochondriacal for years, have drifted from ordinary hypochondriasis to insane melancholia, rarely recover from the latter development.

All hallucinations of the senses are unfavourable in melancholia as in all non-acute insanity; so is a long-continued suicidal tendency, a symptom very likely to recur even when apparent convalescence has taken place. Long and persistent refusal of food with delusions that it is poisoned is a bad sign, and so is picking of the face and hands, though the writer has known one lady, in whose case this was a marked symptom, recover after seven years. It is a popular idea that religious melancholia is unfavourable. This is not correct. The particular character of the delusion depends on the bent of the patient's mind. The clergyman thinks he is to be eternally lost; the city man thinks that his business is ruined, that his family are going to the workhouse and he to prison. But both recover, things being equal, the one as quickly as the other.

In pronouncing a prognosis concerning male patients between the age of twenty-five and fifty-five, whether the insanity presents the symptoms of mania or melancholia, we must always bear in mind, if we see them in an early stage, that the disorder may turn out to be general paralysis. It is often preceded by melancholic ideas, and these may last for a considerable time, and be looked upon as an attack of melancholia. They may pass away in due course, and perfect recovery apparently ensue, to be followed at a later date by maniacal excitement and all the usual train of exalted delusions. It is most difficult to diagnose some cases of general paralysis in the initial stage, and it is as well to guard one's prognosis in this direction.

We may also be deceived by recurring attacks. A patient is suffering from melancholia which progresses satisfactorily and recovery ensues after a hopeful and gradual amendment; but in no long time it is followed by symptoms of excitement and a violent attack of mania has to be treated, to be followed again by recovery. Then, after a longer or shorter time, the melancholia again makes its appearance, and this cycle goes on frequently through life in ever recurring sequence. When this sequence is once established the prognosis is most unfavourable.

Passing from states of mental excitement or depression, we come to those of mental weakness or dementia. This may be either *primary* or *secondary*, the latter being the sequel of other forms of insanity or of organic disease of the brain, or epileptic or apoplectic seizures.

Primary dementia may be divided into the *acute* and the *chronic*, the former being curable, the latter not. *Acute primary dementia* is a variety of insanity which occurs in young persons, and, although it is very acute and requires much care and skilled treatment, it generally terminates in recovery. Such patients appear utterly lost and demented; they will not converse, but sit in motionless stupor, or wag their heads, or snap their jaws in some silly automatic fashion, stopping perhaps if sharply spoken to and then commencing again. They require to be fed, washed, and dressed, like young children; they can do nothing for themselves. The circulation is very feeble, and the hands are blue with cold, even in the hottest weather. Nothing can look more utterly unpromising and hopeless than the condition of these patients, yet the prognosis is good, and as a rule they recover. We may entertain good hope if they are young, for the curable form of dementia generally attacks those at the ages of puberty or adolescence between thirteen and twenty-five years. In the writer's experience, this form only occurs in patients between these ages. The prognosis is good if the onset is recent, and the sufferer is at once subjected to appropriate treatment. When recovery takes place, if we question the patient, and he remembers anything of the early part of the attack, we generally find that there have been no strictly melancholic ideas or feelings at any stage of the disorder. This form generally has its origin in some fright or shock, and the prognosis is favourable if we can trace it to some known and adequate cause.

Primary dementia in people more advanced in life is of very different omen, and most unfavourable is the prognosis. It may come on very suddenly, the chief symptom being a marked and rapidly increasing loss of memory. This may show itself without any other mental symptoms, but, if severe and growing quickly, it renders a patient at once unfit for the ordinary affairs of life. The cause in a great number of instances, especially in women, is alcohol. Women do not exhibit delirium tremens as men do, and the secret tipplers—and these are the majority—do not drink enough at a time to produce it, but the common result of their drinking is this loss of memory, and with it, frequently, a certain amount of paralysis of arms and legs. Total abstinence sometimes, though rarely, cures these patients in a marvellous and unexpected manner; both the mental and bodily symptoms disappear, to return, unfortunately, in the majority of cases when the woman returns to her evil habit. Our prognosis that she will do this, if she has the chance, is about the most certain that we can pronounce. The prognosis as to recovery at all is, as a rule, very unfavourable. The memory once lost rarely returns, whatever may be the cause of its impairment. Primary dementia comes on very frequently after epileptic attacks when the latter are numerous and frequent. Everything here will depend on the frequency. If they are infrequent, and only occur one at a time, the mental disturbance may be very slight and completely pass away before the next seizure. If frequent, the mind will become more and more obscured and demented, and here, too, the loss of memory will be very noticeable. Inasmuch as chronic epilepsy in adults is a most intractable disorder, it follows that the prognosis is necessarily bad. Primary dementia is also found in connection with syphilis, and here also the prognosis is bad, for with the most antisyphilitic treatment the result is seldom favourable when the disease has advanced to the extent of destroying the mind. Apoplectic effusions, tumours, and softening may all equally produce dementia, and are all of evil omen. Besides this, we find senile dementia, the childishness and loss of memory of old age, a natural decay of brain power, of which there is no cure. Sometimes, too, we meet with a similar dementia coming on, apparently without cause, in persons who are not in advanced age, but of sixty years or so. This is a premature old age, occurring in minds which have never been strong, and without work or worry are nevertheless worn out before their time. It need hardly be said that hope of cure there is none.

Secondary dementia may follow attacks of acute delirium where the latter has lasted long; if convalescence is retarded, and great exhaustion has supervened, a demented condition may be the result, and may continue for some time, gradually passing away with returning health, and requiring probably change of air and scene. The prognosis is not unfavourable if the individual is young, and has not had any or many previous attacks. The converse is unfavourable, especially where there is a history of strong hereditary taint. We may hope for recovery if there is progressive improvement, however slow, but if months go on, and the patient does not wake up, or improves up to a certain point and then stops, remaining weak-minded and vacuous, content to remain in an asylum without wishing to leave, and indifferent as to his future, the worst is to be feared. There is a form of dementia not uncommon amongst young people, the course of which is after this fashion. In the beginning there occurs a somewhat sudden attack of mania. It runs an ordinary course, being possibly somewhat protracted; recovery then takes place, though it may not be quite so perfect as one could wish. After a year or two of convalescence, more or less satisfactory, another attack of acute insanity comes on, and when the patient emerges from it, he does not go forward to recovery, but slides gradually into a chronic and incurable condition of dementia. This is the history of a number of the young demented patients, especially males, to be found in every asylum. They all have a bad hereditary history and all masturbate, men and women. The friends try to lay the insanity to this cause and urge its prevention. But prevention of the habit does not cure such persons; the prognosis in every such case is of the most gloomy character. This secondary dementia rarely follows melancholia for the reasons already stated. Melancholia may exist for a long time, nay, indeed, become chronic, but the mental faculties are retained, and if the sufferer can be diverted from his gloom and self-absorption, and induced to turn his thoughts to some other subject and converse thereon, it will be found that his memory is as good as ever, that nothing has escaped his observation, and that his criticism of what goes on around him is wonderfully keen.

If we apply to the various clinical insanities the principles laid down at the commencement, we see why the prognosis in each is good or bad. For example, in **puerperal insanity** the prognosis is highly favourable. Clouston states that out of 60 cases 45 recovered, a proportion of 75 per cent. Bevan Lewis' record of recoveries reaches 80 per cent. Here we have an acute disorder occurring for the most part in young women, due to a definite cause and coming on rapidly. Even here the prognosis will be affected by the age of the patient, and will be less favourable when it is over thirty, and there have been former attacks. Heredity bears a large part in the causation, yet even with this inherited predisposition 75 to 80 per cent. recover. So, too, the prognosis in the **insanity of pregnancy** is good though not so good as in the last. We find here a well-defined cause producing melancholia, which, like most melancholia, passes away with time and treatment. In the **insanity of lactation** the strength is exhausted, and the weakened brain upset, the attack ranging from simple melancholia to acute delirium. The prognosis will depend somewhat on the rapidity of the onset, cases which come on slowly and gradually after a long period of suckling being less likely to recover. The recovery rate according to Clouston is even higher than in puerperal insanity, being 77.5 per cent. Bevan Lewis, however, gives it as only 65.6 per cent. In **alcoholic insanity** the prognosis is good or bad according as the drinking has been prolonged and chronic or not. The young man who has had few or no previous attacks recovers from his delirium. For the old tippler, male or female, there is but little hope. In **phthisical insanity** the prognosis is bad, the brain disturbance being complicated by severe bodily disease. So, too, is the **insanity of epilepsy.** The melancholia of the **climacteric** is for the most part a curable complaint, unless the bodily strength is too far reduced. It is a question whether any insanity merits to be classed as uterine or ovarian. But the prognosis in what is so called must be based on the principles already laid down.

It should never be forgotten that in a vast majority of recent cases of insanity a favourable prognosis must depend upon treatment being early. Statistics from every source prove that on early treatment depends recovery, and perfect recovery. The poor are far better off in this respect than the rich. The latter will avoid proper treatment as long as possible: hence the records of private asylums cannot show the percentage of recoveries to which the physicians of our public asylums can point. This is a fact strongly to be impressed upon the friends of every insane patient. G. FIELDING BLANDFORD.

PROGRESSIVE PARALYSIS. (*See* GENERAL PARALYSIS.)

PSELAPHESIS, PSELAPHIA (ψηλαφάω, I grope or feel). A feeling or searching about with the fingers, as in delirium. (Fr. *psélaphèse;* Ger. *Touchiren.*)

PSEUDACUSIS (ψευδής, false; ἀκοή, a sound or noise). False or deceptive hearing. Hallucination or illusion of hearing. (Ger. *Gehörstäuschung.*)

PSEUDÆSTHESIS (ψευδής, false; αἴσθησις, feeling). False or deceptive feeling. Imaginary sense of touch in organs long removed, as after amputation. (Fr. *pseudaesthésie;* Ger. *Gefühlstäuschung.*)

PSEUDAPHIA (ψευδής, false; ἁφή, touch). The same as pseudæsthesia.

PSEUDOBLEPSIS (ψευδής, false; βλέψις, a beholding). Hallucination or illusion of vision. (Fr. *pseudoblepsie;* Ger. *Falschsehen.*)

PSEUDOCHROMÆSTHESIA (ψευδής, false; χρῶμα, colour; αἴσθησις, sensation). Anomaly in the perception of visual sensations, in which the vowels in words appear coloured, each having a different tint. Their combination gives to each word a particular colour depending on the arrangement of the vowels in the word. Sometimes the word is seen black as usual, but soon this perception revives the idea of a colour such as red for *a*, rose for *e*, white for *i*, &c. The memory of, or the hearing, the word revives the idea of its colour, independent of any visual sensation cause by the objective presentation. (Littré).

PSEUDOCHROMIA.—False perception of colour.

PSEUDOGEUSIA, PSEUDOGEUSTIA (ψευδής, false; γεῦσις, taste). A false perception of taste. Taste hallucination.

PSEUDO-HYPERTROPHIC PARALYSIS.—This disease is occasionally associated with imbecility, according to Duchenne.

PSEUDOMANIA (ψευδής, false; μανία, madness). A state of mind in which a person accuses himself of crimes of which he is innocent. It is often connected with habitual lying or inordinate vanity.

PSEUDOMNESIA (ψευδής, false; μνῆσις, memory). An affection of memory observed in some mental conditions in which a person believes he remembers facts that never existed.

PSEUDONARCOTISM (ψευδής, false; ναρκόω, I stupefy). A nervous condition, having somewhat the appearance of narcotism, sometimes met with at the menstrual periods and at the menopause. Hysterical narcotism.

PSEUDONOMANIA (ψευδής; μανία). A morbid propensity for lying. A form of moral insanity.

PSEUDOPSIA (ψευδής; ὄψ, the eye, sight). False vision. Visual hallucination or illusion.

PSEUDOSMIA (ψευδής, false; ὀσμή, odour). A false or exaggerated sense of smell. (Fr. *pseudosmie*; Ger. *Geruchstäuschung*.)

PSYCHAGOGIA (ψυχή, the mind; ἄγω, I lead). Mental excitement produced by certain impressions. (Fr. and Ger. *psychagogie*.)

PSYCHAGOGICA (ψυχή, the mind; ἄγω, I lead). Medicines which restore consciousness or restore the mind, as in syncope. (Fr. *psychagogique*; Ger. *psychagogisch*.)

PSYCHALGIA (ψυχή, the mind; ἄλγος, pain). A name devised for melancholia owing to its supposed analogy to neuralgia. Literally mental pain.

PSYCHE (ψυχή, the breath; the mind or soul as usually understood; a butterfly, on account of its transformation from the caterpillar, becomes an image of the soul.). At a later period of antiquity it was used to personify the soul of man. See the beautiful myth related by Apuleius. Her beauty excited the envy of Venus, who ordered Amor to inspire Psyche with love for a contemptible man. The sequel is well known. Eventually she overcame the jealousy of the goddess, and having become immortal, was united with Amor for ever.

PSYCHEISM (ψυχή, the mind). Another term for the somnolent condition induced by manipulation, &c., called animal magnetism or mesmerism.

PSYCHENTONIA (ψυχή, the mind; ἔντασις, tension). Mental over-exertion. (Fr. *psychentonie*.)

PSYCHIATER (ψυχή, the mind; ἰατρός, a physician). A mental physician. The Medico-psychological Association of Great Britain and Ireland adopts for its motto, ψυχῆς ἰατρός.

PSYCHIATERIA, PSYCHIATRIA (ψυχή, the soul; ἰατρεία, healing). The treatment of mental diseases. (Fr. *psychiatrie*; Ger. *Seelenheilkunde*.)

PSYCHIATRIE (Ger.). Psychological Medicine.

PSYCHIC FORCE.—A supposed "force" to which the phenomena of spiritualism were assigned by Mr. Crookes, F.R.S., in 1871.

PSYCHIC PARALYSIS.—A paralysis such as hysterical hemiplegia, where no organic central lesion is known to be the cause of the paresis.

PSYCHICAL. Of or belonging to the mind; **P. blindness**, mind or soul-blindness; **P. deafness**, word-deafness.

PSYCHICAL EXALTATION. (*See* Exaltation, Mental).

PSYCHICAL REMEDIES.—The employment of the mind and its faculties in the treatment of bodily disease. Psychotherapeutics. (*See* Hypnotism and Suggestion.)

PSYCHICAL RESEARCH, SOCIETY FOR.—The object of this Society is to investigate in a systematic manner that large group of debatable phenomena designated by such terms as mesmeric, psychical, and spiritualistic. It is thought that amidst much illusion and deception, an important body of remarkable phenomena, which are *primâ facie* inexplicable on any generally recognised hypothesis, would be, if incontestably established, of the highest possible value. It includes an examination of the nature and extent of any influence which may be exerted by one mind upon another, apart from any generally recognised mode or perception. It is the aim of the Society to approach these various problems without prejudice or prepossession of any kind, and in the same spirit of exact and unimpassioned inquiry which has enabled science to solve so many problems, once not less obscure, nor less hotly debated (*Proceedings* of the Society, vol. i. p. 3). Among the prominent members (past or present) of the Society are, Prof. Sidgwick, the late Prof. Balfour Stewart, the late Prof. Adams, Lord Rayleigh, Mr. Arthur, J. Balfour, Prof. Alex. Macalister, Mr. Alfred Russel Wallace, Prof. Barrett, Prof. Oliver Lodge, Dr. Lockhart Robertson, Prof. Ch. Richet, the late Mr. Edmund Gurney, and Dr. A. T. Myers. Hon. Secretaries, Mr. F. W. H. Myers, and Mr. Frank Podmore. Assistant Secretary, E. T. Bennett, 19 Buckingham Street, Adelphi, W.C.

PSYCHLAMPSIA or **PSYCLAMPSIA** (ψυχή, the mind; ἐκλάμπειν, I shine). A name for mania, proposed by Clouston to show the analogy between it and chorea or eclampsia. He calls it a mental chorea or eclampsia.

PSYCHOCOMA (ψυχή, the mind; κῶμα, deep sleep). Mental stupor. (*See* Stupor, Mental.)

PSYCHODOMETER (ψυχή, mind; ὁδός, a way; μέτρον, a measure). An instrument for measuring the rapidity of psychic events.

PSYCHOGENESIS.—The law of psychogenesis is the elimination of the incongruous in mental development and progress. It is the assimilation or incorporation of life with life. It is a common principle which sweeps through the whole range of mental evolution, alike in the individual and the race. It applies to the simpler inferences of perceptual experience, and to the more complex judgment in matters intellectual, æsthetic and moral (Prof. Lloyd Morgan).

PSYCHOKINESIA (ψυχή, mind; κινέω, I move). Defective inhibition; impulsive insanity.

PSYCHOLOGY (ψυχή, the soul; λόγος, a description). Science of mind. (Fr. *psychologie*; Ger. *Psychologie*.)

PSYCHOMETRY (ψυχή, the mind; μέτρον, measure). The measurement of sense-relations of mental phenomena.

PSYCHOMOTOR (ψυχή, the mind; *moveo*, I move). Term applied to cortical centres, supposed to cause voluntary movements, but now rarely employed.

PSYCHONEUROSES (ψυχή, the mind; νεῦρον, a nerve). Mental diseases.

PSYCHONEUROSIS, VASOMOTOR.—A special form of insanity described by Reich as occurring in a child whose mother had been frightened during pregnancy.

PSYCHONOSEMA (ψυχή, the mind; νόσημα, a disease). Mental disease. (Fr. *psychonosème*; Ger. *Seelenkrankheit*.)

PSYCHONOSOLOGY (ψυχή, the mind; νόσος, disease; λόγος, a description). The doctrine of mental diseases. (Fr. *psychonosologie*; Ger. *die Lehre von den Seelenkrankheiten*.)

PSYCHOPANNYCHIA (ψυχή, the mind; παννύχιος, all night long). The repose or sleep of the soul after the death of the body. (Fr. *psychopannychie*; Ger. *Seelenschlaf*.)

PSYCHOPARESIS (ψυχή, the mind; πάρεσις, weakness). Mental enfeeblement.

PSYCHOPATHIST.—A mental physician; an alienist.

PSYCHO-PATHOLOGY.—(Forensic) Science which treats of the legal aspect of insanity, *i.e.*, the rights and responsibilities of lunatics.

PSYCHOPATHY (ψυχή, the mind; πάθος, a disease). Mental disease. (L. *Psychopathia*; Fr. *psychopathie*; Ger. *Gemüthskrankheit*.)

PSYCHOPHYSIC LAW.—The law expressing the relation between a change of intensity in the stimulus, and the resulting change in the sensation.

PSYCHOPHYSICAL ACTIVITY.—The activity of a hypothetical substratum which fills up the time between stimulus and apperception. It is a variety of psycho-physical movement (*q.v.*).

PSYCHO-PHYSICAL METHODS.—I. The following suggestions are made with a view of getting data beyond those which are strictly necessary for diagnosis, since such data would be extremely valuable, both from the psychological standpoint and as a basis for determining the function of diseased parts, should the case come to autopsy.

The above title is employed in a *general* as well as a *special* sense. In the latter, it is intended to supplement the article on Reaction-Time by Professor Jastrow, by detailing the particular methods employed at the present time in the investigation of time relations of mental phenomena, &c.

How to Observe.—Patients should be away from all distractions, in a room apart and at ease—as a rule, either sitting or lying down, and with the mind placid, a condition which of course is difficult to secure in a large number of mental cases. Experiments should rarely last an hour, as the attention is easily fatigued. Successive observations should be made at the same time of day. For experiments not involving the eyes, it is best to have the patient thoroughly blindfolded.

Records.—May be written, or (in some cases, *e.g.*, areas of anæsthesia) delineated on an outline of the body, such as may be copied from any work on anatomy.

In progressive disease, a careful study of one patient has more value than a casual study of several.

Beginning with the Skin Sensations.—Is the sense of contact anywhere absent? Where? If present, test "discriminative sensibility" with compasses. (For a table of normal discriminations in various regions see Foster's "Text-book of Physiology" under "Tactile Sensations.") Compasses should be made of a substance non-conductive of heat, and slightly blunted at the points, like the rounded end of a small needle. The best form is that where one point is fixed and the other slides along an arm (at right angles to the first point) on which a scale is marked so that the distance between the points is easily read off. (See "Æsthesiometer," by J. Jastrow, *American Journal of Psychology*, vol. i. p. 552.)

Sense of Locality.—The patient to touch a spot on his body which the observer is touching or has touched.

Temperature-sense. — Discrimination of differences. Two objects—preferably thermometers with large bulbs—the temperature of which is known, are applied successively to the same spot on the body, and the patient required to distinguish between them.

Sensibility to Heat and Cold.—Test by applying metal points suitably warmed or cooled. If these sensations are dull, the area stimulated must often be large, a square inch or more, to get any reaction at all. (Refer to "Eine neue Methode der Temperatursinnprüfung," Dr. A. Goldscheider, *Archiv für Psychiatrie und Nervenkrankheiten*, Bd. xviii. Heft 3, 1887. "Research on the Temperature-sense," H. H. Donaldson, *Mind*, No. xxxix. 1885.)

Those cases in which the sensation for one sort of temperature-stimulus remains while that for the other is absent, are specially important.

Motion on the Skin.—By drawing a point up or down the skin of a limb, to determine whether the direction can be recognised. (Refer to "Motor Sensations of the Skin," by G. Stanley Hall and H. H. Donaldson, *Mind*, No. xl., 1886.)

Pressure. — By placing weights successively on the same spot, the patient to detect the difference between any pair of weights. Such weights can easily be made by loading paper cartridge-shells with various charges of shot.

Tickling.—It is specially important to determine the conditions under which this disappears.

Muscle-sense. — Discrimination of weights. Weights to be lifted and thus distinguished. Mr. Francis Galton has a set of weights for this purpose. (*See* "On Apparatus for Testing the Delicacy of Muscular and other Senses in Different Persons," by Francis Galton, F.R.S., *Jour. of the Anthropol. Inst.*, May 1883. A brief account of this is given in "A Descriptive List of Anthropometric Apparatus, &c.," published by the Cambridge Scientific Instrument Co., Cambridge, England. Refer to Weber's *Tastsinn und Gemeingefühl*. Müller und Schermann, "Ueber die psychologischen Grundlagen der Vergleichung gehobener Gewichte," Pflüger's *Archiv*, Bd. xlv. 1889.)

With paper cartridge-shells filled with shot, the more elegant apparatus of Galton can be fairly imitated.

Position of Limbs.—To imitate with a sound limb the position in which the affected limb is placed, or the reverse—eyes closed.

Clonus, Knee-jerk.—(*See* "The Variations of the Normal Knee-jerk and their Relations to the Activity of the Central Nervous System," Dr. Warren P. Lombard, *American Journal of Psychology*, vol. i. 1887.)

Vision.—Ophthalmoscopic data. Pupillary reactions. In case of paralysis of the external ocular muscles, test the subjective sensations of motion on attempted movement of the paralysed muscles.

Field of vision.

Field for various colours. For this some sort of perimeter is needed.

Colour-blindness. Some system of coloured wools is the simplest device for this purpose.

Visualisation (*q.v.*), number-forms, &c. (*See* "Inquiries into the Human Faculty and its Development," Francis Galton, F.R.S., Macmillan & Co., 1883.)

Hearing.—Limits of audition, by means of a small whistle. (*See* "Descriptive List.")

Coloured sounds. Associations of certain colours with given tones. (Refer to *Zwangmässige Lichtempfindungen*; Lehmann & Bleuler. "Inquiries into Human Faculty, &c.," Francis Galton.)

Time-sense. — Repetition and maintenance of a given *tempo*. This involves the use by some device of which a graphic record can be obtained — a revolving drum, for example. (Refer to a series of articles in Wundt's *Philos. Studien*, under the title "Zeitsinn.")

Smell.—Its delicacy, by means of standard solutions of graded strength.

Taste.—Test different portions of the tongue for bitter, sweet, acid, and salt. For bitter and sweet the test can now be made with accuracy. (*See* "Note on the Specific Energy of the Nerves of Taste," by W. H. Howell and J. H. Kastle, *Studies from the Biological Laboratory of the Johns Hopkins University*, Baltimore, vol. iv. 1887.)

Equilibrium-sense. — Special susceptibility to dizziness on whirling, &c. These facts bear on the functions of the semicircular canals. (*See* "The Sense of Dizziness in Deaf Mutes," *American Journal of Otology*, Boston, 1882, by W. James.)

Reaction-time. — To get valuable results, some apparatus is needed. The simplest is that described by Joseph W. Warren, M.D., in a paper "On the Effect of Pure Alcohol on the Reaction Time, with a Description of a New Chronoscope," *Journal of Physiology*, vol. viii. 1887.*

Dr. Warren employs a chronoscope which he names the Bowditch Neuramœbimeter, or "nerve-reply measurer," a term which scarcely does it justice, as its range is very wide (Fig. 1).

The apparatus consists of certain appliances, including (1) the standard tuning-fork (*F*); (2) the recording magnet of Deprèz (*M*); (3) the adjustable holder (*H*, *H'*). The following description is taken from Dr. Warren's article: "The tuning-fork carries on one arm a little brass plate whose edges are turned up to hold a strip of smoked cardboard (115 × 28 mm.), the other arm being balanced by another brass plate, which is held in place by a screw clamp. The fork is attached in the usual manner to a wooden carriage, which slides in grooves on the larger base board. This board has an upright block at the end, held in place by a large screw which permits some movement for adjustment. In the centre of the block is an elliptical

* We are indebted to Prof. M. Foster for permission to reproduce Figs. 1 and 2.

FIG. 1.

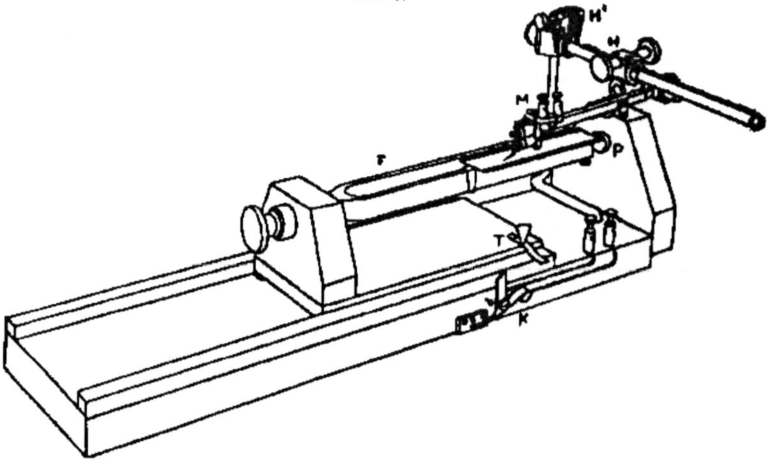

plug (*P*) or spreader, which can be set by a rod at the back. This plug is so placed as to allow the fork to be pushed up to the head board when the long axis is perpendicular. If the fork be pulled with the spreader in this position, the record is a straight line. Turning the spreader through an angle of 90° forces the prongs apart, and the fork begins to vibrate when the pull removes it from the plug, the record changing from a straight line to an undulating one. At the left a brass rod runs up to carry the adjustable holder, which in turn carries the writing magnet. On the base board (*K*) is seen a key to which wires go from the binding posts, and which may be opened by the brass strip or tongue (*T*), whose position on the slide can be varied by the set-screw. To ensure a good electrical contact, the key is faced with platinum, and has a small spring (*S*) to keep it open or shut as the case may be. Evidently, the entire arrangement for mounting and using the fork and magnet is so simple, that a very moderate ability to use tools will suffice for its construction." Dr. Warren adds that "the working of the instrument is equally simple. A card suitably smoked is placed upon the plate as it stands drawn away from the magnet. The key (*K*) is opened, and the plug (*P*) turned so as to have its long axis perpendicular. Then the magnet is lifted by pressing on the spring (*H'*), and held while the fork is pushed home. The magnet now drops on to the card and is adjusted, the plug is turned to spread the tuning-fork, and the key is closed. While the left hand holds the head board, the right pulls the fork which records its vibrations by the scratcher of the writing magnet, and also in passing opens the key (*K*) when the tongue (*T*) reaches it. We shall have then a record of the vibrations of the tuning-fork whose legibility will depend on the speed with which the fork is pulled. If we connect the wires from a battery with the writing magnet and the binding posts in such a way that the key will break its circuit, we shall be able to indicate the instant of opening the key in the record; for the magnet will lose its magnetism, and the pen will change its position, and this will cause a change of level in the vibrations recorded by the tuning-fork. If, after a brief interval, a current of electricity should pass again through the magnet, the pen would return to its former position, and another change of level in the record of vibrations would occur; the number of vibrations from the beginning of the first change of level to the beginning of the return, gives us the *measure of the time* which elapsed from breaking the circuit until it was closed again. In the apparatus described a standard tuning-fork (100 vibrations to the second) is used. The load changes the rate of vibration somewhat, and for exact time-measurements, a comparison must be made with some other standard (pendulum). Obviously, the opening of the key (*K*) may be adapted to giving a variety of signals dependent upon breaking an electric current, and we may thus signal to *any of the senses of the percipient*, or stimulate nerve or muscle directly, and a reply may be given by any object which undergoes such changes on account of the stimulation as to cause an electric current to pass anew through the writing magnet. The application of the Bowditch Neuramœbimeter is thus seen to be very extended. Although this instrument is not quite so simple as that of Exner and Obersteiner,* it has certain very important advantages besides a greater variety in its applications."

Many details in regard to the practical working of the apparatus employed by Dr. Warren in connection with the galvanic battery† are not necessary for our present purpose, but the diagram below (Fig. 2) shows the arrangement of the apparatus.

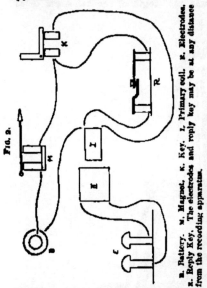

FIG. 2.

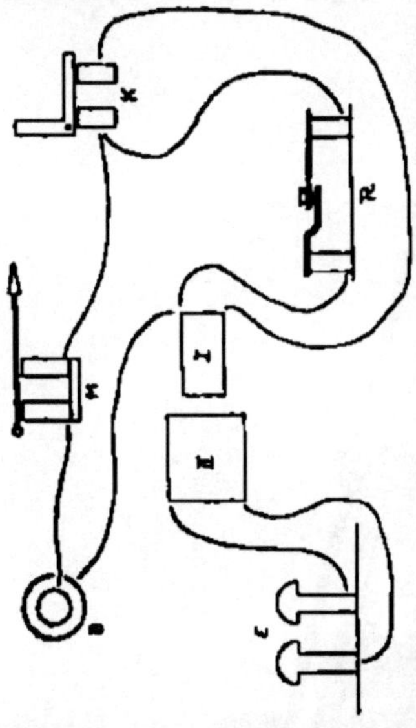

B. Battery. M. Magnet. K. Key. I. Primary coil. E. Electrodes. R. Reply Key. The electrodes and reply key may be at any distance from the recording apparatus.

The primary factors of all chronoscopes are *signal* and *reaction*. The particular mode of registering the period of time which has elapsed between these two recorded factors has been variously carried out by different observers. Hence chronographs have been adopted according to preference. By some Marey's Chronograph* is preferred.

The nature of the mental process involved in experiments in reaction-time has given rise to much difference of opinion. Professor James has always maintained that the opinion originally held by Wundt is not tenable. Wundt distinguished "between two stages in the conscious reception of an impression, calling one *perception*, and the other *apperception*, and likening the one to the mere entrance of an object into the periphery of the field of vision, and the other to its coming to occupy the focus or point of view. Professor James,† on the contrary, holds that *inattentive awareness* of an object and *attention* to it are equivalents for perception and apperception. Then there is, according to Wundt, the conscious volition to react, thus making three successive elements in the psychophysical process. The succession of conscious feelings during the stage in question, James denies. According to him, it is a process of central excitement and discharge, with which doubtless some feeling co-exists, but what feeling we cannot tell, because it is so fugitive. . . . The feeling can be nothing but the mere sense of a reflex discharge. *The reaction whose time is measured is, in short, a reflex action pure and simple, and not a psychic act.* A foregoing psychic condition is, it is true, a pre-requisite for this reflex action. . . . . The tract from the sense-organ which receives the stimulus into the motor-centre which discharges the reaction, already tingling with premonitory innervation, is raised to such a pitch of heightened irritability by the expectant attention, that the signal is instantaneously sufficient to cause the overflow. . . . . "Expectant attention" is but the subjective name for what objectively is a partial stimulation of a certain pathway, the pathway from the centre for the signal to that for the discharge.‡ Wundt has more recently adopted the same view of the nature of the psychic process, namely, that there is neither apperception nor will, but that they are merely *brain reflexes due to practice*.§ Cattell's conclusions are in accord with those of Professor James.

The "Hipp Chronoscope" is a somewhat costly instrument, to be used only

* "Ueber eine neue einfache Methode zur Bestimmung der psychischen Leistungsfähigkeit des Gehirnes Geisteskranken," *Archiv für pathol. Anat.* 1874, Bx. 427. S. Exner has contributed "Experimentelle Untersuchung der einfachsten psychischen Processe," Pflüger's *Archiv f. d. ges. Physiol.*, vii. 601. E. Kraepelin has contributed "Ueber die Einwirkung einiger medicamentöser Stoffe auf die Dauer einfacher psychischen Vorgänge"; Zweite Abtheilung, "Ueber die Einwirkung von Æthylalkohol," Wundt's *Philos. Studien*, Bd. i. 573.

† The time which elapses between the stimulation of one or two fingers of the left hand by an induction shock, and the closing of a simple key by the right hand which rests upon it, is recorded on a card.

* *Cf.* "La Méthode Graphique," part ii. chap. ii.

† "The Principles of Psychology." By William James, Professor of Psychology in Harvard University. 2 vols. London: Macmillan. 1890.

‡ *Op. cit.*, vol. i. p. 91.

§ "Physiol. Psych.," 3rd edition (1887), vol. ii. p. 266. See also Lange's experiments, *Philosophische Studien*, vol. iv. p. 479 (1888).

with great caution. The conditions attending its use have been given by Prof. J. McK. Cattell, of New York, in his article "Psychometrische Untersuchungen," which appeared in Wundt's Journal, *Philosophische Studien*, vols. iii. and iv., 1886–87.

Quite recently Prof. Jastrow has stated that a large amount of work in regard to time-measurements of mental processes has been done with the Hipp Chronoscope. The objections to its use are the difficulty of regulating it and "the possible sacrifice of accuracy to convenience." He succeeded, however, after many trials in accurately determining the error of the

FIG. 3.

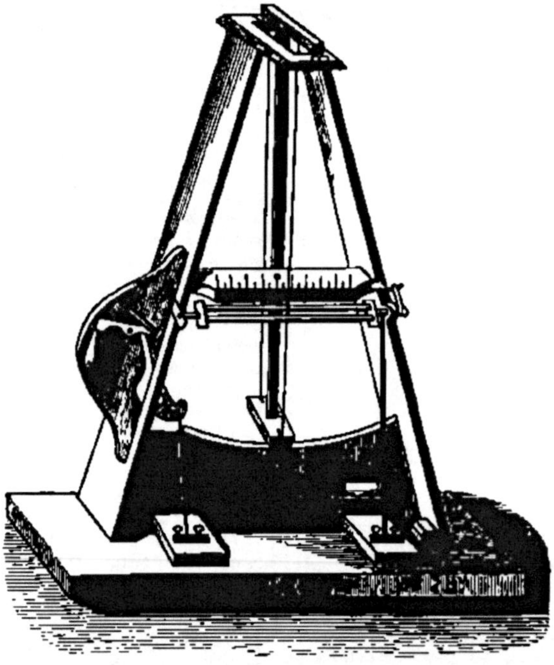

instrument, by means of apparatus constructed for the purpose. The maximum error during six months was .005 seconds, and the average error about .002 seconds. He concludes with stating that the apparatus thus modified "has proved itself so easy of manipulation, and so time-saving, that its use is confidently recommended to experimental psychologists."*

Mr. Galton has introduced an apparatus for measuring reaction-time which has the merit of great simplicity. He calls it the A-form Chronoscope. The description which follows (Fig. 3)* is given by the inventor himself:—

It measures the interval between a signal and the response to it, by the space traversed by an oscillating pendulum when measured along a chord. The pendulum is always released at the same angle of 18° from the vertical, and the graduations are made on a chord of the arc through which it swings, situated at a vertical distance of 800 millimetres from the point of suspension. In this case, the length of the half-chord or of 800 × tan 18°, is equal to 259.9 millimetres. The graduations show the space travelled across from the starting-point, at the close of each hundredth of the time required to perform a single oscillation. The places for the alternate graduations are given in the subjoined table, which has been calculated for the purpose, and may be useful in other ways, but the times to which the entries there refer, are counted

* *American Journal of Psychology*, Dec. 1891, p. 211, art. "Studies from the Laboratory of Experimental Psychology of the University of Wisconsin."

* See the *Journal of the Anthropological Institute*, Aug. 1889. Mr. Groves, 89 Bolsover Street, W., is the maker, and has supplied a number of instruments to hospital laboratories.

from the vertical position of the pendulum, and are reckoned up to − 50 on the one side, and to + 50 on the other. The value of the decimal is only approximate; it had, in many cases, to be obtained by graphical interpolation. If the pendulum is of such a length as to beat seconds, the graduations, as below, will be for hundredths of a second; if made to beat half-seconds (which is the case in the instruments now made), the interval between each alternate graduation will stand for a hundredth of a second. The graduations are numbered on the bar of the instrument, starting from the point whence the pendulum is released, which counts as zero.

T = the time of a single oscillation. Angle of oscillation 18° on either side of the vertical. The distances are measured upon a chord that lies 800 millimetres vertically below the point of suspension. The decimals are only approximately correct.

$\frac{T}{100}$	Distances from vertical.	$\frac{T}{100}$	Distances from vertical.
0	0	26	185.9
2	15.7	28	197.0
4	31.3	30	207.4
6	46.8	32	216.2
8	62.2	34	224.8
10	77.6	36	232.7
12	92.3	38	239.8
14	107.0	40	246.4
16	121.5	42	251.2
18	135.2	44	255.1
20	148.5	46	257.9
22	161.5	48	259.5
24	174.0	50	259.9

A pendulum must have considerable inertia in order to keep good time; on the other hand, it is impossible to give a sudden check to the motion of a body that has considerable inertia without a serious jar. Therefore it is not the pendulum that has to be sudddenly checked in this apparatus, but a thread that is stretched parallel to it, by an elastic band both above and below. As the pendulum oscillates the thread swings with it, and the thread passes between a pair of light bars that lie just below the graduated chord, and are parallel to it. On pressing a key, these bars revolve round an axis common to both, through a little more than a quarter of a circle. They thus nip the thread and hold it tight, while no jar is communicated to the pendulum. The signal either for sight or for sound is mechanically effected by the detent at the moment when it is pushed down to release the pendulum. The pendulum may also be released, without giving any signal. A sound-signal is made by releasing the hammer which strikes the detent. This produces the sound-signal and at the same time releases the pendulum. The sight-signal is produced by pressing a key at the back which changes the colour of the disc and at the same time, releases the pendulum.

Mr. Galton prefers this instrument to one he formerly used, the action of which depends upon a falling rod.

It may be serviceable to state some details respecting the laboratory of psychology in the University of Pennsylvania where Professor Cattell has hitherto worked.* Similar apparatus may be seen at most of the Universities in the United States, including Harvard University, where Professor James fills the chair of psychology, and Clark University where Dr. Sanford is instructor in psychology.

The laboratory possesses apparatus which measures mental times conveniently and accurately. The chronoscope in use is an improvement on one described in *Mind* (No. 42). The mean variation of the apparatus is now under one-thousandth of a second. New pieces have been made for the production of sound, light, and electric stimuli. Apparatus for measuring the rate of movement and other purposes has been added. The observer is placed in a compartment separated from the experimenter and measuring apparatus. With this apparatus researches are being carried out in several directions. Professor Dolley is measuring the rate at which the nervous impulse travels, using two different methods. In one series of experiments an electrical stimulus is applied to different parts of the body, and a reaction is made either with the hand or foot. The rate of transmission in the motor and sensory tracts of the spinal cord has thus been determined. In a second series of experiments two stimuli are given at different parts of the body, and the interval between them adjusted until the observer seems to perceive them simultaneously. Professor Fullerton is carrying on a research to determine the rate at which a simple sensation fades from memory. A stimulus is allowed to work on the sense organ for one second, and after an interval of one second, a stimulus, slightly different in intensity is given for one second, and the least noticeable difference in intensity is determined by the method of right and wrong cases. The interval between the stimuli is then altered, and it is determined how much greater the difference between the stimuli must be in order that

* Prof. Cattell has now removed to Columbia College, New York.

it may be noticeable. The rate of forgetting is thus measured in terms of the stimulus. Intervals varying from one second to three minutes have been used. For these experiments a new apparatus was constructed, and it was discovered that when sensations of light are successive and last for one second, the least noticeable difference in intensity is not about one-hundredth as is supposed, but much the same as for the other senses under like conditions. The rate, extent and force of movement are the subject of a somewhat extended investigation. The least noticeable difference in motion has never been studied in the same way as the like difference in passive sensation. Yet it would seem to merit such study even more, owing to the importance and obscurity of the "sense of effort." The laboratory possesses apparatus for studying the time, intensity and area of stimulation needed to produce the just noticeable sensation and a given amount of sensation. These mental magnitudes are correlated so that one may be treated as the function of the other. The results of studying the relation of time to intensity have been published in *Brain* (pt. 31), it being found that the time which coloured light must work on the retina in order that it may be seen, increases in arithmetical progression as the intensity of the light decreases in geometrical progression. The laboratory has a valuable collection of Kœnig's apparatus for the study of hearing and the elements of music, and a spectrophotometer, a perimeter and other pieces for the study of vision.*

In conclusion the writer may observe that it would yield the best results if any one interested in work of this nature would settle on some single topic and pursue that specially.

HENRY H. DONALDSON.

[*References.*—In addition to references given, see especially A Laboratory Course in Physiological Psychology, by Edmund C. Sanford, Ph.D., The American Journal of Psychology, edited by G. Stanley Hall, April 1891, *et seq.*, and the following literature cited:—*Dermal sensations:* Weber, Tastsinn und Gemeingefühl; Wagner, Handwörterbuch der Physiologie, vol. iii. pt. 2; Funke, Hermann's Handbuch der Physiologie, vol. iii. pt. 2. *Sensations of temperature:* Blix, Zeitschrift für Biologie, Bd. xx. h. 2, 1884; Goldscheider, Neue Thatsachen über die Hautsinnesnerven; Du Bois-Reymond's Archiv, Supplement, Bd. 1885, pp. 1–110; Fechner, Elemente der Psychophysik, vol. ii. pp. 201–211. *Sensations of pressure:* Beaunis, Eléments de physiologie humaine, ii. 579; Eulenberg, Berliner klin. Wochensch., 1869, No. 44; Reference Handbook of the Medical Sciences, vol. i. p. 85; Aubert and Kammler, Moleschott's Untersuchungen, v. 145; Blaschko, Zur Lehre von den Druckempfindungen, Verhandl. d. Berliner Physiol. Gesell. Sitz., 27 März 1885. *Static and kinaesthesic senses:* Aubert, Physiologische Studien über die Orientierung (trans. with comments of Delage's Études Expérimentales sur les illusions statiques et dynamiques de direction, &c., Tübingen, 1888, p. 41. *Sensation of rotation and progressive motion:* Aubert, trans. above cited; Mach, Bewegungs-Empfindungen, Leipzig, 1875; Brown, On Sensations of Motion, Nature, vol. xl. 1889, p. 449. *Innervation sense:* Wundt, Physiologische Psychologie, i. 397; Sternberg, Zur Lehre von den Vorstellungen über die Lage unserer Glieder; Pflüger's Archiv, xxxvii. 1885, 1; Loeb, ibid., xlvi. 1–46; James, Psychology, ii. 516; C. L. Franklin, Amer. Jour. Psychol., ii. 653; Ferrier, Functions of the Brain, p. 380; Funke, op. cit. *Sensations of motion:* Goldscheider, Untersuchungen über den Muskelsinn; Du Bois-Reymond's Archiv, 1889, pp. 369, 540. *Sensations of resistance:* Goldscheider, *op. cit.* *Bilateral asymmetries of position and motion:* Hall and Hartwell, Mind, vol. ix.; Loeb, Pflüger's Archiv, xli. 1887; *ibid.* xlvi. 1890, 1–46. *Taste:* Kittmayer, Geschmacksprüfungen, Göttingen Diss. 1885; Oehrwall, Untersuchungen über den Geschmackssinn, Skandinav. Archiv f. Physiol., Bd. ii. 1890, pp. 1–69, and Dr. Sanford's abstract in Zeitschrift f. Psych., Bd. i. 1890, p. 141; Bailey and Nichols, The Delicacy of the Sense of Taste, Nature, xxxvii. 1887–8, 557; Lombroso und Ottolenghi, Die Sinne der Verbrecher, Zeitsch. f. Psych., Bd. ii. 1891, pp. 343–48; Camerer, Die Methode der richtigen u. falschen Fälle angewendet auf den Geschmacksinn, Zeitsch. f. Biol., xxi. 570; Keppler, Das Unterscheidungsvermögen des Geschmacksinnes f. Concentrationsdifferenzen der schmeckbaren Körper, Pflüger's Archiv ii. 1869, 449. *Smell:* The olfactometer of Zwaardemaker can be obtained at Utrecht (Mechanicker Harting Bank) at 1.50 mk.; see his paper, Die Bestimmung der Geruchsschärfe, Berlin. klin. Wochensch., xxv. 1888, 47, p. 950, abst. in Brit. Med. Journ., 1888, ii. 1295; Bailey and Nichols, The Sense of Smell, Nature, xxxv. 1886–87, 74; Lombroso and Ottolenghi, *op. cit.*; Du Bois-Reymond's Archiv, 1886, pp. 321–57; Hermann's Handbuch, iii. (pt. 2), pp. 225–86. *Hearing:* For special instruments see Hensen, Physiologie des Gehörs; Hermann's Handbuch, iii. (pt. 2), pp. 119–120; Jacobson, Du Bois-Reymond, Archiv, 1888, 189; Starke, Wundt's Philos.-Studien, iii. 1886, 266; *ibid.* v. 1889, 157; Helmholtz, Sensations of Tone, Eng. trans. by Ellis; Wundt, Phys. Psych. (under this head the references are too numerous to cite); see Sanford's second article, The Amer. Jour. of Psychology, Dec. 1891, pp. 307–322.]

* The foregoing account is condensed from a description given in *The American Journal of Psychology*, April 1890, p. 281, under the heading of "Psychology at the University of Pennsylvania."—[ED.].

11. In the absence of complicated and expensive apparatus designed *ad hoc*, the observer may advantageously employ the ordinary apparatus current in the physiological laboratory—viz., clockwork and cylinder covered with smoked paper, chronograph, and Marey's tympana.

(1) The *clockwork and cylinder* is ordinary physiological use is the most expensive item (£10 to £20); but it is the most universally useful as regards all kinds of records and time-measurements, and should therefore appear as a matter of

course in the furniture of a neurological laboratory. A very convenient form is that in which the clockwork bears three axes, upon any one of which the smoked cylinder is placed, giving speeds of approximately 270, 45, and 7½ mm. per second (for still slower records it is convenient to have a separate clockwork carrying a cylinder on the one hour axis (£1 to £2)).

(2) The *chronograph* (£3 to £4) is required to control the rate of movement of the smoked surface. In its simplest form it is a tuning-fork or reed (10 to 100 vibrations per second), marking the undulations against the smoked surface by means of a light style, or as a more handy arrangement, it consists of (*a*) a reed with a platinum wire dipping in and out of mercury, kept in vibration by an electro-magnet; (*b*) second electro-magnet marking vibrations against the smoked surface; (*c*) a battery; and (*d*) wires joining the two electro-magnets, mercury pool and battery into one circuit. For reaction timing we may employ the cylinder on the quick axis (270 mm. per second), and mark time in hundredths of a second by tuning-fork or reed; or when very numerous records are desired on the same paper, it is sufficient to take the medium speed (45 mm. per second) and mark time with a reed of 20 per second.

(3) *Tympana* in the form of miniature kettle-drums, with drum-heads of elastic membrane, and joined by india-rubber tubing, are useful for time-signalling as well as for other purposes. The recording tympanum carries a lever which marks against the smoked surface. Or, if desired, the chronographic signal may be employed with two keys in its circuit, one the question key, to make the circuit with application of tactile, auditory, or visual stimulus, the other, the answer key, to indicate sensation by breaking the circuit. The reaction-times given in the figure below are taken in this way.

A still simpler device is formed by a straight slip of wood or metal working in a vertical plane on a horizontal axis, and marking against the cylinder as usual, with stops to prevent excessive movement. This is easily adapted to give the ordinary reaction-times to touch, to hearing, and to sight, and by using two such slips side by side, the time of discrimination or that of volitional choice can be determined. Practically it is most convenient to rest the two slips across a closed india-rubber tube in connection with a recording tambour.

Touch.—The observer, blindfolded, rests his finger on the lever, and has to remove it in response to a tap; the interval on the smoked surface between the marks of tap and removal gives the reaction-time.

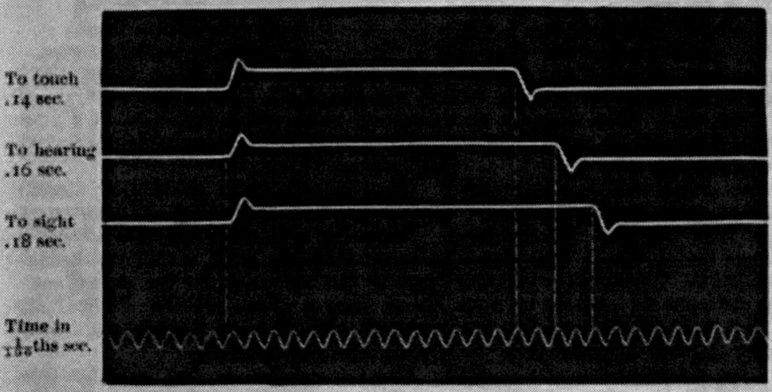

Hearing.—The observer has to move the lever in response to a tap upon it; the interval gives the time as before.

Sight.—A signal fixed to the lever is raised and made visible by its movement (which must be made soundless); the subject taps the lever as soon as he sees it; reaction-time marked as usual.

The following "directions to students" in use in the physiological laboratory of St. Mary's Hospital, will sufficiently explain the principle upon which reaction-times are taken, and in accordance with which the conditions of response may be adjusted to measure the shortest time required to discriminate between two sensations (discrimination-time or dilemma), or the shortest time required to choose between two volitional acts (volition-time). In the first case the hand of a blindfolded person, on whom the simple reaction-time to touch has been determined to be, say 0.15 second, is stimulated on the little finger or on the thumb, with the understanding that only one of these stimuli is to be signalled; the reaction-time is now found to be, say 0.17 second, from which the conclusion is drawn that 0.02 second was the discrimination-time —*i.e.*, that required to distinguish between the two sensations. In the second case the experiment is conducted with two signals (in this case the tympanum method will be found most convenient), on the understanding that one signal is to be used when the little finger is touched and the other when the thumb is touched; the total time, say 0.20 second, under these conditions, is considered to be the sum of 0.15, the simple reaction-time, *plus* 0.02, the discrimination-time, *plus* 0.03, the volition-time. The experiments may be still further complicated in a variety of ways, to measure the time of recognition of letters, numbers, words, simple ideas, &c. The following are taken from the "directions to students" alluded to above, and are carried out with the reaction-timer already described, *i.e.*, a slip of wood (or for discrimination two slips of wood) across a tube attached to a recording tympanum, and with the cylinder on the middle rate axis. Two persons cooperate in the observations, one as operator and one as subject.

Measure the simple reaction-time with tactile, auditory, and visual sensations.

Tactile. — The subject, blindfolded, places a finger on the lever. The operator taps the finger. The subject responds by pressing the lever as soon as he feels the tap. The interval between the two marks on the smoked cylinder gives the measure of the reaction-time to a tactile stimulus.

Auditory. — The subject, blindfolded, places his hand ready to press the lever. The operator strikes the lever so as to make a sharp sound. The subject responds by pressing the lever as soon as he hears the sound. Reaction-time as before.

Visual.—(The butt end of the lever is painted white; the rest of the apparatus and the movements of the operator are hidden by a screen). The lever is depressed quickly and quietly. The subject responds as soon as he sees the white end move down. Reaction-time as before.

Take an average of ten observations in each case.

Measure the discrimination-time. A double lever is now used.

Tactile. — The subject, blindfolded, places an index finger of each hand on each lever, it being agreed that he is to react only to a touch on one side; sometimes one, sometimes the other, finger is tapped by the operator. Take the average of ten responses made in succession without mistake.

Auditory.—A single lever is struck, now with a small bell, now with a bit of wood. The subject, blindfolded, has to answer only to one or other of these two sounds. Take average as before.

Visual.—(The butt ends of the two levers are painted of different colours.) The subject has to signal the movement of one or other of them as agreed upon. Average as before.

The result = simple reaction-time
+ discrimination-time.

Measure the volition-time.

Repeat the previous series of observations, but with the understanding that the left hand is to be used to signal touch, sound or sight in connection with the left hand lever, and the right hand for differing stimuli of these three kinds in connection with the right-hand lever. Averages to be taken as before.

The result = simple reaction-time
+ discrimination-time
+ choice or volition-time.

In connection with these observations of reaction-times (which presumably are cerebral) measure the lost time of a true reflex act (which is presumably bulbar) as follows:—

Fix a fine thread to one of your eyelids and to the lever of a bell crank myograph.

From the secondary coil take a wire to a large electrode fixed to any convenient part of the body, and for the second electrode take a silver chloride silver wire covered with chamois leather and moistened with salt solution.

Use the cylinder on the quickest axis, or else use a shooting myograph, placing the trigger key in the primary circuit.

Press the silver electrode against the conjunctiva of the lower lid; select by trial a suitable strength of shock; see that the thread from the upper eyelid is kept tight and that the trigger key is shut; let off the apparatus, and measure the interval between the moment when the conjunctiva is stimulated and the moment when the upper eyelid moves. You will find it to be about five-hundredths of a second.

A. D. Waller.

xxx. The instrument chosen for the inquiries carried on at the Wakefield Asylum was one of a series of anthropometric apparatus made by the Cambridge Scientific Instrument Co., and designed by Mr. Francis Galton, with certain modifications introduced by the writer. We have found it to be a most valuable, simple, and exact instrument, well adapted for the purpose in view.

The instrument consists of a solid, upright, square standard of pitch pine about 5ft. 10in. in height, supported on a firm tripod of the same material, fitted with levelling screws. To the summit of this standard is adapted a simple arrangement for the suspension and release of a graduated rod which should hang from this support in a perfectly vertical position, and not in contact with any of the other fittings of the instrument. This position of the rod is readily secured by the levelling screws of the tripod. Astride the rod at its upper end is a brass weight, which descends a certain distance with the falling rod. A little more than half way down the standard, a rectangular piece of teak* is screwed vertically, and at right angles to its long axis, supporting a small electro-magnet, to which is adapted (as an armature) a spring stirrup which clamps the falling rod on the breaking of an electric circuit. The further end of this cross piece supports a horizontal slab or table on which rests the hand of the person to be tested.

For a **sound signal** the metal weight astride the rod is caught by a teak diaphragm projecting from the standard after a definite descent of the rod; or, if an *electric* signal be required, an arrangement is adapted to this diaphragm, whereby an electric circuit is broken by the impact of the weight.

The rod itself is concealed from the subject to be tested by a projecting ledge of pine wood, which lies parallel with it and betwixt it and the subject; and to this ledge is fitted, at a convenient height for the eye, a brass plate with a small slit or window. A lengthened slit in the rod corresponds to this window in its position of rest; but, as the rod falls, the window is shut off, and a sight signal thus given. The window in the brass plate can be adjusted vertically.

The rod hangs free within the stirrup clamp, which, being attached by a horizontal spiral spring, effects on the release of the stirrup the clamping of the rod. The base of the stirrup is kept fixed as an armature to the electro-magnet, either by the induced magnetism of an electric current, or by the simple arrangement of a cord attaching it to a bell-crank lever, whose vertical arm is fixed by a steel spring placed below it. If this latter arrangement be adopted, pressure on the horizontal arm of the lever releases it from the spring, and the stirrup clamp closes upon the rod. It need scarcely be added that this mechanical arrangement should be discarded whenever an electric circuit is available. It will be useful to describe more particularly the *rod and its release, the signalling, the clamp.*

* Mahogany or teak.

The Rod.—This consists of a strip of box-wood* about three feet in length, graduated along its edge in hundredths of a second up to thirty divisions; hence, it fails to register a longer interval than three-tenths of a second. This limitation in the measurable period was a serious defect, which has been completely remedied by a modified arrangement whereby the period may be extended indefinitely. It is unnecessary to detail here the author's new arrangement, since the results given (see REACTION-TIME) were chiefly obtained by the shorter registry of the older instrument. In the original instrument the rod was suspended by a horizontal bar, which, on the turning of a milled head by an assistant, swung round and released the rod. An appreciable click was often thus induced *preceding* the true sound signal. To obviate this the writer has substituted a straight bar electro-magnet, and the rod suspended therefrom was released, on breaking the electric circuit, with absolute silence. The button for breaking the circuit was placed on the top edge of the teak cross-piece, so that the operator could, whilst seated in front of the instrument, start the rod and read off the register without the assistant's aid.

The Signal.—For a *sound* signal we have attached to the upper end of the standard an electric bell which rings when the weight falls on the diaphragm.

For a *sight* signal we have added a small brass table supporting a candle shaded from draught, which slides into a slot in the standard, and can be drawn out immediately opposite the small window already indicated. The light can be adjusted vertically by a screw. We have found this arrangement essential for securing a fairly uniform intensity of stimulus.

The Clamp.—The stirrup, as before stated, is held in position by an electro-magnet, which in our instrument will, with a single Bunsen cell, support a weight of over 3¼ lbs. The circuit for clamping the rod passes to a small contact-breaker on the teak table. So that the depression of a button here effects the clamping of the falling rod, whilst the mechanical arrangement of bell-crank lever may be utilised with advantage for drawing the armature back into contact.

The steel base of the stirrup is fitted with rubber where it comes sharply into contact with the rod. This rubber is apt

* Either box- or lancewood may be utilised for this purpose.

to loosen, and is best secured by two stout ligatures. The hempen cord securing the base of the stirrup to the bell-crank lever should also be replaced by strong catgut. The most essential features to be secured in the use of this instrument are its solidity, steadiness, simplicity of arrangement, good levelling adjustments, the silent release of the rod, uniformity in the intensity of the stimulus, secure clamping of rod, arrangement for checking momentum and rebound of rod.

The Test.—The individual to be examined sits with his hand comfortably resting on the small teak slab, the forefinger gently applied to the button, the depression of which breaks the circuit to the electro-magnet. The operator sits in front of the instrument, and reads off from time to time the extent of fall of the rod. An assistant, if preferred, stands behind the instrument, and, pressing upon the button fixed betwixt the two binding screws (on the top edge of the teak cross-piece), breaks contact, and releases the rod attached to the upper electro-magnet; and, after the fall of the rod, he releases it again by drawing back the stirrup armature, and suspends the rod in its former position on the magnet. Or, if the old arrangement be preferred, the assistant stands behind and suspends or releases the rod from the horizontal bar by turning the milled-head screw to the right or left respectively.

In the test for an *acoustic stimulus* the individual with his forefinger resting on the button is told to listen for the signal and depress the key *as quickly as possible* when he hears it. In the test for *optical stimuli* the candle-flame is brought on a level with the small slit in the brass plate. With his finger still on the button, he is directed to keep his eye fixed upon the light, and *instantly* depress the button when the light disappears. The upper edge of the stirrup armature is exactly opposite the zero line of the rod, at the moment when the sound and sight signals are given, so that the further fall of the rod is read off in hundredths of a second at the time when it is clamped by the stirrup.* (*See* REACTION-TIME IN CERTAIN FORMS OF INSANITY.)

W. BEVAN LEWIS.

PSYCHO-PHYSICAL MOVEMENT.—The movement of either an imponderable or ponderable agent, upon which all psychical processes are supposed to depend. Fechner postulates a ponderable substance as the medium of psychical phenomena.

PSYCHO-PHYSICAL TIME.—This expression is used in psychometry for the time occupied during the fourth of Exner's seven processes, which occupy Reaction-time (*q.v.*). Reaction-time is the interval between the instant when the external stimulus begins to act on the end-organ of sense and the resulting movement of some member of the body; the fourth process, or psycho-physical time, is the time occupied in transmission of the sensory excitation into the motor impulse in the brain. This time is further subdivided into three parts, occupied by three processes, as follows: (*a*) Perception simple. This is the mere perception that the subject is in some way affected; (*b*) Apperception or discernment-time, which, as the name implies, is the time occupied in clearly discerning the nature of the affection; (*c*) Will-time—the time occupied in deciding on the motor impulse. Either of these times can be reduced by experiment. The measurement of psycho-physical time is obtained by directly finding the whole reaction-time, then measuring the time exclusive of psycho-physical time and finding the difference. (*See* REACTION-TIME.)

PSYCHO-PHYSICS.—Experimental psychology. Fechner divides it into outer and inner psychophysics; the former (*äussere Psychophysik*) comprising stimulus and apperception; and the latter (*innere Psychophysik*) including the process which intervenes between stimulus and apperception; it connotes mental function.

Psycho-physical Laws.—Under the heading of "Psycho-Physical Methods" a practical account of these methods is given, and to this article the reader is referred for a description of the instruments employed. Theory and practice go hand in hand together, and the results must be ultilised in the direction of formulating *general laws* with regard to sensibility. Researches are directed to, (1) absolute, and (2) comparative sensibility. Of the former, the sense of touch has been the most thoroughly investigated, little having been done with regard to the other senses. The latter (2), however, has been much more the object of psycho-physical research, and observers have been able to arrive at general conclusions and to formulate certain laws. The first general law with regard to comparative sensibility was pronounced by Weber, and, although it has been expressed in different manners and has often been modified, and although it has been contradicted, it

* The Cambridge Instrument Company inform the Editor that since they supplied Dr. Bevan Lewis with the instrument he has described, they have made some improvements, but their new apparatus is the same in principle.

has nevertheless proved to hold good in all cases.

Weber's law is this: The sense-impressions produced by two pairs of stimuli remain the same, provided that the difference in each of the two sets increases or decreases in the same proportion. For example, the difference between a stimulus which may be expressed by 100 and increases by 1, and between another stimulus which may be expressed by 200 and increases by 2, or is expressed by 400 and increases by 4, would be perceived as one and the same sense-impression.

On this law has been based the science of psycho-physics, on which we have the greatest authority in Fechner, who by his methods of arranging psycho-physical experiments and of utilising their results, has proved Weber's law to hold good for all kinds of sensibility. Fechner's methods* are: (1) Methode der eben merklichen Unterschiede; (2) Methode der richtigen und falschen Fälle; (3) Methode der mittleren Fehler.

(1) The method of ascertaining differences of sensation which are just distinguishable.—This may be done—*e.g.*, by comparing the difference between two weights; if the difference is great, it is easily distinguished; but if it is not great enough, it will barely be distinguished, or even not at all. The method consists in finding that difference which just becomes appreciable, and this difference is reciprocal to the sensibility—*i.e.*, if the appreciable difference is great, the sensibility is small, and *vice versâ*.

(2) Method of right and wrong cases.—It consists in testing the sensibility—*e.g.*, by weights or light, constantly varying the amount of the former and the intensity of the latter. Cases in which the difference is correctly appreciated are called "right" cases; those in which it is not recognised or appreciated are called "wrong cases." From these results is ascertained the mean difference, which, as before, is reciprocal to the sensibility. This method yields very good results, but a very great number of observations must be made.

(3) Method of ascertaining the mean error.—It consists—*e.g.*, in trying to find from a number of weights one which is equal to a given weight previously determined, or to draw a line equal to a given line. The difference between the actual weight or line, and those erroneously chosen or drawn by the person making the experiment, as being equal to the former, serves to determine the mean error, which again is reciprocal to the sensibility.

Each one of these three methods may be applied to all spheres of sensibility, but it must be understood that one method is more suitable for one kind, another for another kind of sense-organ.

We refer the reader to Fechner's "Elemente der Psychophysik," 1889, and Wundt's "Grundzüge der Physiologischen Psychologie" (trans. into French, 1886), and to a treatise by Dr. Georg Elias Müller, of Göttingen, in the "Bibliothek für Wissenschaft und Litteratur" (vol. xxiii.), entitled "Kritische Beiträge zur Grundlegung der Psychophysik."

PSYCHORRHYTHM (ψυχή, the mind; ῥυθμός, a measured movement). Alternating mental conditions. (*See* FOLIE CIRCULAIRE.)

PSYCHOSES (ψυχή, the soul). The name for mental affections as a class. Used very loosely for mental phenomena, states of consciousness, thoughts, ideas, &c. German alienists restrict the meaning of psychose (sing.) to healthy states of mind, whilst they employ psychosen (plur.) in the sense of abnormal mental conditions.

PSYCHOSES, FULMINATING (ψυχή; *fulmen*, lightning). Mental affections characterised by explosive outbreaks.

PSYCHOSIN.—The cerebroside of sphingosin. (*See* BRAIN, CHEMISTRY OF, p. 149.)

PSYCHOSIS.—A mental affection. (Fr. *psychose;* Ger. *Gemütskrankheit.*)

PSYCHOSIS; OR, THE NEURAL ACT CORRESPONDING TO MENTAL PHENOMENA.—In studying mental action the physiologist must necessarily confine his descriptions to physical facts, and observe the physical signs accompanying mental action. All expression of mental states is by movement; we begin by studying these signs. The general means of studying movements and classifying them, is described under "MOVEMENTS" (*q.v.*), and the early signs of mental action in the child are given under "EVOLUTION;" the general mental capacity of an individual may be studied by observation of these signs. In the following table the properties of neural action necessary to certain mental states are indicated.

The table (p. 1026) illustrates the advantage of the scientific **method of studying mental action**, as well as the convenience of the metaphysician's methods. The metaphysician names, or labels, an almost in-

* The term "methods" is used in two senses: first, in regard to the practical means adopted as regards apparatus, &c.; secondly, the principles according to which certain experiments should be conducted, and the results utilised.

 Psychosis

numerable list of "mental activities," but does not necessarily give us exact means by which we can observe and determine them. These are said by the physiologist to correspond roughly to various aggregations of a few observable physical phenomena—*i.e.*, certain modes of action among nerve-centres similar to those found among the modes of action and growth in the cellular elements of other living things.

Intellectual Faculties or Modes of Action.

Physical Conditions.*	Instinct.	Intelligence.	Will.	Memory.	Imitation.	Thinking.	Emotion.
1. Spontaneous action	P.	P.	—	—	—	P.	P.
2. Impressionability	P.	P.	P.	P.	P.	P.	A.
3. Controllability of spontaneity	—	P.	P.	—	P.	—	A.
4. Retentiveness	P.	P.	P	P.	P.	P.	—
5. Diatactic action	—	P.	—	—	P.	P.	—
6. Delayed expression	—	P.	P.	P.	—	P.	A.
7. Reinforcement	—	—	—	—	—	—	P.
8. Double action	—	P.	—	P.	—	—	—
9. Compound cerebration	A.	P.	P.	—	—	P.	A.
10. Uniform series of acts	P.	—	—	—	—	—	—

P.—present. A.—absent.

Spontaneity.—An essential character of brain action giving aptness for mental function is spontaneity. That is spontaneous action of many small centres, or centres governing small movements; this is shown to be a marked character of the infant brain, it is nearly lost in the adult for movements, but reverts in some conditions—*e.g.*, fatigue and emotion, chorea, delirium. It seems that as evolution advances spontaneous action of the centres for movements decreases, but that it remains for mental action, and leads to new thoughts, spontaneous and vague uncontrolled thinking.

Controllability of Spontaneous Action is seen in evolution of the infant and when action is temporarily inhibited by sight of an object, this is commonly followed by acts not previously performed; it is probable that some (diatactic action) neural arrangement for action among the cells is formed during the quiet time by the sight of the object.

Delayed Expression.—Here we have retentiveness, the physical impression received by the centres through the senses is left as a diatactic union among them; the impress is strong enough just to form such union ready for subsequent action. The remaining physiological properties of the brain necessary to mental function are sufficiently described for present purposes under Movements (*q.v.*).

We now commence the study of brain action in displaying mental function with certain facts and observations before us, and have mainly to consider the theory put forward, and its fitness for describing various well-known mental phenomena. Further evidence as to the usefulness of the hypothesis may be found in the suitability of the same modes of observing, describing and arguing as applied to general conditions of the nerve-system and to mental action. Lastly it will be seen that the theory and methods used are in harmony with the laws of evolution which have so greatly aided biological research. To study subjective conditions, is to study our own mind, not those observed.

Hypothesis.—The hypothesis is that every mental act depends upon the formation and action of a certain combination among the nerve-cells.

The neural state corresponding to mental action depends on the special centres called successively into co-action, and the ratios of their action. When we see a series of movements we infer activity and discharge of force from a number of nerve-centres corresponding. In obeying a word of command, in catching a ball, sound and sight are respectively the stimuli preparing particular groups of nerve-centres for action. We assume as our hypothesis that such actions are due to some kind of functional union of the centres produced by the stimulus received through the senses antecedent to the movement. The act of getting the nerve-centres ready for action is here supposed to be the formation of some kind of union among them for the passage of nerve-currents through the cells which govern the particular combinations of the resultant movements. Examples of unions among nerve-centres are seen in the symmetrical movements of the eyelids and mobile features of the face—we infer that the centres for the two sides of the face usually form a functional union because the sight or sound which precedes a change of facial expression is usually followed by equal and synchronous movement on either side. This hypothesis of functional unions for action we have illustrated by examples of facts seen in cellular growth. The term "functional union for action," or

* These physical conditions are referred to in the text by quoting the numbers as given in the table.

"is union," simply applies to the co-action, or synchronous action for a certain period of time, on a single occasion, or many occasions, or uniformly within our experience—of a certain number of like-living elements.

The evidence as to the functional union occurring is the combination of action, or the series of combinations. We observe the combination of movements, and infer combination of action in the centres. The term "functional union" is convenient; it involves a theory—we must explain rather than define the meaning of the term; it is an inference from the time of the acts; it is probably the outcome of the common impressionability of the subjects.

As evidence that some kind of physical union among the centres is formed we refer to the following facts:—Repetition makes all actions quicker and more precise; they follow more readily and certainly upon the same stimulus. Practice makes the actions precise and perfect.

It is assumed here that a mental act is not due to the function of one mass of brain which does nothing but produce that one act, but the outcome of the particular set or combination of cells which happen at the moment to act together, the union of cells for such act being temporary, though capable of recurring. It has been shown that one group of cells acting together produces one particular movement, and it is believed that similarly one group of cells can produce one particular act of mind—the particular thought thus depends upon the particular group of cells acting. It is also believed that groups of cells can be caused to act together in mental acts, as for certain movements, by a very slight stimulus of sound or sight.

The expression of a thought consists in the motor action of a group of cells; the thought (act of psychosis) consists in the formation of the union of cells whose motor, or efferent action, produces expression of the thought. Thought precedes and is known by subsequent movement; thought is a part of the cause of the movement, and must correspond to some physical (it may be temporary) arrangement among the cells. We do not know what the "arrangement" may be, but, as it leads to associated movements, we suppose that it consists of associations among cells. Thus, "thinking" is the getting ready for action; it is the molecular or functional formation or arrangement of unions among nerve cells. A special combination or series of movements may occur, and these may not be called up again till some special stimulus recurs—*i.e.*, a special associated action of cells or union among them does not recur till that special stimulus recurs. These associations, ties, or unions among cells may be dissolved.

The mental function of nerve-centres appears to be merely the faculty for the formation of combinations for action; it is a form of impressionability, such that forces acting through the senses can produce unions among the centres, controlling the special centres in the union, and deciding how long the union shall last, whether it be quickly dissolved or rendered permanent.

Diatactic Action and Compound Cerebration.—This formation of unions among nerve-centres previous to sending efferent currents to muscles, and thus producing movements and visible expression, we have termed "diatactic action" (*διατασσω*, to get ready for action).

This diatactic action is inferred to exist as the neural change or activity corresponding to a "thought;" it is exactly the same, so far as we know, as the getting ready for a co-ordinated motor action.

The analogy between the motor (or efferent) action of nerve-centres, as expressed by movements and the hypothetical diatactic unions supposed to be the neural representation of thoughts, is shown in the following table. The facts placed in parallel columns are usually found to co-exist, or to follow one another rapidly:—

Motor Expression.	Conditions of Mental Faculty.
1. Much spontaneous action controllable through senses.	Capacity for intelligent thought.
2. Visible impressions cause many combined actions	and many thoughts.
3. Identical impressions followed by similar actions	and similar thoughts.
4. Inherited tendency to certain actions	and to recurrence of certain thoughts.
5. Uniform work causes more fatigue than variety.	A change of subject of thought is recreative.
6. Variations of work do not necessarily cause more bodily waste.	Variations of thought not necessarily followed by signs of brain fatigue.
7. Permanent reflex actions.	Permanent fixed thoughts, easily called up.
8. Fixed lines of motor action.	Uniform lines of thought.
9. Habits of movement.	Habits of thought.
10. Untrained movements are irregular.	Untrained thoughts are irregular.
11. In somnolence, gradual subsidence of movement	and of thought.

12.	In passion, a spreading area of movement not controlled from without.	A rapid flow of uncontrolled thoughts.
13.	Certain movements cannot co-exist.	Certain thoughts cannot co-exist.

Psychosis.—Writers on mental science define and illustrate the **law of adhesiveness.** Those scientific thinkers who accept the generalisation of evolution will find in the writer's "Law of Syntrophy" some evidence of a widely spread, if not universal, mode of action, both in growth and modes of action of nerve-centres, embracing the modes of neural action which lead to adhesiveness.

The Law of Syntrophy.—When the attributes of action in a living thing have for a time been controlled by a force acting upon it, and that force causes its action, then the impressions made may be followed by action similar to that which occurred during the period of stimulation. Any force producing synchronous action among like living elements is usually followed by subsequent synchronous action among them. The law of syntrophy states that, when such a union has been brought about by some force, as an impression made upon them, then the same force acting again is usually followed by action in the same group or union of elements.

This law of syntrophy is of course only a generalisation from observed facts, many of which occur among conditions of vegetable and animal growth, and their enumeration here would be out of place; suffice it to say we have arranged and classified a catalogue of such facts in support of this theory.*

This law of syntrophy, like other laws of nature, is only a generalisation of experience; it is based on observation, and shows that synchronous action may result from the like stimulation of similar living subjects. Now, the nerve-centres are similar subjects of nutrition, and their special co-action, or, as we commonly call it, union, may be similarly brought about. It is suggested that a "diatactic union of nerve-centres" may be formed by coincident stimulation, and is not necessarily due to organic union of the nerve-centres by nerve-fibres. Why a certain diatactic union is formed by one sight impression, a second union by another sight impression, we do not know, but this is the inference drawn from observed facts.

See a boy looking earnestly at an object that interests him, he gazes at it and is motionless; when spoken to he begins to talk of it and to describe it, saying what he thinks about it. The boy while looking at the object is supposed to be thinking about it, acts of psychosis are supposed to be taking place in his brain, his brain is being got ready for the subsequent speech. We cannot see what is going on in his brain, but when he tells us what he thinks about the object we have an expression by movement of that which occurred in his brain during his quiet time. The words he now says are the outcome of certain movements of his body produced by currents from those groups of nerve-cells which were being prepared by the impression following the sight of the object. The words that come out depend upon the special cells previously arranged into unions. The inference is that during that wonderful "quiet time," while he gazed motionless at the object, the light reflected from the object gets the brain ready, preparing diatactic unions among his centres. In such a case the expression of what took place in the brain might be delayed; he does not speak describing his thoughts till he is questioned—the acts of psychosis and their expression may be separated by an interval of time, the impression produced upon the brain is not expressed till it is again stimulated by our interrogations.

A boy learns his lessons from a book at night and says it in school next morning; while looking at his book his sight of the book results in certain arrangements among his nerve-cells (A B C), such that next day when told to say his lesson we have expression by movement in the words produced by movements of *a b c*. If that has happened in the boy's brain which the teacher wished for during evening preparation, impressions were produced making functional arrangements among the centres; the expression of such impressions is delayed till the time for saying the lesson; then, the word of command is followed by expression of the brain action, and if the lesson be successful, the brain impressions are rendered firmer and stronger.

We observe our travelling companion, his eyes are directed towards a particular advertisement at several stations; subsequently he speaks to us of the subject matter of that advertisment. Such action in our companion indicates intelligence. During the time of our journey an impression must have been made upon his centres by the sight of the advertisement, this was a functional union of centres (theory) formed by light, "a getting ready," a change molecular in kind, seated

* See author's work on "Mental Faculty," Cambridge University Press.

in certain nerve-centres, occurring at the time of the impression by light, not at that time followed by efferent nerve-currents from centres to muscles. Such may be called an act of psychosis without expression at the time.

Instinct.—(1) Spontaneity. (2) Impressionability. (4) Retentiveness. (10) Uniform series of actions.

Instinct as a mental character is indicated by certain actions which result in an impression upon the animal, and such action is looked upon by some as an indication of intelligence. The nerve arrangements for instinct are congenital, or constructed previous to an individual existence, or as the result of impressions upon the ancestry. It seems that certain groups of nerve-cells tend to co-act in a diatactic union either spontaneously or upon the occurrence of certain stimuli. An infant breathes on coming into contact with the air, the act is due to the construction of the nerve system, making the centres for certain movements tend to co-act; the action may even begin spontaneously (1). The chick pecks (10) his way out of the shell without any apparent stimulus to action, but picks up food better off the dark ground (2). The infant's lips begin to move when in want of food, even before they touch the breast. The continuance of these special neural arrangements shows the high degree of retentiveness (4) in the brain; they are very fixed and permanent. The actions of instinct are usually a uniform series of movements (10). The congenital faculty of instinct does not involve aptitude for intelligence and compound cerebration. A capacity for imitation is a special and high class form of instinct, but this latter does not necessarily imply special capacity of impressionability. There may be no known differences in the neural arrangements for instinct and intelligence, but there are great differences in the relations of their action to their necessary antecedents.

Intelligence.—Brain characters: (1) Spontaneity. (2) Impressionability to external forces. (3) Controllability of spontaneity. (4) Retentiveness. (5) Diatactic action. (6) Delayed expression. (8) Double action. (9) Compound cerebration.

Intelligence as a term may be incapable of formal definition, but we may indicate the modes of brain action necessary to the display of this faculty. Aptitude for intelligence necessitates spontaneity, this being capable of control through the senses (see EVOLUTION) (1, 2, 3, 5). Later, adapted action following a period of inhibition (6), or control of spontaneity, shows the occurrence of compound cerebration (9). We think it will be found that the physiologist's studies of intelligence are observations and inferences on compound cerebration, its history and causation; this is the great character of brain action, giving capacity for thought; illustrations are given under explanation of the processes of logic. Adapted action indicating compound cerebration is very suggestive of the higher character of intelligence as compared with instinct, memory, imitation. Of course an act of memory or imitation may lead to compound cerebration and intelligent and adapted action.

These signs of intelligence are not found at birth, we do not find that impressions received are retained (4); memory and retentiveness are later acquisitions; further, in the earliest stages, there seems no evidence of double action in the brain (8); we do not see a stimulus to action leave any definite impression on the brain which produced it.

Want of spontaneity, or absence of controllability of the spontaneity may lead to defective intelligence; it is well to try and define the physical defect of a brain leading to defective psychosis.

Will or **Volition.**—(2) Impressionability. (3) Controllability of spontaneity. (4) Retentiveness. (6) Delayed expression. (9) Compound cerebration.

Volition is absent in the infant, it is present in a variable degree in man. Will is indicated by voluntary action (see VOLUNTARY MOVEMENTS). This kind of mental action is often independent of any strong present impression, and is due rather to past or antecedent impressions (4), or to inherited impression and training. Volition or will, as a neural act, may be delayed in its expression (6), the mind is made up, its visible action may be deferred. To the physiologist, will does not appear to be some essential unknown force acting upon nerve-centres stimulating them to action. Physical health promotes strength of will; to exercise will strongly against present impressions from without leads to the signs of fatigue, as is readily seen in children. It is due to the intrinsic force or diatactic unions formed by past impression, and as in all such cases may be very persistent, but easily exhausted for a time though apt to recur. Spontaneity (micro-psychosis) is antithetical to the display of will; capacity of compound cerebration favours it.

Emotion.—(7) Reinforcement. (6) No delayed expression. (1) Spontaneity.

Here we may group the more prominent signs of emotion of various kinds, so as to consider the characters in which they are distinguished from more direct indications of intellectual activity. Let us look at the expressions of mental excitement—speech becomes more and more rapid (7), words are frequently repeated, so that though utterance is constant, the vocabulary becomes very limited. There is much movement in the parts of the face, the area of movement increasing (7); but unless the condition pass on to what is called an explosion of passion, expression in the face remains symmetrical. The individual is not easily controlled in action through the senses; these signs are well marked in mania, the action shows much spontaneity both for movement and psychosis (1).

The signs of exhaustion follow.

"Mental excitement" is a condition known to every one by numerous and rapid actions involving many small parts, the area of action tending to increase from cerebral reinforcement. There is diminished impressionability to control. The action following upon stimulation is different from the normal in many cases. The signs of strong emotional conditions may be illustrated by reference to passion, excess of laughter, emotional crying, hysterical attacks.

Memory.—(2) Impressionability. (4) Retentiveness. (6) Delayed expression. (8) Double action.

Memory as a mental faculty is known to us by the relations of the antecedent force which impressed the brain to the outcome of action (4). It appears that when an impression is produced upon the brain (2) the subsequent expression in memory is due to a union among cells having been produced by that impression which may long remain inactive (6); the expression may be by word or gesture. The antecedent force which produced the neural impression may have had a double action (8), an immediate efferent current producing movement and a later or delayed outcome. Thus a special facial gesture may recur upon sight of a well-known object; recurrence of the impression strengthens the certainty with which the act recurs or is remembered, the effect of the impress is "cumulative." Too large a number of acts of memory may lessen the faculty of spontaneous thinking.

Imitation. — (2) Impressionability. (3) Controllability. (4) Retentiveness. (5) Diatactic action.

The objects of imitation are postures and movements in other men; sight of action in another man is followed by action of the parts seen moving. The impression received stimulates the nerve-centres corresponding to those acting in the party imitated; it appears that common impressions in the past upon the ancestors of both subjects leads to this impressionability. Imitation is analogous to instinct in depending upon congenital neural arrangements, and not necessitating compound cerebration; it differs from instinct in being stimulated by an object similar to itself, in which character it appears to be a higher form of impressionability.

We have explained our hypothesis as to the neural processes corresponding to the expression of mental states and mental activities, we must now consider the diatactic neural action corresponding to a *train of thought* under the name compound cerebration. This is the hypothesis: "In the mode of brain action termed compound cerebration one diatactic union may by its activity stimulate another to action, and thus a series or train of activities, in part the result of past impressions, may occur, ending in some visible expression." A careful study of the motor signs of mental acts has led us to frame this hypothesis. It appears that a primary stimulus may produce a diatactic union *ABC*, the stimulus from this a union *BDE*, followed by *EFG*, and finally *GHK*, which, sending efferent currents to muscles, produces action in *ghk* as a visible expression of the outcome of the train (series of acts) of thought.

Compound Cerebration.—Intellectual effort, trains of thought, and the higher modes of thinking, must correspond to neural acts highly adapted and controlled. It is this association of past neural impressions and present stimulation that we have now to study, under the term compound cerebration. This kind of neural action is believed to occur when we see specially adapted action slightly delayed after its stimulation, but well adapted to the circumstances. Compound cerebration is in part due to previous impressions, in part to present forces; it is to some extent expressed in the selection and use of words. Among persons whose antecedents and inheritance are similar, there is an average or normal for the outcome of compound cerebration, which we should expect to see follow a certain impression.

In evolution the capacity for diatactic action precedes the appearance of adapted action and compound cerebration. Diatactic unions when formed may cohere and produce larger unions, or may be connected in serial order, so that a fixed series of neural diatactic unions act in fixed order of succession on a certain stimulus.

Brief evidence of some neural process, such as compound cerebration, is given in the following table:

Observed Facts.	*Methods of Thought.*
Spontaneity being quelled, a period of quiescence precedes adapted action.	A period of time is required for thinking out a subject previous to a new line of action.
The acquisition of new modes of expression is followed by signs of fatigue.	Persistent thinking is followed by fatigue.
Visible development consists of series of acts of growth and movement resulting in final action well adapted to circumstances.	Mental development consists in the formation of trains of thought leading to certain results.

The mental philosopher says, "Human knowledge consists of mind and matter—*i.e.*, the subjective world and the objective world." We would rather say that we study diatactic neural action in relation to objects, and objects in action and to physical forces. We are not here concerned with consciousness or any form of subjective feeling, but it may be remarked in passing that the subjective impressions probably correspond to the formation of a neural diatactic union occurring in every mental act. Prof. Bain says: "The primary attributes of intellect are retentiveness and consciousness of difference and agreement." Romanes indicates "choice" as a criterion or character analogous to those of mind, and instances examples of choice in the amœba which retains certain particles of food and rejects others.

It is thus desirable that we should describe the neural processes which, according to our hypothesis, correspond to the increase of judgment or making comparisons. This will be dealt with in speaking of the physiological process corresponding to the processes of logic.

Thinking, or the exercise of intellect, may be said to be present in any man capable of conducting a train of thought, and expressing inferences or results of thought by words or other mode of expression. The mental processes in a correct mode of thinking have been defined by the logician; we may begin by studying the neural processes corresponding to the logician's use of the terms, "proposition," "syllogism."

The consideration of a proposition may be represented by two diatactic unions in coincident activity; should they remain co-active the unions corresponding to subject and predicate become coherent and the proposition is granted as true. The possibility of cohesion of these diatactic unions depends upon their previous coincident activity—*i.e.*, past experience. Speaking of the terms predicable in psychology, we use those which connote facts in the body of the living man; abstract terms connote expression by his nervemuscular action—*e.g.*, kindness, joy, &c. Such diatactic unions result from impressions produced by sight of movements and postures in others. Examples may be drawn from motor action showing that certain nerve-centres cannot be in coincident action. It is difficult to perform the acts of stroking with one hand and patting with the other, or to move the feet and hands at different ratio. The "energetic hand posture" on one side, and the nervous posture on the other, do not usually coexist.

Logician's Definitions.	*Physiologist's Equivalent.*
Term—the simplest result of thought.	A diatactic neural union—the simplest representation of a thought.
Proposition—implies coexistence of two terms.	Two diatactic unions must be brought into co-activity.
Syllogism—two premises or propositions with one term common to both.	Three diatactic unions are rendered active in pairs in succession.
The proposition is accepted or denied.	Unions representing "terms" cohere permanently; or, they will not cohere permanently.
Abstract terms predicable of man.	Unions the results of impressions by sight of nervo-muscular action.
Mental comparison.	Two unions rendered temporarily co-active, they either cohere or not, according to past impressions received.

A Line of Thought or Argument.—(1) Spontaneity. (2) Impressionability. (4) Retentiveness. (5) Diatactic action. (6) Delayed expression. (9) Compound cerebration.

Thinking is represented in neural action by a series of diatactic unions due to compound cerebration, partly sequential to past impressions, and it may be in part due to present stimulus. A child sees an object, and thinks about it; he sees a knife, and leaves it alone, taking scissors instead, so as not to cut himself. The stages of thought are a compound series of neural acts ending in visible movement. Any great amount of reinforcement may lead to mental confusion, hence emotion is antithetical to quiet and correct thought. Spontaneous thought is apt to be vague, as contrasted

FIG. 1.

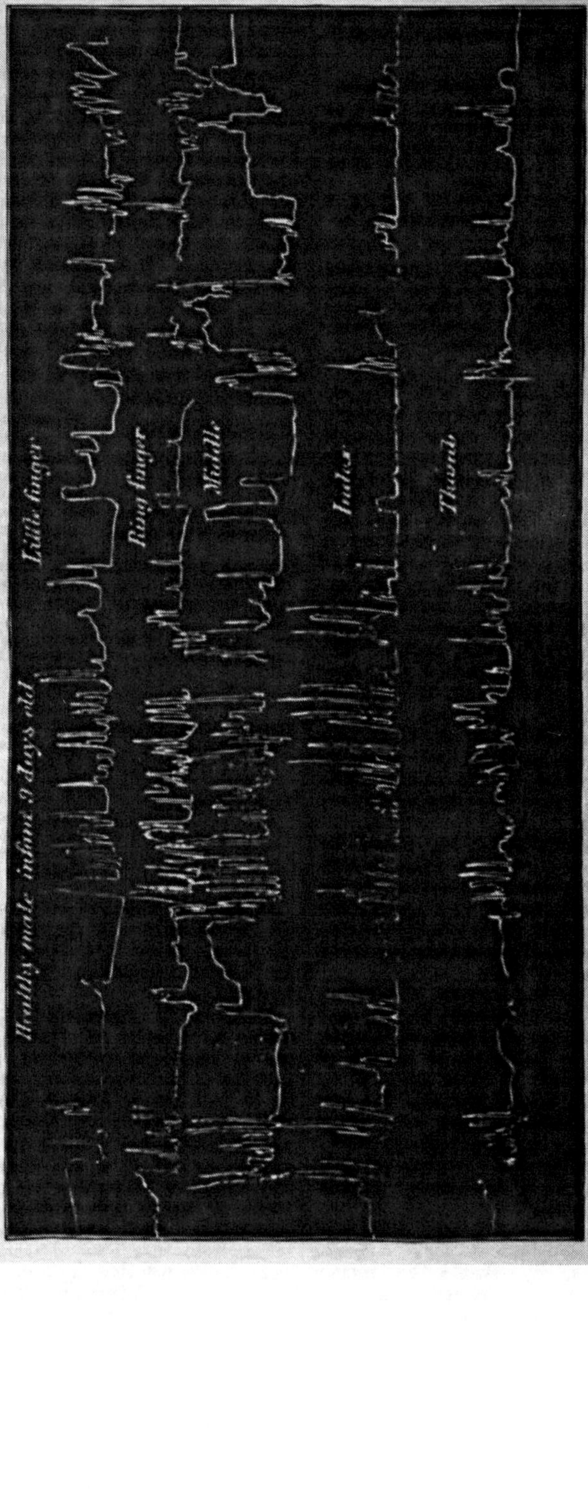

Tracings of the spontaneous movements of an infant's hand during fifteen minutes—Microkinesis.

FIG. 2.

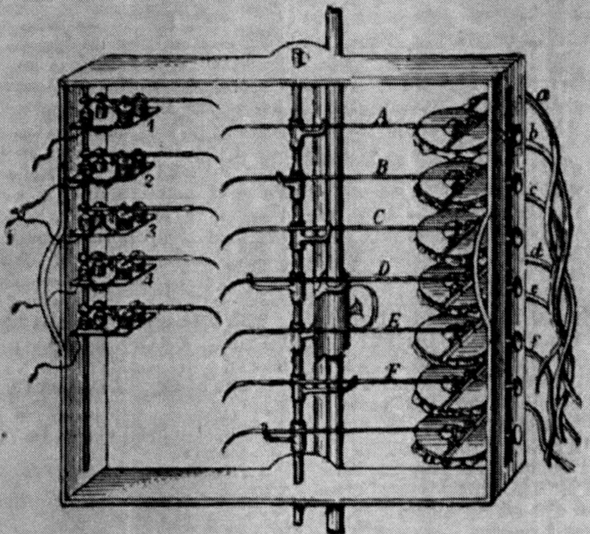

Frame supporting the recording tambours for taking tracings.

FIG. 3.

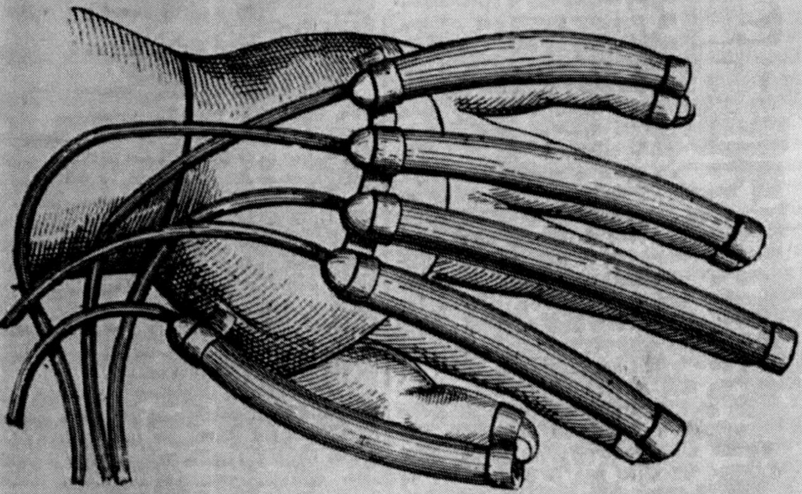

India-rubber motor gauntlet ; each finger-tube is connected with a recording tambour by a flexible tube, and its movements are recorded in the tracing (see *Journal of Physiology*, 1883 and 1887). The apparatus used is now in the South Kensington Museum.

with thinking due to knowledge the result of experience or impressions from without.

Normal and Abnormal Mental Action.—Normal mental action may be briefly defined as that which in a large average of cases is usual under the special circumstances; this necessarily varies with the age, and social and educational position of the man. Normal mental action may be said to be such as is in "harmony with the environment." To be in "harmony" is to be in concord or agreement, and the use of the term connotes at least two similar things compared as to action. In the mental action which is said to be harmonious with the environment, it is the intrinsic forces (or results of former impression) which are compared in action with the forces at present acting upon the brain. They tend to similar action or otherwise. The present environment of the brain is mainly the sum of the forces or stimuli incident to it, calling into action the diatactic neural unions which have previously been formed in it as intrinsic conditions. Harmony or discord in action depends upon whether the forces now stimulating its action are similar to those which built up its present tendencies to action; if the tendencies thus formed are similar to the action at present stimulated, this is harmony.

Harmony with the environment is due to the fact that the outcome or sequence of past impressions is similar to that stimulated at the present by forces around. Spontaneous action being solely produced by past or inherited impressions, is less likely to be in harmony with the environment, than action controlled by present conditions. Thus microkinesis may be compared with adapted action. The value we put upon a particular mental act depends in part upon the value we put upon its relation to surrounding things and forces; if it have no relation to the environment, it will probably produce no internal impression, and will probably not be preserved. It is the expression of mental acts adapted by the environment, and impressing it, that are most useful, and are preserved.

A marked feature of normal mental action is its variation. In an imbecile there are few variations of action, and but few brain centres acting separately. A farm labourer has a vocabulary of about 300 words, Shakespeare employed about 15,000; the variability of mental acts is a fair criterion of mental activity.

Conclusion. — This brief account of the working of our hypothesis of the neural action corresponding to mental acts, may serve to show that it is possible to study psychology as a department of pure physiology, and to describe mental facts in terms connoting brain properties, such as may be observed and compared with other modes of vital action. Clinical descriptions thus given appear useful for the advancement of medical knowledge, and enable us to avoid speaking of physical conditions as if they were ever produced by immaterial causes. The value of mental action is not to be estimated in foot-pounds, because it does not depend upon the quantity of force, but upon the control of its distribution by past and present impressions upon the nerve-centres. FRANCIS WARNER.

PSYCHOSIS TRAUMATICA.—Mental affection following injury. (*See* TRAUMATISM AND INSANITY.)

PSYCHOSOMATIATRIA (ψυχή, the mind; σῶμα, body; ἰατρεία, a healing). A medicine for mind and body. (Fr. *psychosomiatrie.*)

PSYCHOTHERAPEIA, PSYCHOTHERAPEUTICS (ψυχή, the mind; θεραπεύω, I attend the sick). Treatment of disease by the influence of the mind on the body.

PSYCHROPHOBIA (ψυχρός, cold; φοβέω, I fear). Excessive dread of cold, especially cold water. (Fr. *psychrophobie.*)

PTYALISM (πτύαλον, spittle). Excessive secretion and escape of saliva; sometimes observed in mental disorders. (*See* SALIVATION.)

PUBESCENT INSANITY. (*See* DEVELOPMENTAL INSANITIES.)

PUERPERAL INSANITY.—Under this head we propose considering the insanity of pregnancy, of parturition, and of the post-parturient period. There is no special form of insanity which is to be distinguished as puerperal insanity, for though the various symptoms of mental disorder may appear in certain relationships more commonly with puerperal conditions than with others, yet there is nothing really special as to the form of the disorder, and we meet with mania, melancholia, dementia, or delusional insanity at this period.

First we shall consider the whole subject, and later enter into the more special questions, for it will be found that to a great extent causes which may at one time lead to one form of the disorder may at another start one of the other forms; puerperal insanity resulting in one case, and insanity of pregnancy in another.

Etiology.—Neurotic heredity is a very common cause, and in some cases there is a direct transmission of a tendency to break down at the reproductive times. In these cases a direct inheritance of the neurosis and the powerful agency of dread or expectancy combine to precipitate the attack. Bodily conditions, more than moral or intellectual distress, act as exciting causes. General causes of exhaustion, such as frequent pregnancies, are potent. Frequent child-bearing, especially if the mother is in poor circumstances, is dangerous. The age of the woman is important; child-bearing is more dangerous if not within ordinary physiological limits. Thus first pregnancies after thirty are specially so, and again pregnancies taking place about the menopause after years of absence of pregnancy are dangerous. Alcoholic intemperance is a factor in some cases, though less common than might have been expected.

We do not find that albuminuria or convulsive attacks are peculiarly dangerous, and but little if any special danger arises from severe sickness or other allied troubles during the pregnancy. We shall consider septic conditions and their influence later.

There is no special relationship between the time of the year and the attacks, and there is but little difference as to the social state of the patients; the general opinion is that it is more common among the rich than among the poor, and that luxurious living and indolence are really dangerous conditions in neurotic persons.

Among the most powerful psychical causes must be mentioned previous attacks; a woman who has had one attack is specially liable to other attacks if the pregnancy follow quickly on recovery from the former attack, and also if the symptoms and surroundings of the patient are similar in the two pregnancies.

Thus, some women suffer more when pregnant with boys than with girls, and *vice versâ*, and it may happen that insanity accompanies only the one or the other sex. Epilepsy also may occur during the pregnancy with children of one sex but not with that of the other.

Worry and anxiety may play some part in the production of puerperal insanity, but it is not the worry of poverty, as the disorder is less common in the poor than the rich. Illegitimate pregnancy seems to be more dangerous, as might be expected, in some classes and in some cases than in others; it is more dangerous, we believe, directly as it affects the social status of the individual and as it interferes with rest and general nutrition during the pregnancy. Grief, such as caused by the death of husband, or of other children, is occasionally a cause; the birth of twins is among the poor a grave cause of depression, and may act as a contributing cause. Fright or shock, and causes which lead the mother to suspect some injury to the child, have also been rarely given as predisposing conditions. We believe that the administration of anæsthetics has been a direct exciting cause of puerperal insanity in some cases. We have met with several such in which insanity has only occurred when these have been given, normal recovery taking place in the same woman delivered without their use.

Insanity of Pregnancy.—This is less common than any of the other disorders which occur at this period. It is most commonly associated with some very distinct neurosis in the individual herself, as well as in her family. Thus, a daughter of an insane mother who herself has had insanity of adolescence or has been an hysterical girl, is very likely to develop in a more or less marked degree the disorder to which we now refer. Illegitimate pregnancy may be a contributing cause, but is less common than might be expected. As a rule, the symptoms are of a more or less melancholic type, with loss of mental power, of will and energy, and with a feeling that there is some bodily ailment present from which she will not recover, or that she will not get over the pregnancy. There may be a special dislike and distrust of the husband and aversion to the other children; there may be infanticidal tendencies. It is common to meet with a history of previous pregnancies and of previous attacks of insanity associated with them. We have frequently met with such histories as the following:—A woman has an attack of post-partum insanity from which she recovers; she has another attack of the same nature followed by another pregnancy during which she develops insanity, which may pass off during the pregnancy, or which may pass from the first into the second group of cases, being first an attack of insanity of pregnancy, but later one of ordinary puerperal insanity.

The insanity of pregnancy may be only an accentuation of the *longings* of that period; thus, while one woman takes only a diet of apples, another prefers pickles, and there may yet be more strange tastes, such as for coal or slate pencil. These may be of little importance in themselves, but if the longing be for alcohol there is no knowing to what this may lead. We are sure that these longings may represent neuroses, as we have seen them most pronounced in the members of nervous families; we have seen the offspring of such pregnancies develop insanity, while other children of the same parents have escaped.

The insanity of pregnancy occurs specially at two periods, (*a*) **before the fourth month**, and (*b*) **after that time**.

The cases occurring before the fourth month are the more hopeful. They frequently pass off with the sickness or at the coming on of the so-called "quickening." The symptoms vary from the simple hysterical to the profoundly melancholic, there being generally a good deal of moral disorder and tendency to cause disturbance in the home relationships. If these cases are placed under favourable conditions, for a time being separated from husband and old surroundings, the symptoms will probably pass off about the fourth month. There is no indication for the production of abortion as this will probably do no good.

A certain number of patients get through the earlier period of pregnancy without trouble, but during the later months become sleepless, restless, timid and impressed by the fear that some evil is going to happen; they suspect their husbands of infidelity, fancy that they are going to be abandoned, or that their children are to be taken from them. Gradually more pronounced melancholia may appear so that the patient has to be put under control, and this is better done early, for it is not like the last group of cases which will be pretty certain to get well at a fixed time. These cases pass into the ordinary forms of puerperal insanity (after delivery). It is not at all common for such patients to be relieved by the birth of the child, though during labour there may be a temporary relief to the symptoms.

During delivery the ordinary emotional disturbance may pass beyond all bounds, so that a patient may become quite uncontrollable. We have known several women in this state get out of bed, and rush about the house threatening to injure themselves if the child were not born soon. We have also met with cases of marked hysteria during labour. These symptoms may pass off with delivery, and this is the rule; but in others the symptoms pass into a more organised form of maniacal excitement. It is noteworthy, too, that in some cases in which there has been mental depression during the later months of pregnancy, delivery may take place without any apparent pain, and thus the child may die untended without there being any infanticidal intention.

During delivery, as already stated, some patients who have been depressed become temporarily bright and sane, only to relapse in the course of a few hours. It will appear, then, that with natural labour in specially emotional subjects, there may be maniacal excitement as an exaggeration of the ordinary disturbance, and that this may pass off or may develop into true insanity.

Ephemeral Insanity (Mania Transitoria) after Child-birth.—This state is not much recognised, but is important from a medico-legal point of view, as well as from the physician's stand-point. Some women, especially those who are in weak health, and who belong to a nervously unstable stock, within the first week, generally within the first three days of delivery, become suddenly delirious with rapid small pulse, tremulous tongue, and great restlessness. There may have been a period during which there was a dread of impending evil. This delirious state may have been preceded by a rigor, but this is not very common. The breasts are tense or tender, and the bowels are confined. This state may pass off as rapidly as it came on, being relieved by the onset of the milk, or by a free action of the bowels. It must be remembered that in this state the mother may injure herself or her child, and in the latter case she may be quite unconscious of the act which she has done. It is well to remember that there may be a temporary relief from the mental disorder which may recur, to run the ordinary course of puerperal insanity. Or this may start a form of delirious mania hardly to be distinguished from septic puerperal insanity.

Ordinary Puerperal Insanity.—The causes already considered require to be referred to rather more in detail before proceeding to the consideration of the forms of the disorder and its course. Hereditary neuroses are very commonly met with in these cases, and play a very important part. Insanity follows the birth of first children more than other deliveries, but it must not be forgotten that one quarter of such cases do not recover, and so do not run the same risk again, and a certain proportion of first cases die, yet these facts being taken into consideration the first deliveries are the most dangerous. Child-bearing begun after thirty is in our experience specially dangerous. As far as the nature of the delivery is concerned, we do not think that instrumental labour affects the risk to any appreciable degree; the majority of our cases have been delivered naturally and rapidly. There is some increase in the danger if the labour has been very prolonged, and if there has been excess of hæmorrhage. The occurrence of twins has been a not uncommon condition, but we are not in a position to state whether this was in greater proportion than might be naturally expected in the proper proportion of such cases.

Drink adds a slightly increased danger to these cases, but here again intemperance is so commonly associated with neurotic heredity that we feel it hard to decide what part it really plays in the production of the insanity. The next causes to be specially referred to are septic. It was originally thought by Sir J. Simpson that albuminuria was common in puerperal insanity. This has not been our experience, but Dr. Campbell Clark has recently reported his experience, which showed a rather large proportion of cases in which some albumen was found in the urine. Therefore the relationship of the insanity to renal complications remains undecided. We believe that convulsions may be a cause of mental disorder, and these generally are associated with albuminuria.

It is necessary for us to point out that there are different modes of blood-poisoning which may be in action. Thus the source may be purely external, such as alcohol or scarlet fever poison; or it may arise from within, as in the sepsis due to retention of the uterine discharges; or the source of poisoning may be double, as seen in some cases in which alcoholism or uræmia is associated with suppression of lochia or of milk. Suffice it to say, that from whatever source derived, blood-poisoning may be directly related to puerperal insanity. We believe that neurotic patients are specially liable to some septic influences, and we know that depressing nervous conditions will conduce to the development of blood-poisoning in suitable conditions, such as the puerperal period. We shall later refer to the special symptoms met with in septic puerperal insanity which support our views. We fear that at present the statistics of puerperal insanity are defective, as to complete them we need the experience of the general practitioner, the general physician, as well as the specialist, for a very large number of cases occurring in private practice are never seen by the last named.

If blood-poisoning be the cause, the symptoms develop within a few days of the delivery, and there is generally marked increase of temperature, which is variable in its elevation. There may or may not be rigors. The general aspect is similar to that met with in delirium tremens or in acute delirious mania. The milk and lochia are generally arrested, though this is not universally the case. There may be the development of secondary trouble, such as pneumonia, local abscesses and the like.

We have done no more here than state the symptoms as they occur, leaving it till later to discuss them in more detail. The use of chloroform has in some instances been followed by nervous troubles in such peculiar circumstances as to make us believe that it may, in some cases, be at least a partial cause of the insanity.

Moral Causes. — As already stated, these are not so common in puerperal insanity as might be expected, yet they do in some cases act as partial causes of the disorder. Dread of the delivery, especially when a former delivery has been followed by physical or mental disorder, is very powerful for evil, and in the same way a previous attack of insanity in the patient or a near relation may have the same effect; desertion by the father of the child, or his death, the death of a child, or other cause of grief may do much to prepare the way for an attack. The shock of labour itself, or the shock or fright produced by foolish or brutal acts perpetrated at the time of delivery are of serious importance. Thus we have seen a woman so frightened by the sight of the placenta that she could not sleep, and passed into a maniacal state. A drunken nurse, or a violent or drunken husband has been seen to cause the same, and we think it worth recording that in a fair number of patients who have recovered, there has been a history that their mental disorder was started by a terrifying dream. In some, no doubt, the dream was part of the unhealthy nervous process already begun. The causes may be predisposing or exciting; simple or mixed; single or combined; and in the great majority of cases there are predisposing influences, which are stimulated into action by more than one exciting cause.

To sum up: the causes most commonly met with are, hereditary tendencies to neurosis, advanced age at first pregnancy, frequent pregnancy, especially in those who are nervously degenerate, previous nervous illnesses; the sex of the child may exert an influence; so may the nature of the labour, the occurrence of eclampsia, blood-poisoning, or the weakness of flooding; and besides, there are certain depressing moral influences, such as shock, which may directly tend to produce the disorder.

The **forms** which puerperal insanity may assume are almost as manifold as the names given to mental diseases. We have seen every variety, from exaggerated hysteria to general paralysis of the insane, but there are certain pretty well recognised forms which it may be well especially to refer to, as they are the more common. We have already spoken of the ephemeral mania, which may be associated with the influx of milk; but there is also a type of hysterical mania which is not very uncommon. This is generally met with in primiparæ of nervous or weakly stock. The labour being perfectly natural, all going well for several days, querulousness is noticed and intolerance of husband or child; then there are emotional displays of a markedly hysterical type, sleeplessness, constipation and capriciousness about food follow. The symptoms may not go beyond this, but for some days they may cause the utmost anxiety; for there is no rule by which to tell whether the case will remain in this state or develop into one of the more advanced forms. The best treatment is absolute quiet, the friends not being allowed access, the baby is to be weaned, the bowels are to be freely relieved, and all the general antiseptic and other measures usual are to be followed carefully, seeing particularly that the breasts are tended and the lochial discharge removed; we believe it is often good at this period to give some diffusible stimulant, such as champagne or brandy and soda water. A week, as a rule, suffices to clear up these cases. We have known one woman have several similar short attacks in recurring pregnancies.

The next form to be noticed is the ordinary puerperal mania. This may depend on the development of the last class, or may be in some way connected with blood-poisoning. In these cases the symptoms generally come on with the same sort of moral disorder and emotional disturbance as the last, although it is more common to meet with a history of slight depression. The patient may have been found crying, and when pressed as to the cause has said that she felt she was going to die, or was going to be taken from her home and her baby. This depression may slowly pass into a state of discontent with those about her, and at this period the nurse is almost sure to be blamed both by patient and friends.

The maniacal onset generally occurs within the first fourteen days after delivery, but it may occur later, and be due to exhaustion. There is little or no increase of temperature. The appetite is generally bad or variable; the skin is pale, not discoloured or flushed; the tongue is tremulous, the bowels confined; the milk may be present or absent; the lochial discharge may be present or absent; the general strength fails rapidly; the sleep is wanting or broken, often disturbed by dreams; there is jealousy and irritability, loss of power of attention, and feeling of restlessness; there may be eroticism and mistakes as to personal identity, and as to that of friends. These symptoms may be followed by or associated with hallucinations or delusions. There are often spectral hallucinations, and hallucinations of smell are frequent, the (skin) feeling may also be morbidly affected; hearing is at times disturbed, but not quite so commonly as the other senses already referred to. Sugar may be present in the urine for a time.

In such a case as that already described, the symptoms will vary, there being many lulls which mislead the friends into the belief that recovery has taken place, but as a rule the cases pass from the more acute stage through a more or less chronic stage of excitement, before any real improvement takes place. Thus after, say six or eight weeks, of acute mania, the patient begins to eat and drink well, to sleep better, to get stouter, but at the same time there is a marked dissatisfaction with her past treatment by her friends. She accuses nurses, doctors and others of unkindness, and expresses a general discontent. This stage often lasts a few weeks, and may become permanent, or it may pass off altogether, or may further pass into one of placid fatness and weakness of mind, which may be recovered from, or may become lasting. In many cases there is apathy associated with amenorrhœa, and in this state it is well, if possible, to try the effect of return to home surroundings and duties, even including cohabitation, precautions against pregnancy being taken.

The general course of these attacks is first, slight depression, followed by excitement, which may vary greatly in degree from time to time. This may be followed by a return to general health without any mental gain for a time. Although about 75 per cent. of these cases recover, some die from secondary affections, or from sudden exhaustion, and some remain permanently weak-minded, deluded, or unstable. It is to be noted that though most of the cases which recover do so within the first nine months, yet a few ultimately get well after from one to three years of apparently hopeless dementia.

The next group to be referred to contains those cases which depend on septic causes, and we repeat that there are some neurotic people who seem to be predisposed to blood-poisoning by their neurosis:

conditions of vital depression and expectancy will lead to serious danger. It is rare to meet with a case of puerperal insanity which depends solely on septic causes. In septic cases the symptoms come on, as a rule, within a short time of delivery, with or without rigors, with variable increase in temperature, cessation of the lochia and the milk; but one or all of these symptoms may be modified. The tendency of the symptoms is to start without any initial depression. There is a near approach to delirium in the excitement, and the confusion of the senses also resembles this more than mania. The ordinary symptoms of puerperal septicæmia may be masked. There may be no complaint of lung trouble, though pneumonia may be present. It seems to us that a very considerable number of patients with some septic troubles following delivery and associated with mental disorder, recover; more, in fact, than we should have expected, looking at the gravity of the complication; there may be in such cases a tendency to secondary deposits of pus, and there may be active delirium, delirious mania, with refusal to take food, great restlessness, sleeplessness, and violence. The refusal of food is one of the most dangerous symptoms, and one for which steps have to be taken at once if life is to be saved. The progress of these cases is generally rapid, so that little is to be done beyond the utmost care as to general measures and feeding. We have known the mental symptoms relieved by the occurrence of some localised septic complication. It may be necessary to use hypnotics, but in all cases these must be given with great caution, and we prefer to give stimulants as well, if not instead of these. Chloral or sulphonal is of use, but we do not think that hyoscyamine should be tried, as the depressing effects are serious, and a further distaste for food may arise from the dryness of the throat. If the patient get over the blood-poisoning there may follow a period of mental disorder of a maniacal type, or, what is more common, a period of partial mental weakness with or without stupor may follow. In the state of mania the ordinary measures will have to be tried, but it is noteworthy that most of these patients are very hard to be managed, and are erotic, obscene, and filthy, and so are unfit for home treatment. In the stage of stupor or dementia, time and suitably adapted changes are to be tried, the visits of friends often being useful, and as soon as all signs of suicidal or destructive tendencies have passed the patient ought to be tried at home, under precautions.

The greatest difficulty in cases of this kind is to distinguish between true septic mania and acute delirious mania, and it is only after very careful study of all the points in the case that this can be made certain. It is not of very great importance, from the physician's point of view, as the treatment will be similar in both conditions, but the friends greatly prefer "blood-poisoning" to "insanity."

In the first place the septic cases frequently arise in association with other bodily symptoms, such as rigors, suppression of discharges, sallowness of complexion, sweating and the like. The tongue is often covered with a white fur and is tremulous. The onset has not, as a rule, followed any special moral trouble, but may have been quite sudden or connected only with symptoms of sepsis, the mental disorder coming on later. In acute delirious mania, it is more common to get a history of a fright or sudden cause of mental disorder followed by mental depression, which may have lasted only a few hours, but was well marked. There may be neither rigors nor suppression of the discharges, or this suppression may follow the first symptoms of the insanity. The skin is pale rather than sallow, with a tendency to a flush of the cheeks; the tongue very rapidly gets dry and brown out of proportion to the amount of recorded temperature. This latter symptom can only give indefinite help, for in both the temperature is raised and uncertain, but in septic cases the temperature is likely to be higher and more irregular, rising at night, while in acute delirious mania the temperature is little above 101°, yet the patient has the aspect of extreme febrile disorder. In both, we believe that large doses of quinine and a free supply of alcoholic stimulants are the proper treatment, yet with all care the majority die.

Instead of maniacal excitement there may be excitement of the melancholic type. Thus, a patient with or without any real cause for anxiety becomes emotional or depressed, full of foreboding, sleepless, and with distaste for food; then passes into a state of terror that something is going to be done to her child, her husband or herself. There is a tendency, which rapidly develops, to resist every attempt to do anything for her, and it is common to meet with patients who repeat over and over again the same piteously monotonous sentence, such as that she does "not know what to do," or that it was "not her fault." With this there may or may not be active attempts at escape or self-injury; nothing that can be done seems to give any rest, and the case is for a time an example of resistive melancholia. These cases are tedious, and require constant feeding and care as to their bodily functions, and little in the way of change of surroundings or stimulation effects any good. Waiting and painstaking care are often rewarded by a return to health, and hope need not be given up for two years at least. This is generally preceded by return of the menses, which are almost always absent during the disordered stage, and return of sleep and appetite and improved general circulation, as seen in better nutrition and healthier complexion. In these cases from time to time the husband and children should be allowed to see the patient. At the end of a few months change should be tried, from one asylum or home to another. In some of these cases the bodily wasting is such that massage may be tried.

In other cases the melancholia is less active, but there may be more marked delusions, and these cases are, as a rule, untrustworthy and suicidal. They often have hallucinations of their senses, and may be led to desperate acts. In some there are ideas of ruin or unworthiness, sleeplessness of a passive kind is also common, and food may be refused. Here again, time and steady care with endeavour to excite interest in the outside and family world are useful, but from six to twelve months is usually required before the mental health is restored. Menstruation is generally absent for some time. In some of these cases, as in those of mania, there may be a period of careless indifference to home and its surroundings, which may render it well that the patient should be sent there on trial.

In nearly all ordinary cases of puerperal insanity there is a period of apathy; this may be the initial or terminal symptom of the attack. A mother may be careless about her child and her husband without having any really melancholic feeling. This state varies from simple indifference to the most profound stupor, and the different cases must be treated on different plans. Thus, in the simpler cases removal from home for a few weeks will suffice, while in others the removal to asylum care is necessary.

These cases are as curable as the others, but take from four to twelve months as a rule. All varieties of stupor may be represented during this period.

There remain still to be considered cases in which the disorder is more generalised, in which something allied to primary delusional insanity arises. In our experience patients, who, as it were, are saturated with neurosis, and in whom puerperal conditions only act as the exciting causes of disorder, may, after delivery, develop, rapidly or slowly, symptoms of suspicion and doubt; they may then become solitary, dissatisfied, and later, after separating from home ties, they may be discovered to have all sorts of sensory perversions and delusions. In some cases the patient has ideas of persecution, ideas that conspiracies are being formed against her, fancies that the husband is unfaithful—this is a very common idea—ideas that the children are not hers, or that they are being affected or infected in some way. It is almost endless to attempt to describe the forms which this disorder may assume. We believe that if seen early and sent away from home, under proper conditions and with a suitable companion, recovery may often follow in such cases, but there is a proportion of these cases in which nothing makes any difference, and who once having broken down never recover.

The duration of the symptoms and their complete organisation make the prognosis unfavourable. In these cases the bodily health is good, and the patients may live at least as long as ordinary persons.

In the last place, we must record the fact, which we believe has not been generally recognised, that general paralysis of the insane may arise after pregnancy and childbirth without any other apparent cause. In these cases we have known at least four women who, after leading healthy lives, and without special or general predisposing causes, have slowly developed mental weakness, fits of an epileptiform nature, tremulousness, loss of expression, and the rest of the ordinary symptoms of general paralysis of the insane. In one such case the patient had a remission, during which she again became pregnant. It is noteworthy that in some female general paralytics the menses will continue up to the end. We believe the tendency in these cases is rapidly to dementia, and that there is little risk of extravagance, though eroticism is not uncommon. The prognosis in these cases is bad.

As already said, every form of mental disorder may be met with in puerperal insanity; in asylums every form of chronic insanity may be met with which has had this for its cause, and it is not necessary to give in any detail notes of such cases, but it is well to state that in patients who have become insane at such periods and recovered, there may be a tendency to finally break down at the climacteric, instead of, as might be expected, gaining increased stability. And again, cases of chronic puerperal insanity do not often get well at the climacteric, yet a few of the cases of melancholia will thus almost suddenly recover. Some patients who have had attacks of puerperal insanity never have recurrences, but others have attacks with each returning pregnancy. Patients who have had attacks of puerperal insanity are often rendered more liable to break down from other causes, and others are never the same in habits and mode of action as before the illness. There are a certain number of patients who are morally perverse after one or more such attacks.

Puerperal insanity, then, is variable in its symptoms, is liable to recur, is fairly curable, but is not uncommonly associated with grave dangers to life.

Insanity of Lactation.—This is arbitrarily fixed as mental disorder following six weeks or later after delivery. This is like the other forms already considered, there being no special causes needing to be named. It is not infrequently associated with weaning, so that we prefer to divide the cases into those in which the disorder follows immediately on weaning, and those in which the insanity seems to develop out of the physical exhaustion of suckling, commonly associated with other causes of vital depression. The former class presents cases in which there is commonly mental depression with one or other of the forms of delusions of dread, fear, jealousy and suspicion. There will be often ideas related to the reproductive organs, fancies that people are trying to influence or mesmerise them and the like. There may be very suicidal tendencies, and it is in such cases that infanticidal ideas as well as acts are commonly met with. There is generally amenorrhœa with complaints that "feeling is dead;" complaints of weight or pains in vertex or occiput, and an utter inability to care for children or husband. There is often an extension of this, so that the patient believes herself forsaken of God. These cases need very careful watching, and are rarely fit for home treatment, asylums being the only safe place for them. Tonics, baths and change of scene and absence from home are generally followed by recovery in from three to six months.

In the other cases in which there is physical exhaustion as the chief cause of breakdown, the patient may often be treated at the seaside with nurses, the great thing being change from home and abundant food and rest. In these latter cases death from phthisis or some secondary cause is to be guarded against.

There is no special form of insanity following lactation; the symptoms may be those of mania, melancholia, dementia, stupor, or may from the outset be delusional. In nearly all cases there is marked physical exhaustion. The symptoms may come on at any time after delivery from six weeks up to one year or more. It is much more common among the poor than the well-to-do. It is frequent in those predisposed by hereditary weakness; it is common, too, in those who have had other attacks of insanity, such as puerperal insanity or the insanity of pregnancy; it is not uncommonly met with in patients, who from one cause or another approached or passed through their puerperal period in an exhausted state; it appears in some cases to depend on prolonged or repeated suckling, or on over-nursing, as with twins; while in some cases weaning seems to be the real active excitant. The state of the uterus may also have an influence. Thus, subinvolution is not uncommon, and with this there may be metrorrhagia or leucorrhœa. It has been supposed that there is more danger at the time representing the first return of the menstrual period after delivery, but we have no experience to confirm this opinion. In a few cases mammary abscesses have acted as exciting causes.

The onset of the disease may be quite sudden, but as a rule sleeplessness and dread are among the earliest symptoms, and the mothers may continue, greatly to the danger of their children, to suckle while still suffering from the earlier symptoms of mental disorder. The duration of the disease varies from three months to eighteen months or more. The symptoms may pass from initial melancholia through maniacal excitement, to partial dementia, to be slowly replaced by health. There is almost always a period of dull apathy, in which the patient may become fat, sleepy, and indolent, while there is also absence of menstruation. These symptoms may pass off rapidly with a return to home cares and surroundings. In our experience nearly 80 per cent. of these cases recover, 5 to 8 per cent. die, the rest remaining more or less permanently deranged. The ordinary course of the disorder is as follows:—

A woman rendered physically weak from some cause when still suckling becomes emotional, sleepless, irritable, and hard to deal with. She may make accusations against those near her, may be generally complaining. This state may pass slowly or almost suddenly into one of profound disturbance of feeling, in which she may kill herself or her children, or may impulsively attack husband or nurse. She may develop hallucinations of any of her senses, but we believe that hallucinations of sight and of smell are specially common; she may refuse food and rapidly lose strength, till her case is rendered serious from simple exhaustion. The melancholia may last for a longer or shorter time, and may vary greatly in degree from time to time, there often appearing breaks in the clouds before its final dissipation. In some cases, instead of melancholia there is an outbreak of maniacal excitement with impulsive violence, and often there is great eroticism. With either of the forms of disorder it is common to meet with special aversion to or delusions about the husband. The form in which stupor is present is hardly to be distinguished from profound melancholia. In all cases the prognosis is decidedly good unless there be some secondary bodily disease. The treatment is one of feeding and tonics, with change of scene and surroundings for some time, tonics such as the more simple forms of iron in effervescent form, cod-liver oil, peptonised milk, cocoa, soups, with a fair amount of stimulant. We prefer malt liquor as a rule to wine. Attention to the bowels is necessary, and a return to home as soon as delusions have passed away.

George H. Savage.

PULSE IN INSANITY.—There are few diseases, either mental or bodily, into which a consideration of the pulse does not enter as an element of greater or less importance, either in connection with the diagnosis, prognosis, or treatment, and so it occurs in the insane that from each of these points of view some information is to be derived by close examination. The cardio-vascular system is doubtless affected in some way by every transient thought, by every voluntary effort, a point demonstrated by the experiments of Mosso, who was able to show by means of the plethysmograph, that during active commentalisation the amount of blood passing to the arm was appreciably diminished, and at the same time it was observed that the radial pulse became considerably smaller and more frequent. The relative condition of the pulse in the carotid and radial arteries during intellectual effort has been studied by Gley, who observed that at this period the carotid pulse became more frequent and exhibited the condition of dicrotism, which was not present in the radial artery at the same time, an observation which would indicate a dilatation of the encephalic vessels, causing a more rapid circulation of the intracranial blood to supply the increased demand for nutritive material made by the hemispherical ganglia during the period of active cellular metabolism. These physiological experiments have their parallel in the realms of pathology, since it has been shown by Mendel that in certain maniacal conditions occurring in the course of general paralysis, a corresponding change to that described by Gley occurs, and it has been maintained by Milner Fothergill that this comparative increase in the vascular areas of the cerebro-spinal system leads to a distinct accentuation of the aortic second sound. It is thus rational to assume that the condition of the pulse, indicating as it does the volume and rapidity of the blood current, and the pressure under which the circulation is proceeding, should in a measure be a guide to some at least of the various forms of altered mental condition which occur in the insane, inasmuch as, on the one hand, transient changes in the central nervous system produce demonstrable changes in the pulse form, and on the other hand, changes in the blood supply of nervous matter can be clinically and experimentally shown to influence its susceptibility to stimuli.

Hypnotism.—In order perhaps the more fully to demonstrate the close relationship which exists between the psychical condition and the circulatory apparatus, attention may be drawn to their relative states in the various stages of hypnotism. Dr. Brugia has shown that during the lethargic condition, the sphygmographic line rises, while during catalepsy and somnambulism it falls, and during the latter stage it is possible to diminish the pulse rate considerably. A similar variation has been shown by Tamburini and Sepilli to exist by making use of the plethysmograph, the conclusion being that during the lethargic state of hypnotism vascular dilatation is present, while during the cataleptic stage vascular contraction is the rule, facts of very considerable significance when considered along with the allied conditions which occur in insanity.

Neurasthenia and Hypochondriasis.— In the condition of so-called neurasthenia or nervous weakness, which may practically be regarded as a functional disease of the nervous system, on the borderland of insanity, the typical pulse-tracing to be obtained is one showing a varying degree of low tension, and the sphygmograph is claimed to be of service, not only in determining the degree of nervous exhaustion present in any individual case by estimation of the tension, but also to discriminate between fictitious and real improvement. Dr. Webber,* from the examination of a large number of cases, has suggested the use of the sphygmograph as a means of arriving at a prognosis in neurasthenia, having observed that if, when a case comes under observation, the pulse tension be not much diminished, the probability is that the patient is merely temporarily "run down," and will readily respond to appropriate treatment, the pulse again resuming its normal degree of tension; if, however, the pulse be of markedly low tension, the prognosis is not so good, and if the tension be not permanently raised, then no reliable improvement takes place. It is difficult in these cases exactly to determine whether the pulse tension be raised secondarily to the improvement in the nervous system, or *vice versâ*, but it is interesting to observe how closely comparable this low tension pulse with its associated symptoms in the condition of nervous exhaustion, is to that which obtains in the muscular exhaustion of fatigue, resulting from prolonged convulsions.

Schüle considers neurasthenia to be a form of hypochondriasis, and apparently, as regards their pulse form, a relationship seems borne out. In the pure form of hypochondriasis the pulse tension is almost invariably low, and it would appear that this low tension may stand in some part as a cause of the mental condition, since where the blood-pressure is habitually low, it can scarcely be that the tissue nutrition is maintained at a high level, and in this imperfect nutrition the cerebro-spinal system must necessarily suffer. Dr. Broadbent has described a well-marked case of this disease in which pulse tension was continually low, and in which, in addition, the condition called agoraphobia was developed at a later period.

Hysteria and Hysterical Insanity.—The vascular disturbance in hysteria varies within the widest limits, and with it the pulse and sphygmographic tracings. In many cases the pulse is characterised chiefly by its extreme mobility in response to the various emotions, and in these a low tension pulse may not unfrequently be observed, but probably the more characteristic form of pulse in hysteria is that showing increased tension, the result of arterial spasm, probably the cause of the excessive flow of urine of low specific gravity so frequently observed in this disease, and possibly also associated in some way with the condition of hemianæsthesia. Dr. Weir Mitchell has recorded the case of a female in whom arterial spasm was so marked as to render the radial pulse exceedingly small, hard, thin, and wiry.

Insanity associated with Cardiac Disease.—Without here entering into any detail as to the various forms of insanity connected in some way with organic disease of the heart, it is important to observe that a consideration of the pulse may suggest in some cases, the possible origin of the mental symptoms, and in others may materially modify the prognosis. In cases of maniacal delirium of cardiac origin an examination of the pulse not unfrequently reveals the failure of cardiac compensation for some mitral lesion by its irregularity in rhythm and force, its tendency to intermittence, its weak percussion stroke, and its easy compressibility, points which not only tend to establish the character of the case, but which at the same time suggest the treatment and means of arriving at a prognosis.

Again, amongst the numerous cases of simple melancholia, or those on the borderland between this condition and hypochondriacal melancholia, there is a distinct class of cases to be recognised whose mental condition is in all probability based on a pre-existing cardiac mitral lesion, most frequently a stenosis, in which mental exacerbations are coincident with the failure of compensation which occurs from time to time; in these cases the pulse presents the usual characters indicative of this condition, and it is to be observed that, as in many cases of uncomplicated melancholia, here also associated with the cardiac phenomena, the pulse is mostly well sustained between the beats. Again, in the expansive form of insanity, which sometimes occurs as a concomitant or sequence of aortic disease, and simulates in these points general paralysis in its grandiose form, assistance in the differential diagnosis is sometimes to be derived from a consideration of the pulse, since a sphygmographic tracing typical of the second stage in general paralysis differs markedly from that characteristic of aortic regurgitation, the forms of aortic disease said to be most frequently associated with this kind of insanity.

The alteration of the pulse which occurs in the forms of mental disease occasionally associated with acute endo- and pericarditic lesions, varies within wide limits; it is, however, usually of low tension, and although in many acute cases of insanity

* *Boston Med. and Surg. Journal*, 1888.

and delirium of this kind, the pulse must enter largely into the diagnosis and immediate prognosis, it can scarcely be said to have any features peculiarly its own to be considered here.

Insanity associated with Pulmonary Lesions.—Of the cases of acute delirious mania in which acute bodily disease has been an eminently prominent factor in causation, pulmonary inflammation, in the form of acute pneumonia, seems to occupy a leading place. In this form of insanity the pulse is of the typical febrile character, of fairly good percussive stroke, and fully or even hyper-dicrotic, rapid and mobile, the respiratory line being usually uneven, its alterations in the course of the case are necessarily the main guide to treatment, and while diminution in rapidity accompanied by increased tension is associated with a favourable termination, it is observed that a very rapid pulse of low percussion stroke is to be regarded as an unfavourable element in prognosis, and an indication for cardiac tonics and stimulants, as many of the patients are apt to die from simple cardiac failure.

Another form of pulmonary lesion frequently associated with mental disease, of which in many cases it may be regarded as a distinct element in causation, resulting in a definite series of symptoms, is phthisis, and it might be readily imagined, in a wasting disease such as this, associated with anæmia, and frequently elevation of temperature, that the pulse would rather tend to be feeble and dicrotic. This, however, would appear to be rarely the case, unless excavation is proceeding rapidly, with considerable variations in temperature. When, however, the physical disease is advancing rapidly, the mental symptoms are usually much improved, they being most prominent as a rule in the earlier stages, and at this period the pulse very frequently presents the signs of considerable tension, the exact significance of which is not at present known, but it is noteworthy, that classed according to mental symptoms, a large number of these cases come under the clinical heading of melancholia, a form of mental disease frequently associated with increased tension. The condition of increased tension in the systemic arteries in phthisis, however, occurs in cases other than those requiring asylum treatment. Emphysema is a form of pulmonary disease which has been recognised by some authorities as a causative factor in mental disease, chiefly melancholic, though, as suggested by Griesinger, it may be that the mental and bodily conditions are merely associated senile changes. In these cases there is probably a general fibrotic change which involves both lungs and systemic vessels, with the result that the pulse exhibits characters closely allied to the "senile pulse" of Marey, a sphygmographic tracing showing a fairly high percussion stroke, according to the condition of the heart, a well marked pre-dicrotic wave, and a somewhat gradual line of descent, indicating considerable pressure in the vessels with some impeded outflow into the veins.

Melancholia (Fig. 1).—Melancholia is an example of a form of mental disease in which a very varied form of pulse may be found, more particularly is this so as regards tension. MM. Ball and Jennings have shown that in chronic morphinism, when the mental condition is one of the intensest misery, the pulse tension is invariably high, and this tension is reduced coincidently with the recurrence of mental comfort, when an additional dose of morphia is administered. Dr. Haig has remarked on the resemblance of this melancholic condition in chronic morphinism to certain cases of melancholia associated with the so-called uric-acid headache, in which there is a markedly high tension pulse, and he suggests that opium in all these cases produces the increased sense of well-being by its action on uric acid, and by this means on pulse tension and cerebral circulation. However this may be, it is established that a fair proportion of melancholiacs present a slow pulse of high physiological or pathological degree of tension, a point upon which stress has been laid by Dr. Broadbent, who has regarded it as possibly the cause of the mental condition, or at least the index of the state of system on which the mental condition depends. It is noteworthy that the anæmia, which is so frequently present in young melancholiacs, does not at all prevent the recurrence of a high tension pulse, since anæmia by itself is not unfrequently associated with increased tension.

On the other hand, however, a certain but smaller percentage of cases of melancholia is associated with a pulse tending towards the opposite extreme of tension, that is a pulse of low tension and compressible, and somewhat more rapid than in the former condition, mobile and readily affected by transient emotions. Melancholia associated with a very low tension pulse is stated by Dr. Broadbent to be of worse prognosis than the reverse condition.

Chronic Melancholia.—In cases of melancholia, of which chronicity is a marked feature, the high tension pulse is almost invariable, though it has, as a rule, but little resemblance to the form of high tension pulse associated with cirrhotic Bright's disease, unless this condition be also present, because the cardiac percussion stroke is weak, and results in a low line of ascent, while the line of descent, forming a wide angle with it, gradually reaches its lowest point; the presence or absence of the pre-dicrotic wave in this form of pulse depending chiefly on the degree of force of the cardiac contractions. The whole pulse is usually small, and indicates a sluggishness of the circulation, resulting from, on the one hand, enfeebled *vis a tergo*, and on the other, some obstruction to the peripheral outflow.

Melancholia Attonita.—In this form of melancholia the vessels also show signs of contraction, and the pulse in the stage of apathy or immobility presents many of the features of the pulsus tardus, pointing to a difficulty in the outflow of blood into the veins, and in addition, a feebly acting heart: the pulse to the finger is weak, owing to the fact that its variations in magnitude are slight and slow. Any mental improvement in these cases is associated with a corresponding change in the pulse, the line of ascent becomes higher, and the tension is diminished, while the volume is increased, and the pulse becomes more rapid, indicating that with the changed mental condition the heart is acting more strongly and the peripheral resistance is diminished.

Senile Melancholia. — The changes which occur in the vessels and other tissues associated with the incidence of senility are necessarily the chief factors in the production of the familiar, tense "senile pulse," which regularly occurs in the forms of mental disease which are apt to arise at this epoch. Not unfrequently, however, in addition to the ordinary pulse change, which is the inevitable concomitant of old age, increased tension over and above this may be brought about by gouty or renal disease, in which the impairment of cerebral blood-supply is presumably increased temporarily or permanently.

Ecstasy.—In the condition of ecstasy, or phreno-plexia of Guislain, where the patient is almost perfectly immovable, and the expression is fixed, and graphically represents one of the forms of emotion, and the muscles are in a state of excessive tension, the pulse does not usually show any marked degree of tension, but is frequently somewhat accelerated, and tends to be more or less dicrotic, the heart factor producing a fairly good line of ascent. It is possible that the tendency to dicrotism in these cases is to be associated with the strong and prolonged muscular strain, which is such a marked feature.

Stuporose conditions.—In some forms of insanity the whole disease is characterised by the condition of stupor, while in others this merely occurs as a passing phase of longer or shorter duration. In the former class, many authorities agree in characterising the pulse as essentially feeble, a point which is certainly true as regards the alteration of the volume of the pulse. But on examination with the sphygmograph, as has been shown by Greenlees and the writer, it is to be observed that the vessel is full between the beats, and the line of descent is therefore well sustained, a condition which inevitably points to the fact that there must be a considerable degree of tension within the vessel; a pre-dicrotic wave may in addition be present, provided the cardiac factor be sufficiently active, and thus a tendency to the formation of a plateau may be evident. That increased tension should be observed in a mental disease such as this is somewhat surprising, until considered together with the observations of Aldridge with the ophthalmoscope, who has shown that in this form of insanity the retinal vessels are straight and attenuated and the choroids pale, and of the writer who has been able to demonstrate that at least in a certain percentage of these cases an actual diminution in the calibre of the vessels at the base of the brain is present. It is evident that arterial stenosis, such as these observations suggest, may account for the condition of increased tension so frequently observed in stuporose conditions, and also for the cardiac complication referred to by Mabille and other authors. That this increased pulse tension is of considerable importance, as indicative of a physical condition definitely associated with this peculiar form of mental disease, is evidenced by the fact that a change inevitably occurs in the pulse, with that in the mental condition, either as a causative, concomitant or sequential alteration, so that when mental health is established, the signs of tension previously present are removed, the cardiac factor becoming more active, the aortic notch and dicrotic wave more obvious, and the outflow into the veins more rapid.

In the stuporose stage of the mental state or states which Kahlbaum would call "Katatonia" (Figs. 5 and 6), the sphygmographic tracings give evidence of difficulty of peripheral outflow, as shown in the mental disease exhibiting this phase, and the condition of tension rapidly subsides when the stage of lucidity occurs.

Intermittent Stupor.—The change which occurs in the pulse becomes most marked in cases of intermittent stupor, sphygmographic tracings taken during the stupor stage showing a striking contrast to those taken during the stage of lucidity, as regards tension. It is noteworthy that the arterial tension observed in the stupor stage can be considerably reduced by amyl nitrite, and that in certain cases a corresponding degree of mental improvement occurs during the action of the drug. Correlative conditions suggestive of the return to mental health and of arterial spasm are a possible explanation of the condition.

Aprosexia.—This is a name introduced by Dr. Guye to indicate the inability to fix attention on any definite, more or less abstract subject, not unfrequently associated with chronic disease of the nose and naso-pharynx, and inasmuch as the leading symptoms are dulness and incapacity for work or movement, resulting in advanced cases in a semi-stupid condition, there would appear some reason for classifying it with the stuporose conditions under consideration, and the more so since it is observed that it is associated in most cases with a pulse of excessive tension. Guye has suggested that the mental condition is due to the incomplete removal of the products of tissue changes, and it is possible that it may be a condition allied to that described by Dr. Haig as connected with the uric-acid excretion.

Mania.—It is by some authorities admitted, or even demanded, that a condition of vascular turgescence and hyperæmia is essential to functional nervous hyper-activity, whether that activity be manifested in the normal direction of health or on the abnormal lines of disease, and therefore it has been premised that, in states of mental exaltation and excitement generally, cerebral hyperæmia is invariably present, a postulate which it would appear impossible to admit when it is considered that a degree of malnutrition of nerve-cells, in the first instance, usually leads to their increased activity, whence results a period of excitement. This change is strictly comparable to what has been shown to occur in the case of the muscular system by Sterson and Schmoulewitch, who demonstrated that when experimental anæmia is induced in muscles, their irritability is increased, in fact, a state of "irritable weakness" and adynamic activity is brought about, just as in the case of the nervous system. That a hyperæmic condition of the nervous centre in this form of mental disease is not at any rate universal, is suggested by the fact that medicinal agents increasing the blood pressure and pulse tension not unfrequently result in diminution or abolition of maniacal excitement.

Acute Delirious Mania (*Délire aigu*) (Figs. 3 and 4).—It is in this form of mania, probably, that the pulse condition is most markedly altered, doubtless to a large extent on account of the increase of body temperature, which may be considerable. It is the form of insanity in which there is the nearest approach to the typical febrile pulse. The pulse is invariably rapid, and this acceleration may reach to as much as 150 per minute; it is usually perfectly regular in rhythm, but not always so in force, and invariably of low tension; a sphygmographic tracing exhibits the following points: the line of ascent is practically vertical, and about the average height, the apex is acute, and the line of descent falls rapidly to the aortic notch, which may or may not sink below the base line, the pulse being usually fully and sometimes hyper-dicrotic. In the later stages of the disease, if it be not arrested, the pulse becomes altered by enfeeblement of the cardiac factor, and the condition of so-called typhomania is brought about. If, however, on the other hand, improvement commence, the change which occurs in the pulse is even more marked than that of the mental condition, the line of ascent indicates a good cardiac impulse, the line of descent becomes more gradual in its slope, and shows the development of a small pre-dicrotic wave. The aortic notch and dicrotic wave, on the other hand, become slight in development, the rapidity of the pulse is reduced, and the tension raised considerably. There are few mental diseases in which the pulse is of greater value in immediate prognosis and treatment, and it is observed that the artificial raising of the tension, in addition to cardiac stimulation, in some cases will produce a degree of mental improvement, and even though this do not occur it undoubtedly tends to avert the tendency to heart failure, so great a danger in this form of mental disease.

Acute Mania.—In the more or less intense excitement which occurs in this form of mental disorder, many observations have been made on the pulse and circulatory system in attempt to localise in time a causative or concomitant alteration which may be of service in throwing light on this abstruse condition. That some change occurs in the blood vascular system is evidenced by the striking pallor of the face, and other alterations of a similar nature. Clifford

Allbutt has suggested, from ophthalmoscopic observation of 51 cases, that the condition of mania is accompanied by anæmia of the fundus, and Griesinger has observed that the cardiac sounds are muffled during the maniacal attack, and clear in the intervals of lucidity, an observation difficult of absolute decision in many cases on account of the mental condition of the patient. As regards the actual condition of the pulse in acute mania, various observers have differed considerably, Dr. Howard stating that there is rarely any marked disturbance other than that which would be caused by any one indulging in the violent and incessant movements peculiar to mania: and doubtless, as Dr. Hack Tuke has observed, it is difficult to know how much the pulse alterations are due to muscular exercise, and how much to the disease itself. However this may be, it is a matter of clinical observation that the condition of mania is very frequently associated with a pulse of abnormally low tension, just as probably the more frequent form of pulse in melancholia is one of increased tension; and moreover, mania of even short duration is able to reduce a pulse of previously high tension, as is seen in the maniacal attacks of general paralysis, to one of complete dicrotism, a point of the greatest importance, as suggesting the most frequent cause of sudden death which is apt to occur in this disease; a view which would appear more tenable than that of Griesinger, who lays stress on the occurrence of apoplectiform collapse. The sphygmographic tracing to be obtained in these cases varies with the degree and duration of the excitement, but usually shows a line of ascent about the average height and vertical, the apex is generally acute, and the line of descent falls directly and suddenly down to the aortic notch, which along with the dicrotic wave, is well marked; this former may reach the respiratory line, but rarely goes beyond it to any extent. There are, nevertheless, cases in which a fairly distinct pre-dicrotic wave occurs, and persists for a considerable time, the line of descent however falling rapidly afterwards. If the maniacal condition be of prolonged duration, the line of ascent becomes considerably shortened, and the condition of full dicrotism obtains, while to the finger the pulse is small, feeble, and almost flickering in character. Raising the tension and increasing the vigour of the cardiac factor in these cases by medicinal agents, certainly sometimes diminishes, or completely quiets the maniacal excitement, as has been shown by Dr. Mickle, while in cases in which this most desirable result is not brought about, the tendency to sudden death during or as a result of excitement, is considerably diminished, and in addition, with the elevation of the blood pressure, nutrition is considerably improved, a point scarcely less important than the immediate return to mental health.

That there is some value in this artificial elevation of the pulse tension is suggested by the fact that mental improvement in cases of acute mania is invariably accompanied by increased pulse tension, resulting in a sphygmographic tracing in which the line of descent is well sustained.

The rapidity of the pulse in mania varies within wide limits, inasmuch as it may be only slightly increased, or may reach 120, or even more. It would appear that this rapidity of pulse is not necessarily proportionate to the degree of excitement of the patient, as suggested by Guislain, but has closer relationship to the duration of the illness, degree of tension, and other factors. Any great frequency would naturally suggest the possibility of the form of acute mania known to be associated with exophthalmic goitre.

Chronic Mania.—Although in a chronic disease, which presents features of such great variety as this, it could scarcely be expected that a uniform character of pulse would be found, it is remarkable with what great frequency the tension is of abnormal height, and this, as far as can be ascertained, independently of history or physical manifestations of such poisons as alcohol or syphilis. The occurrence of this form of pulse in chronic mania is of interest in connection with the observations of Dr. Burman, who found that the average weight of the heart was somewhat increased in the older cases of mania. In chronic and recurrent alcoholic mania, this condition of increased tension is an almost constant feature, resulting in a deliberate, forcible, and well sustained pulse.

General Paralysis.—The pulse and circulatory system in this form of mental disease have received considerable attention from time to time, chiefly owing no doubt to the fact that it is one of the most definite forms of mental disease with which the physician is brought into contact. In the earlier stage Spitzka states that the pulse frequently shows very high tension in the active forms of the disease, but, however, modifies this statement considerably by adding that in a large number of patients it is normal. Some truth appears to exist in both these statements, inasmuch as the pulse in the first stage varies within the same limits as the normal pulse as regards tension, but as the disease progresses with its mental and bodily symptoms the tension almost invariably increases. In the early stage then the sphygmographic tracing may show features indicating a low state of arterial tension, with ready outflow from the arterial system, and it may possibly be that this condition occurs most frequently in that class of cases in whom, coincident with the mental breakdown at the commencement of the attack, there is also considerable physical debility (Fig. 7). In another class of cases, however, the pulse shows distinctly a much higher arterial tension, and it is the form of tracing obtained from these cases that has been regarded as the typical pulse of the early stage of general paralysis, and represented as such by Dr. Thompson (Fig. 8). The line of ascent is slightly oblique and short, the primary ventricular wave never forms an acute angle, but usually one more nearly approaching to the right angle. The line of descent is of considerable length and has a gradual slope, and presents no traces (Thompson), or slight traces, of the aortic notch and dicrotic wave, and the only point calling for special notice is the occurrence in this line of a "number of wavelets" such as almost invariably occur in a pulse of fairly high tension, in which the pre-dicrotic wave does not reach a pathological degree of prominence, and the dicrotic wave is as such scarcely definable.

In comparing these two sphygmograms, both of which represent the condition of the pulse which may occur in the early stage of general paralysis, it is readily seen what very opposite conditions are at work in their production; in the former a fairly active heart with diminished arterial tension, and in the latter a less active heart with increased arterial tension, the latter being shown by the increase of the apical angle and the marked want of prominence of the dicrotic wave; but even this evidence of tension rapidly disappears, and a fully dicrotic condition may be brought about, if during this stage the patient become temporarily acutely maniacal, a point which would tend to indicate that the degree of tension previously present was due to a persistent spasm of the vessels, a view which is generally assented to. It is thus seen that during the early stage of uncomplicated general paralysis, the pulse may present almost any feature from complete dicrotism to a considerable degree of tension, the latter not usually exceeding what must be termed the physiological limits, though the cardiac factor is almost invariably somewhat at fault, producing a feebler line of ascent than normal. It has been suggested that the sphygmographic tracings in this early stage of general paralysis may be of some service in the differential diagnosis between the syphilitic and non-syphilitic forms of general paralysis, the force of the disease in the former being spent presumably on the blood-vessels, some proportionate increase in pulse tension may be expected to occur. There is, however, scarcely evidence to indicate that this takes place, and in many cases it would almost appear that rather the reverse obtains, possibly explicable by the condition of debility of not unfrequent occurrence in patients suffering from syphilis.

The typical line of progress in the march of the disease is now towards increased tension, as is shown by sphygmograms taken during the second and more typical stage of general paralysis (Figs. 9 and 10). The line of ascent becomes somewhat less slanting than formerly, and is also longer, the apex varies a little but tends to form a plateau, owing to the very marked prominence of the pre-dicrotic wave. From this point the line of descent falls rapidly to the aortic notch, which varies a little as regards its prominence, cases sometimes occurring in which the aortic notch reaches quite down to the respiratory line, and is followed by a well-marked dicrotic wave. In these latter, the condition of actual tension present in the first and early second stage has been replaced by what has been called by Dr. Broadbent virtual tension, and it is more particularly in these cases that, though the pressure required for tracing is generally considerable, the average occlusion pressure as pointed out by Dr. Bevan Lewis is low, and it is in this point that the pulse in the second stage of general paralysis chiefly differs from that which occurs typically in chronic Bright's disease, to which it is apparently so nearly allied. The typical pulse of the second stage of general paralysis would indicate that the heart at first is fairly active, but not hypertrophied to any great extent, a point which has been suggested by the clinical observation of Dr. Milner Fothergill, but which Dr. Burman, on post-mortem grounds, did not uphold, though the actual figures given by the latter rather indicate that what hypertrophy may exist in these cases when uncomplicated is comparatively slight. The tension, however, on the vessel wall is shown by the sphygmographic tracings to be considerable, owing probably to some interference with the outflow of blood from the arterioles and capillaries, this being brought about by a pathological alteration in the coats of the vessels interfering with their elasticity. That this change is to some extent muscular rather than fibrous is suggested by the fact that in many cases the signs of tension may be completely removed by amyl nitrite. The condition of virtual tension which is apt to appear in sphygmographic tracings during the second stage apparently points to a secondary degeneration of the vessel walls, and the subsequent dilatation of their lumen, a condition which has been shown by the writer to occur in the cerebral basal vessels in some cases of general paralysis, and combined with this it is probable some relative cardiac failure is necessary to produce this form of pulse. Although the form of pulse varies considerably, as do the details of the line of mental and bodily progress of the disease towards its termination, it would appear that as a rule the cardiac factor diminishes in force and vigour, and in the most advanced condition the line of ascent is slightly oblique and short, and the line of descent has only a low elevation, and is of gradual slope. Evidence of increased tension may be present even at a late period in the disease, and the effect of continued convulsions is to reduce the tension considerably, and slightly increase the rapidity. In connection with the subject of general paralysis, it is of interest to note how frequently the high tension pulse as it occurs in the second stage is to be observed in cases of simple coarse spinal disease such as locomotor ataxy.

Epileptic Insanity.—In connection with epilepsy it is a noticeable fact of frequent observation that in a certain proportion of cases there is a co-existing cardiac disturbance, and it is believed by many authorities that in some cases the relationship is causal, owing to a disturbance of the cerebral circulation, while in others that it is a secondary lesion as a result of the strain put upon the heart during each epileptic paroxysm, in other cases, again, it may be merely a concurrent condition, possibly in congenital cases, both diseases being related in some way to a common cause, and in addition it seems probable that there are cases of epilepsy in which the seat of the discharging lesion is intimately associated with the nucleus of the vagus nerve. Each of these conditions requires consideration in a study of the pulse in epileptics. Dr. Brown-Séquard has reckoned a weak and slow acting heart among the causes of epilepsy, but also admits the reverse condition as a causal condition. He in addition makes use of the pulse as an important element in differential diagnosis of cases of *petit mal* from those of simple syncope, in that in the former the pulse does not lose so much in frequency and force as it does in the latter. Dr. George Thompson suggests the lax condition of the arterial wall as of most frequent occurrence in epilepsy, this condition being more exaggerated in the epileptic status. Dr. Haig has drawn attention to a relationship which he believes to exist between epilepsy and a form of migrainous headache, which he considers is due to uric acid in the blood, and has shown that some epileptic fits are preceded by a diminished and accompanied by an excessive excretion of this acid. It would appear that for convenience of description the varying conditions of the pulse in epileptics may be arranged into five groups.

(1) **A class of epileptics** in whom there is present a **cardiac lesion of congenital origin** of the nature of a malformation, and in whom as a concomitant or resultant condition epilepsy exists. Owing to the not unfrequent occurrence of epilepsy in congenital heart disease, many authorities hold that the epilepsy is a secondary condition, owing to a disturbance in the cerebral circulation, resulting from the cardiac lesion. In these cases the pulse varies somewhat in accordance with the heart condition which is present, and the state of the heart as regards compensation; not unfrequently, however, the sphygmographic tracings show a considerable degree of tension, owing probably to some difficulty in the peripheral outflow into the veins. It is evident, however, that no single tracing could be looked upon as typical of the series.

(2) **A class of epileptics, fairly active, and otherwise healthy,** in whom dementia has not proceeded to any great extent, and in whom the heart hypertrophies slightly in accommodation for the intense strain thrown on it from time to time in the occurrence of epileptic attacks. In these the arteries are lax, and the heart is irritable and mobile, and the sphygmographic tracings present the following characters: The line of ascent is of average height and vertical, the apex is sharply acute, and the line of descent is not very long, the outflow into the veins being rapid; the tidal wave is slight if present, and the aortic notch and the dicrotic wave are well marked, and the pulse tends to be somewhat more rapid than normal. If the fits in epileptics of this class be preceded by a pre-convulsive stage of stupor, the pulse tension is usually raised at this period, but the highest pulse tension which can be re-

sion, its
nd the oc
ementia
, the mo
associated
nd Imb
cases of c
of impe
in the
is signs of
teresting
eciles, as

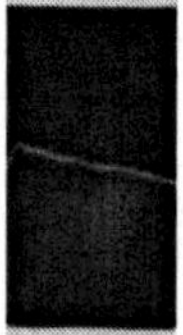

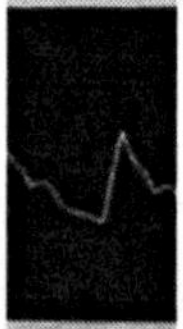

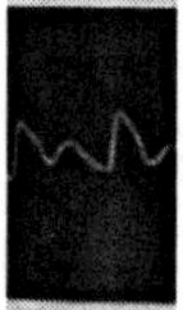

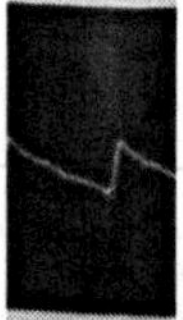

FIG.

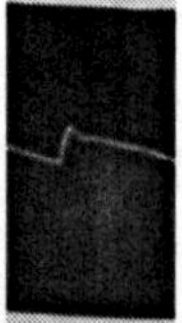

3, 4, 5 an
own ; Fig
ournal of
Lewis ; Fig

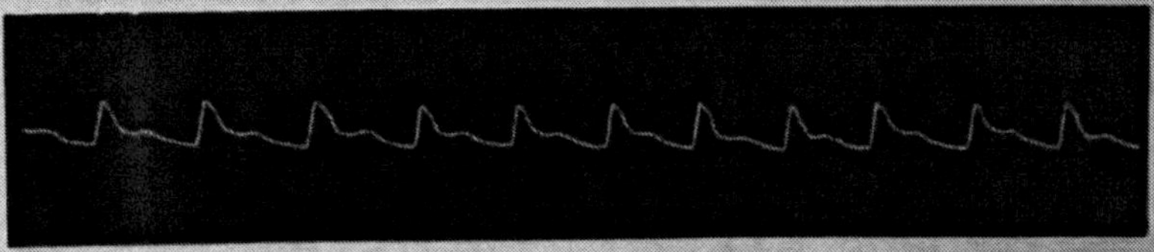

FIG. 6.—Mental stupor (B). Same pulse during period of lucidity.

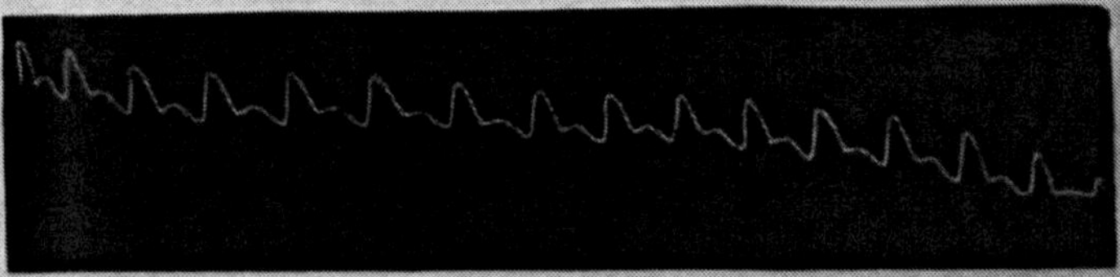

FIG. 7.—General paralysis (A). First stage.

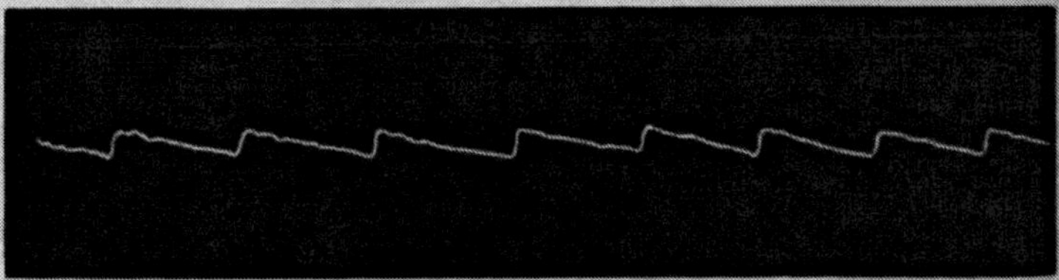

FIG. 8.—General paralysis (B). First stage.

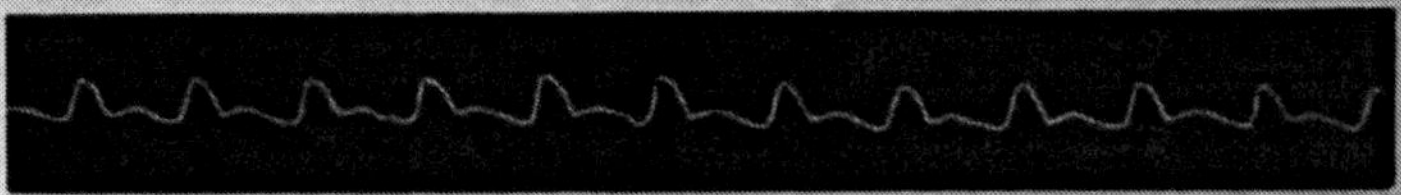

FIG. 9.—General paralysis (C). Second stage.

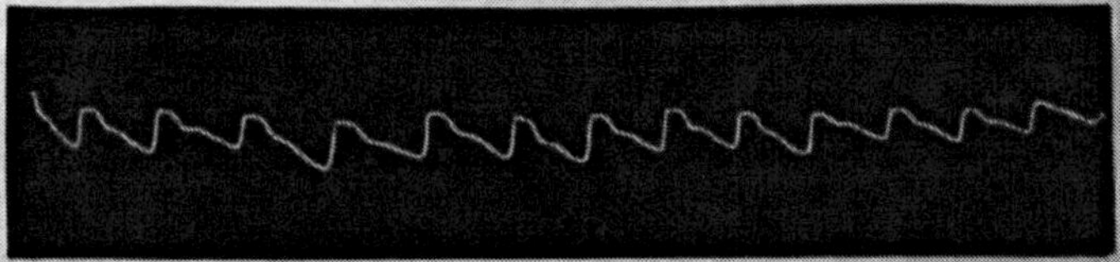

FIG. 10.—General paralysis (D). Second stage.

J. R. WHITWELL.

PUNNING IN MANIA.—In the excitement and exaltation of mania, rapid verbal association is often a marked feature, and clever puns are sometimes made —but oftener the reverse.

PUPILS, THE REACTIONS OF THE, in HEALTH and DISEASE.—The size of the pupils in a healthy subject is dependent chiefly on the intensity of the light to which the eyes are exposed. They are large in dull light, small in bright light. They become contracted during accommodation and convergence and dilated again when the muscular efforts are relaxed.

The normal pupil has three distinct reactions, the first and second of which are reflexes, the third is an associated action.

(1) **Reflex Contraction on Exposure to Light.**—This may be brought about by light falling upon the eye under examination, or upon its fellow, and to differentiate between these two reactions, the terms *direct* and *consensual* are used; the former signifies the alteration in the pupil of the lighted eye, the latter the

movement excited simultaneously in the opposite pupil. In this reflex act the optic is the afferent, and the third (motor oculi) the efferent nerve, and the centre, situated in the grey matter beneath the aqueduct of Sylvius, is that part of the third nerve nucleus, near its anterior limit, which specially controls the sphincter iridis. The impulse travels centripetally by the optic nerve, and, at the chiasma, in consequence of the decussation of the fibres, extends along each optic tract to the corpora quadrigemina. Thence, by way of Meynert's fibres, it reaches the oculo-motor nuclei, and becoming an efferent impulse, passes down the trunk of the third nerve, to the ciliary ganglion, and thence along the ciliary nerves to the iris. The centre of each third nerve receiving an equal stimulus, an equal contraction occurs in the two pupils—*i.e.*, the consensual and direct reactions are equal. Clinical observations and anatomical researches indicate that the consensual reaction of the pupil *may* be brought about in a way other than that just mentioned. In the rabbit's brain it has been shown that the oculo-motor nerve has a double origin, part crossed, part uncrossed (Gudden), and although the crossed origin has not been actually proved in man, it is very probable that it exists. Transverse fibres crossing the middle line between the two third nerve nuclei are figured by several writers. Thus it is readily conceivable that an impulse reaching the nucleus of one side should cross directly to that of the other side. It has been asserted recently by good authorities that the optic nerve contains special fibres whose function is to convey the impressions which give rise to these pupil reflexes and that these fibres are not directly concerned in vision. By some it is stated that these pupillary fibres can be distinguished microscopically. In the nerve trunk they run with the fibres supplying the macular part of the retina and appear to be less readily damaged by disease than are the visual fibres. Bechterew holds that these pupillary fibres do not cross at the optic commissure but pass to the oculo-motor nucleus of the same side by entering the grey matter surrounding the third ventricle; however, there is not as yet sufficient anatomical evidence to establish this view.

(2) **Reflex Dilatation.**—The centre for this, often described as the skin-reflex, is stated to be in the medulla oblongata (Salkowski) or beneath the corpora quadrigemina to the outer side of the centre for the light-reflex (Gowers.) The path of the afferent impulses varies greatly, and may be along almost any cutaneous nerves, spinal or cranial, or some of the nerves of special sense. Pinching or pricking the skin of the face, neck, arm or leg, will excite the reflex, and loud noises have been known to induce it (Westphal) in persons under chloroform. It also occurs in emotional states as anger or fright. The efferent (motor) impulses reach the eye generally by way of the cervical and upper dorsal spinal cord (where the cilio-spinal centre of Budge is situated), the two first dorsal nerves, the cervical sympathetic, the cavernous plexus, the branches of the fifth nerve, and the ciliary ganglion. It seems unlikely, however, that this constitutes the only path along which efferent impulses may pass, for the reaction is retained after complete division of the cervical sympathetic.

(3) **Contraction in Association with Accommodation, and Convergence of the Visual Axes.**—This narrowing of the pupil, the object of which is to cut off the light rays which would traverse the peripheral parts of the lens, is more intimately connected with convergence of the optic axes than with accommodation. A good deal of evidence has been adduced in favour of the existence of a special centre for the three associated movements, accommodation, convergence, and pupillary contraction, and at least one clinical case has been recorded (Eales) which almost proves that in man such a centre is present, although it has not yet been accurately localised. In dogs, as shown by the experiments of Hensen and Völckers, the centres controlling the ciliary muscle, the sphincter iridis, and the internal rectus muscle, are situated close together in the posterior part of the floor of the third ventricle; and these observers regard this region as the probable centre for the associated action of the three muscles, internal rectus, ciliary muscle, and sphincter of the iris.

There are in addition, some pupillary movements, which should probably be regarded as associated with other cerebral centres, as, for example, the respiratory centre, and others again in which no such association is likely. Dilatation of the pupil, sometimes considerable in degree, occurs with each deep expiration or inspiration. The pupil is also subject to minute and ever-recurring alterations in size. This unceasing movement is called hippus, or the unrest of the pupil (Laqueur), and is ascribed to the influence of the multitudinous sensory and other impressions to which the reflex centres are constantly exposed. It has been stated that in very excitable people the effect of psychical and sensory stimuli is manifest in the unduly wide pupils so often seen in such individuals. During sleep, when reaction to outside stimuli is almost nil, the pupils are contracted.

Alterations in Size of Pupils.—The two pupils are of equal size in the great majority of healthy people; exceptionally however, marked inequality is present, without any local conditions, such as posterior synechiæ, to explain it, and in eyes with perfect vision. If inequality of pupils (anisocoria), due to disease, be present, the most sluggish is usually the pathological pupil. There is no standard size for the pupil, but an average can be obtained by the measurement under similar conditions as regards light, &c., of the pupils of a large number of healthy individuals. Even on this point, however, the figures published by different observers do not entirely agree. In adults an average size of 4 mm. in good daylight is probably nearly correct. The measurement should be made with the accommodation at rest—*i.e.*, with the eye gazing into the distance. Speaking generally, the pupils are larger in children than in adults, and in young than in old persons. It was formerly held, and by good authorities, that the pupils of myopic eyes were, as a general rule, wider than those of emmetropic or hypermetropic eyes, and the explanation given was that in myopic eyes accommodative efforts are seldom required. It seems doubtful, however, if such is really the case. Hutchinson thinks that there "is a relationship between the size of the pupils and the state of the patient's nerve tone, due allowance being made for age and other circumstances. If the tone be low the pupils are large. The size of the pupils is almost in inverse ratio with that of the arteries."

Mydriasis is the term used to denote abnormal dilation of the pupil; three varieties are recognised. (1) **Artificial**, produced by drugs, such as atropine, which are hence called mydriatics; (2) **Paralytic**, generally due to disease of the pupil-contracting centre or fibres; (3) **Spasmodic**, caused by irritation of the pupil-dilating centre or fibres by disease.

Paralytic Mydriasis (Iridoplegia.)—This condition of pupil may result from a lesion situated in the nucleus of the third nerve or in any part of the nerve between its nucleus and the iris. Disease of the ciliary ganglion through which the nerve fibres pass on their way to the sphincter iridis, gives rise to this symptom, although in such a case the dilating fibres to the iris, or at least some of them, might also be affected. Damage to the extreme peripheral filaments supplying the iris, as in some cases of intra-ocular disease, also leads to this form of mydriasis. Any interruption in the transmission of stimuli from the retina to the third nerve centre gives rise to the condition, and this may occur even though the pupil-contracting centres and fibres be nearly or quite healthy. The pupil in paralytic mydriasis is moderately dilated; this dilatation can be increased to the maximum by mydriatics, but only a medium contraction can be effected by myotics; the reflex dilatation to sensory stimuli is retained, but the other reactions may vary; if the lesion be situated in the oculo-motor nucleus or in the course of the third nerve, reflex action to light, direct and consensual, and associated action with convergence are lost; if the lesion be in the afferent path—*i.e.*, between the retina and the centre, the efferent tracts being healthy, the direct contraction of the pupil to light is lost, but the consensual reaction and the associated reaction are unaffected.

Paralytic mydriasis is met with in tumour or other forms of disease at the base of the brain, which destroy the third nerve in any part of its course between the inter-peduncular space and the sphenoidal fissure through which it leaves the intra-cranial cavity. New growths in the meninges or bones of the basis cranii, disease (thrombosis) of the cavernous sinus, or tubercle at the base are among such causes. Destruction of the third nerve-nucleus will of course give rise to this condition. In instances like the above, in which the whole nerve is affected, the pupil symptom will be accompanied by paralysis of the other ocular muscles supplied by this nerve; there will be ptosis, divergent strabismus with loss or impairment of upward, downward, and inward rotation of the globe, and cycloplegia.

In general paralysis of the insane (*see* Eye), in epilepsy, in cerebral hæmorrhage, in orbital disease (tumour or abscess), damaging the ciliary nerves, in increased intra-ocular pressure, as in glaucoma of any variety, this pupillary condition may be present. In hæmorrhage from the middle meningeal artery unilateral mydriasis on the same side as the hæmorrhage, occurs in about 50 per cent. of the cases, and is thus a valuable symptom in regard to trephining. Paralytic mydriasis due to interruption in the afferent fibres is met with in optic atrophy and other lesions, such as injury to the nerve by perforating wounds, or by fracture of the bones at the apex of the orbit.

Spasmodic Mydriasis, or Irritation Mydriasis, is a condition concerning which our knowledge is more limited. Belief in the presence of radial or dilator muscle-fibres in the iris renders discussion of the pupillary condition, which would result from spasm of them, comparatively easy. There seems, however, scarcely a doubt that in man such fibres do not exist, and hence it is no longer accurate to speak of spasmodic mydriasis. The alternative term is a better one, and should be held to signify mydriasis induced by irritation of the nerves which inhibit the action of the sphincter of the pupil. This condition is recognised (Lesser), and is to be distinguished from paralytic mydriasis by a moderately dilated pupil, which does not become larger in response to sensory stimuli (reflex dilatation lost); its reaction to light and with convergence are retained although diminished in degree. Mydriatics dilate this pupil to the maximum, but its contraction under the influence of myotics is less than normal.

Irritation mydriasis may be present in the early stages of disease of the cervical spinal cord, as tumours or meningitis, or of disease in the course of the cervical sympathetic, by which irritation but not paralysis of the pupil-dilating fibres is caused. It also occurs in some conditions of mental disturbance, acute mania, melancholia with excitement, &c. It has been stated to accompany severe intestinal irritation.

Myosis is the name applied to any abnormally small pupil. Here also three forms are recognised:—

(1) **Artificial**, due to the action of drugs, such as Calabar bean, which are hence termed myotics; (2) **Paralytic**, due to paralysis of the pupil-dilating centre or fibres; (3) **Spasmodic**, due to irritation of the pupil-contracting centre or nerve-fibres, giving rise to spasm of the circular muscle of the iris.

Paralytic Myosis.—This condition is induced by any pathological process preventing the transmission of impulses which in health are inhibitory to the action of the sphincter pupillæ—*i.e.*, impulses travelling along the pupil-dilating fibres (*see* page 1053). In order that the term shall be correct (just as in using the term spasmodic mydriasis) the paralysis must be understood to refer to loss of nerve power only, and in no wise to a dilator muscle in the iris. The pupil in this condition is moderately contracted, it does not react to sensory stimuli (reflex dilatation lost), but retains its reactions to light and with convergence. It is further contracted by myotics and dilates but partially to mydriatics.

Paralytic myosis is met with in tabes dorsalis and in general paralysis of the insane (*see* Eye). It is sometimes spoken of as the "spinal pupil," and has to be distinguished clinically from the Argyll-Robertson pupil. In the former the pupil is contracted but not very small, and retains its reactions, both reflex and associated; the lesion is then in the medulla oblongata or the spinal cord (cilio-spinal centre). In the latter the reaction of the pupil to light is lost, the associated action with convergence is retained, and the lesion is probably in Meynert's fibres.

In spinal cord disease, above the first dorsal vertebra, disease in the neck, such as goître and other tumours, aneurism, enlarged glands, &c., this form of myosis may be present and results from interference in the efferent path of the pupil dilating impulses in the cord or cervical sympathetic. In injuries to the spinal cord or sympathetic in the neck the condition found is stated by Hutchinson, jun., to be not so much an active contraction of the pupil, as loss of dilatation in full light.

Spasmodic Myosis, or Irritation Myosis.—Disease which gives rise to this condition acts as an irritant to the centres from which impulses travel to the sphincter of the pupil, or to the nerve fibres in their course. It is doubtful if myosis due to spasm is ever more than a temporary condition, and one about which we have not as yet much accurate knowledge. Spasm of the ciliary muscle is not uncommonly met with and easily recognised. In some of these cases the pupils are unduly small, and there is doubtless spasm of the sphincter iridis as well, but the association is not constant. In this condition the pupil does not generally contract to light, neither does it dilate when shaded. The associated action with convergence is lost. It dilates widely to mydriatics, and becomes still further contracted under the influence of myotics.

The contraction of pupil which is spoken of as *congestion myosis*, and which is seen in the early stages of inflammatory conditions of the anterior parts of the eye (generally slight injuries to the cornea), may be here referred to. The explanation generally given that it is due to an increased vascularity of the iris is probably in the main correct, though it may be said with equal probability to be partly a reflex contraction.

Spasmodic myosis is met with more frequently than the paralytic form. It is a nearly constant symptom of the early stage of inflammatory intra-cranial affections, as, for example, meningitis of all kinds, and marks the onset of inflammatory reaction after injuries to the cortex and deeper parts of the brain. In cerebral hæmorrhage, myosis is at first present (Berthold.) It may be caused by intracranial tumours in the neighbourhood of the origin of the third nerves, or in the course of the nerves, and would then probably be followed by paralytic mydriasis. It has been noted at the beginning of hysterical and epileptic seizures and is a sign of poisoning by certain drugs—*e.g.*, opium, Calabar bean, tobacco.

J. B. Lawford.

PURSUIT, IDEAS OF. (*See* Persecution Mania.)

PYROMANIA (πῦρ, fire). **Synonyms.**—*Monomanie incendiaire* (Fr.); *Feuerlust*, *Brandstiftungsmonomanie*, or *lust*, or *trieb* (Ger.).

Definition.—A morbid impulse to burn.

Historical.—The mental condition to which has been attached the term pyromania is more frequently alluded to, and more fully treated in foreign than in English psychological literature. This is doubtless owing to the fact that it is a condition not specially recognised by English jurists or in English courts of law. In offences like arson the question of responsibility is rarely raised, the cases seldom attract attention, no interest is felt in the accused, and conviction and imprisonment follow as a matter of course. In the past no inconsiderable number of incendiaries have been found insane whilst undergoing sentence, and transferred from penal restraint to asylum custody. The method of inquiring into the mental condition of such cases before trial might be improved upon. As has been said, it is to foreign psychologists that we owe most of our knowledge on the subject of pyromania. Some have maintained that it is an instinctive insanity characterised by intermittent irresistible impulse, some that it is a reasoning insanity, whilst others have contended that it is the accidental result of some recognised form of mental disorder.

Platner did not describe pyromania as such, although he mentions most of the facts upon which it was afterwards founded—viz., the Feuerlust or delight in seeing a fire, characteristic of imbeciles, the disturbances of sexual development, more especially in the case of young females, and also the apparent want of motive in many of the incendiary acts. According to Platner one of the causes of incendiarism is "amentia occulta," by which he designates a condition of mind where the intellect remains unaffected, whilst the feelings and conduct are disordered. Henke regarded the frequent disposition to incendiarism amongst young people as often consequent upon irregular bodily conditions, especially irregular organic development at the time of puberty or just before. Meckel was the first to use the term impulsive incendiarism (*Brandstiftungstrieb*) and to describe it as a new disorder. Vogel did not look on impulsive incendiarism as a mental disease if criminal motives were present; he allowed, however, that when irresistible impulse existed with absence of motive, it arose from a morbid mental disorder. Masius was far from accepting the doctrine of an instinctive incendiary monomania, and declared that impulses to fire-raising frequently occur in connection with some of the well-known forms of insanity—*e.g.*, idiocy and melancholia, but that a greater number are due to criminal motives. Fleming also rejected the instinctive theory, and considered that the propensity to incendiarism originated almost always from normal motives—*e.g.*, revenge, hatred, &c. He found in some cases a morbid mental condition which, however, possessed no special features. He disallows the influence of puberty, and regards the incendiary act as merely the accidental outcome of a morbid mental state. Meyer held somewhat similar views on the subject. Casper too denies the existence of a special incendiary insanity. He believes that fire-raising perpetrated either with or without motive is always a criminal act; and unless there is clear evidence of a disordered mind, it should always be punished as a crime. Jessen, who wrote largely on the subject, admits its existence as a reasoning monomania, but demurs to its occurrence in an instinctive form. Griesinger adopts the same conclusion. He states that it is due to a diseased mental condition, especially melancholia, or to a spasmodic neurosis, such as epilepsy, or associated with derangements of the sexual organs. In France the doctrine of instinctive monomania was founded by Esquirol, and applied to incendiarism by Georget. Marc was the first to use the term pyromania. He states that genuine pyromania is chiefly manifested in young persons between the ages of twelve and twenty, and is generally the result of abnormal development of the sexual organs. Morel regarded it as an instinctive form of insanity in some children with hereditary predisposition. Motet says that impulsive incendiarism is found in all forms of insanity, yet not as a blind instinct in such cases. He affirms that in genuine pyromaniacs, in whom there is a real appetite, the real satisfaction of which is eagerly sought after, there is the irresistibleness of a morbid impulse. Moussel concludes that there exists a mental disease which is essentially characterised by an impulse to burn. This impulse, if not irresistible, is unique, and seems to spring of its own accord from the unconscious victim. He also excludes cases of real insanity, stating that by real pyromaniacs he means persons who set fire to things, not on account of sensorial perversions or delirious conceptions, but impelled to do so by an overpowering impulse. Lasègue and Tardieu have dealt with the subject in connection with imbecility, and Giraud and Rousseau have added to the literature of the question by contributing a number of interesting cases bearing more particularly on the association of incendiarism with disorders of the sexual functions. Marro found that in incendiaries lesions of sensibility are frequent, and religious sentiment remarkably prevalent. He was struck with the large proportion of cases mentally alienated. Such is a brief *résumé* of the views entertained by various observers on the subject of pyromania. No doubt is cast upon its existence, but a decided difference of opinion is expressed as to whether it exists alone without other symptoms of insanity. As a rule English observers appear to agree with the views held by many of the German writers—viz., that it is not a disease *per se*, but the result of some of the well-known forms of insanity, and this view we are inclined to support.

Criminal Class.—Amongst a considerable number of incendiaries who have come under our own observation, a large proportion belonged to the epileptic and weak-minded class, others were truly insane, whilst a few possessed characteristics of an essentially criminal nature—viz., an inferior cranial development, a low state of moral feeling, a capacity for alcoholic indulgence, and an unscrupulous perseverance towards the gratification of their animal instincts. One man who answers to this description set fire to a stackyard, for which he underwent a term of penal servitude; shortly after his release he returned to the same place, and again fired the stackyard, because the owner had given evidence against him at his first trial. He affirmed that the long term of imprisonment, to which he was sentenced for his crime, was more than counterbalanced by the great loss the farmer sustained by the burning of his stacks. Allusion has been made to Morel's opinion, that pyromania occurs as an instinctive form of insanity in some children, with hereditary predisposition. There are certain children, more or less weak-minded although not imbecile, who suffer from moral defect, the result of an inherited neurosis. They are prone to lying, to stealing, and to acts of cruelty, in which they seem to take a special delight; occasionally they develop a propensity for incendiarism. Of a morally perverse nature, they exhibit a passion for playing with fire, simply because it is forbidden them to go near it. Dr. Savage instances the case of a boy who set fire to every house he was sent to, after being there a short time. Sometimes the act is committed out of spite or malice, at other times from wantonness or for the mere pleasure of seeing a blaze. This propensity may be instinctive in the sense that such children display a powerful instinct to destroy, but it can hardly be regarded as characteristic, for they are as likely to prove destructive in other ways as opportunity offers. Pyromania, therefore, in this class does not appear to be a form of mental disorder *per se*, but rather the outcome of a primary moral insanity.

Puberty.—In many cases, if the development of the mental symptoms be traced, it will be found that they tend to become intensified at the age of, or after, puberty, the result being that some become truly insane, others criminal, few do well. From them the ranks of the older incendiaries are largely recruited, and amongst them the advocates of the independent existence of pyromania find many of their clients.

Genuine pyromaniacs are usually described as young persons, for the most part dwellers in the country; badly developed, of defective intelligence, hereditarily tainted with insanity or epilepsy, and presenting anomalies in character, habits, and feelings; having, as a rule, no delusions, no motive for their crimes, but imbued with an irresistible impulse to burn. We have met with incendiaries to whom the above description generally applies. In some cases repeated questioning has elicited a reason for their criminal doings, —*e.g.*, a feeling of revenge, or desire to get into prison, to avoid want and exposure. An outstanding feature in these cases is their remarkable forgetfulness, and it is almost always a difficult matter to arrive at a satisfactory explanation with them, for, as a rule, they possess unlimited capacity for lying and deceit, and their invariable answer to all queries is, "I don't know." Owing to this pretended want of memory, it is sometimes by no means an easy task to deduce the measure of their responsibility. The cunning displayed by them, the precautions taken to avoid discovery, and the presence of motive without clear evidence of insanity, will stamp the act as criminal. In the absence of motive, an examination into their antecedents may reveal a history of hereditary neurosis, or of infantile convulsions, of previous indulgence in drink, and also of a period of unrest and mental inquietude before the commission of the crime. The establishment of such and similar symptoms will afford a more solid basis for the plea of irresponsibility being raised than the advancement of the mere dictum of intermittent irresistible impulse.

In the case of females, especially young girls, attention should be directed to derangements of the reproductive organs. Pyromania often appears at the beginning of the sexual life, and just as sly stealing seems to be characteristic of the mental disturbances arising from pregnancy, so fire-raising appears to be a feature of the nervous disorders attendant on the establishment of menstruation. Puberty is a critical period when weak systems succumb, as at each recurring epoch there are nervous changes which exercise a disturbing influence on the system generally. The occurrence of incendiarism dependent on the altered mental conditions coincident with the evolution of puberty has been frequently observed and described, amongst others by Rousseau who relates (*Ann. Méd. Psych.* 1881) the case of a young girl who suffered from headache, general malaise, great anxiety, and abdominal pain. Her nights were disturbed by voices whispering, "Set on fire, set on fire." She resisted for some time, but yielded to the delusional promptings on the day of her first menstrual flow, and again at her third menstruation; both dates coincided exactly.

In this class of cases the presumption that the incendiarism has been the result of disease, will be strengthened by the presence of such symptoms as vertigo, epistaxis, and derangement or suppression of the menses, by the complication of epilepsy or chorea, and by the occurrence of such physical signs as glandular swellings and cutaneous eruptions. Anæsthesia also may be present.

Such physical signs as glandular swellings and cutaneous eruptions are worthy of note. The mental symptoms may vary from hysterical excitability and irritability to depression and stupor, but in the generality of cases a tendency to sadness and melancholia will be found. When a motive exists with absence of mental derangement the act should be regarded as criminal; on the other hand, the presence of mental aberration with or without motive will indicate that the patient is suffering from the insanity of pubescence or adolescent insanity, and is therefore irresponsible.

Such cases — *i.e.*, of pyromania amongst young females — seem to be of much rarer occurrence in this country than on the Continent, where they are not infrequently observed. This probably arises partly from the fact that they are rarely suspected and partly that they are treated with leniency if arrested. Whatever may be the reason, an examination of the English prison blue-books affords evidence that females are rarely connected with arson in this country. During twenty-two years only six females were received into Broadmoor asylum charged with incendiarism, the youngest of whom was twenty-one years of age at the date of her trial.

Motives.—The most common motives for arson may be enumerated as revenge, fear, anger, hatred, and nostalgia. These states of feeling may be aggravated by drink, which, in this as in other forms of crime, plays a conspicuous part, and by exercising its pernicious influence on the brain tends to weaken the powers of self-control in many individuals who might otherwise hold in check their revengeful passions. In the case of one prisoner, a young man who came under our observation, the combined effects of drink and passion led to his attempting to set on fire his father's dwelling-house whilst the family were asleep. He had been refused some slight request, and whilst under the influence of alcohol, adopted this means of revenging himself. In this instance the prisoner was sane.

The element of revenge is also a powerful incentive to arson amongst weak-minded individuals, who, by reason of real or fancied wrongs, seek to wreak their vengeance on those who they fancy have injured them; or who, driven by distress and want, whilst wandering aimlessly about the country, set fire to isolated stacks and outhouses, in order that, by so doing, they may find shelter in prison. Men of this type sometimes enlist as soldiers; as a rule they turn out worthless characters, who find the salutary restraints imposed by discipline more than they care to submit to, and who, in order to obtain their discharge, occasionally, amongst other offences, commit arson, preferring penal to military discipline. Of 83 men tried in 1863 by court-martial, 8 or nearly 10 per cent. were incendiaries. Acts of fire-raising committed by men such as these may be regarded as essentially criminal, for although a certain amount of weak-mindedness may be proved to exist, it is not of sufficient importance as, taking the nature of the act and the existent motive into consideration, to warrant the question of responsibility being raised.

Associated Forms of Insanity.—The association of pyromania with the various recognised forms of insanity has now to be considered. In the course of 22 years (1864-86) 103 persons, who had committed incendiarism, were admitted into Broadmoor asylum; 95 were males, and only 8 females. The percentages to the total number of persons admitted for all offences are—males, 7.5 per cent; females, 2 per cent; total, 6.2 per cent. The annexed figures show approximately the nature of the psychical condition observed in connection with these cases.

	Males.	Females.	Total.
Imbecility (congenital) .	35	1	36
Epilepsy " .	4	0	4
General paralysis . .	6	0	6
Mania, acute (usually *a potu*)	5	1	6
Mania, recurrent . .	4	0	4
Mania, chronic . .	6	1	7
Melancholia . . .	17	4	21
Monomania . . .	8	1	9
Dementia . . .	10	0	10
	95	8	103

This table indicates that incendiarism occurs most frequently among *congenital imbeciles* and *melancholiacs*. The ages of the male congenital imbeciles averaged 20-25 years; that of the female congenital imbecile was 21 years; all the rest of the women exceeded 30 years of age at the date of the commission of the crime which led to their incarceration.

There are not a few imbeciles who are dangerous to society, and who are prone to commit offences, some of which are of an incendiary character. This obtains also in the case of true *idiots*. Some are quiet, others peevish and irritable, given to acts of violence, and addicted to masturbation. In some instances the fire-raising is perpetrated for the mere pleasure of seeing a blaze, in others from childish mischief or imbecile spite. One imbecile on being questioned as to his motives will stoutly deny any knowledge of the crime, and endeavour to cast the blame on some other person; another will take keen pleasure in detailing the number and describing the effects of the fires he has caused. Sometimes these poor creatures become the too facile tools of other individuals more designing than themselves, and by whom they are incited to crime. Simplicity and asymmetry of the cerebral convolutions are pathological appearances which have been noticed in those incendiaries.

Epileptics are more given to crimes of violence than to such offences as arson, yet instances of incendiarism do occur amongst this class. For the most part the culprits are of the congenital type, and revenge is almost always the exciting cause. The presence of epilepsy in cases of incendiarism is an important factor in determining the mental condition of the accused.

This crime is rarely committed by *general paralytics*. The Broadmoor records show six cases—one patient who set fire to several ricks gave as his reason for so doing, that he wished "to clean the stackyard."

In the various phases of *mania*, more particularly mania *a potu*, pyromania may be developed. In such cases it is frequently associated with delusions of persecution.

Next to congenital imbeciles, persons suffering from *melancholia* supply the greatest number of insane incendiaries. Under this heading will be found many of the class described in connection with the disorders of puberty. In some cases, the fire-raising seems to be resorted to for the purpose of relieving the intense feeling of anxiety and general uneasiness which pervades the mind, and comparative mental ease has been known to follow the morbid depression of acute melancholia after the commission of the crime. This feeling was experienced by one of the Broadmoor inmates, who set fire to several stacks of straw whilst labouring under acute mental distress, brought on by domestic troubles. He afterwards declared that he felt relieved in mind after the act was committed. In other cases, a prominent feature is the presence of religious delusions, which frequently have a direct bearing on the incendiary act. This was curiously illustrated in another of the Broadmoor cases. The patient's father had died; this event was the exciting cause of his mental malady. He conceived the idea that it was possible to communicate with his father's spirit by writing. With this view he posted the letter, and inserted with it, in the letter box, some matches and several pieces of straw, believing, that if the letter were then and there consumed, the smoke would waft the message to its destination.

Closely allied with the subject of incendiarism in melancholia, is the consideration of those cases where the act is an accompaniment of *monomania*; here, too, it is frequently associated with religious delusions and characteristic sensory hallucinations. In one case the crime was due to the patient being constantly tormented by an intolerable smell of burning and the noise of the crackling of fire; his sense of taste was also affected. Other cases have been observed where hallucinations of sight were present, and one patient declared he was burned with hot irons during the night.

In *dements* the arson is invariably of an aimless character.

In conclusion, we find that pyromania occurs amongst certain children. In such cases it does not appear to be the result of a specific instinctive monomania, but to be due to a primary *moral defect* of hereditary origin. It is a condition frequently observed at the onset of, or after the development of puberty, when it is associated with the nervous disorders arising from the changes in the reproductive system at that period. Incendiarism is a crime frequently perpetrated by weak-minded individuals from various motives, and for which they ought to be held responsible.

It is associated with various recognised forms of insanity, especially imbecility and melancholia.

Responsibility.—There are not sufficient grounds for supposing that pyromania is a disease *per se*, an instinctive monomania characterised by intermittent irresistible impulse. It is requisite that some other evidence of insanity be forthcoming, in order that the incendiary may be held irresponsible for his misdeeds.

When a motive is present without definite symptoms of a disordered mind, the incendiary act should be regarded as criminal.

With or without motive, if evidence of insanity exists, the accused should be held irresponsible.

Each case ought to be judged according to its individual psychological peculiarities.

The following extract from Griesinger thus appropriately sums up the subject: "The grand question *in foro* in all such cases must ever be to ascertain whether there existed a state of disease which limited, or could have limited, the liberty of the individual; sometimes the symptoms of undoubted mental disease can be clearly distinguished—a dominant feeling of anxiety, hallucinations, states of hysterical exaltation; in other cases, the actual existence of a nervous disease, epilepsy, or chorea, renders probable the assumption that the accused has been subject to some passing mental aberration" (p. 271).

John Baker.

[*References.*—Bucknill and Tuke, Psychological Medicine. Taylor, Medical Jurisprudence. Jessen, Die Brandstiftungen in Affecten u. Geistesstörungen. Griesinger on Mental Diseases. Motet, Jaccoud's Dictionnaire de Médecine et de Chirurgie. Montjel, Archives de Neurologie, vol. xiii., 1887. Tardieu, Médecine Légale. Marro, I Caratteri dei Delinquenti. Rousseau, Ann. Méd.-Psych., 1881. Journal of Mental Science—viz., Savage, Moral Insanity, July 1881; North, Insanity and Crime, July 1886; Campbell Clark, The Sexual and Reproductive Functions, October 1888; English Prison Blue-books.

PYROPHOBIA (πῦρ, fire; φόβος, fear). Morbid dread of fire.

Q

QUEEN ADELAIDE'S FUND.—This fund was established in 1839 for the benefit of such patients as might be discharged cured from the Pauper Lunatic Asylum at Hanwell, then the only county asylum for Middlesex. It was formed by private donations and legacies, and accumulations were invested and a portion thereof applied towards the foundation "of a separate fund called Queen Victoria Fund," for the benefit of patients at Colney Hatch Asylum, then the second Middlesex asylum. In view of the Local Government Act, 1888, a scheme was approved by the Charity Commissioners dated December 10, 1889, consolidating the charities and endowments, and directing that the income should be applied for the benefit "of lunatics maintained at any time during their period of detention in any asylum for the reception of pauper lunatics at the cost of any parish, extra-parochial place or liberty, mentioned in the second schedule hereto, being situate either wholly or partially within the limits of the county of Middlesex, as defined at the date of the creation of the charity."

[For these particulars we are indebted to Mr. J. W. Palmer, Clerk to the London County Asylum, Hanwell.]

QUERULANTENWAHN (Ger.).—A form of so-called paranoia in which there exists in a patient an insuppressible and fanatic craving for going to law in order to get redress for some wrong which he believes done to him.

Individuals who fall victims to this disorder are always strongly predisposed; in their youth they are extremely egotistical, and are the kind of people who "know everything better." *Querulantenwahn* differs from other forms of paranoia in so far as the wrong which the patient is suffering or has suffered may not be quite imaginary—*e.g.*, some law-suit has been decided against him. This event is the exciting cause of *Querulantenwahn* in a predisposed individual; not being capable of appreciating the real state of affairs and acknowledging that he himself is to blame for what he suffers, he appeals from the higher to the highest courts. The more he fails, the more he becomes convinced that enormous wrong is being done to him, and with growing passion he plunges into other law-suits to enforce his rights. Feeling that not only the judges but even his own lawyers are conspiring against him, he takes his legal affairs into his own hand, often acquiring a considerable knowledge of the law. Thus he becomes a plague to the courts of justice, and a terror to judges and lawyers, as well as to his friends and neighbours, because, egotist as he is, he is most sensitive to even harmless words and actions referring to himself, while he, in his morbid passion, is not ashamed of using any, even illegal, means to injure his supposed enemies. Beyond all this, he neglects his family, his business, and his money matters, spending everything on his insane hobby, and gradually going down the road to ruin. Unfortunately, it is only when he has lost everything he possesses that the true condition of things is recognised, and steps are taken to prevent further legal proceedings and to render him harmless.

An individual labouring under this disorder is mostly quite logical in his reasonings and conclusions, only he starts from a wrong premiss, and, as the most important morbid element, there is a complete absence of capability of recognising that other people have equal rights with the patient. This form of "paranoia" (Verrücktheit) has occasionally been observed in connection with phthisis and mitral stenosis (Griesinger, Kraepelin). (*See* PARANOIA.)

QUININE.—Physiological and **Therapeutical** effect. Quinine lessens protoplasmic and amœboid movement, makes the enlarged spleen shrink, lessens outwanderings of leucocytes, augments the red hæmacytes in size, but lessens their power of giving up oxygen, and the conversion of oxygen into ozone by hæmoglobin, thus lessening the ozonising action of the blood; it also lessens excretion or formation of uric acid; but in fever increases the appetite, blood circulation and pressure, quickens respiration, lessens tissue change. Contrary effects follow large doses.

Action in Disease.—As to the theory of its action in disease; it may control inflammation by restraining diapedesis of leucocytes. It may control high temperature by lessening the ozonising action of the blood and thus checking oxidation, and also abate febrile temperature by dilating the contracted cutaneous vessels, thus increasing the discharge of heat; while by its influence, just referred to, in lessening the formation of heat it also reinforces the cooling effect, as is shown by the lessened expiration of carbonic acid under the influence of quinine, which also checks over-fermentation, as in the digestive canal, and checks sepsis and microbic life.

In the insane, as in the sane, quinine may be used beneficially for its corroborant or tonic, or indirect sedative effects. It may rightly be employed as a specific in malarial fever; for various other maladies making periodic rhythmic attacks, such as periodical or malarial neuralgia, epilepsy, diarrhœa, dysentery, hæmaturia, intermittent headache; or to relieve neuralgia, and especially of the supra-orbital type, even when not of periodic or of malarial nature; or as antipyretic in fevers, inflammations, and phthisis. Also in rheumatism, lumbago, excessive sweat of chronic phthisis, cutaneous diseases of malnutrition, the pallor of townsfolk; and to counteract losses of blood, profuse secretions, or pathological discharges.

For those who are pyrexial, feeble, exhausted, cachectic, or in advanced organic cerebro-spinal disease or phthisis; in moderate doses, and with the adjunct of tepid sponging of the whole frame, it is the most valuable and safest antipyretic we have used.

It is one of the best tonic and corroborant agents for thin, or weak, or pallid exhausted insane persons. In small doses it improves their appetite, digestion, and circulation, gives tone and force to the nervous system, stimulating sluggish or feeble brain function, increasing the reflex action of the spinal cord, and adding fire to the sinking vital flame. Hence, in all forms of melancholia, or stuporous insanity and its congeners, it acts well, even at early stages. But great doses act the contrary way, and are hurtful.

In mental diseases, larger doses have also been employed to act on the coexistent states of the cerebral and spinal system. Thus the congestive condition and tendencies of general paralysis have been treated by full doses of quinine, although theoretically benefit is hardly to be expected. In stuporous insanity, also, full doses have been given; sometimes apparent good effect follows the employment of moderate quantities.

Where the insanity is based on malarial intoxication of blood and tissues, and hence deranged action of brain, quinine may have conspicuous success, as we have observed in several patients who had been saturated with malaria in India, or who had been brought thence with mental disease and latent malarial conditions of the system. One such case we published in the *Practitioner* in November 1881. It is that of a young soldier who had several attacks of ague, and some time after the last attack became strange in manner, wandered away without object, and was irritable, sullen, talked incoherently, and was disposed to be violent. During more than half a year the mental perversion persisted and became worse, the patient also muttering and talking to himself, being at times noisy, mischievous, and even passing motions in bed. Still later, he was noisy and restless at night, filthy and obscene in language, or threatening, destructive, and inclined to violence; still later, morose, impudent even to effrontery, irrelevant and incoherent in statement, sometimes excited, defiant—he was the subject of delusions of being followed and annoyed. At last he was mentally dull, confused, amnesic, slept badly, had but little appreciative perception of time, place, or surroundings. The face had become sallow, muddy, lemon-hued, œdema swelled the feet and legs, the urine was albumen-free, heart and pulse failed, lungs evinced disease, the spleen enlarged, the body-weight sank, the hæmacytes showed malarial changes microscopically; and, after failure of other treatment, the whole complex of symptoms, psychic and somatic, steadily and rapidly disappeared in a few weeks under quinine, at first in full and then in moderate or small doses.

W. J. Mickle.

R

RABIES (Lat. *rabies*, rage or madness). Madness occurring after the bite of a rabid animal. In an animal inoculated with the poison of rabies three stages are generally noticed; those of restlessness, outbursts of excitement and fury, and finally depression, exhaustion, and paralysis, ending in death. (Fr. *la rage*; Ger. *Hundswuth*.) (*See* Hydrophobia.)

RABIES CANINA.—Rabies produced by the bite of a dog, wolf, or fox; also rabies in the dog, &c.

RABIES FELINA.—Rabies from cat bite; also rabies in the cat, &c.

RABIES MEPHITICA.—The result of a skunk bite, which is nearly always fatal.

RAGE (Fr.). Hydrophobia of animals.

RAILWAY BRAIN. — Under this term cases of obscure nervous disease following railway accidents have been described. Many such cases are probably hysterical. Their chief importance is in connection with medico-legal practice. (*See* Hysteria and Shock.)

RAILWAY SPINE.—A peculiar class of symptoms attributed to affection of the spinal cord following railway accidents, &c. It includes spinal rigidity and irritation, sensory disturbances, and various manifestations of neurasthenia. (*See* Shock, and Hystero-Epilepsy.)

RAMOLLISSEMENT (Fr. *ramollir*, to soften again). This term is applied to softening of any tissue, but by English pathologists is usually confined to softening of the brain and spinal cord.

RAPHANIA; or, **RHAPHANIA.**—An affection produced by eating the seeds of the wild charlock or *Raphanus raphanistrum*. Also a synonym for Ergotism (*q.v.*).

RAPTUS MELANCHOLICUS (*rapio*, I seize; melancholia, *q.v.*). A term for the sudden and impulsive acts of suicide or homicide sometimes observed in melancholiacs. Also used as a synonym of Ecstasy.

RASEREI (Ger.). Furious insanity, delirium.

RATIONALISM (*ratio*, reason). An ambiguous word meaning the doctrine of following the dictates of reason. Rationalism is, according to Descartes, belief in those things only which can be presented to the mind so clearly and distinctly that they admit of no doubt. This definition is essentially anti-theological, and it is in this sense that the word is used to-day. In psychological medicine the term may be applied to the treatment of patients, especially those labouring under delusions, by an appeal to reason, and by advancing actual proof that the belief held by the patient is absurd and illogical.

RAVERY.—Delirium.

REACTION-TIME IN CERTAIN FORMS OF INSANITY.—The simple reaction-time, which is the basis of all other measurements of psycho-physical operations, has been the subject of inquiry at the hands of numerous observers; and we have the conclusions arrived at by such authorities as Helmholtz, Donders, Wundt, Exner, Hirsch, and others, with respect to the *normal* reaction-time to acoustic, visual, tactual, or gustatory stimuli, as well as the variations observed under diverse physiological conditions, or alterations in the intensity or nature of stimulus applied. It is the object of the present article to summarise results obtained in certain forms of mental disease, explaining the instrument and method adopted, and giving the bare facts without any attempt at their further elucidation. The method adopted was similar in every respect to that employed for results already given by us, and the tabulated records embrace amongst fresh cases many of those published in a previous work.

Simple as the mechanism is, which we have described under "Psycho-physical Methods" (*q.v.*), we find it absolutely necessary when dealing with the insane to observe several precautions which it may be of interest to note here.

First, as regards the patient, he should be told precisely, beforehand, what he is to expect, and what he is expected to do. Let him listen to the electric signal, and, by a few preliminary trials, accustom him to respond quickly thereto. Instruct him to keep his finger on the contact breaker at slight tension so that *no time be lost* in breaking circuit. In certain subjects it is needful to insist frequently upon keeping the attention on the bell and responding as quickly as possible.

The room where such observations are carried on should be as absolutely quiet as practicable; voices in conversation, the chiming of a clock, the bark of a dog, movements of others in the same room, objects passing to and fro within the field of vision, such as birds in a cage, will utterly vitiate the results obtained in many of this class of patients. If such accidental circumstances intervene, the register should be regarded as doubtful or discarded.

So vagrant becomes the attention of many from visual impressions, that it is occasionally necessary, when testing the reaction to acoustic stimuli, to blindfold the eyes, and it is equally essential, when testing the reaction to visual stimuli, to maintain the most absolute silence.

Each case must be treated on its own merits, but it is often fatal to our results to arouse by any stray remark the slightest emotional disturbance in our patients; in fact, the attention should be directed solely to the experiments in hand. The operator and assistant should remain quite immobile whilst the signal is being awaited. A little acquaintance with these tests, personally applied, readily suffices to show how distracting these slight movements and sounds are, and this applies with far greater force to the insane, and particularly to certain forms of mental ailment. The slightest preliminary click in the release of the rod is distinctly misleading, and should at once be rectified. This, however, never occurs with the armature suspension.

After a series of preliminary trials, when it is obvious our subject has accustomed himself to respond properly, a series of test trials should be taken. We never exceed twenty trials with these subjects, since, beyond this number, a large proportion of cases betray some exhaustion from the sustained attention requisite; an average is struck from their total, and the maximum and minimum delay also recorded.

Table I. (p. 1064) is a list of the reaction-time to visual and acoustic stimuli in some typical cases of **general paralysis.**

In the earlier stage of this disease, when maniacal excitement predominates with the obtrusive egoism engendered by the extravagant nature of their delusive concepts, there is often some difficulty in keeping our patient's attention on the signal. It is often necessary to take advantage of this feature to induce him to regard the trial as a "test of skill," when even acutely maniacal subjects can be satisfactorily dealt with. In this early stage of general paralysis, remarkably little if any delay characterises the response to an *acoustic* stimulus. A glance at the table referred to will at once indicate that the reaction to acoustic stimuli averaged eighteen-hundredths of a second for the early stage attended with excitement, and this is the average for *healthy* subjects, according to Donders and Von Wittich. An exception occurs in the case of W. R., where the response occupied twenty-two-hundredths. The remaining cases were all instances of more advanced disease, dementia and negative emotional states being the more prevalent feature. These patients were carefully selected to exclude sources of fallacy, and whenever a

Table I.—Reaction-Time in General Paralysis.

		Acoustic Stimulus. Sec.	Optic Stimulus. Sec.
T. C.	Heavy, demented, but attentive	.249	.247
C. A.	Calm, sluggish, unobtrusive	.198	.260
E. D.	Advanced dementia, with excitement and egoism	.246	.255
S. M.	Calm, dull, heavy, demented	.194	.248
J. N.	Heavy and demented, depressed, much paresis	.203	.272
J. M.	Calm, subdued, demented	.178	.246
F. L.	Heavy, demented	.259	.277
C. P.	Depressed, obscure egoism, sluggish	.211	.270
T. R.	Cheerful, calm, slight dementia, no optimism	.248	.300
J. S.	Early excitement, garrulous, optimistic	.195	.267
T. B.	Early stage, slight mental enfeeblement	.172	.257
W. W.	Sub-acute mania, grandiose, noisy, and obtrusive	.174	.204
C. E.	Noisy, boisterous, maniacal, egoistic	.189	.270
W. T.	Garrulous, maniacal, incoherent, optimistic	.164	?
W. R.	Mania, garrulous, obtrusively egoistic	.221	.230
J. R.	Sub-acute mania, grandiose, egoistic	.186	.212
T. S.	Tremulous with excitement, optimistic, notable paresis	.189	.271
W. L.	Wild, maniacal, incoherent, extravagant optimism	.183	.188
T. P.	Maniacal, garrulous, egoistic	.165	.250
R. C.	Calm, notable bulbar paralysis, much optimism	.195	.232

fugitive attention was betrayed, or such enfeeblement as rendered the test doubtful, the case was excluded from the category. The *average* reaction-time of this latter class to acoustic stimuli rose to twenty-one-hundredths of a second, several ranging to twenty-four and twenty-six-hundredths.

Tested for their reaction to a *sight* signal, these subjects, with few exceptions, betrayed a decided delay beyond the normal standard. The greater number of observers* give nineteen-hundredths of a second, or even less, as the normal reaction-time to visual stimuli. Hankel has certainly overstated it at twenty-two-hundredths. Taking nineteen-hundredths as the standard in health *cæt. par.*, we find notable delay in these cases of general paralysis where the average reaction-time for the whole series of cases was twenty-five-hundredths. However, several cases ranged as high as twenty-seven-hundredths and upwards. Upon the whole it may be stated that in earlier stages of general paralysis the reaction-time to visual stimuli is more uniformly delayed, and that later on both visual and acoustic stimuli show a retardation in the response.

The Reaction-time in Chronic Alcoholic Insanity.—Table II. (p. 1065) exhibits the more important cases examined.

In all these cases of chronic alcoholic insanity, with (in the majority of instances) systematised delusions of persecution, delay in the reaction-time is noted for both acoustic and optic stimuli, but especially so with the latter. On analysing the results given above it will be found that for acoustic stimuli the average reaction-time was twenty-one-hundredths, and for optic stimuli twenty-six-hundredths. A proportion of *one-fifth* of the series registered above twenty-four-hundredths for a sound signal, and *one-third* of these cases gave over twenty-seven-hundredths as the time of their response to an optic stimulus. A few cases exceeded these limits, and being estimated by a special method (the rod being graduated up to thirty-hundredths only), were found to exceed thirty-two-hundredths for sound, and forty-eight-hundredths for sight, the maximum attained.

The Reaction-time in Epileptic Insanity.—The individuals selected for the test comprised those cases only of chronic epilepsy of many years' duration, where mental enfeeblement was not so far advanced as to introduce any notable fallacy into the results obtained; and for the same reason, the trial was made during an inter-paroxysmal period, some days subsequent to the last epileptic seizure. Table III. (p. 1065), although short, will suffice to establish the more important facts observed.

The average reaction-time for sound in the above series is twenty-three-hundredths, and for an optic stimulus twenty-six-hundredths. One case tested by another method gave as high a register as forty-hundredths. Those who are familiar with the special features of epileptic insanity need scarcely be reminded that such subjects, beyond all other instances of mental derangement, lend themselves most readily to inquiries which have as their object the *physiological* condition of

* *E.g.*, Auerbach, Von Kries, Von Wittich, Donders, Wundt, and Exner.

Table II.—Reaction-Time in Chronic Alcoholic Insanity.

		Acoustic Stimulus. Sec.	Optic Stimulus. Sec.
W. J.	Calm, attentive, grossly deluded	.155	.217
J. M.[1]	Chronic alcoholism, delusions of persecution	.153	.212
H. W.	Chronic alcoholism, delusions, violent	.176	.265
J. C.	Slight mania, hallucinations, suspicious, tremulous	.181	.253
W. W.	Chronic alcoholism, demented, morbus Brightii	.180	.250
H. G.	Dangerous, homicidal, delusions of persecution	.189	.218
J. C.	Slight dementia, with considerable excitement	.189	.253
R. B.	Chronic alcoholism, hypochondriasis, suspicious	.197	.266
E. L.	Chronic alcoholism, hallucinations, suspicious	.195	.256
B. C.	Delusions of persecution, vindictive, violent	.199	.287
W. F.	Calm, amnesic, demented, and grossly deluded	.198	.264
W. N.	Slight mania, deluded, suspicious, irrational	.206	.242
J. J.[1]	Hallucinations, delusions of persecution	.206	.262
D. F.	Tremulous from excitement, timid, suspicious, deluded	.215	.286
J. F.	Noisy, obtrusive, maniacal, egoistic	.218	.265
G. A.	Suspicious, deluded, reticent, and grim	.211	.254
J. M.[2]	Extreme depression, suicidal, suspicious	.211	.245
W. S.	Tabetic, deluded, treacherous, homicidal	.216	.251
G. M.	Mania *a potu*, excited, voluble	.219	.250
W. H.	Demented, maniacal, grandiose, and egoistic	.228	.296
S. M.	Alcoholic paraplegia, amnesia, deluded	.228	.254
J. N.	Sub-acute mania, amnesia, suspicious, hostile	.225	.276
J. J.[2]	Maniacal, wild, boisterous, recurrent excitement	.222	.297
J. J.[3]	Delusions of persecution, grim, treacherous, homicidal	.228	.236
J. G.	Delusions of persecution, querulous, suspicious	.220	.277
J. R.	Advanced dementia, delusions, depression	.230	.241
J. W.	Dementia, much enfeeblement of memory, apathetic	.230	.275
A. K.	Calm, inobtrusive, demented	.241	.270
J. T.	Suspicious, deluded, hostile, treacherous	.243	.259
J. B.	Degraded, maniacal, vicious, and repulsive	.244	.300
J. K.	Calm, demented, amnesic, deluded	.270	.300
W. M.	Dementia with much excitement, deluded	.300	?
T. C.	Demented, degraded, much paresis	.300	?

Table III.—Reaction-Time in Epileptic Insanity.

		Acoustic Stimulus. Sec.	Optic Stimulus. Sec.
F. P.	Calm, apathetic, slight imbecility, sluggish	.189	.235
J. W. S.	Dementia, sluggish and apathetic	.189	.251
G. A.	Mild imbecility, querulous, suspicious, hypochondriacal	.188	.235
J. D.	Mental enfeeblement with excitement	.192	.211
J. J. M.	Depression with dementia, sluggish	.200	.232
B. L.	Dementia, deluded, suspicious, hostile, violent	.219	.295
J. V.	Notable suspicion, gross delusion, maniacal, violent	.211	.257
J. I.	Dementia with excitement and delusions	.220	.258
M. C.	Hemiplegia with contractures, querulous, often suspicious, violent	.223	.251
W. H.	Dementia, apathy, negative states	.223	.262
R. H.	Advanced dementia, torpor	.240	.265
T. O. M.	Dementia with excitement	.252	.269
W. W.	Maniacal at times and violent, mental enfeeblement	.260	.294
L. D.	Dementia with much depression	.270	.275
A. D.	Profound dementia, great torpor, and apathy	.285	.297
S. F.	Bright aspect, lively, excitable, but childish and most unstable	.281	.300
R. T. R.	Bright and lively in aspect, but of sluggish intelligence	.297	.294

the patient. The eagerness with which they one and all submit to the test was sufficient evidence that their whole attention, so far as possible, would be concentred upon a quick response to the signal. It will be evident, however, on examining Table III. (given above), that all except three cases exceed the normal reaction-time for a sound signal, some registering as high as twenty-eight-hundredths or twenty-nine-hundredths. One case only can be assigned to the normal reaction limits for an optic stimulus. Most of the others range high; and, in the case of A. D., B. L., W. W., R. T. R., S. F., we find nearly three-tenths of a second registered in all alike. We have therefore in these cases a retardation of the normal reaction-time beyond that noted in general paralysis or in alcoholic insanity, the comparative results being as follows:

Average Reaction-Time for a Series of Cases.

	Acoustic.	Optic.
General Paralysis	.19	.23
Alcoholic Insanity	.21	.25*
Epileptic Insanity	.23	.26†

So far, therefore, as the above results are concerned they confirm the view already expressed by the writer, and which may be repeated here:—"It will be apparent, from the observations on *healthy subjects*, that, whereas from twelve-hundredths to eighteen-hundredths of a second formed the limit of variability for *acoustic stimuli*, and fifteen-hundredths to twenty-two-hundredths* for *visual stimuli*; in the *insane*, the former is only exceptionally below twenty-hundredths, and the latter rises from twenty-four-hundredths to thirty-hundredths of a second."†

Table IV.—Insanity of the Adolescent Period.

		Acoustic Stimulus. Sec.	Optic Stimulus. Sec.
M. D.	Maniacal, vicious, impulsive, degraded	.277	.295
J. T.	Egoistic, obtrusive, impulsive	.243	.259
F. N.	Maniacal, obtrusively egoistic	.239	.264
F. W.	Egoistic, exalted notions, impulsive	.242	.300
J. B. S.	Exalted notions, gradually advancing mental enfeeblement	.246	.282
W. S.	Convalescing from recent maniacal seizure	.159	.260
E. M.	Chronic mental enfeeblement following upon adolescent insanity	.261	.287

In all these cases it is to be noted that sexual perversion existed, the vice of masturbation having been for years practised. The same remark applies to the following typical instances of hypochondriacal melancholia occurring in individuals at the fourth and fifth decades of life:

Table V.—Hypochondriacal Melancholia.

		Acoustic Stimulus. Sec.	Optic Stimulus. Sec.
A. H.	Depressed, suicidal, craving for sympathy, visceral hypochondriasis	.202	.270
J. D. H.	Acute melancholic distress, numerous subjective ailments, loss of self-confidence, timidity, and distrust	.180	.267
G. R.	Fanciful, importunate, "visceral" hallucinations	.233	.290
R. R.	Self-distrust, importunate, introspective	.245	.266
G. A.	Hypochondriasis	.211	.254
J. H.	Morbid depression, fretful, querulous, numerous fanciful visceral ailments	.212	.274
J. M.	Fitful, explosive, melancholic states, visceral ailments (imaginary), numerous subjective perversions	.204	.218
J. W.	Greatly depressed, fretful, deluded	.239	.249
T. E.	Reticent, gloomy, morose, introspective, and hypochondriacal	.267	.274
R. W.	Much depressed, fanciful, and obtrusively querulous	.290	.300

An instance of hypochondriacal melancholia in an aged subject, J. W., aged seventy, gave as the reaction-time for *sound* 1.360 (or 136-hundredths of a second) as estimated by another method; whilst his reaction-time for a *sight* signal was twenty-seven-hundredths of a second. This was a reversal of the order hitherto obtained, and was quite exceptional in our experience. The greatest care was observed to detect any possible fallacy, but in almost every trial this subject responded to the sound signal after a delay of from one to one and a half seconds.

* One-third of the cases range above .27.

† One-third of the cases range above .29.

* This, as previously stated, is too wide a margin, nineteen-hundredths being more correct.

† "Text-book of Mental Diseases, 1889," p. 136.

Table VI.—Results in Other Forms of Insanity.

		Acoustic Stimulus. Sec.	Optic Stimulus. Sec.
T. H.	Chronic mania, deluded, very incoherent	.215	.258
W. R.	,, ,, much mental enfeeblement	.271	.284
J. L.	,, ,, ,, ,, ,,	.252	.256
J. W.[1]	,, ,, ,, ,, ,,	.251	.288
T. G.	,, ,, delusions, incoherence	.268	.294
R. T.	,, ,, ,, ,,	.257	.288
G. P.	Chronic melancholia, suicidal	.224	.273
J. G.	,, ,, delusional	.271	.282
R. W.	,, ,, ,, hypochondriacal	.290	.300
J. M. B.	,, ,, impulsive, suicidal	.210	.250
T. H.	,, ,, apathetic, reticent	.204	.258
J. W.[2]	Recurrent mania	.268	.289
W. W.	,, ,,	.176	.260
J. W.[3]	,, ,,	.284	.300
J. G.	Maniacal excitement, simple, garrulous, and incoherent	.300	.300
W. H. Mcl.	Acute mania	.226	.226
K. R.	Mania superadded to congenital defect	.223	.252
J. D.	Chronic brain atrophy, dementia, depression	.235	.262
B. J.	,, ,, ,, ,, ,,	.186	.236
M. H. L.	Amnesia after puerperal eclampsia	.228	.252
J. F.	Amnesia, dementia, depression	.199	.239
G. Mcl.	Slight dementia, posterior spinal sclerosis	.172	.251
J. E.	Mania, optimism, egoism, tabetic	.136	.215
S. W.	Profound melancholic depression, timid, deluded	.292	.298
W. W.	Dementia with excitement	.221	.247
C. P.	Chronic melancholia, delusions of persecution	.181	.213
C. W.	Simple melancholia of mild type	.188	.221
S. S.	,, ,, convalescing	.180	.180
W. P.	,, ,, ,,	.178	.199
J. H. B.	,, ,, ,,	.139	.205
E. H.	,, ,, ,,	.189	.188
C. K.	Monomania of pride	.146	.241
W. H.	Simple maniacal excitement	.187	.236
M. R.	Chronic melancholia—mild type	.195	.252
J. H.	Mania of suspicion	.171	.223
W. H. S.	Excitement superadded to congenital defect	.232	.280
M. E. B.	Delusional insanity	.195	.232

W. Bevan Lewis.

REACTION-TIME (in the Sane.)—The study of the **time-relations of mental phenomena** has in recent years acquired considerable importance. Improvements in specialised methods and apparatus, the introduction of rigid analyses of mental processes along the lines suggested by physiological science and the comparative study of mind, have resulted in a body of facts and generalisations which, though destined to much revision and modification, may be subjected to an orderly and critical exposition.

Analysis of a Simple Reaction.—The simple reaction may be defined as the signalling by a predesignated movement that an expected stimulus has been perceived. We are informed that a bell is about to strike, and that as soon as the sound is heard we are to press a key; the time intervening between the striking of the bell and the pressure of the key is "a simple reaction-time." In this process we distinguish as physiological factors, (*a*) the impression of the sense-organ, (*b*) the passage of the impulse along afferent nerves (and, it may be, spinal cord, together with delays whenever the impulse enters cells) to the brain, (*c*) the passage of the return efferent impulse from the brain to spinal cord, and nerve and muscle, and (*d*) the contraction of the muscle. The factor thus unaccounted for, the transformation of the sensory into the motor impulse, is the central or psychological factor, of which we have regrettably little knowledge. It is, however, the variations of this factor and the influences by which its time relations are favourably or unfavourably affected that will, to a great extent, occupy us in the present article. (*a*) The **inertia of sense-organs** has been determined by measuring how rapidly sense-impressions may follow one another without fusing—*e.g.*, in the rate of rotation of a disc with coloured sectors, or of a toothed wheel held against the finger. This determination would include the time of stimulation and of recovery of the sense-organ, and thus measure a longer interval than the one sought. On the other hand, if we expose an impression for the minimum time during which it can be recognised, the recognition will take place upon the basis of the after-image, and the determination be shorter than the one sought. For clear optical impressions well illuminated, the former process varies between 25 and 40σ;* the latter may be as brief as 5σ. For other senses and under other conditions very different results would be found. (*b*) The **rate of a nervous impulse** may be preliminarily accepted from experiments upon the lower animals as well as upon man, as 110 feet per second, under normal conditions, for both sensory and motor nerves. (*c*) The **latent time of the muscle** and (*d*) the time of **its contraction** have been determined upon the lower animals, and would form a slight and constant factor in the reaction. With these facts in view, it has been estimated that in a reaction from eye to hand, requiring 150σ, the central process and the remaining processes occupy about equal times. The rate of this simplest voluntary act is thus relatively slow; for if men were to form a line by grasping one another's outstretched hands, it would take about three minutes to pass a hand pressure along a mile of such a human telegraph.

Conditions affecting Simple Reaction-Times.—The influences affecting reaction-times may be considered as—

(*A*) **Objective**, or affecting the condition of the experiment, and

(*B*) **Subjective**, or affecting the attitude of the reactor.

Under (*A*) we may consider (1) **the nature of the impression.** The reaction-time will vary according to the sense-organ stimulated; averages of large numbers of determinations give for hearing 138σ, touch 148σ, sight 185σ. This order is quite constant, and the long time of visual reactions is to be referred to the long inertia period of that sense as well as to the fact that it requires a more precise accommodation to the stimulus than the others. If the eye be electrically stimulated the reaction-time is some 30σ shorter. The reaction to a contact upon the skin is a quicker process than to a temperature impression, and cold is reacted to in a considerably shorter time than heat. The senses of taste and smell have a much longer period of reaction, and the time seems different for different types of taste and smell; for smell, oil of roses 273σ, camphor 321σ, musk 319σ, ether 255σ; it takes most time to taste quinine, least to taste sugar, and an intermediate time for salt and acid. The chief factor in the differences above noted would seem to be the mode of action of the sense stimulation; the slow chemical processes acting upon the relatively inaccessible sense-organs of the tongue and nose require most time; the probably chemical stimulation of the retina being next in order, and the mechanical processes of contact and sound consuming least time. Within the same sense the more sensitive portions and those most accustomed to be stimulated lead to the quickest reactions; stimulation on the front of the hand is reacted to more quickly than on the back; on the fovea more quickly than on the outlying portions of the retina.

An important factor is (2) **the intensity of the stimulus**, the law being that within limits the time decreases as the intensity increases. Berger and Cattell varied a light from 7 to 23, to 123, to 315, to 1000 units, and to two greater degrees of intensity, and found a decrease in time from 210σ to 184σ to 174σ, to 170σ to 169σ to 156σ to 148σ. For sound, as a ball fell from the heights of 60, 160, 300, and 560 millimetres, the reaction-times were 151σ, 146σ, 127σ, and 123σ. For four degrees of electrical touch-excitations 173σ, 159σ, 154σ, and 145σ. Wundt and Exner find corroborative results.

(3) **The mode of reaction may affect** the reaction-time; simple movements and those made familiar by practice will be more quickly executed than complex and unfamiliar ones. Reacting by uttering a sound was found longer (by 16σ and by 30σ) than reacting by moving the finger; and a movement of the thumb or little finger is at the outset less prompt than a movement of the forefinger. In the experiment of Ewald, in which the stimulus was given in the very key by which the reaction (consisting in the very natural movement of drawing the finger away) was to be made a very brief time, 90σ, was found, and the process seemed to lose something of its voluntary character.

(*B*) The more important **subjective** factors refer in the main to the **expectation** and the **attention**. We begin with:

(1) The **subject's foreknowledge** of the experiment, formulating the law that the more definite this foreknowledge the quicker the reaction. If we experiment once with a preparatory signal preceding the stimulus by a regular interval, and again without such a means of fixing the precise *time* of the impression, we shall find the second time longer than the first; Wundt 175σ and 266σ; Martius 127σ and 178σ, Dwelshavers 193σ and 266σ. The

* The sign σ stands for the one-thousandth of a second (.001 sec.).

most favourable interval between signal and stimulus seems to be from one to two seconds. If we inform the subject of the nature, but not of the *intensity* of the stimulus, and vary that irregularly, the time is lengthened—with the intensity of the sound foreknown, 121σ; with it irregularly varied, 203σ.

(2) The effect of **distraction** has been studied by having a disturbing noise in the room or by imposing a mental task while reacting. Wundt's reaction-time lengthened from 189σ to 313σ (weak sound) and from 158σ to 203σ (strong sound) by the former means; while Cattell's reaction was lengthened by 30σ when attempting mental addition during reactions. Some persons are very sensitive to disturbances, others (and especially those with whom the reacting process is almost automatic) not at all so.

(3) An important distinction is the **direction of the attention** first brought forward by N. Lange—if the attention be focussed upon the expected stimulus, the reaction is *sensory*; if the attention be focussed upon the intended movement the reaction is *motor*. The latter is found to be the shorter—to sound, Lange, 227σ and 133σ; Münsterberg, 162σ and 120σ; Martius, 161σ and 141σ; to sight, Lange, 290σ and 113σ; to touch, 213σ and 108σ. This change in the attitude of the subject seems to modify the central process involved; it is also important in the explanation of divergent results obtained before this distinction was taken into account.

(4) **Practice and Fatigue.**—These influences are quite generally observed, but their extent is very various. They are most marked in processes that are complicated and not thoroughly learned. The effect of practice is most marked at first; later the stage of constant times no longer affected by practice or by a period of disuse sets in.

(5) **Individual Variations.**—The general fact here to be noticed is that different individuals require different times for the performance of the same operations. It was this fact brought to notice by the astronomers that called attention to mental differences, and the term "personal equation" used by them to denote such differences has been given a wider meaning. Such differences seem to be greater in complicated than in simple tasks. Though correlation of personal characteristics with a quick or slow reaction-time would be premature, it may be noted that the time in children is longer than in adults, that in extreme age the time is also long, and that the educated react more quickly than the uneducated.

(6) **Variations under Abnormal Conditions.**—While lengthening of the reaction-time has been observed as the result of headache or indisposition, the more systematic observations relate to the action of drugs. We may here cite the researches of Kraepelin showing that the effect of amyl, ether, and chloroform is sudden lengthening of the reaction-times (from 185σ to 298σ), reaching a maximum in a very few minutes, and followed by a rather long period of slightly shorter than the normal times (170σ); the effect of alcohol was a brief period of shortened times followed by a long period of lengthened times. A strong dose increases the extent of both phases of the effect, but the manner of taking the drug seems also of importance. A long reaction-time amongst the insane has been frequently observed (especially in melancholia), but the field for individual variation is here very large. Obersteiner cites a case of general paralysis, in the incipient stages of which the time was 166σ, in a more advanced stage 281σ, in a most advanced stage 451σ. Abnormal variations of reaction-times have also been observed in hypnotised subjects.

Analysis of Complex Reactions.—When, instead of reacting in a prescribed way to a single expected stimulus, the reaction depends upon and varies with the stimulus, the process is an ADAPTIVE reaction; for example, let there be two stimuli, say a red or a blue colour, and if red appears let the right hand press the key, and if blue appears let the left hand do so. The additional processes here involved above those of the simple reaction are thus a more specific recognition of the stimulus and a choice between movements. Thus Donders and his pupils (1865-68), who first performed experiments of this kind, with a simple reaction-time of 201σ, react with the right hand to a red light, with the left to a white light in 355σ. Cattell performs a similar reaction in 340σ, his simple reaction-time being 146σ. The next step would naturally be to determine how much of the additional time is needed for the distinction, how much for the choice; but it is doubtful whether we can signal the appreciation of a distinction except by showing it in the resulting movement, and we cannot execute a choice except on the basis of some distinction. A favourite mode of attempting such an analysis is by reacting to only one of a group of impressions passing all others without reaction; this "incomplete" form of reaction is interesting and useful for comparative purposes, but while it is admitted that the recognition of the stimulus as the one to be reacted to is in itself a distinction, though an easy one, it seems quite as plausible to regard the choice between action and non-action as an easy form of choice.

Cattell and Berger with simple reaction-times of 146σ and 150σ, perform the "incomplete" reaction (*i.e.*, react if the one colour appears, but do nothing if the other colour appears) in 306σ and 277σ, the adaptive in 340σ and 295σ; Donders' times for the three processes are 201σ, 237σ, and 284σ.

Another mode of measuring the "distinction-time" is to ask the subject not to react as soon as he appreciates the presence of the stimulus, but only after he has appreciated some detail—*e.g.*, not to react when a colour appears, but only when he knows what the colour is. This leaves everything to the subject himself, and the difference between this and the simple reaction may be large or small according as the tendency of the subject leads him to make the distinction somewhat before or somewhat after pressing the key. Friederich makes this "subjective" distinction between colours in 267σ (simple reaction-time 175σ), but both Tigerstedt and Tischer find only about half this difference in a closely similar experiment. While utilising all these methods for studying the influences to which these times are subject, it seems best, in view of the fact that the variations in the "incomplete" and "subjective" times found by different observers are so great as compared to the variation in adaptive times, not to decide what portion of the time is needed for distinction, what for choice.

Conditions affecting Complex Reactions.—Amongst the variety of conditions affecting complex reactions we will begin with—

(1) **The Number of Distinctions and of Choices.**—A variation in the range of distinction while leaving the choice the same is effected in the incomplete and subjective reactions. Cattell reacts to a colour when either that or one other colour may appear, in 306σ, when either that or one of nine others, in 313σ. Friederich makes a subjective distinction between two colours in 267σ, between four colours in 296σ. Six of Tischer's subjects recognise one of two sounds in 146σ (simple reaction 114σ), one of three in 164σ, one of four in 178σ, one of five in 194σ. For adaptive reactions involving increase in the number of distinctions and of choices, Merkel's ten subjects react with the several fingers to one of two visual impressions in 276σ (simple reaction, 188σ), to one of three in 330σ, to one of four in 394σ, to one of five in 445σ, to one of six in 489σ, to one of seven in 526σ, to one of eight in 562σ, to one of nine in 581σ, to one of ten in 588σ. When the movements are naturally associated with the impressions the increase in time with the increase in number of modes of reaction is less marked; thus, in reacting by naming words, a process that habit has rendered familiar, there is but an increase of 10σ in naming one of twenty above naming one of two words; but an increase of 60σ for naming pictures, and of 163σ for naming colours under like conditions. A further important result is that the increase affects the choice more than it does the distinction, and in general the faculty of making complex distinctions is easier and earlier of acquisition than the faculty of utilising and indicating these in one's reactions.

(2) A condition allowing of almost endless variation is the **specific nature of the impression and reaction.** All the types of reaction above cited may be regarded as illustrating this point, but including other variations as well. A few typical results are the following: (*a*) **The more closely alike the impressions, the longer the distinction.** As two sounds originate from positions nearer the median plane, it takes longer to decide whether the sound comes from the right or the left; at three points the additional time above the simple reaction-time was 17σ, 78σ, 137σ. (*b*) When the reaction is to take place to one of two impressions different in intensity and not to the other, **the time is shorter when that one is the more intense of the two.** (*c*) **The complexity of the impression is an important factor.** Pictures are recognised more quickly than letters; letters more quickly than words; English words (by an English-speaking person) more quickly than German words. As numbers increase from one to six places, the time of recognising them increases. (*d*) Again, different qualities of sensation vary in the ease of their perception. Salt is recognised more quickly than acid; acid more quickly than sugar; sugar more quickly than bitter (adaptive reactions 384σ, 394σ, 409σ, 456σ).

(3) **The fore-knowledge of the subject** may be varied by having the impression any one of a more or less extended group. Thus if either a light or a foreknown letter was to appear, the light was reacted in 190σ, but if either a light or a one to three-place number, the reaction was 297σ. Münsterberg reacts with the

five fingers to five Latin declensional endings in 465σ; to five German declensional forms, each finger reacting to one of three words, in 688σ; and to five general categories, each finger reacting to one of an indefinite group of words, in 893σ. The less definite the range of possible impressions the longer the reaction-time. The mode of reaction has a like influence as in simple reactions, except that—

(4) **The association of stimulus with movement** plays a more important part. When that association is natural, as in naming, the time is relatively short. Again, when the thing named is one that we are accustomed to name, as a letter (424σ) or a word (409σ), the time is shorter than when not, as a picture (545σ), or a colour (601σ), though the relation of the recognition-times is quite the reverse. Again, when the name is one that we are accustomed to speak (*i.e.*, in the vernacular), it takes less time than when the association is less familiar, as in a foreign tongue. Cattell has measured one's familiarity with foreign languages very successfully by this method.

An important difference between the laboratory experiment and equivalent mental processes in daily life, is that in the latter case—

(5) **An overlapping of mental processes** takes place. The processes take place not serially, but in part overlap. The influence of this distinction may be tested by comparing the time per word of reading 100 words, 255σ, or letters 224σ, with the time of reading one word 430σ, or one letter 424σ. Cattell has experimented by reading letters through a slit in a screen as they moved across the field; and found that as the width of the slit increased, and so the number of letters visible at one time increased, the time of reading a letter decreased. The fact that we can thus to some extent do several things at once appears as the result of observation as well as of experiment, and emphasises the difference between isolated and continuous mental operations.

We may finally consider, under—

(6) **Miscellaneous variations**, a few points already noticed in simple reactions. The generalisations respecting practice and fatigue are equally true of complex reactions. Berger has measured the time of reading Latin words in the several classes of a German Gymnasium, and shown a decrease in time as the pupils advance in class; that this is the result of practice rather than of general development appears from the fact that the time of naming colours shows no such regular difference. The individual variations occur as in simple reactions, and are probably greater in extent. Complex reactions are similarly subject to the action of drugs, the distinction being especially different under such circumstances. These times have been measured in a few cases of insanity, and shown to be very considerably longer than in normal persons.

Association Times.—A great variety of reactions may be viewed as responses to questions; the appearance of the stimulus being equivalent to the question "What in certain respects is this impression?" and the answer, whether indicated by a name or a movement, is the reaction. From this point of view the association between question and answer is deserving of special study.

We will consider first those cases in which—

(1) **The answer is limited to a single one**, and (*a*) the arriving at the answer involves nothing more than an *act of memory*. Thus the naming of objects in a foreign tongue, translation of words, simple addition and multiplication, answers to geographical and miscellaneous questions, would be here pertinent, and a few such results may be cited. Cattell names a picture in German in 644, in English in 545σ; translates words from English to German in 323σ, from German to English in 281σ. Vintschgau multiplies numbers from 1 × 1 to 9 × 9 in 233σ. Given a city to name the country in which it is situated requires 462σ; given a month to name its season, 310σ; to name the following month, 389σ, the preceding month, 832σ; given an author to tell in what language he wrote, 350σ; given an eminent man to tell his sphere of activity, 368σ. In the next type of association the attainment of the answer involves (*b*) an act of *judgment or comparison*; such a judgment being, not a deliberate decision, but the selection under the stress of an immediate response of some one factor as the deciding one. Thus, Cattell decides which is the greater of two eminent men in 558σ. Münsterberg answers a miscellaneous group of such comparisons in 947σ, or 99σ longer than the same process without comparison. The comparison may be extended to more than two terms, as in asking which is greatest, best, and so on of a group of objects.

(2) We pass next to questions admitting of **more than a single answer**, the answer being determined by the mental peculiarities of the individual. The question becomes more general, and the answer chosen from a more or less extended class. Thus, Cattell, when given a country, names

a city in it in 346σ; given a season, names a month in it in 435σ; given a language, names an author writing in that language in 519σ; given an author, names one of his works in 763σ. Answers involving a more extended selection are the following: Given a general term, to name a particular instance under it, 537σ; given a picture, to name some detail of it, 447σ; given a quality, to name an object possessing that quality, 351σ; given an intransitive verb, to find an appropriate subject, 527σ; given a transitive verb, to find an object, 379σ.

Before passing on we may conveniently consider a few typical generalisations suggested by the above results. In the **first** place, the reactions here studied vary considerably in character. Thus, easy and quick reactions under various headings are the following:—To name the country in which a given city is situated, "Paris," 278σ; to give the language in which an author wrote, "Shakespeare," 258σ; "Which has the more agreeable odour, cloves or violets?" "Who is greater, Virgil or Ovid?" 600–800σ; to name a "German wine," "a number between ten and four" (450–600σ). Correspondingly difficult and long reactions are "Geneva," 485σ; "Plautus," 478σ; "Which is healthier, swimming or dancing?" "Which is more difficult, physics or chemistry?" 1200–1500σ; to name "a beast of the desert," "a French writer," 1200–1500σ. **Secondly**, the effect of the foreknowledge of the subject again appears. In multiplying numbers from 1×1 to 9×9, where the smaller number always stood first, the multiplication by 9, 8, and 7 took least time because then the first number gave the subject a more definite foreknowledge of the number to follow. Again, Münsterberg precedes the asking of a question by a series of words, from amongst which a pair is to be selected for comparison—thus: "Apples, pears, cherries, peaches, plums, grapes, dates, figs, raisins; which do you like better, grapes or cherries?"—and finds that this hint of the nature of the question shortens the time from 947σ to 676σ. Furthermore, Cattell asked the question once for a series of terms, varying only the term in each case, while Münsterberg varies the entire question each time; accordingly, the foreknowledge of the general nature of the question makes the former's time considerably shorter than the latter's. **Thirdly**, the overlapping of mental processes may also be illustrated in associations. Münsterberg finds that it takes less time to answer a question consisting of two others than to answer those two separately—*e.g.*, 1049σ to name the most important German river, 992σ to decide which is more westerly, Berlin or the Rhine; but only 1855σ (or 176σ less than the sum of the two) to answer by the word "Rhine" the question, "Which is more westerly Berlin or the most important German river." **Finally**, it is here shown that the bond of association is often stronger in one direction than in the reverse. Thus, not only is it easier to pass from the special to the general than from the general to the special (Cattell, 374σ and 433σ; Trautscholdt, 757σ and 947σ), but it takes longer to recall that May precedes June than that June follows May; longer to go back and find a subject for a verb than to go forward and find an object for it; longer, when given a quality, to find an object having that quality than to recall a quality for a given object.

(3) **Unlimited Associations.**—Here the task is simply to name any word suggested by a given word, and the result depends very greatly upon the associative habits of the individual. For a variety of such associations Münsterberg finds a time of 896σ, Trautscholdt of 1024σ. (We may calculate the time needed for associating the word by subtracting from the total time the time needed to repeat a word; in the latter case the "pure association-time" thus found was 727σ.) These times vary greatly with the particular association, and it may be stated that the variation increases as the task becomes more complex and more dependent upon individual differences. Short associations were "gold-silver," 390σ; "storm-wind," 368σ. Long ones, "God-fearing," 1132; "throne-king," 1437σ. Trautscholdt classifies the associations into those suggested by the sound of the word, by the sense-qualities of the object denoted by the word, and by logical relations, and finds 1033σ, 1028σ, and 989σ as average times for the three classes. Cattell and Berger find the association-times to concrete nouns 374σ, to less concrete nouns 462σ, to abstract nouns 570σ, to verbs 501σ, all being "*pure* association-times."

Many of the influences to which less complex reactions are subject are also true of association-times; practice, fatigue, the taking of drugs, individual variations, have all been more or less successfully investigated, but the great variability of the reactions makes a concise and conclusive statement of the results impracticable.

The facts thus briefly reviewed by no means exhaust the field of investigation; but with an increase in our power of analysis, and of subjecting mental states to experimental methods, the study of the time-relations of mental phenomena, already fertile in suggestions and results, will increase in interest and importance.

JOSEPH JASTROW.

[*References.*—In addition to those given in other articles, especially Wundt, Fechner, Exner, and Cattell, see: The Time-relations of Mental Phenomena, by Professor Jastrow, 1890. General.—Sergi, La Psychologie Physiologique, 1888. Buccola, La legge del tempo nei fenomeni del pensiero, 1883. Ladd, Elements of Physiological Psychology, 1887 and 1890. Kraepelin, Die Neueste Literatur auf dem Gebiete der psychischen Zeitmessung, Biologisches Centralblatt, vol. iii. pp. 53–63. Fricke, Ueber psychische Zeitmessung, Idem, vol. viii. pp. 673–690; ix. pp. 234–256, 437–448, 467–469. Ribot, German Psychology of To-day (translation), 1886, pp. 250–287. Donders, Die Schnelligkeit Psychischer Processe, Du Bois-Reymond's Archiv, 1868, pp. 657–681. Jastrow, An Easy Method of Measuring the Time of Mental Processes, Science, September 10, 1886. Simple Reactions. Preyer, Grenzen des Empfindungsvermögens, &c., 1868. V. Wittich, Bemerkungen zu Preyer's Abhandlung, Pflüger's Archiv, vol. ii. pp. 329–350. Baxt, Ueber die Zeit, welche nöthig ist damit ein Gesichtseindruck zum Bewusstsein Kommt, &c., idem, iv. pp. 325–336. Adaptive Reactions. Münsterberg, Beiträge zur Experimentellen Psychologie, pp. 64–188. Kries, Ueber Unterscheidungszeiten, Vierteljahrschrift für wissenschaftliche Philosophie, xi. pp. 1–23. Tigerstedt and Bergqvist, Zur Kenntniss der Apperceptionsdauer zusammengesetzter Gesichtsvorstellungen, Zeitschrift fur Biologie, xix. pp. 5–44. Merkel, Die zeitlichen Verhältnisse der Willensthätigkeit, Wundt's Studien, vol. ii. pp. 73–127. Association Times. Vintschgau, Die physiologische Zeit einer Kopfmultiplication von zwei einziffrigen Zahlen, Pflüger's Archiv, xxxvii. pp. 127–202, 45–53. Trautscholdt, Experimentelle Untersuchungen über die Association der Vorstellungen, Wundt's Studien, i. pp. 213, 250; i. 14, 45. Galton, Inquiries into Human Faculty, pp. 182–203.]

REASON, DISORDERS OF.—Popular term for mental disorders.

REASONING INSANITY.—Insanity where the reasoning power is still present. Moral insanity, &c. (Fr. *folie raisonnante.*)

REASONING MANIA, REASONING MELANCHOLIA, REASONING MONOMANIA.—These terms are given to each particular form of insanity, mania, melancholia, monomania, respectively, when still accompanied by reasoning power, though the ordinary mental symptoms are evident.

RECOVERIES. (*See* STATISTICS.)

RECTAL FEEDING. — There are, among the insane, many cases in which the administration of food by means of enemata is essential to the preservation of life. Setting aside those in which it is necessary for surgical, or special medical, reasons, persistent refusal of food frequently co-exists with so much irritability of stomach that a sufficient quantity of food cannot be administered by the stomach-pump or nose-tube to maintain life, and we have to rely upon the power which the intestines possess of absorbing and applying such liquid food in digestible form as may be introduced into them.

In this way patients may be kept alive, and in tolerable health, for weeks, or even months, without a particle of nutriment being taken by the mouth; and, even in minor cases, it is frequently a distinct advantage to give rest to the stomach when that organ is unduly irritable.

The food should consist of beef-tea or milk, with peptones, and the addition or not, of a small quantity of whisky. The beef-tea should be made fresh by placing in one quart of cold water one pound of shredded lean beef, and macerating on the hob for two hours, or until the quantity has been reduced one-half.

To this should be added ten grains of pepsine, and thirty minims of diluted hydrochloric acid.

Four ounces of this mixture should be given every three or four hours, or a smaller quantity more frequently. It may be varied by the substitution of milk, to a pint of which has been added two drachms of Benger's Liquor Pancreaticus, and twenty grains of bicarbonate of soda.

These enemata must, of course, be given warm.

In most cases the addition of half an ounce of whisky to each enema is distinctly beneficial.

There are various forms of peptonised meat which may be used as enemata or suppositories, but it is obviously better to rely upon home-made productions, the composition of which is accurately known.

The mode of using the enemata should be as follows:—

After the bowels have been cleared by an aperient or an enema, the patient should be placed upon the left side or the back on a bed, and the oiled nozzle of a four-ounce brass syringe, charged with the nutritive fluid, inserted into the rectum, and there kept for some moments after its contents have been discharged.

The enema will then be usually retained without difficulty, but there are cases in which it may be necessary to plug the anus.

A much larger quantity than four ounces may be retained by using a flexible tube, which should be passed for eight or ten inches up the intestine, and the nutritive enema slowly and gently introduced either by means of a syringe or by pouring into the tube by a funnel.

FREDERICK NEEDHAM.

RECURRENT INSANITY. — The term recurrent is more especially applied to mania, in those cases in which there are repeated returns of the attack. It may be applied to melancholia also. The recurrence is referred to in the description of forms of insanity, and does not call for a special article.

RECURRING UTTERANCES.—A term applied to the verbal repetitions made at every attempt to speak by one who is the subject of motor aphasia. (*See* APHASIA, POST APOPLECTIC INSANITY.) They are either the last words uttered, or the words a patient was about to express when taken ill (Hughlings Jackson). As the lesion involves the motor speech area of the left side, the opposite corresponding centre must be the one to originate these, and, as Gowers points out, the right hemisphere must ordinarily therefore take part in normal speech. In the early stages of the illness new word-processes cannot be voluntarily originated, but the residual disposition of those last energised by the will leads to the stimulation of the right motor speech centre at every attempt to speak. The loss of speech from disease of the left motor region is not a complete loss of speech, but a loss of *voluntary* speech (H. Jackson). When speech is being slowly regained by the right hemisphere, many of the recurrences of utterance will be found to have been due to the defective voluntary influence, and to a tendency to the re-energising of nerve processes recently in activity—consonants will be repeated instead of the proper consonants being uttered, and those which occurred in the recurring utterances will be cropping up in wrong places. Ultimately, almost complete recovery may occur, and there may remain only slight and occasional errors in the form of words with a difficulty in finding the word desired and a tendency to use wrong words. (Gowers.)

REFLECTION (*reflecto*, I turn again). Meditation or the turning over in the mind a series of thoughts that follow each other. (Ger. *Nachdenken.*)

REFLEX ACTION (Physiological).—Although what are generally known as reflexes are to a great extent independent of mental influence, and therefore hardly come under the classification of psychological phenomena, yet there are some which do not differ essentially from the general class, which must be taken into consideration in the study of functional irregularities of the machinery of thought. It is impossible to draw a sharp line between the simple reflex action, in which the centre of transference between the afferent and efferent impulses is in the spinal cord or medulla, as, for instance, the spasmodic twitching of the leg or foot when the sole is tickled, and the infinitely more complex processes which we term mental, but which owe their initiation to as distinct a provoking impression through the nerves of sense as in the other case, and which usually eventuate in some form of purposive muscular activity. As a rule the term "reflex action" is confined to those motor or other results which are immediate, and which impress us as being comparatively mechanical; for where there is a time-interval beyond that required for mere conduction between the peripheral stimulus and the muscular contraction, there is obviously opportunity for the exercise of judgment, and a distinctly psychological process intervenes and supplants or varies the more automatic method of transference. The intervention may be of the simplest description, and may not occupy more than a moment of time, and bring about no appreciable variation of reflex result; or it may be prolonged and of infinite complexity, so that the primary sensory impulse may be varied to such a degree by the higher nerve centres as to take the form of an efferent impulse of a very different character from that which would have been brought about in the more direct manner, or, again, the primary stimulus may be inhibited and no consequent movement may follow.

In considering the bearing of the phenomena of reflex action upon psychology it is well to bear in mind that as the nervous mechanism becomes more complex, actions which originally were performed independently of cerebral influence become subject to the action of the higher mental centres, and as we go up the scale of animal life we find a constant emergence of non-intelligent reflex actions, which apparently differ scarcely at all from the movements among plants, into the region of intelligent choice of alternation which we call mental. Thus, the newly hatched snapping turtle will snap indiscriminately at everything which comes between its eyes and the light, whereas a dog, when provoked, even though its inclination may be to bite, will weigh the circumstances, and will refrain if it perceives that its welfare may be affected adversely by such action.

Seeing that the first effects, in all cases, of the intervention of the cerebral centres between the afferent and efferent currents is one of temporary arrest of action, and that the functions of what we regard as the higher parts of the nervous organism are in a large measure inhibitory, it becomes well worth while to consider what becomes of the energy represented by the afferent current when its immediate return is arrested or deflected by the exercise of the higher nervous faculties.

Quite low down in the animal scale intervention of cerebral phenomena in the reflexes which have to do with self-preservation and reproduction, take the form of desire or appetence, and the whole organism is thereby stimulated towards the accomplishment of acts which are required for the sustenance of the individual or the continuance of the race.

The strength of appetite as an inducement to action is too well known to require comment, but it is worth while to observe that the acts consequent on such appetites as those mentioned are often still, even among the higher animals and mankind, dependent, for their successful achievement, upon the primary reflexes of which they are a development. Thus, the ingestion of food and the accomplishing of the sexual act are neither of them completed without becoming subject to automatic nervous processes beyond the control of the will.

In these and other reflexes where desire is a prominent factor, it is, of course, initiated and intensified by influences *ab extra* acting in certain special ways through the organs of sense.

Recognising the enormous influence of appetite in calling forth and swaying the bodily and mental activities in all animals, and bearing in mind the continuity of the chain of physiological relationship which connects together all living beings, it becomes obvious that it would be very unsafe to ignore, in dealing with normal or perverted mental processes, any important facts in the natural history of appetence. And especially must we consider the nature of those influences which, at one time unconsciously, but now more or less with the mental cognisance, kindle into life these imperious and powerful motive forces, which, even when the mind retains its balance, will impel to action, setting at nought the inhibitory action of conscience and the will, and which, when higher inhibitory centres are weakened or paralysed, may dominate the whole economy with disastrous results.

There can be no doubt that in man and the higher animals, in spite of changed environment and consequent alteration of habit and structure, certain of the reflexes which were appropriate to former conditions of life remain as vestiges, just as do the traces of organs which at one time had important duties to perform. The seats of specialised sensation which were a necessary part of the chain of causation in the performance of life duties of our remote progenitors still respond in some degree to appropriate stimuli, even although their functions have long been out of date. Thus, the writer's experiments have shown that the titillation of the palms of the hands and soles of the feet of young infants at once sets to work the grasping muscles of the fingers and toes, which in the new-born ape are so vitally necessary in enabling it to cling to its dam.

It is noteworthy that not only does this response of the reflex apparatus to appropriate stimuli in this instance persist long after the need of the instinct has ceased, but also that there is found remaining a very considerable degree of the muscular power which among arboreal beings is necessary to render it efficient. Thus experiments have shown that some infants of a few days old can sustain their whole weight by the grasping power of the fingers for two minutes and upwards (*see* figure, p. 1076). This is important as proving that we may have accompanying a vestigial reflex of any kind a persistence of other attributes which were once appropriate and necessary, but which now may be useless, and in some cases even a source of danger.

Reflexes which do not work in the same simple manner as the above, but which proceed to action *via* the appetites and emotions, are also continued in part, even when the animal has so changed in accordance with evolutionary law that their appropriateness is a thing of the past. Indeed, it seems probable that the deeper reflex processes, such as the pleasure or desire intervening between an external stimulus and the movements towards which it tends, are, from the fact that they are more central, and therefore sheltered from the stress of changed environment, of a more persistent nature than those on the peripheral receptive surface, where the wear and tear is greater, and where the plasticity necessary to ensure a ready adaptation to new surroundings must be always a prominent feature. It is evident that these deeper vestigial impressions partake of the nature of *ideas*, and ideas which at one time were the habitual precursors of acts which may from altered habits of life have become inappropriate, and therefore vicious.

It is obvious that in the study of mental (and moral) pathology such possible vestigial reflexes deserve serious consideration, for it is more than probable that they may have an immense influence in causing certain morbid lines of thought

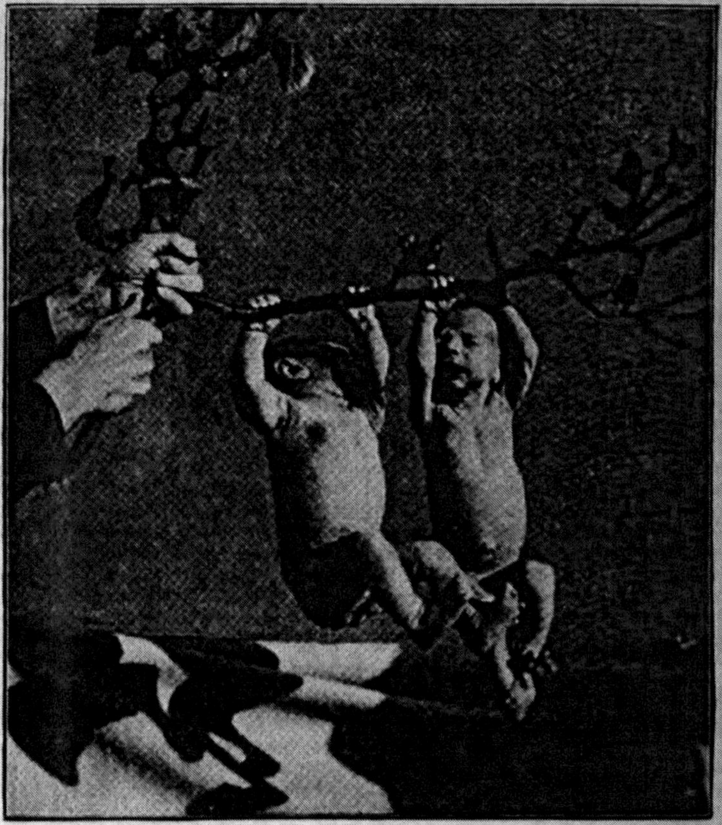

Infants suspended from branch of tree.

and action in the insane and those whose powers of mental and moral restraint are weak or perverted. LOUIS ROBINSON.

REFLEXES. (*See* GENERAL PARALYSIS.)

REFUSAL OF FOOD. A common symptom in insanity, especially in melancholia. (*See* FEEDING, FORCIBLE.)

REGICIDES.—We describe by this name, for want of a more exact term, the fanatics who, without belonging to any sect or any conspiracy, have assassinated, or tried to assassinate, a monarch or one of the great men of the day.

It is expedient at the outset to distinguish between *true* and *false* regicides.

The **true** regicides are those who, prompted by some special idea, make an actual attempt on the life of some political or religious leader.

The **false** regicides are those who make a sham attempt in order to attract attention, and so arrive at obtaining redress for more or less imaginary grievances. These latter are in reality only calculating persons with ideas of persecution (*persecutés raisonnants*). We are not concerned with them here (Mariotti, Perin, &c.).

The true regicides in their turn fall into two categories:

(1) The **mad regicides,** whom some sudden frenzy prompts to strike at a king. These are simply regicides who have become so accidentally—madmen in reality rather than regicides, and among whom are met all the types of madmen, from the simple visionary (*vésanique*) to the epileptics acting under the influence of their hallucinations or their unconscious impulses. Apart from the fact of their crime, which renders them suddenly celebrated, these individuals do not, as so many sick persons, afford special interest (Margaret Nicholson, Charlotte Carle-

migellix, Anne Neil, Robert Maclean, &c.)

(2) **The typical regicides**, the most important, those whom in this study we have especially in our mind, and of whose nature we are going briefly to speak.

Typical Regicides.—The typical regicides are essentially, from a clinical point of view, persons of ill-balanced or degenerate brain. That is to say, they almost always have inherited morbid tendencies, and are the bearers of intellectual and physical stigmata of degeneration. Some even have for the moving spring of their actions strongly marked psychopathic antecedents.

One thing especially distinguishes them as regards the temperament of the mind; that is, mysticism. We mean by that a half-instinctive tendency to become over-excited on matters of politics or religion. It is particularly to be noted that this mysticism is commonly hereditary with them (Charlotte Corday, Staaps, Karl Sand, John Wilkes Booth, Orsini, Nobiling, Passanante, Guiteau, &c. &c.).

Such is the true nature of regicides. They are persons of ill-balanced mind, intelligent for the most part, but of weak will and morbid instability, who lead the most aimless and unsettled existence till the day when their temperament makes them espouse with ardour the political or religious quarrel that the occasion happens to bring into notice. Then their imagination becomes over-heated, and by a more or less long initiation, they end by transforming party questions into truly frenzied ideas.

The frenzy of regicides is an *essentially mystic delirium*, either religious, or religious and political, or, in certain instances, political only. In its habitual form, this mysticism finds expression in *the belief in a mission to be fulfilled, a mission that most commonly has been inspired by God, and which is to be crowned by martyrdom*. In the ideas that constitute it there is nothing absurd or incoherent; on the contrary, they are generally based on a logical and likely principle (Balthazar Gérard, Pierre Barrière, Jean Châtel, Charles Ridicoux, Ravaillac, Aimée Cécile Renault, Charlotte Corday, Staaps, La Sahla, Karl Sand, Guiteau, Hillairaud, &c. &c.).

Hallucinations may accompany this frenzy, but when they are present, they are of a peculiar nature. They are genuine *visions*, analogous to those of hysteric frenzy and of ecstasy. They are *intermittent*, occurring especially *at night during sleep*, and sometimes seeming to mingle with *dreams*. The type of this kind is that of Jaques Clément: "One night, when Jaques Clément was in bed, God sent him his angel in a vision, who, in a bright light, appeared to him and showed him a naked sword, with these words, 'Brother Jaques, I am a messenger from Almighty God, and come to announce to you that by your hand the tyrant of France is to be put to death; reflect then, and know that the martyr's crown, too, is prepared for you!' Having said this, the angel disappeared" (Palma Cayet).

The crime of the regicide is not a sudden or blind act; it is, on the contrary, a well-considered and, for a longer or shorter time, premeditated act. Often, even, it has been preceded by a period of conscious obsession that has ended in annihilation of the will, and during which the regicide, a mystic always, sometimes invokes Heaven in order to seek there an inspiration.

Be that as it may, when the act has been decided upon, the regicide hesitates no more, he goes straight to the end thenceforth with the boldness of a convinced person. Proud of his mission and his part, he strikes at his victim in broad daylight, in public, in an ostensible and almost theatrical manner. Hence, he rarely makes use of poison; frequently he has resort to the dagger or to firearms, and, far from fleeing after the crime is accomplished, he seems to put himself in evidence as if he had performed some great deed.

Laschi maintained that suicide is of frequent occurrence with regicides immediately after the crime. Such is not the case, and it may be said that it is the exception (de Pâris l'Ainé, Sand, Nobiling). What is true is that a tendency to suicide is frequently met with in such persons, but at any moment whatever of their existence as one of the consequences of their morbid organisation. As regards the *indirect suicide*, alleged by certain regicides, and particularly by Passanante, as the determining cause of their crime, it has nothing to do with facts of this kind. In indirect suicide the madman kills a person in order to obtain death, his only end; with regicides, the criminal accepts death in order to kill another, his only object. It is not to suicide that he aspires, but to *martyrdom*. The distinction here is essential.

This idea that they are suffering martyrdom for an heroic act and with a view of obtaining happiness in heaven and celebrity on earth explains the behaviour of regicides after the crime. It accounts for their proud, haughty, and declamatory bearing in the courts of justice; it explains especially their courage and stoicism in the face of death. All indeed, men and women, political or religious fanatics, from Mucius Scaevola, burning his right hand coolly in the fire in order to punish it for having struck at another than Porsenna, from William Parry and Balthasar Gérard in 1584, to Charlotte Corday, Staaps, Sand, and Guiteau, without speaking of Damiens, of whom Michelet could say that he was the most striking example in physiology of what a man may suffer without dying, all have endured without complaint, and almost with indifference, the most horrible tortures, like the martyrs whom in this point they resemble.

Among the **causes** that induced the crime of regicides there must be named first in order a predisposition, most commonly hereditary, that makes them from their birth of ill-balanced minds and thus subject to all accidental influences—as regards these they may to a great extent be summed up in the operation of the surrounding mental atmosphere: Spirit of the time, monastic life, important events, exciting preaching and reading, former or recent examples, &c. &c. The surrounding mental atmosphere gives besides a special colouring to the frenzied ideas in accordance with the spirit and the tendencies of the epoch. That is why in the present day, instead of invoking the interests of heaven or the realm as formerly, most of the regicides put forward socialism or anarchy (Max Hoedel, Nobiling, Passanante, Olivia Moncusi, Otero Gonzales, Baffier, Gallot, &c.).

What we know of the nature of regicides and the motive power of their actions, enables us to comprehend *à priori* that they cannot have **accomplices.** At all times, however, people have tried to see in them, not madmen of any degree whatever, but the instruments of a sect or a party. From this there have resulted grave historical errors, notably in the cases of Jaques Clément and Ravaillac. In reality, with the typical regicides, save with rare exceptions, as in the cases of Fieschi and Orsini, the crime is the act of one person only. It has been conceived, meditated, and executed as the act of a madman is conceived, meditated, and executed.

To sum up, we see that *regicides are hereditarily ill-balanced or degenerate persons of mystic temperament, who, led astray by some political or religious frenzy, which is complicated sometimes by hallucinations, imagine themselves called to the double part of justiciary and martyr, and under the influence of an obsession which they are not able to resist, they strike at one of the great persons of the day in the name of Heaven, their country, or humanity.*

The practical question to be asked from this study is the following: **What is to be done with regicides?** Formerly, and in spite of the vague idea one had of their insanity, they were condemned to the most terrible punishment, that for parricides, not only for the purpose of punishing them, but also to constitute an example. In our own time physicians have almost always been in disagreement regarding them, and in consequence of this disagreement they have suffered the full penalty of the law. Very few have escaped with their lives, but the number of them. sufficient to show that regicides, when they survive, fall into madness and dementia. This is what happened especially in the cases of La Sahla, Passanante, and Galeote. After that, can their morbid predisposition be denied?

We repeat, therefore, What is to be done with regicides?

It is not allowable that, in a question of this kind, one should be chiefly concerned with the idea of constituting an example. Besides, the means would be badly chosen, for nothing helps so much to make regicides as the martyrdom of a regicide. On the other hand, to pardon them is hardly more practicable: the case of La Sahla is sufficient to establish that.

There can be no doubt that one must place oneself on scientific ground, judging always, not the crime, but the criminal. In that manner it is easy to draw a conclusion in each case.

Where the regicide is manifestly the victim of frenzy and of hallucinations, as Jaques Clément, Ravaillac, Staaps, Guiteau, &c., there is no room for hesitation, and confinement in a lunatic asylum becomes imperative. It is, moreover, the thing the regicide dreads most; such treatment breaks his pride, because he considers it a disgrace to be treated as an insane person, *he* a hero and a martyr! If one wanted to constitute an example, this would assuredly be a better one.

As regards the other regicides, those whom Laschi calls regicides from inclination, and who are in reality insane, although to a less degree, one must be guided by the special case. As a general principle, these individuals being unbalanced and their act an abnormal one, it shows how dangerous they may become to society. The solution that is most conformable to the principles of science and the public interest would be to place them for the necessary period and with medico-legal safeguards in one of those asylums for the criminal insane which in England and Ireland have long been established, and which the great majority of specialists in France and Italy demand as intermediate between the prison and the asylum properly speaking.

E. RÉGIS.

REGISTERED HOSPITALS.—Legally, a hospital means in England and Wales any hospital or part of a hospital or other house or institution (not being an asylum) wherein lunatics are received and supported wholly or partially by voluntary contributions, or by any charitable bequest or gift, or by applying the excess of payment of some patients for or towards the support, provision, or benefit of other patients. If registered, as these institutions are and have been since the passing of the Act (1845) 8 & 9 Vic. c. 100, s. 43, they are called registered hospitals.

"After the passing of this Act (or immediately after the establishment of such hospital, as the case may be) the superintendent shall apply to the Commissioners to have such hospital registered, and thereupon such hospital shall be registered in a book to be kept for that purpose by the Commissioners."

Under the recent Act (1890), 53 Vic. c. 5, s. 230, it is enacted that every hospital for the reception of lunatics shall have a medical practitioner resident therein as the superintendent and medical officer thereof. When application is made for registration, the Commissioners inspect the hospital, or employ persons to report to them thereon. If they are of opinion that the application should be acceded to, they are to make a report to a Secretary of State, who shall finally determine upon the application; if this be granted, the Commissioners issue a provisional certificate of registration. Within three months the managing committee are obliged to frame regulations for the hospital and submit them to the Secretary of State for approval; if this is obtained, the Commissioners issue a complete certificate, specifying therein the number of patients of each sex who may be received in the hospital. A superintendent who receives or detains a patient in the hospital contrary to the provisions of the Lunacy Act or the terms of the certificate of registration shall be guilty of a misdemeanour (s. 231).

Other sections enact that the regulations for the time being in force shall be hung up in the visitors' room in the hospital, and a copy of them sent to the Commissioners. No building which is not shown on the plans sent to the Commissioners shall be deemed part of the hospital for the reception of patients; infraction of this rule subjecting the superintendent to a penalty as guilty of a misdemeanour. The accounts of the hospital must be audited once a year by an accountant approved by the Commissioners, and printed; further, the form in which the accounts are to be reported may be prescribed by the Commissioners.

With regard to pensions, it is enacted that the managing committee may grant to any officer or servant who is incapacitated by confirmed illness, age, or infirmity, or has been an officer or servant in the hospital for not less than fifteen years, and is not less than fifty years old, such superannuation allowance, not exceeding two-thirds of the salary of the superannuated person, with the value of the lodgings, rations, or other allowances enjoyed by him, as the committee think fit.

Certain disqualifications in regard to the members of the managing committee are insisted upon: (*a*) Any medical or other officer of the hospital, (*b*) any person who is interested in or participates in the profits of any contract with or work done for the managing committee of the hospital, but so that this disqualification shall not extend to a person who is a member of a corporate company which has entered into a contract with or done work for the managing committee.

Lastly, if the Commissioners are of opinion that the regulations of the hospital are not properly carried out, they, after giving due notice, and after the expiration of six months, are empowered, with the consent of the Secretary of State, to close the hospital.

Bethlem Royal Hospital.—We have already given a brief account of this hospital. (*See* BETHLEM ROYAL HOSPITAL.)

Bethel Hospital, Norwich. — This institution was founded in 1713 by Mrs. Mary Chapman, widow of the Rev. S. Chapman, rector of Thorpe, near Norwich. Its care and government were committed by her to a master, under the direction of seven trustees. By her will she endowed it with the rents of all her real estates in Norfolk or elsewhere, and her residuary personal property, amounting to about £3500, to which bequests and donations have been since added from time to time, to the amount of upwards of £11,000. The money is invested in the names of the trustees, either in the funds or on mortgage. Unfortunately, abuses of various kinds were committed in the hospital through the default of the master. The foundress, in consequence, resided for some years in the house, and practically directed it herself.

The primary objects of the charity are declared in her will to be "Such persons as are afflicted with lunacy or madness (not such as are fools or idiots from their birth), and are poor inhabitants of the city of Norwich, or elsewhere, to be from time to time put into the house by appointment under writing of her said trustees, or major part of them, always preferring such persons as are inhabitants of the city of Norwich." It is provided that should there not be a sufficient number of distempered persons in the city of Norwich whom the trustees shall judge fit and proper objects to partake of the charity, they are empowered to put into the house any persons in the county of Norfolk, or elsewhere, afflicted with lunacy, whose relations or friends may desire to place them in the hospital. Very low sums are paid by the friends of patients for their maintenance.

A Royal Charter was granted to the hospital in the fifth year of the reign of George III., under which the board of governors now act.

There are about two acres of ground, including the site for the hospital. The chief officers of the institution are a visiting physician, medical superintendent, a master and matron.

The general style of architecture is that of a plain brick building with no pretensions to ornament; there have been additions and alterations from time to time in the original building.

Lunatics above the pauper class, and belonging to the city of Norwich, are provided for on such terms as their friends can afford, some free, and others from the nominal rate of 1s. up to 20s. per week. Cases are admitted from beyond the city at 20s. and up to 30s. per week. The weekly cost per head is 16s. 3*d.* as returned to the Commissioners; the total cost, exclusive of structural additions and alterations, being 18s. 6*d.*

St. Luke's Hospital.—This hospital originated in the good intentions of a few persons who desired to make further provision for indigent lunatics. We are not aware that among the motives which led to this step there was any intention to reform the treatment then in vogue. Buildings were found in Upper Moorfields, in a locality called Windmill Hill, and formed part of a leasehold estate held under the Corporation of the City of London. The hospital was opened July 30, 1751. The accommodation proved to be insufficient, and in consequence land formerly known by the name of The Bowling Green, in Old Street Road, was obtained. Upon this spot St. Luke's now stands, the first stone being laid July 30, 1782. The expense of the building was about £50,000. In 1787 there were 110 patients, now there are 200.

The institution is under the direction and control of governors, and the qualification for the office is the payment of thirty guineas to the treasurer. The general management is placed in the committee, annually appointed by the court of governors, which committee appoints a house committee, the members of which attend weekly at the hospital.

The funds of the hospital are derived from patients, charitable subscriptions, donations, and bequests. the property of the hospital being vested in the public funds.

The cost per head per week is at the present time £1 4s. exclusive of building repairs, rates and taxes.

The terms of admission are as follows: Cases in which the patient has been insane twelve months, or has been discharged uncured from a similar institution, are ineligible, except on payment of 21s. per week. Idiots, persons suffering from epilepsy, or under the age of twelve or above seventy, or being pregnant, are not eligible under any circumstances. Patients other than free cases are admitted at 14s., 21s., or 30s. per week, according to the nature of the case and the circumstances of the friends. The medical staff consists of a consulting physician, a resident medical superintendent, an assistant medical officer, and a qualified clinical assistant.*

Manchester Royal Lunatic Hospital.—This hospital, which is connected with the Manchester Royal Infirmary, and was originally contiguous to it, was opened in 1766, the building having cost £15,000, which was raised by voluntary contributions. The object of its foundation was to make provision for poor lunatics, to lessen the expense of their maintenance, to assist persons of middling fortune, and supply a hospital for lunatics on moderate terms, the lowest weekly charge being fixed at 7s. In 1845 it was removed to Cheadle, nine miles from Manchester, in the county of Chester. An entirely new building was erected. The two institutions remained under the control of the same body of trustees or governors. The land and building cost £30,208, and with villas built and general extension of the main building, the cost was about £60,000, raised by private benevolence.

* Some of the above information has been obtained from Dr. Mickley, the Medical Superintendent of St. Luke's.

It was opened August 25, 1849. After the expiration of three years the payments of patients enabled the governors to dispense with contributions from the public.

The Manchester Royal Lunatic Hospital is designed for patients of the middle and higher classes. It is the desire of the governors to relieve those persons whose position in life disqualifies them from coming on the rates and being admitted into county asylums, but who are unable to pay at private asylum rates. When the income exceeds the expenditure the surplus is to be applied to the diminution of the rates of payment made by poor patients or in otherwise increasing the usefulness of the institution.

Mr. Mould, the medical superintendent, has introduced the treatment of patients in separate villas to a very large extent and with very beneficial results. A very interesting account of this important work was given by Mr. Mould himself in his presidential address in 1880.*

In this address he observed :—"Some eighteen years since, with the liberal aid and cordial co-operation of the committee of visitors, I established in connection with the Royal Hospital at Cheadle, three villa or cottage residences, built in the asylum grounds; and subsequently, in addition, rented ordinary dwelling-houses, with suitable surroundings, for the purpose of placing in them patients who, I believe, from their chronic or convalescing condition, would derive benefit from the change from the ordinary routine of asylum ward-life. All asylum physicians constantly experience the injurious effect a large number of chronic cases collected together have upon the comfort and convenience in the treatment of the more acute cases, and the serious interference with the means of classification; and it is generally accepted that the greater freedom you can accord a patient, consistent with safety, the less irritation and excitement there is; and it constantly occurs that a patient who is noisy and troublesome in a hospital ward amongst numbers of others settles down into comparative quiescence in a cottage house with its more home-like freedom. I do not of course claim originality in the placing of cottages in the grounds of an asylum for the treatment of patients, as it was adopted years ago by Dr. Bucknill, at the Devon Asylum; but I venture to urge the adaptation of it outside the grounds of the asylum as a practical solution of the increasing difficulty now existent in providing sufficient accommodation for patients of both the private and pauper class. Ordinary dwelling-houses are taken either on lease or at an annual rent as may be the most convenient, and would, of course, revert to their original use without any deterioration in value, if not required for patients. They vary in annual value from £8 to £350. They are readily and efficiently worked by the asylum's staff, and, in my opinion, if such houses were attached to the county asylums as well as the existing hospitals for the insane, to be rented when convenient, and to be built when not, they would relieve the State from the cost of a very large number of patients, whose friends could and would very gladly pay moderate and remunerative rates for such separate accommodation. The extra trouble and responsibility thrown upon the medical superintendent would be met by a small quarterly charge made upon each patient, which though little in itself, would amount in the aggregate to a fair sum. County asylums would of course obtain money from the rates for the purpose of providing and furnishing such buildings as we have described for the treatment of private patients; but in the case of hospitals the State should be empowered to advance money at a low rate of interest, as is now done to other public bodies, and in this way provide accommodation for a class of patients whose urgent need has hitherto been supplied by public benevolence or private enterprise."

Mr. Mould concludes his account of the treatment of patients by means of villas or cottages by the following statement:

"In this way more than one half of the patients at least reside outside the main building, and many more might be so placed with advantage, if the necessary accommodation could be readily obtained. This system requires constant and vigilant supervision, and the immediate temporary removal to the hospital of any patient requiring more active treatment" (*Jour. Ment. Sci.*, October 1880, p. 340).

Since the period above referred to, the system has been still further extended, and when Cheadle was visited by members of the association in March 1890, a very favourable impression was produced upon the visitors.

The general management of the institution is vested in a committee elected annually by the trustees of the Manchester Royal Infirmary, and out of their own body. The medical superintendent is the

* Delivered at the annual meeting of the Medico-Psychological Association, July 30, 1880 (*Jour. Ment. Sci.*, Oct. 1880, p. 327).

sole responsible master and manager of the whole establishment.

The terms vary according to the accommodation, that is, rooms and attendance required, and the pecuniary means of the patients.

The usual terms are twenty-five shillings, one guinea and a half, two guineas, three guineas, four guineas, six guineas a week, and some pay even higher; but these latter are wealthy, and require large separate accommodation and service.

Some patients are received without any charge, others at from ten to twenty shillings per week, and fully three-fifths of the whole number of patients pay one guinea and a half per week *and under*. As the institution in all its departments is self-supporting, the number of patients paying the lower rates of board is of necessity regulated by the surplus arising from the payments made by the wealthier patients. Those paying the highest rates have of course the separate rooms and attendance they specially pay for; but all who pay the lower rates, and whose social position and mental condition allow of it have the full advantage of association with and of the comforts and conveniences of those who pay the higher, both in the main hospital building and in the various houses in the immediate neighbourhood and at the seaside, without extra charge being made.

The York Lunatic Hospital, or York Asylum.—This institution was opened in the year 1777, and is situated in that part of the city of York called Bootham. A public meeting was held at York in 1772, summoned by Archbishop Drummond and 24 gentlemen of the county, at which a liberal sum of money was subscribed. The class of patients in view were those of limited incomes, and it was not till 1784 that accommodation was provided for persons in more affluent circumstances. A charitable fund was founded in 1789 by Mr. Thomas Lupton, and another in 1843 by Dr. Wake, for many years visiting physician to the institution.

The York Asylum is under the management of a body of governors consisting of the Lord Mayor of York, the governor of the Merchants' Company, York, the Mayor of Doncaster, and all benefactors of £20 and upwards.

At the Annual General Court of Governors, four of their number are appointed auditors, quarterly courts appoint seven governors to form the managing committee for the ensuing quarter, and visitors are appointed for the male and female wards.

The number of acres is [illegible] of pasture and farm.

Sources of income are payments of patients' donations and legacies, the produce of the land and rent of a farm, and the interest assigns from the Lupton and Wake funds.

The rates of payment and number of patients on December 31, 1891, were as follows:—

39 patients from £1 to £4 4s. per week each inclusive; 16 from 10s. to 19s. partially maintained from Lupton's Fund; 4 from 5s. to 9s.; 13 from £20 16s. to £190 each per annum; 1 wholly maintained from Lupton's Fund; 55 city paupers at 14s. per week. Total, 128.

The contrast between the condition in which this excellent asylum has long been, and its unsatisfactory state at an early period of its history, is so gratifying, and redounds so greatly to the credit of the modern management of the institution, that it is only right to quote the description given by Dr. Conolly of its former condition:—"Among the ill-conducted asylums of this country at the time when Pinel's great work of reformation was effected in France, the worst seems to have been that of the city of York, which had been founded in 1777, and had soon become a scene of mercenary intrigue and mismanagement. At a much later period it had arrived at the perfection of whatever was wrong and detestable."

The Retreat, York.—In 1791, a female patient confined in the old York Asylum, and a member of the Society of Friends, was treated in such a way as to attract grave suspicions of ill-treatment, but her relations were refused admission. It was thought by William Tuke desirable under these circumstances to project a new asylum at York, one which should be conducted in a humane manner, and with proper regard to the feelings of the patients' friends. The proposal took a definite form at a meeting of this community in the spring of 1792, and at midsummer a "retired habitation" was "instituted," bearing the name of "The Retreat," the first instance in which the term was applied to an asylum for the insane. Ground was purchased in the neighbourhood of the city, amounting to eleven acres, and a building of modest pretensions was erected. It still remains, and forms the centre of a very much larger establishment. It was surrounded by airing courts, gardens, and fields. A few years afterwards, a small separate institution, desired for a limited number of convalescent patients, was established, within an easy distance of the original building. The

"Appendage," as it was called, was occupied for about thirteen years.

From the earliest period occupation on the farm was introduced, and regarded as highly important to the health and recovery of the patients.

The methods of restraint, when regarded as absolutely necessary, were of a simple character. The idea of employing chains was abhorrent to those who conducted the Retreat, although they were to be found in use many years afterwards at St. Luke's and at Bethlem Hospital.

The result of the humane treatment here pursued was so satisfactory that it became the cradle of the reform of the general and medical treatment of mental disorders.

Constitution, Government, and Management.—The government of the Retreat is vested by the trust deed in a general meeting of subscribers and directors held annually at York. Forty subscribers were originally nominated as directors. They and their successors, duly appointed, together with any other donors, subscribers, and agents appointed by any qualified meeting, constitute the general meeting and continue the directors of the institution, in whom the government of it is perpetually to vest and remain.

The committee, of which the treasurer is *ex officio* a member, meet at the Retreat every month, and oftener if required, for the transaction of business; amongst other things, they admit and discharge patients, and sanction the necessary current expenditure of the establishment.

The main sources of income consist of the payments of the patients, the great deficiency which would arise from the low payment of some being counterbalanced by the higher scale of payment by others; when, however, the income falls below the expenditure, or when there is a special outlay upon the building, donations and annual subscriptions must be relied upon.

The rates of payment vary from fourteen shillings to seven guineas per week.

Officers, Attendants, &c.—The officers attached to the Retreat are: a medical superintendent, one visiting medical officer, and two assistant medical officers, a steward, and a matron. The number of attendants necessarily varies with the proportion of the higher class patients in the asylum.*

* It is to the Editor of this work an interesting circumstance that the centenary of this institution is celebrated this year at York, and that the superintendent of the Retreat, Dr. Robert Baker, is elected to preside over the annual meeting of the Medico-Psychological Association, which, in honour of the event, meets at the York Retreat.

The average weekly cost per head is £1 15*s*. 6*d*.

The number of acres is 34.

During the past eighteen years no addition has been made to "The Retreat" main building, but many decided improvements have been made. But although the main building has not been added to, the following villas have been erected, and one (Belle Vue) has been purchased: The East Villa, at a cost of £1900; Gentlemen's Lodge, accommodating 30 patients, £12,000; West Villa, providing for 15 ladies, £4000 (including electric lighting, £400). Belle Vue House was bought for the sum of £4000. Gainsborough House, Scarboro', is leased at £90 a year as a seaside residence.*

Wonford House, Exeter.—Wonford House dates back, under the name of St. Thomas's Hospital, to an earlier period. The first proposal for founding a hospital for the insane was laid before the Grand Jury of the County of Devon at their meeting at the Castle of Exeter, March 16, 1795, as follows:

"*Outline of a Plan for a Lunatic Asylum.*—This institution is intended to relieve the most helpless and pitiable class of mortals who cannot, consistently with the care of the patients, be received into the county hospital. This relief may be afforded without affecting the present hospital as to its regulations and expenses, it being proposed that the lunatic asylum should be a distinct and independent institution, standing on its own foundation, and supported by separate and distinct means.

"The patients of the lunatic asylum, by a weekly payment suited to their circumstances, will render annual subscriptions unnecessary. The experiment has been tried in several parts of the kingdom, and has answered the most sanguine expectations."

The grand jury having passed a resolution approving of the above proposal, a subscription was opened, and at a meeting of subscribers held at Exeter, July 29, 1795, a series of resolutions were adopted in accordance with the foregoing proposal.

It was not, however, until 1799 that sufficient funds were in hand, and a suitable house and estate purchased. The hospital was opened for the reception of patients July 1, 1801, and on July 18 the first patient was received. The institution was subsequently registered as St. Thomas's Hospital.

Government.—It was governed by a

* Dr. Baker has kindly supplied us with these particulars.

committee of management, consisting of donors of twenty guineas and upwards, and of ten members elected annually by the governors. For many years the medical staff consisted of two visiting physicians and a resident medical officer, but about ten years ago the visiting physicians were abolished, and the medical superintendent became the sole responsible head under the committee.

The hospital remained on its original site of Bowhill House, in the district of St. Thomas, until 1869, when it was transferred to its present site, a mile and a half from Exeter, on the rising ground to the east of the city, a beautiful and healthy situation. The estate purchased then consisted of about twenty acres; and on this was erected the present hospital, afterwards called Wonford House, a name taken from a neighbouring village. It is also the name of the hundred in which Exeter itself is situated.

During the last few years forty additional acres of land have been purchased. A comfortable house, with garden, accommodating fifteen to twenty patients has also been secured at Dawlish as a sea-side residence and sanatorium.

The hospital has accommodation for between 130 and 140 patients. They belong to the upper and middle classes, and consist of (1) those who can pay remunerative rates of board; (2) those of the same social position, but unable to pay the full charges, and admitted by the committee after careful consideration, at various reduced rates, according to circumstances. The full rate is £2 7*s.* per week. About three-fifths of the patients pay less than this. At present five are received free of charge; twenty-two pay from ten shillings to £1 a week, and forty-eight more at various rates, between twenty-seven and forty-seven shillings; the remaining fifty patients pay the full rate or more.*

The average cost of maintenance, exclusive of additions or repairs to building, rates and taxes, is about £1 15*s.* weekly.

St. Andrew's Hospital for Mental Diseases, Northampton.—It appears that this institution originated in two benefactions of £100 each by an anonymous donor in 1804 and 1807, who presented these sums to the Governors of the General Infirmary at Northampton, in trust, to apply the same towards the building of a lunatic asylum. It was decided to establish a hospital separate from the infirmary for the reception of 120 private and pauper patients, to be under the management of a committee, and maintained independently of the county rate. Earl Spencer, the Marquis of Northampton, Earl Fitzwilliam, the Bouverie, and others assisted in the undertaking. The institution is supported by donations, legacies, and the payments of the more opulent patients.

The management of the institution is vested in the governors, who consist of benefactors of £30; the Lord-Lieutenant of the county for the time being is president. At the annual meeting the directors choose a committee of management, which meets at least once a month.

The number of acres is 105.

The rates of payment are as follows: 1st class, £2 2*s.* and upwards; 2nd class, £1 5*s.* a week and upwards, according to the requirements of each case. Patients are assisted in their payments at the discretion of the committee, the number so helped in 1891 being 87, a large proportion of whom were free.

The reception of pauper patients was discontinued in the year 1876, and the hospital is now entirely devoted to the care and treatment of patients of the upper and middle classes. There is no endowment, the hospital being supported by the payments of patients.

There is accommodation for 350, including detached villas on the hospital estate, and houses at Moulton Park. Moulton Park is an estate of 450 acres, two and a half miles distant from and belonging to the hospital, and is used for the occupation in farm, garden, and dairy work for the patients who reside there.

There is also a seaside mansion and estate leased by the hospital near Conway, called Benarth Hall, to which patients are regularly sent for the benefit of their health and change of scene. The estate is situated on the estuary of the River Conway, and the patients have the sporting rights over more than 500 acres.

Coton Hill Institution, near Stafford.—Although the present building was opened in 1854, there was an institution intended for paupers as well as patients of the higher and middle classes, which was opened in 1818, under the Act 48 Geo. III. c. 96.

The foundation of this original charity arose out of a legacy left to the Stafford General Infirmary for the purpose of adding wards for insane patients to that institution. But it was agreed to erect a separate asylum. Patients were admitted at rates of payment varying from 2*s.* 6*d.* to 10*s.* or 12*s.* per week, according to their means. The surplus payments derived from the patients of the independent

* We are indebted to Dr. Murry Deas for the particulars here given.

classes were an important source of income, and considerably diminished the charge for pauper patients. This appropriation of the funds was taken into consideration in 1846, and it was directed that in future the savings of the hospital should be placed to the credit of the charitable fund in accordance with the original agreement. Lord Ashley's Act (1845) rendered it necessary to extend and remodel the institution. After many plans were considered and discarded, it was decided to dissever the connection between the county and the voluntary part of the institution, and to erect upon an extended scale a suitable building for the various classes of private patients. Great difficulty had been experienced in the working of a large mixed establishment. It was decided, therefore, that certain additions should be made to the county asylum, to adapt it for the reception of an increased number of pauper patients. The committee decided upon the present site for the building, land being placed at their disposal by the late Earl Talbot.

In spite of the liberal help afforded, assisted by a public meeting held in November 1851, and the funds at the disposal of the committee, it was found impossible to finish the building. The arrangements were, however, completed, and it was decided to open the institution as soon as practicable, the sum required being raised upon mortgage. This has unfortunately crippled the action of the governors, a considerable debt having been incurred. The institution stands in the centre of an elevated plot of land of 38 acres in extent, and can accommodate 140 patients (both sexes). The private patients were removed from the county asylum to the new building in May 1854.

The government of the institution is vested in president, vice-president, and a general committee qualified and elected from the body of subscribers.

The sources of income are derived from the annual subscriptions and the payments of patients.

The original main building, with the chapel in the grounds, cost £30,374. Since 1854, when the place was opened, the following additions have been made, namely, two galleries, one each side of the main building, two semi-detached villas and three lodges in the ground, and a large recreation hall and theatre were added to the main building in 1889, and opened in 1890. These additions have cost £7791, making the total cost of the hospital £38,165. There are surrounding it 31 acres of land, garden, &c., for which £6000 was paid. In addition to this, about 81 acres generally are rented for farming purposes.

The average weekly cost per head was, in 1891, £1 13s. 7*d.*

The object of this hospital has from the first been to a great extent charitable. Some 92 of the patients at the present time pay for their board less than the average cost, and 26 of these pay less than £1 per week. It may be added that there are still some few cases that have been in the asylum since 1854, paying the nominal sums of 4*s.* 6*d.* and 7*s.* 6*d.* per week.

The number of patients that can be accommodated is 140. There are two classes of insane patients for whom this hospital is designed—(1) patients in more or less affluent circumstances who shall contribute according to the accommodation required, such weekly sum as may be agreed upon; (2) patients in such circumstances, although not paupers, who shall be received at such reduced rates of payment as the committee upon consideration of their circumstances may determine, the deficiency being made up out of the surplus moneys received from the patients of the first class beyond their actual cost, assisted by annual subscriptions, donations, and legacies.

Government.—The real estate and funds of the institution are vested in five trustees.

The general direction and management of the institution are vested in the president, vice-presidents, and a general committee, qualified and elected.

The immediate control of the institution is under the direction of the resident medical superintendent, who is responsible to the committee.

A president and six vice-presidents are elected for life.

Annual subscribers of two guineas and upwards, and all donors of twenty guineas and upwards at one payment, are governors of the institution, and privileged to vote in the election of the general committee.

The president and vice-presidents are members of the general and house committees.

The court of quarter sessions of the county of Stafford may appoint any number not exceeding 24 of the Justices of the county to be visitors of the institution.*

Lincoln Lunatic Hospital (**The Lawn**).—This institution was opened for the reception of patients, April 26, 1820, the funds having been furnished by donations from the nobility and gentry connected with the county of Lincoln, who

* We are indebted to Dr. Hewson, the Medical Superintendent of Coton Hill, for many of the foregoing particulars.

in consequence became "governors of the lunatic asylum for the county." The object was to enable patients to be admitted at lower rates than elsewhere.

We believe that the origin of this hospital was really due to a donation of £100 from Paul Parnell, Esq., a surgeon in Lincoln.

The government of the hospital was vested in a board of governors, the qualification being a donation of twenty guineas or an annual subscription of not less than two.

Unfortunately, the building was very faulty in construction, and the airing courts consisted of damp, small, and cheerless enclosures situate on the north side of the building. The grounds to the south, commanding a beautiful prospect, were, strange to say, scarcely used by the patients. Since 1847 all this has been altered, and the south side of the building, formerly used by patients under restraint, consists of cheerful and well-furnished day-rooms. There are about nine acres of land belonging to the institution.

Previous to January 1, 1854, the rates of payment were for first class patients, 21s. per week; for second class patients, 15s. per week; for third class patients, 10s. per week. These terms were raised to 30s., 20s., and 12s. per week, partly in consequence of the removal of the pauper lunatics. The terms are now 30s. weekly and upwards, but they may be lowered by the committee to a smaller sum when they think proper.*

It was in this institution that absolute non-restraint was first introduced as a system. This was done gradually through the exertions of Mr. Gardiner Hill and Dr. Charlesworth, the last use of restraint being in the year 1837.

The following table is of interest as showing the gradual change in regard to restraint at the Lincoln Asylum:

Year.	Total Number in the House.	Total Number Restrained.	Total Number of instances of Restraint.	Total Number of Hours under Restraint.
1829	72	39	1,727	20,424
1830	92	54	2,364	27,113
1831	70	40	1,004	10,839
1832	81	55	1,401	15,671
1833	87	44	1,109	12,003
1834	109	45	647	6,597
1835	108	28	323	2,874
1836	115	12	39	334
1837	130	2	3	28

* Dr. Russell, the medical superintendent, has supplied us with these particulars.

Warneford Hospital ([illegible]), **Headington Hill, Oxford.**—It is stated that some of the governors of the Radcliffe Infirmary, especially Dr. [illegible], President of Corpus Christi College, originated this hospital by their praiseworthy exertions.

A number of propositions were adopted at a meeting of the governors of the infirmary held April 28, 1813. The necessary funds were obtained as follows: The trustees of the Radcliffe Infirmary granted at different periods the sum of £2700; corporate, testamentary, and individual contributions raised the amount to about £20,000. The site fixed upon was Headington Hill.

The asylum was opened on July 10, 1826, as "The Oxford Lunatic Asylum." The institution has twenty-two acres of ground, ten of which are laid out as a garden and cricket-field, the other twelve being kitchen garden and grass land.

It is intended for the care and treatment of patients of both sexes belonging to the middle and upper classes of society. The situation on Headington Hill, about a mile and a half from Oxford, is very healthy. The buildings, to which large additions have been recently made, are substantial and are comfortably furnished, and are well adapted for the successful treatment of the inmates.

The management is under the control of a committee. The staff consists of a medical superintendent, assistant medical officer, chaplain, and matron, all of whom, with the exception of the chaplain, are resident. There is a private chapel within the grounds.

The ordinary terms are two guineas a week, but many of the patients pay less. The average cost of each patient (exclusive of building repairs, rates and taxes, and extraordinary expenses) is £1 7s. 10d. per week.

There is accommodation for 100 patients, 50 of each sex. There are at present 80 patients, vacancies being in the new wing for male patients, which was opened a short time ago.

No person in a state of idiocy or suffering from epilepsy or paralysis is admissible.

The annual income is aided by the rents and interest of the real estates, and of a mortgage given by the late Dr. Warneford, in honour of whom, on the grant of a new charter some years ago, its name was changed from the "Radcliffe Asylum" to that of the "Warneford Lunatic Asylum." He lived long, and was a warm friend and munificent benefactor of the institution,* his donations exceeding the value of £70,000.

Nottingham Lunatic Hospital (The Coppice).—"The Coppice" is a registered hospital for the insane, situate about two miles from Nottingham Market Place and the Midland and Great Northern Railway Stations. It was originally promoted and brought into operation by gentlemen connected with the Nottingham General Hospital. Donations and subscriptions for the purchase of land and building an asylum were commenced in 1789, and had accumulated, in 1809, to about £6000. It was then decided by the subscribers, in conjunction with the county and borough of Nottingham, to build an asylum at Sneinton, near Nottingham, to be called the General Lunatic Asylum for the County and Town of Nottingham, for the reception of private and pauper patients. It was opened on February 13, 1812, and afterwards was from time to time enlarged to meet the increasing number of applications for admission. The accommodation being still found inadequate, it was decided, on the recommendation of the Commissioners in Lunacy, to separate the private from the pauper patients, and to build a new asylum for the former. Terms having been equitably arranged, and a suitable site found at a convenient distance from Nottingham, the present hospital for sixty patients was built and furnished at a cost of about £20,000, leaving a balance of about £10,000 in the hands of the trustees, as an endowment fund for charitable purposes. The first stone of the new building was laid on October 30, 1857, by the Duke of Newcastle, the then president, and it was opened for the reception of patients by Dr. W. B. Tate,† the present medical superintendent, on August 1, 1859, on which day thirty private patients were transferred to the hospital from the asylum at Sneinton. Since its opening the hospital has been enlarged by the addition of wings, the cost of which and furnishing was about £10,000. It will now accommodate about 100 patients, all of whom pay, for their medical treatment and maintenance, sums varying from 10s. to £2 a week. It is exclusively for the reception of private patients of the middle class. The property of the hospital is vested in trustees, and it is managed by a committee of gentlemen of the county and town of Nottingham who are subscribers to it, and are chosen yearly. The endowment fund and annual subscriptions amount to about £800 a year, whereby the committee are enabled to admit a certain number of deserving cases belonging to the county and town of Nottingham at reduced rates of payment. The site is an elevation facing the south, and commanding an extensive view of the surrounding country. Mr. T. C. Hine, of Nottingham, was the architect.

The weekly rate of cost per head is £1 11s., exclusive of any charge for lodging. Dr. Tate informs us that, although there are patients paying only 10s. a week, the hospital will not in future take any at so low a rate.

Barnwood House, Gloucester.*—In January 1857 a general meeting of the surviving subscribers to the Gloucester Lunatic Asylum was held at Gloucester, and appointed a committee to act on their behalf in all matters affecting the interest of the trust. In the report of this committee it is stated that the sale of the subscribers' interest in the county asylum had been completed for £13,000. With that sum at their disposal and other sums amounting to £6500 they entered into an agreement in the month of May to purchase, from the County of Gloucester Bank, *Barnwood House*, with its gardens, pleasure ground, and lands, amounting to forty-eight acres, which purchase was completed on February 8, 1858. Plans were submitted to the committee for the adaptation of the house to the purposes of an asylum, involving extensive additions. These plans were adopted.

The establishment was registered as a hospital for the insane January 1, 1860. The Commissioners in Lunacy made their first visit on the 17th, and stated in their report that the building afforded excellent accommodation for the upper as well as the middle class patients.

The first general meeting of the supporters of the institution was held January 30, 1860, Earl Ducie, lord-lieutenant of the county, presiding.

A general committee of management was appointed. This asylum has well fulfilled the object for which it was established. Additions have constantly been made to its size in improving the character of the accommodation. The average weekly cost of maintenance is just under £2.

Holloway Sanatorium, St. Ann's Heath, Virginia Water.—This hospital,

* We are indebted for these particulars to the Medical Superintendent of the Warneford Asylum, Dr. J. Bywater Ward.

† To whom we are indebted for these particulars.

* This account is derived from information supplied by the late superintendent, Dr. Needham.

founded by the late Mr. Thomas Holloway, was opened June 12, 1885. It is a registered hospital for the care and cure of the insane and nervous invalids of the upper and upper-middle classes at moderate rates of payment.

The charge for board, &c., varies from £2 2*s.* to £3 3*s.* a week and upwards, according to the requirements of the case, at the discretion of the committee. One-fourth at least of the total number of patients are maintained at weekly rates of 25*s.* or under. Payment for one quarter must be made at the time of admission; subsequent payments must be made quarterly and in advance. For each patient or boarder there must be furnished an obligation for payment of board, &c., to be signed by two responsible persons; fourteen days are allowed for signatures to be obtained for this document after a patient has been admitted.

Lady companions live with the lady patients. Gentlemen companions live with the gentlemen patients. The assistant medical officers, four in number, also lunch and dine and spend much of their time with the patients. One of the assistant medical officers is a fully qualified medical woman. Lectures and practical tuition on special and general nursing are given to the staff, and trained nurses and attendants are sent out to nurse cases at their own homes.

A seaside branch at Brighton has been established. It is fitted with all modern sanitary improvements.

St. Ann's Heath is situated on the Bagshot sands formation. The building is surrounded by its own pleasure grounds. It is close to the Virginia Water Station, twenty miles from London.

We observe from the auditor's report, dated January 1892, that the income from maintenance accounts during the previous twelve months amounted to £42,905 4*s.* 8*d.* and that the expenditure (less repayments by patients, &c.) was £33,088 16*s.* 2*d.*, leaving a surplus revenue of £9816 8*s.* 6*d.* The average number of patients and boarders during the year was 347; average weekly income per patient, £2 8*s.* 11*d.*; average weekly expenditure per patient, £2 0*s.* 7*d.*, leaving an average weekly surplus per patient of 8*s.* 4*d.* The number of patients and boarders at the end of the year (1891) was 340.*

The Average Weekly Cost per Head in Registered Hospitals (including everything except the charges for building, repairs, rates and [illegible]) [illegible] lows:

	£	s.	d.
Bethlem Royal Hospital	[illegible]	[illegible]	[illegible]
Bethel Hospital, Norwich . . .	[illegible]	[illegible]	[illegible]
St. Luke's Hospital . . .	[illegible]	[illegible]	[illegible]
Wonford House, Exeter . . .	[illegible]	[illegible]	[illegible]
The Retreat, York	[illegible]	[illegible]	[illegible]
York Lunatic Hospital . . .	[illegible]	[illegible]	[illegible]
Nottingham Lunatic Hospital .	[illegible]	[illegible]	[illegible]
Warneford Asylum, Oxford . .	[illegible]	[illegible]	[illegible]
Lincoln Lunatic Hospital . .	[illegible]	[illegible]	[illegible]
Manchester Royal Lunatic Hospital ([illegible])			
Barnwood House	[illegible]	[illegible]	[illegible]
St. Andrew's Hospital, Northampton	[illegible]	[illegible]	[illegible]
Coton Hill, Stafford . . .	[illegible]	[illegible]	[illegible]
Holloway Sanatorium . . .	[illegible]	[illegible]	7

The foregoing institutions for the insane form a complete list of Registered Hospitals. There are also registered under "The Idiots Act, 1886," the Eastern Counties Idiot Asylum, Essex Hall, Colchester, Essex; the Royal Albert Asylum for Idiots, Lancaster; and the Asylum for Idiots, Earlswood, Redhill, Surrey. These are referred to at pp. 551–552.

There are, further, the military and naval hospitals, not included under "Registered" hospitals, namely, the Royal Military Hospital, Netley, Hants, and the Royal Naval Hospital, Yarmouth, Norfolk.

Lastly, there is the State Criminal Asylum, Broadmoor, Crowthorne, Berks, which, like the military and naval hospitals, stands apart from the hospitals which are called "Registered." It was erected in 1863 in conformity with the Act 23 & 24 Vic. c. 75, entitled "to make better provision for the Custody and Care of Criminal Lunatics," passed in 1860. This is a most important and successful institution, and has been and is under excellent management. For a somewhat detailed account of this asylum, the editor may refer to "Chapters in the History of the Insane in the British Isles," 1882, pp. 265–284. THE EDITOR.

RELAPSES. (*See* STATISTICS.)

RELIGION, Relations of, to INSANITY.—Religion may be defined for present purposes as the relations of man to a supernatural being or beings, rightly or wrongly believed to exist. The connections of such a belief with insanity are far-reaching and complicated; they will be best dealt with under the following heads. Religion may, on the one hand, produce unsoundness of mind, or, on the contrary, hinder its development; secondly, it may cause certain symptoms of insanity, or modify them; finally, it may be employed as a means of moral prevention and treatment.

(1) Like all the so-called moral causes of insanity, the influence of religion can

* The particulars of the account of the Holloway Sanatorium are derived from information received from Dr. Rees Philipps, the medical superintendent.

hardly be stated with accuracy. Statistics are of little use, for countries which differ as to religion, differ also in those other conditions of civilisation which are potent factors in the causation of unsoundness of mind. This would obviously be the case, if figures were equally available for study in Mahommedan and heathen nations as in Europe. Even such scanty means of comparison as asylum statistics in Turkey and Egypt afford are rendered of no avail, by the much smaller number of the insane placed under confinement in those lands than in Christendom. Any comparison between Christian countries of different faith is liable to similar fallacies. Schüle, for instance, points out that the relative preponderance of Protestant over Catholic admissions into Illenau is probably due to the fact that the former are proportionately more numerous in the towns, the rural population being mainly Catholic. One inference only seems to us deducible from statistical tables of the relative proportion of insanity among Catholics, Protestants, and Jews, in some of the German provinces, Switzerland, and Denmark. The religion of the majority of each nation or district will be found to contribute relatively more persons to the ranks of the insane than the religion of the minority; a result which may be naturally accounted for by observing that the minority usually belong to a higher social stratum than the majority of the population. But in the case of very small religious bodies, such as the Mennonites and Jews in Germany, this rule is reversed, and insanity is more frequent proportionately among their members, owing apparently to the influence of consanguineous marriages.

If we leave statistics, and consider the matter *à priori*, it would at first sight seem as if the effect of religion must be exclusively beneficial, and have considerable influence in preventing insanity. The precept, "Walk before me, and be perfect," which stands at the origin of all the monotheistic religions of the world, contains explicitly or implicitly every moral element which could be appealed to for such a purpose. The consciousness of responsibility in the presence of an all-seeing judge will restrain the passions, and urge to wholesome industry, with a sanction that no less far-reaching belief can equal; the sense that he can always turn to an ever-present father and friend should give to one who leans upon his God a constant support in the loneliest and most sorely tried life; lastly, to the Christian the example of his Master, who chose a life of poverty, ending in ignominy and apparent failure, is the surest comfort in the troubles and disappointments which must be the lot of all.

We believe this estimate of the influence of religion is the true one, and that every religion, however widely it may differ from our standard of the truth, if it enforces the precepts of morality, is a source of strength to the sound mind that sincerely accepts it. An agent which can effect so much good must, however, be equally potent for harm. The mind on which religion acts may be abnormal, in which case it is not wonderful, as an old author puts it, "that the light should be painful to sick eyes, which to healthy ones is delightful." Or the fault may lie in the application of religion, like a drug which can save life, but is equally able to destroy it, if given inopportunely or excessively. For the characters of religion which we have just enumerated may all be exaggerated into potent causes of insanity. The sense of responsibility to omniscient justice may pass into a belief in condemnation irrevocable and inevitable; the habit of communing with God may easily grow into self-contemplation and ecstasy; the repression of the lower part of human nature may be strained into practices ruinous to health of mind and body. The common factor in all these exaggerations is *fanaticism*, which looks only at one side of religion, and commits the fallacy of supposing that the dependence of man upon a higher being must supersede all those other duties which, on the contrary, derive therefrom their greatest sanction. As one of the natural growths of an ill-balanced mind, fanaticism is closely akin to the other manifestations of the insane temperament; and this accounts for the fanatical habit of mind that is so often associated with the hereditary neuroses, above all with epilepsy. Overstrained and one-sided religious views are, however, not so often the primary cause of an attack of insanity, as its first symptoms, though symptoms which in turn act as causes of further evil and intensify the disease. For instance, an endeavour to study the mystery of existence and solve the problem of evil has been rightly denounced as highly dangerous to mental health; yet it is recognised as an early symptom ("Grübelsucht") of an otherwise deranged mind. Or again, a case of melancholia in which religious delusions seem at first sight to have been the cause of all the troubles, will be found, if traced from the beginning, to have originated in disordered bodily health.

But the influence of religion as an exciting cause of insanity is far more important in its action on masses of men than on individuals. Religious excitement, culminating in insanity, prevailed endemically about the chief shrines of heathen antiquity, and among the worshippers of Cybele and Bacchus, and still continues among the dervishes and fakirs of Eastern countries. In all Christian communities epidemics of the same kind, of varying gravity and extent, have from time to time occurred, such as the Flagellants of the middle ages, the Camisards and Convulsionnaires of France in the last century, and the Revivalists of Ireland and America almost in our own days. The last is particularly interesting, because its characters can be studied in the excellent description given by Archdeacon Stopford ("The Work and the Counter-Work," Dublin, 1859). He considered all the cases of morbid religious excitement in Belfast as "clearly and unmistakably hysterical"; but he tells us that physicians recognised characters differing from the ordinary type of hysteria. The proportion of what we should now term hystero-epilepsy and of catalepsy seems to have been considerable, and on a very brief and limited inquiry he met with more than twenty cases of positive insanity of an hysterical kind, and usually with erotic symptoms. The main point of medical interest appears to be that these cases of insanity are developed out of, and among, a much larger number of neuroses of vaguer character. We are able to confirm this by our own observation, happily on a very small scale, of the fanatical excitement of an obscure sect—"the Army of the Lord"—where, we believe, only two cases of insanity occurred out of many hysterical ones. It is remarkable that Stopford was informed by an American alienist, that one revival in the United States had been free from any instances of these evil results, which were so common on other occasions; and it is even more striking that we have so very little evidence of insanity among the vast audiences which followed the great preachers of the middle ages, or Wesley in later times. Even Whitefield's preaching seems to have been usually free from any such manifestation, though on at least one occasion (at Cambuslang), among many instances of bodily manifestations, like those of an Irish revival, some cases of positive insanity occurred. It is clear that some other factor is at work in the epidemics we have described, besides appeals, however impassioned, to the conscience, and even to the emotions. This injurious element appears to consist in encouraging cries and groans, dancing, contortions; in short, bodily manifestations [illegible] which are propagated by imitation. [illegible] further light is thrown on these [illegible] epidemics by the analogous results of indiscriminate hypnotism, as practised by non-professional exhibitors, which have been recorded of late years, hysteria having been occasionally evolved among many instances of somnambulism, catalepsy, and other neurotic states.

(2) We need not dwell at any length upon the influence of religion in producing special symptoms of insanity, or in modifying those caused in some other manner. It will be obvious that a delusion which is to account for the morbid feelings of a lunatic, must be constructed by him out of his previous beliefs; and that many religious delusions must therefore be confined to the members of particular religious bodies. It may not be uninteresting for us to mention as an example of this, that we have only met with one Catholic "unpardonable sinner," a type relatively far more numerous among other melancholiacs in this country. For this reason it is often difficult to fathom the delusions of persons whose religion is unfamiliar to us; and care is needed lest we set down to insanity what may be due to religious convictions or practices we do not understand. The religious delusions of the insane have of course the general characters of their unsoundness of mind; being exalted in the maniacal, depressed in melancholiacs, inconsistent and wild in general paralytics, and systematised in chronic lunacy. But there are some varieties of religious insanity which are uniform and characteristic enough to be typical. Such are the mixture of erotic and religious excitement in many epileptics; the simple belief in perdition common in amenorrhœal melancholia; and the manner in which insane masturbators will assert that they are heroes and martyrs, under some special dispensation of Providence.

(3) The way in which religion is to be employed in the prevention and treatment of insanity may be deduced from what we have said of their ætiological relations. If we can control the education of children of insane temperament and unsound family history, the religious training should not be neglected. Such children are naturally attracted by the emotional side of religion; let its moral aspect be the more earnestly pressed. Above all, we should constantly urge upon them that belief in a higher power does not exclude duties to self and to others, but rather invests such offices with a higher motive and sanction. Singularity should

be repressed most effectually by gentle ridicule and humour; and wholesome activity should be used to prevent reverie and self-contemplation.

In the treatment of insanity, religious influence plays an important part. Like all other moral treatment, it will be generally injurious when the disease is advancing or at its height; but it is often most useful when improvement has once begun, and the mind is seeking for support. Much may even be done by religion to humanise chronic and incurable lunatics, to give them rational interests in life, and make them more resigned to fancied grievances, and to the calamity which has overtaken them. The main lines of management will here be the same as in the prevention of insanity; but they can only be applied successfully by one of training and experience. We cannot too earnestly add our protest to those of Griesinger and Maudsley against any attempt to wield religious influence by those who have not been completely trained to use a weapon so potent for good or ill.

J. R. GASQUET.

RELIGIOUS DISEASES.—Diseases of the nervous system arising from excess of religious emotion. (*See* CONVULSIONNAIRE.)

RELIGIOUS INSANITY.—A female patient above sixty years of age, at present in Bethlem Hospital, under the care of Dr. Percy Smith, is an excellent example of the exalted variety of religious insanity—theomania. She asserts that when she speaks it is not herself, but God's voice which is heard. She says she has visions from God, and that she is in the hospital simply for the purpose of converting the inmates. The power of the devil has recently ceased. She says she could not be happier, and is, in fact, in a state of ecstasy. She believes that God will avenge her cause, and bring vengeance upon those who force her to do anything against her will. This patient labours under chronic diabetes.

Under the heads of DELUSION and MELANCHOLIA, the subject of Religious Melancholy, with or without marked delusions, has already been treated. Under DEMONOMANIA, we have referred to theomania and caco-demonomania. It is necessary, however, to describe in more detail the extraordinary religious aberrations under which a number of insane persons labour, whether of an exalted or depressed character. Esquirol stated (writing in 1824) that indifference in religion had become so great in France that forms of insanity caused by religious fanaticism or mysticism were no longer observed, or at least had almost entirely disappeared. Such cannot be said to be the case at the present day even in France; much less does it apply to Great Britain and the United States. From the latter country we have a very lucid description of the religious delusions of the insane, contributed by Prof. Henry M. Hurd, M.D., who read a paper under this title at the International Medical Congress, held at Washington in 1887. We proceed to give a *résumé* of his article.

The patient may either have the delusion that he is under the especial patronage of the deity, nay, possibly, deity itself; or the very reverse, an outcast, the object of the wrath of God, and altogether too wicked to obtain His mercy. Hence there are to be found in asylums "Gods," "Messiahs," "Kings of Kings," and "Lords of Lords," while at the other end of the pole, figure "devils" and the like.

Religious delusions may be classified according as they :—

(1) **Accompany the Mental Development of Over-stimulated and Injudiciously Educated Children.**—The usual form of the delusion is morbid fear, and when the youth fails to derive from religion the emotional satisfaction which he expects, he fancies that he has neglected some religious duty, and he is before long overwhelmed by remorse for imaginary sins.

(2) **Characterise the Insanity of Pubescence.**—Here the mental depression and hebetude which so frequently occur at this age occasion the fear of death and future punishment, leading to the desire to perform some religious act either as a penance or as the means of procuring peace of mind and solace.

(3) **Are Caused by Self-abuse.**—The patient is self-conscious and introspective; is scrupulous in religious observances; and frequently falls into the delusion that he has committed the unpardonable sin. Mental weakness follows in a considerable number of cases; auditory hallucinations, visions, trances, and ecstasies are common. Suicide is likely to take the form of self-immolation, immediately connected with religious delusions. Fearful mutilation of the person may occur.

(4) **Are associated with (so-called) Paranoia.**—Sexual excitability is often associated with misapprehended religious duty. This combination in a neurotic subject has repeatedly led to extravagant ideas and the foundation of fanatical sects. Johanna Southcote is a type of one variety. Texts of Scripture are applied personally, and nothing is too absurd for adoption under the guise of superior spirituality.

(5) **Are associated with Epilepsy, Dementia, and General Paralysis.**—Dr. Hurd denies that the delusions which accompany epilepsy are generally of a religious character, and holds that the religious acts to which they are certainly remarkably prone are generally the result of a previous religious education, and are continued from force of habit after the development of mental disease. "There is never or rarely any sense of religious fear or unworthiness, but rather a sense of satisfaction in the performance of religious duties. . . . . Occasionally, in the dementia which follows religious melancholia, there is an abiding, habitual sense of religious unworthiness and spiritual deadness. In general paralysis, on the other hand, there may be extravagant delusions of religious importance, which closely resemble those developed in acute or chronic mania, and are due to the rapid flow of ideas through the brain, and are a part of the general cerebral excitement."

(6) **Are observed in Melancholia and Climacteric Insanity.**—The enormous influence of certain forms of religious training must be taken into account. Delusions of unworthiness are frequently only the crystallised form of the tenets which have been inculcated from childhood. It is but too true that the mental sufferings of the religious melancholiac exceed in intensity, by a long way, those of the other forms of mental disease. He is in the peculiar condition of believing that he merits all the tortures he endures, and that it will be redoubled, and justly so, in the world to come. In unison with the amazing inconsistency which characterises the lunatic, he frequently anticipates the awful sufferings of limitless duration by terminating his life.

(7) **Arise in Chronic Mania, or Toxic Insanity.**—These delusions are usually of an exalted character. They are not always developed in persons of religious antecedents, even when assuming a devotional form. Assumptions of religious superiority are not felt by such patients to be incongruous. Again, a patient believes that he must expiate his sins on the Cross. Another hears the Almighty's voice commanding him to do this or that, and he may succeed in deluding many others as well as himself.

Course and Determination of Religious Delusions.—As they are frequently associated with the insanity of pubescence, the study of developmental insanities (*q.v.*) bears especially upon the subject of this article. "The religious delusions which accompany masturbatic insanity are not necessarily incurable. They are, however, liable to become persistent, and are not readily amenable to treatment. They may be considered incurable whenever the patient has reached the stage of religious extravagance, which is surely indicative of mental deterioration. The religious delusions of paranoia are essentially incurable, being the legitimate development of a mental 'twist,' and the outgrowth of an abnormal personality. They eventually become thoroughly assimilated by the mind and integral part of its constitution. During the stage of persecution they may at times pass from the mind, but after the stage of transformation they cannot. The religious delusions of epilepsy, general paralysis, chronic mania, alcoholic and toxic insanity require little special mention. They are the débris of decay, and the broken fragments of a hopeless wreck. The religious delusions of melancholia are more curable. They mark deep-seated disease, but the prognosis is not hopeless." (*loc. cit.*) THE EDITOR.

REMITTENT INSANITY occurs when there is a distinct remission of the symptoms followed by a period of exacerbation. Such alternate periods of abeyance or cessation of the malady and relapse are frequently observed in general paralysis. Esquirol says, "I have often seen during the first month after the commencement of the attack, a very marked remission take place, after which the disorder returns with increased intensity" ("Maladies mentales," vol. i. p. 42). "Melancholia is much more frequently remittent than continuous or intermittent, and there are very few labouring under this form of insanity who are not worse every other day; some enjoy a marked remission every evening and after dinner, while some are worse on waking from sleep in the morning" (p. 439). Again he says: "Remittent insanity offers some very remarkable anomalies, either in its character or in the duration of the remission. In some cases it is only the transition or transformation from one form of mental disorder to another; thus a patient passes three months as a melancholiac, the three following months as a maniac, and lastly, about four months as a dement, and this successively, sometimes in a regular manner; but others with great variation. A lady, aged fifty-two, is melancholy for one year, and maniacal and hysterical for another year. In other instances the remission only presents a sensible diminution of the symptoms of the same form of insanity" (p. 78).

RENAL AFFECTIONS AND INSANITY. (*See* BRIGHT'S DISEASE and DIABETES.)

RESISTIVE MELANCHOLIA.—The marked feature of many cases of melancholia is the extreme resistance to anything the patient is wished to do. Its chief importance is in connection with feeding (*q.v.*).

RESPONSIBILITY. (*See* CRIMINAL RESPONSIBILITY.)

RESTRAINT. (*See* HISTORICAL SKETCH OF THE INSANE, and TREATMENT.)

RETINITIS PARALYTICA.—An abnormality of the retina described by Klein, and chiefly found in general paralytics. (*See* EYE SYMPTOMS IN INSANITY.)

REVERIE.—When the controlling power of the will over the thoughts and feelings is removed, the sequence of ideas depends either on new sensorial impressions or on subjective suggestions, the result of previous states of ideation. In the latter case, which is the condition of reverie, the attention is so engrossed that objective stimuli make no impression on the mind unless strong enough to enforce attention. (Fr. *rêverie.*)

RHABDOMANTIA (ῥάβδος, a rod; μαντεία, a prophesying). Term for the supposed manifestations derived from the use of the divining rod. The art is allied to that of clairvoyance, &c. (Fr. *rhabdomantie.*)

RHACHIASMUS (ῥάχις, the spine). Dr. M. Hall gave this name to the spasmodic action of the muscles at the back of the neck, which occurs early in epilepsy. (Fr. *rhachiasma.*)

RHEMBASMUS (ῥέμβω, I wander about, or am distracted). Has been used for a wandering state of mind, and for somnambulism. (Fr. *rhembasme.*)

RHEUMATIC FEVER AND INSANITY.—Though there are some grounds for believing that rheumatic fever may depend on or be associated with changes in the nervous system, it cannot be considered to be a neurosis; yet there are some very distinct relationships between acute rheumatism and mental disorder. On several occasions we have met with marked moral changes in patients after recovery from rheumatic fever. This may occur in patients who have had high fever and delirium; in those who have had heart complications, or in those in whom the disease appeared to have run a simple and uncomplicated course.

We believe it is most common in those who have suffered with delirium, and that it is in fact the direct result of some brain affection. Symptoms may vary from slight moral change to well-marked mental disorder.

We have met with several patients, mostly women, who have ceased to perform their domestic duties, and have caused family discord in consequence of their changed habits, the industrious mother becoming indolent and negligent of her duties. It is certain, too, that some persons who before rheumatic fever were sober and truthful, after it became intemperate and untruthful. In some the chief symptom is either forgetfulness or neglect of simple and necessary work, so that the patients lose their situations and lie in bed.

There may be loss of interest, loss of will power, loss of affection on the one hand, and loss of control with moral defect on the other. This partial mental weakness may be temporary or may be permanent, not leading to any progressive degradation, but leaving the patient mentally crippled for life.

In some cases mental disorder has followed the heart disease so common in rheumatic fever, and though in our experience melancholic conditions have been the most common, yet we have met with several cases of acute mania in which great restlessness and excitement have followed close on endocarditis or pericarditis. Dr. Julius Mickle has fully studied the relationship of insanity to heart disease in his Gulstonian Lectures.

In the next place, we will refer to the so-called cases of metastasis to the brain, during the course of rheumatic fever; serious delirium may appear, and at the same time the joint affection may disappear; in these cases there generally is great increase of temperature; the delirium and the rapid exhaustion resemble in many particulars acute delirious mania, and both diseases often end fatally; but the rheumatic disease is generally associated with a much higher temperature than that met with in acute delirious mania, in which the temperature rarely rises above 103°.

The alternation between the brain affection and the joint affection is noteworthy, as in the cases to be considered later this alternation is the essential symptom. After the acute delirious stage of rheumatic fever true delirious mania may arise, or more or less well-marked attacks of insanity may follow, or a period of partial weakmindedness very similar to that met with after continued fevers may be present, the rheumatic fever starting mental disorder which does not pass off with the rheumatic symptom.

In some cases a true alternation between rheumatic fever and mental disorder occurs; for example, a patient suffering from an ordinary attack of rheumatic fever suddenly loses all joint affection and becomes maniacal. Such alternations have in our experience been more common among women than among men, and do not seem to be specially related to neurotic heredity.

The alternations may follow any of the forms of treatment, and do not depend on the medication. A patient may suddenly become maniacal, and the mania may run a course of several months, and may pass off without any special complication, but as a rule there is almost always a return of the rheumatic fever before the recovery. In one case we have seen two well marked recurrences of the rheumatic fever alternating with two attacks of mania, in the end subacute rheumatism coming on before mental convalescence. Melancholia, or any other form of mental disorder may alternate with rheumatic fever, but we believe mania to be much the more common.

Nearly all such cases recover.

No special form of treatment directed to the rheumatic state seems in any way to affect the mental disorder. In some cases of insanity with the onset of rheumatic fever the mental symptoms may pass off either for a time or permanently. Only for a time if the insanity belong to the chronic or degenerative types, and more permanently if it occur in patients already improving from acute mental disorders.

GEO. H. SAVAGE.

RHINOLEREMA, RHINOLERESIS (ῥίς (ῥινός), the nose; λήρημα, λήρησις, a silly action or saying). Terms for "delirium nasi" or depraved sense of smell. (Fr. *rhinolérème;* Ger. *Delirium der Nase.*)

RIBS, FRACTURES OF.—In former days when there was much scandal in connection with the management of lunatic asylums, fractures of the ribs were often heard of; in the present day such occurrences are infrequent. It is stated by some authorities that owing to nutritive changes the bones are more brittle in the insane than in healthy individuals; the ribs are also so exposed to violence when force has to be used, that fractures of those bones are more common among the insane than among healthy individuals. (*See* BONE DEGENERATION.)

RIGIDITY.—In psychological medicine rigidity of limbs is met with most often in catalepsy and hysteria (*q.v.*). There is also a general rigidity in melancholia with stupor. Rigidity is also observed in paralytic idiocy and insanity, and sometimes the early and late rigidity in hemiplegia is complicated with mental disorder.

RISUS SARDONICUS (*risus*, a laugh; *sardonicus*, connected with the herb Sardonia, which was said to draw up the features of the eater). A distortion of the features, said to resemble a grin, caused by spasm of the muscles of the face. It is observed in tetanus. The unilateral form has been observed in hysteria (*q.v.*).

ROYAL ASYLUMS IN SCOTLAND.—These institutions were founded by the exertions and benevolence of private individuals, before legislative enactments compelled the erection of asylums for pauper lunatics. They are also called "Chartered Asylums," because each has a Royal Charter of Incorporation. Prior to the Lunacy Act (Scotland, 1857), all these establishments received pauper as well as private patients; but, owing to the erection of District (County) Asylums, there now is a tendency to reserve them, in whole or in part, for the insane of the middle classes. It has been felt that the charity of the founders should not form a grant in aid of the ratepayers, to relieve them of the obligations imposed by the law.

The Royal Asylums are seven in number, and were all opened about the beginning of the century. The oldest is at Montrose, where action was first taken in 1779. It was built on the Links near the town in 1781. The death of the poet Ferguson (1774), in deplorable circumstances in the "City Bedlam," of Edinburgh, moved Dr. Andrew Duncan to persist for more than a quarter of a century in advocating the erection of an asylum for the insane, specially for such as belonged to the cultured classes, and those who were in straitened circumstances.

After years of unsuccessful effort, the Edinburgh Royal Asylum was at length opened in 1813, for patients who were able to pay for the accommodation afforded. In 1806 only £223 had been subscribed, but a grant of £2000 was obtained from Government; and it is noteworthy that this was the only aid given by the Government to these asylums. However, the money so obtained was spent in purchasing ground at Morningside, and voluntary contributions enabled the managers to build the East House as above stated. In 1842, the West House was opened for the reception of pauper patients belonging to Edinburgh; and the history of the institution, designed as a *national charity*, and conducted successfully to its present eminence, can best be followed by perusal of an interesting memorandum by Sir Arthur Mitchell, K.C.B., published in the Twenty-fifth Report of the Commissioners in Lunacy for Scotland.

Of the seven Royal Asylums, five were built by public subscription, and two were endowed out of funds left for charitable purposes. There is reason to believe that no country, proportionately to its population, has voluntarily done so much for the care of the insane, during the period in which laws were chaotic on the subject. It is to be regretted that the benevolence towards this class of sufferers which marked the early years of the present century should have diminished with its progress; and it is to be hoped that the institutions inherited from that time will yet provide for the accommodation of all the private patients for whom only low rates of board can be paid. There is at present a marked effort being made to compass this end. Thirty years ago the directors of Murray's Royal Asylum at Perth, decided that it would be contrary to the constitution of the institution to receive paupers; while, at the same time, they were empowered to receive local patients not belonging to that class at such unremunerative rates as they thought fit. Lately, the Glasgow Royal Asylum has been similarly set apart for the admission of private patients only; and the Royal Edinburgh Asylum, after a full and impartial legal inquiry, has been freed from the incubus of maintaining pauper patients for less than they cost.

In 1855 it was found that the total capital expenditure made by the several chartered asylums for land, buildings, and furniture amounted to £352,632. That figure has been steadily increased year by year, mainly out of surplus revenue, derived from the profits on keeping the richer class of patients, until the total sum now stands at £929,473. This is exclusive of the new houses at Morningside and the extension at Aberdeen, which are expected to cost £80,000 and £50,000 respectively.

The Elgin District Asylum was also built in a remarkably public-spirited manner. Although it does not rank as a Royal Asylum, it was built before the passing of the Lunacy Act of 1857, on ground given by the Trustees of Gray's Hospital, the county agreeing to a voluntary assessment to defray the expense of the building. It was opened in the year 1835.

It should also be noted that prior to 1855 great exertions were made to erect an asylum at Inverness, and subscriptions were obtained to the amount of £5000. In consequence of the prospect of the provision of district asylums, however, the money was ultimately returned to the subscribers.

On reviewing the present position of the Royal Asylums it may be stated that they generally fulfil their important functions with success. "They are distributed over the country so as to make them fairly convenient, as regards locality, for supplying the accommodation required." That they command the confidence of the public is evident by these figures:—In 1857 there were 652 private patients in Royal Asylums and 231 in licensed houses (called in Scotland private asylums). In 1890 there were 1402 in Royal Asylums and 152 in licensed houses. The private asylums of Scotland are now retained for the higher classes; and those which formerly received patients at low rates are practically extinct. It yet remains for the Royal Asylums to provide for the accommodation of all the indigent private insane, and to obviate the necessity of submitting those who can only pay such rates as £30 a year to pauper conditions. This is a matter for public consideration, which should be placed in the forefront of lunacy administration. The directors or managers of the Royal Asylums have not only a trust to conserve, but are also bound to enlarge the limitations of that trust by fostering the spirit of Scottish independence in avoiding in so far as is possible the stigma of pauperism.

From what has been said above, it will be evident that the writer entertains an invincible objection to *mixed asylums*, if by that term it be understood that middle class private and pauper patients live under one roof and use recreation grounds common to both. There are indeed valid arguments in favour of the managers of Royal Asylums undertaking the charge of private and pauper patients in separate buildings and separate grounds; and experience has proved that, in the latest developments of asylum administration, this system is capable of the best results.

Aberdeen.—Founded in connection with the infirmary, under the same managers; built by voluntary contributions; opened in 1800; now rebuilt, and disjoined from the infirmary, which had been unduly benefiting by the joint management; consists of three main buildings:—(1) The pauper house, containing both pauper and private patients at low rates; (2) The detached establishment for private patients paying over £60 per annum; (3) An estate and mansion in the county, some miles away, principally occupied by working patients. Extent of grounds, 330 acres. Accommodation provided for 230 private and 450 pauper patients. The charitable area of the institution includes Aberdeenshire. Lowest rates for paupers, £26; for private patients, £28 per annum. Income from board paid by patients assisted by a small charitable fund—total £20,500 in 1890. Lectures on mental diseases during the summer session of the university.

Dumfries.—The Crichton Royal Institution was founded by the widow and other trustees of the late Mr. James Crichton, of Friars Carse, whose name it bears, and the residue of whose estate was devoted to its endowment. Its affairs are administered by a board regulated by their Act of Incorporation, 4 Vict. 3rd July 1840, and consisting of the successors of the original trustees of Mr. Crichton, and of noblemen and gentlemen holding official positions in the county of Dumfries, whose trusteeship is *ex officio*, and five elected directors holding office for a term of three years each. The institution was opened in 1839, when its first house, now reserved for patients of the higher class, was completed. A second house, principally devoted to patients of an intermediate class, was opened in 1849. This house also accommodates patients sent by the parochial boards of the three southern counties. The rates of board for patients in the first house range from an ordinary minimum of £70 upwards. For patients of the intermediate class in the second house the rates are from £25 to £52 per annum. There is a charitable fund in connection with both houses of the institution from which grants are made to persons in straitened circumstances belonging to the three southern counties to assist them in maintaining their relatives, inmates of the institution. These grants vary according to circumstances from £10 to £50 in each case. There are usually about fifty patients on this fund whose rate of board is thus reduced to a merely nominal sum. Besides the first and second houses mentioned above, there are several detached villas, formerly mansions, on neighbouring residential properties which have been purchased by the institution. The grounds have thus been extended to 665 acres. The accommodation is now about 1000 beds, of which about 300 are required for the pauper lunatics of the district, leaving about 700 available for private patients. Besides the purchase of land, there has been expended in buildings to date a sum of £130,000. The annual revenue is £45,000.

Dundee.—Founded in connection with the infirmary, and under the same managers, in 1805. Built by voluntary subscriptions and opened in 1820. Now disjoined from the infirmary and rebuilt in 1882. The old asylum had become too small, and was surrounded by the town. Consists of one modern building in the country. Extent of grounds 290 acres. Accommodation provided for 80 private, and 320 pauper patients. The charitable area of the institution includes the counties of Forfar and Fife. Lowest rates for paupers £28 12s., for private patients £25 per annum. Income from board paid by patients £11,700 per annum.

Edinburgh.—Built by voluntary contributions, aided by a small Government grant. Opened in 1813. Managed by *ex officio* directors and a medical board. Consists of three main buildings:—

(1) The East House for private patients at an ordinary minimum rate of £84 per annum. This is the original establishment, repeatedly enlarged and altered. It is soon to be replaced by a new building, now in process of construction, on a newly purchased estate of 62 acres lying to the west of the old asylum property. Great pains have been taken by Mr. Sydney Mitchell, the architect, to make it attractive, cheerful, and devoid of any prisonlike characteristics; to make the plan meet all modern ideas and requirements. The idea underlying the design of this building is to adapt its various wards and villas to the varying mental condition of the patients who are to inhabit it; from the padded room suitable for the deliriously maniacal patient, to the attractive separate villa suitable to the quiet and convalescent. Every effort has been made to remove the hurtful prejudice of the public against asylums, by making this one a true hospital for the treatment of this special disease with none of the repulsive features of the older buildings.

The site is richly wooded with old timber; part of it is on Easter Craiglockhart hill; the views include some of the finest near Edinburgh. The design provides for central building with four wards for each sex, with private parlours, dining-rooms, drawing-rooms, billiard-rooms, library and great central hall. This part of the asylum will accommodate about 100 patients, who will consist of the more recent, dangerous, troublesome and dirty class, along with some quietly dements cases. The wards occupy the ground and first floor, while the second floor is entirely occupied by bedrooms. The different wards are differently constructed to suit different classes of patients. On the estate at various distances from the main building there are six villas, two of which are hospitals. The general character of these villas is that of private houses for the well-to-do classes of society. The head of each is to be an educated and responsible official.

(2) The West House, opened in 1842, for paupers and patients at low rates of board.

(3) Craig House, for patients of the higher classes, purchased in 1879. Besides these, several smaller villas and cottages.

Extent of grounds, 120 acres. Accommodation provided for 344 private and 500 pauper patients. The charitable area of the asylum includes all Scotland. It is a national institution. Lowest rates for paupers, £31; for private patients, £28 10s. per annum. Income from board paid by patients aided by charitable funds (now amounting to £15,600), £46,000 per annum. Lectures on mental diseases during the summer session of the university.

Glasgow.—Founded in 1810. Built by voluntary contributions and opened in 1814. Rebuilt on a better site and on a more extended scale in 1842. Under the management of directors representing the subscribers and various public bodies in the city. The physician superintendent is also a director. It consists of two main buildings. The building called the East House was designed for pauper patients, while the West House has always been reserved for the higher class of private patients. For nearly two years no paupers have been admitted, and those now resident are only retained until their respective parishes can remove them to the rate-provided asylums at present being erected. The accommodation thus gained will be devoted to private patients at the lowest possible rates of board. Of 333 private patients, resident at the beginning of 1892, 111 pay £40 a year, and 34 pay £30 a year or less. Extent of grounds 66 acres. Accommodation will be provided for about 460 private patients by this recent arrangement. The charitable area of the institution has no limit, but is chiefly exercised in the West of Scotland. Lowest rates for private patients £30 per annum, and less in exceptional cases. Income from board paid by patients, £28,000 per annum. No endowment. Lectures on mental diseases during the summer session of the university.

Montrose. — Founded in connection with the infirmary; but with the infirmary and dispensary *subsidiary to the asylum.* The infirmary continues to benefit by this long-continued connection. Built by voluntary subscription. Opened in 1782. Rebuilt in the country in 1857. The managers, fifty in number, are self-elected, with a few *ex officio*. The asylum consists of three main buildings. (1) The main asylum containing patients at moderate rates of board. (2) The hospital, opened in 1891, for sick and infirm cases. (3) A separate villa for ladies at the higher rates. Extent of grounds, 270 acres. Accommodation provided for 80 private, and 480 pauper patients. The charitable area of the asylum extends to the counties of Forfar and Kincardine. Lowest rates for paupers, £28 12s., for private patients £25 per annum. Income from the board paid by patients, £16,903 per annum.

Perth.—Founded by the trustees of the late James Murray, Esq., whose name it bears. Managed by directors self-elected and *ex officio* in terms of the charter. Opened in 1827. Consists of two main buildings. (1) The original institution, enlarged in 1839, and further enlarged and modernised in 1889. (2) A neighbouring mansion house for quiet and convalescent patients of the higher class. Several houses in the vicinity, the Highlands and St. Andrews, are also occupied by patients. Extent of grounds, 63 acres. Accommodation for 136 private patients. The charitable area of the institution is limited to Perthshire. Lowest rate for local patients, £52 per annum. This is modified by the directors in special cases with the result that out of 104 patients resident at present, 17 pay less than that rate, the actual minimum being £30 per annum. The income is derived from board-rates paid by patients—the total for 1891 being £10,100.

A. R. Urquhart.

RUNNING AMUCK.—A term originally used by Anglo-Indians and others to denote the exhilarated state of intoxication accompanied by frenzy induced by the abuse of certain forms of cannabis (notably the *cannabis sativa* or *indica*, Indian hemp) by the natives of India, the Malayan Archipelago, Arabia, and Western Africa. Under the influence of large quantities of this drug they become so excited that they rush blindly and furiously about the streets with knives or other weapons, shouting "amuck! amuck!" ("kill! kill!"), indiscriminately attacking passers by, and even committing murder. European soldiers have, under the influence of this intoxicant, presented the same symptoms of impulsive destructiveness, and in one recently recorded instance a private succeeded in killing a number of his comrades and others before being shot down. In India the plant is known as bhang, subjee, or sidhee, and that prepared for sale, dried, and from which the resin has been extracted is popularly called gunjah. In Arabia the leaves and capsules, without the stalks, are known as haschish, and it was with this that Hassan, the subah of Nishapour, used to stupefy his victims before murdering them, whence the name *assassin*. In Western Africa it is known as dakka or diamba. The former word has travelled south, and is used by the Hottentots of the northern parts of the Cape Colony for the leaves of a native species of hemp which they smoke, and which induces first an excitable frenzy and later a stuporous narcotism like that of opium.

The term "to run amuck" has been popularised into a colloquialism for the action of one who talks or writes on a subject of which he is totally ignorant, or who runs foul of sense or popular opinion.

"Frontless and satire-proof he scours the streets,
And runs an Indian muck at all he meets."
DRYDEN.

"Satire's my weapon, but I'm too discreet
To run amuck and tilt at all I meet."
POPE.

It is also fancifully used to denote the blind impulsive aggressiveness of epileptic furor.

RUSSIA, PROVISION FOR THE INSANE IN.—The facts which serve to illustrate the condition of the insane in Russia during various periods of history, to illustrate the gradual amelioration of their condition of life, provision made for them by the organisation of institutions adapted to the management and treatment of mentally affected individuals, as also various statistical information concerning the insane, &c.—such facts have only quite recently been subjected to scientific investigation. Facts serving to illustrate various data pertaining to the above-mentioned questions were principally worked out in 1887 by the initiation of the first Congress of Psychiatry in Russia. It is precisely these facts and data which have been utilised for the present sketch.

Owing to the state of ignorance which prevailed during the Middle Ages in Russia, as also to a great extent in other European countries, it could hardly be expected that any correct idea concerning the insane as invalids that ought to undergo proper treatment, could be at all conceived. In Russia one group—the so-called "yourodivie," which were according to all probability no other than imbeciles or idiots—were regarded with special honour by the lower classes, and were accordingly surrounded with a kind of halo of sanctity, and therefore set apart from the mass. Others, principally hysterical women (so-called "klikoushy"), were looked upon as being possessed by the devil, and were therefore pursued by the people and tortured.

In the Middle Ages, when religion exercised a paramount influence on social life, philanthropy being centred in the clergy, the solicitude for the insane, as also for the poor, for pilgrims, &c., was left to the charge of the monks and priests. Such solicitude was even regarded as their direct duty, as we learn from an authentic statute of the Grand Duke Wladimir, the Saint (eleventh century), which was later corroborated in the sixteenth and seventeenth centuries.

The radical reform which was introduced in the government administration, as also in the whole social condition of Russia, by Peter the Great, affected the insane, inasmuch as the Emperor caused cases of insanity occurring amongst the nobility to be brought before the Senate. This ukase (1722) or ordinance, specially introduced with the intention of organising a criterion of the capacity of the nobility to serve in the army, to govern their estates, and to enter into matrimony, has in great measure influenced the legislation of the present day in Russia as concerns the acknowledgment of the legal rights of the insane. The maintenance of the insane in monasteries, under the charge of the monks and the clergy, was corroborated by an ukase of Peter the Great (1725).

The primary ordinances concerning the establishment of special institutions for providing for the insane appeared in the reign of Catherine II., in 1762: the preceding year a similar ukase had been already issued by her predecessor, Peter III., but had not been put in practice. However, the new ordinance of Catherine II. could not be immediately brought into action, it being of great importance beforehand to obtain information concerning similar institutions in other countries of Europe. It was only in 1776 that the first "mad house" in Russia was erected in Novgorod. During the reign of the same empress (Catherine II.), only three years later in 1799, a "mad house" was erected also in St. Petersburg, on the very spot on which later (1784) was established the Obouchow Hospital, which exists to the present day. Dating from that time the organisation of various institutions for the insane in many towns of the extensive Russian Empire can be easily traced, such institutions being erected principally in the capital either by direct order of the Government, or of various administrative departments.

The beneficial endeavours on behalf of the provision for the insane, made greater progress in St. Petersburg than in other towns, the capital being the great centre of the administration, and therefore under specially favourable conditions. Thus, during the reign of the Emperor Nicholas I., in 1832, the inauguration of the hospital of Miséricorde took place; it being originally destined for the accommodation of 120 patients, and organised according to the model of the best asylums for the insane existing at that time in England; later the hospital of Miséricorde was very much enlarged and reformed. In its time that hospital, owing to its admirable organisation and regulations, was accounted one of the best for the insane, and stood on a level with the best of the kind in Europe.

Endeavours towards providing for the insane in St. Petersburg were unanimously approved of during the first half of the present century. At that period was founded the hospital of St. Nicholas (1856). In the year 1859, a section for insane military officers and soldiers with their families was organised, according to the highest then known standard for providing for the insane; this section was confided to the charge of the Imperial Medico-Chirurgical Academy. It was in this section that Professor Balinsky undertook, for the first time in Russia, a course of lectures on psychiatry. A clinic for the insane was established several years later (1866) at the Medico-Chirurgical Academy. This clinic, endowed with profuse materials for scientific investigations, has proved itself to have been a nursery for rearing a number of competent specialists in the domain of medical psychology, who in course of time have successfully occupied posts as directors in various asylums for the insane in Russia. During the same period several private asylums for the insane were also established, amongst which the first was organised in 1847, by Dr. Leidesdorf, who latterly occupied the post of professor at Vienna. In 1870, a new exemplary asylum was inaugurated out of the private funds of the Czarevitch, the present Emperor, Alexander III.; this hospital was originally intended for as many as 120 patients. During the following years the town administration undertook the task of placing the incurable insane in various asylums and sections of almshouses. In 1885, a special asylum was established for the incurables—the hospital of St. Panteleimon containing from 500 to 600 patients.

At the present time (January 1, 1889), St Petersburg possesses accommodation for the insane as follows:—

	Beds.
In hospitals and asylums pertaining to the town administration	1370
In the hospital of Miséricorde	250
In the hospital of the Emperor Alexander III.	280
In the clinics of the military hospitals .	200
In private asylums	145
Total . . .	2245

The number of inhabitants of St. Petersburg, according to the census (made during one day, December 15, 1888), amounted to a total of 975,368; therefore one bed for the insane is provided for every 434 inhabitants.

The duty of providing for the insane in the extensive Russian Empire, was, at the latter end of the last century, centred in the "Board of Public Assistance." Measures were then taken by this Board for gradually establishing asylums for the insane in various government towns. The most ancient of these is the Rogdestwensky Hospital in Moscow, established towards the end of the last century, and rebuilt in 1812, after the conflagration of Moscow. By the middle of our century, nearly fifty of our government towns, including Siberia, possessed asylums of public assistance. According to official data in 1852, these asylums contained 2554 insane, the yearly maintenance of each of these patients amounting to the sum of 89 roubles 82 copecks (£12). Under such conditions the maintenance of each patient could hardly be satisfactory, and as early as 1840, the Minister of the Interior endeavoured to procure means for the better provision of the insane, both as to quantity, as also to quality; however, the difficulty of the question to be solved was such that no radical reform could be possibly undertaken at the time.

In 1869 the Minister of the Interior established an asylum for the insane in Kazan. Owing to the insufficiency of medical specialists, and to the lack of scientific knowledge of psychiatry, it is not until quite recently that a system of providing for the insane in Russia has been thoroughly undertaken; previously the insane were looked upon as unfortunate beings who should be taken care of, but at the same time who should be kept under strict control as dangerous to the public safety. Owing to this fact, in the majority of asylums established by the Board of Public Assistance the sections for the insane bore the character rather of prisons than of asylums for curing the mentally affected. In these wards the patients were all huddled together, no difference whatever being made for the acute or chronic forms, for curable or incurable patients, or even imbeciles. The care of these sections was nearly always entrusted to such medical men as were considered deficient in ability for practising their profession, or who had in some way or other proved themselves guilty of breaking the law of the land.

It was only during the beneficial reforms of the reign of Alexander II., owing to which the local administration in the provinces of Russia underwent a radical reform, that rapid progress was made in the mode of providing for the insane. Thus, beginning from 1860 in a whole range of governments of the provinces of Russia were organised rural municipalities (*semstvo*)—an institution based on a system of election, in which case the deputies are chosen amongst the local inhabitants—mostly landowners thoroughly acquainted with the wants of the province in which they live, and personally interested in its welfare. It was to the solicitude of these rural municipalities that the government entrusted the task of providing for the sick and the insane amongst the local inhabitants. These municipalities having undertaken to carry out the instructions to place in the asylums all persons suffering from insanity, and requiring proper treatment and care, the old buildings of the Board of Public Assistance proved very shortly to be overcrowded with patients, and it became expedient to build new asylums.

Taking into consideration the enormous expense which such buildings incur, the government decided to come to the aid of the rural municipalities. Thus, in 1879 the Minister of the Interior issued an order by which the government endowed the municipalities with a fund of fifty per cent. of the total expenses laid out by them for the amelioration of the asylums for the insane.

Dating from that time great efforts were directed towards the improvement of the system of providing for the insane; willing and able supporters of such improvements manifested themselves at the beginning of 1880, amongst a considerable contingent of young Russian medical psychologists, endowed with thorough scientific knowledge of their task; a fact most certainly to be attributed to the successful teaching of psychiatry in the Medical Academy of St. Petersburg and at the Universities of Moscow, Kazan, Charkoff, Kiew, Warsaw, and Dorpat. Some of the rural municipalities endeavouring to forward the improvement in the system of provision for the insane in their districts, undertook to send doctors of their staff to the universities of the empire, with the intention of affording them the opportunity of acquiring a thorough knowledge of the best systems of the treatment of the insane. At the same time plans of projected asylums for the insane were subjected to the examination of specialists belonging to the Association of Medical Psychologists at St. Petersburg.

Measures were also taken to entirely separate the insane from other groups of patients by the inauguration of establishments specially adapted to the regulation of professional workshops, of agricultural labour and to the transfer of the chronic patients to the colonies. These beneficial reforms rendered it possible to adopt in such asylums to a wide extent the system of "non-restraint," to obtain a great percentage of convalescence amongst the patients, to introduce a regular system of statistical information, &c. However, the realisation of such beneficial reforms even in the present day is to be found only in a small number of rural municipalities; more than in any other governments we find that these beneficial reforms have been partially realised in the improvement in various ways of the condition of the insane in the governments of Twer, Saratow, Tauride, Poltawa, also partially in the governments of Riazan and Novgorod. In many other governments unfortunately, asylums for the insane, even in the present day, form only a certain section of the municipal general hospitals for the various groups of patients. Lastly, in an immense portion of the Russian Empire, for instance in Siberia, in the Western Provinces of European Russia, such asylums have not yet been introduced and mentally affected patients are all confined together in the badly organised asylums of the old Board of Public Assistance system introduced before the above-mentioned reform took place. In general we are bound to state the fact that the above-mentioned reform of the provision for the insane is very slowly advancing in the rural districts of the Russian Empire; in fact it may be said to be still at an early period of the carrying out of such desirable reforms.

Undoubtedly the general number of asylums and wards for the insane in the empire is yearly increasing, and, according to the latest official data (the statistical returns of the Medical Department of the Ministry of the Interior, 1887), there exist already 85 asylums for the insane with accommodation for 9125 patients to the general number of 110 millions of inhabitants of the Russian Empire.

For the purpose of being better able to estimate such data, it is, of course, indispensable to be acquainted with the total number of the insane in Russia. Unfortunately, however, taking into consideration the natural difficulties which hinder any attempt to conduct satisfactory statistical tables in so vast an empire as Russia, we must own to the fact that at the present time correct data do not and cannot possibly exist. This most important question has been partially solved by statistical information obtained by the former director of the medical department, the late Dr. Mamonoff. According to the reports of the conscription committee, the number of the insane and epileptic could be ascertained through the examination of recruits in 1876, 1877, and 1878. The percentage of insane and epileptics existing amongst a given number of young men of twenty years old become clearly exhibited by these reports. Thus it has become obvious that out of a number of 754,362 recruits claimed by the conscription committee to be examined by the medical inspectors, 3072 young men were rejected by the Commissioners owing to their being affected with various forms of insanity. It follows that the number of cases of insanity is, approximately, 4 to a ratio of 1000 recruits; while the number of epileptics was 1.7 to 1000 recruits. In these cases there was great disparity in the returns as regards various districts of Russia. The greatest percentage of cases of mental affections was to be found in the Baltic provinces—namely, in the government of Esthonia, 12.8 to 1000; of Livonia, 7.9; of Courland, 6.2; also in the northern governments of Novgorod, 6.9, and Olonetz, 5.6; in the western governments of Vilna, 5.8; and the governments of the Vistula, from 5.4 to 4.4. The average percentage of cases of mental affections is to be found in the government of Pskow, Moskow, Toula, Kief, and Bessarabia. The minimum percentage (less than 4 to 1000) fell to the lot of the governments of Central and Southern Russia.

Undoubtedly it is impossible to judge of the extent of cases of insanity amongst the whole population of Russia by the percentage of insanity obtained from the examination of recruits of a known age. It is probable that the actual proportion of the mentally affected in Russia is considerably less than the above-mentioned average. This is clearly proved, independently of general conclusions, by various private data collected in separate governments of Russia. For instance, in the government of Courland, according to the returns obtained by the Medical Inspector-General, the number of the insane (in the year 1884) was estimated at 1 in 400; in the government of Livonia (1881), 1 in 884; in the government of Perm (1881), 1 in 1120; of Oufa, 1 in 788; in the government of Esthonia (1878), 1 in 530. In the government of Moscow (1886) the total number of the insane (not counting the town of Moscow) was estimated at 1662.

According to the census of 1882, in the government of Moscow (without counting the town of Moscow itself) the number of inhabitants was reckoned at 1,287,509; therefore there appears a ratio of 1 in 774.

It is needless to add that such data cannot be looked upon as infallible; and besides, owing to their bearing only a partial signification, therefore, the above-mentioned statistical returns cannot on any account be used as a basis for any statistical information as regards the whole population of Russia. However, in the absence of other more accurate statistics, even such scant returns can be taken into serious consideration.

Recently the members of the Medico-Psychological Association of St. Petersburg, as also those of the First Congress of Russian Medical Psychologists, firmly insisted on and pointed out the extreme necessity of obtaining a definite knowledge of the general percentage of the insane in our fatherland. For, to facilitate the furtherance of such information, there exists already a series of statistical tables, with questions demanding exact answers to the same. We may therefore cherish the hope that in some not far off future we shall fully possess the means of resolving in a satisfactory manner this most difficult problem. J. Mierzejewski.

S

SACER MORBUS (*sacer*, sacred; *morbus*, a disease). An old name for epilepsy.

SAINT AVERTIN.—The patron saint of lunatics; so-called from the French *avertineux* (lunatics). St. Avertin's disease is a name given to epilepsy.

SAINT DYMPHNA.—The tutelar saint of those afflicted with insanity. She was said to be a native of Britain and a woman of high rank, and is supposed to have been murdered at Gheel, in Belgium, by her own father, who was insane. St. Dymphna's disease is a term used for insanity. (*See* GHEEL.)

SAINT HUBERT'S DISEASE.—A synonym of Hydrophobia. St. Hubert was the patron saint of huntsmen, and those descended from his race were supposed to possess the power of curing the bite of mad dogs.

SAINT JOHN'S EVIL.—A synonym of Epilepsy.

SAINT MATHURIN'S DISEASE.—A name given either to epilepsy or insanity. St. Mathurin was the patron saint of idiots and fools.

SAINT VITUS'S DANCE. (*See* CHOREA.) A psychopathy of hysterical origin, spreading by imitation, at one time widely prevalent in Germany and the Low Countries. For its cure an annual procession of jumping and dancing performers was made on Whit Tuesday to a chapel in Ulm dedicated to St. Vitus, who was supposed to have the power of healing all nervous and hysterical affections.

> "At Strasbourg hundreds of folk began
> To dance and leap, both maid and man;
> In open market, lane, or street,
> They skipped along, nor cared to eat
> Until their plague had ceased to fright us,
> 'Twas called the dance of holy Vitus."
>
> Translation from an old German chronicle (Jan von Königshaven).

SAINT VITUS'S DANCE AND INSANITY. (*See* CHOREA.)

SALAAM CONVULSIONS. (*See* ECLAMPSIA NUTANS.)

SALICYLIC ACID.—The actions of salicylic acid and salicylate of soda upon the nervous system are very nearly the same, and any slight difference that may be observed is probably due to the greater solubility and consequently more rapid absorption of the sodium salt. When combined with powerful bases, such as quinine, the effect of the compound may be due to the base rather than the acid, and we need not consider such compounds here.

The toxic effect of salicylic acid or of sodium salicylate, for in this article we shall use the names indiscriminately, is exerted both on the functions of sensation and motion, and its effects appear to be due partly to a peripheral and partly to a central action. The most marked symptoms of its action are very much like those produced by quinine, namely, ringing in the ears and a certain amount of deafness. These are sometimes accompanied by fulness in the head, actual headache, giddiness, and sometimes by sickness and vomiting, which may be due to a local irritant action of the drug on the stomach, but which may possibly also have to a certain extent a central origin. When the administration of the drug ceases, these symptoms quickly pass off, but with large doses numbness and loss of sensation, with or without itching in the extremities, hallucinations of sight, nervous excitability, drowsiness, delirium, and unconsciousness have been observed. Indications of paralysis sometimes appear in the form of strabismus, ptosis, and difficulty in moving the legs, while sudden starts or twitchings of the muscles or tremor occur. Although ringing in the ears is usually the first symptom to attract attention, yet the optic nerve frequently shows signs of affection before the auditory. The first indication of such an affection in our experience has been the appearance of spectra whenever the eyes were shut. These frequently take the form of disagreeable faces, but they disappear whenever the eyes are opened. In other people the ocular spectra persist while the eyes are open. In one of our patients the administration of sodium salicylate caused large patches of red and green colour, but without any distinct form, to appear before the eyes while open. In another patient actual hallucinations taking definite form occurred, and he saw processions of people going round his bed. At first we mistook these hallucinations for the delirium of fever, but there was no high fever to account for delirium. The visions ceased when the salicylate was discontinued. The delirium varies in character—may sometimes be gay and sometimes melancholy or frightened, and may alternate with unconciousness, either partial or complete. As a rule the delirium is not violent.* The exact *modus operandi* of salicylic acid in producing these symptoms has not been precisely made out. We observe, however, that they may be classed as (1) irritation with (2) diminished activity of the normal functions, both of the central and peripheral nervous system. Thus, in the case of the optic nerve, we have diminution of the visual power with subjective sensations of colour or form amounting to actual hallucinations. In the case of the auditory nerve we have deafness more or less complete, with buzzing or ringing in the ears. In the case of nerves of general sensation we have itching, and more or less complete anæsthesia. In the case of the motor functions we have twitching, starting, tremor, and occasional paralyses. The delirium is probably, to some extent, dependent upon the false impressions conveyed to the cerebrum by the nerves of sense, but in all probability the cerebrum itself is also affected by the drug. On post-mortem examination, in cases of poisoning by salicylic acid, both in animals and man, considerable congestion of the membranes of the brain has been found with ecchymoses. A similar condition has been found in the internal ear, and in addition to great congestion and ecchymoses, exudation of yellowish red fluid has been found. In animals and in patients the tympanum has shown indications of inflammation, and fluid has been found in the tympanic cavity. The labyrinth appears also to be affected, as high tones are not so readily heard, and the hearing of a tuning-fork through the bones of the head is also impaired. The retinal vessels appear usually to be contracted. On the skin eruptions of various kinds have been observed, some of them having a character like urticaria. Although in these cases no microscopic examination has been made of the skin, yet we may probably be correct in assuming that the pathological anatomy of urticaria, due to salicylic acid, is like that of urticaria due to other causes, and in it distension of the vessels of the skin has been found with great numbers of leucocytes in the meshes of connective tissue and surrounding the blood and lymphatic vessels. The disorders of sight, hearing, and general sensation, usually disappear very quickly after the drug has been discontinued, and this fact seems to indicate that they are probably due in great measure to disturbances of the circulation, although we must not forget that the salicylic acid probably has an action upon the nerve structures themselves. Occasionally the deafness due to salicylic acid is more permanent, and this would point to changes in the ear from inflammation or extravasation caused by the drug, and remaining after its complete elimination from the body. The treatment of these effects of salicylic acid or salicylate of soda is based on the idea that they are due to congestion, and therefore ergot has been administered with the idea of contracting the vessels. This has been administered either in the form of infusion or Bonjean's extract, one part of this being given to ten parts of salicylate of soda. In deafness remaining after the medicine has been discontinued the cold compresses, ice-bags, the local application of tincture of iodine round the ear, or abstraction of blood by leeches, has been recommended, and if necessary the tympanum should be punctured. In more chronic cases the regular use of air douches, the introduction of the chloride of ammonium vapour into the middle ear, and the injection of a few drops of 3 per cent. solution of chloral hydrate has been found useful. The dose required to produce toxic effects appears to vary very greatly indeed in different individuals. Persistent singing in the ears has been produced by as little as fifteen grains of salicylate of soda in divided doses. Severe symptoms of delirium have usually been consequent on the administration of large doses, such as twenty grains of salicylic acid every three hours. Yet doses of twenty grains of salicylate of soda have frequently been given every two hours in acute rheumatism without injurious effects. The unpleasant effects of salicylic acid or salicylate of soda on the nervous system are supposed by some to be due in great measure, if not entirely, to impurities, and it has been stated that similar symptoms are either not produced at all or only to a much slighter extent by salicylic acid or salicylate of soda of vegetable origin.

T. LAUDER BRUNTON.

* In one case salicylate of soda has appeared to produce double consciousness. The patient, a man of great ability and mental power, was suffering from orchitis following influenza. On awaking during the night, drenched with perspiration, he had the feeling that the one person, wet and cold, was in duty bound to attend to the swollen and painful testicles of the other person. As he sat up to do this he got warmer, and the exertion seemed to make the two personalities come nearer and nearer together until they united.

SALIVATION (*saliva*, spittle).—**Definition.**—A symptomatic disorder, either central or peripheral in its origin, characterised by hyper-activity in the functions of the salivary glands. The term salivation is used to denote an excessive secretion of saliva from whatever cause, and is employed indiscriminately as a synonym of ptyalism (πτύαλον, spittle), sialorrhœa (σίαλον, saliva; ῥέω, I flow), and flow of saliva. The amount of saliva normally secreted by an adult in the twenty-four hours is about 1500 grammes, but this quantity is rarely constant, a large number of external factors being able to induce sialorrhœa temporarily, such as cold, cutaneous irritation, &c., while various articles of food, such as mustard, ginger, pepper, &c., may bring about the same effect. Excessive masticatory movements, too, can cause a copious flow of saliva, as we have on several occasions been able to prove by making patients masticate substances other than food stuffs, such as india-rubber; here the salivation is purely mechanical in origin. All these cases of sialorrhœa are accidental and not pathological.

Before treating of salivation as a symptom in nervous disease it is necessary to mention that there may exist at times an apparent ptyalism, a false sialorrhœa, the recognition of which is important. Thus, during sleep in weak patients or in individuals who breathe with their mouths open (especially children with adenoid vegetations of the nasopharynx), and in whom the head is inclined forwards, the saliva often dribbles out of the corners of the mouth, though the salivary secretion is not increased, but is on the contrary less abundant during the night. In the same way we may see in absent-minded individuals, and especially in old people, the saliva escaping from an imperfectly closed mouth. As for ptyalism in cretins and idiots we shall deal with it in a special paragraph. After having thus eliminated the sources of error by which we may be misled, chiefly when measuring the quantity of saliva secreted *per diem*, we may consider the phenomena of actual salivation, and we shall here treat of it as coincident with certain nervous conditions. The relations between the flow of saliva and the modifications of the nervous system with which they appear to be connected are not always perfectly clear, and this form of sialorrhœa has been called *sympathetic ptyalism*.

Symptoms.—It will perhaps be of advantage primarily to describe the general symptomatology of salivation as found uniformly in all cases, and to mention the pathogenic results arrived at from observation and experimental research. During salivation the quantity of fluid secreted is increased in variable proportions according to circumstances; we have frequently obtained quantities of two, three, and even five litres, but as in most cases a certain amount of the saliva is swallowed by the patient, the numbers given are less than the actual amount. The saliva in cases now under consideration is generally transparent and not opalescent as in ptyalism due to causes other than nervous disorder. The consistence of the secretion is less tenacious than in the normal condition, and it is the less viscous the greater the quantity secreted. The density of the liquid produced has not attracted the attention of observers; according to the investigations of Tubini it is diminished in sialorrhœa. The saliva is usually without any smell, a fact which distinguishes this type again from the salivation present in other forms of disease. Although the chemical characters of the saliva in pathological cases have been well studied, a good many particulars still remain to be cleared up. The *reaction* of the saliva in nervous or sympathetic sialorrhœa is generally slightly alkaline; moreover, it is now admitted that the substance which gives to the mixed saliva its acidity is furnished by the buccal mucus. The *chemical composition* of the saliva when secreted in excess shows first of all that the quantity of water is considerably increased; moreover, we generally find an abundance of fats, and lastly albumen. This last-named substance we know is not found in normal human saliva, it is only present in lesions of the medulla oblongata, as we shall show later on; it is absent, too, in functional affections and organic disease of the brain. *Microscopical* examination does not show any anomaly worth mentioning, save perhaps that there may be a large or small number of micro-organisms. The loss of saliva is accompanied by various functional disturbances. Some patients get rid of the saliva by continuous spitting, others allow it constantly to dribble from the corners of their half-open mouths. During the night, according to whether the salivation takes place consciously (spitting), or unconsciously (dribbling), the patient wakes up to spit and suffers from insomnia, or he is not inconvenienced, and the dribbling continues incessantly. This persistent and abundant loss of saliva always entails suffering on the whole organism, and for two reasons: it is, first, the loss of a fluid containing valuable inorganic substances, which exhausts the patient, and secondly the non-utilisation of a necessary digestive medium which causes dyspepsia.

The **course and duration** of salivation are variable according to the causes which produce it, a fact which we shall consider later, when reviewing the principal nervous disorders which originate this morbid disposition. It may be temporary, chronic, and also intermittent.

A brief consideration of the *mechanism of salivary secretion* will help us to understand the influence of nervous disorders on the production of salivation, and in the short description we are about to give we shall specially avail ourselves of the results arrived at by François Franck, who has experimentally investigated the influence of the brain on the salivary secretion. Above all we would briefly remind the reader of the fact that the researches of Ludwig, Claude Bernard, Schiff and Vulpian have unmistakably marked out the efferent channels and actions of the nervous influence. We know that the centripetal (sensory) nerves are principally represented by the lingual and glosso-pharyngeal. The vascular centrifugal nerves come from the sympathetic, and the glandular centripetal nerves from the chorda tympani. The nervous system acts at one and the same time on the vascular apparatus and on the secretory apparatus, and experiment has shown the independent action of the nervous system on each of these two factors of secretion. The same organs, however, may be influenced positively (*excito-sécrétoire*), or negatively (*fréno-sécrétoire*), but we have not been able as yet to determine the special nerve tracts for each of these modifications. Less is known as to the nerve centres for salivary secretion. Some physiologists place it in the medulla. Claude Bernard has shown that puncture of the pons produces an abundant secretion in the submaxillary gland, and that puncture of the floor of the fourth ventricle in front of the diabetic point also causes salivation. Beaunis has observed in the rabbit abundant salivation on electric cauterisation in the region of the third ventricle. Eckart has shown that stimulation in the region of the origin of the facial nerve produces salivation. On the other hand, having regard to the common observation that pure cerebral representations (ideas, emotions) act on the salivary secretion, the question is raised how far direct experiments are able to reproduce these secretory functions of the cerebrum. Bochefontaine in 1876 investigated the amount of salivary flow under the influence of stimulation of various points of the cerebral surface, and repeated his experiments in 1883. He found that salivation was produced in consequence of stimulation of the angular gyrus as well as of other points, and he draws the conclusion that the brain itself as a whole influences the secretion of saliva. Is there not, however, a *direct* cerebral influence which brings into play actual centres of salivation, or are the effects due to some kind of reflex action, that is to say, has the stimulation no other effect, such as the production of subjective phenomena of gustation which on their part cause salivation? François Franck, to whose experience we shall have to return when treating of epilepsy, thinks that cortical localisation of salivation is out of the question, but he believes that ptyalism following stimulation of the brain is due to "a central epileptic influence."

It will now be well to consider the salivation of different neuropathic conditions, and we shall study it (*a*) in the nervous diseases strictly so-called, and (*b*) in mental disorders.

(*a*) Salivation may be observed in central nervous diseases (of the cerebrum, medulla, &c.) and in peripheral nervous affections (lesions of the trifacial and facial). It may occur in *neurasthenia*, a fact to which, to our knowledge, due importance has not been given. We have had an opportunity of observing some cases in which this symptom showed itself with peculiar character. In one patient who presented most of the symptoms of neurasthenia, and especially the characteristic headache, salivation appeared in crises coincident with the exacerbations of the cephalalgia, and we have met with this same intermittent form in several other patients. It is necessary to add that among this class of patients the salivation is often attributed to the gastric disorders from which they so frequently suffer. In *hysteria* salivation is somewhat rare, and we have not had many instances among the large number of hysterical patients who frequent Professor Charcot's *clinique*. If it occurs in these it presents itself with extraordinary intensity. Tanquerel des Planches, who has collected a great number of cases of sialorrhœa, maintains that this affection appears in hysterical women in consequence of moral emotions, or after the ingestion of cold or acid beverages, or after the inhalation of strong scents. We have probably also to deal with hysteria in a case reported by Rayer, that of a young lady who suffered from ptyalism which returned for several years at regular intervals; and a case observed by Gilles de la Tourette appears to belong to the category in which the intense character of salivation peculiar to hysterical patients showed itself. We may add that we have tried the influence of suggestion on some of Professor Charcot's hystero-epileptic patients who had been thrown into the condition of *grand hypnotisme*, but we obtained spitting rather than an actual excess of saliva (hypercrinia). In *epilepsy*, Albertoni, in 1876 and 1879, satisfactorily proved that salivation is indeed a secretion, and he has completed his investigations experimentally by counting the drops of saliva flowing out from a tube which he introduced into Wharton's duct. François Franck has studied the mechanism of salivation in its relation to the phases of an epileptic attack. For this purpose he made a tracing of the salivary flow, together with that of the convulsions, and demonstrated that actual salivation does not take place during the tonic phase of the attack, the slight flow of saliva observed in that stage being due to mechanical expulsion. In the clonic phase alone actual hyper-secretion occurs, which increases as the convulsions become more violent. If we examine the course of the salivation in a series of attacks we find that it becomes less marked, and may even cease after a certain number of seizures, reappearing however after an interval of rest. Féré (1890) has also studied salivation in epileptics, and has made various experiments on his patients. He found that the salivary secretion was increased during the period of the attack, but decreased as the attacks became more frequent, disappearing altogether after a certain number of seizures; he tried the effect of the injection of pilocarpine and found that the salivary function became exhausted after a period of hyper-activity. *Local affections of the brain* may produce salivation. A certain number of cases of cerebral hemiplegia, produced either by hæmorrhage or by focal softening, have been recorded, in which sialorrhœa formed an important symptom. Here we may remind the reader of the case of hemiplegia with sialorrhœa, in which Ebstein first tried the subcutaneous injection of atropine for the purpose of arresting the excessive salivary flow. Salivation may present itself also in lesions of the medulla. It has always been found in labio-glosso-laryngeal paralysis, in which however it may have been only apparent, due to the non-closure of the lips as well as to the difficulty of deglutition. In the same way salivation is met with as a frequent symptom in cases of bulbar tumour, and in pseudo-bulbar paralysis. *Neuralgia and neuritis of the trifacial* are said by most authors to produce salivation, a fact which is indisputable, so far as neuralgia, especially of the superior and inferior maxillary divisions is concerned, but which is far less certain with regard to neuritis; in fact Adamkiewicz has recently (1890) published a very complete record of paralysis of the trifacial, in which he does not mention any disorders of salivation, a circumstance which it is easy to understand from a physiological standpoint. In *facial paralysis* salivation deserves mention on account of its diagnostic value. If in these cases ptyalism appears it indicates that the nervous lesion, which is the cause of the paralysis, is seated above the medulla. If the paralysis is caused by a lesion of the facial nerve the secretion of saliva may, on the contrary, be arrested on the paralysed side in consequence of the pathological condition of the salivary secretory fibres which are contained in certain branches of the facial (chorda tympani, lesser superficial petrosal). If salivation exists in a case of facial paralysis in which the orbicularis palpebrarum is also affected, we may make the diagnosis of focal cerebral lesion.

(*b*) Alienists have for a long period noticed and described the frequency of disorders of the salivary secretion *in the insane and idiots*. These modifications are due to different causes according to the form of mental affection in which they occur.

Diminution in the quantity of saliva is very difficult to observe and estimate. It is only found in certain forms of melancholia, and even then not frequently. The increase of salivary secretion is very frequently to be found, but in order to be appreciated it must be very considerable. There is, moreover, especially in these cases, the liability to error already mentioned. The flow of saliva from the mouth may indeed occur either because the patients do not pay any attention to deglutition, as in dements, idiots, &c., or because the patient is prevented swallowing by an exc ss of saliva. Nevertheless authorities agree as to the existence of ptyalism in certain cases of mental disorder, a subject we shall consider concurrently with the prognostic value of this symptom.

The practical researches mentioned above have demonstrated to a certain point that stimulation of the cerebral cortex in general, and stimulation of certain parts of the brain in particular, produce an increased salivary secretion; they explain why such an increase of saliva is observed (Krafft-Ebing) in affections connected with lesions of the "fore-brain." We may here mention that salivation is easily produced by moral excitement, so that it is not surprising to find the salivary function influenced by a permanent mental disorder. As François Franck remarks, the general expression "to make one's mouth water" corresponds perfectly to a phenomenon in which an emotion produces an actual increase of secretion. In analysing this fact we are able to construct a logical series at the commencement of which stands an impression of taste which, connected with a former sensation, produces by a reflex act the secretory reaction; the latter may present itself later, independently of the special cause which originally produced it. The more or less conscious recollection of the former sensation registered in the cerebral cells may be called up again by various associations of ideas, having their starting-point in visual, auditory, or olfactory impressions, which again recall the gustatory impressions formerly perceived. Up to this point we remain in the region of fact, material in so far as the secretory reaction is the result of the recollection of a sensation previously produced by an external impression. By a species of cerebral education, however, it may happen that sensations completely independent of the gustatory sensation—a general desire to possess something—may be accompanied by a similar salivary reaction. If we neglect the phases through which the phenomenon has passed, in order to consider the fact alone of a cerebral influence without any connection with an actual gustatory influence, we come to the conclusion that there is a direct action of the brain on the salivary secretion. By constructing the logical series, however, we are always able to go back to a gustatory impression, stored up as a recollection in certain cerebral cells, which are in a condition to react to impressions other than gustatory, and produce an increase of secretion.

After this psychological explanation let us look at the opinions of investigators into the occurrence of salivation in the insane. Esquirol attributed ptyalism to spasm; Fodéré to over-excitation; and both say that it is especially met with in *maniacal conditions*. Morel, Krafft-Ebing, and Dagonet hold the same views. Berthier attributes spitting in the insane to three causes—(1) agitation, (2) hallucinatory disorders, and (3) gastric disorders; but he confounds spitting and ptyalism, two undoubtedly distinctly different phenomena, one of which may exist without the other. It is very difficult to appreciate whether we have to deal with true salivation when we encounter a case of excessive spitting, but generally when ptyalism is present the voluntary ejection of saliva is absent. The latter condition is of great clinical importance, because it almost always indicates a chronic condition. We find it not only in agitated mental states, as Berthier believes, but frequently also in melancholia, in which it is a symptom that the mental affection is passing over into a chronic form. In *persecution mania* we find it most frequently associated with hallucinations of taste, the patient endeavouring to get rid of the poisons introduced into his mouth by his enemies. We must also take into account the gastric disorders so frequent in insanity, and especially in conditions of melancholia.

The value of ptyalism as a **means of prognosis** is great, a fact of which we may easily convince ourselves by the observation of certain mental conditions, such as mania or melancholia, with or without periodical exacerbations. In cases of this kind when ptyalism appears a return of the attack may at the same time be observed, the end of which was, on the other hand, indicated by a diminution in the amount of salivary secretion. Like spitting, but in a much less degree, salivation indicates generally the transition into a chronic state, and in all cases is a sign of the gravity of the affection and an indication of its long duration.

Ptyalism has in certain cases been described as a crisis of insanity, and Perfect, Roflinck, Pinel, Esquirol, and Baillou have furnished examples of this. Foville reports the case of a female patient who suffered from intermittent dementia, and recovered several times through spontaneous ptyalism. Thore reports a case of a high degree of mental stupor, in which a very abundant sialorrhœa appeared, which was followed by rapid recovery.

Starck, lastly, believes ptyalism to be of use as a **means of diagnosis**, founding his view on the difference between the saliva secreted under the influence of the tri-facial and facial nerves, in case it is thin and aqueous, and that secreted under the influence of the sympathetic, when it is viscid and stringy. He believes that when salivation is present, we may deduce from the nature of the saliva which point of the nervous system is affected. As yet, however, no definite conclusion can be drawn from this tempting hypothesis.

Ptyalism in *dementia* is of little interest. Most frequently it is associated with paralysis of the tongue and lips, the latter being continually kept half open. The flow of saliva may in all respects be compared with incontinence of urine and fæces, which occurs in the same patients in consequence of atonia of the sphincters through the failure of will power. At the commencement of secondary dementia we very frequently observe as one of the first symptoms of decline a slight increase in the salivary secretion. It may easily be imagined that the buccal sphincter being weak, and acting unlike the vesical and anal sphincters under the influence of reflex action, is the first to give way; we therefore have to deal with simple incontinence of saliva, so to speak, and not with actual hypersecretion. Various authors interested in idiocy, particularly Séguin, have observed in this affection an increase of the salivary secretion. Séguin even attributes the insensibility of the mouth and tongue partly to a kind of maceration of these parts in the liquid saliva, comparing the process to that which happens when we keep one part of the body for a long time in a bath. Whether in idiocy we have to deal with simple incontinence of saliva or actual hypersecretion is at present undetermined. According to our own investigations and personal observations, there exists in many cases a decided hypersecretion. Certain incurable idiots slobber to an extraordinary degree, actually soaking themselves with fluid, while others not less incurable slobber but little, and then only when the mouth is constantly kept open. On the other hand, we have seen in some of these patients the salivary incontinence ceasing at the time when the intellect and the will first showed signs of development under the influence of treatment, whilst in other patients we have found salivation to remain absolutely incurable in spite of local and general treatment. Lastly, we are frequently unable to attribute the salivation to a feeble tonicity of the labial sphincter, because idiots are to be met with who cease to slobber while incontinence of urine and fæces persists. There must therefore be some other reason than want of tone of the lips or weakening of the will of the patient, and we then have to take into consideration some lesion of the centres on which salivation depends.

PAUL BLOCQ.

SALTATIO, SALTATIO SANCTI VITI (*salto*, I dance). Synonyms of Chorea Magna.

SALTATORIC SPASM (*saltator*, a dancer). A name given to a rare form of clonic spasm in the legs which comes on when the patient attempts to stand, causing springing or jumping movements. It is more frequent in males, and in some there has been an antecedent history of functional nerve disturbance, epilepsy, &c., while in others depressing physical or mental influences have preceded its occurrence. The onset of the affection is sudden, and the spasms affect the flexors and extensors of the legs alternately, and with great rapidity in severe cases; there is no loss of power in the limbs, sensation is apparently unaffected, and there are no concurrent nerve disturbances, though Bamberger relates a case in which palpitation, dyspnœa, pupillary inequality, and unilateral facial spasm coexisted. The affection, after lasting some months, gradually disappears. Its pathology is obscure, and its treatment unsatisfactory (Gowers). (For further information on this subject see Bamberger, Wien. Med. Wochenschr., 1859; Erlenmeyer, Centralblt. f. Nervenkr., 1887; Frey. Arch. f. Psych., Bd. vi., 1875; Guttman, Berl. Med. Wochenschr., 1867, and Arch. f. Psych., Bd. v., 1876; Kollman, Deut. Med. Wochenschr., 1883, No. 40, and 1884, No. 4; and Gowers, Lancet, ii. 1877; especially the last-named, who discusses the probable pathology of the malady at length.)

SALVATELLA (*salus*, health). The name of the vein of the little finger. It receives its name because it was believed in olden times that blood-letting from it was efficacious in the treatment of melancholia. (Fr. *salvatelle*; Ger. *Salvatella*.)

SANGUINE TEMPERAMENT. (*See* TEMPERAMENTS.)

SARDONIC LAUGH. (*See* RISUS SARDONICUS.)

SATURNINE INSANITY. (*See* LEAD.)

SATYRIASIS.—This word denotes a condition of morbid excitement of the sexual functions in the male, with an irresistible tendency to repeat the act frequently. To this irresistible impulse we find sometimes superadded insane ideas, hallucinations, and disorders of general sensibility. The same morbid condition, when occurring in the female, has received the name of nymphomania. In order not to repeat ourselves, we refer the reader to the article treating of nymphomania, which comprises the whole question.

Satyriasis must be regarded more as a symptom than a special and distinct affection. It appears, in fact, as a symptom in the course of various maladies, but in a transitory form, and its duration is very short. In other cases, but only as an exception, its duration is long, and its course chronic.

Its pathological causes are manifold. Lesions of brain or spinal cord, encephalitis, myelitis, hæmorrhage, softening, tumour, traumatism, and compression; diseases dating from intra-uterine life or from early childhood, and followed by intellectual and physical disorders; deformity of the vertebral column seems to be frequently connected with a disposition to sexual excitement. Satyriasis also may occur at the commencement of various forms of mental disorder, as mania, congestive mania, general paralysis, epilepsy, moral insanity, and all varieties of mental degeneration; in affections of the skin of the genital organs, in cases of parasites and tumours of the rectum, and also as a consequence of toxic action of various medicines, *e.g.*, cantharides.

Among the **predisposing** causes it is sufficient to mention a vicious life and immoral books and pictures, especially if the intellectual life is limited. In degenerated individuals, whose imagination is much more developed than their power of judgment, the sexual appetite predominates over all other desires and wants, and for such the distance between desire and act is very short; thus certain crimes arise which have become much more frequent of late years. They are all the work of individuals with a limited intellect, and all bear the distinct character of imitation. The individual has read about or seen the scene which he reproduces. His brain, apparently gifted with fairly normal faculties, is unable to resist the sexual impulse; and there is at the time no thought of the responsibility which justice afterwards will claim from him. In some patients the insane ideas and the morbid impulse have their common cause in the brain as well as in the genital organs. This, however, does not hold good for all cases, for there are differences. Extreme abstinence, as well as the abuse of sexual intercourse, may produce satyriasis. The authors on this subject have described at great length the disorders and murders of Gilles de Retz, of the Marquess de Sade, and other well-known lunatics. The disorder is quite as evident in the case of the curate of Cours as in the tormented existence of the monks in Egypt, and in the monasteries everywhere, the history of which tells of the passionate struggles with the evil one. In the former case insanity and vice co-operate; in the latter, prolonged abstinence and mysticism produce alienation. *Régime* influences the want of intercourse more than climate. The sexual appetite differs according to race, mode of living, and education. Toxic agents, like alcohol, opium, and haschisch, increase at first, but diminish and extinguish it afterwards.

Symptoms.—Satyriasis shows itself by libidinous ideas, obscene language, and lascivious gestures and attitudes, showing the morbid proclivity to sexual acts, which nothing except a material obstacle can restrain. The intensity and the course of the phenomena, as well as the termination, depend on the principal disease. The frequent repetition of the act may in the long run produce exhaustion, and death may occur in coma; a case, however, which is rare. The symptoms mentioned occur frequently at the commencement of various mental disorders, and of paralysis agitans, and are of short duration; but it may also happen that in degenerated individuals they reappear like attacks of mental disorder of intermittent form.

Medico-Legal.—Satyriasis deserves attention from a medico-legal point of view with regard to the responsibility of the patient. Generally, it is not found in confirmed insanity, in dementia, or in epilepsy, and it varies at the commencement of general paralysis, of moral insanity, and in the less advanced states of mental degeneration. In studying these various categories of patients it is often difficult to say whether we have before us a lunatic or a perverted individual. The act committed by the patient is at first sight in no way different from the action of a vicious person. When we are obliged to make a distinction between the two, we have to examine their whole existences in their daily manifestations, and then, although certain lunatics and certain criminals present, on our first examination, numerous points of similarity from a social and criminal point of view, it is found possible to separate them.

Sexual excitement connected with satyriasis may develop a tendency to pæderasty. All pæderasts are not lunatics, and with many it is an acquired vice, deserving to be punished at the hands of justice.

Treatment.—A patient suffering from satyriasis must in any case be sequestrated, in his own interests and in those of society, and this measure must be taken as soon as possible in order to avoid accidents. In the first period of general paralysis there exists occasionally sexual excitement, which may bring trouble and scandal into conjugal life.

The treatment of the first symptoms of satyriasis may be successful. Bromide of potassium, bromide of camphor, prolonged baths, and saline purgatives are the best remedies. The principal indication is to cure the disease of which satyriasis is a symptom. In every individual, especially in the young, physical strength must be developed, and the mind must be directed to healthy studies. Satyriasis is often the result of the want of employment so frequent among the wealthy classes, especially when art and literature exercise a pernicious influence by indelicate representations and descriptions.

Gustave Bouchereau.

[*References.*—Sauvage, Nosologie méthodique Londe, Dictionnaire, vol. iii. Marc, De la folie. Morel, Traité des maladies mentales. Motet, Dictionnaire, Jaccoud. Dechambre, Dictionnaire encyclopédique.]

SAUTEUSE (Fr.). Literally dancer. (*See* CONVULSIONNAIRES.)

SCABIOPHOBIA, (*scabies ; φοβέω*, I fear). Morbid fear of, or erroneous belief that one is affected with, scabies.

SCANDINAVIA, PROVISION FOR THE INSANE IN.

Sweden.*—The first traces of any kind of care for the insane in Sweden is to be found in the Middle Ages, "Houses of the Holy Ghost," religious establishments under the management of the Roman Catholic priests, originally destined for the lodging and nursing of the sick poor, but receiving some insane patients also.

During the Reformation (1527) all monasteries were confiscated, except those which acted in accordance with the "Houses of the Holy Ghost." These were by-and-by transformed into asylums and hospitals which were partly occupied by the insane. The largest of these asylums was founded in 1531, by Gustavus I., on the "Riddarholm" at Stockholm; it was in 1551 removed to Danviken, in the vicinity of the capital, and more recently, in 1861, to Konradsberg, and has been erected for 109 patients according to the latest views of asylum construction.

As the general care for the sick poor was by degrees improved, one or more establishments for this purpose were founded within every county. Connected with these were arranged small wards for the insane. These, however, were soon found to be insufficient and defective, and at the beginning of the century the treatment of the insane began to make greater strides in consequence of the increased knowledge of psychological medicine.

Small county hospitals were therefore abolished, and larger special asylums for the insane were erected in several counties. (Central Hospitals, 1832.) More recently this division has also been abandoned, and the asylums are now opened to patients from any part of the whole country. The supreme government of the asylums, from the year 1837 to 1876, was vested in delegates from the "Serafimer Order," the duties of which were subsequently taken over by the Royal Medical College. In the year 1858 a common law for all asylums came into operation.

* Contributed by Dr. Thure Björck, Lund.

The asylums in Sweden which are altogether public are as follows:

	Patients.
Stockholm (Konradsberg)	265
Upsala	400
Nykoeping	70
Vadstena	360
Vexioe	220
Wisby	30
Malmoe	175
Lund	354
Goeteborg (Flisingen)	170
Kristinehamn	290
Hernoesand	[illegible]

In the course of 1890 were opened: (1) A new building for incurables (700) in connection with the asylums at Lund; (2) A new asylum in the vicinity of Piteaa for 300 patients. Most of these asylums are up to the modern requirements of psychological medicine, and afford the opportunity of occupying the patients in large gardens, and with suitable agricultural labour.

The statistics for 1887 give the number of insane as 6885, and of idiots as 4984 in a population of 4,700,000. Idiots with dangerous tendencies are confined in public asylums, but for the most part idiots are placed by the municipal authorities under their charge in special schools. There exist fourteen schools of this description, in all for 343 idiots, with subvention from the State. Moreover, five workhouses for adult idiots have been founded (1857). These establishments are for the most part due to the energy of Professor Kjellberg, in 1856 medical superintendent of the asylum at Upsala, who has done much to forward the claims of psychological medicine in Sweden.

Clinical lectures on psychiatry are given at the Universities of Upsala, Stockholm, and Lund, and every medical student is obliged to be on duty in an asylum for two months before he can be admitted for the final medical examination.

Norway.*—Even in the early ages of Norwegian history mention is made of mental diseases. The notorious King Sigurrd Jorsalfar (1130) suffered from melancholia with hallucinations; while the state of unbridled fury mentioned by the sagas, or mythological traditions of the North, and known as "Berserkgang," in the opinion of the historian Munch, was a periodical insanity, the subjects of which were under the influence of an uncontrollable homicidal and destructive impulse; those thus afflicted sought by vows to the deities to be freed from their

* Contributed by Dr. M. Holmboe, Rotvold, Norway.

malady. At a later period the persecution of sorceresses showed the extent to which the demonopathy of witchcraft had taken root in the northern as in the southern countries of Europe. Besides this we know little or nothing about the condition of the insane in past ages. No public provident care for them existed; they were, it seems, under the care of their relatives, or allowed to roam about at their own free will. Later the prisons became the receptacles of the more dangerous section when relatives and friends were incapable of properly taking care of them.

The first sign that the welfare of the insane was regarded as a State concern was given by the royal rescript issued in 1736, enjoining that in all the chief hospitals of the kingdom one or two rooms should be set apart for the reception and safe custody of the insane poor, "that they should not easily break out therefrom." In accordance with this rescript, reception rooms were by degrees arranged in the hospitals of Oslo, Bergen, Throndhjem, Christianssand, Stavanger, Arendal, and in the district of Hedemarken. These rooms were called "Dollhuse," or "Daare-kister;" they were destined only for the detention of the most dangerous of the insane, and their arrangement and accommodation were dismal and defective.

The agitation on behalf of an improvement in the condition of the insane which arose about the beginning of the century in most civilised nations, in a short time also reached Norway. In 1824 the attention of the Storthing (Parliament) was called to the wretched state of some of the above-mentioned madhouses, and it was demanded of the Government that they should appoint a committee for the investigation of this matter, and in the next year a commission was constituted, the result of whose investigations was made public in 1828, by an account written by one of its members, Fr. Holst, professor of medicine. He clearly demonstrated the defective and unsuitable state of the above-mentioned houses, and proposed the founding of a number of new establishments for the treatment of the insane at the public expense. A long period, however, elapsed before any public benefit resulted from these proposals, financial difficulties in all probability causing the delay.

It was not before the year 1843 that the matter was taken in hand again by the physician, H. Major. In eloquent terms he described the wretched condition in which the insane lived, and the unjustifiable, and very often cruel, treatment to which they were subjected. His warm and energetic appeal succeeded in raising a strong opinion in favour of an improvement in the treatment of the insane; and the result was the first step towards the amelioration of their condition—the founding of the first State asylum for the insane, at Gaustad, near Christiania (opened in 1855), and the passing of the Norwegian Lunacy Law by the Storthing in 1848. By this law, which is still in force, every asylum and other establishment for the custody of the insane must obtain royal authority, and the conditions under which such is granted are merely that a modernised and humane method of treatment shall be carried out. Patients are to be employed in becoming labour, are to live together socially, are to have exercise in the open air; isolated confinement and mechanical restraint are only to be resorted to for a short time and when the state of the patient makes it absolutely necessary; the association of the insane with criminals is interdicted. Every lunatic asylum has to be directed by an authorised physician, and his management is controlled by a committee appointed by the Government, among the members of which one at least must be a physician. The insane placed with private families are also to be under the supervision of physicians; and no patient is to be secluded without notice of the matter being given to a physician, who has to investigate the necessity and advisability thereof. The expenses for the care of the insane poor are charged upon the towns and counties.

The successful working of the asylum at Gaustad, and the important literary productions as to the cause and spread of mental disease in Norway published by its physicians, Sandberg and L. Dahl, effectively maintained and promoted the public interest in the improvement of the condition of the insane. By degrees the Storthing voted sums of money for the building of two new State asylums, adapted to the demands of our time—Rotvold, near Throndhjem (opened in 1872), and Eg, near Christianssand (opened in 1881). Besides these, several of the older establishments above named have undergone considerable improvement, and still exist as municipal asylums. At Bergen a new municipal asylum is in course of construction.

The census of 1865 shows that there were in Norway 2039 idiots, 3156 cases of acquired mental disease, or a total of 5195 insane. This gives a proportionate ratio to the population of idiots 1.835, of acquired mental diseases 1.529, and of the total number of insane 1.327 per 1000. A comparison with past enumerations shows that there is a relative increase in the number of those suffering from acquired mental disease, while there is a decrease in the number of idiots. The last census of 1875 made the number of insane to be 4568, or a proportion of 1.398 per 1000; but, no distinction being made between idiocy and acquired mental disease, these numbers are unfavourable for comparison with past enumerations. From all the computations made, it appears that mental disease is more prevalent in the southern parts of the country, less widely distributed in the north.

At the present time Norway has eleven lunatic asylums in use, with the following average number of insane (in 1887):—(*a*) asylums founded and managed by the State—Gaustad 324, Eg 242, Rotvold 224, or a total of 790; (*b*) municipal asylums and those founded by charitable associations—Christiania 108, Oslo 40, Christianssand 24, Stavanger 8, Bergen 65, Throndhjem 80, or a total of 325; (*c*) private asylums—Rosenbergs 160, Mollemdal 63 (both at Bergen), a total of 223. Thus, taken as a whole, the asylums of Norway accommodate 1338 insane, the accommodation, however, being frequently inadequate, and in view of providing for this, some asylums (Christianssand, Gaustad, and Rotvold) have endeavoured to place dements without dangerous tendencies in private families residing in their vicinity, under the constant supervision of their several physicians. This system is mainly in vogue at Rotvold, where at present 70 insane are placed out in this manner. For idiots three private educational establishments, with subventions from the State, have been founded, two at Christiania, one near Bergen.

At the Norwegian University psychological medicine is not yet recognised as a distinct branch of medical education. Courses of clinical lectures on mental diseases are given every year by the superintendent physician of Ganstad Asylum to a limited number of medical students.

[*References.*—P. A. Munch, Det norske Folks Historie. 1852–53. Fr. Holst, Beretning fra en etc. i Aaret 1825, naadigst nedsat kongelig Kommission. H. Major, Indberetning om Sindssygeforholdene i Norge i 1846. L. Dahl, Bidrag til Kundskab om de Sindssyge i Norge den 31. December 1865. Sandberg, Gaustad, 1855–70.]

[NOTE.—Since the foregoing article was written Dr. Habgood, senior assistant medical officer, Kent County Asylum, Maidstone, has contributed an article to the *Journal of Mental Science*, January 1892, the result of a visit to the Norway asylums. Referring to the preponderance of melancholia over mania in that country, he observes that "the distribution of a small population over a large tract of country, the mountainous character of that country, the monotony of life, the lack of amusement, the phlegmatic character of the race, in contrast to the crowded condition of the people, the high tension of living, and the excitement of city life which prevail in England, probably explain the difference between the two countries. The small number—1.9 per cent. of the admissions (being 6.4 less than in England)—of those suffering from general paralysis might be explained in the same manner." He states that the eleven asylums (three Government, six municipal, and two private) are under the control of the Medical Department of the Ministry of Justice. The King appoints the superintendent of the Government asylums. While speaking favourably of the New Municipal Asylum at Bergen, Dr. Habgood observes that the rooms used for the seclusion of maniacal cases with destructive propensities contained nothing but a heap of straw, the patient himself being naked. Observation is carried on through lantern-lights in the roof by an attendant who walks up and down on a place provided on the roof. "The medical officers defend the method by arguing that it is useless to give clothes and bedding to those who will not only not use them, but destroy them as fast as they are supplied."—ED.]

Denmark.—In former times the care of the insane was considered to be a private matter, and the first disposition on the part of the State to interest itself in their condition was manifested by the fact that Christian IV. ordered in the year 1632 the construction of *daarekiste* in connection with the "pest-house" at Copenhagen. Originally this pest-house was a *domus leprosorum*; later it was used for the common epidemic diseases under the name of *St. Hans Hospital*. In the course of the following century similar rooms of confinement were arranged in connection with the common hospitals of nearly the whole kingdom. The purpose of these establishments, however, was the protection of the community from the insane, not the amelioration of the condition of the insane themselves. The veritable reform of Danish psychiatry is to be dated from the year 1808, when the city of Copenhagen bought "Bidstrupgaard," in the vicinity of Roskilde, about sixteen (English) miles from the capital, and built on the spot an asylum, which was ready for occupation in 1816, and was therefore one of the earliest established asylums of the Continent. Its official name was converted into St. Hans Hospital, with the addition of "Claude Rosset's Stiftelse," in memory of a French emigrant who enriched the asylum with an endowment.

In 1820 the asylum of Schleswig was founded, at that time belonging to the Danish monarchy. Originally built after designs by Esquirol, it has lately been considerably enlarged, and is now under the German Government.

The next period of importance in the history of Danish psychiatry is the beginning of the fourth decade of this century, when a philanthropic and scientific reformation was started by the late Dr. Hübertz and Dr. Selmer, leading to a total re-organisation of the lunatic establishments of the country in accordance with modern principles. These efforts resulted in the foundation of the first provincial asylum near Aarhus on Jylland, in 1852, of which Selmer became the medical superintendent; and next, in 1858, Oringe, in the vicinity of Vordingborg (Sjælland), and the rebuilding of St. Hans Hospital (1860). The latter, which previously had given room, in addition to the insane, to some old and infirm sick poor, was arranged only for the purpose of cure. More recently it has become necessary to build several houses for incurables. The St. Hans Hospital admits only the insane of Copenhagen; it is now unfortunately too small, and will be further enlarged. It has been superintended since 1863 by Professor Steenberg, renowned for his researches in syphilitic cerebral disorders, until the present month (March 1892), when he died. In addition to the enlargement of the asylum for the capital, it has been necessary, during the past ten years, to erect new asylums for the rest of the country (Viborg, 1877, for incurables; Middelfort, 1888). The ward for insane patients at the "Communal Hospital" in Copenhagen, which is connected with a ward for diseases of the nervous system, is intended for the provisional admission of the insane of the capital, and for the observation of criminals. It has of late been enlarged to the extent of fifty-five beds. In the abovementioned asylums the number of patients is as follows:

	Patients.
St. Hans Hospital	990*
Aarhus	540
Oringe	450
Viborg	340
Middelfort	400

Besides these asylums, some of the old establishments were chiefly erected as workhouses, and they are still in use for the reception of insane patients—namely:

	Patients.
Roskilde	with about 50
Holbæk	" " 12
Soro	" " 35
Stege	" " 74
Saxkoebing	" " 88
Mariager	" " 30

* There will be an additional separate building, providing for 250 patients.

Spread over the country there are to be found single patients or a small number of insane under private care, but no true private asylums. This is in all probability because the public asylums are open to patients of the higher classes, who pay an extra fee.

The census of 1880 gave the number of 3,263 insane, a proportion to the population of 1.6 per 1000. Besides these there were recorded 2602 idiots (1.3 per 1000). Only about one-tenth of the idiots are confined in special "schools," partly public, partly private, with assistance from the State.

Clinical lectures on mental diseases are given in the ward for the insane in the Communal Hospital. Moreover, an opportunity is granted for junior assistant-physicians to be on duty for some months in the asylums.

From the statistical report on mental diseases in asylums in Scandinavia presented to the International Medical Congress at Copenhagen in 1884 by Prof. Steenberg, we find that the number of insane in Finland was at that time 4400, or 21.2 per 10,000, a higher proportion than in Norway, Sweden, or Denmark. In 1771, forty beds for the insane were provided in the old leper hospital Sjählo; but it was not until the foundation of an asylum at Lappvik in 1841 that an attempt was made to treat the insane. At the same date some cells were set apart for this class in all the hospitals in the country, where the authorities were obliged to place lunatics in the neighbourhood for treatment. In 1884 there were two old asylums (Sjählo and Lappvik), five reception houses, and an entirely new hospital at Kuopio; subsequently, also, at Kexholm and at Tammarfors.

In the most recent publication having reference to the insane in Denmark * it is stated that there were at the beginning of 1890 a little more than 1000 patients in the asylums of Copenhagen, which would be about the whole number in this town. As the population is somewhat over 300,000, the rate would be about one insane to every 300 inhabitants. If this scale were applied to the rest of the country, whose population is exactly six times as large, the total number of the insane would be 6000, but this figure is certainly too high. A metropolitan population produces more lunatics than a rural population; instances need only be given of the greater number of cases of general paralysis among the

* "Denmark; its Medical Organisation, Hygiene, and Demography" (presented to the Seventh International Congress of Hygiene and Demography, London, 1891).

former than the latter. In 1889 these represented one-seventh of the patients sent to the asylums from Copenhagen, which, in proportion to the population, is nearly nine times as many as from the rest of the country, but how great the difference is altogether can scarcely be determined.* From the returns made in 1860, 1870, 1880, and approximately in 1890, of the number of insane in Denmark, it appears that in the first twenty years "the number has been steadily and gradually increasing; in the first decade with 578, and in the second with 809. Presuming (what everything tends to prove) that this increase has also continued at the same rate in the third decade, the number given by the recent census of 1890 will be about 4300. This number would be too low, just as the figures, 6000, obtained by judging from the number of insane in Copenhagen, were too high. The correct number must be between these—namely, 5150, or about one to each 390 inhabitants. Of these it is known that a little above 1000 are found in Copenhagen. The rest, about 4150, would therefore reside in the country."

It is stated in the same document, with regard to inebriety as the cause of insanity, that it stands at 10.2 per cent. of the admissions taking the whole of Denmark. In Copenhagen it is 11.5 per cent.—in other words, one-tenth of the individuals admitted into asylums have themselves caused their disease through drink.†

With regard to restraint, it is observed: "Conolly's endeavours to do away with the mechanical restraint reached this country a little more than twenty years ago, and for several years this system was consistently carried out, but by-and-by less *doctrinaire* opinions became prevalent. It is not only by doing away with the abuse of mechanical restraint that the striving for liberty manifests itself, but also by making the wards more open, and the life in them less restrained." ‡

With regard to the number of imbeciles (including idiots), statistics were obtained in 1845, but, as in all other countries, they must have been very imperfect, and the same remark applies to census returns in subsequent years. In 1888–89 more accurate information was obtained, with the result that 3907 of the population were found to be idiotic or feeble-minded. It is stated that the actual number of imbeciles may be estimated at about 5000, and that while the imbecile rate for the whole country is, according to the figures, 18 per 10,000 inhabitants, it is in fact nearer 25 per 10,000. It is observed that the social condition appears to have no influence upon the distribution of imbecility in the agricultural classes. Of all the cases there were about 85 per cent. congenital. With regard to their care it appears that Dr. Hüberts took up the idea of improving their education at the time that Guggenbühl was prominently before the world. Only a small proportion of imbeciles in Denmark are cared for in asylums; the rest are at home or in workhouses, and are not subject to official inspection. In order to advance from the existing inadequate provision for imbeciles in this country, it will be necessary to be content to wait for many years. Such is a statement by Dr. Chr. Keller, who has an institution for 500 imbeciles. The first Danish imbecile institution was opened in 1855 at Gamle Bakkehus, in the vicinity of Copenhagen. The institution was removed in 1860 to a more suitable building, and accommodates 60 imbeciles. It is called "The Institution for the Care of Feeble-minded Children." A large building is about to be opened, which will accommodate 460. It is situate at Ebberödgwaard. The superintendent is Dr. Friis.*

KNUD PONTOPPIDAN.

* *Op. cit.* p. 399. † *Op. cit.* p. 405. ‡ *Op. cit.* p. 410.

* *Op. cit.* p. 413.

SCAPHOCEPHALIC IDIOCY. (*See* IDIOCY, FORMS OF.)

SCAPHOCEPHALUS (σκάφη, a boat; κεφαλή, the head). A form of head sometimes noticed in congenital idiocy, in which the shape is like the keel of a boat upside down. The head is out of all proportion larger in the antero-posterior diameter than in the transverse.

SCARLATINA. (*See* POST-FEBRILE INSANITY.)

SCATOPHAGIA (σκατός, excrement; φαγεῖν, to eat). Synonym of Coprophagia (*q.v.*). (Ger. *Skatophagie*, *q.v.*)

SCHEINBILD (Ger.). An illusion.

SCHLAFGÄNGER (Ger.). A somnambulist.

SCHLAFSUCHT, SCHLAFKRANKHEIT (Ger.). Abnormal somnolency, narcolepsy.

SCHOOLS, ASYLUM. (*See* TREATMENT.)

SCHWANGERSCHAFTSWAHN (Ger.). Puerperal insanity.

SCHWERMUTH (Ger.). A term for melancholia.

SCILLOCEPHALUS (*scilla*, the squill; κεφαλή, the head). Term for a small peaked head, seen sometimes in idiots. (Fr. *scillocéphale.*)

SCLERENCEPHALIA (σκληρός, hard; ἐγκέφαλος, the brain). Induration of the brain. Cerebral sclerosis.

SCOTLAND, ASYLUMS IN. (*See* GREAT BRITAIN, INSANITY IN; and ROYAL SCOTTISH ASYLUMS.)

SCOTTISH LUNACY LAW.*

From the earliest records it would appear that the Sovereign, as *pater patriae*, was the natural and legal guardian of the insane.† The ward and custody of the property of lunatics were deputed to tutors, appointed after cognition by inquest. These were selected as being kinsmen of lawful age, men of judgment, discretion, and rule. By a statute of Robert I., in the beginning of the fourteenth century, the custody of persons of furious mind was devolved upon their relations, and, failing them, upon the sheriff of the county. According to Sir Thomas Craig, there was a distinction between the "fatuous" and the "furious." The custody of the former was committed to the nearest agnate‡ (nearest male relative on the father's side), while that of the latter belonged to the Crown, as having the sole power of coercing with fetters. Legal procedure was more definitely settled by the statute of 1474, cap. 67, which was amended by the Act of 1585, cap. 18; and these statutes continued to regulate the appointment of *tutors-at-law* until 1868, when the Court of Session Act (31 & 32 Vict. cap. 100) was passed, and provided for *cognition of the insane* as described under that heading.

Another class of guardians to lunatics are termed *tutors-dative*. This process has fallen into disuse for many years, and has now merely an antiquarian interest.

Judicial factors, or **curators bonis,** are at the present time by far the most important functionaries in this department. They are appointed by the Court of Session or by the sheriffs under the regulations described under *curatory of the insane*. The practice seems to have originated in the *nobile officium* inherent in the Court of Session as the supreme court of equity in Scotland. The nomination of judicial factors has now practically superseded the more ancient procedure, so that the cumbrous and costly process of cognition has become almost extinct.

There is another remedy provided by the law of Scotland for the protection of silly, imbecile, or facile persons who are lavish, improvident, or careless in the management of their property. This procedure is called **interdiction,** which has been defined as "a legal restraint laid upon those who, either through their profuseness or the extreme facility of their tempers, are too easily induced to make hurtful conveyances, by which they are disabled from signing any deed to their prejudice without the consent of curators, who are called interdictors." Interdiction may be either (*a*) voluntary or (*b*) judicial.

(*a*) **Voluntary interdiction.** — This was of frequent occurrence in ancient times. An Act passed in 1581 regulated it in some measure, and it was formally sanctioned in the seventeenth century. Voluntary interdiction proceeds upon execution of a deed, or bond of interdiction, narrating the weakness of the grantor as the cause, declaring confidence in persons to be named (the interdictors), which binds the party not to alienate "his lands, teinds, heritages, annual rents, life rents, reversions, tacks, or others; nor to grant dispositions or assignations, nor bonds, obligations, or contracts; nor to become cautioner for sums of money, or to perform acts and deeds," without the concurrence of his interdictors. There must be a valid cause, or the deed may be set aside by the courts. Prodigality and injury to the family must be conjoined with mental weakness and facility. But the cause may be scarcely referred to in the bond. It is imperative that the bond be recorded in the register known as the "Books of Council and Session,"* whereby it is held to be published to the lieges and made patent to all.

(*b*) **Judicial interdiction** is obtained by decree of the Supreme Court, after proof being led as to the facility and weakness. In modern practice, the relations may institute proceedings for interdiction when the defects of the *prodigus* are not sufficiently marked for cognition or curatory. Or it may proceed from the *nobile officium* of the Court themselves, when they perceive that a party to any suit before them is liable to imposition, from an extreme profuseness and facility of temper.† This not being an *actio popularis*, neither the Lord Advocate nor the public can interfere. The summons states that the person is "of weak and facile disposition, easily imposed on and liable to do deeds to his own lesion and prejudice." The Court will name interdictors without whose consent there would be no power of alienating heritage or of contracting debts, if the action be unopposed. If the Court proceeds to proof, the defender must appear; and, if the interdiction is granted, it is published

* *See also* CURATORY and COGNITION.
† Craig, Jus. Feudale, lib. ii. cap. 20.
‡ Adopted from the Roman Law.

* General Register of Inhibitions (31 & 32 Vict. c. 64, s. 16).
† Report of proceedings under a brieve of idiotry: Duncan v. Yoolow, by L. Colquhoun, 1837.

and registered. The interdictors must be of perfect age and sane mind. They have no trust, no management. Their duties are rather negative than positive, as they do not originate deeds, but merely adhibit their consent. The interdiction terminates by sentence of Court; by death; if statements in the original deed are false; if re-convalescence can be declared. Voluntary interdiction cannot be recalled by the person interdicted without the consent of his interdictors, and if there be a failure of a quorum of these he must apply for others. But there are so many exceptions and limitations to the bond of interdiction that it is not often in use. For instance, it only affects heritage and no other property. Rational and onerous deeds, moderate and reasonable tradesmen's accounts, are also excepted. Moreover, the whole system of interdiction may be rendered futile by imprisonment for non-payment of debt*—for the Courts will not grant relief, although the party interdicted may have to burden his lands.

Besides these remedies, which have reference, chiefly, though not exclusively, to the future protection of persons of deficient capacity, a retrospective remedy is provided by the action of **Reduction** on the ground of insanity, or idiocy, or facility, fraud, and lesion as the case may be. And this last remedy seems to reach all those causes by which an individual may be injured by the weakness of his intellect, even where the defect is not so grave as to render him a proper subject for curatory or interdiction. Of course, it has been decided by the highest authority that even insane persons can execute valid deeds, but the circumstances under which this subject is considered will be found detailed under the head of *Civil Incapacity.*

We have seen that it was the policy of the law of Scotland, from a very early period, to entrust the persons of lunatics to the care of their relatives. This policy in a modified form is continued to the present day. As a general rule, the law takes no special cognizance of insane persons, unless their seclusion or protection is necessitated, or their property is endangered. It was only towards the close of the reign of George III.† that the Legislature directed its attention to the devising of securities for the due regulation of the custody and treatment of the person of unsound mind. It is unnecessary to go into detail as to the history of the circumstances which brought about the report of the Commissioners appointed to inquire into the lunatic asylums of Scotland, bearing date 1857. A *résumé* of the laws enacted consequent on that report will sufficiently describe the machinery by which the personal care and control of the insane are governed.

[Explanatory Note.—Throughout the following *résumé* of the Lunacy Acts it will be understood that there is a uniformity of procedure as regards pauper and non-pauper lunatics, except where specially noted. The terms used are briefly defined (also in 20 & 21 Vict. c. 71, s. 3) as follows:—The "Board" means the General Board of Commissioners in Lunacy, Scotland; "Secretary," means the secretary of the Board; "District Board" means the Board chosen by the County Council to manage the lunacy affairs of the district; "Public Asylums" means all asylums erected without view to pecuniary gain; "District Asylum" means the asylum erected and maintained under the provisions of the Acts by the district board; "Private Asylum" means an asylum for the reception of more than one lunatic kept for pecuniary gain; "Lunatic" means any person who, in the opinion of two properly qualified medical persons, is a lunatic, an insane person, an idiot, or a person of unsound mind; "Pauper Lunatic" includes any lunatic towards the expense of whose maintenance any allowance is made by a parochial board; "Medical Person" means any person registered as a practitioner in medicine or surgery pursuant to the Act 21 & 22 Vict. c. 90; "Judicial Factor" means *factor loco tutoris, factor loco absentis, curator bonis, tutor dative,* or tutor at law by reason of service, having charge of a lunatic; "Sheriff" includes sheriff-substitutes; "Superintendent" means the person having the charge of any asylum, including proprietors of private asylums, or licensed houses, and those having pecuniary interest therein, also the governor of a poorhouse where lunatics are kept: the word "Month" means a calendar month; "Private" patient means non-pauper.]

Board of Lunacy.—The General Board of Lunacy for Scotland is composed of five commissioners. The chairman and two legal commissioners are unpaid; the two medical commissioners are paid.* The Board is aided by a secretary, clerks, and two deputy commissioners, who are all paid under statutory regulations. The meetings of the Board, their powers and their duties, are regulated by the various Acts of Parliament, the titles of which are appended to this article. The commissioners serve under an oath, may derive no profit for discharging their duties, and are specially exempted from personal responsibility.† The paid commissioners are required to devote their whole time to the duties of their office. Generally speaking, the Board have the regulation of all matters in relation to lunatics and asylums, the

* But see Debtors Act, 1880 (43 & 44 Vict. c. 34); and Civil Imprisonment Act, 1882 (45 & 46 Vict. c. 42).

† 55 Geo. III. c. 69; 9 Geo. IV. cap. 34; 4 & 5 Vict. cap. 60; all of which are repealed.

* There is no statutory reason for this arrangement of legal and medical commissioners.

† 29 & 30 Vict. c. 52, s. 23.

superintendence of all affairs arising out of the Lunacy Acts. They are also authorised, with the concurrence of the Lord Advocate or Solicitor-General, to institute inquiries, summon witnesses and examine them on oath relative to any case falling under the provisions of the Lunacy Acts.* It is also competent for them to authorise search of records as to whether any particular person has been confined as a lunatic within twelve months.† The Board is, moreover, endowed with powers to require asylum accommodation to be provided ‡ to their satisfaction, and to alter or vary the lunacy districts, subject to the sanction of the Secretary of State for Scotland,§ and to take steps for the adequate accommodation of pauper lunatics in any district.‖ They are empowered¶ to inspect lunatics in private houses,** where the person is not kept for gain, but whose case may require confinement, or coercion, and who may have been detained for more than a year, or who has been subjected to harsh treatment; but only with the consent of a Secretary of State or the Lord Advocate. If removal should appear necessary, however, the Board must apply to the sheriff for an order. It is also specially enacted†† that the commissioners may take the assistance of such medical persons as may be required for the purposes of the Lunacy Acts. As the Board is empowered to enforce such rules and regulations as they may make, a statutory penalty is fixed for any infringement or violation.‡‡ The secretary is required by the Act to keep the books, minutes, and accounts of the Board, and to make annual returns as to lunatics and asylums.§§ He is aided by a staff of clerks. Finally, on the 1st day of February of each year a report is presented to the Secretary of State, regarding the lunacy affairs of Scotland.

Inspection of Asylums and Single Patients.—A most important duty of the paid commissioners is the inspection, at least twice a year, of all asylums (chartered,‖‖ district, parochial and private), all lunatic wards of poorhouses, the Lunatic Department of H.M. Prison at Perth, and the training schools for imbecile

* 20 & 21 Vict. c. 71, s. 11.
† 20 & 21 Vict. c. 71, s. 40.
‡ 20 & 21 Vict. c. 71, ss. 51, 52.
§ 50 & 51 Vict. c. 39, s. 1.
‖ 25 & 26 Vict. c. 54, s. 9.
¶ 29 & 30 Vict. c. 51, s. 14.
** *I.e.*, detained without the sanction of the Board.
†† 20 & 21 Vict. c. 71, s. 20.
‡‡ 29 & 30 Vict. c. 51, s. 20.
§§ 29 & 30 Vict. c. 51, s. 15.
‖‖ Included under the head of Public Asylums, and usually termed "Royal Asylums" (*q.v.*).

children. They are specially enjoined* to inquire into the condition of the lunatics, to record in the "Patients' Book" the general state of health of the patients, what coercion has been imposed, remarks on any special cases, and the particulars of the management of the asylum. They are empowered to visit by night or by day, and to record all inspections, stated and occasional, in a book to be kept by them.

In addition to these inspections by the commissioners, the Secretary of State may order a special visitation, and asylums are subject to the scrutiny of the Sheriff† and three of the justices of the peace specially appointed.‡ A section of the Act§ seldom put in force provides for the appointment of district inspectors by the district boards. The entries made in the patients' book on the occasions of these inspections must be copied and transmitted to the Board within eight days under a penalty for neglect.‖

The *Deputy Commissioners*, of whom there are two, are chiefly occupied in visiting lunatics in private dwellings.¶ They are deputed with such powers of the commissioners as the Board directs, and are by statute medical persons.**

Access.—Access of friends and others to lunatics is provided for by the statutes ordaining †† that the minister (clergyman) of any parish in which an asylum is situated, or the minister of any church to which a patient belongs, or any relative of a patient, or any member of the parochial board liable for the maintenance of a pauper patient has liberty to visit any such patient in an asylum, subject to the general regulations imposed by the superintendent. These regulations must have the sanction of the Board of Lunacy. Under a special instruction from the Board, the superintendent of the asylum must intimate to them any refusal of access within two days, whether it be complained of or not; and by statute an entry of the refusal must be made in the register of the asylum. The decision of the Board is made final; and an order can be obtained from the Board for access to a patient by a relative or friend for themselves, or for any medical or other person whom they may desire to have admitted. There is also provision ‡‡ for the access of

* 20 & 21 Vict. c. 71, s. 17.
† 20 & 21 Vict. c. 71, s. 25.
‡ 20 & 21 Vict. c. 71, s. 26.
§ 20 & 21 Vict. c. 71, s. 70.
‖ 20 & 21 Vict. c. 71, s. 17.
¶ See Boarding-out.
** 20 & 21 Vict. c. 71, s. 21; also 29 & 30 Vict. c. 51, s. 3.
†† 20 & 21 Vict. c. 71, ss. 47, 48.
‡‡ 20 & 21 Vict. c. 71, s. 79.

parties having an interest in the maintenance of a pauper lunatic, by warrant of the sheriff, in any investigation regarding his settlement.*

Letters.—Patients can only communicate by letter with the sanction of the superintendent; but† any letters addressed to the Board, or their secretary, or one of the commissioners, must be forwarded unopened. And any letter from the Board, or their secretary, or one of the commissioners, addressed to a patient, must be delivered unopened if marked "private." But if it appears to the Board that the contents of the letter are of such a nature that the superintendent should be made acquainted therewith, a copy will be transmitted to him.

Asylums.—There are various classes of asylums for the reception of lunatics recognised by the law.

(1) Royal, chartered, or public asylums.
(2) District asylums.
(3) Parochial asylums.
(4) Lunatic wards of poorhouses.
(5) Criminal asylums.
(6) Private asylums.
(7) Training institutions for idiots.

(1) *The chartered asylums* are charitable institutions built from legacies, or funds derived from donations, and from any profits that may accrue. They are managed by directors elected and *ex officio*, and nearly all receive both private and pauper patients. Where they have been established (all before the passing of the Lunacy Act) they have usually undertaken the work of district asylums. It was found to be unnecessary to build district asylums for certain counties where chartered asylums existed. They are supported by the payments made by the patients, either as private patients or as paupers under contract with district boards. The district boards are empowered‡ to contract with asylums existing prior to 1858, for the reception and maintenance of paupers belonging to the district, subject to the decision of the General Board. There are at present seven chartered asylums in Scotland, and at five of them paupers are received on these terms. Statutory powers have been conferred on the royal asylums to borrow money, and to grant pensions to officials.§

* The legal residence or establishment of a person, in a particular parish, town, or locality, which entitles him to maintenance of a pauper, and subjects the parish or town to his support.

† 29 & 30 Vict. c. 51, s. 16.

‡ 20 & 21 Vict. c. 71, s. 59.

§ 29 & 30 Vict. c. 51, ss. 25, 26. See ROYAL ASYLUMS.

(2 & 3) *District and Parochial Asylums.*—These were called into existence by the Acts now under consideration, and are built by assessment.* The inmates are paupers, with a comparatively small number of private patients, who have the same accommodation as pauper lunatics, and are a little above the pauper class. But these are only admitted† if the whole space be not occupied by paupers.

Parochial asylums are institutions which existed prior to 1857. No parochial asylum was called into existence by these Acts. Parochial asylums were permitted to be *continued* by 21 & 22 Vict. c. 89. They are not built by assessment, but out of the poor rate.

The whole of Scotland is divided into districts,‡ which may be varied or altered, subject to the approval of the Board. For each district a district board is chosen from and by the county council,§—and the included town councils—which has succeeded to the powers and duties of the commissioners of supply.‖ The Board may require a district board to provide an asylum after having inquired into the necessities of the district,¶ and the asylum so erected is vested in the district board, which acquires, holds, and administers it. Full powers are given to sell old or to provide new asylums,** or even to dissolve the district board †† where no district asylum is required.

The expense of providing, altering, and repairing district asylums is reported by the district board to the General Board, and the assessment is levied on counties and burghs according to the real rents.‡‡ District boards have power, subject to the approval of the Board, to make contracts for the maintenance of the lunatics of the district with any public, private, district, or parochial asylum,§§ to buy up the right of accommodation in asylums,‖‖ to acquire additional grounds,¶¶ to borrow money on the security of the assessments,*** under statutory regulations.†††

* 20 & 21 Vict. c. 71, ss. 54, 55.

† 20 & 21 Vict. c. 71, s. 80.

‡ 20 & 21 Vict. c. 71, s. 49.

§ 52 & 53 Vict. c. 50, s. 11; 40 & 41 Vict. c. 53, s. 61, &c.

‖ Commissioners appointed to assess the land tax, &c.

¶ 20 & 21 Vict. c. 71, ss. 51, 52; 25 & 26 Vict. c. 54, s. 9.

** 20 & 21 Vict. c. 71, s. 53.

†† 25 & 26 Vict. c. 54, s. 12.

‡‡ 20 & 21 Vict. c. 71, ss. 54, 55.

§§ 25 & 26 Vict. c. 54, s. 8.

‖‖ 20 & 21 Vict. c. 71, s. 58.

¶¶ 25 & 26 Vict. c. 54, s. 11. Also Lands Clauses Consolidation (Scotland) Act, 1845.

*** 20 & 21 Vict. c. 71, ss. 61, 62.

††† 20 & 21 Vict. c. 71, ss. 63, 64, 65, 66; and 25 & 26 Vict. c. 54, s. 13.

In brief, the State lays on them the duty of providing asylum accommodation for the pauper lunatics of their district, and of furnishing annual and special statements* to the General Board regarding their proceedings. The charge for pauper lunatics detained in asylums under agreement with the district board is fixed at a weekly sum, with the approbation of the General Board, and the district board is bound to keep books and accounts in such manner as the General Board directs from time to time.† It is enacted that every pauper lunatic shall be sent to a district asylum,‡ unless other arrangements have been made with the consent of the General Board. There are now ten district and six parochial asylums, and, owing to the policy of the Board, no pauper lunatic has been admitted into a private asylum for many years. By a recent Act§ the General Board have the power, on the application of the county council, burgh magistrates, or the parochial board of any parish or combination interested, to alter or vary the districts, and to regulate the whole matters arising out of such alteration, with the sanction of the Secretary of State for Scotland (*vide supra*).

(4) *Lunatic Wards of Poorhouses.*—This is an important feature in the lunacy laws—viz., that special wards in poorhouses may be licensed by the Board‖ for the reception of lunatics, for the maintenance of whom the Government subvention is payable. Moreover, no patient is admitted without the sanction of the Board; and, by statute, only those who are not dangerous, and do not require curative treatment, are admissible to these wards. The result of this is that they are a relief to the over-crowding of the lunatic asylums by the removal of incurable and inoffensive patients. Sometimes these are admitted from their homes direct, under the order of the sheriff, and with the sanction of the Board; but the great majority are transferred from the asylums.¶

(5) *Criminal Asylum at Perth.*—This is established in connection with her Majesty's General Prison, and is regulated by special Acts.** It is a separate building, and contains all the criminal lunatics in Scotland except those who may have been removed to the ordinary asylums,†† or have been discharged. Provision has been made* for criminals found insane as bar to trial, or acquitted on the ground of insanity, or becoming insane in confinement. An important section† deals with the liberation of criminal lunatics under proper precautions and regulations. In case these are infringed, warrant is issued by any principal Secretary of State for the custody and removal of the person as if no liberation had been granted.

(6) *Private Asylums.*—In former days there were many private asylums, especially in the neighbourhood of Musselburgh, but the policy pursued has limited these to a few houses for the better class of patients. They are five in number, exclusive of the specially licensed houses to be mentioned hereafter. All private asylums are licensed by the Board‡ to the superintendent of the asylum, after consideration of his qualifications and of the plan of the proposed asylum. Any alteration must be described, even if the total number of patients is not to be increased. The licence costs not less than fifteen pounds, and lasts for no longer than thirteen months.§ If the renewal of a licence be refused it may be continued for three months,‖ and if application for transfer is made, provision exists for that purpose. There is a penalty, not exceeding £100 or a year's imprisonment, attached to the offence of receiving a lunatic in an unlicensed house, or of sending him thither.¶

(7) *Training Institutions for Imbecile Children.*—These may be licensed by the Board without any fee, in the name of the superintendent for the time being. They must be supported in whole or in part by private subscription. There are at present two institutions of this nature; in addition to Dr. Ireland's training school for imbeciles, which is also inspected by the Board.

Private Dwellings.—These are of two kinds, (*a*) where not more than four patients are received; (*b*) and where not more than one patient is received.

(*a*) The Board grant special licences for the reception of not more than four lunatics to occupiers of houses without the payment of any fee.** The holders of these licences are subject to the same provisions as proprietors of private asylums.††

* 20 & 21 Vict. c. 41, s. 67.
† 20 & 21 Vict. c. 71, ss. 73, 74.
‡ 20 & 21 Vict. c. 71, s. 95.
§ 50 & 51 Vict. c. 39.
‖ 21 & 22 Vict. c. 89, s. 1; and 25 & 26 Vict. c. 54, ss. 3, 4.
¶ 25 & 26 Vict. c. 54, ss. 4, 14.
** 23 & 24 Vict. c. 105; and 40 & 41 Vict. c. 53.
†† 25 & 26 Vict. c. 54, s. 23: 34 & 35 Vict. c. 55, s. 4.

* 20 & 21 Vict. c. 71, ss. 87, 88, 89; 25 & 26 Vict. c. 54, ss. 19, 20, 21; and 34 & 35 Vict. c. 55, ss. 2, 3.
† 34 & 35 Vict. c. 55, s. 2.
‡ 20 & 21 Vict. c. 71, s. 27.
§ 20 & 21 Vict. c. 71, s. 28.
‖ 20 & 21 Vict. c. 71, ss. 29, 30.
¶ 20 & 21 Vict. c. 71, s. 39.
** 25 & 26 Vict. c. 54, s. 5.
†† Except in so far as exempted by the Board.

Sanction for reception and detention of a lunatic is given by the Board under a special form, and any one concerned in the disposal of a lunatic in one of these houses without the sanction of the Board is liable to a penalty not exceeding £10. The patients in these houses are visited by the commissioners or deputy commissioners, and a continuous record of their condition is kept. They are reported to the Board on arrival and departure, just as if they were in an asylum. Notice of reception and departure of every boarder, not being a lunatic, is to be given to the Board within three days. This by regulation of the Board.

(*b*) The reception of lunatics as single patients is governed by statute, so that any one detaining or aiding in detaining any person who on inquiry is found to be a lunatic, without the order of the sheriff or the sanction of the Board, is liable in a penalty not exceeding £20.* But fourteen days are allowed in which to make application for an order or a sanction. In case of a pauper the inspector must make application, and the sheriff may grant his order on the production of one medical certificate. Visitation is made by the commissioners or deputy commissioners, the medical attendant, and (if a pauper) by the inspector of poor (relieving officer). The medical attendant visits at least once a quarter, and the inspector of poor at least twice a year. The deputy commissioners visit as nearly as can be once a year. A record of visits is kept in a book designed for the purpose, and false entries are subject to a penalty of £10.

There is an important reservation which legalises the position of insane persons who may have been received into temporary residence, not exceeding six months, and under a medical certificate stating that the malady is not confirmed.

This is an important part of the lunacy system of Scotland, fully referred to under BOARDING-OUT (*q.v.*). Briefly, all lunatics in private dwellings who are paupers are under the control of the Board, and also all those under *curators bonis*, or who are kept for gain, or whose malady is of more than a year's duration and who are confined to the house or otherwise under any form of coercion. The dealing of the Board with these cases is intimate and constant. The statutes require a report in the circumstances detailed above, whether the patient be pauper or not, or dangerous or not, and occasionally the attention of the public is directed to this by public advertisement. It is important to note that claims on the contribution (£90,500) from imperial funds in aid of the cost of maintenance of pauper lunatics is admitted only if the Board are satisfied that the patients are properly provided for.

* 29 & 30 Vict. c. 51. s. 13.

Having now referred to the different circumstances in which lunatics may be placed for care and treatment, it becomes necessary to refer in detail to the procedure for their admission, detention, transfer, or liberation.

The detention of a lunatic in an asylum can only be secured by the order of a sheriff. The schedule in use* sets forth a petition to the sheriff supported by a statement and two medical certificates. This procedure † rests on the idea that the step is one which involves a loss of personal liberty, and accordingly the officials who are entrusted with the power of taking away personal liberty for other causes than lunacy are authorised to admit patients into an asylum. The sheriff is the judge; that is to say, he may refuse his order or call for further evidence, &c., and, whether the person in question be rich or poor, the procedure is the same. First, then, some person, who has to state the relationship in which he stands to the patient, must petition the sheriff to grant his order, and must make a statement of particulars. This is accompanied by two medical certificates granted by properly qualified medical persons, and bearing that they have separately examined the patient and found him to be a lunatic, and a fit and proper person to be placed in an asylum. Facts supporting these opinions, observed by the certifiers, must be given. A certificate must not be founded only on facts communicated by others. The petition should be signed after the statement and certificates. On these documents being presented to the sheriff, he considers them as he would any other petition which craves him to interpose his authority; and he may refuse to grant an order. If granted, the order must be acted on within fourteen days or it falls to the ground, and the date of the petition must not be more than fourteen days after the dates of the medical certificates.‡

But if, as is very probable, the circumstances do not permit of the delay which is implied in getting the sheriff's order, a certificate of emergency § granted by a qualified medical person authorises the detention of the lunatic for three

* Schedule C, 20 & 21 Vict. c. 74.

† 25 & 26 Vict. c. 54. s. 14.

‡ See Discharge or Removal, *infra*.

§ 25 & 26 Vict. c. 54. s. 14; and 29 & 30 Vict. c. 51. s. 4.

days, thus permitting of ready access to asylum treatment. By special instruction of the Board, a written request from the person desiring to place the lunatic in the asylum should accompany the certificate of emergency and be addressed to the superintendent. But if the order of the sheriff be not obtained before the expiry of the three days, the lunatic must be discharged, as his detention becomes illegal. There is no limitation as to who shall sign the petition, except in the case of paupers, when it must be done by* the inspector of poor. The primary duty of the inspector of poor, however, on learning of the presence of an unintimated pauper lunatic in his parish, is to report the fact to the Board and to the parochial board, under a statutory penalty of £10 in case of failure. He must also observe the same rule when made aware of a lunatic in an asylum becoming chargeable to his parish, and must similarly intimate when the chargeability of the pauper is transferred to another parish.

The settlement of pauper lunatics is often much disputed. The statutes distinctly state that a pauper lunatic is to be held to belong to the parish of his legal settlement† at the time of the sheriff's order granted in his case. By the next section it is provided that the parish of settlement is to be liable in payment of expenses subject to the decision of the sheriff in assessing them. But if the lunatic has adequate estate, it must bear the expense of maintenance, &c. If the lunatic is a pauper, the expense will be defrayed by the parish in which he was found, and from which he was sent. The sheriff is empowered ‡ to certify the amount of expenses, and his finding is not subject to review. Notice must be given to the parish of settlement by the parish disbursing these expenses.

The order for admission into an asylum costs § five shillings for a non-pauper, and half a crown for a pauper lunatic. These fees are remitted by the sheriff clerk ‖ to the Board, and are at present applied in reduction of the estimate of the Board's expenses. And whatever ¶ balance of moneys over receipts for such fees, licences, &c., may be necessary, is voted by Parliament. The sheriff clerk is also bound to send notice to the

* 20 & 21 Vict. c. 71, s. 112; and 25 & 26 Vict. c. 54, s. 18.

† 20 & 21 Vict. c. 71, s. 75, *et seq.*

‡ 20 & 21 Vict. c. 71, s. 78.

§ 20 & 21 Vict. c. 71, s. 31; and 29 & 30 Vict. c. 51, s. 22.

‖ 20 & 21 Vict. c. 71, s. 32.

¶ 20 & 21 Vict. c. 71, s. 33.

Board as to each order within seven days from the granting of the order, under a penalty not exceeding £10.* The sheriff's order is granted by the sheriff of the county in which the lunatic is found, or in which the asylum is situated, and the procedure is governed by the undernoted sections.† The order and medical certificates may be amended, if incorrect or defective, within twenty-one days after admission, but these amendments must obtain the sanction of the Board, or they may refer the matter to the sheriff for recall should he decide on that course.‡

The **medical certificates** § must not be granted by persons having immediate or pecuniary interest in the asylum in which the lunatic is placed; nor can a medical officer of any asylum grant a certificate of insanity for the reception of any lunatic, not a pauper, into such asylum, except the certificate of emergency. Heavy penalties are attached to the offences of granting a certificate without examination or of granting it falsely. Unqualified medical persons are specially debarred from practising under the Lunacy Acts; and precautions are taken to prevent any qualified medical person granting lunacy certificates with reference to an asylum in which he has pecuniary interest or concern.‖

If any action at law be raised against a medical person in respect of a lunacy certificate under these Acts, it must be initiated within a year of the date of liberation of the person who alleges injury, and the Lord Ordinary tries the case without a jury.¶

On the admission of a patient to an asylum it becomes the duty of the superintendent to report upon the physical condition of the person so admitted within three days, by regulation of the Board. And by statute it is enacted** that copies of the orders, medical certificates, petition, and statement shall be transmitted to the Board by the superintendent within fourteen clear days but after two clear days from the day of admission. With these copies must be sent a notice of admission and a report as to the mental and bodily condition of the lunatic by the medical attendant of the asylum. This must be in the prescribed

* 20 & 21 Vict. c. 71, s. 37.

† 25 & 26 Vict. c. 54, s. 14; 29 & 30 Vict. c. 51, ss. 4, 5, 6, 7.

‡ 29 & 30 Vict. c. 39, s. 5.

§ 25 & 26 Vict. c. 54, s. 14; and schedule D, 20 & 21 Vict. c. 71.

‖ 20 & 21 Vict. c. 71, s. 71.

¶ 29 & 30 Vict. c. 52, s. 24.

** 20 & 21 Vict. c. 71, s. 37.

form,* and failure to transmit is punishable by fine of £20.

In every asylum licensed for 100 patients a medical person must be resident,† and in every asylum licensed for more than 50 a medical person must visit daily. Rules are also laid down as to the visiting of smaller asylums by medical persons. It is a statutory duty of the superintendent to keep a register of lunatics in which particulars are entered according to schedule.‡ The formalities of admission may be delayed by the distance at which the lunatic is found from the asylum, and the law has provided a remedy § for that in the case of Orkney and Shetland. Another part of the statutes deals ‖ with the difficulty of conveying dangerous lunatics from remote localities. It provides for a justice of the peace, on sworn credible information, granting a warrant for safe custody and transmission to the nearest town in which a sheriff or sheriff substitute resides.

There is a small class of lunatics, not criminal, but dangerous or offensive to decency, who are dealt with after apprehension under a special clause.¶ The sheriff may, in such a case, on the application of the procurator fiscal (public prosecutor) or the inspector of poor or any person, accompanied by a medical certificate so describing the lunatic, commit him to safe custody. The sheriff thereupon causes notice to be given in the local newspapers of such a commitment, and that it is intended to inquire into the condition of the lunatic on a day named. If lunacy is shown to exist, the sheriff ** issues an order for removal to an asylum, and detention there until recovery takes place, or until two medical men approved by him certify that the lunatic may be discharged without risk of injury to himself or the public.

Voluntary patients are also admitted under a special section.†† These patients are desirous of submitting themselves to treatment, but their mental state is not such as renders it legal to grant certificates of insanity. They can only be received on the previous assent of one of the commissioners, which is given in the form of a sanction to the superintendent to keep and entertain the patient as a boarder. It is necessary that the commissioner should have the patient's written application before he grants the sanction. It is also enacted that all voluntary patients must be produced to the commissioners at their visits, and none can be detained for more than three days after having given notice of intention to leave the asylum, unless in the interval the sheriff's order be obtained subject to all the regulations aforesaid.*

The penalties for maltreatment are set forth by statute;† and, by the rule of the Board, the superintendent is obliged to give immediate notice to the procurator fiscal if a patient has been seriously hurt. The fiscal then investigates the case, and takes action if so advised.

Moreover, all attendants must be notified to the Board on arrival and departure, and the reasons for their departure must be specified. The Board keeps a register of attendants, and when an attendant, against whose name an evil report stands,‡ is engaged, the superintendent engaging him is notified by the secretary as to the facts, and must say if he intends to retain the services of the person referred to. This is governed by special instructions from the Board, and gives some security against maltreatment; which is further regulated by an instruction to the effect that the procurator fiscal must be made aware of any maltreatment of a serious nature within twelve hours, and precautions must be taken to prevent any incriminated party from leaving the asylum.

Improper detention is provided for under the statutory regulations above detailed, and any patient, on liberation from asylum control, who considers himself to have been unjustly confined, may get without charge a copy of the order, petition, and certificates on which he was confined.§ Since the passing of these Acts there has been but one action in Scotland on account of illegal detention, and

* Schedule F, 20 & 21 Vict. c. 71.

† 20 & 21 Vict. c. 71, ss. 45, 46.

‡ Schedule I, 20 & 21 Vict. c. 71.

§ 25 & 26 Vict. c. 54, s. 14.

‖ 20 & 21 Vict. c. 71, s. 90.

¶ 25 & 26 Vict. c. 54, s. 15.

** That is, if the inspector of the parish does not within twenty-four hours undertake to the satisfaction of the sheriff to provide for the safe custody of the lunatic.

†† 29 & 30 Vict. c. 51, s. 15.

* The Board have recently referred at length to the position of voluntary patients in asylums. They state that no person should be received or kept in an asylum as a voluntary patient unless he fully understands and appreciates the voluntary nature of his residence. Should it be necessary, for the safety of the patient, that he should be certified, the Board recommend that he should be removed on that step to another asylum, if there has been no marked change in the mental state since admission. And the Board also indicate that the superintendent should regard voluntary and certified patients with an equal feeling of responsibility.

† 20 & 21 Vict. c. 71, s. 99.

‡ That is, notice of dismissal from an asylum for serious misconduct has been received.

§ 20 & 21 Vict. c. 71, s. 94.

it was not instigated by the patient himself.

Discharge or Removal.—The sheriff's order is not granted without limit as to time. It remains in force although the patient may be absent from the asylum * temporarily. The lunatic may have been absent on pass or by having escaped for twenty-eight days, or may have been absent for three months under the personal care of the asylum officials, or may have been absent for a specified time on probation with the consent of the Board.† But if these periods have been exceeded, or if the superintendent or medical attendant fail to grant a statutory certificate ‡ after the expiry of three years from the date of the order,§ or if the superintendent give notice of the discharge of the lunatic, then the sheriff's order remains no longer in force—the authority for the detention of the person as lunatic lapses.

Pauper lunatics may be discharged by authority of the parochial board, at a duly constituted meeting, if a certified copy of the minute be left with the superintendent of the asylum, and if the patient be not a dangerous lunatic, either detained as such or certified by the superintendent as such.‖ Strict regulations are laid down for the protection of lunatics so removed.¶

Liberation on probation ** is granted on the application of the person at whose instance a lunatic is detained, the nearest known relative, or the inspector of poor of the parish, or by the Board, without an order by the sheriff. The Board fixes the time and regulations under which the probation is authorised, but the period is limited to twelve months, and it is specially enacted that the conditions on which probationary discharge is granted shall not be altered.††

* 29 & 30 Vict. c. 51, s. 6.

† 25 & 26 Vict. c. 54, s. 16.

‡ *I.e.*, that the detention of the lunatic is necessary and proper, either for his own welfare or the safety of the public, in the last fortnight of December of each year, or on the 1st day of January.

§ 29 & 30 Vict. c. 51, s. 7. "*In no case shall the sheriff's order remain in force longer than the first day of January first occurring after the expiry of three years from the date on which it was granted; or than the first day of January in each succeeding year, unless the superintendent or medical attendant of the asylum, on each of the first days of January, or within fourteen clear days immediately* preceding, *grant and transmit to the Board a certificate, on soul and conscience, that the detention of the lunatic is necessary and proper, either for his own welfare or the safety of the public.*"

‖ 29 & 30 Vict. c. 51, s. 9.

¶ 29 & 30 Vict. c. 51, ss. 10, 11.

** 25 & 26 Vict. c. 54, s. 16.

†† 25 & 26 Vict. c. 54, s. 16; 29 & 30 Vict. c. 51, s. 8.

Recovery * of a lunatic, in so far that he may be safely liberated without risk of injury to himself or others, must be intimated to the Board by the superintendent of the asylum, and also to the person at whose instance the lunatic was detained, or to the nearest known relative, or to the inspector of poor. If these do not remove the person, the Board may order his discharge forthwith, and the expenses will be borne by the parish liable.†

The liberation of a lunatic is provided for by statute in the following manner:‡—Any person who may have procured two certificates from medical persons approved by the sheriff, and who in consequence may have obtained an order of liberation from the sheriff, may procure the liberation of the lunatic. The Board may similarly grant an order for liberation, but with this difference—the certificate laid before the sheriff may be to the effect that the lunatic has recovered or may be liberated without risk of injury to himself or others, while the certificates on which the Board can act must be of absolute recovery. The facts of these removals must be entered in the register and transmitted to the Board. Lunatics detained by courts of law§ cannot be released under this section without the authority of the Court or the warrant of a principal Secretary of State. Should an attempt be made to remove a dangerous lunatic the case must be reported by the superintendent to the procurator fiscal.‖

Lunatics may be **transferred** from one asylum to another under various circumstances.¶ Should certificates be granted by two medical persons that an asylum is unsuitable for the confinement of any lunatic, the procurator fiscal or one of the commissioners may make application to the sheriff for an order for removal to another asylum, and, when such is granted, intimation to the responsible parties must be made.** If the superintendent of any asylum shall show good cause to the Board, they may grant authority for the transfer of patients from one building to another without any additional sheriff's

* 25 & 26 Vict. c. 54, s. 17.

† 25 & 26 Vict. c. 54, ss. 17, 18. The superintendent of an asylum has no longer any statutory authority to detain a patient after he ceases to be a lunatic.

‡ 20 & 21 Vict. c. 71, s. 92.

§ 20 & 21 Vict. c. 71, s. 93.

‖ 29 & 30 Vict. c. 51, s. 12.

¶ 20 & 21 Vict. c. 71, s. 91.

** 20 & 21 Vict. c. 71, s. 44. This section refers only to the transfer of the patients from one building to another, as when the licence of a private asylum is transferred (see 25 & 26 Vict. c. 54, s. 16), which gives authority for transfer of a patient and for probation.

order. But due intimation must be given to the parties interested, and notice must be made to the Board regarding the patients so transferred.* The usual form of transfer is an authorisation from the Board granted on the application of the nearest known relative or inspector of poor, or the person at whose instance the lunatic was confined. This application is accompanied by a statement and a medical certificate, and the effect of the authority for transfer is to continue the original sheriff's order in the asylum to which the lunatic is conveyed as if no such change had taken place.

Escape.—By a regulation of the Board all escapes must be reported to the Board within fourteen days from the date of escape. By a recent Act† the commissioners have the power to authorise an application to be made to the sheriff for a warrant to retake a lunatic who may have escaped from Scotland to England or Ireland. This warrant is sufficient authority for any justice of the peace in England or Ireland to countersign the same, and such warrant may then be legally executed in the countries named. The question as to whether the police have power to arrest a lunatic under a sheriff's order has not been decided in the law courts.

The **death** of a lunatic must be entered in a register kept for that purpose,‡ and notified to the responsible parties and to the Board. By special instruction of the Board every case of sudden or unexpected death, or death under suspicious circumstances, is to be at once intimated to the procurator fiscal and to the Board.

Restraint and seclusion, as well as the compulsory use of the shower bath, must be entered in a register kept for the purpose. By a special instruction of the Board restraint is defined as follows: Whenever a patient is made to wear an article of dress, or is placed in any apparatus which is fastened so as to prevent the patient from putting it off without assistance, and which restricts the movements of the patient and the use of his hands and feet, it is restraint. And whenever a patient is placed by day in any room or locality alone, and with the door of exit locked or fastened, or held in such a way as to prevent the egress of the patient, it is seclusion.

The **statistics** of insanity in Scotland, as officially reported by the General Board of Lunacy for 1890, may be briefly summed up as follows:

* 25 & 26 Vict. c. 54, s. 16.
† 52 & 53 Vict. c. 41, s. 79.
‡ 20 & 21 Vict. c. 71, s. 97.

The number of lunatics [illegible] the official cognisance of the Board was 12,595; 10,539 of these were maintained by parochial rates, 1945 from private sources, and 57 at the expense of the State. The royal and district asylums contained 5589 pauper and 1527 private patients. The poorhouse wards contained 882 paupers, besides 1517 in parochial asylums. There were 152 private patients in private asylums, but no paupers. Private dwellings accommodated 124 private and 2489 pauper lunatics. The lunatic department of H.M. prison at Perth contained 57 lunatics, the training institutions 142 private and 116 pauper idiots and imbeciles.

During the year 522 private and 2213 pauper patients were received into establishments by direct admission (sheriffs' orders), while there were 30 private and 321 pauper transfers; 98 voluntary patients were admitted, the total number of such cases resident on January 1, 1891, being 61. 199 private patients and 975 paupers were discharged recovered. Those unrecovered were removed as follows: By friends 114, by minute of parochial boards 328, by escape 17, after probation 46, on expiry of emergency certificate 1, by warrant of sheriff 35, by being placed in Perth prison as a Queen's pleasure lunatic 1, total 542. The deaths numbered 140 and 638 for private and pauper patients respectively. 105 cases were discharged on statutory probation, exclusive of those sent out on trial for twenty-eight days.

These figures show a great increase since the Board was first constituted. The number of those under cognisance has, in fact, doubled. The development of the lunacy administration of Scotland has proceeded upon the lines indicated by the undermentioned Acts of Parliament, and is set forth in detail in the annual reports of the General Board of Lunacy.

Lunacy Acts, Scotland.

Lunacy:

20 & 21 Vict. c. 71. An Act for the regulation of the care and treatment of lunatics, and for the provision, maintenance, and regulation of lunatic asylums in Scotland. 1857.

21 & 22 Vict. c. 89. An Act to amend the act of last session. 1858.

25 & 26 Vict. c. 54. An Act to make further provision respecting lunacy. 1862.

27 & 28 Vict. c. 59. An Act as to deputy commissioners and others. 1864.

29 & 30 Vict. c. 51. An Act to amend the Acts relating to lunacy. 1866.

30 & 31 Vict. c. 55. An Act to enlarge for the present year the time within which

certain certificates regarding lunatics may be granted. 1867.

34 & 35 Vict. c. 55. An Act to amend the law relating to dangerous and criminal lunatics. 1871.

50 & 51 Vict. c. 39. An Act relative to lunacy districts. 1887.

52 & 53 Vict. c. 41. An Act to amend the Acts relating to lunatics (certain sections applicable to Scotland). 1889.

52 & 53 Vict. c. 50. An Act to amend the laws relating to Local Government. 1889.

Also references in these:

Assessments:

14 & 15 Vict. c. 23. An Act to authorise the advance of money. 1851.

17 & 18 Vict. c. 91. An Act for the valuation of lands and heritages. 1854.

20 & 21 Vict. c. 58. Valuation of Lands Amendment Act. 1857.

31 & 32 Vict. c. 82. County General Assessment Act. 1868.

Prisons:

23 & 24 Vict. c. 105. The Prisons Administration Act. 1860.

40 & 41 Vict. c. 53. The Prisons Act. 1877.

Court of Session:

13 & 14 Vict. c. 36. An Act to facilitate procedure in the Court of Session. 1850.

20 & 21 Vict. c. 56. An Act to regulate the distribution of business in the Court of Session. 1857.

31 & 32 Vict. c. 100. (Cognition, s. 101.) To amend the procedure in the Court of Session. 1868.

Factors:

12 & 13 Vict. c. 51. The Pupils Protection Act. 1849.

43 & 44 Vict. c. 4. Judicial Factors Act. 1880.

52 & 53 Vict. c. 39. Judicial Factors Act. 1889.

Also the various Acts of Sederunt of the Court of Session bearing on these Court of Session and Factors Acts, published yearly in the Parliament House Book.

Drunkards:

42 & 43 Vict. c. 19. The Habitual Drunkards Act. 1879.

51 & 52 Vict. c. 19. The Inebriates Act. 1888. A. R. URQUHART.

SCYTHIAN DISEASE.—Disease said to be not infrequent in the Caucasus, and occasionally seen elsewhere, characterised by atrophy of the male reproductive organs in adults, followed by mental abnormity, leading to the assumption of the dress and habits of women. (Billings.)

SEASONS, EFFECTS OF. (*See* STATISTICS.)

SEBASTOMANIA (σεβαστός, worshipped; μανία, madness). A term for religious insanity.

SECLUSION. (*See* TREATMENT.)

SECONDARY SENSATIONS (Ger. *Secundärempfindungen*; Fr. *audition colorée*).—There are people with whom every sensation of sound is accompanied by a sensation of light. If, for instance, a bell is rung in the vicinity of such a person (colour-hearer), he not only hears the sound as such, but at the same time observes a red colour; if he hears the letter *a* (German *a*) pronounced, he has the impression of a blue colour.

Such sensations for which the physical cause seems inadequate (a sensation of light produced by sound) are called **secondary sensations**; primary and secondary sensations together are designated as **dual sensations**.

In addition to (1) sensations of colour accompanying sensations of sound (**sound photisms**), other secondary sensations have been observed, namely: (2) Sensations of sound from perception through light (**light phonisms**); (3) Sensations of colour from perception through taste (**taste photisms**); (4) Sensations of colour from perception through smell (**odour photisms**); (5) Sensations of colour from perception of pain, temperature, and touch (**pain photisms, &c.**).

In **sensations of colour caused by musical sounds** the shade is determined by the pitch, the lighter shades corresponding usually to a high pitch, the darker to a low pitch. The colours representing different tones vary with different persons. The scale of colours corresponding to the scale of musical sounds passes most frequently from dark brown or dark red, through red and yellow to white. In isolated cases, however, the lower notes give colours quite different from the higher; thus, D produces a brownish violet, A, a Prussian blue, A_1, an ochre, C_4, a whitish yellow.

The overtones (partial tones) of a sound often cause, in addition to the photism of the fundamental tone, special photisms which can be separated from each other even when the acoustic impression appears as a single sound. By representing the partial tones of a sound on a coloured top, Nussbaumer, a colour-hearer, was able to imitate the photism of the entire sound.

Entire musical selections usually make the impression only of the single sounds with which the photisms come and go. Often, however, an entire combination of sounds, a melody, and especially a particular key, appears in a fixed colour, so that, for instance, a whole piece of music seems dark blue because it is written in E flat. With many persons sounds from different instruments produce different colours, so that all notes of a cornet are yellow (light or dark according to the pitch), while those from a flute seem blue.

Noises also have corresponding photisms. These are generally brown or gray; other colours, red especially, are less frequent.

Most *sound photisms* are projected on externality, not, however, on the field of vision as ordinary sensations of light, but on the field of hearing; they are localised just as the sound itself is. Thus the sound and its accompanying photism produced by a guitar seem, in the opinion of the colour-hearer, to come from the string struck; the bright photism of a note from a fife appears to come out of the fife, &c. If the sound itself is falsely localised (ringing in the ears referred to externality) the same occurs with the photism. In a few rare cases sound photisms are always localised in the head.

The **limitation in space** of sound photisms is even more uncertain than their localisation, but the photisms of higher and less sonorous sounds have, other things being equal, more definite boundaries than those from lower and more sonorous ones; their expansion, too, is much less. In a few cases the colour phenomena assume definite forms and appear as flames, as brilliant drops, and the like. The photisms of simultaneously occurring sounds often unite to form a single colour; under other circumstances the different single colours are sharply differentiated from each other. The latter often occurs with discords, while the colours from sounds which accord easily unite.

The **duration** of photisms is exactly the same as that of the sounds which produce them. The sensation of colour and form referred to a definite locality lasts just as long as the sound is heard. If the first sound is replaced by a second, the photism is, in the same moment, correspondingly changed.

The photisms of the *sounds* of *speech* occupy a peculiar position. Of all photisms those for vowels are most frequent. It may be stated as a rule that *e* and *a* (German *i* and *e*) give light colours, *o* and *u* (long) darker, while *a*, as in "are," sometimes gives darker colours, sometimes lighter, *e* (long) gives a great preponderance of white. The higher vowels have, therefore, like the higher musical tones, lighter shades, the lower darker. Other than these no rules can be given for the photisms of the vowel sounds.

For the *consonants* colour sensations are much rarer. They are, if present at all, usually very weak, of a greyish colour, and are only exceptionally strongly coloured.

Photisms for *entire words* [illegible] they are usually of several colours, which correspond to the colours of the sounds composing the word. Although the pronunciation of a word progresses in time, in the mind of the colour-hearer the photisms of the entire word are blended to form a simple image, that is, from the succession in time of the sound impressions results a juxtaposition in space of their photisms; thus, for the author, the word "country" consists of a brownish part (*ou*), and a smaller white part (*y*), which are connected with each other from left to right. Word photisms are often of a single colour, which, generally, corresponds to the principal vowel or the principal syllable—"Rudolph," for example, may be green with a person whose photism for *u* is green.

Names of *persons, months, days of the week*, and *numbers* often produce ideas of a single colour. These do not always correspond to the colours of the component parts, and, therefore, differ in principle from sound photisms proper. Perhaps they are due simply to the influence of the constant involuntary association of ideas. In isolated instances the colour image for the sound of a name can be easily separated from the colour impression for the corresponding conception (conceptions, too, produce sensations of colour); thus, with the author, the photism for the word "Friday" is white, the day itself is thought of as blue. These single-colour ideas for numbers, names, &c., seem to follow no well-defined rule.

The photism of an *entire speech* depends, first, on the voice of the speaker, then on the language, that is, on the predominance of particular sounds (vowels or consonants). The photisms of the words follow each other so quickly that it is generally impossible to fix the attention on them, while the voice remains about the same throughout and so determines the impression.

Not sound alone, but all sense perceptions produce sensations of colour. There are people who have a photism with every taste, with every smell. On account of the infrequency of taste and smell photisms it is at present impossible to give with certainty any general rules concerning them. Agreeable, delicate tastes and smells, however, seem to produce the more agreeable and delicate shades of colour; disagreeable sensations cause correspondingly disagreeable colours. Green, a colour rare in other forms of photisms, occurs comparatively often in taste photisms. With these taste and smell photisms, more important, probably, than the colour itself is its transferency, its distinctness, and its saturation.

Taste photisms are nearly always referred to that part of the oral cavity which receives the sensation. With *odours* the colour is referred not only to the nose itself, but the space surrounding the person and the fragrant body—that is, the immediate neighbourhood of the body seems filled with the colour.

In photisms of **cutaneous sensibility** the general law seems to prevail that the sensation produced depends upon the extent of cutaneous surface receiving the impression; thus, if but a point is touched, the photism is brighter than when a surface is affected. Pain generally gives strong, even brilliant colours. Red and yellow predominate also in these photisms.

With some persons sensations of sound are produced by the **sight of certain forms and colours** (*phonisms*). Phonisms are usually very slight noises, rarely loud sounds. Since these are very uncommon, not much can be said concerning them.

The disagreeable sensations which many people experience from a screeching sound have been described as **secondary sensations of general feeling.**

With most colour-hearers these secondary sensations invariably accompany the primary sensations. The former may be blended with associated ideas of the primary perceptions; thus, a colour-hearer may conceive Adam as blue because the photism of the word "Adam" is blue, &c. In an article in the *Musical World*, entitled "Scales and Colours," Grant Allen examines Haydn's "Creation," and finds that, according to the key, chaos is composed in dark and gloomy colours, light in white, &c. In the autumn of 1883 a long discussion over this subject was carried on in the *Standard*.

From the examination of a few exquisite colour-hearers, Bleuler and Lehmann conclude that photisms have no influence upon the function of the eyes, phonisms no influence upon the function of the ears. Urbantschitsch, on the contrary, found, by examining a great number of persons (not colour-hearers), that looking at certain colours increases the capacity for hearing certain sounds; that a high note of a tuning-fork seems higher when one looks at red, blue, green, or yellow, but lower if at violet. The apparent contradiction in the observations of Urbantschitsch and Bleuler and Lehmann seems to indicate that these observers investigated different phenomena.

Laws.—The individual testimony of different persons concerning secondary sensations presents no general conformity. A few laws, however, seem well established: (1) Photisms light in colour are produced by sounds of high quality, intense pain, sharply defined sensation of touch, small forms, pointed forms; dark photisms from opposite conditions; (2) High phonisms are produced by bright light, well-defined outlines, small forms, pointed forms; low phonisms from opposite conditions; (3) Photisms with well-defined forms, small photisms, pointed photisms are produced by sounds of high pitch; (4) Red, yellow, and brown are frequent photism colours, violet and green are rare, while blue stands between these extremes.

Frequency. — Secondary sensations occur more frequently than is generally supposed. Bleuler and Lehmann found such sensations in 76 persons out of 596 (12¾ per cent.). A disposition to secondary sensations seems to be present with most persons, for such expressions as "clear tones," "pointed tones" ("spitze Töne"), "dull sounds," &c., are found in all languages, are understood by everybody, and are in harmony with rules given for secondary sensations. Wundt ("Physiologische Psychologie") ascribes to these a chief part in the formation of language.

Secondary sensations are transmissible by **heredity.** Entire families of colour-hearers are known. A connection with nervous and mental disease is unproved.

Many **theories** have been suggested to explain colour-hearing. Some of these will not bear even the most superficial criticism, and all are incapable of positive proof. The explanation commonly offered, that colour-hearing is due to a simple association of ideas which constantly occur together, is certainly false. The regularity with which light colours predominate for high notes, &c., is on this theory unexplainable.

The colours appearing in photisms differ but slightly from the ordinary colours perceived by the eye. It must be noticed, however, that these photism-colours usually appear as pure colour sensations, separated from all ideas of matter which are associated with every coloured surface. They can best be compared with coloured flames, or with evening red in a cloudless sky. Photism colours have been observed, although very rarely, which optically have never been perceived, which indeed are, optically, inconceivable; for example, the author's photism for the German modified *u* (ü) is a mixture of light red and yellow and a little blue without producing a trace of green.

The surroundings of photisms—that is, the field on which they appear—are not black, but a neutral ground free from every colour.

The **transitions** from one photism to another frequently correspond to similar changes in common colours; thus for a colour-hearer *a* (in "father") may be blue, *o* (in "bone") yellow, and the sound between these two *oa* (a in "water"), green. Mixtures of colours frequently occur and follow the ordinary laws which govern the mixing of pigments; for example, the simple photism of a word of two syllables may be orange, because the vowel of the first syllable appears red, and that of the second, yellow.

The **colour sensations caused by optic impressions** differ somewhat from ordinary secondary sensations. These occur very infrequently, are usually less exactly defined than other photisms, yet always clear enough to admit of description. One rule only can be stated for these: pointed and small bodies produce lighter colours than blunt and larger bodies. Perhaps the colour phenomena are photisms of form-phonisms—that is, tertiary sensations.

Bearing a certain relation to secondary sensations, but perhaps differing in nature from them, are **impressions of form for general ideas** (as for piety), especially for a series, for a succession of numbers, musical scales, days of the week, &c. Such "form ideas" are more frequent than photisms, but appear with colour-hearers to be very pronounced. Francis Galton in his work, "Enquiries into Human Faculty and its Development" (1883), devoted considerable attention to these "numberl forms" and similar phenomena. With these ideas a certain, though unconscious process of reflection cannot be excluded.

E. Bleuler.

[*References.*—The first observations of secondary sensations were published by Pick in Mendel's Neurologisches Centralblatt, 1887, p. 536, and by Lussana, Sur l'audition colorée, Arch. Italiennes de Biologie, 1883. Further, the following publications are of importance: Nussbaumer, Wiener med. Wochenschrift, 1873, Nos. 1–3. Bleuler and Lehmann, Zwangsmässige Lichtempfindungen durch Schall und verwandte Erscheinungen, Leipzig, 1881 (report of seventy-seven cases). Francis Galton, Enquiries into Human Faculty and its Development, Macmillan & Co., 1883. Rochas, in La Nature, 1885, April, May, September. Girandeau, De l'audition colorée, in l'Encéphale, 1885, p. 589. Baratoux, Audition colorée, in Progrès médic., 1887. Steinbrügge, Ueber secundäre Sinnesempfindungen, Wiesbaden, 1887 (preliminary report of 442 cases). Urbantschitsch, Sitzungsbericht der Gesellschaft der Aerzte in Wien, Oct. 1, 1887. Münchner med. Wochenschrift, Oct. 25, 1887, p. 845. Suarez de Mendoza, L'audition colorée, Paris, 1890.]

SECONDARY V[illegible].—A synonym for Secondary D[illegible] insanity.

SEDATIVES.—Under this heading we shall include sedatives proper, hypnotics or soporifics, narcotics. Before considering these in detail we must first say a few words on sleep, and the general means at our disposal for inducing it.

The activities of the body during sleep are, as a whole, lowered, the pulse-rate is diminished, the breathing less frequent, the movements of the stomach and intestines less. There is less heat produced, secretion is not so free. Most striking of all, however, is the quiescence of the central nervous system, which shows itself in the cord and lower centres generally by an impaired reflex excitability* (of which, indeed, the above phenomena are, to a great extent, the expression), and in the brain by abolition, at times perhaps complete, of the more complex workings of the cortex. A sleeping man has been likened to a being which has suffered extirpation of its cerebral hemispheres, and at any rate these organs are not functionally in evidence. It is generally accepted that the brain during sleep contains less blood than in the waking state.

The object of sleep is repair, and for this the vital activities which still persist are, in health, wholly sufficient.

Sleep varies much in health—i.e., in degree; and this not only among different individuals, but also for the same individual at different times. Each spell of sleep, moreover, has its own curve of intensity. At the beginning, the dip into sleep is greatest, and is to be measured by fathoms, then the curve rises rapidly again, and thence on, till the awakening, sleep is comparatively light, the organism is in shallow waters. The ultimate causes of sleep it is unnecessary to consider. They are still obscure. It is sufficient for us that we have in sleep another instance of periodicity belonging essentially to all organisms, and that the capacity for sleep, though it may suffer great modification by disease, is never abolished completely. We must always bear this in mind in our treatment of sleeplessness, viz., that the organism before us is still capable of sleep if we can only find out and remove the disturbing elements. It is necessary that we should remember further that sleep is one thing and unconsciousness another,

* This is true generally in spite of the fact that certain local mechanisms appear to be in a state of excitation—*cf.* the closure of the eyelids and the contracted state of the pupils (Landois, "Physiology"); and that certain reflexes appear to be more easily started during sleep—*e.g.*, glottic spasm in laryngismus stridulus and catarrhal croup.

and that we seek sleep, not for the sake of unconsciousness, but for the sake of rest and repair. But repair demands the activities of the vital processes. Hence we must always aim at procuring sleep at least cost; *i.e.*, with least interference of these processes.

For all functions, periodic in their nature, there is, if interference be called for, a right and a wrong time to interfere.

This holds pre-eminently for sleep, and more particularly for those cases in which we aim at obtaining sleep of the most natural kind possible. It may be stated as an axiom that the more gentle the means employed to induce sleep, the more natural will be the sleep induced; and further, that the more gentle the means employed, the more careful must we be to select the right time for their use. This is the meaning of the formula "hora somni sumendus"; viz., that the adjuvant must come in at that moment when the organism is itself moving sleepwards.

In studying the problem of sleep procuring we shall do best to examine the natural phenomena of sleep in health, and to imitate these as far as possible. The physiology of the bedroom is the withdrawal of the organism from disturbing influences, light, sound, and the maintenance of the temperature of the body by means of a minimum of heat production. The therapeutics of the sick chamber will require the more careful exclusion of external stimuli, and the question of an extra blanket, or a hot bottle to the feet, may have to be considered. Soporifics of this class will include all and every means at our disposal for *removing* the irritant, external or internal, which is preventing sleep. It is not necessary to specify further.

Next it is recognised in physiology that the prolonged and uniform application of certain stimuli of small degree of intensity promotes sleep. Thus the monotone of a voice, the stroking of the hand, or playing with the hair, have frequently the required soothing effect. These means have their value in sickness also, and accordingly we recognise that the *addition* of *certain* stimuli, defined as above, gives us a new class of soporifics. It is certain that the phenomena of hypnotism depend to some extent upon this engaging of the consciousness by gentle and continuous stimulation. The phenomena of Braidism, for instance, are of this kind. Heidenhain considers that in such we have to deal with the inhibition of the activity of the cells of the cortex cerebri.

For further information on this subject see HYPNOTISM.

Before leaving this class it may, perhaps, be well to mention the value in some cases of a small quantity of light food shortly before sleeping time. This is sometimes of undoubted value, and it may be that the explanation of its action falls in here, for in it we have the addition of a slight stimulus to the organs of digestion; possibly also the slight afflux of blood to the site of stimulation is a further element in causing sleep, since it must to some extent withdraw from the brain.

Should the organism not respond to these simpler means we must examine the nervous system peripherally and centrally, for it may be that an abnormal state is at fault, and not abnormal stimulation. If peripheral, *e.g.*, pruritus (without external cause), a neuralgia, with inflamed nerve-trunk or nerve-ending, then we shall look among local analgesics (*e.g.*, heat or warmth, cocaine, &c.) for the required soporific. If central, or if we are unable to combat the local trouble by local means, then our remedies must be such as influence the central nervous system. To this class more properly belong the remedies known as somnifacients, soporifics, hypnotics, and narcotics.

At the outset we must put the question, Is there a distinction between hypnotics and narcotics? Dujardin-Beaumetz answers in the affirmative. He holds that for the drug to be hypnotic it must imitate the natural condition of sleep by effecting a lowered intra-cranial pressure, and that drugs which, though bringing about unconsciousness, do not lower cerebral pressure, or which increase it, cannot claim to be hypnotics. On this line he separates chloral as a hypnotic from opium as a narcotic. Whether this position can be maintained is doubtful. In disease we are certainly familiar with loss of consciousness in association with raised intra-cranial pressure; *e.g.*, the coma of apoplexy. But we are also familiar with unconsciousness as the result of a toxæmia; *e.g.*, the coma of uræmia. And though such unconscious states differ strikingly from natural sleep, yet in the different forms of artificial or drugged sleep it is probable that these two factors—quantity of blood, including blood pressure, and quality of blood—do each play a part. To dissociate these factors, however, in any given case is very difficult, and it will therefore be safest not to attempt any such absolute separation.

It will be convenient to arrange in groups the drugs employed as sleep producers. In this we shall follow Schmiedeberg ("Grundriss der Arzneimittellehre," 1888).

The first group includes the bromides of potassium, sodium, ammonium, and lithium. It is included in the larger class of salts, of which chloride of sodium may be taken as the structural type.

Potassium bromide is the best known member of the group, and the following statements will refer to it.*

It is a general depressant to the tissues; the frequency and force of the heart's action are lowered; the temperature (in toxic doses) is decidedly lowered; the nervo-muscular system is generally affected—thus the muscles are relaxed, sensation is impaired both general and special (skin, sight, hearing), in particular the mucous membrane of the soft palate and fauces is benumbed; reflex irritability of the spinal cord as a whole is lessened; sexual vigour may be impaired or abolished (it is to be noted that the sexual act is in part a skin reflex: Gowers); the receptivity of the brain is diminished—*cf.* lowering of sensation; the motor area is less easily roused into action (this has been shown by direct irritation of the motor area in dogs); the finer workings of the cortical cells are interfered with; there is mental apathy even to hebetude; the memory is impaired. The stress of the action of the drug falls, indeed, upon the nervous system, and though all parts of this system suffer from the drug, yet it appears to be the sensory nerves, the sensory portions of the spinal cord, and the cortex cerebri which suffer most. The action on the cortex cerebri is much less marked for animals than for man, but then our means of testing the cortex cerebri in animals is very defective. From the above list of symptoms we would single out the following: first, *diminished reflex excitability of the fauces*, because it is an early symptom and marks the point when the patient is coming under the influence of the drug; secondly, *the influence on the sexual function*, because this also appears early, and because undue sexual excitement plays so important a part in the genesis of mental affections; thirdly, the *lowering of cerebral (cortical) activity*, motor and sensory, because it is the direct application of this action which makes the value of the drug in the controlling of the cortical explosions of epilepsy, and in the treatment of cerebral excitement of all kinds, especially epileptic. In these latter states bromides promote sleep by rendering the brain less sensitive to disturbing influences. It is probable that the patient is permitted to go to sleep rather than actually put to sleep. It is difficult to ascertain to what [illegible] element is active in [illegible] salts, to what extent the [illegible] is certain on the one hand [illegible] undergoes but little decomposition [illegible] the tissues, therefore acts as such, [illegible] the other hand that, on man, potassium bromide acts quite differently from the equivalent dose of potassium carbonate or potassium sulphate. It may indeed be true that potassium salts in general are depressant, but it is certain that the sedative action of the special salt, potassium bromide, is largely, if not chiefly, attributable to the bromine. Experiments on animals with potassium salts give results which closely resemble each other; so much so that it is clear that the potassium rules the effect; but, after all, these tests are very coarse as compared with the delicate tests which we can apply clinically, and it is clinical evidence which establishes the special sedative action of potassium bromide.

Sodium Bromide.—On man therapeutic and toxic doses of this salt yield effects like those of potassium bromide; thus, in epilepsy, the psycho-motor centres are controlled, and in the insomnia of excitement the patient is calmed and sleep promoted. Reflex excitability is diminished. This is most evident in the condition of the soft palate and fauces. These effects must be due to the bromine element, since neither on man nor on animals are we able to determine any positive action as belonging to sodium salts as such.

In the molecule of bromide of sodium the percentage of bromine is greater than in that of bromide of potassium in the proportion of 20 to 17.

Bromide of Ammonium acts therapeutically like the potassium and sodium salts, but we have reason to believe that it is less depressant than the potassium salt. Experiments on animals show that ammonium salts as a class exert a stimulant action on the organism. This appears as an early effect, but it does not last, and in the later stages these salts are depressant like potassium salts. Clinically there is not much evidence in favour of even a transient stimulant action of bromide of ammonium, but the probability is great that the salt, if not noticeably stimulant, is yet less depressant than the potassium salt.

The percentage of bromine in the molecule is practically the same as that in bromide of sodium.

Bromide of Lithium has also been introduced into practice; it is said by Weir Mitchell to act in smaller doses, and

* Some of the symptoms here given do not appear except for very large and continuous dosing.

to be efficient in some cases of epilepsy which have not yielded to potassium bromide, also to be a more powerful agent in insomnia. Weight for weight there is much more bromine in the lithium salt than in any other salt of bromine, the percentage of bromine in the molecule being 92 per cent.

Bromide of Calcium has a similar action to potassium bromide; it has been given in doses of 15 to 30 grains; it is said not to depress.

Bromide of Strontium has been recommended by Laborde, G. Sée, Dujardin-Beaumetz. It is said to be well borne by the stomach. In epilepsy as much as 150 grains have been given *pro die*.

Bromide of Rubidium has been employed, and also, for cheapness, a compound of this salt with bromide of ammonium—a double salt (Laufenauer). These preparations are said to have been used with good results as substitutes for bromide of potassium.

Bromide of Cæsium is said to possess similar properties to the rubidium compound.

Bromide of Gold.—Goubert has reported most enthusiastically on the use of this salt in the treatment of epilepsy. He speaks from a ten years' experience. The salt used by him is probably the tribromide, $AuBr_3$, since it is given in solution in water. The doses are *per diem* $\frac{1}{10}$–$\frac{1}{16}$ grain for children, $\frac{1}{8}$–$\frac{1}{4}$ grain for adults. Symptoms of bromism are said not to occur. (Note the very small dosage.)

Ferric Bromide (Fe_2Br_6) has been recommended by Dr. Hecquet, formerly physician to the Abbeville Hospital, as of value in all those cases in which it is desired to soothe without depressing or to strengthen without exciting. The compound is said to be well borne even by irritable stomachs. It is given either in solution or in lozenge form, dose 3 to 5 grains. Dr. Hecquet gives preference to the ferric over the ferrous salt ($FeBr_2$). It will be of interest to observe to what extent this salt will be available as a sedative in the treatment, *e.g.*, of epilepsy and cerebral excitement among anæmics.

Ethylene or Ethene Bromide ($C_2H_4Br_2$).—This compound has recently been brought before us as a sedative in epilepsy by Dr. Julius Donath, of Budapesth. The theory of the action is that the radicle C_2H_4 is burnt up in the body and liberates bromine, which, acting *in statu nascendi*, exerts its sedative action under the most favourable conditions. Dr. Donath holds that the bromine is *the* sedative factor in the action of bromides. Ethylene bromide, a liquid, is given in oily emulsion or in solution in rectified spirits. Dose 1.5 to 3 grains twice or thrice daily. The results obtained are encouraging. (*Therap. Monats.*, June 1891.)

Monobromide of Camphor, $C_{10}H_{15}(Br)O$, is obtained by replacing one atom of hydrogen in the molecule of camphor by an atom of bromine; its action is depressant like that of bromides generally, but it is liable to irritate the stomach, and cannot claim any special advantages. The dose is gr. ij–x in pill with curd soap or Canada balsam.

Hydrobromic Acid has been employed as a substitute for potassium bromide, but though it appears to possess similar properties, and to have the advantage of a less tendency to produce bromism, yet it is rarely used, and its position is not definitely determined. It is very acid and very irritant to the stomach, and requires free dilution. As a soporific one drachm, divided into two or three separate doses, each well diluted, may be given at bedtime.

It cannot be said that the relative value of the bromides has yet been established. Theoretically, on the view that the bromine is the active element, the order of efficiency should be as follows: Lithium bromide, and then the ammonium, sodium, potassium, and rubidium salts in descending scale. Clinical experience, according to some observers, favours this view, but, according to others, it does not; thus the potassium salt is held on good authority to be a more efficient cerebral sedative than sodium bromide, the difference being attributed to the depressant action of the potassium. Others, whilst admitting the superiority of the potassium salt in the treatment of epilepsy, regard the sodium salt as the more efficient hypnotic. More recently, M. Féré (*Annuaire de Thérapeutique*, February 1892) has endeavoured to establish the relative poisonous action of a long list of bromides, but his list has reference to lethal doses, and the results obtained we can hardly accept as final, even from a toxicological point of view.

Dosage.—Bromide of potassium is a safe drug, and may be given without fear up to one-drachm doses, and these repeated four times a day if necessary. As a hypnotic and sedative in cases of great excitement it may be given even more frequently (Clouston). Of course, smaller doses, gr. xv–xxx, should be first tried.

Sodium and ammonium bromides may be given in similar doses. The sodium salt is being extensively administered, and is frequently given up to drachm doses.

Lithium bromide is efficient in half the dose of the potassium salt (Weir Mitchell).

The combination of two or more bromides in the dose was advocated by Brown-Séquard in the treatment of epilepsy; he considered it more efficient than the same total dose of any one bromide. Erlenmeyer recommends a combination in the following proportions: Potassium and sodium bromides of each one part, ammonium bromide one-half part. Combinations such as these will undoubtedly succeed sometimes when the single bromide fails.

Bromides are frequently combined with cannabis indica, or conium, or hyoscyamus; this is especially recommended by Clouston and Eccheverria. The former speaks most highly of tincture of cannabis indica thus administered.

The efficacy of the combination of chloral with bromides is universally recognised. Ten to twenty-five grains of chloral with half a drachm to a drachm of bromide of potassium are very useful in cerebral excitement (Clouston). Eccheverria advises the use of ergot of rye with bromide, and Macfarlane the use of ergot of rye and digitalis with the bromide. These latter adjuvants affect powerfully the circulation, ergot contracting the arterioles, and digitalis effecting the same and in addition controlling the heart. In the acute mania which may follow epileptic attacks bromides in half-drachm or drachm doses with half a drachm of tincture of digitalis will be found very useful. [M. Poulet has further recommended the combination of calabar bean, picrotoxine, and belladonna with bromides —*e.g.*, gr. $\frac{1}{4}$ – $\frac{1}{6}$ of sulphate of eserine or $\frac{1}{10}$ – $\frac{1}{50}$ gr. of atropine sulphate. See *Bulletin Général de Thérapeutique*.]

It should be added that the smallest dose of bromide which is adequate must be given, and that if the sodium salt will answer the purpose it should have preference. In the treatment of children the sodium salt is to be preferred (Nothnagel and Rossbach).

It is well known that bromides frequently cause the appearance of acne-form eruptions. This troublesome complaint may in many cases be prevented by the simultaneous administration of arsenic (*e.g.*, ♏v of the liquor arsenicalis, Eccheverria).

One toxic symptom, happily very rare, calls for mention because of its gravity: it is œdema of the glottis. Death has been thus caused, and in other cases it has only been avoided by the performance of tracheotomy. This symptom manifests itself rarely, and hence special heed should be taken during the early administration of the drug, and on the appearance of any roughness of the throat, [illegible] difficulty in swallowing, [illegible] ready to lessen or suspend [illegible] tration. Œdema of the larynx [illegible] even with small doses; it is [illegible] forstell it. We need not [illegible] other symptoms of bromism, [illegible] clude mental torpor, tremor, [illegible] anæmia, wasting, intestinal and [illegible] catarrh.

Bromides are held to be [illegible] tra-indicated by anæmia (*vide* [illegible] mide).

Chloroform and Alcohol [illegible] Schmiedeberg thus names the [illegible] of bodies derived from the [illegible] and possessed of hypnotic or [illegible] powers. The following list includes the more important members of the [illegible] *Alcohol* (and the alcohols), [illegible] ethers), *aldehyde* and especially [illegible] *hyde*, *chloroform*, *chloral hydrate*, [illegible] *amide*, *urethane*, *chloral urethane*, [illegible] *methylal*, *sulphonal*, *tetronal*, [illegible] *hydrate*, *hypnone* (Leech, *Brit. Med. Journ.*, November 1889). The list will [illegible] become much more extensive.

These bodies act upon the nervous system as follows [the sequence of [illegible] in detail is not always the same for the different members of the group ([illegible] berg)]:

(1) Sensibility for impressions, external and internal, is dulled.

(2) Voluntary motor control is impaired; the psychical activities become [illegible]

(3) The impairment of sensibility proceeds to complete extinction; the volitional movement is likewise abolished; the psychical activities are reduced to mere dream-like representations, or even these are lost. In this stage the reflexes generally of the cord and base of the brain are impaired or practically abolished, all except those very stable reflexes, circulatory and respiratory, which still permit of organic life.

(4) The centres respiratory and circulatory become paralysed, and death [illegible].

Stage (3) is the stage of complete narcosis.

The implication of the nervous centres is, as Dr. Leech puts it, in the inverse order of their development: first the cortex cerebri, then the centres of base of brain and cord, then the respiratory and circulatory centres of the medulla.

Important is the influence on the vascular system, which varies greatly with the particular hypnotic employed. Though it is only in the latest stage that the heart gives out, yet vascular tone and blood-pressure always suffer more or less. With some the impairment is scarcely noticeable even for deep narcosis—*e.g.*, urethane

(Schmiedeberg); with others it is very marked—*e.g.*, chloroform, chloral hydrate.

Practically for this group we may disregard the influence exerted upon the peripheral structures, nerve trunk and nerve ending.

We may now consider individually the action of the different members of the group.

Alcohol.—The use of alcohol as a night-cap is well known, though, as a rule, it is only in the milder forms of insomnia that it is effectual. In some cases, however, of the acute delirium of fever it acts very beneficially as a sedative and sleep-giver, and in acute mania it is a recognised mode of treatment. It is an excellent sleep-giver for children, whose nervous systems are readily affected by the unaccustomed influence. It may be given as brandy or whisky or in the form of wines and malt liquors; in acute mania these latter are frequently to be preferred. In connection with this it is of much interest to recall the fact that porter was employed as a soporific in acute mania at the York Retreat early in the present century (Samuel Tuke, "The York Retreat," 1813), and that this treatment gave rise to much comment at the time. In cases where the heart flags and the nervous system is much weakened Anstie prefers wines containing plenty of compound ethers to brandy. In general, whisky is superior to brandy or wines. Strong ale, stout, and porter are highly hypnotic.

Alcohol in its various forms may serve as a vehicle for and adjuvant to the administration of other hypnotics, but the importance of keeping its use well in hand cannot be too much insisted on; it is a drug, and to be used as such. To obtain the best effect from alcohol it should be given in full dose—*e.g.*, ℥ij–℥iij of whisky taken as a draught, warm, not sipping—hot, just as the patient is getting into bed (Whitla).

The higher alcohols of the ethylic series—*e.g.*, propylic, butylic, amylic—are not employed as medicines; they contaminate, however, wines and beers, in particular the cheaper and less carefully prepared sorts, being present as the fusel oils. These contaminants act like alcohol, but they are much more powerful than it, and hence the deleteriousness of crude specimens of beers and wines. Derivatives of these alcohols may be used for anæsthetic or sedative purposes—*e.g.*, amylene, amylene hydrate (*vide infra*).

If alcohol be given at all continuously and in large dose—*e.g.*, six to eight ounces—as in the treatment of the delirium of fever or acute delirious mania, we would urge special attention to the tongue, skin, pulse, respiration, and the delirium itself. Should the tongue become moist and the skin lose its dry, harsh character, the pulse and respiration become slower and the delirium lessen or give way to quiet sleep, then alcohol is doing good; but should there be no improvement in these respects, it will not be wise to push the alcohol beyond the above doses.

Ether finds its chief employment as an anæsthetic and anti-spasmodic stimulant. We need not discuss these actions here, but in full doses by the mouth it often acts as a soporific—*e.g.*, in doses of one drachm. It may be given in the form of a julep with syrup of orange and orange-flower water, or with the further addition of rectified spirits of wine.

Acetic Ether, acetate of ethyl, was long since described as possessed of soporific powers. M. Sédillot gave thirty drops for this purpose, but MM. Trousseau and Pidoux could not confirm this action.

It will be rarely necessary to fall back on ether for soporific purposes.

Chloroform, like ether, ranks as an anæsthetic. It is rarely used as a hypnotic, but in some cases in which violent movements make sleep impossible—*e.g.*, severe cases of chorea—it has been inhaled more or less continuously to keep the patient at rest. It has also been employed in the same way in the treatment of repeated convulsive attacks, but in such cases chloral is far more valuable. Chloroform insensibility sometimes passes into natural sleep after withdrawal of the drug; this is true of ether also. A hypodermic injection of morphia previous to the administration of chloroform ensures a more persistent effect; this combination is in some cases desirable, as advocated by Victor Horsley in operations on the brain. Chloroform may be used as a means of diagnosis in some cases of insanity complicated with hysteria; practically it is not used either as a simple sedative or as a hypnotic.

Paraldehyde $(C_2H_4O)_3$.—This substance is a polymer of aldehyde; chemically it is therefore closely allied to alcohol. It has been much used of late as a hypnotic, in particular by alienists. It shows the generic action of the alcohol group, affecting first the brain, then the cord, then the medulla oblongata. If death take place, it is at the lungs; the action on the circulation is comparatively slight. Quinquaud and Hénocque have maintained that the blood-colouring matter undergoes change by reduction into methæmoglobin, but this is disputed by Hayem, who states that the blood is not affected (Dujardin-Beaumetz, "Nouvelles Médications"). The advantages of paraldehyde are: its relatively slight depressant action on the heart and vascular system, and on the respiratory apparatus; also its slight poisonous action on the tissues, which allows of its administration for long periods without obvious detriment.

The disadvantages are: its unpleasant taste and the unpleasant odour imparted to the breath; the fact that a stage of excitement frequently precedes the hypnosis, this being more marked than for chloral; further, its slighter power over pain as compared with opium, and even with chloral (Loebisch, "Die neueren Arzneimittel").

The sleep of paraldehyde is quiet, and closely resembles physiological sleep.

The drug has been very largely used by alienists, and their verdict is that it is a very valuable hypnotic. Morselli, Krafft-Ebing, Kéraval and Nerkam, S. A. K. Strahan, Clouston, and many others speak in the highest terms of it. It is said to be contra-indicated in advanced cases of phthisis with laryngeal complications, since in these cases it is liable to cause cough, vomiting, and much excitement (v. Noorden, *cf.* Loebisch); also in cases of ulceration of the stomach. Krafft-Ebing insists that the drug is well borne by the tissues; he admits, however, that with prolonged and high dosage it does harm. He himself reports a case in which the symptoms resembled chronic alcoholism, and another case in which delirium and epileptiform attacks occurred during the withdrawal of the drug. These cases do not invalidate the general statement that paraldehyde is well borne.

Dose.—Forty-five minims to 1, 1½, or 2 drachms are given for hypnotic purposes, beginning of course with the smaller dose. Clouston sometimes advances the dose to 3 or 4 drachms. At one asylum a patient, a woman, received with benefit 10 drachms every night. Sleep generally obtains in from five to twenty minutes (Dujardin-Beaumetz). In ordinary asylum practice Strahan advises that a first dose of from 45 minims to 1 drachm should be followed by the same dose if sleep do not set in in five minutes. As a rectal injection 1 to 2.5 drachms may be given.

As vehicles for the drug have been recommended: Olive oil, flavoured with some volatile oil—*e.g.*, of peppermint; mucilage, flavoured with orange peel or cinnamon; spirit in the form of grog or as a spirituous mixture, with vanilla flavouring (Loebisch).

Chloral Hydrate.—[illegible] this body becomes broken [illegible] system with evolution of [illegible] that its action is of this [illegible] tenable; chloral acts as such. [illegible] of its administration the most [illegible] points to be remembered are [illegible] the respiratory and circulatory [illegible] isms (cardiac and vaso-motor) [illegible] markedly affected; in over-dose [illegible] threatening at the lungs and heart; (*b*) that the temperature is [illegible] pressed by toxic dose; (*c*) that [illegible] hypnotic dose the drug has [illegible] power over painful impressions [illegible] reflex excitability; hence, *e.g.*, the [illegible] cough still continues. In lung [illegible] is a point of practical importance, and [illegible] respect of this chloral hydrate, and [illegible] the whole chloral group, contrasts with opium; (*d*) that idiosyncrasy towards the drug is not infrequently manifested.

The chloral sleep of small dose is generally regarded as a refreshing sleep, closely resembling natural sleep; it is considered to be in part the result of anæmia of the brain; in full dose it is possible that the lowering of blood-pressure, which will include a lowering of intra-cranial pressure, may also be a factor.

In giving chloral we must use the drug with caution in low states of vitality generally, but especially if the heart be weak; in this case, indeed, though small doses may still be given—*e.g.*, 15 to 20 grains—large doses are dangerous. In the insomnia of cardiac disease, of mediastinal tumour, of aneurism, in which diseases dyspnœa is prominent, great benefit results from combining chloral hydrate with opium. In cases of obstructed lung circulation—*e.g.*, bronchitis and emphysema—we must watch carefully the effects of the drug. In cases of overdose the usual stimulant and rousing treatment of narcotic poisoning is to be adopted. Artificial respiration may be called for, and as an antidote strychnine may be injected—4 minims of the liq. strychninæ, B.P., repeated every ten to twenty minutes, if necessary (Brunton); but, in addition, it is most essential that the patient should *be kept very warm*. When pain is the cause of sleeplessness chloral, in safe dose, is uncertain; it is greatly surpassed by opium; it may, however, be tried.

When convulsions are present, and by their violence and frequent recurrence are exhausting the patient, chloral is often of the greatest value as a rest giver. In the *status convulsivus vel epilepticus* it is the most valuable drug at our command.

Chloral may be given for long periods without causing much gastric or intestinal derangement; it contrasts in this respect with opium. But, on the other hand, a chloral *habit* or *craving* is rather easily established, and this manifests itself in great depression of the vital powers, the general nutrition suffering, and the tone of the nervous system in particular being much lowered. Among the list of symptoms we note feeble-mindedness, tremor, and sensory impairment; gastro-intestinal disturbance; vaso-motor troubles, including erythematous rashes. Dyspnœa, with præcordial anxiety, and even asphyxia, are recorded. Joint pains are sometimes complained of (Rosenthal, *Wien. med. Pr.*, Sept. 1889). It is to be noted for this as well as for other drugs that prolonged administration does not necessarily establish a *habit* or *craving*.

Children bear chloral well.

Dose.—On account of the susceptibility of some people chloral ought never to be given, as a first dose, in larger quantity than 15 to 20 grains; this for adults. Wood states that this dose should not be repeated oftener than once an hour till the total quantity taken has reached 1 drachm; some hours should then elapse before any more is given, except the case be very urgent. Once the powers of the patient have been gauged the dosing may be less restrained. In cases of great mental excitement, and in delirium tremens, Nothnagel and Rossbach have recommended doses varying between 45 grains and 2 drachms. Constantin Paul in similar states has given 90 grains of chloral in an enema with good results. These higher doses, however, are dangerous, and they ought never to be given as a first dose to any one unaccustomed to the drug. Clouston, after a very extensive experience of the drug, always gives it in small dose—*e.g.*, 10 to 25 grains—along with bromides ("Treatment of Mania," "Mental Diseases"). On the whole, much larger doses are given in asylums than in ordinary practice. Chloral *habitués* sometimes mount up to very big doses—5 drachms (Rosenthal).

Given by the mouth, chloral should be freely diluted because of its pungency; weak syrup forms a good vehicle. By the bowel the same dose may be given as by the mouth, and either as an injection or as a suppository. If given for convulsions the suppository form is best, because there is less likelihood of extrusion during a convulsion; the suppository should be pushed up as high as possible with the finger.

Chloral may be injected hypodermically, but this method has the disadvantage of requiring several syringefuls (the Pravaz syringe), and of causing abscess not infrequently.

For children, from three upwards, suffering from convulsions, the dose may be 5 grains by the mouth or anus; this is to be repeated according to the requirements of the case. The new-born infant may receive 1 to 2 grains by the mouth (Wood).

Chloral hydrate may be very advantageously combined with bromides; also, in certain cases already referred to, with opium.

Bromal Hydrate.—In this compound bromine takes the place of the chlorine of chloral hydrate. The poisonous action of bromal is much greater than of chloral; great excitement precedes (in animals) the production of anæsthesia—the soporific action is not marked. Clinical experience of the drug is still lacking. It has been given in doses of from 3 to 5 *grains*; it should be freely diluted, because very irritant locally.

Butyl Chloral Hydrate, also called croton chloral hydrate, $C_4H_5Cl_3O.H_2O$, represents a chlorine derivative from butylic alcohol, analogous to chloral hydrate, the derivative from ethylic alcohol. Within the tissues the chemical behaviour of butyl chloral hydrate is exactly similar to that of chloral hydrate. As a hypnotic the action of this drug is less marked than for chloral, but given in large doses it is soporific, and the sleep is accompanied by anæsthesia of the head (Liebreich). Its chief use is in the treatment of neuralgic states, especially of the trigeminus nerve, and of insomnia dependent thereon. It is given in 5 to 10 grain doses, frequently repeated if need be. These doses have no direct hypnotic action. V. Mering calls in question the anæsthesia of the fifth nerve, described by Liebreich, but there can be no question as to the value of butyl chloral hydrate in neuralgia of the fifth.

Chloral-Amide.—By the interaction of chloraldehyde and the amide of formic acid this body is obtained. The molecule $C_3Cl_3H_4NO_2$ contains the grouping NH_2. It is possible that the introduction of this will explain the absence of depressant action said to be characteristic of chloralamide as contrasted with chloral hydrate (see Leech, *Brit. Med. Jour.*, Nov. 2, 1889). This new drug has been favourably reported on by Drs. Reichmann, Hagen, and Hüfler, in Germany, also by observers in this country, Hale White, Strahan, and others. The last observer speaks from an experience of over two hundred administrations. It is claimed for chloral amide: (1) that it does not depress the respiration or the circulation; (2) that the temperature is not lowered; (3) that it is serviceable in many cases of sleeplessness from pain; (4) that after-effects and by-effects are rarely witnessed (a little drowsiness the next day has been complained of, and in a few cases there has been slight headache; there has been no gastro-intestinal disturbance). Collapse symptoms have, however, been observed after the administration of chloral-amide, and attributed to the drug (Robinson, *Deutsch. med. Wochenschr.*, No. 49, 1889); also some erythematous eruptions recalling the eruptions of chloral hydrate (Umpfenbach, *Ther. Monats.*, Feb. 1890). Pye-Smith records a case of universal dermatitis after two doses of 40 grains, at intervals of eight hours (*Lancet*, 1890, p. 546). The sleep of chloral-amide is said to be calm and refreshing. Dr. Strahan says that at any time the patient can be roused and made to answer a question, protrude the tongue, or the like. Sleep was obtained by him in nearly every case, "even in patients suffering from extreme maniacal excitement, and in no case where it failed to induce sleep did it excite." He observes that "it may be given to paralytics, whatever their stage." In his opinion it is equal to paraldehyde, "but in no way superior," except in that it is pleasanter to take, and that it does not give any disagreeable odour to the breath.

It is not quite so prompt in its action as chloral, but takes effect in from half an hour to one, two, or even three hours. The average is about an hour. The dose is 30 to 45 grains; 55 grains are quite a safe dose (Strahan). Weak alcoholic solutions are the best to administer, as the drug dissolves readily in spirit. It must *not* be given with alkalies, nor must the solution be hot, as under these conditions it is decomposed. Chloral-amide has a faintly bitter taste.

Chloralimide, with formula $C_2Cl_3NH_3$, must not be confounded with chloral-amide. In the former there are reasons to believe that there is present the group NH (imidogen), not NH_2 (amidogen). The substance, a crystalline solid, insoluble in water, but soluble in alcohol, ether, and chloroform and oils, is very stable. Broken up it yields, weight for weight, more chloroform than either chloral-amide or chloral ammonium, and for this reason Chouy claims that it is more hypnotic than either of these. Inasmuch, however, as it is improbable that chloral compounds act by yielding chloroform within the organism, this theoreti[illegible] be admitted as of much [illegible] testimony is required to [illegible] value. Chloralimide is given [illegible] doses as chloral hydrate, [illegible] pills or wafers, or in alcoholic [illegible] oily emulsion (Merck).

Chloral Ammonium, [illegible] closely allied to chloral [illegible] structure; in the molecule, [illegible] is the group NH_2. The [illegible] given in doses of 15 to 30 [illegible] good effect, and it takes [illegible] depressant hypnotic. It appears, [illegible] to be unstable, slowly breaking [illegible] the solid state; in this it [illegible] chloralimide.

Urethane, or ethylcarbamate, [illegible] belongs to a group of bodies, [illegible] thanes, in which radicles of [illegible] series replace one atom of [illegible] carbamic acid. In the molecule [illegible] amidogen, NH_2, and to this is [illegible] in the case of chloral-amide, the [illegible] of depressant action upon the [illegible] system. The compound occurs in [illegible] form of colourless columnar [illegible] crystals, of nitre-like taste. It is [illegible] soluble in water and most media.

Urethane, as a hypnotic, has the [illegible]tage of being very safe, and for the [illegible] chiefly, that it does not depress the heart. Even in the deeper grades of [illegible] in rabbits there was no appreciable lowering of the blood-pressure (Schmiedeberg). It is specially indicated for children, who bear it well, and it has been employed among these by Otto and König in the treatment of the excitement of the feeble-minded. It is of value in sleeplessness without definite cause, and especially if this occurs in very debilitated states of body, particularly in heart weakness. On the other hand it is not a very certain hypnotic; it fails where pain is the cause of insomnia, or where there exists a disturbing reflex—*e.g.*, cough. Kraepelin obtained good results in melancholia and general paralysis, but in the stage of excitement of the latter disease, also in mania and delirium tremens, he was obliged to turn to paraldehyde. Otto and König confirm his results (Loebisch, "Die neueren Arzneimittel," 1888). On the whole urethane stands as a safe but rather feeble and unreliable hypnotic (Gordon, Needham, *Brit. Med. Jour.*, Nov. 2, 1889). Urethane sleep is, for the *smaller doses*, natural, and the reflexes are but little modified. In dose of 30 to 60 grains there is marked slowing of the pulse, and the breathing is deepened. In general there are neither by- nor after-effects, but with the larger doses there has been complaint of a sense of weight of head and somnolence, also vomiting. There may be some little excitement on first giving the drug.

Dosage.—For children, grains 4 to 8 to 16; for adults, 30 to 60 grains (given in half the total dose at an interval of fifteen to thirty minutes). In exceptional cases, 90 to 120 grains may be given, but the dose must not be carried further. Urethane should be given in 10 per cent. solution, with a little syrup of orange peel, to cover the saline taste. Subcutaneously a 30 per cent. solution may be injected; one to three injections, each containing 4 grains, were effective (Rottenbiller). (*Cf.* Loebisch, *op. cit.*) Tolerance of the drug is rapidly established.

Chloral-urethane, also called ural ($C_5H_8Cl_3O_3N$), is a compound of urethane with chloral (*cf.* chloral-amide). The urethane is held to counteract the depressant influence of the chloral. The drug acts very similarly to urethane; it is given in doses of 30 to 45 grains. At present the reports concerning chloral-urethane are discrepant. Poppi speaks very highly of it, but Hübner and Sticker, and Mairet and Combemale, do not give it unmodified praise.

A preparation known as somnal is, according to Merck, only an alcoholic solution of chloral and urethane—it is a mixture and not a compound; it is given in half-drachm doses.

Acetal, $C_2H_4(C_2H_5O)_2$, has practically ceased to exist as a hypnotic. According to Leech, it has the disadvantage of an unpleasant taste and smell, and no advantages. (For references see *Brit. Med. Jour.*, Nov. 2, 1890.)

Hypnone, $(CH_3)(C_6H_5)CO$, or methyl-phenyl-ketone, is a substance crystalline at 14° C., liquid and oily at 20° C.; it has a peculiar fragrant odour and a pungent creasote-like taste, is but little soluble in water, readily soluble in alcohol, ether, chloroform, and fixed oils; its reaction is neutral. It was introduced as a hypnotic by Dujardin-Beaumetz in 1885. The drug has not made much way, and is not likely to, for the following reasons: It is very uncertain (Dujardin-Beaumetz and Bardet, von Hirt, Rey, Maïret and Combemale, and others); it influences pain very little; is unable to act in cases where cough prevents sleep; the patient soon grows accustomed to it, and the dose needs to be increased; it is very irritating to the stomach, and the blood is said to suffer from its prolonged administration; the blood-pressure and the breathing suffer depression in toxic dose, but in ordinary therapeutic dose this effect is very slight.

Dujardin-Beaumetz and Bardet consider hypnone of special value for the insomnia of alcoholics, and for nervous insomnia. They state that it leaves no after-effect. For the insomnia of morphinism it is useless.

Dose.—Three to six drops, best given diluted with glycerine or almond oil in capsules, or as an emulsion with tincture of orange. Much larger doses have been given in mental affections—viz., up to 17 to 25 minims. Krafft-Ebing gets no result under 10 drops. He speaks well of 15-drop doses, and says that 30 drops may be given.* Hypnone is not adapted for hypodermic injection, according to Krafft-Ebing—*i.e.*, there is no advantage in so using it; but Conolly Norman records good results from the undiluted injections of ♏v–xij.†

Hypnal (mono-chloral antipyrine).—If chloral and antipyrine be brought together in solution, a body separates which, if the mother solutions be dilute, is oily in the first instance, then crystalline, but crystalline at once if the solutions be concentrated. The body is a compound of chloral and antipyrine with definite chemical formula. M. Bonnet, of Dreux, first described it as possessing hypnotic and analgesic properties. M. Bardet, by further experiment, established these statements.

The hypnotic dose is about 15 grains; rarely are 30 grains required. Pain is decidedly influenced according to M. Bardet. The quantity of chloral is 45 per cent., of antipyrine 55 per cent. of the compounded drug, hence the quantities which are efficient of the two components are remarkably small, the action of each being apparently heightened by the other. Hypnal has a saline taste, and is without the irritant action of either compound on the stomach.

M. Bardet has not tried the drug in mental affections; he regards it less as a new drug than as an efficient way of administering chloral and antipyrine (*see* "Nouveaux Remèdes," March 24, 1890).

Hypnal is soluble in about five to six times its weight of water, and is best given in such solution along with an equal volume of simple syrup, to which may be added spirits of wine and tincture of orange peel (*see* Bonnet's formula, "Nouveaux Remèdes," 1890, p. 361).

Methylal, $C_3H_8O_2$, is a limpid, volatile liquid, which in odour resembles acetic acid and, to some extent, chloroform also.

* *Wiener klinische Wochenschrift*, Jan. 16, 1890.

† Consult Loebisch, "Die neueren Arzneimittel," 1888; Dujardin-Beaumetz, "Dictionnaire de Thérapeutique."

It is an anæsthetic, local and general. It may be inhaled or given by the mouth, in doses of 1 to 4 drachms, freely diluted with water and syrup; it acts as a hypnotic (Leech, *Brit. Med. Jour.*, Nov. 1889). The sleep obtained is tranquil and deep, and supervenes quickly; it is, however, of short duration only, a result of the speedy elimination of the drug. The heart is slightly accelerated and the blood-pressure lowered, but in therapeutic dose it does not rank as a cardiac depressant; the respiration is rendered slower. Reflex excitability generally is lessened; also the excitability of the psycho-motor centres. Injected under the skin it may irritate so violently as to produce sloughing, but diluted (1 in 9) it has been used successfully by Krafft-Ebing in the treatment of delirium tremens. He finds that in a few hours a prolonged and quiet sleep is produced. Two injections, each containing about 1.5 grain of pure methylal in solution (1 in 9), would in many cases suffice to give sleep, but often four to five injections during the day are needed.* His results confirm the previous results obtained by Richardson, Personali, Maïret and Combemale; the latter observers made observations on 36 cases of insanity; the doses ranged between 75 and 120 grains. Tolerance of methylal is easily established (*cf.* Dujardin-Beaumetz, "Dictionnaire de Thérapeutique," vol. iv.; H. C. Wood; Leech, *Brit. Med. Jour.*, November 1889).

On account of the high price of the drug, the hypodermic method is to be preferred.

Methylal is very little used now.

Sulphonal, $C_7H_{16}S_2O_4$, is a white crystalline powder very insoluble in cold water, sparingly in boiling water, fairly soluble in alcohol and ether. It is without taste or odour. Sulphonal has been extensively used as a hypnotic, and with, on the whole, excellent results. It does not depress the heart or give rise to serious effects (Krafft-Ebing). Leech places sulphonal thus in relation to some other hypnotics—(1) sulphonal, (2) amylene hydrate, (3) paraldehyde, (4) urethane, (5) methylal; but not one of these, he says, equals chloral hydrate in the certainty of its effects. Rabbas and Garnier speak very highly of sulphonal; Clouston, on the other hand, places it far behind paraldehyde. Umpfenbach holds that, for certainty of action combined with safety, sulphonal does not present any advantages over chloral in the treatment of the insane. One objection to sulphonal is the, so-called, delayed or deferred action, the patient not sleeping during the night after the [illegible] of the drug, but sleeping [illegible] very drowsy the next day. In [illegible] cases after-effects are [illegible] fulness in the head, giddiness, slight ataxia of the limbs, difficulty of speech; in some rare cases vomiting has occurred (Knoblauch, J. M. Stewart, Umpfenbach). In most of these cases these effects have resulted from large doses, but Knoblauch lays more stress on the prolonged use of sulphonal as causal, and Umpfenbach also refers to this cumulative action. A few cases of rash, scarlatiniform or measly, have been observed during sulphonal administration (Schotten).

Tolerance is not easily established; some, indeed, have stated that patients do not grow accustomed to the drug. If tolerance do occur, a break in the administration will re-establish its efficacy. Of late two cases of sulphonal habit—*i.e.*, craving—"amounting to a perfect mania," have been recorded by Dr. Gilbert, of Baden-Baden, and cases of toxic symptoms have been more frequently described.

Dose.—15 to 30 grains in soup or warm milk, one or two hours before bed-time; the gritty crystalline powder should be rubbed up finely in a mortar, else it hangs about the gums and teeth. Sulphonal thus powdered may also be given in beer, or mixed up with the food (Krafft-Ebing). More recently the method has been adopted of pouring boiling water on to the dose, say half or two-thirds of a tumblerful of water, and allowing this to cool just sufficiently to make it drinkable. The sulphonal dissolves in the boiling water, and has not time to separate out before it is taken. Sleep follows this mode of administration in from fifteen to twenty minutes. Sulphonal may also be given in cachet or tabloid form; it then acts more slowly, viz., in from one to two hours.

Very large doses of sulphonal have been taken without bad effects, and Krafft-Ebing records the administration by mistake of 150 grains, with no other effect than a prolonged sleep of twenty hours, and some giddiness on awakening. Given in small doses, 7 to 8 grains several times a day, it quiets the patient and favours sleep. Erlenmeyer considers that the dose should never exceed 30 grains.

Tetronal is a body having the same structure as sulphonal, but differing in the replacement of two methyl groupings by two of ethyl. It is said to be a more powerful hypnotic than sulphonal, and that this increase of power is due to the excess of ethyl groupings, of which there are four in all, whence the name. It occurs in tabular crystals and plates, which

* *Wiener klinische Wochenschrift*, Jan. 16, 1890.

are but sparingly soluble in water, but freely soluble in alcohol and fairly so in ether. They possess a camphoraceous taste.

Halfway between tetronal and sulphonal is a body containing three molecules of ethyl in all and one of methyl: it is called **trional**, and it is said to be intermediate between sulphonal and tetronal in its activity (*Brit. Med. Journ.*, vol. i. 1890, p. 87). Trional forms tabular crystals rather more soluble in water than tetronal, 1 in 320 parts, freely soluble in alcohol and ether. The dose of tetronal is gr. x–xx, but Schultze recommends gr. xv–lx of either tetronal or trional. Either may be given in suspension like sulphonal, or in cachet, or in a large quantity of warm water, or in soup. If the terms tetronal and trional are to stand, it would be well to call sulphonal dional, and so place the three in relation. Tetronal and trional are still insufficiently examined clinically, but there is no doubt that they come near to sulphonal in therapeutic value. Schultze considers that trional has the advantage over tetronal, and that the former is equal, if not in some respects, superior to sulphonal (*Therap. Monats.*, Oct. 1891).

Amylene Hydrate ($C_5H_{12}O$). — This substance is tertiary amyl alcohol, the molecular grouping being different from that of the primary amyl alcohol of fermentation, the chief constituent of fusel oil. It is a colourless mobile liquid with high boiling-point. The odour is pungent, the taste unpleasant; it is ethereal and camphor-like; it dissolves in 18 parts of water, in alcohol in all proportions. In toxic dose amylene hydrate kills by arrest of respiration and then of the heart, but these centres are the last to give way. The cortex cerebri first suffers, then the centres of the base of the brain and cord with abolition of the reflexes. The drug therefore resembles essentially alcohol in its mode of action. Hypnosis occurs at a stage when the respiration and heart are *practically unaffected*. Mering has studied exhaustively the effects on man: he finds that doses of 45 to 75 grains cause a refreshing sleep of five to twelve hours, without any preliminary stage of excitement. Cases of the insomnia of over-strung nerves, the sleeplessness of old age, of convalescence from acute disease, of delirium tremens, &c., are well treated by it. For the insomnia of pain it is less reliable. Mering advises in such cases that it should be combined with opium. Nausea, vomiting, headache do not follow the use of amylene hydrate. Mering places the drug between chloral hydrate and paraldehyde. He says that 15 grains of chloral are equivalent to 30 grains of amylene hydrate and to 45 grains of paraldehyde. It has the advantage over paraldehyde in taste, and over chloral in that it does not depress the heart. It should be diluted some 10 times if given by the mouth. The extract of liquorice is a useful corrigens. Beer is an excellent vehicle. As a rectal injection it should be administered with water and mucilage, diluted some 12 to 15 times. The appetite is liable to suffer, and the stomach is sometimes upset by the drug. The peculiarity of the durability of the effects of amylene hydrate, as compared with ordinary alcohol, is probably to be explained in part by its higher boiling-point. (*Cf.* Loebisch, *op. cit.*)

The results of more recent experience confirm in general Mering's statements. Jastrowitz, among others, speaks strongly in favour of the drug; he finds it very useful in the treatment of the sleeplessness of morphinists. Dietz speaks highly of it in nervous affections.*

Piscidia Erythrina (Jamaica Dogwood).—The rind of the root of this tree is employed either as such, dose 60 grains, or as tincture, or liquid extract, dose of either one-half to two drachms. Water with some flavouring is the vehicle. Krafft-Ebing considers that 2 to 3 teaspoonfuls of the fluid extract are required for hypnotic effects.

Piscidia is generally regarded as a substitute for opium; it raises blood-pressure and retards the pulse, but dilates the pupil (Brunton). Krafft-Ebing, however, regards it as more allied to simple sedatives—*e.g.*, the bromides. He thinks it deserves the name "vegetable bromine."† Sleep is brought about, according to him, indirectly as the result of a benumbing influence on the cortex cerebri. Neither headache nor constipation is produced.

Drs. Scott and McGrath have found it useful in nervous excitement. Senator has used it with advantage in cases of neuralgia of the head. Piscidia has of late fallen into comparative disuse. A few years ago it was much prescribed in London.

Opium and its Alkaloids.—The principal alkaloid of opium is morphia; the similarity of action between the mother drug and morphia depends on the preponderance of morphia. The action of morphia is a twofold one: it paralyses the functions of the cortex cerebri on the one hand; it causes an increased reflex excitability of the central nervous system on the other hand. The first effect is

* Boas, *Deutsch. Med. Wochenschr.*, Jan. 9, 1890.

† *Wiener Klin. Wochenschr.*, Jan. 1890.

narcotic, the other is convulsant. Of the other alkaloids of opium, some show the double action of morphia, but in these the narcotic influence is less and the tetanic influence relatively greater; this differentiation culminates in thebain, which is a pure convulsant, and belongs to the strychnine group. (It must be understood that the tetanic stage ultimately gives way to a paralytic stage.) This twofold effect, narcotic and convulsant, is witnessed alike in man and the lower animals, but, whereas in man the cerebral effects are most pronounced, in the vertebrates farthest from man—*e.g.*, frogs—it is the phenomena of an increased reflex excitability which are most striking.

In detail, the effects of opium and morphia on man * and the higher animals include, first, a diminished perception of pain (whilst the sense of touch remains unaffected) and a lowered reflex excitability, as is evidenced, *e.g.*, in respect of cough. Schmiedeberg, whose description we closely follow, points out that, whilst these effects occur without there being, at first sight, any apparent affection of the cortex cerebri, yet the heaviness and sleepiness which soon set in suggest that from the very outset the receptive centres of the brain are depressed in their functions. The occurrence in certain cases of vivid imagining and mental excitement during the waking state as well as immediately preceding sleep has been interpreted by some as due to actual stimulation of certain parts of the brain, but it is possible that these flights of fancy, which may amount to hallucinations, are the result of a withdrawal of control, a loss of balance by subtraction rather than by addition (*cf.* Schmiedeberg), though against this view is the fact of the smallness of the dose, which in some cases will suffice to excite. The next effect is sleep, at first slight, and from which the patient can be easily roused; then more deep, and not to be interrupted except by powerful stimulation; then the unconsciousness deepens, and a state of coma supervenes, in which the excitability of the cortex cerebri is practically annulled. The benumbing influence of opium ultimately spreads to the medulla oblongata and specially influences respiration; death takes place by asphyxia.

In animals the vascular system suffers no diminution of tone except in the deepest stages of narcosis; but in man local vascular dilatation, as of the face and surface of the body, may show itself even with therapeutic doses, and probably [illegible] on the vascular dilatation are the appearance of a sense of warmth, the outbreak of perspiration, sudaminal eruptions, itching of the surface. The fall of temperature noted in animals poisoned by morphia is probably due to the excessive loss of heat by the surface (Brunton and Cash). When, at a later stage, the vessels generally are relaxed, the flushed face becomes pale; and, still later, when the breathing has become much impaired, a livid tint supervenes. Schmiedeberg suggests whether the capillaries of the brain are not also congested at the same time as those of the face; but the teaching of Horsley and Schäfer is that the brain under the influence of a moderate dose of morphia bleeds much less than in the natural state.* The heart is one of the mechanisms most resisting to the influence of opium (Nothnagel and Rossbach). The pulse is in the early stage increased in frequency; later it becomes slower and increased both in fulness and in force; in the end it may again become more frequent, and it then becomes weak also. Blood-pressure is lowered to a variable extent by large doses of opium, but we may remember that, practically, opium and morphia do not, in therapeutic dose, depress the heart and vascular system.

The condition of the pupil is not constant even for man; it is very variable indeed for animals. All that can be said with certainty is that the contraction is not due to peripheral action. Peripheral action on muscle and nerve may be disregarded. The activities of the stomach are diminished and appetite is checked. The action upon the intestinal tract is not sufficiently explained, but what we do know is that peristaltic action is lessened, that the secretion of the bowel and its appendages is diminished, and that constipation results. The amount of urine is generally diminished.

Of these effects of opium, it is important to note: (*a*) the influence over pain; (*b*) the quieting of cough; (*c*) the non-depressant action on the heart and vessels (indeed, opium in therapeutic dose may rank as a cardiac stimulant); (*d*) the production of anorexia and constipation, with their disturbing action on assimilation in general.

The sleep obtained by opium is not very refreshing; it is in many instances light and disturbed by exciting dreams. It is frequently followed by fulness in the head and a dull listless feeling.

Opium is eminently a drug for temporary use; if given for any length of time,

* Man is without exception far more sensitive to opium than all other animals (Nothnagel and Rossbach).

* "Brain Surgery," Brit. Med. Assoc., 1886.

it invariably does harm by its effects on [illegible]. Its influence over pain makes it of the greatest service when this is the cause of insomnia. The like holds in cases of sleeplessness from irritative coughs, but where there is much secretion within the bronchial tubes, opium is contra-indicated. In relation to pain and cough, opium contrasts with the chloroform, chloral hydrate, and alcohol groups generally. The influence on the urine is a somewhat uncertain one, but there is no doubt that the dangers of opium administration in kidney disease—*e.g.*, the contracted kidney—have been overstated. The presence of albumen should, however, in all cases make us more watchful in the use of opium and morphia. On account of its non-depressant, even stimulant, action on the heart, opium is never contra-indicated by cardiac disease; indeed, it forms one of the most valuable drugs we possess in the treatment of heart pain, and of heart distress generally—*e.g.*, dyspnœa. In the startings from sleep of heart disease morphia gives great relief. Balfour points out that "mental aberration of a more or less violent character" may occur in the course of aortic disease. He thinks it is mostly occasioned by anæmia, and he finds that full hypnotic doses of morphia, given subcutaneously, are of great benefit.

Opium is found of great use in mental states of worry, fret, apprehension; it is in such cases that some practitioners insist on the value of opium as against morphia. Sir Andrew Clark speaks of the advantage of *whole* opium in such cases for the purpose of "taking the gristle off the nerves."

For simple insomnia, independent of pain or cough or heart disease, it is not usual to have recourse to opium, and more especially if the insomnia be habitual—for such it is, however, always available as an occasional dose—though other drugs are to be preferred.

For the insomnia which frequently precedes the establishment of mental disease opium may be employed, and here it may, according to Clouston, act as prophylactic by a timely interruption of a sleeplessness which threatens to become a habit. In these cases, however, there appears to be no special indication for opium rather than for bromides or chloral.

In established mental disease the value of opium is much debated. In melancholia Clouston holds it to be harmful; he speaks most emphatically on this point, asserting that "in a series of elaborate experiments which he made it always caused loss of appetite and loss of weight." In acute mania he says that opium should be used only as a temporary placebo, and not continuously. Schüle states broadly that opium is "the plaster splint of the sick mind," and that the general indication for its employment is the presence of a hyperæsthesia with heightened reflex excitability (*cf.* Nothnagel and Rossbach). In melancholias associated with unrest and excitement Nothnagel and Rossbach state that there is a general agreement as to the good effects of opium. They speak more vaguely of its use in other forms of mental disease, but according to them the tendency of late years in the treatment of the insane has been the use of morphia more and chloral less. Krafft-Ebing writes that even now the indications for the use of opium are by no means clear; he finds opium of the greatest value in delirium tremens, in dysthymias, and in commencing melancholias. In anæmic conditions opium, he says, acts disproportionately strongly, and is of doubtful utility. Blandford says that each case of mental disease must be treated on its own merits, and that it is necessary "to experimentalise, so to speak, on each individual," and so determine the use or uselessness of opium. The form of insanity in which, in his experience, opium "does least good and most harm, is acute delirious mania in *sthenic* patients, where there is great excitement with heat of the head," and that it does most good in cases of quiet melancholia. In delirium tremens both opium and morphia (as hypodermic injections) have been much employed, and very large doses have been given. Some give preference to the morphia hypodermic, others to opium in substance and by the mouth. Of late it has been maintained that this disease is best treated by a simple expectant dietetic treatment (*cf.* Nothnagel and Rossbach). If employed it is probable that the hypodermic method is the best, because the surest, since we know so little about the absorptive powers of the alimentary tract of an alcoholic. The delirium of alcohol and also that of fever have been treated beneficially by combining tartar emetic or tincture of aconite with opium. It is obvious that this treatment is indicated chiefly in sthenic cases.

The action of **morphia** is similar to, but not the exact equivalent of, opium. The difference in this action is difficult to express. Practical men state somewhat vaguely that opium, in its calming effects on the nervous system, acts more *smoothly* than morphia; by this they imply that the other alkaloids of opium modify or *round* the action of the morphia. The difference is a clinical experience and not a scientific finding. Besides this primary difference, opium differs from morphia, it is said, in being more constipating, and more liable to cause headache and nausea, but more stimulant and more diaphoretic.

Nothnagel and Rossbach consider that the controversy as to the choice between opium and morphia must be regarded as decided in favour of the morphia. They refer to the subcutaneous administration of morphia, and certainly this method has the advantage of greater precision.

Administration.—Opium, as a hypnotic, may be given as powder or extract, or in the form of one of its numerous preparations. These are really special formulæ adapted to meet special morbid conditions—*e.g.*, of the intestinal tract, of the respiratory organs, &c. Opium by the mouth generally requires one to two hours to develop its effects. Morphia in the form of one of its salts may be given by the mouth in the place of opium. Some choose the bi-meconate of morphia in preference to the other salts, but it is doubtful whether this has more than a theoretic advantage.

Opium or morphia may be given per rectum if need be, and either as an injection or as a suppository.

Or morphia may be administered hypodermically, and this plan has been largely adopted in the treatment of the insane. Thus employed the narcotic action is more rapid and more lasting, and the alimentary tract is less affected in the way of anorexia and constipation. A small piece of ice with smooth surface dipped in salt and applied firmly for about thirty seconds is the best means of producing anæsthesia in cases where the slight pain of the puncture is dreaded.

Whether the subcutaneous or oral method be adopted, opium or morphia may be given either in occasional big doses to meet occasional urgent symptoms, or systematically and in ascending doses. Schüle, Wolff, Voisin, have urged the systematic use of morphia injections in rising dose till the patient is calmed. In elderly people, in general, the dose should be smaller, and this holds in particular for cases of general paralysis of the insane (Nothnagel and Rossbach).

Dose.—Tolerance of opium and morphia soon becomes established, and for this reason, and the disastrous nature of the opium habit, the drugs must always be kept well in hand. Idiosyncrasy is sometimes manifested with regard to opium, the smallest doses exciting and not soothing. Age is a very important element. The hypodermic method is not suitable for children.

Of opium it is unnecess[illegible] the doses of all the prepara[illegible] suffice to give those of the [illegible] tions which may safely b[illegible] with, viz.:

Of the crude opium and o[illegible] ½ gr.–1 gr.; of the tincture, l[illegible] and wine, ♏xv–xx.

Morphia may safely be g[illegible] mouth, to the extent of ¼–½ [illegible] dose, though, according to [illegible] the largest quantity of mor[illegible] should be injected, as a first d[illegible] not exceed one-eighth grain f[illegible] and one-sixth grain for a man.

The above are safe doses, th[illegible] may in cases of idiosyncrasy [illegible] unrest or excitement instead [illegible] ing.

Of the other alkaloids of opi[illegible] be said in general that the stat[illegible] observers are very conflicting, [illegible] this variance is probably the res[illegible] difficulty there is in securing reli[illegible] parations. So far as observatio[illegible] the present goes, there is no r[illegible] believe that in papaverine, or [illegible] or codeine, we have drugs posses[illegible] advantages over morphia, excep[illegible] Krafft-Ebing puts it, those of "[illegible] price and weaker action."

Convulsant action is more pro[illegible] for these alkaloids than for morphia.

Codeine is obtainable in a pur[illegible], and, in combination with phosphori[illegible], it is adapted for hypodermic in[illegible] because it is so little irritant. Fron[illegible] claims that it produces less headache, giddiness, and vomiting than morphia (*Wiener Klin. Wochenschr.*, 1890, No. 3, p. 45). It must be given in about twice the dose of morphia.

Hyoscyamine and Hyoscine.—From the Hyoscyamus niger, an alkaloid hyoscyamine is obtained; it is crystallisable, and is isomeric with atropine. In addition there is present an amorphous alkaloid which is likewise isomeric with atropine; it has been named hyoscine. Commercial hyoscyamine is said to consist largely of hyoscine.

The whole plant hyoscyamus certainly resembles in its action the whole plant belladonna, and this resemblance holds to a considerable extent for the active principles of the plants, atropine on the one hand, hyoscyamine and hyoscine on the other. In a case of acute mania the action of the two alkaloids, hyoscyamine and atropine, appeared to be identical (Ringer, *Practitioner*, March 1877). This question of the precise relative value of these plants, and of their active principles needs further investigation, but as it now stands it may be said that hyoscyamus and its active principles are credited with less delirious action and more soporific action than belladonna and its derivatives.

From experiments with crystallised hyoscyamine Dr. J. C. Shaw concludes that the drug acts exactly like atropine upon the heart and vessels, increasing the frequency of the pulse with, in the first instance, rise, but subsequent fall, of blood-pressure. Dr. Laurent, from a careful study, comes to the same conclusions (Dupuy, "Les Alcaloides," 1890). In fact, the only differences admitted are that the delirium produced is more subdued than for atropine, and that there is a greater tendency to sleep. The mydriatic action of hyoscyamine is less than that of atropine, according to Shaw.

Hyoscine, according to Wood, differs from atropine, and therefore from hyoscyamine also, in its effect upon the heart—*i.e.*, it does not depress the heart to any degree, nor does it paralyse the vagi; the pulse rate is somewhat diminished. Other observers maintain that it acts upon the heart like atropine—*e.g.*, Kobert (*see also* Dupuy, "Les Alcaloides"). The probability is that the substances used have not always been identical. Hyoscine is generally admitted to be a much more decided soporific than hyoscyamine.

The advantage of hyoscine as a soporific is its freedom from after-effects. Some dryness of the throat may occur, and sometimes there is headache, but the alimentary tract is not upset, and in particular there is no constipation. It is in this that the drug has such an advantage over opium. (Atropine, it will be remembered, is held to act in small doses as a laxative, and Laurent states that hyoscyamine acts similarly.)

Hyoscyamine, or by preference hyoscine, is used in the treatment of acute mania and of insomnia accompanied by delirious excitement, whether in the insane or not (Wood). Mitchell, Bruce, and Tirard say that kidney disease does not contra-indicate hyoscine; and Bruce, that he has used it with benefit in exceedingly feeble states of the heart. Both alkaloids have been largely tried by alienists: hyoscyamine by Robert Lawson, Clouston, Savage, Gnauck, Fronmüller, hyoscine by Gnauck, Claussen, Krafft-Ebing, Magnan, and others. Hyoscine is generally given as hydrochlorate or as hydrobromate.

Hyoscyamine may be given in doses by the mouth of $\frac{1}{8}$ to $\frac{1}{6}$ and up to $\frac{1}{3}$ grain. Gnauck allows the administration of crystalline hyoscyamine *subcutaneously* up to $\frac{1}{4}$ grain as the maximum dose, but the doses $\frac{1}{30}$ to $\frac{1}{15}$ grain, advocated by Browne, should be exceeded with caution, and as initial dose it would be well to begin with $\frac{1}{100}$ grain.

Hyoscine by the mouth may be given in doses of $\frac{1}{150}$ to $\frac{1}{100}$ grain, mounting up if need be to $\frac{1}{50}$ or $\frac{1}{30}$ grain, or even to $\frac{1}{30}$ grain of the hydrochlorate of hyoscine. Hypodermically the dose should vary from $\frac{1}{150}$ to $\frac{1}{50}$ grain. Very marked idiosyncrasy is, according to Wood, not infrequent. Drs. Ramadier and Sérieux (*Bulletin Général de Thérap.*, Jan. 1892), after two years' experience with hyoscine hydrochlorate at the Vaucluse Asylum, speak highly of its value in the treatment of mania, in all its varieties, alcoholic, epileptic, &c. They consider the subcutaneous administration the best, but counsel that the dose should begin with $\frac{1}{200}$ grain or even $\frac{1}{300}$ if the patient be weakly.

Merck's preparations of hyoscyamine and hyoscine are to be advised.

Caustic alkalies should not be given with either, since they decompose the alkaloids. This fact we owe more especially to Garrod, who showed the inefficiency of hyoscine as a mydriatic after admixture with caustic alkalies.

Sulphate of Duboisine, obtained from the Duboisia myoporoides, has of late been employed in cases of mental excitement. The alkaloid duboisine is regarded as identical with hyoscine and isomeric with hyoscyamine and atropine. Max Lewald and Vladimir Preininger speak to the value of duboisine, but there seems no reason to prefer it to hyoscine or to an equivalent dose of hyoscyamine. The actual quantities used by the above observers are 0.002 gramme, or about $\frac{1}{33}$ grain; they counsel that this dose should not be exceeded. We would advise that for the present at least the same caution should be observed as for hyoscine, and a very much smaller dose, viz., $\frac{1}{300}$ grain be commenced with (*vide Therap. Monats.*, December 1891).

Cannabis Indica, or Indian Hemp (Gunjah, Bang, are Indian names for the dried plant; Haschish is the Arab name given either to the plant itself or a preparation of which Indian hemp is the chief constituent). Indian hemp contains a volatile alkaloid, cannabinin, the qualities of which have not been thoroughly determined; also a base, strychnine-like in its action, tetano-cannabin (it is not known whether all varieties of Indian hemp contain this), and further an amorphous, resinoid, bitter substance, cannabinon, which is the special, active substance of the hemp. Cannabinon, or the crude hemp, acts chiefly upon the cerebrum, causing exaltation of the psychic functions; the excitement is mostly pleasing, the ideas flow easily, hallucinations of sight or hearing may be present, and forced movements of various kinds (motor hallucinations) are often executed. At times the merriment is very boisterous; at times there is delirium. Mental depression may follow, and the distress be very great. Sleep is the next event, but before it sets in there may be much impairment of sensation, preceded or accompanied by sensations of pins and needles; the anæsthesia may be almost complete and hold for both tactile and painful impressions; muscular sense may be lost. The effect on the breathing and circulation is but slight. The pupils are dilated, but they contract to light.

Cannabis indica has been much employed as a hypnotic and as a sedative. Dr. Russell Reynolds, speaking from an experience of thirty years, states that it is of much value in the treatment of senile insomnia, in which there may be wandering and great restlessness (fidgetiness) at night, whilst during the day the patient may be quite rational. "In this class of cases there is nothing comparable in utility to a moderate dose of Indian hemp—viz., ¼ to ⅓ grain of the extract at bedtime." In alcoholic delirium it is very uncertain; in melancholia it is sometimes of service by converting the depression into exaltation. In the treatment of night restlessness of patients with "general paralysis" it is very useful; also in the insomnia of "temper disease," whether in children or adults, it is eminently useful. Dr. Reynolds has found it of no use in acute mania, but on the other hand Dr. Clouston has found it of the greatest service when combined with bromide of potassium.

In the treatment of neuralgia, especially of the fifth, and of sleeplessness the result of such, cannabis indica is most valuable. It is very valuable in migraine.

Dose. — Rosenthal advocates cannabis indica, the extract prepared according to the recent method, in doses of from 1 to 3 grains in the treatment of the opium habit. The more recent extract is, according to him, less liable to fungus than the older preparation (*Wien. Med. Presse*, September 15, 1889). A preparation, the tannate of cannabin, has been recently introduced and much praised as a hypnotic by Fronmüller. Krafft-Ebing finds it very uncertain. Wood speaks to the same effect.

The simple officinal extract appears to be very variable in composition, and from this result the discrepancies in the observed effects. Dr. [illegible] stress on the importan[illegible] drug. According to [illegible] in the form of extrac[illegible] gr. ⅛ in the first in[illegible] gr. $\frac{1}{10}$ for a child; it m[illegible] sequently. The dose[illegible] by Fronmüller, viz. [illegible] represent a much we[illegible] that of the B.P. T[illegible] whole the best prep[illegible] Dr. Reynolds (20 m[illegible] extract); he advises[illegible] it should be made o[illegible] that it should be ad[illegible] bread-crumbs as d[illegible] minimum dose which must not be [illegible] in less than four to six hours, [illegible] may be increased by one drop every [illegible] or fourth day until relief is obtained [illegible] the drug proved useless. It should be noted that according to his scale of doses the quantity of the B.P. tincture to be begun with would be 4 minims. Given in a mixture the resin is liable to separate out unequally.

Cannabinon is given in the same dose as the officinal extract. The tannate of cannabin, introduced by Merck, is recommended by Fronmüller in doses of 5 to 10 grains. The substance is a yellowish brown powder insoluble in water and in ether, soluble in alcohol; it is inodorous, rather bitter, and tastes somewhat like tannin. The drug is said not to intoxicate and not to constipate. It may be given in powder simply or with the addition of a little sugar. (*Bullet. de Thérap.*, 1883, p. 334.)

Conium (Hemlock). — The officinal species of this genus is the Conium maculatum. Two alkaloids are present in the plant, coniïne and methyl-coniïne. The former alkaloid, $C_8H_{17}N$, is in the pure state quite colourless (Merck), liquid, volatile, and possessed of a peculiar penetrating odour; it is unstable. It forms a number of salts, of which the hydrobromate is well adapted for therapeutic use, since it is fairly stable and forms well-defined crystals which are sufficiently soluble in water. The action of coniïne closely resembles that of curare, poisoning, as it does, the motor nerve-endings throughout the body. The sympathetic motor fibres are paralysed more slowly than the cerebro-spinal. The terminations of the efferent fibres of the vagus are also paralysed, and in this respect the drug contrasts with curare, which is without influence upon them. (Pelissard, Jolyet, Cahours; *see* Dujardin-Beaumetz, "Dictionnaire de Thérap.") Sensory nerves are affected to some extent; thus, numbness, formication are complained of, but the action is slight, and is slow in appearing, and with a massive dose motor paralysis may exist without any apparent sensory failure. The topical application of either coniine or conium (the whole drug) causes some local anæsthesia.

The influence on the cerebral nervous system, in particular the brain, is much less definite than that on the peripheral system; still, there does appear to be some benumbing action on the brain when large doses are taken—*e.g.*, thinking becomes very laborious, and a state of cerebral vacuity is present (Dujardin-Beaumetz). Schmiedeberg speaks of a slight cerebral narcosis, and, among the older records, Pereira states that an actual condition of coma has been occasioned. Special sensibility may suffer—*e.g.*, vision. Along with the impairment of sight there is dilatation of the pupils and some ptosis. The affection of sight will in part be the result of the internal ocular paralysis.

According to some observers, the spinal cord is also slightly affected, its functions depressed; occasionally, convulsions are witnessed which are not the result of asphyxia. On the whole, it is certain that the central nervous system is relatively unaffected.

Conium kills by respiratory paralysis. The influence on the circulation is still uncertain. In toxic doses the temperature is lowered. The urine frequently shows the presence of much mucus (catarrhal state of the urinary passages). Sweating of the skin, and sometimes skin eruptions, are produced.

Use.—In mental diseases conium has been extensively employed—*e.g.*, mania and hysterical excitement; some alienists speak well of it when given in full doses. The indications for its use, however, are by no means clear, and we are disposed to regard it as a sedative of secondary value, the more so on account of the uncertainty of its preparations.

In motor excitement, chorea, tetanus, it has been employed, and in the former affection it is easy to demonstrate its power to control the movements, though this action appears to be palliative and not curative. It might be found useful in the motor restlessness of the insane. The employment of conium in spasmodic lung affections, asthma, whooping-cough, does not belong here.

In neuralgias, tic douloureux, sciatica, conium has its advocates. Dujardin-Beaumetz insists on the much greater efficacy of conium when introduced subcutaneously, and that in this respect the parallelism to curare is maintained, though less strikingly. The dose for injection should be $\frac{1}{6}$ to $\frac{1}{3}$ grain of the hydrobromate of coniine. He recommends the following solution:

	Grms.
Crystallised coniine hydrobromate .	0.5
Alcohol	1.5
Cherry laurel water . . .	23.0

Of this solution a Pravaz syringeful would contain $\frac{1}{3}$ grain of the salt. By the mouth $2\frac{1}{4}$ grains (0.15 gramme) of the hydrobromate of coniine may be given in the twenty-four hours.

Of the whole drug, conium, the succus is generally regarded as the most efficient preparation, though H. C. Wood has frequently found it inoperative. Large doses must be given—*e.g.*, two drachms to half an ounce—but even these doses rapidly become tolerated; thus, in one case, a child suffering from chorea received hourly, except when asleep, seven drachms of the succus conii (Ringer, "Therapeutics"). Dujardin-Beaumetz finds the alcoholic extract of the seeds the best preparation of the whole drug. The alkaloid coniine being volatile and unstable, we should be prepared to find that specimens which have been kept may be almost wholly inert or exceedingly variable in their activity. We must remember, moreover, that the proportions of coniine and of methyl coniine in the plant are variable, and that the alkaloid methyl coniine differs from coniine by acting more powerfully on the spinal cord; hence, that different specimens would act differently. At Bethlem Hospital the succus conii has been given by Dr. Savage continuously, in doses ranging from two drachms to two ounces, without causing any bad symptoms; the cases were of recurrent mania. These doses, even the larger ones, were given thrice daily.

Calabar Bean, the dried seed of Physostigma venenosum, is a spinal sedative, but it influences the brain also. The active principle is an alkaloid, physostigmine, also called eserine; but there is present in the brain another alkaloid, calabarine, whose action, strychnine-like, opposes that of physostigmine. The influence of the latter predominates, however. Physostigmine occurs in colourless crystals slightly soluble in water, freely soluble in ether; it forms various salts—*e.g.*, the sulphate, hydrobromate, salicylate, borate.

The action of physostigmine is upon muscular tissue, striped and plain, as shown by twitchings of the skeletal muscles, contractions of the stomach, spleen, uterus, bladder, and pupil; the latter action finds practical application. The blood-pressure rises (action on heart and vaso-motor fibres). There may be dyspnœa. The respirations are first accelerated, then retarded. Further, it causes increase of glandular secretions—*e.g.*, mucous, salivary, lachrymal, cutaneous, &c. It acts also on the central nervous system, in particular the cord, causing paralysis, general and, if the dose be sufficient, complete; death results from arrest of respiration. Physostigmine paralysis is of spinal origin, and the brain does not share in the production of this symptom; the posterior limits suffer before the anterior. Death results from the invasion of the medulla by the paralysis. Sensation if affected is so secondarily. The peripheral nerves, motor and sensory, practically escape. Preceding the paralysis a period of great excitement may occur; this has been especially witnessed in experiments on cats, the animals running wildly about; guinea-pigs may exhibit the same. The excitement has been attributed to the dyspnœa caused by the drug, but, as Dr. Brunton states, this can hardly be the whole explanation, and we must infer *that there is direct cerebral stimulation.* In confirmation of this we find, from experiments on animals, predisposed to epileptiform attacks, by Brown-Séquard's method, that physostigmine increases the liability to convulsive seizures, and the same has been observed in respect of epileptic patients, the attacks becoming more frequent.

When Calabar bean, not its active principle physostigmine, is administered, discordant results are frequent; thus, convulsions probably of spinal origin, and like those produced by strychnine, may occur; it is held that these are caused by the calabarine present.

Therapeutic Use.—In tetanus physostigmine would seem to be directly indicated, and by several observers successful cases are recorded. To be serviceable here it must be given freely in quantity sufficient to produce paralysis, and must be pushed indeed to such an extent that but a little more would permanently arrest breathing (Ringer, "Therapeutics"). Dr. Eben Watson gave 72 grains of a spirituous extract in twenty-four hours; and one of the writers of this article gave $2\frac{1}{2}$ grains of the watery extract every hour for thirty-six hours (for a short time four grains were given hourly: Ringer's "Therapeutics"). In chorea the value of physostigmine is not established. In paraplegia and locomotor ataxy the drug has been employed.

In general paralysis of the insane Calabar bean has been repeatedly tried. Sir James Crichton Browne speaks [illegible] it, and he is even quoted as having [illegible] two cases by means of it. This [illegible] is, however, an entire misrepre[illegible] for in a letter to the *Journal of* [illegible] *Science*, April 1875, p. 152, he [illegible] "While claiming for the Calabar [illegible] a valuable power of modifying and [illegible] ing the progress of that mos[illegible] ent malady, I have never sugge[illegible] it should be regarded as a cure." [illegible] observers confirm Sir Crichton [illegible] as to the modifying influence of [illegible] stigma on general paralysis. B[illegible] recent and extended trials with the [illegible] at the Wakefield Asylum have yie[illegible] different results.

Dose.—The large doses which [illegible] given in the treatment of a critical [illegible] like tetanus have been mentioned [illegible] it must be added that the plan of [illegible] istration in this disease should be, [illegible] doses at short intervals—*e.g.*, h[illegible] that the drug may be withheld [illegible] symptoms of collapse or of [illegible] appear.

In the treatment of chronic spin[illegible] tions or of general paralysis sma[illegible] should be employed, but they sh[illegible] continued for long periods; thus, [illegible] Crichton Browne's cases, doses [illegible] grain of the extract were given [illegible] ously for from nine to twelve [illegible] Doses of $\frac{1}{50}$—$\frac{1}{10}$ grain every two [illegible] hours may also be tried in the[illegible] plaints (Ringer, "Therapeutics"). [illegible] sostigma, as the officinal extract, [illegible] given in the above doses, either [illegible] mouth, or by rectum; or, dilut[illegible] water (*e.g.*, $\frac{1}{5}$ grain in 10 minims), [illegible] be injected subcutaneously.

If the salts of physostigmine be [illegible] istered—*e.g.*, sulphate or salicyl[illegible] dose, by the mouth, is $\frac{1}{60}$—$\frac{1}{30}$ gr[illegible] may be increased to $\frac{1}{12}$; hypoderm[illegible] $\frac{1}{120}$—$\frac{1}{50}$ grain. If we use these salts [illegible] alkaloid in the treatment of tet[illegible] must push the drug by repetition [illegible] dose till an effect is produced.

Boldine is an alkaloid obtained [illegible] the leaves of the Peumus boldus, of [illegible] (nat. order, Monimiaceæ). It is [illegible] slightly soluble in water; freely solu[illegible] alcohol, ether, and chloroform; it is [illegible] possess feeble narcotic powers. In [illegible] plant, however, another active princ[illegible] glucoside, has been found; it has [illegible] named boldo-glucine.

Boldo-glucine possesses decided [illegible] notic powers, and it is held that the [illegible] plant acts as a hypnotic by means of [illegible] glucine chiefly. A certain amount of [illegible] incoordination precedes sleep. In [illegible] dose death takes place by asphyxia [illegible] heart also is weakened; the temperature is slightly lowered (Laborde: Dupuy, "Les Alcaloides").

Of the glucoside, doses of 2 to 8 grammes (30 grains to 2 drachms) have been given in draughts, capsules, or rectal injections. M. Magnan treated successfully, at St. Anne's Asylum, a case of insomnia with horrific hallucinations; he gave 30 grains of the plant. Dr. Juranville mentions ten similar cases. The sleep is said to be natural and not to be accompanied by anæsthesia (*Brit. Med. Journ.*, 1888, vol. i. p. 918). Dr. Laborde states that there is some anæsthesia (*loc. cit.*). It cannot be said that the drug has been thoroughly investigated (Leech).

SYDNEY RINGER.
HARRINGTON SAINSBURY.

SELENIASIS, SELENIASMUS (σελήνη, the moon). Literally, the moon-disease; lunacy. (Fr. *séléniase;* Ger. *Mondsucht.*)

SELENOBLETUS (σελήνη; βλητός, stricken). Moonstruck. Supposed disease from exposure to the moon's influence. Lunatic. (Fr. *sélénoblète.*)

SELENOGAMIA (σελήνη; γάμος, marriage). A synonym of Somnambulism. Literally, wedded to the moon.

SELENOPLEGE, SELENOPLEXIA (σελήνη; πληγή, a stroke). "Apoplexia" from exposure to the moon's influence. (Fr. *sélénoplexie.*)

SELF-MUTILATION. — The interest which naturally attaches to those strangely mysterious cases of self-mutilation, self-torture, and self-dismemberment of various parts of the body which are sometimes met with in medical practice, and not unfrequently by the alienist physician, both within and out of asylums, will probably be intensified, and possibly some additional light may be thrown upon the obscurity which surrounds the whole subject, by an endeavour to trace some of the motives which have prompted to the commission of the acts at various periods of history, and under various religious conditions.

Cases of the kind are on record from the earliest ages; by the Levitical law priests were forbidden to make any cuttings in their flesh, showing that the custom then prevailed. Many, perhaps most, of those self-inflicted tortures have at all times had their origin in unduly exaggerated religious fervour, enthusiasm, or fanaticism, and the custom of inflicting self-injury probably had its birth in the peculiar religious beliefs of Orientals in the remoter East.

Believing, as they did, the material body to be essentially corrupt, the handiwork of an evil spirit, they sought communion with Deity, by extirpating its passions and desires.

Dean Milman says regarding this common Oriental belief, "The principle of the purity of mind and malignity of matter is the parent of all that asceticism which from earliest ages pervaded the old religions of the East."

In Thibet, in India, in China, in Siam, and in Mahomedan Asia, the Lama, the Faquir, the Bonze, the Dervish, are all examples.

These fanatics have withdrawn from the society of man in order to abstract the pure mind from the dominion of corrupting matter.

Under each of these systems the perfection of human nature was estrangement from the influence of the senses which were enslaved to the material elements of the world.

An approximation to the essence of the Deity was sought to be attained by a total secession from the interests, the thoughts, the passions, the common being and nature of man.

The practical operation of this elementary principle of Eastern religion has deeply influenced the whole history of man, but it had made no progress in Europe till after the introduction of Christianity.

The manner in which it allied itself with a system to the original nature and design of which it appears altogether foreign, forms an important chapter in the history of Christianity.

The worship of Cybele was orgiastic; there was an inward frenzy helped on by wild music and dancing, the supposed working of a divine influence upon the soul. The priests of Cybele were seen in devotees and females of excitable temperament. The vulgar beheld them with awe, as manifestly possessed with divinity. The philosophers despised them as impostors.

Atys, in a paroxysm of false devotion, mutilated himself to qualify for the priesthood of Cybele.

"He plunged into the Phrygian forest dark
Wherein the mighty goddess [Cybele] dwells,
And by a zealot frenzy stung,
Shore with a flint his sex away,
Which madly on the ground he flung."

His feelings when he comes to the consciousness of his condition are the subject of the famous poem of Catullus.

Origen, a father of the Church, whose Christianity had a strong Oriental tinge, made himself an eunuch on the strength of a liberal understanding of St. Matthew xix. 12. Probably, also, his bitter grief and remorse, as recorded in his "sad and doleful lamentations after his fall, in the days of Severus," may have helped to conduce to the act, being betrayed into making sacrifice as the only alternative left to him of having his hitherto undefiled body polluted by miscreants.

We have in the monastic flagellations of the Christian Church instances of self-torture as an expiation for sin.

Sometimes self-torture arose from a desire to conciliate malignant powers supposed to delight in the pain of their votaries; thus, the priests of Baal, who, failing to bring fire from heaven by their enchantments, cut themselves with knives and lancets until the blood gushed out upon them (1 Kings xviii. 28).

The worshippers of Moloch ("horrid king besmeared with blood") made their children pass through the fire in his honour. The Hindoo prostrates himself before the car of Juggernaut.

Sometimes the motive for self-torture has been remorse, self-hatred; the offending senses or members must be chastened for their sins.

The Gadarene demoniac expresses the sense of his misery, and the terrible bondage under which he had come, by a blind rage against himself as the true author of his evil, wounding and cutting himself with stones. Such persons are described in the Gospels as grievously possessed by devils or evil spirits.

Sometimes the motive for which self-torture is undergone is simply to show endurance of pain and strength of will, as by the American Indians, and by Mucius Scevola, in the Roman legend, who burnt his hand in a brazier of live coals to convince Porsena that no amount of pain could subdue his spirit.

Other motives conduce to self-mutilation. Thus, the convict, if opportunity serves him, will mutilate, or even dismember, himself to avoid the performance of his allotted task, or to excite sympathy. Individual cases are to be found in our criminal reports.

In a quaint treatise on mutilation and demembration by Sir Alexander Seton, a Scotch lawyer of the seventeenth century, he defines mutilation to be the cessation and prevention of the office and distinct operation of a member, albeit no particle of it be cut off; and by demembration he understands the cutting off of a member.

In speaking of *castratio viridium*, he says it is one of the most atrocious demembrations, and when a man does it himself he is *sui homicida*, and so punishable with death and confiscation of goods, and its equivalent if one suffered himself willingly to be castrated by another.

All the states of mind leading to self-mutilation, self-torture, &c., hitherto considered, are compatible with comparative sanity, although they are to insanity near akin, and generally indicate more or less mental derangement.

Of actual insanity leading to self-mutilation Herodotus records a notable example in the Spartan king, Cleomenes. The Lacedæmonians had invited Cleomenes back to Sparta, offering him his former dignity. After indulging in wild and extravagant enterprises, immediately on his return he was seized with madness; he struck every citizen he met in the face with his sceptre. This extravagant behaviour induced his friends to confine him in a pair of stocks. Seeing himself on some occasions left with only one person to guard him, he demanded a sword. The man at first refused to obey him, but, finding him persist in his request, the man, being a helot, gave him one. Cleomenes, as soon as he received the sword, began to cut the flesh off his legs. He ascended to his thighs, from his thighs to his loins, till at length, making gashes in his belly, he died.

Of St. Francis of Assisi it was said that he had divinely received the stigmata, or marks of the Saviour's passion, on hands and feet. The question has been much debated whether these marks were self-inflicted from fanatical motives.

A similar imitation of the crucifixion is told of certain French devotees of the last century.

Orgiastic paroxysms of intense devotion have at different times found their way into Christianity, and perverted its pure and peaceful spirit into a visionary frantic enthusiasm, where the mild and rational faith has been too calm for persons brooding over their internal emotions.

In the present day it is found that, although instances of self-injury are not unfrequent, probably the intention of those inflicting them is more commonly suicidal in character, whereas instances of wilful self-mutilation for its own sake are much more rare. An investigation into the various causes leading to the act is attended with so much the greater interest on that account.

The usual difficulty presents itself in investigating the origin of cases of this kind that occurs in the investigation of many other forms of mental disease, or perhaps it exists in even a greater degree, owing to the condition of mind to which the patient is frequently reduced before being brought to an asylum after the injury, or to the difficulty of obtaining reliable evidence as to the mental condition of the patient before, at the time of, and immediately subsequent to the infliction; and we are often baffled by obstinate and persistent taciturnity or by stupor, the associate of the melancholic condition.

The task of investigation becomes easier, however, when we find the mutilative act the direct result of **hallucination** affecting the special senses, or **delusion** evidently conducing to it.

Patients labouring under those forms of mental disorder, being sometimes talkative and communicative, will readily admit that the act has been committed owing to hearing a voice from heaven commanding them to do it, or by terror at seeing a vision, and in the frenzy produced thereby, being impelled to self-mutilation or injury. The act may be induced by fear of loathsome disease, produced by a perverted sense of smell, or of poison by diseased sense of taste.

The number of publicly recorded cases of self-mutilation is not great; it therefore becomes of the more importance when well-authenticated facts are ascertained with regard to causation in cases of the kind that they should be brought under the notice of the profession through the usual channels.

Before proceeding with the narrative of several cases which have during recent years come under the notice of the writer, reference may be made to the importance of the subject in its general as well as in its medico-legal aspect, and with this object in view also attention is called to two cases which were published in the *Journal of Mental Science* for April 1882.

In the first of these, reported by Dr. Howden, of Montrose, a tendency to self-mutilation was shown to exist in several members of the same family, and the injury inflicted was similar in character in each member, although it does not appear that one was even aware of the act which had been perpetrated by the other many years before. One member imagined that God had ordered her to mutilate herself, and she accordingly attempted to pull out her tongue, and, on being restrained, she succeeded in biting a large piece off. A brother of the foregoing patient had succeeded in gouging out one of his eyes. In a subsequent attack the first-named patient believed that God had ordered her to burn herself, in order to purify her soul, which would then appear in heaven of pure gold. She subsequently succeeded in injuring her body internally and in gouging her eyes out.

The second case, that of a farmer named Brooks, is of peculiar interest medico-legally, for this man, in whom insanity does not seem even to have been suspected, not only inflicted an injury upon his own person, but he succeeded in getting a jury to believe the false story he told with regard to the manner of its infliction, and was thus the means of causing two neighbouring farmers, who were perfectly innocent of the crime with which they were charged by Brooks, to be sentenced each to ten years' penal servitude. What mental state he was in, or what moral or other obliquity existed in Brooks to account for his conduct, is not shown by this account.

In connection with the **medico-legal** aspect of this subject, the writer would also briefly remark upon those curious cases, sometimes causing much anxiety, which are occasionally met with, especially among the more educated classes, where circumstantial statements are made with regard to supposed injuries said to be self-inflicted, of which there is no evidence. A remarkable, although extreme, instance of this kind occurred many years ago in the case of an eminent scientific man who had been educated as a surgeon. This gentleman laboured under occasional maniacal attacks, alternating with extreme depression. He informed the writer, when visiting him one morning in his bedroom, that, in the course of the preceding night, he had dislocated his ankle- and hip-joint on one side, and broken both bones of the leg on the other. As if this were not enough, he spoke also of a wound in the temporal artery. He gave evidence of his own firm belief in the existence of those injuries by having carefully and accurately bandaged all the parts named for them respectively, and for this purpose he had torn his sheets into bandages, and he resisted, with evident anxiety, the removal of those bandages, whereupon not the smallest sign of any injury was found to exist.

Cases in which the mutilative act was occasioned by **hallucination**.—The first of these to be narrated was that of a lady, concerning whom the accounts heard were of a very alarming and unusual character. They were somewhat as follows: That if she were left alone, or free from restraint for even a single instant, some dire tragedy would certainly ensue; that if her hands were allowed to be free for one moment, she would gouge out her eyes with her fingers, pull out her tongue, or do something else equally dreadful. She was reported to have occupied a "locked bed" every night for a very lengthened period, and to have seldom been without some form of restraint for many days together. It was further reported concerning her that self-injury was attempted in every possible way; that she necessarily had an attendant to watch her at all times, whilst frequently and for long periods she had required more than one.

She was admitted into the Crichton Royal Institution in October 1875, and the entries in the case-book on December 2, 1875, regarding her proved the correctness of the foregoing history. There occurs the following entry in the case-book:

This is a very bad case, in which little or no improvement has taken place. The patient an hour and a half after admission gouged out her right eye, which now presents a horrible wreck. She refuses her food, and has to be fed artificially three times a day. Restraint is employed to prevent her gouging out the other eye, as she is on the *qui vive* to get an opportunity of doing herself injury.

In 1880 this patient was examined by the writer, and the following was her mental and bodily condition:

A greatly reduced, exhausted, and emaciated frame, cachectic and hollow features and worn facial appearance; the right eye is wanting, the hair is grizzled and grey, and there are marked facial lines; the cause of the repeated mutilative attempts of which she has been guilty, and to which she has still a determined tendency, is hallucination of the senses both of hearing and vision, whilst the other special senses are markedly disordered as well. She hears voices commanding her to do the acts referred to; she sees her children burning in the fire, shrieks with terror, and tries to push in her head beside them. She says she feels she is not worthy to live, because she is so diseased and wicked that she is a burden to herself, and she refuses her food because it is poisoned.

Under careful nursing and nourishing with generous diet and a moderate amount of stimulant she gradually improved, and it became possible to entirely discontinue the use of restraint, and the last report in the case-book referring to the year 1883 was as follows:

From the time of the last entry to the present the improvement then reported has been well maintained, and restraint of any kind has never again been found necessary. Although still subject to the same hallucinations and delusions they are well under control, and do not influence her conduct in the same manner as previously. She is never without supervision, but she is allowed a considerable amount of liberty to admit of her taking healthful exercise. She attends and enjoys the various amusements, and she joins with spirit and animation at times into the dances, she plays the piano, and altogether leads a life of as much composure and comfort as can be expected in a case of the kind, in which recovery cannot be hoped for.

A very marked case of self-injury, the direct result of aural hallucination, occurred in A. B., a patient in a metropolitan asylum. This patient not only heard voices in the manner peculiar to such cases, but he was in the habit of shouting at the top of his voice up to the skies, and asking questions to which he professed to receive direct replies; on one occasion, in reply to a question put in this manner, he received an order to mutilate his throat, whereupon, having obtained surreptitious access to the shoemaker's shop, he secured a knife, and carried out the order; fortunately, surgical aid was at hand, and his life was saved.

Prichard, in his work on insanity (p. 113), describes a case in which the patient habitually wounded his hands, wrists, and arms with needles and pins; the blood poured copiously, dropping from his elbows when his arms were bare.

The following are cases of sexual self-mutilation; similar ones are given in Krafft-Ebing's "Psychopathia Sexualis," by Moll, and by some of the French authors, more particularly in their systematic works on mental diseases.

An officer in the Indian service, who had been many years resident in the East, and had come to acquire many Eastern languages and ways, in a fit of religious enthusiasm and excitement removed the testes and part of the scrotum. The determination with which he carried his mutilation into effect is shown by the fact that, the knife which he used being a very blunt one, the patient was occupied two hours in doing it. It subsequently transpired that he removed the testes under the impression that he must become an eunuch to enable him to preach to and convert tribes in Northern India. He said that he would do the same again; that he was quite justified in doing it. He evidently gloried in the idea and spoke openly on the subject. He died insane recently.

The following case of sexual self-mutilation was admitted into the Southern Counties Asylum in 1883: W. B., eighteen years of age, a tall and handsome farm servant, single, by religious persuasion a Presbyterian. He has had no previous attacks of mental disease; he has been four days insane; the cause of his insanity is not known; he is stated to be neither epileptic nor suicidal, but dangerous to others. No member of the family is known to have been insane. The facts indicating insanity as given in the medical certificate for admission are: Violent in his conduct at times, has fixed delusions, prays that he may be delivered from his enemies, states that his medical attendant is in league with others in plotting against him. His mother states that he believes himself to be the "Apostle Paul," and that he is being persecuted; he refuses food from her, saying that she wants to drug him, and deliver him to his enemies.

The following particulars were ascertained with regard to the seriously mutilated condition in which he was found on admission:

On March 6, 1883, whilst employed as a farm servant, he told his fellow-servants, who were then at dinner, that he was going home to his father's house about two miles off, but it appears that instead of doing so, when alone in a field a short distance off, he, with a sharp pen-knife, completely and cleanly removed the whole of the penis. The hæmorrhage ensuing from the wound was very great, and feeling alarmed about it, he went to some running water near at hand, and bathed the wound; the water being very cold at the time, it seems to have assisted in arresting the hæmorrhage.

The lad's master soon after found him lying in a field with marks of blood about him, and had him conveyed home. On his medical attendant visiting him he found him quite rational at the time, but he seemed much dejected, and expressed his regret several times to his mother and medical attendant for what he had done. The hæmorrhage had ceased, there had been oozing from the cut surface, but the lad's mother had applied cobwebs, which caused a clot to form and this had arrested the oozing.

When questioned, he admitted that he had masturbated, and when asked why he had so mutilated himself he said that he considered he was only doing his duty, and following out the spirit of Scriptural injunction: "If thy right hand offend thee cut it off." He had been reading some quack publications on nervous debility, and also Salvation Army publications, which roused within him strong convictions of his wickedness, and an impulse came upon him that he ought to do something. So he got his Bible, and happening to open it at Leviticus he believed it to be his duty to do what he did, but he remarked if he had opened his Bible at any other place he would not have done so.

For some time after admission there was much taciturnity, depression, and stupor, with absolute refusal of food, and he had to be fed with the stomach pump. He also tore the surgical dressing from his wound, and had to be constantly watched to prevent this. This condition was followed by excitement, an exalted and religiously exhilarated frame of mind, during which he sang and repeated psalms and hymns by night and day. This was succeeded by a gradual return to his normal mental condition, in which he now remains, the wound having healed by granulation over its entire surface.

The following is a case possessing interest from the fact that self-mutilation and attempted self-mutilation were always sought to be effected by the same agent, namely, "fire," although, unfortunately, from the extreme taciturnity which characterised the case, the reason, first, why self-mutilation was so persistently attempted at all, and, secondly, why the particular agent employed was "fire," could not be ascertained.

The lady in question was a patient in West Malling Place, Kent. Two and a half years previously to her admission there, and whilst in an acutely melancholic state, she thrust her right hand into the fire, and it became necessary to amputate some portion of it, the hand remaining permanently contracted and disfigured.

Throughout the year 1882 she made repeated attempts to do the same, undeterred by her previous experience of pain and suffering. She also tried to set fire to herself with a candle and to get possession of matches.

The patient died in the year 1887 of well-marked organic brain disease. She had pin point pupils followed by continuous convulsions and paralysis.

In going round the wards of almost any asylum for the insane cases are continually encountered of what may be described as minor self-mutilations. A patient is met with here and there who inflicts severe punishment upon his own head or body with his clenched fists, causing extensive ecchymosis or even wounding. Another, again, in a maniacal or excited state, will cause self-injury or laceration by dashing himself against walls, or by throwing himself upon the ground. Some of these injuries are undoubtedly self-inflicted for supposed sin or other cause, but a large proportion of the minor mutilations, such as biting the nails into the quick, picking the skin of the face, or head, or hands, arms or body, with finger-nails, needles, pins, glass, &c., into sores more or less extensive, are self-inflicted by patients in a state of dementia who do not reflect or reason upon what they are doing, and the mischievous propensities probably arise simply from nervous, fidgety, restless habits, generating a desire to be doing something, or possibly in some cases originating in an irritable state of the skin. JAMES ADAM.

SENILE DEMENTIA, SENILE INSANITY, SENILITY.—Mental maladies of, and the mental weakness from, old age, commencing at various ages in different persons. (*See* DEMENTIA; OLD AGE.)

SENSATION. — Psychologically considered, sensations are merely modes of our being affected mentally through our sense organs; these sensations are built up by synthetic and other processes into presentations of sense, and we then perceive "things" as having qualities revealed by our mental states. (*See* PHILOSOPHY OF MIND.)

SENSATIONS, SUBJECTIVE. (*See* HALLUCINATIONS.)

SENSE.—The faculty by which impressions are received so as to affect the mind. The senses usually enumerated are sight, hearing, touch, smell, and taste, but to these a sixth must be added, namely, muscular sense.

SENSES, DISORDERS OF. (*See* HALLUCINATIONS; ILLUSIONS; SMELL, HALLUCINATIONS OF.)

SENSIBILITY. — The power living parts possess of receiving conscious impressions from external objects. It is termed "organic" when impressions are unconsciously received.

SENSITIVE.—Capable of receiving conscious impressions. It is also used to express the state of mind of any one easily or deeply affected by impressions so slight as to be out of proportion to the effect produced.

SENSITORIUM, SENSORIUM COMMUNE. — The seat of sensation in the brain. (*See* BRAIN, PHYSIOLOGY OF.)

SENSUS COMMUNIS. — Literally, "common feeling." It is the tone of consciousness at any moment, and is made up of the general result of mingling of nervous impulses of indefinite origin and great variety from all parts of the body pouring into the central nervous system. Among the stimuli are the changes in the blood and blood-vessels, the presence of extractives, &c., in the blood, the movements of the various bodily organs, &c. The characteristic of the sensus communis is the entire absence of [illegible] feelings composing it.

SENTIMENTAL TEMPERAMENT.—Lotze's alternative name for the [illegible] cholic temperament. (*See* [illegible].)

SENTIMENTS. (*See* [illegible].)

SERICUM.—The Arabian physicians prescribed sericum for a bad memory, and as a general nervine tonic and cordial. Avicenna in this agreed with Serapion, and gave it with musk. It formed an ingredient in the electuary of Mesue (Syrian), which was administered as a remedy in insanity. A London physician, the author of "A Discourse on the Nature, Cause, and Cure of Melancholy and Vapours," published in the early part of the eighteenth century, recommended it, among other restoratives, in melancholia, "toasted." Passing from its internal administration, Moses Charras ("Royal Pharmacopœia") lauds its fragrance and its beautiful texture as affecting the senses. A special influence has been attributed to it in this connection, and is by Grant Allen accounted for, psychologically, by the soft and voluminous character of the material. An old French author (anonymous) writes of "ce tissu charmant qui inspiroit aux dieux un amour éperdu, et aux hommes la fureur et la rage des plaisirs effrénés," and which in the form of "la ceinture de la mère de l'amour," possessed "la vertu des philtres." Moll has recently referred to its aphrodisiac properties; metaphorically, Shakespeare ("2 Hen. V.") does the same.

Recognising a subtle connoisseurs in the material, the Roman Senate, in the reign of Tiberius, enacted, "Ne vestis serica viros fœdaret" (Tacit. "Ann." ii. 33; Dion. Cass. lvii. 15; Suidas v. [illegible]). Stringent measures were taken in subsequent reigns against its use. Christian writers denounced it — *e.g.*, Clemens Alexand. ("Pædag." ii. 10), Tertullian ("De Pallio"). The virtuous wife, according to Plutarch, ought not to wear it ("Conj. Præc." vol. vi. 550, ed. Reiske). See references to sericum, including the *Coa Vestis*, in Tibullus, Horace, Ovid, &c. The psychology of clothes receives curious illustrations from this study, and is a deeper subject than appears at first sight. The psychical relations between sensory impressions and particular textures are not unimportant in mental affections, and deserve more study than they have received.

SEX, INFLUENCE OF, IN INSANITY.—Aretæus, the Greek physician of the first century, and Cœlius Aurelianus, a writer of uncertain age and country, taught that men are more subject to insanity than women. Esquirol, who appears to have been the first who applied statistics to the matter, showed elaborately that more women are insane than men, the proportion being thirty-eight women to thirty-seven men.* Georget, Haslam, and others confirmed this conclusion. Burrows, even before Esquirol, had said that more women were insane than men in large towns, but that it was not so in the country. Parchappe made an important step in advance by pointing out that in order to form an accurate estimate of the sexual incidence of insanity we must consider the admissions to asylums, and not the actual number of inmates, the latter being affected by the varying rates of mortality and recovery in the two sexes. He considered the admissions to various large asylums (Bethlem, Bicêtre, Salpêtrière, Charenton, Turin, &c.), and found that, with the very marked exception of Bicêtre and Salpêtrière, the admissions of men exceeded those of women. He concluded that the solution of the question was still doubtful.† A few years later Thurnam made a more accurate and decisive investigation than any that had gone before.‡ He showed that the probability of recovery is greater in women than in men, the recoveries of women exceeding those of men by from 4 to 28 per cent. He showed also that there is a still greater difference in the rate of mortality, the mortality of men being 50 and sometimes nearly 90 per cent. greater than that of women—*i.e.*, nearly double. In 1844, in England and Wales, there were 9053 male inmates of asylums to 9701 females, the admissions of women in London greatly predominating over those of men, in comparison with the country. In 24 asylums out of 32 (including a total of 71,800 admissions), Thurnam found a decided excess of men among admissions, the average excess being 13.7 per cent. In a very large number of British asylums (including 67,876 admissions) there were about 36 men to 32 women. In France more women become insane relatively to men than in England. Thurnam also observed that a larger proportion of women become insane relatively to men among the lower classes than among the higher. He concluded that "in nearly all points of view women have an advantage over men in reference to insanity; for not only do they appear to be less liable than men to mental derangement, but, when the subjects of it, the probability of their recovery is on the whole greater, and that of death considerably less. On the other hand, the probability of a relapse, or of a recurrence of the disorder, is somewhat greater in women than in men." Dr. Jarvis, a few years later, after examining the statistics of asylums in Great Britain, Ireland, France, Belgium, and America, came to the similar conclusion that "males are somewhat more liable to insanity than females."*

* "Maladies mentales," 1838.

† "Recherches statistiques sur les Causes de l'Aliénation mentale." Rouen, 1839.

‡ "Observations and Essays on the Statistics of Insanity." London, 1845.

If we look to the gross number of lunatics in the various countries of Europe, we shall find on the whole that throughout the century, as Esquirol showed, the women are more numerous than the men. There are, however, notable exceptions; according to Haushofer, male lunatics are more numerous in Germany, Denmark, Norway, and Russia. In Italy in 1888 there were 11,895 male lunatics to 10,529 female, being a proportionately greater increase among the men than among the women, but to a very slight extent.

A relatively greater increase of male lunatics does not, however, seem to be the rule in Europe, and for this country at least Thurnam's results can no longer be accepted. In Bethlem from 1786 to 1794 there were 4992 men to 4882 women admitted, a very obvious excess of men. At the middle of the present century Thurnam found it necessary to examine the proportion of admissions in order to show the excess of males. In the early days of the Lunacy Commission (*i.e.*, thirty years ago) the rate of increase of insanity to population was greater among males than among females (as Mr. Noel Humphreys has pointed out); in recent years the rate of increase among females has slightly exceeded that among males. At the present time not only is the female population of our asylums in excess of the male, but the admissions of women are in excess of the admissions of men. During the ten years 1878–87, the total number of admissions of women to the public and private asylums of England and Wales was 69,560, as against 66,918 men; this shows an increase of women, producing equality of the sexes. If we turn to the report of the lunacy commissioners of England and Wales for 1890 we find a larger proportion of female admissions. During that year 8466 women were admitted to the county and borough asylums to 7690 men; in the registered hospitals and licensed houses the excess of women was equally well marked, and the grand total of admissions for 1890 was 10,025 women as against 9109 men. Some

* "On the Comparative Liability of Males and Females to Insanity." 1850.

deduction must be made when we take into consideration the slight excess of women in the general population, and the greater frequency of recurrence of insanity in women, but, even with these deductions, there is no doubt that the incidence of insanity in this country is now greater on women than on men.

In the United States of America and in the English colonies (as in foreign countries generally) there is an excess of male lunatics. The statistics for the United States are still very imperfect, but in Pennsylvania, where they receive most attention, the excess is very clear; thus, during 1889, an average year, there were 1017 admissions of men to 836 of women. In New South Wales the number of insane persons on the official registers at the end of the year 1890 was 1966 men and 1196 women. At the Cape, at the same time, the European and coloured inmates of the asylums numbered 335 men and 240 women, the excess of men being nearly as well marked among the white as among the black population.

While there is some variation in different countries as to the proportion of male and female lunatics, nearly everywhere there are more male than female idiots. The statistics are not altogether reliable, but there seems to be no doubt as to this general result. Thus, in France, in 1866, while there were 24,190 male lunatics and 26,536 female, there were 22,736 male idiots to 17,217 female idiots. The admissions of idiots to asylums recorded by the Lunacy Commissioners were, during 1890, 165 males to 71 females; and the total number of persons in establishments for idiots was 955 males to 478 females. The number of admissions here shows a ratio very closely approximating to that stated some years ago by Langdon Down as that in which the sexes are affected—*e.g.*, 2.1 to 0.9. Microcephales are said to be more commonly male than female. Cretinism also, unlike goitre, is more common in males in the proportion (according to Lunier, writing in Jaccoud's "Dictionnaire") of 5 to 4, varying, however, according to region.

If we turn to the causes of insanity, we find that the most frequent causes, according to French statistics, fell as under:

Men.	*Women.*
Alcoholic excess.	Love and jealousy.
Venereal excess.	Religion.
Loss of fortune.	Destitution and misery.
Love and jealousy.	Loss of fortune.
Destitution and misery.	Violent emotions.
Pride.	Loss of a loved person.
Violent emotions.	Venereal excess.
Deceived ambition.	Pride.
Religion.	Alcoholic excess.
Loss of a loved person.	Deceived ambition.

According to another classification of French statistics, the results are somewhat similar, except that loss of fortune, destitution, and misery, being combined as pecuniary causes, come at the head of the list on the women's side, and before love on the men's.

During the ten years 1878–87, 136,478 persons (66,918 men and 69,560 women) were admitted into all classes of asylums in England and Wales. If we consider the causes of their insanity, the proportion per cent. to total number admitted during the ten years was as follows:

	M.	F.
Alcoholic intemperance . .	19.8	7.2
Various bodily diseases and disorders	11.1	10.5
Domestic troubles (including loss of relations and friends)	4.2	9.7
Adverse circumstances (including business anxieties, and pecuniary difficulties)	8.2	3.7
Parturition and the puerperal state	—	6.7
Mental anxiety, "worry," and overwork	6.6	5.5
Accident or injury . . .	5.2	1.0
Religious excitement . . .	2.5	2.9
Love affairs (including seduction)	0.7	2.5
Fright and nervous shock .	0.9	1.9
Sexual intemperance . . .	1.0	0.6
Venereal disease	0.6	0.2
Self-abuse (sexual) . . .	2.1	0.3
Over-exertion	0.7	0.4
Sunstroke	2.3	0.2
Pregnancy	—	1.0
Lactation	—	2.2
Uterine and ovarian disorders	—	2.3
Puberty	0.2	0.6
Change of life	—	4.0
Fevers	0.7	0.5
Privation and starvation .	1.7	2.1
Old age	3.8	4.6
Other ascertained causes existed in	2.3	1.0
And the causes were unknown in	21.3	22.1
There had been previous attacks in	14.3	18.9
Hereditary influence was ascertained in	19.0	22.1
Congenital defect was ascertained in	5.1	3.5

On the whole it may be said that causes acting on the brain are more common in men; moral and emotional causes are more common in women; excesses, both intellectual and sensual, are more common causes in men.

If we turn to the consideration of the prevalence of special forms of insanity in the sexes, the subject becomes somewhat more complex, but certain conclusions seem to be fairly clear. States of exaltation, speaking generally, belong to early age; "mental exaltation," as Clouston remarks, "is perfectly natural in childhood. It is, in fact, the physiological state of brain at that period." States of depression belong to a somewhat more advanced age. Mania, in both men and women, is more common than melancholia. Both mania and melancholia seem to be more common on the whole in women than in men, but the preponderance of female over male melancholiacs is much more marked than in the case of the maniacal. Progressive insanity with systematised delusions (*délire des persécutions*) is much more common in women; thus, Garnier finds it in 2.16 per cent. of male lunatics, in 8.64 per cent. of female lunatics. It is worthy of note that while melancholia (as well as *folie du doute* in the widest sense) is commoner in women, hypochondria is unquestionably much commoner in men; thus, Michea found sixty male hypochondriacs to twenty-one female.

Garnier ("La Folie à Paris," 1890) gives the following results of his experience at the Paris Préfecture de Police as to the relative frequence of various types of insanity in men and women during the years 1886–88. He adopts Magnan's classification, and is dealing with 8139 persons (4831 men and 3308 women); they are here averaged in the order of frequency for both sexes combined.

	M.	F.
Alcoholism (acute, sub-acute, chronic)	1813	376
Mental degeneration (idiocy, imbecility, psychic debility, hereditary degeneration)	821	644
General paralysis	711	288
Intellectual enfeeblement (due to hæmorrhage, softening, or tumour)	548	438
Melancholia	179	509
Mania and maniacal excitement	210	321
Epilepsy	294	169
Senile dementia	150	287
Chronic monomania (progressive systematic psychosis)	105	276

Thus the order of frequency in men is: alcoholism, mental degeneration, general paralysis, intellectual enfeeblement, epilepsy, mania, melancholia, senile dementia, chronic insanity. In women it is: mental degeneration, melancholia, intellectual alcoholism, mania, general paralysis, senile dementia, chronic insanity, epilepsy. On the whole these results seem to correspond with those usually found in large urban populations.

While most forms of mental disorder are fairly stationary as to their relative frequency in the sexes, there are two exceptions: alcoholic insanity and general paralysis have a tendency to progress, to change their relative positions in the sexes, and also to some extent to vary in various countries. While alcoholic insanity always stands at the head of the list so far as men are concerned, its exact percentage among men varies considerably in different countries, as does also its relative frequency among women. In England there is, comparatively, a small difference between men and women, as may be seen from the table of causes already given; and in both sexes alcoholism may be said to be the most frequent cause of insanity. The figures given by Bevan Lewis correspond very closely with this general table: of 464 subjects of alcoholic insanity studied by him, 344 were men and 120 women. In Paris (according to Garnier's recent statistics) alcoholic insanity is, as we have seen, extremely common among men but comparatively rare in women, while in both it is increasing. Taking the two sexes together, alcoholic insanity in Paris has doubled in fifteen years, but among women, taken separately, it has more than doubled; so that while alcoholism in men is increasing at a tremendous rate, the difference between the sexes is decreasing. It is worthy of note—and the fact has as yet scarcely attracted sufficient attention—that while in men alcohol tends to affect the brain, in women it tends to affect the cord and nerves. Rayer, among 170 cases of delirium tremens, found only 7 women; Bang, at Copenhagen, found only 1 woman to 455 men; Hœgh-Gueldberg, 1 woman to 172 men; Clifford Allbutt in 1882 said that he had never seen delirium tremens in a woman, while he regarded spinal symptoms in women as common and specifically alcoholic; and Broadbent at a meeting of the British Medical Association spoke to the same effect. Lancereaux, who has given special attention to this matter, states that alcoholic muscular paralysis is found in only 3 men to 12 women. Ball finds that sexual excitement is a more frequent complication of dipsomania in women than in men.

General paralysis, which by its ætiology

to some extent as well as by the character of its symptoms is related to alcoholism, resembles it also by its frequency and rate of progression in the sexes. Its increase among both men and women in England has been noted by Savage and many others. In Germany the growing proportion of women among general paralytics has been noted by Mendel, Sander, and others; the proportion was formerly 1 woman to 5 men; it is now 1 to 3. Siemerling, who does not consider that the statistics of the Charité, in Berlin, show any real increase of general paralysis in women, admits it for men; he finds a sexual difference in the symptoms, which are on the whole quicker in women, with a tendency to delusions often of a sexual character. In France the increase of general paralysis in both sexes is well marked. Garnier finds that in Paris it has nearly doubled in men during fifteen years, and in women considerably more than doubled during the same period; so that there is 1 woman to 2½ men. This *maladie du siècle*, as it has been called, is the disease of great urban centres; it is largely the result of nervous over-strain in efforts for which the organism is not naturally adapted or sufficiently equipped, and it is not difficult to account for its growing frequency among women who are thrown into the competitive struggle for existence. A detailed consideration of the sexual incidence of nervous diseases cannot be entered into here. It may be said generally that gross lesions of the nervous system are more common in men, and so-called "functional" disorders more common in women. (*See* STATISTICS OF INSANITY.) HAVELOCK ELLIS.

[*Reference.*—For some details under this head, see H. Campbell's Differences in the Nervous Organisation of Men and Women. 1891.]

SEXUAL INSANITY. (*See* EROTOMANIA.) Includes satyriasis and nymphomania.

SEXUAL PERVERSION. — The term "perverse sexual feeling" (*conträre Sexualempfindung*) was first used by Westphal (in *Archiv f. Psych.*) to express a condition which had already received attention from Casper and others, and which is described as consisting of an innate perversion or "inversion" of the sexual feelings with consciousness of its morbid nature. It is maintained that in this condition a passion for the sex to which the sufferer belongs, instead of the normal inclination to the opposite sex, exists; and that this is a state which is innate—*i.e.*, appears as early as the dawn of sexual feelings, and remains constant; is in fact, *quâ* the individual, a physiological state. The [illegible]
view, which seems [illegible]
untenable, is derived [illegible]
statements of persons [illegible]
the symptoms of sexual [illegible]
unhappy creatures, for [illegible]
"Urnings"* was invented [illegible]
man lawyer who wrote on [illegible]
personal experience, claims [illegible]
number of the human [illegible]
this abnormal appetite, and [illegible]
have the power throughout [illegible]
nising each other when they [illegible]
is to be observed that the [illegible]
confessions of persons [illegible]
disturbance of any kind [illegible]
untrustworthy. Any man who [illegible]
to sexual depravity in whatever [illegible]
the period of puberty, and [illegible]
indulge in it, will be disposed [illegible]
he had been led by a natural [illegible]
And yet how many cases of [illegible]
vity of various sorts occur in [illegible]
are followed by the development [illegible]
ordinary sexual passion. A [illegible]
argument is derived from the [illegible]
such persons often spring from [illegible]
families—are themselves [illegible]
frequently exhibit temporary [illegible]
nent conditions of degenerative [illegible]
disturbance. It is also [illegible]
sexual passion appears at an [illegible]
early age in such cases. But [illegible]
capable of another interpretation [illegible]
appears to us to be, at least in [illegible]
rity of cases, the true one. In a [illegible]
delicate, or ill brought up child, [illegible]
passion appears early. The [illegible]
at its first appearance is always [illegible]
and is very easily turned in a [illegible]
tion. This occurs in ordinary [illegible]
masturbation. As in [illegible]
other forms of sexual depravity, [illegible]
is more apt to become [illegible]
begins early before the higher [illegible]
have developed, and once the [illegible]
habit of mind is definitely [illegible]
opment of appetite along the [illegible]
may fail to take place. Some [illegible]
nation as this seems more [illegible]
the belief that an individual is [illegible]
the anatomical characteristics of [illegible]
and the mental characteristics of [illegible]
Besides, it brings these cases [illegible]
with that form of sexual [illegible]
which we are most familiar, [illegible]
This view is also borne out by the [illegible]
that these cases are almost [illegible]

* The word "Urning" has no [illegible] Ulrich, who was the Bavarian jurist [illegible] wrote several extraordinary pamphlets [illegible] for people of this kind the legal right of [illegible] with persons of the same sex. The term has [illegible] into general use in Germany.—[Ed.]

plicated with it. Out of seventeen cases of so-called congenital sexual perversion described by Krafft-Ebing, in the third edition of his book on "Sexual Psychopathy," in three or four at most the condition did not seem to have originated in masturbation in early life, and many of the histories are simply accounts of the depraved habits unfortunately common in boyhood carried on into adult life.

Akin to sexual perversion, in the limited sense of the word, are many other aberrations of the venereal appetite, all of which are probably to be regarded as essentially of the same nature and having a similar origin. In these, apparently through some accidental mental association formed in early life, some object not directly connected with the performance of the sexual functions calls up sexual feelings and desires. Such cases in their disgusting details seem hardly worthy of the minute study that has been given to them. For the purpose of the physician it seems sufficient to look upon them as varieties of masturbation. One class, perhaps, deserves special note through its possible importance from a medico-legal point of view. In this form sexual excitement is combined with bloodthirsty tendencies to mutilation, or even murder, or to both. It would seem that in some cases the murderous tendency appears as the equivalent and representative of sexual passion. Some shocking crimes certainly seem to have been due to this association, but here, as in the previously considered cases, we must not hastily assume that a highly abnormal development of the generative feelings necessarily implies congenital perversion. Those who wish to follow up the subject of sexual aberration in its less usual forms will find detailed information in the works of Casper, Westphal, Krafft-Ebing, Tarnowsky, Lombroso, Charcot, Moll, and others.

CONOLLY NORMAN.

SHOCK.—The sudden depression of organic, vital, and nervous power produced by injury either to mind or body.

SHOCK FROM FRIGHT.—It has long been recognised that fright may be a cause of serious disturbance of health, and the phenomena of shock induced by it, like as they are in all respects to those which ensue upon severe physical injury, give evidence of a grave effect upon the nervous system. Isolated cases are to be found recorded in the literature of a former time which show that these facts have been always acknowledged, but larger attention has been paid to the subject in the present, both because of the widened study of nervous diseases, and because of the comparative frequency with which such results are now to be seen. It is not proposed in this article to write a description of the symptoms of shock, for every text-book of surgery has an adequate account of them, and the monograph of Groeningen contains all that there is to be said upon the subject. Rather shall a short account be given of the results, both early and remote, of shock to the nervous system induced by fright, dealing more especially with those symptoms which are indicative of mental or cerebral disturbance. The siege of Strasbourg and the siege of Paris during the last Franco-German war were both productive of many examples of grave nervous disorder, even ending fatally, which clearly had their origin in the terrible circumstances to which the sufferers had been exposed—to wit, the constant bursting of shells, the ever-present sense of danger, the anxiety as to the safety of friends, the inadequacy of the food supply. Happily in this country we have been spared such experiences, but like sources of neurotic disturbance are to be found very often in the events of an ordinary railway collision, where we have in combination everything which is likely to induce great terror—magnitude and violence of the forces, loud noise, shrieks of the injured, and utter helplessness of individual passengers. It is not, therefore, a matter of any surprise to learn that the after-effects of a railway collision may be very serious even when no bodily injury has been inflicted. Of the physical injuries sustained in railway accidents this only need be said, that at no period do they differ from the same injuries sustained in other ways, and the symptoms of shock which accompany and follow them are likewise of the same kind as are ordinarily seen. There is, however, the added element of fright, which is prone to make the symptoms of shock of somewhat longer duration than usual, although there is this compensating advantage, that the infliction of some definite bodily injury—of a broken leg, for example—is frequently antagonistic to the protraction of the after-symptoms of nervous disturbance such as have had their chief origin in fright alone. In other words, it is often to a man's advantage, as far as the mental consequences are concerned, that he should have received some definite local injury, for experience on this point is perfectly clear that he is thereby rendered less liable to suffer from prolonged neurotic disturbance. And the reason for this is to be found in the fact that the bodily injury more or less satisfies the requirements of the patient himself in seeking an explanation, consciously and unconsciously, of the symptoms which were present after the accident, and the natural tendency each day towards recovery from the physical injury provides that element of hope which is so often wanting when the cause of the symptoms is entirely hidden and obscure.

Collapse from fright (and it is of that alone we have to speak here) is met with in various degrees of severity after railway collisions, and we may leave the cases out of account in which there has been some physical injury inevitably associated with and giving rise to shock. The times of onset also differ widely; there may be immediate collapse, or collapse of which the symptoms are delayed, for the simple reason that they have been warded off by the excitement of the scene—warded off, yet not prevented, nay, rather increased by the delay, for the excitement is itself a cause of nervous prostration, which in its turn may make the symptoms not perhaps more pronounced in themselves, but more persistent and less prone to pass quickly away. Thus it is by no means uncommon for a man who has merely felt a little dazed and sick at the time of the accident to break down completely after he reaches home, and then to present the symptoms of ordinary collapse. And from this period may date the beginning of more obvious cerebral and mental disturbance. Soon, or not until after the lapse of a few days, during which the scene of the accident may have been terribly present to him, both in sleep and when awake, repeating, as it were, the terror which originally harmed him, he has an attack of acute uncontrollable hysterical crying. Attacks of this kind are likely to recur, and in the intervals there is prone to be developed a sense of extreme despondency, which is maintained and increased by advancing bodily weakness. For, as a consequence of the accident, whether, as some have suggested, because of molecular disturbance of the cerebro-spinal centres by the physical violence of the collision, or because of a purely dynamical nervous derangement, the accompaniment of fright alone, very considerable digestive disorder is liable to ensue. From this cause, and from a more direct deprivation in all probability of the normal stimulus of healthy nervous tone, the muscular system wastes, and there is inability both to take and to digest food. Extreme bodily weakness is the result, and this general condition of feebleness and prostration, to which nowadays the term neurasthenia is often applied, cannot act otherwise than injuriously upon those [illegible] which have to do with [illegible] both the hysterical [illegible] companying despondency [illegible] increased thereby. A [illegible] obviously been established [illegible] ground for surprise that, as [illegible] outcome of these combined [illegible] despondency should deepen [illegible] lancholia, that there should [illegible] tions at night, or that suicid[illegible] should be displayed. There [illegible] tion, however, that such results [illegible] rare in this country, although [illegible] common elsewhere. Further[illegible] be said of these mental distur[illegible] the time of their continuance [illegible] pearance depends very much [illegible] state of the bodily health, and [illegible] secret of treatment is to [illegible] general nutrition. Do this, and the [illegible] tal disorder may in the vast [illegible] cases be left to take care of itself.

There are yet other manifestations [illegible] cerebral disturbance resulting [illegible] terror which is incidental to [illegible] lisions. Reference has already [illegible] to the dazed sensation which [illegible] experience at the time of the [illegible] It may sometimes present [illegible] and more serious characters. [illegible] be complete and sudden unco[illegible] without any blow upon the head [illegible] dition of almost complete uncon[illegible] may supervene some hours after [illegible] dent. In the state of immedia[illegible] sciousness there is usually [illegible] lessness, and the person is carried [illegible] the scene, and has no subsequent [illegible] tion of what he has gone through [illegible] he has been. This state of [illegible] ness as to the events of the moment [illegible] however, in all instances [illegible] the helplessness of coma. In [illegible] which seems in itself to indicate [illegible] annihilation of the higher faculties [illegible] sensorium, a man may neverthele[illegible] able to perform acts which are [illegible] under perfect cerebral volition and [illegible] He may take himself home, but [illegible] subsequent recollection of how he [illegible] there; or in his unconsciousness of [illegible] really occurred he may give a [illegible] erroneous account both of what happened to himself at the time of the accident [illegible] how he conducted himself afterwards. Cases of this kind have been recorded [illegible] Thorburn, Charcot, and others, and [illegible] view is now very commonly held that [illegible] dazed condition which has been described is very closely allied to, if it be not [illegible] identical with, the state induced [illegible] posive experimental hypnosis. The obser[illegible] vation of several remarkable [illegible] a railway collision ten years and more ago led the writer to suggest that many of the phenomena displayed were akin to those of the hypnotic condition, and this view has received support from many quarters by many observers. To Charcot, it may be said, and to his disciples, more perhaps than to any others, it is that we owe a knowledge of the fact that the phenomena of hypnotism are practically identical with the phenomena of the state which has been here spoken of as not uncommon after railway accidents where fright acts as an all-powerful cause of ill. It has been shown by Charcot, as every student of his works knows, that in this condition of hypnosis, during which it may be assumed that the higher cerebral regions and their combinations are in a state of torpor or temporary inactivity, by the force of "suggestion" the hypnotiser may induce and at his will maintain various abnormal conditions in the hypnotised person, such as hemi-anæsthesia, for example, contortions or pareses, and spastic rigidity of the trunk and limbs. And recognising the fact that accidents accompanied with much terror are prone to be followed by what he and others of his school call "hysterical" disturbances of the nervous system, such as the various anæsthesiæ of non-anatomical distribution, the monoplegiæ and kindred paralytic disorders without gross structural underlying lesion, and recognising also at the same time the hypnotic condition as being caused by fright, Charcot has formulated the theory that, in the state of hypnosis so induced, a local injury to a limb, for example, may act in much the same way as the suggestion of the hypnotiser. In other words, the abnormal sensations of pain, heaviness, and numbness, with stiffness and weakness, which are the result of a blow may suggest to the hypnotised the fixed idea of palsy of the affected part, and "traumatic suggestion" comes thereby, in his view, to play a large part in the production of like symptoms. The works of Charcot himself, of Guinon, and others contain numerous examples of such cases, and, although seemingly not with the same frequency as in France, they are met with in this country. Cases showing almost every conceivable, or described, variety of such neuroses have fallen under the notice of the writer: in some the hypnotic condition has been extreme directly after the accident, and has been accompanied by some special anæsthetic disturbance; in others the state akin to hypnosis has been of later development, and the special symptoms have been likewise delayed. In his judgment and experience, this sequence of events is due to the fact that lapse of time and enfeeblement of the general nutrition during it are necessary to prepare the nervous system for the possible representation of such phenomena. It is not every one who can be purposely hypnotised, as it is not every one who is dazed or rendered unconscious by the sudden terror of a railway collision, but it is conceivable that the nervous system may be reduced to the condition in which such a thing is possible by the long continuance and injurious agency of that vicious circle which has been already named. Suffice it here to say that, whatever view may be taken of the origin of these symptoms, there will be no dispute that the condition of hypnosis itself and the possibility of it, together with the special symptoms which are prone to accompany or follow it, are alike manifestations of cerebral and mental disorder, the result, in the particular instances considered here, of fright, direct or indirect. By the French school they are looked upon as largely "hysterical," but some injustice has been done to Charcot and his followers in attributing to them the view that these cases are hysterical, and hysterical only, using the word as of no more import than is ordinarily meant by it in the case of trivial derangements which have no such deep foundation in serious cerebral disorder.

Passing in the next place to disturbances of a more obviously psychical character, it is to Oppenheim and other German authors to whom the reader must turn for detailed information. In his masterly work on the "Traumatic Neuroses" this author has brought together a series of cases obviously very like those which are met with in this country and in France, but in which, as the result of causes similar to those with which we are familiar here, there ensue the symptoms of much more definite psychical disturbance. Thus, we find a description of cases in which despondency and irritability are prominent, deepening sometimes into hypochondriasis, accompanied by hallucinations, and going on to distinct dementia, weakness of memory, and even delusional insanity. He describes in full detail the various accompanying bodily disorders, the muscular weakness, the altered gait, the feeble speech, the pareses, the loss of sexual desire, the disturbances of the special senses, of the pulse and circulation. With all such things we are perfectly familiar here, and they have been fully described by the writer in another place, but it is certain that we do not meet anything like so often in this country with examples of the mental disorders such as have been described by Oppenheim. There must be some reason for this, to be found either in racial peculiarities and habits, or in the fact that Oppenheim's description is drawn almost entirely from the cases of patients in hospital. It is not inconceivable that the daily record and observation of symptoms and signs of disease in a hospital ward may have a good deal to do with the intensity and perpetuation of complaints of which much less might be thought in other circumstances. Oppenheim's own cases must be studied, and no one will deny that, as they are presented, he has weighty grounds for holding that it is neither in the narrow domain of traumatic hysteria, nor in that of traumatic neurasthenia, that they are to be placed, but that they fall into a special class of their own, of the traumatic neuroses or the traumatic neuro-psychoses. "Traumatic hysteria," "traumatic neurasthenia," "traumatic neuroses"—these three terms cover the different varieties of symptoms which are met with as the result of railway shock or of other accident where there is cause for terror, and, if it is under these three heads that the chief descriptions of them are to be found, there is, it is believed, no very wide difference of opinion about them nor any which is not perfectly explicable. The views, at any rate, which have been expressed here as to the prevalence of mental disorders after severe shock from fright are based on no inconsiderable experience, and support to them is to be found in the experience of asylum physicians throughout the country. And unquestionably the prognosis is distinctly more favourable here than the record of Oppenheim's cases leads one to conclude. The lines of treatment may be sufficiently indicated in a very few words. Rest and the avoidance of work, both bodily and mental, until the general nutrition has been restored; absolute quietude at first and freedom from all mental anxiety afterwards; above all, the avoidance of litigation and the early and amicable settlement of the claim for compensation on account of the injuries sustained. HERBERT W. PAGE.

[*References.*—Groeningen, Ueber den Shock, Wiesbaden, 1885. Charcot, Lectures on Diseases of the Nervous System, vol. iii., 1889, New Sydenham Soc. Trans. Guinon, Les Agents-provocateurs de l'Hystérie, Paris, 1889. Thorburn, A Contribution to the Surgery of the Spinal Cord, London, 1889. Page, Injuries of the Spine and Spinal Cord, 2nd edit., 1885; Railway Injuries, 1891. Berbez, Hystérie et Traumatisme, Thèse de Paris, 1887. Vibert, Étude médico-legal sur les Accidents de Chemin-de-fer, Paris, 1888. Strümpel, Ueber die traumatischen Neurosen, [illegible] Heft 3. Oppenheim, Die [illegible] Berlin, 1889.]

SIALORRHŒA. (*See* [illegible]

SIBYLS, THE (Σίβυλ [illegible]) of gen. being Σιού, of Jove [illegible]. The psychologist cannot [illegible] idea of what a sibyl must [illegible] in her ecstatic state [illegible] Virgil's description of the C[illegible] when Æneas saw her and was [illegible] was a fit time to consult [illegible] "While saying these words [illegible] ance, her colour, are not [illegible] hair uncut, not smooth; [illegible] heaves, and her fierce heart [illegible] fury; she appears larger, and [illegible] with mortal voice, since she is [illegible] the now nearer influence of [illegible]. Her excitement is then [illegible] rageous, and it is only when [illegible] heart is somewhat curbed that [illegible] for her office. We are told [illegible] terrific mysteries, involving [illegible] obscurities, and bellows in her [illegible]

It was the same sibyl who, [illegible] 550 B.C., presented herself so [illegible] to Tarquin, and made him an [illegible] prophetic books, which he [illegible] was glad at last to secure three [illegible] had been burnt.

As is well known, the Christian [illegible] accepted and applied the sibylline [illegible] cies to the advent of Christ. [illegible] says, "We shall speak of '[illegible]' without any distinction whenever we [illegible] have occasion to use their [illegible]" (vol. i. p. 17). The Rev. M. Dods, [illegible] (the editor of Justin Martyr's W[illegible]) observes, "The sibylline oracles [illegible] generally regarded as heathen [illegible] largely interpolated by unscrupulous [illegible] during the early ages of the Church."

If any one visiting the churches in [illegible] has felt surprised at the frequency [illegible] which the painter's brush has [illegible] ployed to depict the sibyls, his [illegible] will be removed when he studies [illegible] ristic writings, and finds how largely [illegible] authors appealed to the authority of [illegible] sibylline leaves.

"The painters, like the poets, have always depicted the sibyls as [illegible] agitated by the convulsions which [illegible] sessed the ancient priestesses. [illegible] however, has given to his sibyls a [illegible] air, an attitude full of serenity, and [illegible] in harmony with the nature of [illegible] oracles, since they were to foretell [illegible] coming of Christ ("Les Galéries [illegible] liques de l'Europe," Rome, p. 395).

The consideration of the character of the sibyls leads us on to that of the whole system of oracular utterances which played so large a part in the history of the ancients. What is true of the former is also true of the priestesses of every shrine. If it be asked whether there are no phenomena familiar to ourselves which closely resemble those described in the classic descriptions of the oracles and seeresses of antiquity, the answer is that there certainly are. Take certain accounts of modern spiritualistic seances.

We are informed by a writer in a recent journal that he does not believe in what is called "spiritualism," and he proceeds to give a narration of a visit he paid to a medium. This modern seeress described the appearance, the age, the time of death, and the general characteristics of the friend of his youth—a young man who died when about thirty years of age. Like the ancient pythoness, she had in the first instance "convulsive spasms," and then passed into a trance. In some other descriptions of the same class of cases the contortions of the limbs and the facial spasms are of a much more pronounced character. In short, attacks of hystero-epilepsy are induced, and in some instances they resemble the striking figures depicted by Paul Richter in his well-known work. The study of these and similar modern phenomena is essential to the psychologist who wishes to understand the character of the sibyls and the heathen oracles in general. To this end the writings of Cicero will be found invaluable.* (*See also* Plato's "Phædrus" in which Socrates discourses on the subject.)

THE EDITOR.

SICCHASIA (σικχαίνω, I feel a loathing for). Loathing or disgust for food, as in pregnancy, melancholia, &c. (Fr. *sicchasie*; Ger. *Ekel*.)

SICK-GIDDINESS. —Seizures compared by Marshall Hall to the effects of a swing on the susceptible medulla oblongata, and regarded by him as intimately related both to sick headache and to epilepsy.

SIDERATION (*sidus*, a star). This term was used by the ancients in two senses: applied to the apoplexy and paralysis supposed to be produced by the influence of the stars, and also to erysipelas of the face and head under the idea of its being due to the influence of the planets.

SIMPLE MANIA. (*See* MANIA, SIMPLE.)

SIMPLE MELANCHOLIA. (*See* MELANCHOLIA, SIMPLE.)

SIMULATION OF HYSTERIA by ORGANIC DISEASE of NERVOUS SYSTEM.—In hysteria there is probably a disturbed or congenitally defective condition of the cerebral substance, involving in all cases the highest nervous centres, and in various examples extending more or less to those which preside over automatic processes. Partial or complete suspension of inhibitory influence would appear to be the most prominent result of the pathological condition, whatever it be, and this is recognised as well in regard to the mental as to the more evidently physical processes belonging to cerebral function. The departures from normal functioning of various organs which occur are apt to simulate those commonly arising from definite alterations of structure, but differ from the latter in the fact that they may often, even when at their worst, be removed instantaneously, usually under the influence of strong emotion. It would seem that the paralysis which is apt to occur as a symptom of hysteria signifies that the power of the highest centres in liberating movement is in abeyance. A loss of power in a limb is diagnosed as of hysterical origin when examination appears to show the absence of such alteration of structure as would explain its occurrence coupled with the fact of its association with emotional symptoms of various kinds, and with a history of other occurrences to which the term hysterical is usually applied.

The grounds upon which any particular condition can safely be relegated to hysteria are therefore manifestly insecure. Emotional disturbance is a frequent and obviously probable *result* of organic disease of the nervous system, and the value of certain physical symptoms accompanying emotional conditions, as tending to support a diagnosis of hysteria, will depend upon the amount of accuracy with which these can be determined to be independent of structural change.

There is a form of **paraplegia** which is easily supposed to be of emotional origin, and the occurrence of which, therefore, along with symptoms of emotional disturbance is, the writer thinks, continually leading to an erroneous diagnosis of hysteria in young women. The patient's gait is observed to become gradually awkward. She walks in an ungainly fashion

* "What authority has this same ecstasy, which you choose to call divine, that enables the madman to foresee things inscrutable to the sage, and which invests with divine senses a man who has lost all his human ones? We Romans preserve with solicitude the verses which the sibyl is reported to have uttered when in an ecstasy,—the interpreter of which is by common *report* believed to have recently uttered certain falsities in the senate" ("De divinatione," ch. 54). Cicero himself doubted whether the sibylline oracles were delivered in a state of ecstasy, on account of their being "far less remarkable for enthusiasm and inspiration than for technicality and labour."

having lost the natural springiness of step. As along with this it is seen that she apparently dances as well as ever, and that the muscles of her lower extremities are well developed, and the general health good, the contradiction is commonly quite enough to suggest that the girl is hysterical, and that she must be treated accordingly. It is found that in going upstairs she drags herself up by clinging strongly to the banisters, appearing unable to lift the foot up, in order to plant it on the stair above. She is sharply admonished, and breaks down in tears. The examination of a number of such cases has shown us that there is a form of muscular atrophy, sometimes of congenital origin, which commences in the ilio-psoas muscle, and may for a more or less lengthy period be confined to that region. Hence the limitation of loss of power to the movement of flexion of the thigh upon the trunk. In the act of dancing this is required only to a small extent, whilst it is most necessary in going upstairs or in stepping upon a chair and lifting the body up. As the muscles which can be tested electrically (the ilio-psoas itself is out of reach) are all found normal, the reflexes probably perfect, the muscular nutrition excellent, the sensory function undisturbed, it is evident that a mistaken diagnosis is very likely to occur.

Another disease which often gives rise to an erroneous diagnosis of hysteria is that which is called **Friedreich's** or **congenital ataxy.** The symptoms are apt to commence insidiously in youth. They include ataxic gait and incoordination of upper extremities, indistinct articulation, nystagmoid movements of the eyes, weakness of muscles of spine, and often lateral curvature. In such cases the knee-jerks are almost always absent. Absence of knee-jerks never, in the writer's experience, arises from hysteria. In conditions of rigid hysterical contracture of the knee-joint it may be impossible for mechanical reasons to evoke the knee-jerk, but simple absence of the phenomenon, no such obstacle being present, is a symptom of structural change.

There is another reflex, the behaviour of which gives valuable information in the diagnosis of hysteria from organic disease of the nervous system. It almost invariably happens that in cases of hysterical paraplegia the contraction produced by tickling the sole of the foot (plantar reflex) is absent, or so slightly present as to be evoked with very great difficulty. The presence of this reflex in a doubtful case becomes, therefore, of considerable weight as pointing to structural disease.

Insular or disseminated [illegible] its early stage, is the [illegible] liable to be diagnosed as [illegible] writer has reason to believe [illegible] at the present time large [illegible] females affected with this [illegible] supposed to be simply "[illegible]

The disease is particularly [illegible] young females—symptoms [illegible] selves about the period of [illegible] is very often a history of [illegible] or long-continued anxiety [illegible] first symptoms. In addition [illegible] few cases of disseminated [illegible] females in which emotional [illegible] not mixed up with those belonging [illegible] tially to the disease. Obviously [illegible] bination of itself causes a peculiar [illegible] to mistakes of diagnosis. [illegible] other sources of error in [illegible] many of the symptoms of [illegible] sclerosis are supposed to suggest [illegible] selves an hysterical origin. [illegible] alleged loss of power in a limb [illegible] parently healthy young female, [illegible] numbness, or "pins-and-needles" [illegible] tion, complaint of loss of sight [illegible] are symptoms familiar enough [illegible] sions of functional trouble. They [illegible] equally modes in which organic [illegible] the kind we are discussing may [illegible] first appearance. These local [illegible] may clear off after a short [illegible] would be the case if they were of [illegible] origin. The girl recovers her [illegible] use of her limb, and nothing [illegible] of the numbness. A little [illegible] loss of sight in the other eye is [illegible] of; a "pins-and-needles" [illegible] scribed in some other part; [illegible] is said to be very weak. The [illegible] the symptoms are of hysterical [illegible] very possibly appear to be [illegible] firmed by this reappearance of [illegible] other situations. Or the patient [illegible] complains of weakness and [illegible] both legs, which increase so that in [illegible] eight weeks she cannot stand. [illegible] comes a rather rapid improvement and she recovers her power completely, [illegible] however, to fail again. After [illegible] and relapses of this kind, the characteristics of confirmed disseminated sclerosis show themselves.

As a rule, though this is not without some notable exceptions, the class of hysterical paraplegia is not difficult of diagnosis by those well acquainted with the symptoms and course of organic disease, the surrounding circumstances, and especially the contradictions palpable in the symptoms leaving one usually in but little doubt. The attitude and condition of the lower limbs may vary exceedingly.

The limbs are most often in a state of perfect flaccidity, a condition of spasticity being comparatively rare. The feet are frequently "dropped." After long disuse it will not unfrequently happen that there are strong adhesions in the joints. Hysterical paralyses are most often complete. The loss of power in disseminated sclerosis is very rarely (except in advanced stages) more than moderate. It is probable that the view still generally held that a shifting of loss of power from one limb to another (such as that which we have described) is really characteristic of hysteria is quite an error. The hysterical woman who has lost all power in her legs will, it is true, very often later on (whilst still paraplegic) lose the power of one arm, usually the left; but she is not prone to lose the power in a limb, then recover it, and then lose it in another. The idea of this shifting of powerlessness being strongly suggestive of hysteria has in all probability arisen from the mistakes in diagnosing as hysteria cases of disseminated sclerosis. This must have been continually occurring before the latter disease had been differentiated. No doubt the hysterical are prone to changes of disorder; at one time, for example, losing the use of a limb or limbs, with or without profound anæsthesia, at another time losing the voice, or closing one eyelid, or contracting a limb, but the shifting about of a state of more or less powerlessness, which we see in disseminated sclerosis, would appear to be *sui generis*, and should save us from error. And equally so with the occurrence of numbness or "pins-and-needles" sensation, sometimes at one part and sometimes at another, which points with considerable distinctness to disseminated sclerosis.

No doubt it is inconceivable that a condition of sclerosis, characterised as it is by overgrowth of connective tissue, can be removed. But it is not difficult to imagine the possible subsidence of the state of hyperæmia, which doubtless precedes the stage of sclerosis.

Where there would appear to be a little more difficulty, in regard to the impairment of sight in one eye, the ophthalmoscope shows no change. But the hysterical patient as a rule, when loss of sight of one eye is in question, is quite blind on that side, whilst the patient with sclerosis has only more or less obscurity of vision. One does not find cases of simple hysteria in which first one eye has lost some amount of vision for a time and recovered, and afterwards the other eye has behaved in a similar fashion. So that this symptom may be taken to point with considerable force to disseminated sclerosis, in which disease an alternation of this kind is very apt to occur. When the ophthalmoscope shows atrophy of disc (and it is remarkable in what a large proportion of cases of disseminated sclerosis some atrophy is to be found—in some a stage of hyperæmia preceding it) experience shows that a diagnosis of functional disorder must be discarded.

The same must be said of nystagmus, a symptom of peculiar value when combined with others about which there might otherwise be some doubt. It is necessary, of course, to remember the possibility of chronic alcoholism producing a temporary nystagmus, but this chance of error ought not to be difficult to avoid.

The tremor on intentional movement is probably of higher diagnostic value than any of the other symptoms of disseminated sclerosis. It is true that in the hysterical a certain clumsiness of movement of the hand when directed to an object is sometimes observed, but, noted carefully, this will probably be found to be dependent upon temporary loss of muscular sense and be rather of the nature of ataxy than of the rhythmical tremor which characterises disseminated sclerosis.

Localised atrophy of muscles with loss of electrical reaction is well known to occur sometimes in the course of disseminated sclerosis, and in a case otherwise open to doubt its presence is undoubtedly of the highest value in determining the organic nature of the condition. But it is not generally known that the localised atrophy may behave like the temporary powerlessness of a limb or limbs, or the shifting numbness. Cases of disseminated sclerosis may be seen in which atrophy of some muscles, with loss of electrical reaction, has cleared off entirely, to be succeeded some time afterwards by a similar lesion in another or the same part.

Disseminated sclerosis is not a new disease, though but recently differentiated. It is highly probable that many symptoms which have come to be considered characteristic of hysteria will, if examined by the light of improved knowledge and experience, be relegated to disseminated sclerosis. T. Buzzard.

SIMULATION OF INSANITY. (*See* Feigned Insanity.)

SIMULTANEOUS INSANITY. (*See* Insanity, Simultaneous; and Communicated Insanity.)

SINGLE PATIENTS.—The question of treating insane persons as "single patients," that is, as patients outside an asylum, has at least two aspects. For the patients may be those whose insanity is recent, acute, and presumably curable, or, on the other hand, the disease may be chronic and incurable, and we have to consider what mode of life will best promote their welfare and happiness, according to the mental state and pecuniary means available for their maintenance. And first of those whose insanity is recent and acute. There are many persons whom we wish, for various reasons, to save from the stigma which, rightly or wrongly, is unquestionably attached to those who have been inmates of an asylum. Many professional men, many fathers of families, may be seriously damaged in position or prospects by such a step, or may even lose the position they hold. Many young men and young girls at the outset of life may suffer great injury if placed in an asylum during an attack of maniacal excitement, which possibly will be of brief duration. Many young mothers break down after their first confinement, but recover rapidly under proper treatment. The reputation of having been in an asylum will never be lost by one of them. If we can cure such patients by private care, we shall confer an inestimable benefit upon them.

What are the curable cases of insanity which can be best treated as single patients? Even very acute mania, or maniacal delirium, is capable of being brought to a successful termination in this way if proper means are adopted. It not unfrequently happens that this very violent mania is only temporary, and it has in this respect obtained the name of **mania transitoria**, from its brief and fleeting nature. Where the symptoms begin almost suddenly without any warning or premonitory stage, and where the cause is also of a brief and sudden character, we can reasonably hope that in a short time they will subside. Individuals of unstable equilibrium are prone to be upset by such causes as shock, fright, or sudden religious excitement, yet the equilibrium, though easily disturbed, is easily regained, and much is often learned from the occurrence of previous attacks and previous recoveries. Other causes also bring about a delirium which may be brief in duration. There is the mania which sometimes arises in the course or towards the decline of acute febrile disease, as measles or scarlatina.

There is the **acute mania caused by drink**, not delirium tremens, but insanity with hallucinations and delusions, often subsiding after a brief treatment.

Violent mania may follow **epileptic attacks**, and pass off quickly. It may be desirable to give all such p[illegible] before sending them to an [illegible] possible to do so with safety [illegible] Besides transient attacks [illegible] are those of acute [illegible] running a course of some weeks [illegible] months, and generally terminat[illegible] ably. They occur for the most part in young people, and there will be a strong wish on the part of relatives [illegible] an asylum. If a suitable house [illegible] such a patient can often be [illegible] nursed through an illness of [illegible] The plan, however, is costly, and [illegible] relatives are willing to incur [illegible] and to follow the physician's orders [illegible] things, an asylum is the only alternative. The treatment can rarely be carried out in a patient's own house; therefore [illegible] must be taken, detached, [illegible] noise, of sufficient size to give [illegible] rooms on the bedroom floor, and with sufficient garden for exercise when the time for it comes. The bedroom must be stripped of furniture, the bed made on the ground, the windows protected by [illegible] nailed across, with sufficient intervals for light and air, and the fire by a guard. The treatment of such a case does not consist of mechanical restraint and fastening in bed by a strait waistcoat. Such patients are not usually dangerous to themselves or others, though they may be violent, noisy, mischievous, and dirty. They require a sufficient staff of intelligent and well-trained attendants under the supervision of an educated person, relative or other. If the expense of all this can be borne, and borne for some time, the malady may be brought to a favourable termination; but it not unfrequently happens that in a few weeks the cost is more than can be met, and recourse is had to an asylum when much money has been spent to little purpose.

Less acute forms of mania, which may be called **acute mania**, as distinguished from acute delirious mania, are not fitted for treatment as single cases. The duration is much longer, the necessity for exercise much greater, and an amount of repression and moral control is urgently demanded which can hardly be applied in a private house. These patients require to be with others, to be subjected to rule and discipline, and if left unchecked in private care there is a risk of their becoming chronic lunatics.

Acute delirious melancholia can hardly be treated in private, though, if death be imminent, as it often is in such cases, it is not wise to remove a patient to die in a few days in an asylum. For purposes of cure, if there be hope of cure, an asylum is necessary. There is certain to be an intense suicidal tendency and a most obstinate refusal of food. The patient will not remain in bed, and requires a warm padded room. All food and medicines have to be administered by force, and for this the staff of an asylum, medical and other, is imperatively demanded. The intense desire for suicide can hardly be dealt with in a private house. Such persons will try to swallow glass or anything they can secrete, will set fire to their dress or the house, throw themselves over the balusters, and, in short, avail themselves of every chance which a private house presents.

Melancholia of a less acute form may often be treated successfully out of an asylum. Patients of this type may indeed refuse their food, but with a passive resistance, allowing themselves to be fed without much difficulty, or feeding themselves under the threat of force being used. So, too, they may be suicidal—that is, they would commit suicide if left entirely alone, but with efficient supervision this can be prevented. It is to be understood that such a person is never to be left alone. Indoors or out, by night or by day, in bed or out of it, he is to be accompanied by a vigilant attendant. He is not to be allowed to fasten himself alone in any place, and all this implies the need of a sufficient staff to carry out such supervision. With it, if the expense can be incurred, a favourable issue is often arrived at, and the plan has the advantage that change of scene can be effected, a move being made after a sufficient sojourn in one place, and great advantage being often derived from such a step. Melancholia, though curable, is generally tedious, so that expense must be calculated in such a case. It is a great pity to place a patient in an asylum just as convalescence is commencing because funds for single care are no longer forthcoming. If this event is likely to happen, it is better to have recourse to the asylum at the outset of the attack.

There is a reason for placing melancholic people in an asylum, and for not treating them as single patients, which is important, and should not be lost sight of. They are often possessed by an intense egotism or self-feeling which prevents their thinking of anything or anybody beside themselves. They imagine that there never was a case like theirs, that they never can get well, that no one can understand the symptoms, and they weary every one around them by ceaseless iteration of their never-ending complaint. Such patients must certainly be removed from their own home, but even if placed as single patients in a family or a doctor's house, they can make themselves the centre and focus of every one's attention, and this increases their egotism and self-importance, and does nothing to cure it. But place one of these in an asylum of, say, a hundred patients, and make him merely the hundredth part of the whole community instead of the one central and principal unit, and a wonderful change often manifests itself in a very short time. He takes his food because all around him are taking theirs, and because, if he refuses it, he knows he will immediately be fed. He gives over talking of his delusions, because the others with whom he sits pay not the slighest attention to him. If he can join in no games or employment, he at any rate sees them going on around him. There are newspapers on the table, and as nobody begs him to read them, or cares whether he does so or not, he takes one up to see what is going on, and so recommences reading. Such persons are not to be cured out of an asylum, and in one they should not sit alone in their own apartments, but should mix with a number of other patients. Neither are melancholiacs the only ones who are egotistical and self-important; many whose malady is mania rather than melancholia are exalted in ideas, thinking themselves high above others in rank or wealth or genius. An asylum is the place to put an end to these high thoughts, which are more likely to be fostered than dispersed by care as single patients.

General paralytics are very unfit for single care. For the most part men—for females are only found in the lower classes—they are at the outset strong, vigorous, and often very violent, and in their violence they are reckless and demented, trying to escape and attacking those about them with no regard for consequences. Moreover, there is no object in trying to save them from the stigma of an asylum, for their malady unfortunately is incurable. They are most difficult to manage in a private house at the commencement of their insanity, requiring very special apartments, and a large staff of attendants. Here and there we may find one in whom the facile and demented state of mind comes on very early. Being by nature of a quiet and easily controlled disposition and weakened by the disease, he can be treated from the first in an ordinary house, though not his own, and he declines gradually in mental and bodily strength till the end is reached. Most paralytics go through this stage, and later can be kept in private, if the friends wish them to die out of an asylum, and can endure them when wet, dirty, and paralysed in an extreme degree.

Young people suffering from **acute primary dementia** can often be managed satisfactorily, and the disorder brought to a happy termination without recourse to an asylum; being young and at the outset of life, this is important. They are neither dangerous to themselves nor to others. They do not refuse their food, though they may require to be washed, dressed, and fed like children. The malady depends so much on the physical condition that the environment is comparatively of less importance, and change of scene may be beneficial when convalescence has commenced.

There are many recent but not acute cases of insanity in which recovery takes place by means of change of scene and removal from home without the aid of an asylum, and without legal restraint. When there is no urgency, it is probable that some such treatment may be adopted in the majority of such cases. In fact, it is often a great satisfaction to friends to try this method, even in an unpromising case, before having recourse to an asylum. Time and money are important considerations. A patient who is not going on well in private care should not be allowed to continue so long that his cure is jeopardised, nor should his means be seriously crippled by the useless expense of these proceedings.

The greater proportion of recent and curable cases of insanity will have to be treated in asylums, and for the majority a good asylum is certainly the best place, the safest, and the cheapest, but there are large numbers of the chronic insane who are able to live comfortably and happily in private families, or in houses of their own under proper supervision, and the law gives ample facilities for their so doing. The selection of a suitable home must depend on a variety of circumstances: on the patient's means, his tastes, habits, and eccentricities. Some require much exercise and long walks; for them the country is preferable to a town. Others like pictures, music, and the moving life and bustle of a town. Some are too peculiar in manner and appearance to walk in streets, and unfrequented country places are better adapted to them. Wherever they are, they should reside, if they be ladies or gentlemen, with educated persons. The chief distinction between life in a family and life in an asylum is that in the former the patient lives with sane instead of insane people. If he is unfit for this, if he is unable to take his meals with the family, and [illegible] bers, he is better off in [illegible] dwell in separate [illegible] meals alone, or with an [illegible] tendant, is not to have [illegible] those in an asylum, but [illegible] disadvantage. Those who [illegible] into their houses should [illegible] them merely as lodgers with [illegible] wait upon them, but as [illegible] ceived into the family, to [illegible] as possible the life of the family, [illegible] mental condition may improve [illegible] and not deteriorate.

The law enacts that single [illegible] must be placed under certificates [illegible] vate patients in asylums, if [illegible] receive them, or take care and [illegible] them, do so "for payment." [illegible] are not necessary if relatives or friends [illegible] charge, and are not paid for so doing. [illegible] the Lunacy Act of 1890 the [illegible] whereby single patients are to be [illegible] under an order of a county court [illegible] magistrate, or justice is in all [illegible] same as that which relates to [illegible] received in hospitals or private [illegible]

G. Fielding Bla[illegible]

SIRIASIS (Σείριος, the dog-star). A name for sunstroke or inflammation of the brain. The dog-star was supposed to have an influence in producing it.

SITOPHOBIA, SITIOPHOBIA (σῖτος or σιτίον, food; φοβέω, I fear). A morbid dread of taking food. (Fr. *sitophobie*.)

SKIN, EXCRETION BY THE.—Ordinary perspiration consists of a mixture of two secretions, the one, more or less fatty, derived from the sebaceous glands; the other, a watery fluid derived from the sweat glands. The secretion from the sebaceous glands is not unlike a concentrated milk, rich in fatty matter, and the sweat derived from the sudiparous glands may be proved to be analogous to a diluted urine.

The sweat is certainly much influenced by mental emotion, and therefore mental states; it would be well if accurate observation were made on the insane as to its variation. On the other hand, the oily matters which lubricate the hair and make the skin supple have not been proved to be affected by mental conditions, but probably are so.

The Sebaceous Secretion.—The only possible way in which the sebaceous secretion can be collected apart from other secretions is in those rather frequent instances in which the little duct leading to the surface of the skin becomes occluded. The secretion then is collected in a cyst, and there is good reason to believe that the contents of these sebaceous cysts represent fairly well the normal secretion.

The author has found the contents of a sebaceous cyst to be of a thick creamy consistence, to have a most decided butyric acid odour, an acid reaction, and to contain cholesterin, butyric and caproic acids. The contents of a cyst examined by C. Schmidt* contained the following:

	Per cent.
Water	31.70
Epithelium and albumin	61.75
Fat	4.16
Butyric acid, Valerianic acid, Caproic acid	1.21
Ash	1.18

Impure sebaceous matter taken from the scalp was investigated by Hoppe-Seyler †; this, rubbed with water and the solution shaken with ether, gave a turbid liquid, which on filtration through filter paper, gave a precipitate with acetic acid, the precipitate agreeing in all its characters with casein; on filtering off the casein and boiling, the liquid is again troubled; it also gives in the cold a precipitate with ferrocyanide of potassium; in short, it gives the reactions of albumin. Sugar is absent.

The waxy secretion of the ear may be considered as that of a highly specialised sebaceous secretion; it has never been obtained free from perspiration residues. Petrequin ‡ and Chevalier give the following as the percentage composition of ear wax:

	Ear wax taken from a middle-aged man.	Ear-wax taken from an old man.
Water	10	11.5
Fat	26	30.5
Potash soap, soluble in alcohol	38	17.0
" " water	14	24.0
Insoluble organic matters	12	17.0

It is because the ear wax contains a large content of soap that it is partly soluble in warm water.

No researches have been made as to the nature of the secretion of the ear in the insane, it is a subject well worthy of research, the more especially since in certain mental diseases there are profound trophic changes in the shape of the external ear.

* *Deutsch. f. klin. Med.*, Bd. v.

† "Physiologische Chemie," Berlin, 1881.

‡ *Compt.-rend.*, t. lxviii., No. 16; t. lxix., 1869.

Perspiration.—The dependance of perspiration upon mental states, the heat or cold of the atmosphere, the general condition of health and its excitement, or repression by drugs, are things of common medical knowledge. Especial interest attaches to the experiments of Luchsinger* and others who have shown how perspiration can be excited by electrical stimulation of the cerebro-spinal and sympathetic nerves. The chief drugs which excite the secretion of the skin are pilocarpin, physostigmin, muscarine, and nicotine; on the other hand, atropine has a distinctly inhibitory effect.

The method of collecting the perspiration in quantity enough to chemically examine it has always been to bring the body to a high temperature by the employment of hot-air baths; in this way A. Kast † was able to collect no less than twenty litres of sweat (of course mixed with some of the sebaceous secretion). Sweat has an acid reaction normally, although Trumpy and Luchsinger have described alkaline sweat produced under certain conditions, as, for example, by pilocarpine; this may be an error, for sweat rapidly putrefies, and any urea changes into ammonic carbonate; hence a sweat may be acid when first secreted, but ammoniacal decomposition sets in, and then the liquid has an alkaline reaction. Sweat contains the following: urea, ether-sulphates, sulphates, phosphates, and chlorides. In a few cases Gamgee and Dewar ‡ have found cystin, and in the sweat of diabetics sugar has been found, for Bizio § and Hoffmann ‖ have each described cases in which they have discovered indigo in sweat. Favre has described a peculiar acid, "sweat acid," to which he ascribes the formula $C_{10}H_{16}N_2O_{13}$, but this requires confirmation. Schottin has recognised benzoic, succinic, and tartaric acids in sweat. Some drugs are certainly eliminated by the perspiration; sulphur is in some degree given off by the skin after taking flowers of sulphur; arsenic has been detected in the sweat of persons taking arsenic, and mercury in the sweat of persons taking mercury. A. Kast has distilled the sweat and recognised phenol in the distillate; to another portion he added hydrochloric acid, and by shaking up with ether and subsequent evaporation of the ether extract and solution in water, he found the solution to give a red colour with Millon's reagent,

* "Die Schweissabsonderung," 1880.

† *Zeit. physiol. Chemie*, xi. pp. 501–507.

‡ *Journ. of Anat. and Physiol.*, vol. v. p. 142.

§ *Wien. Academ. Sitzungsber*, Bd. xxxix. s. 33; *Atti dell' Istituto Veneto di Scienze, lettere ed arti* x.

‖ *Wien. med. Wochenschrift*, 1873, s. 292.

thus indicating the presence of aromatic oxyacids. Jaffes' test showed the presence of skatoxyl. The same observer, operating upon the large quantities of sweat before alluded to, established the relation which exists normally in sweat between the ethereal hydrogen sulphates and the mineral sulphates in the following way:

The liquid was made faintly alkaline by sodium carbonate, excess of absolute alcohol added, the liquid filtered, and the whole evaporated on the water bath to a small bulk. In the concentrated liquid the ethereal sulphuric acid and the mineral sulphuric acid were separately estimated, with the following result: In 200 c.c. of the concentrated sweat (equal to 10 to 12 litres of unconcentrated sweat), sulphuric acid A = 0.2422; ethereal sulphuric acid B = .022; $\frac{B}{A}=\frac{1}{12.009}$. In the urine of the same individuals collected at the same time, in 200 c.c. of urine A = .718; B = .448; $\frac{B}{A}=\frac{1}{16.02}$. By administering 10 grains of salol in three days to the same individuals, the quantity of the ethereal hydrogen sulphates in the urine was much increased; $\frac{B}{A}=\frac{1.339}{1}$, whilst in the sweat $\frac{A}{B}=\frac{1}{9.504}$; in other words, the sweat, unlike the urine, remains fairly constant in composition. With regard to other salts the following relation was shown to exist:

	Chlorides.	Phosphates.	Sulphates.
Sweat . .	1	0.0015	0.009
Urine . .	1	0.1320	0.397

Finke * made some quantitative researches on the amount of perspiration eliminated by three different individuals. The quantity varied considerably even when the temperature and other conditions were equal. At temperatures varying from 13° to 27.5°, and with rest or active exercise, the extremes of the hourly secretion varied from 53.04 to 815.337 grammes, and the quantity of solid matter from 0.923 grammes to 6.967 grammes. The inorganic salts amounted from 0.246 to 0.629 per cent. of the secretion, and the amount was relatively the more considerable, the smaller the content of solid matter. In one research the hourly cutaneous excretion of urea was 0.112, and in the other 0.199 per cent. of the sweat, which would give for [illegible] four hours the large [illegible] grammes to 15.1 grammes [illegible] off by the skin.

In making any experiments [illegible] nation by the skin, such [illegible] different persons are only [illegible] the skin surface is estimated [illegible] been done so seldom that [illegible] number of individuals have been [illegible] no generalisation can be laid [illegible] there is little doubt that if [illegible] only take the trouble to measure [illegible] persons, certain relations will [illegible] exist between some dimensions [illegible] different part of the body which [illegible] enable the surface to be estimated [illegible] only a few leading measurements [illegible]

The relative surfaces of two bodies [illegible] are similar in form are as the [illegible] any similar dimensions, using [illegible] similar in its strictly geometrical [illegible] For example, supposing that two [illegible] hands were precisely similar in [illegible] is to say, that the circumference [illegible] arm throughout bore everywhere [illegible] proportion to the whole length of [illegible] in each case, but that the lengths [illegible] respectively as 1 to 1.3, then the [illegible] surfaces would be as 1.3 to 1, [illegible] say, as 1 to 1.69. But in most cases [illegible] be found that while the general [illegible] the same, the proportion between the length of the limb and the circumference is not the same; in this case the surface varies as the mean circumference multiplied by the length of the limb. To obtain the skin-area, the body may be divided as follows: (a) the head, (b) the trunk, (c) the arms, (d) the legs.

The simplest way of taking the measurements accurately is to have elastic bands which can be put round so as to divide the body into small surfaces; for instance, place a band round the neck and another round the chest, just below the armpits, then the surface between these two bands can be determined by taking measurements at equal distances apart; the mean of these numbers is to be multiplied by their number and their common distance apart.

The whole length of the trunk may be divided into some number of equal parts, and the circumference measured at each of these lines; then the surface will be obtained by adding half the first and last measures to the remaining measures of the trunk, and multiplying the sum by their common distance apart. In the same way with the limbs. The surface of the hands is easiest taken by ripping up a good fitting glove and measuring it. The feet may be divided into small zones by

* Hoppe-Seyler, "Physiol. Chemie," s. 769.

elastic bands, and then these small surfaces are easily measured.

Similar remarks apply to the head and face.* In these inquiries of course the weight of the person, the height, and, if possible, the bulk should also be taken; the latter may be done in a bath; a scale carrying a point, and working with a coarse and a micrometer screw, is so arranged that the point just touches the water, then the person is immersed therein with the exception of the nostrils; the instrument is again adjusted so that the point touches the water. This gives an indication by which the experimenter will know the bulk of the water displaced; if the bath is of irregular shape it will be convenient to find out experimentally the amount of water thus displaced rather than by calculation; that is to say, when the person has retired from the bath, to adjust the liquid to the heights indicated. In all these instances the water must be reduced to the standard temperature of 15°. A. WYNTER BLYTH.

SKULL-MAPPING.—A good method of delineating the skull line in the two directions corresponding respectively to the circumferential line of the horizontal and perpendicular planes at the level of their greatest areas is as follows:

The calvarium having been removed in the ordinary way—care being taken that it is cut at a level about an inch above the superciliary ridges in front and the occipital protuberance behind, and that the line is as straight as possible—the brain and membranes are cleared away, and a strip of lead 17 inches long, ¾ of an inch wide, and of the thickness of half a crown, is laid upon the basis cranii in the direction of its length. The anterior end of the lead must be slit for about 3 inches, so as to enclose the crista galli, and the two strips brought up to the cut margin of the skull anteriorly. The whole length of the lead included in the skull is now to be pressed close down on to the bone, and pushed into all the hollows, bent over the posterior clinoid process and into the foramen magnum, then up the occipital bone to the cut margin posteriorly.

The spare lead is to be bent over forward, and its extremity placed against the tips of the anterior portion, so as to prevent springing.

The position of the torcular Herophili having been marked on the lead with chalk, the strip may be removed bodily, placed on a sheet of paper, and the part which has been in apposition with the skull drawn round with pencil.

A perfect copy of the basis cranii in its median line will be thus obtained; and the same process being carried out with the calvarium, and adapted to the line already drawn, the complete internal antero-posterior circumference will be shown (Fig. II.).

To get the horizontal circumferential line, a ring of bone a quarter or one-third of an inch thick is carefully sawn off just below the line of incision made in removing the calvarium. If properly cut, this ring will lie flat on the table, and should be cleaned and preserved.

By placing this ring on paper and drawing closely round it on both sides, the

FIG. I.

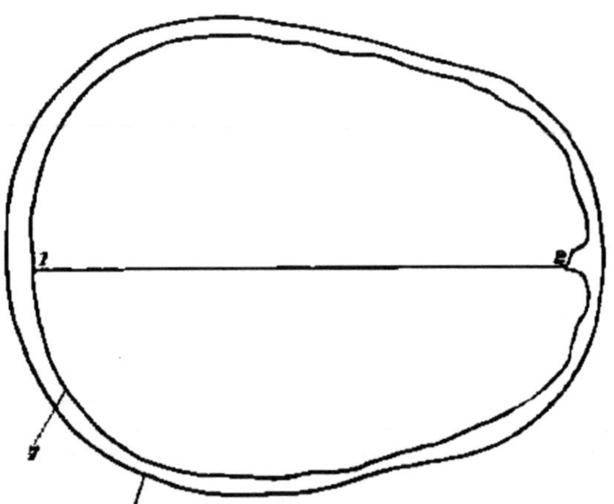

* The writer is indebted to Mr. Henry Law, Mem. Inst. C.E., for the working out of this mathematical scheme.

internal and external circumferential lines of the skull are obtained as shown (Fig. I., 7, 8).

The lines thus taken in the two directions should be drawn on the same piece of paper for purposes of comparison.

A straight line is now drawn on the perpendicular section (Fig. II., 1, 2), from the point corresponding with the torcular Herophili to the frontal bone, and just touching the posterior clinoid process (Fig. II., 3).

From 1 to 2 will constitute the base line of the skull.

If a line be now drawn at right angles to this base line and with its lower extremity touching the anterior margin of the foramen magnum (Fig. II., 4), its upper end (Fig. II., 5) will be found to correspond, almost absolutely, with the highest

FIG. II.

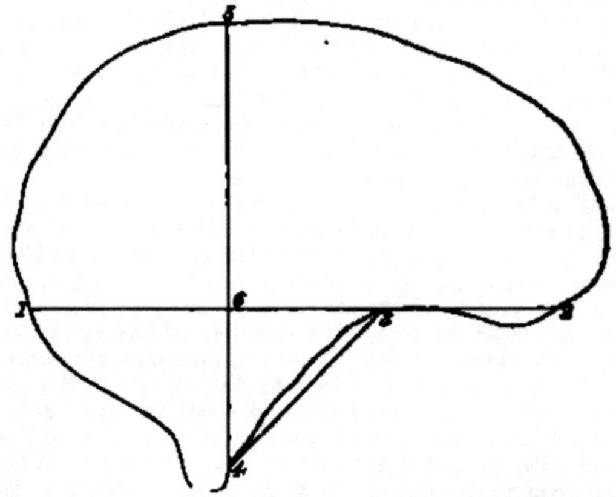

point of the antero-posterior arch of the skull, and to cut the horizontal circumferential line at its point of greatest width.

This line (Fig. II., 4, 5) in the point at which it cuts the base line (1 to 2) determines the relative size of the anterior and posterior portions of the brain, and bears, it is believed, a relation to the degree of intelligence of the individual. The space below the base line is occupied by the cerebellar and ganglionic portions of the brain.

Taking the posterior-clinoid process as a fixed point, the line joining it with the anterior margin of the foramen magnum, and which corresponds pretty nearly with the basilar process of the occipital bone, will be more or less inclined as the line 4, 5, is moved backward or forward; in other words, the angle 4, 3, 2, Fig. II., will be larger or smaller.

The above method [illegible] skull figure is especially [illegible] use of asylum superintendents [illegible] in like positions, and [illegible] which add to the value of [illegible] records. [illegible]

SLAVERING.—Allowing [illegible] flow out of the mouth and down [illegible] chin. (Fr. *bavant*; Ger. *geifern*.)

SLEEP.—The relation of [illegible] medical psychology is important [illegible] ways:

(1) The physiology of sleep; [illegible] state of the mental functions during [illegible]; (3) The mental disturbances which [illegible] arise during sleep; (4) The loss of sleep as a cause and as a consequence of [illegible]; (5) prolonged sleep.

(1) **The Physiology of Sleep.**—[illegible] doubt the investigations and [illegible] made by Mr. Durham and by Mr. Mosso are of great importance in regard to the diminished blood-supply caused by the action of the vaso-motor centre being no longer inhibited by the brain when it becomes fatigued. Although, however, the unrestrained action of the sympathetic appears to be a very plausible explanation of the phenomena of sleep, it is open to doubt whether we may not confound the *post* with the *propter hoc*. Our active mental work during the day undoubtedly induces dilatation of the cerebral vessels. Then the cortical corpuscles become exhausted, and, as there is no longer mental stimulation, the vaso-motor contractions are free to play on the vessels and lessen their calibre. It does not follow, however, that this is the cause, although it is the accompaniment, of sleep. This may be induced by the simple weariness of the corpuscles and by the excretory products

and carbonic acid present in the blood after the activity of the cerebral functions. Dr. Cappie (the subjoined criticism of whose views will be found in the *Journ. of Ment. Sci.*, Ap. 1883), while holding that less blood circulates in the arterial and capillary vessels of the brain, maintains that there must be an exactly corresponding excess of blood in the *veins*. The brain is compressed, and its functions temporarily suspended. Dr. Cappie "believes that the veins of the pia mater become distended from the back flow of blood caused by the atmospheric pressure on the large veins of the neck, and it is the compression on the cortex of the brain by these distended veins that produces sleep. It is not stretching analogy too far to say that that condition of the brain which leads to sleep is similar to the state of a muscle after severe work, and that, just as in the latter case the contractions grow feebler as the excretory products accumulate, so in the brain the supply of nerve-energy gradually fails as the nerve corpuscles become more and more hampered from the same cause. But experiment has shown that exactly in proportion to the depth of sleep there is marked anæmia of the cerebral cortex, a condition which cannot be supposed to result directly from the aggregation of fatigue products in the cerebral corpuscles, since the wide changes in the calibre of the vessels could only be produced by local stimulation or through the agency of the vaso-motor system. There is no reason, *à priori*, why there should not be local vaso-motor centres in the brain just as in the other viscera and tissues, and it is conceivable that such vaso-motor centres may be influenced by the state of the tissues, and so give rise to the changes in the circulation."

A recent writer, Dr. Louis Robinson, after passing these and other theories of sleep in review, including that of periodic brain rhythm, observes that not one of these theories can be accepted and not one of them ignored; that taken together they account for most of the phenomena but that the explanation becomes in consequence a very complicated one.

State of the Eye during Sleep.—Different observers report differently on a point upon which one would have looked for unanimity. Sander* finds that the usual opinion that the eyeballs are directed upwards and inwards is incorrect; he describes the axis of the eyes as parallel, and as if regarding a distant object. It is true that in falling asleep the balls converge and turn upwards, and that this condition will be reproduced when we disturb a person's sleep by trying to raise the lids, and hence, according to Sander, the error, one into which we confess we have fallen. It was one which Sir Charles Bell made, and must be very difficult to avoid. Divergent eyeballs may be observed in profound stupor from cerebral disease. In ordinary mental stupor we have seen them turned upwards and inwards. On arousing a sleeping person, the pupils are seen to dilate, having been contracted during sleep, the more so the profounder the sleep. Dr. Ludwig Plotke has made extensive observations on the pupil in sleep.* He confirms the statements of Sander. Even when the pupil is dilated by atropine it becomes contracted during sleep. The pupil dilates most widely at the moment of waking, and this is not prevented by a strong light. During sleep the cornea becomes dull.

State of the Retina during Sleep.—Dr. Hughlings Jackson has found the disc whiter than normal, the arteries a little smaller, and the veins large, thick and almost plum-coloured. Dr. Cappie naturally claims these appearances as favouring his views.

(2) **State of Mental Functions during Sleep.**—Although it is very doubtful whether in ordinary sleep the whole brain is absolutely free from functional activity, it must be held, in theory at least, that the faculties of the mind are suspended. M. Lemoine observes that however illusory may be the object of the pleasures and pains of sleep, the mind does not the less experience enjoyment or suffer pain—but we here enter at once upon the domain of dreamland, and refer the reader to the article DREAMING.

(3) **Mental Disturbance arising during Sleep.**—(*a*) The most serious mental disturbance which may occur during sleep is an attack of *epileptic mania*. Nocturnal epilepsy must never be overlooked as a possible explanation of unusual or alarming occurrences in the course of sleep.

(*b*) There may be a sudden outbreak of *acute mania* in sleep independently of epilepsy. Two gentlemen conversed together in the evening, and on retiring to rest, A. had no reason to expect what actually happened to B. before morning. He was aroused from sleep by his friend in a state of excitement, threatening his life under the delusion that there were burglars in the house, and that he was connected with them. It transpired that he had piled up various articles of furniture upon the table, and everything was

* *Archiv für Psychiatrie*, Bd. ix. Heft 1.

* *Archiv*, Bd. x. Heft 1.

in wild confusion. He was wide awake. Next day he was removed to an asylum and recovered.

(*c*) *The night terrors* of children. (*See* DEVELOPMENTAL INSANITIES.)

(*d*) *Hallucinations* in a half asleep state occasionally occur and ought to be included in this section. As Dr. Folsom observes, "an hallucination of sight occurring a single time is not uncommon in people in reasonably good health. Frequently repeated, such hallucinations are less rare than is supposed, without any indications of mental or other disease. Occasionally, like flashes of light, they are precursors of headache. I have observed frequent hallucinations of hearing only once, independently of insanity. If of a distressing nature hallucinations of sight and hearing may be a fruitful source of insomnia. They occur beyond the power of the will of the individual to call them up, although it is sometimes able, under some conditions, to cause them to disappear. The hallucinations of sight constitute new arrangements of mental impressions which can be more or less recollected, or they form combinations which seem entirely new. Once I have found two sisters subject to them, and once two sisters, a cousin, and a common grandmother; curiously enough, the different members of the families not knowing each other's peculiarities, which, however, were quite different in kind, until I began my investigations. They had thought them uncanny, and had concealed them." *

(*e*) *Ordinary Sleep-walking or Somnambulism.*—A large number of persons are given to walking in their sleep. Practically however it is an affection peculiar to childhood and youth. It rarely affects idiots and imbeciles.

We proceed to describe the condition of the special senses, general sensation, the motor system, and the mental functions in sleep-walking, based upon a large number of observations.

Sight.—A general opinion prevails that sleep-walkers have their eyelids closed, but are able to see clearly in consequence of the exaltation of the sensory apparatus, and this was the opinion of the late Dr. Guy. In the first place, the eyes are very frequently open. In the second place the visual sense is extremely acute, and the dilated pupil renders it easier to perceive objects with very little light. Thirdly, the sense of touch is exalted, and the sleep-walker saves himself in consequence of this fact from running against furniture, &c. That the subject may write correctly although some object [illegible] him and the paper, [illegible] actually sees what he [illegible] if he is asked to [illegible] dot the letter *i* which he [illegible] may do it accurately, [illegible] removed it is found that [illegible] are not in the right places.

Hearing.—Subjects vary in [illegible] Some do not hear a word [illegible] hear distinctly and respond.

Smell.—The same remark applies [illegible] have a very distinct olfactory [illegible] —*e.g.*, for gas. It would be [illegible] to say in the instance we [illegible] that it was of a subjective [illegible] sociated with a dream.

Taste. — Observations are [illegible] meagre upon this head, but a [illegible] enjoy a meal with apparent [illegible] though not remembering the [illegible] wards.

Tactile Sensibility.—As we [illegible] ready intimated this may be [illegible] sic. On the other hand, the [illegible] employed when carrying the sleep-walker to bed may not be felt, and we [illegible] matter of fact that the subject is [illegible] not aroused thereby.

Anæsthesia.—The somnambulist [illegible] entirely insensible to pain. It is [illegible] to say that this is consistent with [illegible] ness of touch.

Motility.—The ordinary [illegible] of somnambulists, and indeed the [illegible] logy of the word sufficiently [illegible] the muscular system is intact [illegible] of wonderful exploits.

Mentality.—Many of the [illegible] statements made in regard to the [illegible] performances of somnambulists [illegible] careful sifting before they can be [illegible] Facts, however, within our own [illegible] demonstrate that not only ordinary [illegible] tal processes are performed by [illegible] walkers, but that much more [illegible] work may be performed, for example [illegible] blems in Euclid. Lessons may be [illegible] and the scholar find in the morning to his or her surprise that the lesson can be correctly said.

Dreaming.—In all probability a dream immediately precedes and accompanies the action taken by the somnambulist. Somnambulism is an acted dream. In many instances the subject on waking can recall accurately the particular dream, and connect it with the deed which was performed during sleep. Out of the dream [illegible] hallucinations arise, which may determine the character of the act performed.

Speech.—Speaking and singing are by no means uncommon; moreover the somnambulistic musician may play in his

* "Disorders of Sleep: Insomnia." By Charles F. Folsom, M.D. 1890.

sleep on an instrument as well as when he is asleep or awake, or even better.

Medico-legal Relations.—Criminal acts have been performed during sleep, and an expert realises this statement as beyond contradiction. It may be very difficult if not impossible to distinguish between ordinary somnambulism and nocturnal epilepsy. The case of Fraser, the man who took away the life of his boy in his sleep is perhaps the most important case which has found its way into a court of law.*

Treatment.—Decided measures, although anything like cruelty is to be severely condemned, appear to be more effective than any other measure adopted to put a stop to this habit. Boys at school are frequently cured, especially when it assumes the character of an epidemic, by pouring buckets of cold water over them at the commencement of their attacks. A schoolmaster states to us that he has always succeeded by the following method: Shortly before the youthful somnambulist retires to rest his master calls him aside, and speaking in a firm and solemn tone says, "I find you were out of bed and making a disturbance in your room last night." "Sir," he replies, "I was asleep, I know nothing about it." Then the master replies, "I will say nothing about it on this occasion, but such a thing must not occur again." "But sir, I could not help it, I was asleep." "Well," the master replies, "you hear what I say. I would not advise you to let it occur again." Our informant adds, "the boy leaves me, possibly with the feeling that he is being somewhat hardly dealt with, but with an established operative motive for checking the tendency to somnambulism, a motive which doubtless will continue to actuate him even in sleep." This is a philosophical observation; it is in fact adopting the principle of checking and over-mastering one automatic process occurring in sleep by another process more potent. The writer does not wish it to be inferred that moral or corrective means alone are to be employed. On the contrary, it is important to attend to the general health, to administer bromides in some instances, and, more important perhaps than all, to avoid over-tasking the boy or girl with mental work, especially shortly before bedtime.†

(4) **Loss of Sleep as a Cause and Consequence of Insanity.**—*Insomnia* is the indication of a morbid condition. It is also, when prolonged, something more. Loss of sleep may frequently be a cause, or one of several causes, of mental disorder. To remove it is therefore of the greatest consequence in the early treatment of the insane. In a large number of instances it is doubtless the consequence and not the cause of mental trouble. The agony of mind associated with melancholia, or the rapid flow of ideas in acute mania, may render sleep an almost unattainable boon, and in these cases it requires great discrimination to decide when, if at all, to administer hypnotics. (*See* INSOMNIA, and SEDATIVES.)

(5) **Prolonged Sleep.**—A very interesting case has recently been reported from Germany. Dr. Wagner, of Königshütte (O.S.), has sent a preliminary report to Prof. Heidenhain, of which a detailed account will shortly be published. We are indebted to Prof. Heidenhain for permission to make use of it. Dr. Wagner states that the account of the sleeping miner, John Latus, as it appears in the papers is quite true. As senior medical officer to the O.S. Knappschufts-vereins he has frequently visited him at the infirmary in Myslowitz, where Dr. Albers has had the patient under his special care.

The patient, with hereditary taint (the father had hanged himself) had maniacal attacks which marked the onset of an apparently long oncoming psychosis. Shortly after he fell into a state of tetanic rigidity. The whole musculature of the body was of such board-like hardness that one could place him in the standing or recumbent position like a stick. He had to be fed by the œsophageal tube.

This condition was maintained during four months, and throughout this period it was not possible to elicit any response whatever, reaction, or sign of consciousness—the nutrition remaining fairly good.

Then he gradually awakened, but soon began to suffer from an aspiration pneumonia (*Schluck-pneumonie*) which passed on to gangrene. On February 5, 1892, about twenty days after he had awakened, Dr. Wagner operated on account of this gangrene with free resection of ribs. The whole of the lower lobe of the right lung had completely sloughed, and was converted into a liquid of indescribable fetor—extensive sloughs then came away—neither this tissue nor the expectoration ever showed tubercle bacilli. Although the man's powers had suffered terrible

* See *Journal of Mental Science*, 1878, p. 454.

† The writer, anxious to obtain as large a number of cases of spontaneous somnambulism as possible, will supply a printed form of inquiry to any reader who will oblige him by filling it up. Although instances of the activity of the mental functions during sleep, or of acts performed dangerous to others are of especial interest, there is no case so simple as not to possess some statistical value.

depression he yet hoped to bring him through.

At the present time the patient's mind is quite clear, but of the four months' sleep, and of the preceding period, there is absolutely no recollection. Dr. Wagner adds that he has not been able to find any similar case in literature.

Since the foregoing was written this patient has died. The autopsy showed that death was the result of profound exhaustion. The most important condition present was pulmonary gangrene, caused, perhaps, by hypostasis, or by the aspiration of particles of food, with the exception of slight meningitis of very recent date. The brain was perfectly healthy. Deposits of a nature not yet ascertained, were found surrounding the spinal roots of the motor nerves. These deposits have not at the present time been examined.*

A case similar in many respects to that of Dr. Albers was carefully observed by the late Dr. Semélaigne (Paris): The patient, a man of fifty-six, slept for seven months without interruption, then alternating periods of sleep and being awake succeeded, until the longest period of all (the thirty-ninth attack), which lasted fifteen months. When awake, no signs of mental disorder were observed. When asleep he was motionless, absolutely mute, the eyelids closed, the eyes turned upwards. The expression was calm and emotionless. Pulse 60, soft; respiration normal; the temperature 36°.7 (Cent.). He died July 19, 1883, after having slept continuously from April 10, 1882, without sign of returning consciousness. The autopsy revealed adhesions and considerable wasting of the convolutions, especially of the psycho-motor zone.†

THE EDITOR.

[*References.*—Maine de Biran, Nouvelles considérations, sur le Sommeil, les Songes et le Somnambulisme, éd. Cousin. L. F. Alfred Maury, Le Sommeil et les Rêves, quatrième édition, 1878. Albert Lemoine, Du Sommeil au point de Vue Physiologique et Psychologique. John Addington Symonds, Sleep and Dreams, 1851. Robert Macnish, The Philosophy of Sleep, third edition, 1831. Edward Binns, M.D., The Anatomy of Sleep, second edition, 1845. Max Simon, Le Monde des Rêves, 1888. A. E. Durham, Physiology of Sleep, Guy's Hosp. Reps., 1860. C. A. Moore, On Going to Sleep, 1868. J. Cappie, On the Causation of Sleep, 1882. Idem, The Intra-cranial Circulation and its Relation to the Physiology of the Brain, 1890.]

* *Lancet*, April 9, 1892.

† *Annales Méd. Psych.*, Jan. 1885, p. 39. Among the references to cases of prolonged sleep (narcolepsy) given by Semelaigue are "Dict. des Sci. Méd.," t. iv. p. 204; t. xxiii. p. 548; *Journ. de Méd. et de Pharm.*, Oct. 1754, Fév. 1755, Juin 1766; Franck, "Path. Interne," t. iii. p. 31; *Arch. gén. de Méd.*, t. i. p. 734, 1863; et t. i. p. 98, 1866; Legrand du Saulle, *Gaz. des Hôp.*, Nov. 1869; Sandras, "Mal. Nerveuses," t. i. p. [illegible]. [illegible] Gairdner has published a case of "[illegible] Disposition to Sleep" in the *Edin. Med. Journ.*, [illegible] 1871. *Gaz. Hebdom.*, 1884, p. 727.

SLEEP - [illegible] LEPSY. Synonym [illegible]

SMELL, HALLUCINATIONS [illegible] —These may occur in [illegible] ease. The very idea that [illegible] smell badly may have [illegible] ducing the sensation; [illegible] cases, hallucinations may [illegible] pectation.

In mental disease there [illegible] disorders of smell besides [illegible] Thus it has been pointed [illegible] that in a certain number [illegible] general paralysis of the [illegible] power to detect the smell [illegible] common; and we have met [illegible] of recurring insanity in which [illegible] was the first symptom in each [illegible]

Simple hallucinations of [illegible] common than are hallucinations [illegible] other senses.

Hallucinations of smell may [illegible] and isolated in a few rare [illegible] it is much more common to [illegible] *associated* with other hallucinations [illegible] perversions of taste as well [illegible] are often associated. [illegible] cutaneous sensibility too are [illegible] this; thus, a patient may believe [illegible] is a bad smell coming from his [illegible] may also complain of general [illegible] of the skin; in such cases a [illegible] sire to wash (the skin) is common. [illegible] in frequency, in association with [illegible] lucinations of smell we meet [illegible] of sight, and we think that [illegible] of hearing are but rarely so [illegible]

Hallucinations of smell may [illegible] *primary*, leading to other [illegible] mental disorder, or they may be [illegible] brought out, as it were, by the [illegible] from which the patient is already [illegible] ing. In such cases expectancy [illegible] important part allied with [illegible] ideas; thus a person who believes [illegible] to be in hell may complain of the [illegible] ing odour of brimstone.

Hallucinations of smell may be [illegible] or *unpleasant*. It is but rarely, [illegible] that simple hallucinations are [illegible] We have met with hallucinations [illegible] sant association; thus a young [illegible] used to have communion with a [illegible] wife told me that when alone [illegible] he had the most delicious smells, [illegible] at certain other times the [illegible] horrid, when another spirit [illegible]

The hallucinations of smell [illegible] character. Thus they may be [illegible]; this is rarely the case, and then [illegible] bably associated with some organic cause. They are *commonly recurrent*, thus they may recur with each menstrual period, or may be worse at night or early morning. They may be simply diffusive or they may occur in gusts or waves. Gusts of odours occur in some cases of epilepsy.

Hallucinations of smell may depend on the higher central nervous system or on the peripheral sense organs.

We have met with one case in which disease of the temporal bone followed by abscess in the temporo-sphenoidal lobe was connected with hallucinations of smell. Another case, with abscess in the corpus callosum, has also been noticed by Cabanis quoted by Morel. We have met with similar disorder of smell preceding an attack of apoplexy, and we believe it is not very uncommon in other forms of coarse brain lesion; such cases may do something towards defining the olfactory cortical centre. Similar hallucinations may arise from disease of the ethmoid plate;* and it is certain that dryness of mouth and gastro-intestinal catarrh may start these hallucinations.

As far as forms of mental disorder are concerned, we do not know any in which these hallucinations may not be present; they occur in delirious states and may lead to refusal of food; they may arise in melancholia and support the ideas of hell or of burning or torture which is in store for the sufferer; they may give colour to the suspicion of the deluded patient, convincing him that poison is being introduced into his food to kill him, or that some love philtre is being used to cause him to commit some sexual fault. In a few cases of general paralysis with melancholic symptoms of the hypochondriacal type, there are hallucinations of smell; they may be present in epileptic insanity. The smells themselves are, as a rule, very limited in kind. This depends on the restriction in our olfactory powers depending on partial neglect. It is noteworthy that this sense is used but little as a factor of higher mind in civilised man, and many of its perversions appear to be allied to reversions.

The pleasant smells are mostly those of flowers or of artificial scents. The bad odours are acrid or fœtid, the latter being more common. Thus we have smells of fæces, of rotting bodies, of burning, cooking, of electricity or sulphur. There are in some cases connecting links, or associated sensations, so that some complain of "strangling smells," "smells of human blood," &c.

* See "Records of Vienna Asylum Reports," 1858, p. 200.

The most interesting association to our mind, is that met with between hallucinations of smell and perversion of the functions of the reproductive organs. Whether this is a true reversion or not we cannot say, but it is interesting to recall the fact that among the lower animals the sense of smell is nearly related to the reproductive functions, smell acting with them as sight does with the higher animals as a stimulus to passion. In the lower classes there still seems to be a strong feeling in favour of strong scents among the younger women as an attraction. But to return to the occurrence of hallucinations of smell in mental disorders associated with sexual disorders. It is certain that these hallucinations are common in the mental disorders of adolescence, especially those in which masturbation plays a part. Both young men and young women suffering from insanity of adolescence often complain of filthy odours which seem to arise near them, and which they may believe to emanate from their bodies or from their surroundings.

In some cases of puerperal insanity we have met with similar complaints of unpleasant odours; they are particularly common at the climacteric period and may pass off at the menopause.

In one case at least, hallucinations of this nature were present in a patient suffering from ovarian disease, and these persisted till the diseased ovary was removed, since which time, though still insane, the patient has had no smell troubles. This appears to us to be a crucial case. In one or two senile cases of melancholia who complained of suffering in consequence of "the sins of their youth," such hallucinations have been present, but we do not think these due to simple sensations. But in some elderly men with great development of sexual desire we have met with these smell hallucinations, and we think the association is noteworthy. GEORGE H. SAVAGE.

SOCIETIES FOR THE STUDY OF PSYCHOLOGICAL MEDICINE.—These exist in various European countries, and in the United States of America. They are named in the Bibliography appended to this work, together with the periodicals published by their authority. (*See* MEDICO-PSYCHOLOGICAL ASSOCIATION.)

SOCORDIA, or **SECORDIA** (*se*, without; *cor*, heart). Without intellect or understanding. Heartless.

SOFTENING OF THE BRAIN.—A very loose term amongst the laity, meaning with them almost any form of insanity. In medicine it is a pathological state depending on changes in the circulatory system, usually local and with symptoms varying according to the part affected. (*See* GENERAL PARALYSIS.)

SOMNAMBULISM (*somnus*, sleep; *ambulo*, I walk). Walking in one's sleep. (Fr. *somnambulisme*; Ger. *Schlafwandeln.*) It is important to recognise clearly the fact that long prior to the induction of artificial somnambulism physicians met from time to time with cases of spontaneous somnambulism, not merely of the common sleep-walking variety, but presenting phenomena of a remarkable character, and occurring *in the day-time*. Lorry is said to have been the first to have described this abnormal condition. Sauvages recorded cases of this description under the head "Cataleptic Somnambulism." One of these is to be found in the Histoire de l'Académie des Sciences in the year 1742.* A female in a hospital was subject to attacks commencing with a fit of catalepsy lasting about five minutes. She then began to yawn and sit up in bed. Her conversation was animated in an unusual degree, and she directed it to friends whom she supposed to be around her. Her remarks were connected with those which she had made in a similar attack the day before. Her eyes were open, although a number of experiments proved she was fast asleep. There were no signs of feeling or perception when a light was brought so near to the eye as to singe the eyebrows, when a stunning noise was suddenly made near her, when strong ammonia was placed under her eyes or in her mouth, or when a feather or a finger was applied to the cornea, or when snuff was blown into the nostrils or she was pricked with pins. She was able to walk about, avoid coming in contact with the furniture, and would then return to her bed, and again become cataleptic. Sometime afterwards she awoke, and had not the slightest remembrance of what had occurred. In a case recorded by Lorry a woman presented very similar symptoms. The cataleptic condition of the arms and fingers was very marked.

The case described by Dr. Dyce, of Aberdeen, belongs to the same class, and is familiar to those who have studied the subject. A girl aged sixteen began to fall asleep in the evening, and would talk in a coherent manner. She also sang. On one occasion she thought that she was on her way to the Epsom races, and, placing herself on [illegible] room. She answered [illegible] being aroused, dressed [illegible] family, and in one instance [illegible] table for breakfast, [illegible] In this state she was [illegible] was affected by the [illegible] out of the fit of somnambu[illegible] returned home, she asserted [illegible] not been to church. In [illegible] attack, however, she correct[illegible] text and the substance of [illegible] which referred to the [illegible] young men.

In these and many other [illegible] could be quoted on the best [illegible] witness a remarkable condi[illegible] mental sensory and motor [illegible] arising spontaneously, to [illegible] ous names have been appl[illegible] ing as certain symptoms were [illegible] minently marked. If the [illegible] retained for any length of [illegible] position in which they are p[illegible] the case is called one of catalepsy. [illegible] expression is fervid and sugges[illegible] contemplation while unconscio[illegible] rounding objects, the case [illegible] ecstasy. Again, both these [illegible] been employed in association [illegible] somnambulistic condition of the [illegible] and then the compound term "[illegible] somnambulism" or "ecstatic [illegible] bulism" has been employed. The [illegible] mental condition, however, is the [illegible] sleep. In ordinary sleep-walking [illegible] motor centres are awake, and [illegible] is easily performed. In catalepsy [illegible] ecstasy these centres are asleep, [illegible] subject may be totally unable to [illegible] limb. (*See* SLEEP, p. 1172.)

THE [illegible]

SOMNAMBULISME PROVOQ[illegible] French term for the hypnotic sleep.

SOMNIATIO. Dreaming. ([illegible] DREAMING.)

SOMNIATIO MORBOSA. In [illegible] vigilii. Hallucination.

SOMNILOQUISM, SOMNILOQUIUM (*somnus*, sleep; *loquor*, I [illegible]) Talking in one's sleep.

SOMNOLENTIA (*somnus*, [illegible]) Sleepiness, somnolence. (Fr. [illegible]*ment*; Ger. *Schläfrigkeit.*)

SOMNOPATHY (*somnus*, sleep; [illegible], suffering. Magnetic Somnambulism.

SOMNOVIGIL (*somnus*, sleep; [illegible], I watch). Somnambulism.

SOPHOMANIA (σοφός, a wise [illegible]; μανία, madness). A species of [illegible]mania in which the patient [illegible] superior wisdom.

SOPOR. Deep sleep. (Fr. [illegible]*sement*; Ger. *Schläfrigkeit.*)

* This and other instances of spontaneous somnambulism will be found in Dr. Prichard's "Treatise on Insanity and other Disorders affecting the Mind," 1835, pp. 445–452.

SOPORARIUS, SOPORIFEROUS (*sopor*, deep sleep; *fero*, I bring). Having the power of inducing deep sleep.

SOUNDNESS OF MIND. (*See* NON COMPOS MENTIS.)

SOURD MUET. Deaf-mutism.

SOVEREIGN, INSANITY OF. — When the exercise of the royal authority is temporarily interrupted by the insanity of the Sovereign the constitutional method of providing for the administration of the executive power with which he is entrusted is the appointment of a Regent by the two Houses of Parliament. There are two precedents for this course, one in the reign of Henry VI. (1454), the other in the reign of George III. (1788–1810). On the latter occasion select committees to examine the King's physicians touching the state of his health, to inquire into precedents, and to report thereon to the House, were appointed. The Prince of Wales was appointed Regent.

A. WOOD RENTON.

SPACE.—The characteristic of presentations of sense is that they have space form. This distinguishes them from mere sensations.

SPACE, OPEN. (*See* AGORAPHOBIA.)

SPAIN, PROVISION FOR THE INSANE IN.—The early history of the insane in Spain, in so far as it is at present known, begins with the establishment of an asylum at Valencia in 1408. This was accomplished by Fray Gope Gilaberto. It is certain that four special buildings, presumably religious houses, were erected in various parts of the country before the end of the fifteenth century. The honour of taking the initiative in thus providing for the insane has therefore been claimed for Spain, although it is on record that six male patients (*homines mente capti*) were confined in Bethlem Hospital as early as 1403. But it is very probable that in this sphere of charity the Spaniards were following the lead of the Mohammedans, who founded and endowed similar establishments shortly after the proclamation of Islam. The spirit of active philanthropy which impelled Fray Gilaberto to his efforts at Valencia, was also manifest in one of the early caliphs, who not only provided maintenance for the insane inmates of the Morestan at Cairo, but also sought to make existence more tolerable by a daily concert of music. And we may agree with Dr. Lockhart Robertson that the Moor would hardly have left such a monument of ignorant neglect as the Granada Asylum lying under the walls of his much-loved Alhambra; for whatever credit may attach to the pious care of the Middle Ages, the legislation and general arrangements for the protection of the Spanish insane are, at present, probably more defective than in any other civilised state.

Lunacy laws, in the ordinary sense of the term, can hardly be said to exist; and it is only of late years that provision for adequate asylum accommodation has been here and there attempted.

This brief article is designed to present a *résumé* of the **laws dealing with the insane**, and the various projects of successive governments; and also to give some account of the **asylums now open to patients**.

A. **Historical.**—Until about forty years ago the care of the insane was entirely in the hands of private institutions. Some of these date from the Middle Ages, and most of them are under the control of clerical corporations. The earliest recorded foundations were due to the *Beneficencia* (Charitable Corporations), and not to any action of the State or local authorities. The opening of the asylum at Valencia, already alluded to, was followed by King Alfonso V. of Aragon founding the "House of our Lady of Grace," at Saragossa in 1425; by Francisco Ortis founding the Casa del Nuncio at Toledo in 1483; and by similar establishments at Seville* (1436), and at Valladolid (1489). Pinel spoke in terms of high praise of the asylum at Saragossa, but had never visited it. Later accounts of it are distinctly less favourable; but it should be mentioned that the institution referred to by Pinel was burnt in 1808 and replaced by another building.

These fifteenth-century foundations were the only regular lunatic asylums in Spain until a comparatively recent period, and it was only after the Napoleonic wars that modern ideas were introduced and eventually affected the fundamental laws of the country. The levelling principles of the French Revolution were then applied to the complex, mediæval institutions which still persisted. A statute was promulgated in 1822 affecting all charitable properties, and the meagre provisions of this law constitute the foundation of the modern legislation in regard to the insane. It decrees the foundation, in every province, or groups of two or three provinces, of a public asylum for the reception of lunatics of every kind. These asylums are to be managed by the provincial authorities, subject to the supervision of Government. They are to be managed on humane principles.

This law empowers private individuals to establish and conduct asylums, under

* *Cf.* "Don Quixote," part ii. chap. i.

the inspection of the provincial authorities. The rules for admission, treatment of patients, &c., were to be provided by a special regulation which has never yet been issued. The unhappy condition of the country caused this statute to remain a dead letter until 1836, notwithstanding the eloquent remonstrance of Señor Burgos, Minister of Fomento. It was not until 1846 that Dr. Don Pedro Rubio, body physician to Queen Isabella, after a visit to the principal existing asylums, recommended that a Government inquiry into the whole question should be instituted. Great difficulty was experienced in ascertaining the facts; but it appeared that at that time (1847) in all Spain there were sixty-six institutions where insane patients were received. These were classed as follows :—

4 asylums exclusively for the insane;
32 common hospitals;
10 houses of mercy (religious hospitals);
2 hospitals for children and foundlings;
16 gaols;
1 nunnery;
1 convict establishment.

The total number of inmates was 1626; of these 151 were supported by their families, and the others by municipal or individual charity. The number of lunatics living in private care was stated at 5651; but there *is* reason to believe that this should have been much greater.

Dr. Rubio then reported that the state of the insane was most deplorable, and that their condition did not practically differ from what is described in the pages of Cervantes. He found them "worse treated than the most atrocious felons."

Briefly, the outcome of this report was a statute, passed in 1849, which was designed to place all lunatic asylums under the exclusive control of the State. It was supplemented by another law (1852), which emphasised the position previously taken—that, *inter alia*, all asylums were national as opposed to provincial or municipal. Moreover, it was determined to found six national lunatic asylums—in Madrid, Saragossa, Valladolid, Corunna, Granada, Valencia, and Barcelona. But only one of these was erected—at Leganès near Madrid. In 1859 a royal decree was promulgated for the erection of this asylum, and the design was thrown open to competition amongst architects of all countries. In response to the programme then set forth, Dr. Desmaisons of Bordeaux went to Spain and visited the various asylums. His experiences were set forth in a little book, published in 1859—"Des Asiles d'Aliénés en Espagne; Recherches Historiques et Médicales." He specially drew attention [illegible] it is the custom in all [illegible] place the insane, when [illegible] home, for a certain period [illegible] in the lunatic ward of a [illegible] or hospice; and to defer [illegible] an asylum until the prospects [illegible] well-nigh vanished. This [illegible] survives to a great extent; [illegible] the hospital physicians of Spain [illegible] trained in such famous schools [illegible] the condition of the insane [illegible] care continues to be a reproach to [illegible] tendom. The hospital treatment [illegible] sanity in Spain cannot be [illegible] triumphant; the country is moving [illegible] in the same direction as other [illegible] seeking success by similar [illegible] expedients. Dr. Desmaison's [illegible] treats of the history of the Spanish asylums, and he specially refers to the [illegible] tive taken by Spanish subjects in [illegible] lishing similar institutions [illegible] among which the asylum of Rome is [illegible] as a remarkable example.

It is unnecessary to refer in [illegible] the shifting policy of unstable [illegible] ments, which entailed contradictory [illegible] and evanescent attempts to [illegible] the question successfully. The [illegible] point seems to have been reached [illegible] when the Government reverted [illegible] ideas of 1822, and by circular [illegible] provincial assemblies to found [illegible] lums or lunatic establishments in the hospitals of each provincial capital.

Seven out of the fourteen provinces of Spain found means to carry [illegible] effect, and private asylums had been established until, in 1879, the following institutions were reported to be existing:—

1. *National Asylum*, one only.—At Leganès, near Madrid; patients, 579.

2. *Provincial Asylums*, seventeen.—(*a*) Seven wards in seven hospitals devoted to the cure of other diseases; patients, 298. (*b*) Ten asylums, four of which date from the fifteenth century; patients, 2147.

3. *Private Asylums*, eight.—(*a*) Four constituted by Royal order; patients, [illegible]. (*b*) Four licensed by the provincial committees for benevolent institutions; patients, at least 163.

It will, therefore, be recognised that the accommodation for insane patients, according to the latest procurable return, is extremely meagre. Spain, with a population of 16,500,000, provides asylum treatment for less than 4000 lunatics, while nearly one-fourth of that number are placed in private asylums, at least two of which appear to be purely commercial undertakings.

B. **Administrative.**—It is not requisite to present in detail the regulations governing these institutions. They are cumbrous and incomplete.

Although there is no law to compel the proprietors of lunatic asylums to obtain a licence, Dr. Esquerdo positively states that one is never established without the consent of the provincial committee, but such consent is never refused. The circumstances above detailed must make it difficult for a committee to withhold consent; besides, it is to be remembered that all private asylums are subject to the inspection of the provincial committee. By royal decree and subsequent instruction certain returns must be made to the central Government. For instance, the Provincial committee must report upon the origin, character, patrons, administrators, &c., of all benevolent institutions.

The rules regulating the admission, detention, and discharge of patients vary with the bye-laws of each asylum. Except in the case of the one national asylum, they have no statutory force, and may be altered from time to time by the provincial authorities. As a general rule, a judicial sentence, as well as a medical certificate, is required, but this is by no means without exception. The proprietors of most of the private asylums require a medical certificate, "to avoid incurring responsibility." The improper detention of a person in an asylum or elsewhere is punishable by the penal code, and carries very severe sentences. It is a criminal offence. The law of 1849 expressly provides that no one shall be detained in any benevolent institution for a longer period than that necessary for his treatment and relief; but his departure must be preceded by a written licence from the director. If any question arises as to the improper confinement of a person in an asylum, the proof lies with the physician who certified his lunacy rather than with the proprietor of the asylum; and it will be at once evident that judicial sentences are avoided, inasmuch as they mean formal and public "incapacitation," besides another judicial sentence on recovery.

Alcubilla ("Diccionario de la Administracion Española ") states that two certificates are necessary, one a medical statement of the patient's insanity, and another emanating from the municipality, setting forth the pecuniary circumstances of the patient. If he is in poor circumstances the local authorities are empowered to act.

The law provides for the inspection of every class of asylum, and states the authorities empowered to carry out the work of inspection; but it has only the appearance of completeness. Briefly, the Minister of the Interior has direct control over the one national asylum, and also direct control over the provincial committees. The chief of each committee is the civil governor of the province, but his duties are too multifarious and urgent to permit of his undertaking the work of inspecting asylums. It should be noted, however, that by a royal order a ladies' committee of visitation was constituted under the presidency of the Princess of the Asturias in 1875.

But there are now no paid inspectors, and the powers of visitation are only optional, so that the theoretic efficiency of the law is worsted by its practical failure. The country is poor, the Government unstable, and the people demoralised. Until better days dawn for Spain, the condition of the insane will remain an indication of national disaster. Now, however, there are distinct signs of happy augury. The more recent accounts of Spanish asylums show an improvement all along the line.

C. **Establishments.**—The writer has no intention to recapitulate the experiences of those travellers who have described the backward state of Spanish asylums. He prefers to indicate, in few words, what is being done to remove the reproach of the past in face of many and almost insuperable difficulties.

No one who is interested in this subject can visit Madrid without coming in contact with Dr. Esquerdo, who established, unaided, a private asylum of excellent reputation, and whose Spanish courtesy has gained him many friends. The Spaniard's standard of apparent comfort differs so much from our ideas that too much has been made of bare walls and darkened rooms by some authors. The National Asylum at Leganès, too, has been much improved of late years. Of course, there are abominable cells and much restraint; no doubt, the sanitation is imperfect; but, in comparison with the state of matters a generation back, the advance is striking and encouraging.

Perhaps the most remarkable improvement is now taking place at Sevilla. There a new asylum is being built in the country, and the patients are being moved from the old wards in the hospital as the accommodation is completed. A drive of three or four miles, over the most execrable roads, separates the new institution from the town. It is built in pavilions under the French influence, which is as dominant in Spanish psychiatry as in other departments of medicine. Nothing better could be desired for patients of the lower class, and no English county asylum could be more presentable in every detail. Only the quieter classes of patients were in residence at the time referred to (1891). Unfortunately, it is only too probable that the apparatus of restraint will be more in evidence when the building is completed.

A visit to the asylum of Granada revealed no material improvement on the state of the building since Dr. Lockhart Robertson's visit in 1868. It was positively stated that all the insane patients had been removed, and the place seemed to be devoted to children and aged poor. It was impossible to ascertain how this had come about, or whither the lunatics had been removed. The physician in charge could not be found, and there was an evident desire to keep strangers uninformed. This may perhaps be accepted as a good omen, for in former days the asylum at Granada was forced on the attention of every passing tourist, and lunatics in every phase of wretchedness were kept on show.

The only book on insanity written by a Spaniard for Spaniards is the treatise by Dr. D. Juan Giné y Partagas. The Spanish Frenopathic Academy, which resembles our Medico-Psychological Association in constitution, as yet remains a numerically unimportant body.

A. R. Urquhart.

[*References.*—Papers in the Journal of Mental Science: July 1868, A Visit to the Lunatic Hospital at Granada, by Dr. Lockhart Robertson; Oct. 1879, Spanish Asylums, by Dr. Donald Fraser; July 1885, A Glance at Lunacy in Spain, by Dr. Jelly; Notes on Spanish Asylums, by Dr. Sequin; Des Asiles d'Aliénés en Espagne, by Dr. Desmaisons, 1859; Lunacy in Many Lands, by G. A. Tucker, 1887; Report on the Working of the Lunacy Laws in Foreign Countries, Blue Book, 1885.]

SPARAGMUS (σπαράσσω, I tear). A spasm or convulsion; applied to epilepsy. Fr. *sparagme.*)

SPASMOPHILIA (σπασμός, a convulsion; φιλία, love or affection for). Hyperexcitability of the nervous system leading to a tendency to convulsions.

SPASMUS CYNICUS. The Risus Sardonicus (*q.v.*).

SPECIFIC GRAVITY OF BRAIN. (*See* Brain, Specific Gravity of.)

SPECIMENS OF BRAIN OR CORD FOR MICROSCOPE, PREPARATION OF.—For those engaged in the microscopic examination of the brain or spinal cord of persons dying insane, it will save much time and trouble, as well as ensure the satisfactory preparation of sections of nervous tissue, to be in possession of the means which experience [illegible] fitted for the purpose.

Macerating fluids [illegible] isolating nerve structures.

Nitric Acid, 20 per cent. [illegible] small fragments of the tissue [illegible] and leave for twenty-four hours [illegible] well in water, tease, stain, [illegible] glycerine. By this method the [illegible] tissue is rendered softer, and the [illegible] fibres are hardened. The following [illegible] fied fluid may be used:—

Glycerine	[illegible]
Water	[illegible]
Strong nitric acid . .	[illegible]

Mix thoroughly. Place small fragments of the tissue in this fluid, leave [illegible] or four days and then wash well [illegible] distilled water.

Ordinary *Müller's Fluid*, [illegible] *chromic acid* (1 per cent. solution), [illegible] *perosmic acid* (1 per cent. solution) may be used as macerating fluids for [illegible] tissues, small pieces of which are left in a few drops of the medium for two or three days and then teased out. They may then be examined in glycerine, water or saline solution.

The last-named fluid is especially useful for defining the outlines of cells and for fatty tissues, degenerations of [illegible], &c. Tissues should be allowed to macerate for from twelve to twenty-four hours before any attempt is made to tease them out.

Hardening Fluids. *General Directions.*—Cut up the brain, cord or nerve with a sharp knife or razor (taking care to make clean cuts and not to drag or tear the tissue) into blocks about one inch square and half an inch thick, or into cubes, each side of which should measure not more than about three-quarters of an inch, or into short lengths not more than half an inch each. Where tissues are to be hardened rapidly, as in absolute alcohol, the small cubes should always be prepared. These cubes should in most cases be taken from different parts of the brain or cord, but one piece from the surface, with the membranes still attached, should always be included. In cutting up the cord, cut through the dura mater in front but leave the pieces arranged in series by a posterior attachment composed of the uncut dura.

(*a*) The delicate pia mater is best prepared by pinning it down to pieces of cork which are then floated in dilute hardening fluids. Large sections of the whole brain either vertical or longitudinal should never be more than [illegible] to [illegible] in. in thickness; they should be laid in a flat-bottomed dish, or tied to wood or glass plates, with a layer of cotton wadding between the plate and the section, as may be found most convenient.

(*b*) Put the tissues away *at once* in the hardening fluid.

(*c*) Put a piece of rag or some cotton wadding saturated with the hardening fluid in the bottom of a wide-mouthed jar; on this place four or five of the blocks of tissue, or a whole brain section, then a second layer of rag or wadding, a second layer of tissue, and so on, the proportion of tissue to fluid never being greater than one to twenty. Fill the jar with fluid, label distinctly with the name, age and sex of the patient, the organ, the supposed morbid condition, and the date and time at which the hardening process is begun and its nature. Put away in a cool dark place, such as an underground cellar; but immediately before doing so, change the position of the pieces of tissue in the bottle. This is especially necessary when spirit is used.

(*d*) At the end of twenty-four hours pour out the fixing or hardening fluid, carefully wash out the jar and rinse the tissue thoroughly with water to get rid of any blood or other deposit which may have settled on it, and which would if left seriously interfere with the hardening process; add fresh fluid. As a general rule fluids should again be changed at the end of the third day, and then weekly for two or three weeks.

(*e*) Each time the fluid is changed the tissue should be carefully examined and its consistency ascertained. When hardened properly, tissues should be tough and firm, never brittle, as they are apt to become if the hardening process is carried too far or has been done imperfectly.

(*f*) After being hardened slowly, the tissues are removed from the fluid, generally about the end of the second to the eighth week, according to the fluid used, and if not hardened in spirit they are washed for several hours in water until no further yellow colour is given; after which they are transferred to a mixture of equal parts of methylated spirit and water for two days and then to methylated spirit* in which they are left until required. The spirit may become cloudy, in which case it must be changed as often as the cloudiness makes its appearance.

(*g*) It is an extremely difficult matter to give definite instructions as to the fluid to be used in individual cases, but the following general rules will assist materially in determining what hardening fluid should be used.

(1) *Corrosive sublimate solution*—saturated solution—may, in some cases, be used as a preliminary fixing re-agent. It stops putrefactive processes and fixes the protoplasm at once. It or Fleming's solution is most suitable for perfectly fresh material.

(2) Where the brain tissue is hard and firm, and not likely to shrivel on the abstraction of water, and where too it is not thought necessary to keep the blood in the organ, *methylated spirit* may be used. Tissues hardened in spirit are sometimes distorted somewhat; but this method has the advantage, that tissues so hardened are very readily stained with logwood or with the aniline dyes.

(3) When the tissues are very delicate, soft, or œdematous, or when there is much blood in them, use *Müller's fluid*.

Müller's fluid is one of the most useful of all our hardening reagents, especially in the preparation of delicate tissues; it fixes the protoplasm of the cells rather than hardens them, and thus causes but little shrinking of the tissues, so that where the organ is congested, or the tissue delicate, it is invaluable. Take of

Potassium bichromate .	2½ parts
Sodium sulphate . .	1 part
Water	100 parts

Use in the proportion of 1 volume of tissue to 20 of fluid (as with all other methods). Change the fluid at the end of the first, third and seventh days, and then at the end of each week till the end of the fifth; transfer to water for several hours after the tissue has been in the fluid for six or eight weeks, and then again to dilute methylated spirit; leave in this for from twenty-four to forty-eight hours, and then preserve in strong methylated spirit. The great advantages of Müller's fluid are that there is no great danger of over-hardening, and although the process takes a considerable time, the results are almost invariably satisfactory; that the red blood-corpuscles remain unchanged in shape, and take on a greenish tinge; it is not essential that the pieces should be small, and this fluid may be used where it would be inconvenient to cut up the tissue into small cubes. Begin the hardening process as soon as the structures are taken from the body, and carry it on, for the first few days, at any rate, in a cool dark place. The hardening process may be completed by osmic acid or bichromate of ammonia.

Hamilton recommends that where large slices are to be made, the brain should be

* Methylated spirit, as now prepared, always becomes cloudy on the addition of water, so that these instructions only apply to re-distilled spirit, or to the spirit specially provided for scientific purposes.

carefully injected with Müller's fluid, through the carotid or vertebral vessels, which should be injured as little as possible in removing the brain; this should be repeated every day for a week before the brain is cut up.

Müller's fluid and spirit is recommended by Hamilton for hardening nerve-tissues, brain, spinal cord, and retina. It is composed of—

Müller's fluid . . .	3 parts
Methylated spirit . . .	1 part

Cool thoroughly before using, and follow the directions given for hardening with Müller's fluid.

Bichromate of potash may also be used for hardening large pieces of the brain. It must be used in large quantities, to which carbolic acid saturated solution (1 or 2 grains to the ounce) has been added. The fluid is not changed, but is kept saturated by the addition, from time to time, of crystals of the bichromate salt. It hardens tissues slowly, taking from six to eight weeks. Keep in a cool dark place.

Chromic Acid.—Where it is desired to harden nervous tissues more rapidly, a solution of chromic acid, not stronger than one-sixth per cent. may be used. Where this or any of the following chromic-acid compounds are employed, the pieces of tissue should never be more than one-sixth of an inch in thickness, and half an inch in diameter. Use twenty volumes of the fluid to one of the tissue. Change at the end of twenty-four hours, again on the second and third days, and then every third day until the tissue is hard and tough. A careful examination should be made about the eighth day to see that the hardening is progressing properly; for if the tissues be left too long, or if the mixture be too strong, they become exceedingly brittle. Wash well, allowing a stream of water to run over the tissues for several hours; then place in equal parts of methylated spirit and water, leave for twenty-four hours, and transfer to pure methylated spirit.

Erlicki's Fluid.—For hardening brain-tissue to be stained by Weigert's method, Erlicki's fluid may be used:—

Potassium bichromate .	2.5 parts
Cupric sulphate . . .	0.5 "
Water	100 "

At the ordinary temperature this fluid hardens tissues in eight or ten days. At 40° C. tissues are hardened in four or five days. With this fluid, however, the tissues shrink more than with Müller's fluid.

Bichromate of ammonia as a 2 per cent. solution may be used [illegible] complete the hardening of [illegible] tres. Use at least twenty [illegible] fluid to one of tissue; change [illegible] of the first, third, and seventh [illegible] at the end of the second, third [illegible] weeks.

Perosmic acid is extremely [illegible] fixing and hardening small [illegible] delicate tissue, or tissue in which [illegible] sence of fatty degeneration is [illegible]. It is used as a one-sixth to [illegible] even one per cent. solution. The [illegible] allowed to remain in it, carefully [illegible] from the light, for about six [illegible] twenty-four hours according to [illegible] nature. Then transfer it to 75 per cent. spirit, in which it may be kept [illegible] quired; or after being well washed [illegible] tilled water it may be placed at once in [illegible] gum and syrup solution, frozen, [illegible] mounted in acetate of potash.

If Farrants' solution be used [illegible] mounting medium, the glycerine [illegible] continually browned by the acid [illegible] sections before mounting are thoroughly washed in water, or in water and glycerine.

Fleming's fixing solution is [illegible] useful for fixing nuclear figures in [illegible] tissues, and for fixing these tissues generally:

Chromic acid (1 per cent.) .	15 [illegible]
Osmic acid (2 per cent.) . .	4 [illegible]
Glacial acetic acid . . .	1 part

Use 10 to 20 parts of fluid to 1 of tissue. Allow tissues to remain in this for from one to three days; but they may remain for weeks, even, exposed to sunlight, with [illegible] effects. Wash thoroughly in water before cutting. After being fixed in this fluid tissues may be hardened by being passed through 30, 50, 70, and 90 per cent. spirit (one day each), and then into absolute alcohol. Embed in paraffine or celloidin.

Golgi's Hardening and Staining Methods.—The method originally employed by Golgi* has been modified by Kölliker as follows:—The cord is cut into pieces of three to four millimetres long, held together by the membranes. They are then placed in the following mixture: Bichromate of potassium (3 per cent.) 4 parts; perosmic acid (1 per cent.) 1 part. Use 30 parts of fluid to one of tissue, and change after a few hours. At the end of from one to one and a half days the tissue is removed and washed for from a quarter to half an hour in a ½ per cent. solution of nitrate of silver, and

* Hofmann and Schwalbe's "Jahresberichte," Bd. x. "Fortschritte der Medicin," Bd. v. p. [illegible] 1887. *See also Journal of Anatomy*, vol. xxv. p. 443.

then placed in about twenty to forty times its bulk of ¾ per cent. nitrate of silver solution for thirty to forty hours. They may then be preserved in 40 per cent. spirit for three to six weeks, after which they soon become spoiled. On removal, the pieces are ready for cutting and examination.

They may be rapidly embedded in celloidin (one hour in absolute alcohol, and one hour in celloidin), and should be cut at once, as they spoil after about twenty-four hours. The sections are clarified in creosote for a quarter of an hour, then in turpentine, and are mounted in xylol balsam. The silver stains the neuroglia and nerve-cells, especially in embryos and young animals, and brings into prominence all nerve-fibres which possess no nerve-sheath, and exist merely as naked axis cylinders.

Golgi's Original Methods.—The Long Method: Harden tissues for twenty to thirty days in 2 per cent. bichromate of potassium, and then place in .75 per cent. nitrate of silver. The Short Method: Harden for four to five days in 2 per cent. bichromate of potassium, then for twenty-four to thirty hours in 1 per cent. osmic acid (2 parts), and 2 per cent. bichromate of potassium (8 parts). Remove and place in .75 per cent. silver nitrate solution.

Methods of Cutting Sections (For fresh Freezing Method *see* p. 1187).—Of the various freezing methods D. J. Hamilton's is the most perfect, especially as it involves no danger of over freezing. To prepare the tissues proceed as follows:—Remove the hardening fluid from the tissue (especially if spirit has been used) by a prolonged immersion, say for twenty-four hours, in water, which should be constantly changed by allowing a very small stream from the tap to fall into the vessel in which the tissue is being washed. Then transfer to a mixture of gum, B.P. strength,* one part; syrup,† one part. To each of these fluids add three drops of a strong solution of carbolic acid prepared by adding one part of Calvert's No. 4 carbolic acid to two parts of water, or saturate (boiling) with boracic acid, to prevent the formation of fungi. If this be attended to, the tissue may be left soaking in the solution for an indefinite length of time, and at the end will "cut" perfectly, if it has been properly hardened in the first instance. Allow the tissue to remain in this mixture for from twenty-four to forty-eight hours or even longer. The microtome is cooled down to such a point that a drop of gum (B.P. solution) placed on the die or disc is frozen. The tissue which has been soaking in the gum and syrup is taken out with a pair of forceps, carefully dried in a cloth, is put to soak for a few minutes in gum, and then adjusted as required on the surface of the cooled disc; gum is painted around it to keep it in position, and to form with it a firm solid mass, which may be cut in a single section. The mass is frozen just so hard that it will cut like a piece of cheese; when softer than this, it is not sufficiently frozen, when harder, it is very difficult to cut, especially if the sections are of considerable size.

Cutting in Celloidin.—Brain tissue or spinal cord after being hardened is transferred to various grades of spirit, then to absolute alcohol, and placed for twenty-four hours or longer, according to the size of the blocks, in a mixture of equal parts of alcohol and ether. From this the blocks are transferred to a very thin celloidin syrup, made by dissolving shavings of celloidin in equal parts of ether and alcohol, then to a stronger, and lastly, into a good stiff syrup of the same material. Then take a piece of wood (not cork, which gives slightly in the jaws of the clamp) cut across the grain, and pour over this a quantity of ether until no more bubbles make their appearance. Over this prepared surface pour some of the thick celloidin, and on this embed the soaked tissues. Bank well up with the thick celloidin syrup, allowing it to dry for some time until there is a good firm film, add more celloidin, again dry, and then immerse in a large quantity of methylated spirit until the whole is thoroughly hardened. Cut these sections under spirit if possible. In any case have a good drop bottle containing methylated spirit constantly playing on the block of tissue that is being cut.

Hamilton (to whom we owe nearly all the good embedding processes used in the freezing method) has succeeded in combining the celloidin with the gum and sugar method. After the tissue is hardened it is placed (if it has not already been hardened in spirit) in methylated spirit for three or four days, the fluid being changed daily. It is afterwards immersed in a mixture of equal parts of alcohol and ether in which it is left for two days, then from one to four days according to the size of the piece of tissue in a syrup of celloidin dissolved in equal parts of ether and absolute alcohol. Then pour a somewhat

* Gum acacia, 1 lb., is dissolved in 80 ozs. of water.

† The syrup is made by boiling one part of crystallised sugar in one part of distilled water until the whole of the sugar is dissolved.

stronger solution of celloidin into a paper box or a pill box and embed, in the centre of this, the piece of tissue. Allow the fluid to be exposed to the air for some time, until it partially hardens (the longer it is exposed the harder it ultimately becomes), then plunge the whole into strong methylated spirit and leave it until the celloidin is quite hard, the ether has been dissolved out. This mass is now soaked in water for twenty-four hours or longer, in fact, until there is no longer any smell of alcohol, and then in a mixture of gum and syrup in the proportion of one to two. During this latter part of the process the fluid may be kept at a temperature of about 40° C. with advantage, as under these conditions the mixture passes readily into the tissues. The procedure is afterwards just the same as in the ordinary freezing method.

Mounting of Serial Sections (*Celloidin.*)—For mounting serial sections of specimens cut in celloidin we now use Al. Obregia's modification of Weigert's method.

(1) Make a solution of sugar candy in water about as thick as ordinary syrup. To 30 c.c. of this add 20 c.c. of 95 per cent. alcohol and 10 c.c. of a solution of pure dextrine of the consistence of syrup. Spread a thin layer of this over a slide and allow it to dry in a warm place, protecting it from dust; keep for several days.

(2) Dissolve photoxylin, 6 grammes, in a mixture of absolute alcohol 100 c.c., ether (pure), 100 c.c.; allow it to stand, and pour off the clear part. Both this and No. 1 will keep well if preserved in stoppered bottles. Thin celloidin syrup may be used instead of No. 2. Cut pieces of satin cooking paper (which is thin and smooth on one surface and leaves no particles on the sections) the size of the slides and place in a flat dish with the smooth surface upwards, and moisten with 95 per cent. alcohol. Remove the sections with similar paper, and arrange them, spreading them well out on the slips in the dish with a pencil moistened with alcohol. Remove the paper and lay it, with the sections upwards, on folded blotting-paper until all fluid is absorbed, then place the paper, face downwards, on the prepared slide, the sections coming in contact with the dextrine; place blotting-paper over it and press lightly with the finger; when the paper is removed the sections are left on the prepared layer. Then pour solution No. 2 over the slide and wave in the air until all cloudiness disappears.

When the slide is put into pure water the sugar is dissolved, and the whole film comes away from the glass very readily, leaving one side quite [illegible] all processes of staining, [illegible] hydrating may go on [illegible] when both surfaces are [illegible] celloidin film. For brain [illegible] an exceedingly good [illegible] medium is not stained by [illegible] or haematoxylin; it is stained [illegible] colours, which, however, may be [illegible] by means of comparatively [illegible]

The paraffine embedding [illegible] tial where specially thin sections [illegible] quired. Small pieces of tissue [illegible] been well hardened and then [illegible] twenty-four hours in absolute [illegible] immersed in clean, pure turpentine [illegible] in a covered porcelain crucible. [illegible] put into a warm chamber, which [illegible] gradually heated up to the melting [illegible] of the paraffin that is used and [illegible] three to twenty-four hours. It is then transferred directly to melted hard paraffine (melting at about 53° C.). Very delicate objects, such as the cord or brain of an embryo, should be passed through several softer paraffines. The tissue is allowed to soak in the melted paraffine for several hours, and is then transferred to a paper box, a pill box, or metal mould, full of melted paraffine. It is kept in position with warm needles, and is cooled rapidly by floating on water. There should be no turpentine left either in the tissue or in the paraffine. When the specimens are to be stained in bulk they should be taken from 75 per cent. spirit, stained, and then passed through 90 per cent. spirit and absolute alcohol, after which they are treated as above; or they may be taken from the turpentine and first transferred to a mixture of turpentine and paraffine for twenty-four hours, after which they are passed into pure paraffine.

In place of turpentine, benzol or chloroform may be used in paraffine embedding. When the tissues have been in absolute alcohol, either before or after staining, immerse in a small porcelain crucible or test-tube in equal parts of chloroform and alcohol. The specimen, which at first floats, after a time sinks, when the mixture should be replaced by pure chloroform. As soon as the specimen again sinks pour off most of the liquid and add to what remains scraps of solid paraffine; place in a chamber heated to 53° or 54° C., and gradually add more paraffine. Keep the specimen at the above temperature until no smell of chloroform is given off, then embed in a paper boat or metal mould as above described, and cool at once in water.

Sections embedded and cut in paraffine are arranged on the surface of the dried syrup with a camel-hair pencil, flattened out and heated in a warm chamber kept at from 57°–60° C. for ten minutes, when the sections have a tendency to become more perfectly spread out. The paraffine is first removed with good blotting-paper, then with xylol or turpentine, after which the slide is placed in absolute alcohol for a few minutes, and then quickly into photoxylin or celloidin solution; dry for ten minutes; wash in water and stain. To dehydrate afterwards use 95 per cent. spirit, and to clear use pure carbolic crystals, 1 part to xylol (pure) 3 parts.

Sections cut in paraffine may also be fixed on the slide with a mixture of equal parts of filtered whites of egg and glycerine, to which is added a lump of camphor. Apply to the slide with a glass rod and scrape off with another ground-glass slide, in order to leave as thin a layer as possible. Arrange the sections on this, heat to the coagulating point of the albumen, and then proceed as in the previous case.

Carmine staining fluid is especially useful for sections of the central nervous system. To prepare it, take of

Pure carmine	1 part
Strong ammonia . . .	1 „
Water	50 parts

Triturate the carmine in a mortar, add sufficient water to form a paste, and then add the ammonia, when the paste will at once turn from a bright red to almost black if the carmine is pure. Add the rest of the water, and keep the solution in a glass-stoppered bottle, in which is suspended a piece of camphor.

After carefully washing out any of the chromates with water or with a dilute solution of carbonate of soda, a section may be stained rapidly by spreading it out on the glass slide, and running a drop or two of the carmine solution over it; allow it to stand for from three to five minutes, and then wash in water for a couple of seconds, and rapidly transfer to acidulated water (eight drops of acetic acid to a pint basinful of water). This latter part of the operation must never be neglected, as the carmine is held in solution by an alkaline fluid, and is only precipitated in the tissues, when the fluid is rendered acid. Where the stain is properly selective, the nuclei and fully-formed fibrous tissue are stained carmine and a delicate pink respectively. Other formed material remains unstained, or is only slightly tinted. The axis cylinders of medullated nerve fibres are stained brilliant carmine, as are also the nerve-cells of the cord, &c., the latter not so deeply. A more selective stain is obtained by staining the sections slowly in a watery solution. They are afterwards treated in the same way. The sections so stained may be mounted in glycerine or in Farrants' solution, or when it is wished to clear up the section still further it may be mounted in Canada balsam.

Congo Red.—A capital stain for the cord and for nerves is Congo red, as supplied by Messrs. Squire & Sons. Its use was suggested to me by Mr. A. Pringle, who used it as a 1–2 per cent. watery solution, diluted as required; it stains very rapidly. Wash thoroughly, dehydrate with absolute alcohol, clear with clove oil, and mount in Canada balsam. Axis cylinders are distinctly stained, the sheath remains colourless, and all cells and fibrous tissues are pretty deeply stained.

Picro-carmine. — Picro-carmine, or picro-carmine with osmic acid, may also be used, especially when Hamilton & Bramwell's half clearing-up method is used. They recommend that the dehydration of sections of the cord or brain should be effected by means of methylated spirit, and that instead of taking out the whole of the water, enough should be left in to keep the denser parts and tissues of the section slightly opaque. Most beautiful preparations may be obtained by this method.

Gold-staining Method.—An exceedingly useful method for nerve-centres is Beckwith's modification of Freud's gold method. Pieces of the tissues are hardened (not over-hardened) in Erlicki's fluid, and then (though not necessarily) in alcohol; sections are made, rinsed with water, and placed for three or four hours in a 1 per cent. solution of gold chloride; they are again washed with water, treated with a 20 per cent. solution of caustic soda for three minutes, then with a 10 per cent. solution of carbonate of potash for thirty minutes; the superfluous fluid is drained off, and the sections are placed for from five to fifteen minutes in a 10 per cent. solution of iodide of potassium. They are washed in water, dehydrated, and mounted in balsam.

This method gives most beautiful results, picking out the delicate nerve fibrils and axis cylinders in a most remarkable manner. One of the great secrets of success is that the specimens should be put directly into the gold solution, the second that in cutting, sections should be wetted with water instead of with alcohol.

Safranin. — Adamakiewicz's Safranin Method for Nerve-tissues.—First place the sections into water weakly acidulated with nitric acid, then into a tube of concentrated watery solution of safranin until they are well stained, wash in methylated spirit, and then in absolute alcohol acidulated with nitric acid, and then with water similarly acidulated, after which the sections are stained in methyl blue, and dehydrated with alcohol, cleared up with clove oil, and mounted in balsam.

Weigert's Staining Methods.—Stain a section (hardened in Müller's fluid, bichromate of potash or Erlicki's fluid) for twenty-four hours in a concentrated watery solution of acid fuchsin (soda salt of rose aniline sulphate), wash in water, and transfer to an alkaline solution of alcohol with 10 c.c. of a solution made by dissolving 1 gramme of fused caustic potash in 100 c.c. of absolute alcohol, and filtering, for a few seconds until the first sign of the grey nerve-tissue of the section becomes visible; wash in water, "which must not be acid," and dehydrate with absolute alcohol saturated with sodic chloride, to preserve the colour of the section. Clear with oil of cloves, and mount in Canada balsam. In sections prepared in this manner, the medullated nerve-fibres stand out as brilliant red lines or points, even those in the anterior horns of the spinal cord. The sheath or part of the sheath is stained by this method. "The ganglion cells and connective tissue (especially in sclerosis) with those of the pia mater vary in tint from a pale to an exquisite blue, which latter is increased by rinsing the sections in a solution of 1 part of hydrochloric acid to 5 of water, and then washing thoroughly in water, before dehydrating them with alcohol. These tissues can also be stained blue with hæmatoxylin, before or after colouring with the acid fuchsin." For the central nervous system, according to Weigert, this is invaluable, but for peripheral nerves it is of no use. To Weigert also we are indebted for the following method of staining the myelin sheaths of the nerves of the nerve-centres. After the tissues have been thoroughly hardened, and a piece embedded in celloidin, it is transferred to a saturated solution of neutral acetate of copper, diluted with one volume of water, the whole being kept at a temperature of from 35° to 45° C. The tissues become green and the celloidin blueish green. Take of

(A)	Water	90 parts
	Saturated solution of lithium carbonate	1 part
(B)	Hæmatoxylin	1 "
	Absolute alcohol	10 parts

When required, mix equal parts of A. and B., and dilute somewhat. Leave the sections in this solution for any length of time between one and twenty-four hours, taking care to keep the temperature at from 35° to 45° C. Wash [illegible] and transfer to a solution [illegible]

Borax . . .	[illegible]
Ferrocyanide of potassium	[illegible]
Water . . .	[illegible]

Allow the sections to remain [illegible] half an hour to two or three hours [illegible] ing to the thickness of the sections [illegible] intensity of the logwood [illegible] wash well in water, dehydrate [illegible] then clear with xylol and mount [illegible] ada balsam or Dammar [illegible] The sheath takes on a blue [illegible] neuroglia light yellow, and the [illegible] cells brown.

Pal's Modification of Weigert's [illegible] —Pal uses the same hæmatoxylin [illegible] ing fluid, but afterwards transfers the sections (previously washed in a dilute lithium carbonate solution) for about a minute into a quarter per cent. solution of permanganate of potash made fresh as required each time, and then to the following:

Oxalic acid (pure) . . .	[illegible]
Sulphite of potash . . .	[illegible]
Distilled water . . .	[illegible]

for a few seconds until the grey matter loses all colour, the "white" matter remaining pretty deeply stained blue. Wash thoroughly, clear, and mount or give a contrast stain with eosin or picro-carmine.

The Pal-Exner Method.—This method is specially valuable for obtaining sections rapidly. The method of procedure is as follows:—Fresh brain or cord is hardened for two days in ten times its bulk of [illegible] per cent. osmic acid, fresh solution being added on the second day. It is then washed carefully in water, dipped for a short time into absolute alcohol and embedded in celloidin or paraffine. The sections are then put into glycerine, washed in water, stained and differentiated by Pal's method, and mounted in the usual manner.

A method devised by Marchi for the differentiation of degenerated nerve fibres in the cord and brain removed at once from experimental cases, is the following:—

Harden for one week in Müller's fluid or, better still, plunge into hot Müller's fluid (Mott); in the case of the brain use Hamilton's injection method. In the case of freshly killed experimental animals, Dr. Howard Tooth, at Dr. A. E. Wright's suggestion, passes a solution of atropine through the vessels in order to prevent the contraction which takes place when Müller's fluid is injected into the brain. Then cut into thin slices, [illegible] mm. each, and harden for another week or more in a fluid made up of 2 parts Müller's fluid and 1 of 1 per cent. osmic acid. Wash thoroughly in water. Then embed in celloidin in the ordinary fashion, after passing through alcohol and ether. Mount the sections without any further staining in Canada balsam. For the description of this method, which certainly gives admirable results, we are indebted to Prof. Schäfer. Schäfer has devised a capital modification of Pal's method for staining the myelin sheath. Harden for a month in Müller's fluid, cut sections, and then put into Marchi's Müller and osmic acid fluid for twenty-four hours. He stains in the following for a few hours (leave overnight):—

Hæmatoxylin (dissolved in a small quantity of absolute alcohol)	1 grain
Acetic acid	2 c.c.
Distilled water	100 c.c.

The sections become black. Bleach by Pal's method (p. 1186), allowing the sections to remain for as much as ten minutes in the permanganate solution, and then continue the bleaching in oxalic acid.

Ehrlich's triple stain is specially valuable for nerve specimens that are to be photographed.

(A) Hæmatoxylin, 2 grammes, dissolved in water . . . . 100 c.c.
Then add absolute alcohol . . 100 „
Glycerine . . . . . . 100 „
Glacial acetic acid . . . . 100 „
Potash alum to saturation.
(Allow this mixture to stand in the sunlight for three or four weeks.)

(B) Make a saturated solution of rubin s. (One of the basic fuchsin series.)

(C) Make a similar solution of methyl orange. (A good ground stain.)

Stain the sections in equal portions of the logwood (filtered and acidulated when used) and distilled water for from five to fifteen minutes, wash well in distilled water, and then leave in tap water until the desired shade of blue is obtained; or wash with a very dilute solution of ammonia, in which case, however, there is a risk of precipitation. Then stain in a watch glass containing equal proportions of (B) and (C) for from ten to thirty minutes, wash freely in tap water, dehydrate, and mount in Canada balsam. This method is exceedingly useful where good contrasts are required.

Aniline blue black is especially useful for staining sections of the nerve centres, bringing into special prominence the nerve cells which are stained a slaty blue colour (Bevan Lewis).

It is made as follows: Take of

Aniline blue black	1 part
Water	40 parts
Dissolve and add rectified spirit	100 „

Keep in a stoppered bottle, filter a few drops into a watch glass, and add eight or ten volumes of alcohol. Stain the section from a half to three minutes, and mount in Canada balsam. For ordinary tissues use a 1 per cent. watery solution, allow the sections to remain in this for a few minutes, and mount in balsam. If the staining is too deep Stirling recommends soaking the sections for a short time in a 2 per cent. solution of chloral hydrate.

Fresh Sections (Bevan Lewis).—To obtain sections of the fresh brain or cord, dry carefully in the folds of a clean soft cloth, and immerse for a short time in the gum and syrup solution (p. 1184). Freeze in gum on an ether microtome. Cut sections and remove them one by one into cold water, from which spread out on a glass slide at once. With a pipette pour on this a few drops of 2 per cent. osmic acid solution, leave it for one or two minutes, then wash thoroughly in water, and stain on the slide with a 1 per cent. watery solution of aniline blue black for one or two hours. Examine at once, or mount in acetate of potash or glycerine. Sections that are to be mounted in balsam should first be well washed in water and then, protected from the dust, should be allowed to dry thoroughly, after which they are covered with balsam and mounted. GERMAN SIMS WOODHEAD.

SPHAGIASMUS (σφαγή, the throat). One of Marshall Hall's terms for the phenomena characteristic of an epileptic fit (see ODAXESMUS), and specially for the spasm of the neck muscles.

SPHENENCEPHALUS, SPHENOCEPHALUS (σφήν, a wedge; κεφαλή, the head). Wedge-shaped head. (Fr. *sphénocéphale;* Ger. *Keilkopf.*)

SPHYGMOGRAPH, USE OF, IN THE VARIOUS FORMS OF INSANITY.—In the various conditions of insanity the influence of the nervous system upon the heart and circulation is such that in nearly every case the sphygmographic character of the pulse is altered in some way from the normal, and, for purposes of diagnosis as well as prognosis, the instrument is frequently of valuable service. The writer has found that the best form of sphygmograph for asylum work is that known as Dudgeon's, not only because of the ease with which it may be adjusted in excitable cases, but also because it can be used in any position of the patient, whether sitting, standing, or lying; the patient's arm need be bared only above the wrist, and the pressure of the spring on the artery can be increased or diminished at pleasure while the instrument is *in situ*. To obtain reliable records of the influence of different forms of mental alienation on the circulation, we must exclude cases in which cardiac or other physical diseases are known to exist.

In **maniacal conditions**, perhaps from exhausted nerve centres and overstrain of the cardiac muscle, the arterial tension is lowered and the sphygmographic tracing reveals some dicrotism. In the acute forms of mania the line of ascent of the tracing is nearly always perpendicular, the apex sharp, and the descent line short, with a fairly prominent dicrotic wave. The cardiac systole is sudden and sharp, and the *vis a tergo* feeble; the sudden ventricular contraction produces a high ascent line, and, as the systemic arteries are rapidly emptied, the summit of the tracing forms an acute angle, while, as has been noted, the descent line is interrupted by a dicrotism (Fig. 1). In the chronic forms of mania the tracing is not so characteristic, the high upstroke of the acute cases disappears, the line of descent is more prolonged, and is interrupted by several secondary wavelets.

In **melancholia** the pulse, unless in acutely melancholic patients, where it is more rapid than normal, is slow and easily compressed, and the sphygmographic tracing in the larger number indicates a weak and feeble cardiac systole and an imperfect filling of the vessels. The upstroke is short and slanting, and the descent line prolonged considerably, the secondary wavelets being either indistinct and unrecognisable, or not marked at all. The pressure in such cases has to be very low, or the character of the pulse-tracing will be lost (Fig. 2). In stuporous melancholia there is usually arterial tension, the apex of the tracing being prolonged to form a "plateau." Chronic cases generally show a normal tracing, arterial tension may exist, but is never so marked as in some forms of insanity. Senile melancholia is nearly always associated with high tension; its removal by diminishing the peripheral resistance and by strengthening the heart is usually followed by recovery. When senile melancholia is associated with low tension the mental disease is rarely recovered from.*

In **epileptic insanity**, in chronic cases, or in those passing through a rapid succession of fits, such as in the *status epilepticus*, the ascent line of the tracing is seldom high or vertical, the percussion wave is generally rounded, and the line of descent either prolonged with secondary wavelets imperfectly marked, or else short and presenting a dicrotic [illegible] times reaches the [illegible] wave (Figs. 3 and 4). [illegible] of an epileptic at other [illegible] ing to his mental and physical [illegible] but as a rule it presents [illegible] cative of feeble cardiac [illegible] condition of the arterial walls. [illegible] status epilepticus, and during [illegible] scious stage of an epileptic [illegible] nary characters of the pulse-[illegible] lost, and it becomes mono- or [illegible] (Fig. 4).

In **general paralysis** [illegible] certain variations are found in the [illegible] ters of the pulse; these changes [illegible] described as those of high tension, [illegible] to that found in chronic Bright's [illegible] *In the first stage of general* [illegible] cardiac systole is generally [illegible] sudden, there is low arterial [illegible] the descent line of the sphyg[illegible] marked by several undulations [illegible] the result of muscular tremors [illegible] paired nerve impulses. To [illegible] tracing more closely, we note [illegible] upstroke is usually somewhat [illegible] primary wave does not form [illegible] angle, the descent line is of [illegible] fall is gradual, and it presents [illegible] of wavelets ranging from 4 to [illegible] dicrotic wave is not recognisable, [illegible] aortic notch is either imperfect [illegible] exist (Fig. 5). *In the second* [illegible] percussion impulse is moderately [illegible] and evidence of arterial [illegible] marked, the apex in the [illegible] being rounded or ending in a [illegible] line. The tracing shows the [illegible] to be more perpendicular, [illegible] any great height; the wave of [illegible] instead of being rounded, [illegible] horizontally, forming in [illegible] "plateau" of Voisin. In [illegible] tidal wave ascends higher [illegible] mary wave, the aortic notch [illegible] well marked, the dicrotic wave [illegible] and the descent line short [illegible] plateau-like summit is [illegible] the pulse at this stage, and [illegible] high pulse tension, sustaining [illegible] the instrument for some time, [illegible] lation through the systemic [illegible] interfered with, as in Bright's [illegible] where, however, the systole of a hypertrophied left ventricle produces a [illegible] perpendicular percussion line. *In the final stage* of the disease the cardiac [illegible] exhausted, the ventricular systole [illegible] and, the weakened arterial walls [illegible] deficient in tone, the pulse-tracing [illegible] characters not unlike those found [illegible] the first stage. The line of ascent [illegible] and slanting, the percussion apex [illegible]

* Broadbent, "Croonian Lectures," 1887.

pointed, and the descent line short and almost uninterrupted by wavelets (Fig. 7). In general paralysis occurring in females the disease is much more prolonged in its course, and the symptoms are rarely so intense as in males; a low percussion wave and a prolonged "plateau" summit can be obtained in the tracing (Fig. 6).

In **dementia** the heart's action is feeble, and the sphygmograph indicates an imperfect filling of the vessels, probably due to slow evolution of nerve impulses along the vaso-motor nerves from an impoverished nerve centre. The tracing shows a slanted and short line of ascent, apex pointed, descent line prolonged, and in a few cases interrupted by several small undulations (Fig. 8). In senile dementia the upstroke is slanted and not high, the apex prolonged and rounded somewhat, and the descent line interrupted by several small notches, indicating a feeble cardiac condition and tense arterial walls, the result of muscular hypertrophy or atheromatous deposit along the course of the vessels.

Imbecility.—Cases of mental defect, where it is inferred there is an arrest in the development of the encephalon, as well as cases where it is evident a certain amount of cerebral wasting or atrophy exists, present tense arteries, and after a time a strong cardiac systole from hypertrophy of the left ventricle. The condition of the pulse in these cases is identical to that found in fibroid degeneration of the kidney and in aortic stenosis (Figs. 9 and 10). We would suggest that a possible explanation of the high arterial tension existing in cerebral atrophy or congenital deficiency is to be found in a similarity of the morbid anatomy of these conditions and that of cirrhosis of the kidneys. There is a certain amount of tissue destruction in both cases, replaced in the one by serous fluid or the products of inflammation, and in the other by fibroid changes; in both cases pressure is exercised on the arteries within the parts affected; this obstructs the systemic circulation, and to overcome the obstruction first cardiac hypertrophy and finally thickening of the arterial muscular coat results, thus producing the increased arterial tension so common to these closely allied pathological conditions.

In **circular insanity**, in the dull and depressed stage, there is shortening of the ascent line, the apex is more or less rounded, and the line of descent prolonged and wavy, indicating a short and feeble ventricular systole and slight arterial tension; in the excited stage the percussion impulse is high and perpendicular, and the descent line short and interrupted by prominent tidal and dicrotic waves, arterial tension being lowered, and the characters of the tracing bear a likeness to those of acute mania.

T. DUNCAN GREENLEES.

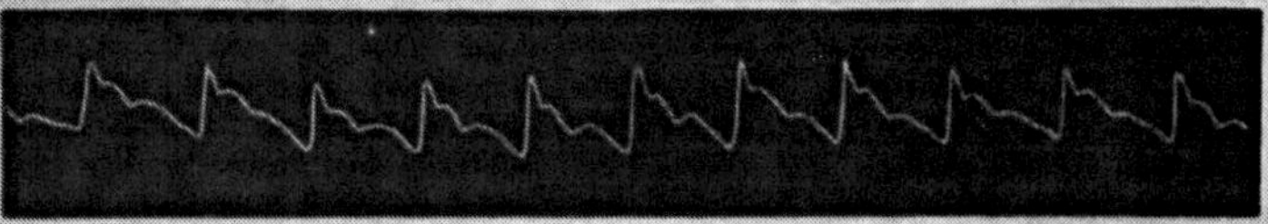

FIG. 1.—Acute mania; pulse 100; pressure used 90 grms.

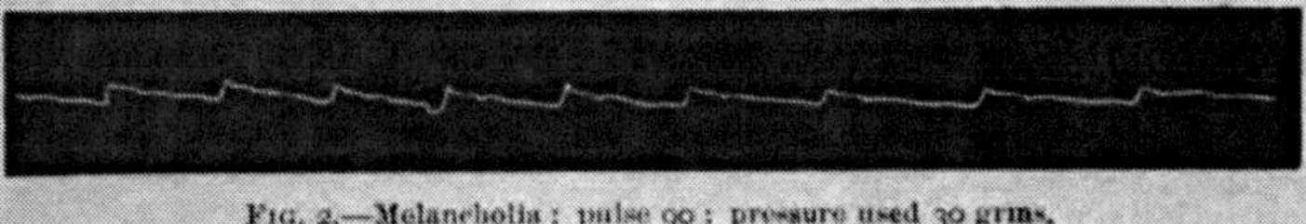

FIG. 2.—Melancholia; pulse 90; pressure used 30 grms.

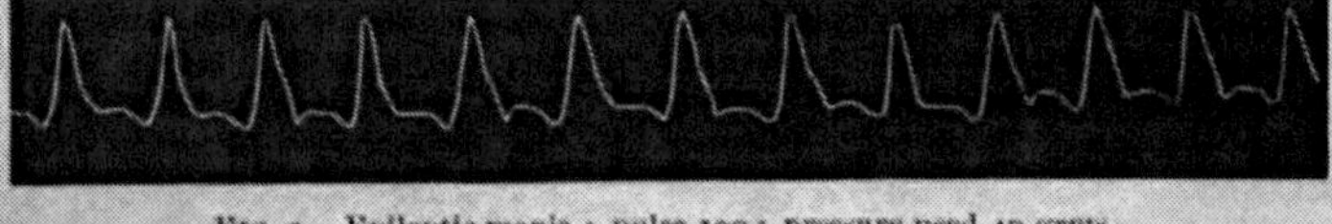

FIG. 3.—Epileptic mania; pulse 100; pressure used 40 grms.

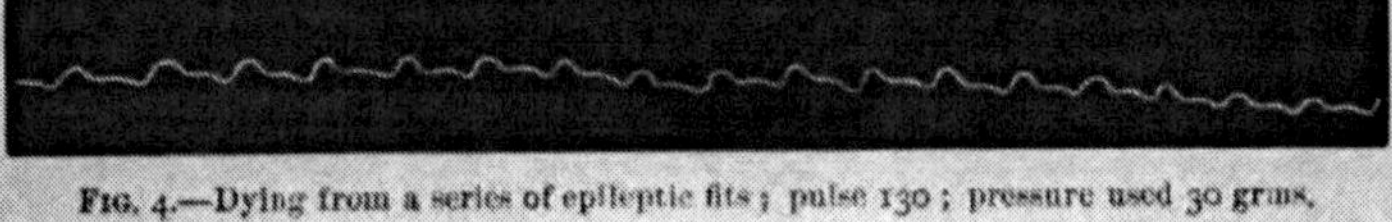

FIG. 4.—Dying from a series of epileptic fits; pulse 130; pressure used 30 grms.

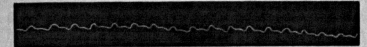

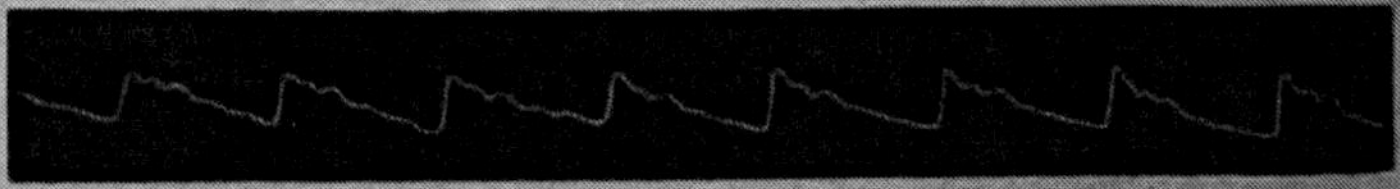

FIG. 5.—General paralysis (1st stage); pulse 80; pressure used 80 grms.

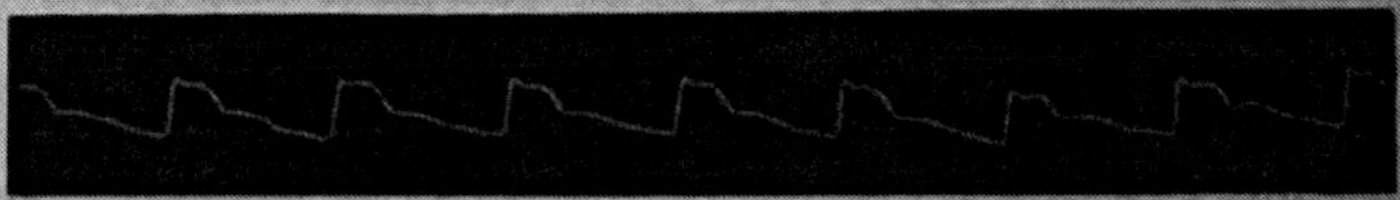

FIG. 6.—General paralysis (2nd stage); pulse 74; pressure used 120 grms.

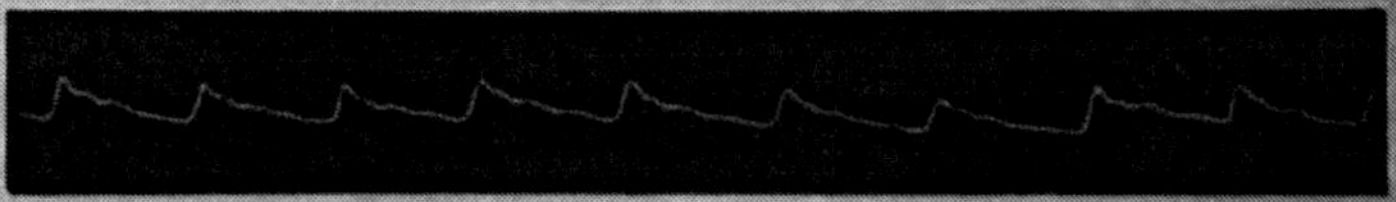

FIG. 7.—General paralysis (last stage); pulse 90; pressure used 40 grms.

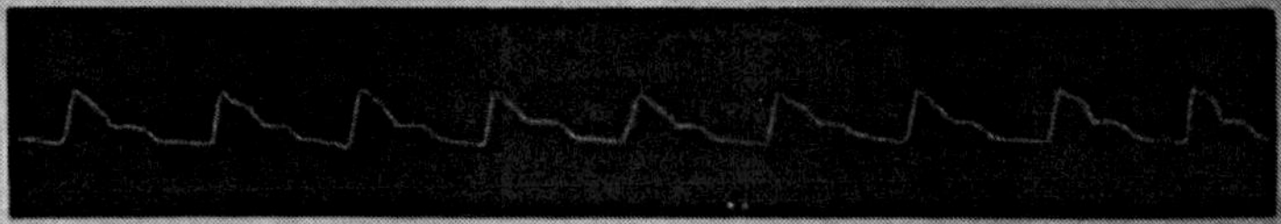

FIG. 8.—Dementia; pulse 86; pressure used 60 grms.

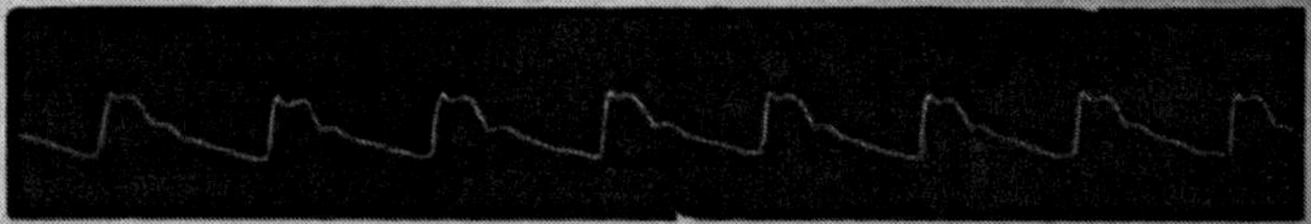

FIG. 9.—Congenital imbecility; pulse 64; pressure used 60 grms.

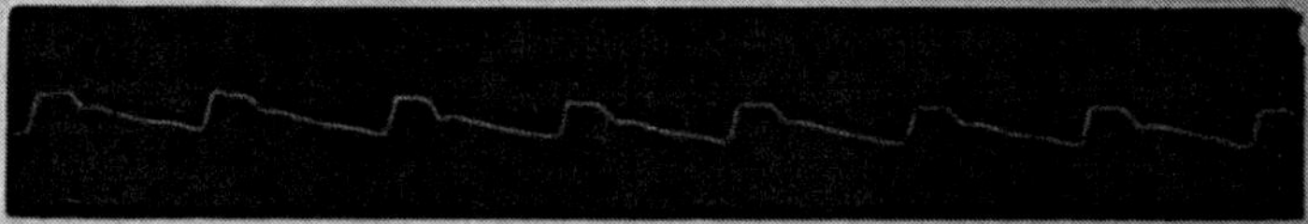

FIG. 10.—Congenital imbecility; pulse 80; pressure used 80 grms.

SPIDER-CELLS. (*See* PATHOLOGY.)

SPINAL CORD, CHANGES OF, IN THE INSANE.—As yet no special changes have been demonstrated as the result of insanity in which no paralytic symptoms have been present. Hence the changes which are most frequently met with depend on general paralysis of the insane or are secondary to some apoplectic attack.

In general paralysis the changes are usually diffused, in some instances chiefly affecting the posterior columns, whereas in others the lateral are more implicated. In these latter the anterior median may also suffer; in some the affection may involve the posterior column on one side, and the lateral, chiefly, on the other. Doubtless some of these changes are secondary to cortical degeneration, but at present it is not easy to trace which depend on primary and which on secondary processes. In some cases of general paralysis the cord is very much and very generally wasted, but in a few cases we have met with enormous increase in size of the cord depending on general interstitial changes. In some cases marked syphilitic changes have been met with in the coats of the arteries.

In secondary dementia depending on old apoplectic attacks, whether due to hæmorrhage or to local softening, changes in the lateral column of the cord may be present. In a few cases of insanity we have met with syringo-myelia, but we have failed to trace any definite relationship between this and the insanity.

In many conditions bony plates have been met with in the dura mater of the cord, but these occur in very different states, such as general paralysis, chronic epilepsy, and chronic recurrent insanity.

Pachymeningitis of the cord may be met with in general paralysis and also in some other conditions of progressive nerve degeneration. Disseminated sclerosis may occur in the insane, but in our opinion it is excessively rare; most of the cases described as such have, in our experience, proved to be cases of general paralysis with spastic symptoms and with changes in the lateral columns of the cord or else cases of developmental general paralysis (Clouston). In some undoubted cases seen in general hospitals, and diagnosed to be suffering from disseminated sclerosis, there have been more or less mental excitement tending to weakness of mind and some paralysis, so that changes may occur in the brain associated with this disease as well as changes in the spinal cord. Besides the changes in the posterior columns and posterior roots which may be present in general paralysis, similar changes may occur in ordinary cases of locomotor ataxy which have become insane. (*See* Locomotor Ataxy.)

In chronic alcoholism there may be present marked general changes in the cord associated, as Bevan Lewis has pointed out, with changes in the general nutrition, a form of general fibrosis which he compares to the changes in Bright's disease.

The accompanying diagrams* show clearly the areas of the cord which are

Fig. 1.

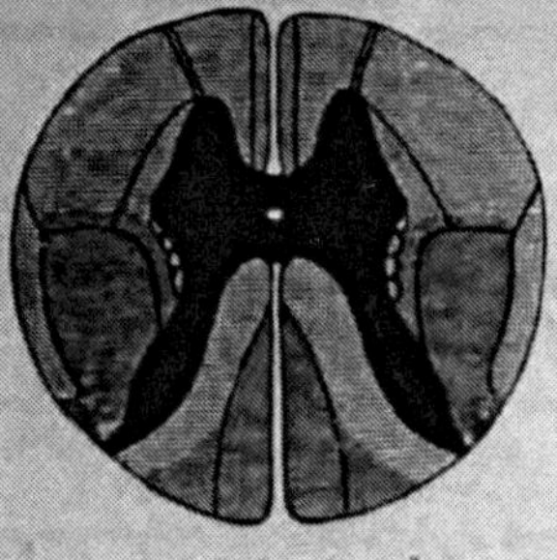

Spinal cord, cervical region; degeneration of lateral and posterior columns.

Fig. 2.

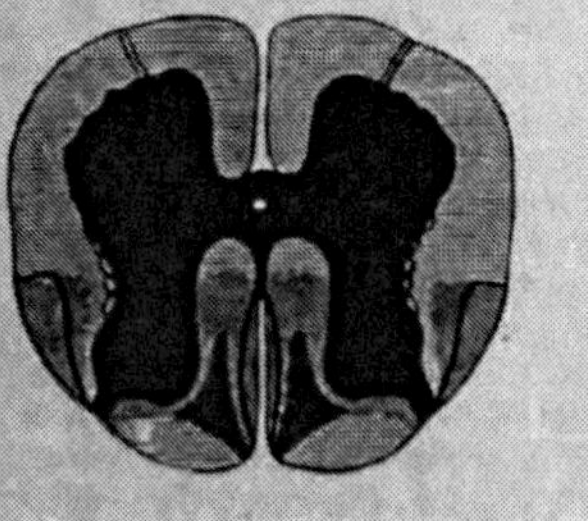

Spinal cord, lumbar region; degeneration of lateral and posterior columns.

* Both diagrams appear in Dr. R. S. Stewart's article in *Journal of Mental Science*, April 1887, "Ataxo-Spasmodic Tabes."

more commonly affected in degeneration of the spinal cord occurring in general paralysis with ataxic symptoms in which the changes are not confined to the posterior columns. (*See* General Paralysis, Pachymeningitis, and Pellagra.)

Geo. H. Savage.

SPORADIC CRETINISM. (*See* Cretinism.)

SPRACHLOSIGKEIT (Ger.). Aphasia; alalia.

STAMMERING.—**Definition.**—The term "stammering" is commonly used as a synonym of "stuttering," and as implying a peculiar and well-known impediment to speech (dependent on a spasmodic affection of one or more of the mechanisms concerned in that function) which checks the speaker in his utterance, and either brings him to a full stop or causes him to prolong or drawl, or to repeat in rapid succession, the letter or syllable at which the check occurs. In a wider sense it may be taken to include various defects of speech, such as the inability, congenital or acquired, to pronounce certain letters or certain combinations of letters, the tendency to hesitate or stumble in utterance, or to transpose letters or syllables, and the habit of interjecting meaningless sounds or words into the pauses which occur in the course of continuous speech.

Causation.—Stammering, in the strict sense of the term, generally first shows itself between the ages of four or five and the time of puberty; but it occasionally arises in adult life, and may then be due to an attack of fever or other acute disease, to hysteria or some other nervous disorder, to nervousness or excitement, or even to temporary soreness of the tongue or lips or other parts engaged in articulation. In most of the latter cases the defect is temporary only. But it is important to bear in mind that confirmed stammerers are apt to have their infirmity aggravated under the influence of similar conditions. Stammering beginning in childhood often undergoes spontaneous improvement as age advances; it is sometimes, but by no means always, of hereditary origin; and it is a curious fact that women rarely suffer from it. The other faults of speech to which reference has been made are due mainly to imperfect training, to bad habits or slovenliness, or to some defect in the relations between the ear and the organs of articulation.

Description.—Articulate speech is a highly complex function. For, apart even from its intellectual relations, and regarding it only as a mechanical act, it involves the perfect command over, and the due co-ordination of, three distinct though correlated mechanisms, namely, those respectively of respiration, of phonation, and of articulation. Of the parts played severally by these three mechanisms, that of respiration is the simplest, inasmuch as it consists solely in keeping the lungs sufficiently charged with air, and so regulating the force of the expiratory blast as to cause the vocal cords to vibrate with due intensity, and to render duly audible the resonances of the mouth and nose on which articulation depends. The function of the larynx is more delicate and complicated; inasmuch as it includes in rapid sequence, according to the requirements of the different literal sounds effected in the mouth, the opening of the rima glottidis so as to allow unvocalised air to pass, and the closing of the glottis for the purpose of producing voice, and the most delicate regulation of the tension of the cords in order to the production of different musical notes. The part played by the true organs of articulation is by far the most complex and varied; for, although articulate sounds are limited in number, their evolution depends on the nicest adjustments of the tongue, lips, palate, fauces, and jaws, and in the utterance of words these are combined in sequences of extraordinary rapidity and variety. It is, as is well known, chiefly in muscular co-ordinations of great complexity and of late acquirement that hitches are liable to occur and to become permanent; among familiar examples of which fact may be enumerated writer's cramp, and the similar affections which are liable to attack the pianoforte-player and the fencer. Stammering would seem to belong to the same category.

The hitch in speech which characterises stammering may occur in connection with any of the mechanisms involved in speaking. It may consist in a sudden momentary arrest of the expiratory act, or in a similar closure of the rima glottidis. But much more frequently the hitch occurs in the organs of articulation themselves, the special features of which depend on the particular letter at which the impediment arises. As a general rule stammering takes place in connection with the explosive consonants; but it is by no means limited to them, for it may occur not only in the utterance of the continuous consonants, but even in that of vowels. In its slightest degree stammering consists in a simple momentary arrest of speech which may be scarcely appreciable by the listener, or in the occasional repetition or reduplication of a letter or syllable. In more marked cases the lips, or the tongue, as the case may be, becomes arrested in [illegible] sary for the evolution [illegible] stammerer is about to [illegible] mains thus for some [illegible] patient is vainly endeavouring [illegible] his speech; or, in place of the [illegible] which under such circumstances [illegible] usually be present, he may [illegible] ing the sound in stuttering [illegible] its worst form the spasm [illegible] main limited to the organs of [illegible] in the patient's violent and [illegible] attempts to speak the spasm [illegible] extend to the muscles of expression [illegible] those of the front of the neck, [illegible] maybe to the extremities. [illegible] portant to observe that even [illegible] and bad stammerers do not always [illegible] mer in equal degree, and may [illegible] not stammer at all. Stammering [illegible] aggravated by anything which [illegible] nervousness or hurry in speech, [illegible] states of health. It is a curious [illegible] stammerers rarely show their impediment when singing or intoning.

Among defects of articulation, which may perhaps be included in the [illegible] stammering, are those which [illegible] certain nervous diseases, such as [illegible] paralysis of the insane and disseminated sclerosis, and the defective enunciation of certain letters for the most part [illegible] from infancy.

The speech of general paralysis is highly characteristic. In its early stages it is marked by a little tremor of the lips which shows itself mainly as the patient is about to articulate, and at the beginning therefore of words and syllables. At this period there may be no appreciable defect of speech, there may be even unwonted deliberation and distinctness of utterance. But by degrees the tremors increase, and then speech obviously suffers. The tremors tend to spread from the lips to the muscles of expression, so that in advanced cases articulation is attended with the development of muscular ripples over the whole face. And the speech becomes more and more hesitating, and more and more marked by a tendency to the repetition of syllables and words, and even to stammering in the strictest sense of the term. Ultimately it becomes unintelligible.

In disseminated sclerosis there is not as a rule any tremor of the lips, but the patient speaks with the so-called scanning or divided utterance. This peculiarity depends largely on the fact that he experiences more or less impairment of power in, or command over, the organs of articulation, and that he speaks with great effort and with more attempt at precision and accuracy than was his wont. As, however, the disease progresses the difficulty of speech increases and he becomes more and more unintelligible; and then, as also in the case of general paralysis, more or less tremor of the lips may come on, there may be more or less obvious stammering, and combinations of letters or even individual letters may become unpronounceable.

In cases of bulbar paralysis speech necessarily becomes defective. Literal sounds gradually fail to be properly enunciated, and the speech may present more or less resemblance to that of general paralysis or disseminated sclerosis. It is an interesting but easily explained fact that, in all these paralytic affections of speech, patients who cannot pronounce combination of letters—that is, words—intelligibly, may often nevertheless be capable of pronouncing individual letters with perfect clearness.

Of defects of speech due to bad habits, imperfect education, and the like it is needless to say much. Among them may be enumerated the habit of interpolating such expressions as "you know," "don't you know," "I mean," and meaningless drawling sounds between one's words; the tendency presented by some persons, and not unusual in aphasic conditions, to transpose letters or syllables; and the inability to pronounce or difficulty in pronouncing certain letters, such especially as *h*, *r*, *s*. Some children are very slow to learn to speak, and, even though they ultimately acquire facility, are long in mastering the pronunciation of certain letters and remain almost unintelligible for years. It is curious that such defaulters are very often bright and intelligent, and present (so far as one can discern) no evidence of defect (structural or functional) beyond this inability to pronounce. Moreover, contrary to the opinions of some, such defects are unconnected with either defective hearing or the want or possession of the musical faculty. In some remarkable cases children even up to the age of ten or twelve habitually make use of only some half-dozen letters.

Treatment.—In treating defects of speech it is important that any local affection, such as soreness of lips or tongue, bad teeth, and the like, should be remedied; for even if it does not cause the defects it helps to accentuate and perpetuate them. For the same reason it is important to attend to the general health. And it need scarcely be added that when defects are traceable to hysteria, to syphilitic affections of the nervous system, or to any other remediable condition, these affections should be expressly treated. For the rest, it is a question of education. Stammering may be largely benefited, and sometimes cured, by careful education. But it is education in which the patient must himself recognise the importance of persistent and systematic work. The stammerer should be taught to speak slowly and deliberately and without excitement, and, when engaged in conversation, never to persist in fruitless or painful efforts to force the word on which he is stammering, but rather at once to stop and then begin the offending word afresh. He should also be made to read or recite aloud for some considerable time daily, uttering his words and their component parts slowly and deliberately and with great distinctness, using, in fact, in their pronunciation more obvious muscular effort than he would be inclined to do in ordinary conversation. He should also be made to practise especially the utterance of those letters or those combinations of letters which he finds it most difficult to evolve, and so to regulate his inspirations as never to permit himself to speak with an insufficient supply of pulmonary air.

With respect to the other defects of speech above referred to, the only mode of dealing with them successfully is also by education; and for this reason it is eminently desirable that children should be taught early to read and speak and recite. In dealing with this subject it must be recollected that, assuming the nervous and muscular mechanism to be sound, the act of speech is purely mechanical; that if the organs of speech be put into certain definite positions, and at the same time respiration and phonation be duly performed, the letters due to such positions cannot fail to be pronounced; and consequently that with very few exceptions every faulty speaker, if he can only be taught to put his organs of articulation into certain positions, cannot avoid pronouncing correctly the letters which he habitually fails to pronounce. But in order to treat such patients successfully it is of course necessary for the teacher and pupil alike to study the details of letter-enunciation. It need scarcely be said, however, that when once bad habits have become ingrained it is exceedingly difficult completely to eradicate them. Even the person who teaches himself in later life to pronounce the letter *h*, which he had heretofore neglected, rarely acquires the power of uttering it without manifest and painful effort.

JOHN S. BRISTOWE.

STATICS OF MIND.—The nature of the products of mind as opposed to the dynamics of mind, that is, the processes on which the products depend.

STATISTICS OF INSANITY.—Accuracy and a correct basis and method of calculation are the only secure foundations of statistics. Accuracy, however great, is useless, if the basis or method be fallacious. On the other hand, however perfect the method, the results are worthless if absolute accuracy be not secured. In no department has there been greater and more misleading error disseminated from neglecting the most elementary principles of statistical science than in psychological medicine.

We commence with:—

(1) **The Method of Calculating the Relative Liability of Different Communities to Insanity.**—For many years statements were made and accepted as to the relative amount of mental disorder in different nations and at different periods of history without the slightest consideration of various sources of fallacy. It was assumed that the numbers of the insane reported in different countries and at different periods were obtained with equal care and facility. This may be laid down as the first source of error. The second fallacy is overlooking the difference in the amount of provision made in asylums for the disordered in mind. The effect of such provision is manifestly to lead to the concentration, registration, and apparent increase of insanity. The third source of fallacy is the oversight of the inevitable accumulation of cases which occurs, due to the excess of admissions over discharges. Fourthly, and arising out of the humane provision for this class, is the decrease in mortality. Lastly, a great mistake made until comparatively recent times is the failure to distinguish between the amount of *existing* and *occurring* insanity. Let us illustrate this by supposing that, in a population of 200,000, 100 become insane every year in England and Wales, and that the mortality of these insane persons is at the rate of 6 per cent. residents. Suppose, again, that the ratio of occurring insanity in Scotland is precisely the same, but that the mortality is 12 per cent. It must be obvious that there will be a much larger number reported at the end of the year in the former than in the latter country. The English would appear to the superficial observer to have a much greater liability to mental disorder than the Scotch. The fact, however, would be that there was an accumulation of cases in consequence of the greater care and better treatment bestowed upon the patients by the English. Yet the fallacy here referred to is one which [illegible] and leads to serious mistakes [illegible] *ing* number of lunatics [illegible] different countries, and in different [illegible] or periods in the same, is [illegible] the test of the liability [illegible] different races, or of the [illegible] different periods.

(2) **Numbers of the Insane in Different Countries, and at Different [illegible] in the Same Countries.**—If we [illegible] take the returns of the number of [illegible] and lunatics in different countries [illegible] should find the ratio to the population vary enormously, and the same [illegible] would be obtained if the reported [illegible] of these classes at one period of [illegible] tory of any one nation were [illegible] with the number alleged to exist [illegible] other period. The main cause of [illegible] widely different statements is [illegible] *imperfect returns* in former as compared with recent periods in the one [illegible] the difference between the perfection of the methods of obtaining statistics [illegible] in more or less civilised countries [illegible] other. Thus, to compare the lunacy statistics of Turkey with those of [illegible] and Wales would be altogether misleading. And again, to compare the statistics of lunacy in England and Wales in [illegible] and 1890 would be equally fallacious. [illegible] 60 years ago it was estimated that in [illegible] there was 1 insane person to every [illegible] of the population. At the present day the estimate is 1 in 1350; but it would be absurd to conclude that any such increase of insanity has really taken place.

Another source of fallacy is the *different mortality-rate* at different periods in establishments for the insane. For example, in England and Wales the mortality, calculated upon the number resident in asylums, was 10.26 per cent. during the 6 years ending 1879, whereas it was only [illegible] per cent. during the 6 years ending [illegible]. If the death-rate had not thus fallen, there would have been above 3000 more deaths in the latter decade than really occurred. From the year 1776 to [illegible] the mortality was 12.12 per cent. of the number resident in asylums in England and Wales. Hence it is obvious that returns of the number of patients without taking into account the death-rate are no proof of a real increase of occurring lunacy. Accumulation necessarily follows upon decreased mortality. Most of the statements made in regard to the increase of insanity fail to take into account this source of fallacy. Nor is account taken of the varying proportion of recoveries and consequent discharge of patients at different periods. The effect of this, however, in leading to mistaken conclusions, is within a comparatively small compass.

In the following observations we take the available statistics of insanity in England and Wales, as found in the Blue-Books.

It is greatly to be regretted that the limit of the past is drawn at the year 1859. Indeed, it is impossible to obtain official returns of admissions exclusive of transfers before 1869. Further, when we restrict our inquiry to absolutely satisfactory returns we are unable to go further back than 1878.

In 1859 (on January 1) there were in England and Wales 36,762 insane and idiotic persons reported by the Commissioners in Lunacy (including those in workhouses).

In 1885 (January 1) there were 79,704. In other words, for every 100 insane in 1859 there were 218 under care in 1885. Making allowance for the increase of the population, there was a rise from 18.674 per 10,000 to 28.984, or 55 per cent.—*i.e.*, a rise from 100 to 155. Taking the quinquennium 1861–65, and also that of 1881–85, there is a rise from 20.8 to 28.6 per 10,000, or an increase of 38 per cent.

If from the foregoing returns the uncertified insane are deducted (*i.e.*, omitting workhouses, and pauper lunatics receiving out-door relief), there were on January 1, 1859, 23,001 patients, and on January 1, 1885, 56,525, that is to say, an increase of 146 per cent. Allowing for increase of population there was a rise of 76 per cent. If quinquennial periods are taken —namely 1861–65 and 1881–85—we find the rise in the certified insane to be 50 per cent.

Such are the figures representing the comparative amount of *existing* lunacy at different periods in England and Wales. We proceed to give the much more important returns of *occurring* lunacy. Here we are restricted to asylums, because no returns can be procured of the number of *admissions* into workhouses, nor the number of out-door patients *becoming* insane. Now, in 1859 there were 9310 admissions into asylums; in 1885 there were as many as 14,774; allowing for increase of population these returns show a ratio per 10,000 of 4.7 in 1859 and 5.3 in 1885, or an increase of 13 per cent. Up to 1878 it is tolerably steady; subsequently the ratio of increase was almost stationary, while during the 5 years 1881–85 it was lower than any of the five years preceding. During this quinquennium the admissions per 10,000 of the population were 5.20, while during the five years 1886–90 *they were almost exactly the same*—viz., 5.25.*

The next point is to deduct the transfers, which, of course, mean nothing in an inquiry into the actual numbers of the insane. As already stated, the Lunacy Commissioners did not report transfers prior to 1869. In that year the admissions of patients into asylums *minus* transfers amounted to 10,617, while in 1885 the corresponding number was 13,557, or an increase of 28 per cent. To show the effect of the elimination of transfers, it should be stated that, when these are included, the rise amounts to 32 per cent. during the same period. If we take series of years, the proportion per 10,000 of the population during 1871–75 was 4.9, while during the quinquennium 1881–85 it rose to 5.2. In deducting transfers, we are free from the disturbing element of a variable quantity, one which may affect the accuracy of the result in either magnifying or minimising the increase.

The next source of fallacy when we are taking the reported admissions into asylums, as representing the number who become insane, is the inclusion of the re-admissions. These are not unimportant, because, although they stand for cases and not different persons, they may tell a tale of the action of the existing causes of insanity at a certain period.

We must, however, eliminate re-admissions for the purpose of ascertaining the number of *persons* who become insane. Obviously, relapses do not convey a correct impression of this proportion of individuals becoming insane at a given period. Now, the ratio of first admissions to 10,000 of the population in 1869 was 4.13, while in 1885 it was 4.21, being a difference of 1.94 per cent. The rise of first admissions between 1880–85 over those between 1870–75 was not as much as 1 patient in 10,000.

We are now prepared to advance a step further. A moment's consideration will show that the only proper test of the increase of mental disease *is the proportion of first attacks to the population* during different periods. First admissions are clearly not identical with first attacks, seeing that a patient may be admitted into an asylum for the first time, and yet have had one or more previous attacks of insanity. In 1876, the year in which these

* The numbers of the insane, &c., in Great Britain and Ireland will be found under these articles. We are not in possession of statistics for 1892, but we may state that for England and Wales there was, on January 1, 1 lunatic or idiot to 335 of the population. The census of 1891, which includes a separate return of the insane, is not yet available for our purpose.

returns were first made, there is some element of doubtful accuracy, and in 1877 no return was made, so that we commence with the following year, 1878, since which the returns have been regularly made. In the last-mentioned year the number of first attacks in England and Wales was 8354, while in 1885 it was 8527. Allowing for increase of population, the number of first attacks per 10,000 living was 3.33 in 1878; in 1879 it was slightly higher, 3.34; in 1880 it was markedly lower, 3.22; in 1881 it rose slightly, viz., to 3.25; in 1882 it was nearly identical; in 1883 there was a fractional rise, viz., to 3.43; in 1884 the number fell exactly to that of 1878; lastly, during 1885 it fell lower, viz., 3.10. Taking the five years 1881–85, the average annual number of first attacks was 3.29; while for 1886–90 the average annual number was 3.46. These figures, so far as they go, are extremely important and interesting, as showing that statistics when carefully handled do not bear out the general opinion that there has been an alarming increase in the number of fresh cases of insanity in proportion to the population, that is to say, so far as first attacks have come under the cognizance of the Lunacy Commissioners.

We are well aware that outside the area of certified lunacy there is a considerable mass of borderland cases, the inclusion of which might seriously affect our deductions. If we allowed ourselves to be influenced by impressions derived from general observations we should be disposed to infer an increase in this class; and if instances of insomnia and neurasthenia were added, we should find it difficult to avoid the conclusion that there has been an increase in affections of the nervous system. While, therefore, not denying the alleged increase of nervous disorders, we consider that the only safe course to pursue is to adhere to statistical returns when grounded on right methods of calculation. So calculating, we maintain that statistics do not support the opinion that a distinctly larger number of persons in proportion to the population become insane than was formerly the case.

(3) **Percentage of Pauper Lunatics to Total Paupers in England and Wales, and of Pauper Lunatics to Population.**—Taking the earliest year in which we are able to procure returns, we find that in 1859 the total number of paupers of all classes on the 1st of January of that year was 1,722,548. The total number of pauper lunatics and idiots at the same date was 31,782, showing a percentage of pauper lunatics to paupers of 1.85. This ratio has gradually [illegible] cent., but, as the ratio of [illegible] the population has [illegible] 2.82 between 1859 and [illegible] consider that this proportion [illegible] number of the accumulated [illegible] proof of an increase of [illegible] in proportion to the population.

Ratio of Pauper Lunatics to Population.—This ratio in 1859 [illegible] while in 1889 it was 1 in 3[illegible]

That there should be a [illegible] last 30 years in the proportion [illegible] lunatics to the population [illegible] being necessarily an increase in [illegible] lunacy must be admitted [illegible] member two circumstances; first, [illegible] insane poor are more carefully [illegible] at the present time, and, secondly, [illegible] ever misleading factor of [illegible] invalidates the inference that [illegible] been an actual increase of insanity [illegible]

(4) **Mode of Calculating the [illegible] tion of Recoveries.**—Some difference of opinion has been held and [illegible] tice been unfortunately pursued [illegible] lating recoveries. They have been [illegible] lated upon the mean number [illegible] institutions, upon the discharges, [illegible] the curable cases, and, lastly, upon the admissions.

(*a*) Were the average duration of [illegible] dence in different institutions [illegible], the recovery-rate might be calculated [illegible] the average number resident [illegible] troducing a source of fallacy in [illegible] the results obtained in various [illegible]. Dr. Conolly adopted this method, [illegible] seems to have overlooked the fact [illegible] the period of time which such a [illegible] embodies is an element in the problem which has to be taken into account.

(*b*) The late Dr. W. Farr, the [illegible] statistician, calculated recoveries on the discharges. Dr. Thurnam has shown [illegible] if the correct mode of calculation is [illegible] which is made on the admissions, it is of great importance to avoid the method of calculating the recoveries on the discharges, seeing that the results are widely different. Thus, at the York Retreat, the recoveries in the course of forty-six years amounted to 46.9 per cent. of the admissions, while, if calculated on the discharges they were 54.6. At the Wakefield Asylum during twenty-three years the recoveries were 44.2 per cent. reckoned on the admissions, and were as high as 50.6 reckoned on the discharges.

(*c*) It is urged by Dr. Mortimer Granville that the true method is to calculate the recoveries upon cases deemed curable. He confesses, however, that "it is curious to notice how closely the percentage gained by this method of computation I suggest, approximates to that obtained by taking the proportion upon the total of 'cases admitted.' This seems to show the wisdom of the method commonly adopted." He also allows that the calculation upon the average number resident offers no advantage over that upon cases admitted.*

(d) On the whole, we consider that the method of calculating recoveries, which is based on the admissions, is a fair one. It is no doubt true that the recoveries in a given year in an asylum, calculated upon the admissions during the same period, include the recoveries of persons who may have been admitted during previous years, and might happen to exceed the admissions of that year; but, on the other hand, it omits recoveries, which will probably occur among the admissions of that year at a subsequent period. There is, therefore, probably very little difference between the calculation and the final results when a series of years is taken. This source of fallacy disappears to a large extent, and would of course be entirely avoided if the admissions terminated, and the record of recoveries was continued for some time afterwards. It has been shown by Dr. Thurnam that the proportion of recoveries is at the minimum (when calculated on the admissions) during the early period of an asylum history, and increases for a considerable time after the opening of an institution. Thus, at the Retreat, York, during the first quinquennium, it was 26.1 per cent.; during the first decennium it was 33.9; during the first fifteen years, 42.5; during the first twenty years it amounted to 46.0; during the first twenty-five years it was 46.8; during the first thirty years it was 46.2; during thirty-five years, 46.0; during forty, 46.5; and during the first forty-five, 47.8 per cent.

At the Hanwell Asylum the recoveries during the first five and one-third years was as low as 19.3 per cent.; during the next ten and one-third years it was 22.2; during the succeeding twelve and one-third years it rose to 23.3.

The rate of recovery, calculated on admissions (minus transfers), in the asylums, registered hospitals, private asylums, and in single houses in England and Wales was, during the ten years 1879 to 1888, 39.91 per cent. In metropolitan and private asylums it was respectively 35.11 and 36.44 per cent. Taking registered hospitals alone it was nearly 50 per cent. (47.34); in county and borough asylums, 40.16.

* "The Care and Cure of the Insane," vol. i. p. 73.

Sir A. Mitchell's statistics* of 1297 patients during the term of twelve years showed a recovery-rate of 65.6 per cent. If re-admissions (499 out of 851 recoveries) are taken into account, the recovery-rate is reduced to 47.3. It must be remembered that there is very little general paralysis in Scotland, and therefore the above high rate of recovery cannot be expected in England and Wales. In the Surrey and Middlesex asylums, during a term of years, the re-admissions amounted to 26.73 per cent. of those discharged recovered, improved, or not improved.†

(5) **Mode of Calculating the Mortality.**—The mortality-rate has been calculated variously upon the admissions, the discharges, and the mean number resident. The last-mentioned method is the correct one. Unfortunately, some of the highest authorities failed to perceive this, and calculated it upon the admissions, or discharges. Such calculations could only be correct if the period of residence were the same in different asylums, and if every case remained in the asylum up to the time of death or recovery. Seeing that the mortality of any community is only accurately exhibited by the proportion of deaths out of a certain number of people, or number living for a specified period, we must obtain the average annual number of deaths to every hundred of the people living one year. Time must, in this instance, be taken into account as all-important. We may go further, and say that "the only strictly accurate, and unequivocal test of the sanitary state of any population, as exhibited by its mortality, is obtained by a *comparison of the deaths at each age, with the average number living at the same age.*"‡

(6) **Mean Number Resident.** — This, the average population, is calculated from a register of the patients in an asylum. Dr. Thurnam has shown that at the Retreat (and there is no reason to regard it as exceptional), the average population for 44 years, when calculated from the number of patients remaining in the asylum at the end of each year, very slightly differed from the results obtained by daily enumerations; while at the York Lunatic Hospital, the average number resident was precisely the same during 21 years, whether reckoned on the number under care at the end of each year, or upon the monthly register. In asylums where the register does not give the number of inmates at longer intervals than a

* *Journal of Mental Science*, 1877.

† Dr. M. Granville's "Care and Cure of the Insane," vol. ii. p. 96.

‡ "Statistics of Insanity," by Dr. Thurnam, p. 15.

month, or a quarter, taking the precise duration of time passed in the institution during the whole period by each patient, and dividing the total by the number of years over which the period extends, is a troublesome, but the only means of obtaining the average number resident. Even the statistician just quoted, who revelled in figures, characterises this method as "almost disheartening."

(7) **Method of calculating Average Duration of Residence.**—The term of years over which the inquiry extends, the number of patients admitted into an asylum, and the average number resident during that term, constitute the data for calculating the average duration of residence. Thus:—

Average number resident.		Years of operation.		Number admitted.		Average duration of residence.
100	×	50	÷	1000	=	5 years

By the multiplication of the average number resident in an asylum by the number of years it has been opened, the years of insane life passed therein are calculated. These "years of residence" (Farr), or "subjective time" (Thurnam), amount in the foregoing illustration to 5000 years, a period which, divided by the number of patients admitted, namely, 1000, yields an average duration of residence in this imaginary asylum of 5 years.

The average duration of residence varies very considerably in different asylums. At the York Lunatic Hospital this amounted, taking the total number admitted for a certain term of years, to 2½ years. Taking the patients who recovered, the period of residence was 8 months; while having regard to those who died, the period extended to 4 years. At the Retreat, York, corresponding periods were as follows:—(*a*) nearly 5 years; (*b*) one year and 4 months; (*c*) nearly 9 years (8.83); more than one-third of those who recovered were discharged within six months of their admission.

In the asylums of Middlesex and Surrey during a term of years, more than half of those who recovered were discharged within six months. A little over one-quarter of the total number recovered between six and twelve months after admission, about one-eighth were discharged in the second year of residence, and nearly half the remainder recovered in the third year.* Sir A. Mitchell states that a large proportion of the recoveries recorded by him in the Scotch asylums occurred in patients under care not longer than from one year to a year [illegible] four per cent. of [illegible] were discharged during [illegible] years.

* Dr. M. Granville's "Care and Cure of the Insane," vol. ii. p. 99.

(8) **Period over which [illegible] Observations should [illegible] Accuracy.**—Seeing that the [illegible] coveries tends to increase [illegible] the opening of an asylum, [illegible] of the number of chronic [illegible] in its earlier years, and that [illegible] cases do not recover until after [illegible] of some years, it is obviously [illegible] comparing the results of treatment [illegible] ferent asylums, to extend the [illegible] observation and comparison [illegible] the history of the first few [illegible] necessity for this precaution [illegible] by the more favourable [illegible] which occurs for some time after [illegible] tablishment of an asylum. [illegible] reasons Dr. Thurnam advises that [illegible] of from twenty to thirty years [illegible] allowed to elapse, and a still longer [illegible] in the case of a small asylum.

The rule may therefore be [illegible] that *the proportion of recoveries,* [illegible] *mean annual mortality, increase* [illegible] *age of an asylum.* Exceptional circum[illegible] stances, such as a difference in [illegible] ment, or an epidemic, may in particular instances affect this formula.

(9) **Conditions affecting the [illegible] tion of Mental Disease whether [illegible] covery or Death.**

(*a*) *Age.*—The chances of recovery [illegible] greatest in the young, putting aside [illegible] of weakness of mind or [illegible] moral obliquity. It must, however, be admitted that a large number of [illegible] pubescent and adolescent insanity [illegible] nate more unfavourably than the [illegible] physician, guided in his prognosis by the general truth, has been led to expect. [illegible]

In regard to the influence of age [illegible] mortality, the latter increases with years, as might be expected, but increases [illegible] rapidly than the mortality of the general population. It is a remarkable circumstance that no tables of mortality bearing on the relation between the age and death of the insane were published before those of Dr. Thurnam, derived from the Retreat and the Lunatic Asylum at York. No tables of asylums for the insane can be regarded as complete unless the age at the origin of the attack of insanity, at admission, the mean number resident at different ages, as also the ages of the patients who recover and die, are given in decennial periods.

(*b*) *Sex.*—Statistics show that more women out of a given number of the population in an asylum recover than men.* That there are exceptions to the rule, especially in some American asylums, must be granted, but special reasons may be given for these departures from the almost universal experience of asylums. Passing on to the influence of sex on mortality, it admits of statistical proof that the advantage is on the side of women, as indeed it is in the community at large, but to a much greater degree than in the population in asylums for the insane. Manifestly it would be very unfair to compare the mortality tables of an institution in which there is a great difference in the proportion of the sexes.

(c) *Previous Condition of Life, Socially and Otherwise.*—It is obvious that the liability to disease and death is much greater among patients taken from the classes of society where intemperance and want are prevalent. So, again, the recovery-rate is lower among the insane from the pauper classes of the community than in the higher classes of society. Nor must it be overlooked that the difference in the dietary in an asylum for the higher and one for the pauper classes would materially affect the termination of the disorder whether in recovery or death.

(d) *Causes of Insanity* (*as affecting Recovery*).—It is manifest that cases of delirium tremens have a much better chance of recovery than cases of sunstroke. These are extreme instances, but they serve to illustrate the important relation between the causes of mental disease and its mode of termination.

(e) *Form of Mental Disorder.*—It is not necessary to prove that a knowledge whether the disorder is in the form of imbecility or acute mania will determine the physician's opinion with regard to the recovery of the patient. Here again it is altogether unfair to compare the results of treatment in institutions receiving totally different classes of patients as respects the form of mental disorder. For example, to draw an inference from the statistics of the termination of the cases admitted into Bethlem Hospital and the Hanwell County Asylum would be altogether unwarrantable.

(f) *Duration of the Attack on Admission.*—This factor is in the highest degree important in the comparison of the results tabulated in the reports of different institutions. The general law may be laid down that the probability of recovery is in inverse ratio to the length of time the patient has laboured under mental disease. After three months' duration the chance of recovery as a general rule diminishes. On the other hand, the liability to death is greater during the early period of the disease.

Dr. Thurnam found that at the Retreat (York) the probability of recovery in cases brought under care within three months of the first attack was as four to one, while it was less than one to four in those cases not admitted until more than twelve months after the attack. This excellent statistician appears to have overlooked the circumstance that the figures on which this statement is based, whilst strictly correct, may be largely explained by the fact that many of the cases admitted a twelve-month after the first attack have been treated elsewhere within three months of its occurrence. The importance of early treatment is not for a moment called in question, but the evidence adduced from those and similar statistics is very unsatisfactory. Notwithstanding this serious source of fallacy, it is desirable to continue the fourfold division in relation to the duration of attack on admission which was introduced by the Retreat. It is as follows:

1st Class. Cases of the first attack, of not more than three months' duration.

2nd Class. Cases of the first attack of more than three but of not more than twelve months' duration.

3rd Class. Cases not of the first attack and not more than twelve months' duration.

4th Class. Cases whether of the first attack or not, and of more than twelve months' duration when admitted.

It is upon this classification that the recoveries and the mean mortality in each class must be calculated.

An inferior division which no doubt commends itself to those asylum officers who dislike the trouble of preparing statistical tables is the twofold division into cases not exceeding twelve months' duration when admitted, and those extending beyond this period.

(g) *Duration of Treatment in Asylum.*—This has already been referred to (§ 7). It is obvious that this factor may greatly affect the results of treatment in regard to the success of a particular asylum. It is only necessary to illustrate this by the effect at Bethlem Hospital of the rule limiting the residence of curable cases to twelve months. As some of these cases subsequently recover at other institutions the reported recoveries of the former are to that extent less than they would have been if no such rule had been in force. Again, in regard to the mortality-rate, the

* In England and Wales the percentage of recoveries, calculated on the admissions, was, from 1880–89 inclusive: Males, 35.47, and females, 43.81.

class of cases admitted for only a year are of the recent class, and therefore are more likely to entail a large mortality.

In a table prepared by Dr. Thurnam, showing the average duration of residence in all cases admitted into certain asylums, he gives the results at various periods from their opening, successively increased by terms of five years. At the end of the first quinquennium such residence was at the Retreat decidedly less than one-half its amount after it had been opened five-and-forty years. At the close of the first decennium it was less than two-thirds. At the end of twenty years the average duration of residence was less than at the close of the forty-five years by more than six months. A table constructed on these lines is essential if we desire to ascertain certain detailed particulars in connection with the residence-rate. A separate statement of the length of residence of every patient admitted into an asylum is obviously necessary before we can demonstrate the fact that it is "by much the lowest in the cases discharged recovered; higher in those which leave improved; higher still in those who died; and highest of all in the cases remaining in the institution at any given time, after a considerable period of operation."*

(10) **Mean Number Resident under Different Circumstances of Sex, Age, Form, and Duration of Disorder.**—The foregoing remarks on the influence of the above-mentioned conditions on the success of various asylums, and consequently the results of treatment, may be supplemented by a few words on the methods employed for ascertaining not only the mean number resident, but its relation to the several factors just enumerated. The monthly register of the asylum should be taken as the basis, and from it must be ascertained the number of months passed in the asylum during a given year by each patient, the figures being arranged in certain periods of life, and according to the fourfold division of time the attack of insanity has lasted at the date of admission, the sex of the patient being also stated. The subjective time in months, obtained from the register for the year in question, is ascertained, and, being divided by twelve, we obtain the mean number resident during the twelve months. Weekly registers yield of course similar results, the divisor being in this instance fifty-two.

(11) **Recoveries.**—In addition to the statistics already given (§ 4) we may add the formula laid [illegible] nam, which, when he [illegible] as too unfavourable, [illegible] quent experience has [illegible] too correct, namely, "[illegible] coveries in asylums which [illegible] lished during any considerable [illegible] say twenty years, a proportion [illegible] less than 40 per cent. of the [illegible] including re-admissions, is [illegible] circumstances to be regarded [illegible] proportion, and one much [illegible] per cent. as a high proportion [illegible] statistics of recovery, however, [illegible] complete without a consideration [illegible] number of relapses.

(12) **Relapses.**—Statistics of the [illegible] Retreat have shown that a relapse [illegible] in two of every three cases in [illegible] had been recovery in the first [illegible] Dr. Thurnam's conclusion from a [illegible] isation of the history of the [illegible] the York Retreat, subsequent [illegible] discharge, was expressed as follows [illegible] round numbers, of 10 persons [illegible] by insanity, 5 recover, and 5 die [illegible] or later during the attack. Of the [illegible] recover not more than 2 remain [illegible] ing the rest of their lives; the [illegible] sustain subsequent attacks, during [illegible] at least 2 of them die."† This [illegible] would be more accurately expressed [illegible] ing regard to the statistics upon [illegible] based, as follows: Of 11 persons [illegible] by insanity, 6 recover, and 5 die sooner or later during the attack. Of the [illegible] recover, not more than 2 remain [illegible] during the rest of their lives; the other 4 sustain subsequent attacks, during which 3 of them die. A very valuable contribution to the life-history of the insane has been made by Sir Arthur Mitchell. He recorded the condition of 1297 patients admitted into Scottish asylums for the first time, and [illegible] asylum before, twelve years afterwards, with this result: 851 recovered, [illegible] not recover, 412 died, 499 were re-admitted, and 273 remained. Now, of the 851 recoveries, 538 *persons* recovered, or 41.5 per cent. of the admissions; of these, 3[illegible] (or 59 per cent. of 538) relapsed for a time, leaving 109 who either remained or died insane. The remaining 429 permanently disappeared as recovered, being 33 per cent. of the original number admitted. As 412 died and 273 remain, 685, or 53 per cent., were accounted for, while 612, or [illegible] per cent., had disappeared at the end of the twelve years. These were traced as far as possible, and it was found that [illegible] had died insane, 78 sane, 94 were living insane, and 197 in a state of [illegible].

* "Statistics of the Retreat," p. 89, Tables 18 and 19; and Appendix I., Table B., Thurnam, *op. cit.* p. 66.

* *Op. cit.* p. 136. † *Op. cit.* p. [illegible]

Although the remaining 201 were not traced it is reasonable to assume that they would terminate in the same proportion. Thus, in twelve years, of 1297 persons—

36.6 per cent. died insane.
31.7 " " are still alive and insane.
31.7 " " are either still alive and sane, or died sane.
———
100.0

Thus, after twelve years there were 68.3 per cent. of those admitted either still living insane or who had died insane. Of the former few would recover, and of those living in a state of sanity some would undoubtedly relapse.* The final result will therefore be less favourable. The writer has elsewhere conjectured that at least 73 per cent. would at death be insane, leaving only 27 per cent. of the total persons admitted likely to die sane.

Very valuable as these statistics are it must be remembered that Dr. Thurnam was able to trace the after-history of every patient who had been at the Retreat *in whom death had occurred*, and that therefore his conclusions, although based on a much smaller number of cases, possess especial value.

(13) **Mortality** (*see* § 5).—The Lunacy Report for England and Wales (1889) gives the annual rate of mortality during ten years ending December 31, 1888; the deaths, calculated on the mean number resident, amounted to 9.70 per cent. In registered hospitals it was 6.56; in provincial licensed houses it was 8.41; in metropolitan licensed houses it was 10.83; in county and borough asylums 9.95; and in the naval and military hospitals and Royal India Asylum, 6.61. At the York Retreat, from its opening to 1891, the annual mortality has been 5.53. Taking the county and borough asylums in Yorkshire, we find that the percentage of deaths on the mean number resident from 1818 to January 1889 was 12.09.

The fall in the rate of mortality in asylums in England and Wales in recent as compared with former years is proved by statistics. We have prepared a table showing the percentage of deaths calculated on the mean number resident during 1818–67, 1868–77, and 1878–87, in the county and borough asylums in Yorkshire. The result is as follows:—The deaths were 13.87 per cent. during 1818–67 and 11.42 during 1868–77, being a decrease between the two periods of 2.45. During 1878–87 the deaths were 11.04, the decrease being slight.

Mr. Noel Humphreys gives a table showing the annual death-rate per cent. of average number resident in the asylums of England and Wales for thirty years, 1859–88, dividing the period into three decades. During 1859–68 the death-rate was 10.31, during 1869–78 it was 10.17, and during 1879–88 it was 9.55.*

The question of the *relative liability of the sane and insane* to death must be now referred to. It may at once be stated that the mortality-rate is higher among the insane than in the sane.

Mr. Humphreys has given a table which shows the annual rate of mortality per 1000 idiots and imbeciles living at different age-periods in the Metropolitan District Asylums for the three years 1886–88 inclusive, compared with the mortality in the general London population, at the same age-periods, and in the same years.

The result is thus summarised by Mr. Humphreys:

"The mean annual death-rate at the age-periods dealt with in the table increased from 42.8 per 1000 among the imbeciles aged 20–40, to 56.8 among those aged 40–60, to 178.2 among those aged 60–80, and to 457.3 per 1000 among those aged upwards of 80 years; or if, on account of the small numbers living over 80 years of age, we treat the numbers aged upwards of 60 years as one age-period, the annual rate of mortality is 195.7 per 1000. The table also shows that, compared with the London rates at the same ages, the mortality of the inmates of the asylums for imbeciles was six times as high in the age-period 20–40, three times as high at 40–60, rather less than three times at 60–80. and not much more than twice as high at 80 and upwards; moreover, it was less than three times as high among all the inmates of these asylums aged upwards of 60 years. Speaking more generally, it may be said that between 20 and 40 years (at which age the bulk of the admissions takes place, and in which period is found a larger proportion of the inmates than in any other) the rate of mortality is six times that which prevails in the general population, whereas at subsequent ages the mortality is less than three times the normal rate among the general population. These metropolitan asylums for imbeciles are mainly filled with chronic and harmless cases, which probably are liable to rates of mortality varying very considerably from those that prevail among the inmates of county asylums" (*op. cit.*).

The class of patients here referred to must be borne in mind.

Taking the whole of England and

* "Contributions to the Statistics of Insanity," by Arthur Mitchell, M.D., LL.D., *Journal of Mental Science*, Jan. 1877.

* Paper read before the Royal Statistical Society, Feb. 18, 1890.

Wales, the annual average mortality at all ages for the thirty years ending 1890 was 22.2 per 1000 for males, and 19.8 for females; the mortality for the ages above twenty was 21.0 per 1000 for males, 19.3 for females. We give the latter period as more nearly corresponding to the period of insane life. The lowest mortality in asylum reports is more than double the foregoing. At the Retreat (York) the average age, at the origin of the disorder, of the patients dying there during a term of years was about 39 years. Now at this age the expectation of life is at least 28 years. The average age at death of these patients was, however, only 56, whereas it should have been 67 (39 + 28) had the mortality-rate been the same as in the population. It was even lower than this at the York asylum, namely, 49½. The following Table* exhibits the high mortality of lunatics at various ages in asylums as compared with that of the general population :—

	Insane Asylums.		General Population.	
	Males.	Females.	Males.	Females.
15–25	8.26	7.87	0.77	0.81
25–35	10.36	7.17	0.55	0.99
35–45	14.35	7.66	1.26	1.20
45–55	14.44	7.36	1.77	1.50
55–65	13.70	10.35	3.06	2.75
65–70	22.41	17.22 }	6.65	5.68
70–75	—	— }		
70 and upwards	31.16	25.76	11.83	11.09
75–85	—	—	14.67	13.39
85–95	—	—	30.72	28.12

Sir Arthur Mitchell has compared the mortality in the Scotch lunatic asylums with that of the general population above the age of ten years, from which it appears that the mean annual death-rate for the latter is 1.7 per cent., as compared with 8.3 per cent. in asylums. His table shows that at all the quinquennial periods between ten and fifty, patients die pretty nearly at the same ratio, excepting between twenty-five and thirty, when the death-rate falls. On the contrary, in the general population, for all the quinquennial periods between ten and fifty it increases in geometrical progression as the ages rise. The death-rate in asylums after the age of fifty rises quinquennially in an irregular manner, while in the general population the rise is rapid and steady.†

* "Manual of Psychological Medicine," 4th edit., p. 133.

† *See* Table in *Journal of Mental Science*, 1879.

(14) **Relative [illegible] Different Ages.**—It is [illegible] to prove, what no one [illegible] fallacy of determining [illegible] comparison of the number [illegible] isting at each period of [illegible] number of individuals existing [illegible] periods in the general population [illegible] must, on the contrary, compare [illegible] and not existing, cases of mental [illegible] at various periods of life, with the [illegible] living at the corresponding periods [illegible] community at large. Recurrent [illegible] ought, strictly speaking, to be [illegible]. Again, cases occurring under ten years [illegible] age are so generally examples of congenital mental defect, that they cannot properly be compared with the population [illegible] the same period, but with the [illegible] births. Further, it is very difficult to ascertain the age of patients at the time of the attack, and consequently it is usual to take the time of admission into asylums. It is evident, however, that the result [illegible] be the throwing forward of the liability [illegible] question to a somewhat later term of life than that which is actually correct. Dr Thurnam was not able to obtain any extensive statistics prepared in accordance with a system theoretically correct. He felt, however, authorised to conclude that "there can be little or no doubt that the period of life most liable to insanity is that of maturity, or from twenty to fifty or sixty years of age. From thirty to forty years of age the liability is usually the greatest; and it decreases with each succeeding decennial period, the decrease being gradual from thirty to sixty years, and after that much more rapid."* At the same time, had the age when the attack first occurred been ascertained, the decade of greatest liability to attack might have been between twenty and thirty years, as is actually the case in the experience at the York Retreat; at any rate, if this is saying too much, large numbers of the cases tabulated as occurring between thirty and forty would be thrown back to the period between twenty and thirty. We have, elsewhere, shown that in American asylums the liability to an attack is greatest between twenty and thirty.

The Tables of the Commissioners in Lunacy indicate a somewhat later age-period for first attacks than we have stated above, the incidence falling most heavily during the decade 35–45.

(15) **Relative Liability to Insanity in Males and Females.**—Although the actual admissions of male and female lunatics into asylums, excluding transfers, showed an excess of the latter during the

* *Op. cit.* p. 164.

seventeen years 1869 to 1885 inclusive,* it is necessary to correct this result by taking the ratio (per 10,000) of admissions to the population, as regards the two sexes.

Up to the year 1879 there was a slight excess of male over female admissions. In 1879 and 1880, however, there was a slight excess in the proportion of female admissions. Taking the mean of the next five years, 1881–85, the male admissions were equal to 5.22 per 10,000 of the population, against 5.18 female admissions, thus showing a very slight excess of males. In the aggregate of the succeeding five years, 1886–90, the reverse was the case; for while the male admissions averaged 5.24 per 10,000 during that period, the female admissions averaged 5.26, showing a slight excess of females. If these two quinquennial periods be taken together, the proportions of the two sexes were almost identical, being 5.23 for males and 5.22 for females.

In the preceding ten years, 1871–80, the male admissions were equal to 5.13, and the female admissions to 4.96, per 10,000 persons living, showing an excess of male admissions, among equal numbers of both sexes living of 3.4 per cent.

We append a tabular statement of the admissions of both sexes from 1881 to 1890 inclusive, separately and in certain terms of years.†

Year.	Admissions per 10,000 of Population.		
	Males.	Females.	Persons.
1881	5.25	5.12	5.18
1882	5.20	5.14	5.17
1883	5.42	5.45	5.44
1884	5.37	5.24	5.30
1885	4.86	4.95	4.91
1886	4.98	4.88	4.93
1887	5.21	5.07	5.14
1888	5.23	5.24	5.24
1889	5.21	5.37	5.29
1890	5.55	5.71	5.63
5 years, 1881–85	5.22	5.18	5.20
5 years, 1886–90	5.24	5.26	5.25
10 years, 1881–90	5.23	5.22	5.22

These statistics appear to show that, while working the admissions of the two sexes upon the population reduces the apparently large excess of female over male admissions, there has been occasionally, and during the last three years uniformly, a slightly greater number of admissions of female lunatics. The natural inference would be that with the increased tendency of women to enter into intellectual pursuits and to take part in political life, there had been injurious results in the direction of mental disorder. It may be so, and there would be nothing remarkable in the circumstance that the relative liability of the sexes to insanity had undergone a marked change in the course of recent years. It remains to be seen whether the returns of coming years will be in accordance with those which we have given, or whether circumstances of which we are ignorant have temporarily interfered with former experience, and so may not be of a lasting character.

(16) **Cases as distinguished from Persons.**—The importance of this distinction will be obvious to any one who will take pains to calculate the recoveries of patients admitted into asylums, with and without regard to this distinction. If of 100 cases discharged recovered one-third consists of the same persons who have recovered more than once, it is obvious that although the number of recoveries is correctly reported, a much too favourable impression is conveyed as regards the number of persons restored to health and enabled to take their place in the world. For a detailed notice of this source of fallacy, and the proper mode of calculating the recoveries on admission, see CURABILITY OF INSANITY.

(17) **Relative Frequency of the Various Forms of Mental Disorder.**—In consequence of the personal equation which influences the classification of mental disorders, the reports of asylums vary to a certain extent in this matter, even when the tabular arrangement is similar, and the difficulty is increased when such statement greatly differs in its divisions. Recent efforts which have been made, dating from the action first taken at the Antwerp Congress of Mental Medicine, and culminating in the resolution unanimously adopted at the Paris Congress in 1889, will tend, it is hoped, to minimise these divergent systems, but we fear a complete unanimity is impossible. In the meantime we must content ourselves with the statistical tables of the forms of mental disorder admitted into British asylums, which are at hand.

Taking, in the first instance, the 43rd Report of the Commissioners in Lunacy, we find that of 14,336 patients (private and pauper) admitted into county and borough asylums, registered hospitals, naval and military hospitals, State asylums, and licensed houses, during one year (1887), the proportion per cent. was divided as

* Fortieth Report of the Commissioners in Lunacy, 1886 (Table III.).

† See SEX, INFLUENCE OF, IN INSANITY.

follows between the forms of mental disorders adopted by the Lunacy Board :—

	Male.	Female.	Total.
Mania	46.1	52.1	49.1
Melancholia . . .	21.1	28.6	24.9
Dementia { Ordinary	13.9	8.3	11.1
Dementia { Senile .	4.7	3.4	4.0
Congenital insanity (including idiocy and other mental defects from birth or infancy) . . .	6.3	4.2	5.3
Other forms of insanity	7.9	3.4	5.6
	100	100	100

The late Dr. Boyd prepared an elaborate table based on a large number of first admissions into the Somerset County Asylum, the result being the following proportions per cent. :—Mania, 42.9; melancholia, 18.4; dementia, 10.6; monomania (delusional insanity), 5.3; general paralysis, 5.1; moral insanity, 1.1; epilepsy, 10.9; delirium tremens, 1.4. We omit idiocy (4.3) because it can bear no relation to the frequency of congenital defect. As to age, Dr. Boyd's figures confirmed the observation of Esquirol, that "insanity may be divided into imbecility of childhood, mania and monomania for youth, melancholia for mature age, and dementia for advanced life." From a large number of asylum returns which we threw together some years ago, melancholia appeared to be much more frequent than in Dr. Boyd's table. Thus, of 100 admissions, half were cases of acute and chronic mania; melancholia, 30; dementia, 11; monomania, 9. From a Table in the same report (p. 52) we note that the proportion (per cent.) of epileptics and paralytics, admitted into the same institution, during the same period, to the total number of patients admitted was: Epileptics, 9; general paralytics, also 9. In both, the male sex predominated; thus, in the former there were 10.9 males against 7.1 females, and in the latter 15 against 3.3 per cent.

(18) **Causation.**—As the Lunacy Commissioners adopt a classification of the causes of insanity, which is fairly workable, and have collected together a large number of returns from English asylums, it is desirable to give the results here for what they are worth. As is well known, the entries made by the friends of patients in the statutory "statement" are extremely unreliable and constantly confound cause and *effect*, the Commissioners state that they have not [illegible] but upon statements verified by the medical officers of the asylum. ([illegible] p. 1205.)

(a) *Condition in Reference to Marriage.* — Two sources of fallacy at least may vitiate the inference drawn from such figures in regard to the number of patients in a state of celibacy. In the first place it may be the mental condition of an individual which has prevented marriage, and not celibacy which has caused or favoured his mental condition. It is extremely difficult to distinguish the sequence of the two events, celibacy and insanity, in a statistical inquiry. Secondly, there is the fallacy arising from taking the condition in regard to marriage of the insane without comparing it with the proportion of unmarried, married and widowed, in the general population. Thus, the condition, in 1881, of the population of England and Wales, aged twenty and upwards, was in respect to marriage as follows :—

—	Unmarried.	Married.	Widowed.
	per cent.	per cent.	per cent.
Males .	27.12	66.09	6.79
Females .	25.85	60.55	13.60
Total . .	26.45	63.19	10.36

If with these figures the corresponding condition of the insane admitted into asylums be compared, it will be found that the proportion of celibates is much greater in the latter. It is true that the proportion of married persons between twenty-five and forty, a term of life in which there are so large a number of admissions into asylums, is less than between twenty and upwards, and that hence a slight allowance should be made on this account, probably to the extent of 7 per cent. What the Table in the Lunacy Commissioners' Report (1889), in regard to the condition of patients admitted into the asylums of England and Wales, shows, is that, at marriageable ages, and in proportion to the population, considerably more single than married or widowed persons are admitted (p. 48). The general conclusion from a study of the whole subject leads to the conclusion that celibacy is more likely to favour mental disease than the married condition. At the same time the result cannot be absolutely stated in figures on account of the impossibility of measuring the extent of the source of fallacy first mentioned.

Table showing the Causes of Insanity in Patients Admitted into the Asylums and Registered Hospitals in England and Wales during the Ten Years, 1878 to 1887.

Causes of Insanity.	Proportion per cent. to the Admissions.		
	Male.	Female.	Total.
Moral:			
Domestic trouble (including loss of relatives and friends)	4.2	9.7	7.0
Adverse circumstances (including business anxieties and pecuniary difficulties)	8.2	3.7	5.9
Mental anxiety and "worry" (not included under the above two heads) and overwork	6.6	5.5	6.0
Religious excitement	2.5	2.9	2.7
Love affairs (including seduction)	0.7	2.5	1.6
Fright and nervous shock	0.9	1.9	1.4
Physical:			
Intemperance in drink	19.8	7.2	13.4
Intemperance (sexual)	1.0	0.6	0.7
Venereal disease	0.8	0.2	0.5
Self-abuse (sexual)	2.1	0.2	1.2
Over-exertion	0.7	0.4	0.5
Sunstroke	2.3	0.2	1.2
Accident or injury	5.2	1.0	3.0
Pregnancy	—	1.0	0.5
Parturition and the puerperal state	—	6.7	3.4
Lactation	—	2.2	1.1
Uterine and ovarian diseases	—	2.3	1.2
Puberty	0.2	0.6	0.4
Change of life	—	4.0	2.0
Fevers	0.7	0.5	0.6
Privations and starvation	1.7	2.1	1.9
Old age	3.8	4.6	4.2
Other bodily diseases or disorders	11.1	10.5	10.8
Previous attacks	14.3	18.9	16.6
Hereditary influence ascertained	19.0	22.1	20.5
Congenital defect ascertained	5.1	3.5	4.3
Other ascertained causes	2.3	1.0	1.7
Unknown	21.3	20.1	20.7

The above table is based upon 136,478 admissions (male, 66,918; female, 69,560). These totals represent the entire number of instances in which the several causes (either alone or in combination with other causes) were stated to have produced the mental disorder. The aggregate of these totals (including "unknown") of course exceeds the whole number of patients admitted. The excess is owing to combinations (*see* Forty-third Report of the Commissioners, 1889, p. 67).

(*b*) *Moral and Physical Causes.*—Much has been written on the relative influence of moral and physical causes in the production of insanity. The real difficulty lies in determining the area of the one and the other. Many causes are of a mixed character—partaking of both the moral and physical. For the sake of uniformity it is better to follow the classification of causes adapted by the Commissioners in Lunacy, given in the foregoing Table. It may be pointed out, however, that "privation and starvation," tabulated under physical causes, contain a strong element of moral agency as well, and other similar combinations might be mentioned.

Moral causes have been regarded by the French school, and some English writers, as in the majority. On the other hand, at the York Retreat, the physical are in excess of the moral causes to a considerable extent. So at the York Asylum. The same result is reached in the statistics prepared by Dr. Earle. In the annexed causation table the physical causes, even after omitting previous attacks, amount to 75 per cent., and the moral to only 25 per cent. If, then, statistics may be trusted, moral causes exert decidedly less influence than physical causes.

Dr. Major has, in the annual reports of the West Riding Asylum, attempted to improve upon the ordinary mode of tabulating the causes of insanity. He combines the causes of the attacks in a manner shown in the following Table in which the factor of alcoholic excess is present in all instances, but is in many combined with other causes:

	Males.	Females.	Total.	Percentage on Admissions.
Alcoholic excess (singly) . . .	30	5	35	7.5
Alcoholic excess with hereditary tendency to insanity . . .	14	5	19	4.0
Alcoholic excess with other physical causes .	9	4	13	2.7
Alcoholic excess combined with moral causes .	13	1	14	3.0
	66	15	81	17.2

The importance of endeavouring to differentiate the causes of attacks of insanity in the foregoing way is obvious, and it is to be regretted that so few of those who prepare asylum statistics take, in this respect, as much trouble as Dr. Major has done.

(*c*) *Predisposing and Exciting Causes.*—In the annual report of the Commissioners in Lunacy, from which the causation table is extracted, separate columns are given, indicating the number of instances in which the cause is supposed to have been predisposing, and the number in which it is supposed to have been exciting. It is no doubt very difficult in many instances to distinguish between these two classes, and some writers have rejected the distinction as worthless. At the same time there are many cases in which the distinction is very clear. Thus, the individual who has a strong hereditary taint has, it must be allowed, a predisposition to mental disorder. Subject this person and one who comes of a perfectly healthy stock, to a reverse of fortune or other calamity; the former will probably succumb and the latter escape the overthrow of reason. The exciting cause is altogether distinct from the predisposing one. It must be admitted that the predisposing causes are the more important of the two.

(*d*) *Occupation.*—The Commissioners (Table xiv.) give the professions or occupations of the population of England and Wales, and of the patients admitted into asylums during the year. It is doubtful, however, whether it is safe to draw inferences from these figures, and we therefore do not give them.

(*e*) *Moon.*—The [illegible] influence of this [illegible] established by careful [illegible] experience of the York [illegible] brought to bear upon this [illegible] result has been entirely [illegible] Moon.)

(*f*) *Civilisation.* — It may [illegible] without danger of contradiction [illegible] proportion of idiots and [illegible] population in uncivilised [illegible] than in those who are civilised [illegible] same time there are many [illegible] the actual number [illegible] latter should be vastly [illegible] the former without a correspon[illegible] ence in the liability to mental [illegible] If we consider only this liability [illegible] recommend savages to remain [illegible] but on the other hand we should [illegible] recommend the class corresponding [illegible] savages (city-arabs, &c.) in [illegible] community to enter the ranks [illegible] cated and well-fed classes.

Age and *sex* fall under [illegible] we have already considered [illegible] liabilities (p. 1202).

Heredity is discussed at length [illegible] article by Dr. Mercier under [illegible] In the Cause-Table of the Commissioners [illegible] it stands at 20.5 per cent. of the [illegible] sions, but the reluctance of the [illegible] of patients to give information [illegible] painful point, leaves the proportion [illegible] doubtedly far too low.

Conclusion.—In concluding [illegible] we would acknowledge the great [illegible] rendered to the statistics of [illegible] Mr. Noel Humphreys' contribution [illegible] a difficult inquiry in his paper [illegible] referred to. Notwithstanding the [illegible] culty arising from the imperfect [illegible] given in the Reports of the Lunacy Com[illegible] missioners, he has concentrated all [illegible] able knowledge and brought it up [illegible] recent a period as possible. His [illegible] confirms the conclusion arrived at by [illegible] writer, that statistics fail to [illegible] real increase in occurring insanity. [illegible] other points upon which this article [illegible] his figures are, without exception, [illegible] accord. It is further reassuring [illegible] principles laid down by Dr. Thurnam [illegible] regard to the preparation of [illegible] of insanity, and to which the [illegible] repeatedly expressed his indebtedness, [illegible] entirely borne out. THE [illegible]

[*References.*—Blue Books of the Commissioners in Lunacy. Farr, Report on the Mortality of [illegible] tics, Royal Stat. Soc. Journ., 1841. Thurnam, [illegible] tistics of Insanity, 1844. Lockhart [illegible] Alleged Increase of Insanity, Journal of [illegible] Science, 1869 and 1871. Hack Tuke, [illegible] and its Prevention (Appendices), 1876; [illegible] Alleged Increase of Insanity, Journal of [illegible]

Science, Oct. 1886; Idem, The Past and Present Provision for the Insane Poor in Yorkshire, with Suggestions for the Future Provision for this Class, 1889. N. Humphreys, Statistics of Insanity in England, with special reference to evidence of its alleged increasing prevalence, Royal Statistical Society Journ. 1890. Mortimer Granville, Care and Cure of the Insane, 2 vols.]

STATUS EPILEPTICUS.—A name given to a rapid succession of epileptic fits without intervening consciousness. It is a rare but dangerous symptom especially if with deepening coma the intervals between the fits become shorter. The temperature is said by Bourneville to rise in some cases as high as 105° to 107°, and death is caused by collapse, or the occurrence of meningitis. Recovery may however take place. Sir James Crichton-Browne has recommended the inhalation of amyl nitrite. Chloral, *per anum*, with subcutaneous injections of morphia, and spinal icebags appear to be the most efficacious.

STEHLSUCHT.—The German term for kleptomania.

STEIFSUCHT (Ger.). Catalepsy or tetanus.

STIGMATA (στίγμα, a hole or mark made by an instrument, a brand-mark). In pathology applied to small red spots on the skin either natural or acquired. They are of interest in psychological medicine owing to cases such as that of Louise Lateau, the Belgian girl, where these red spots seem to have appeared on parts of the body to which the mind had been intensely directed. Brewer ("Dictionary of Phrase and Fable") gives a list of men and women who have claimed to be able to show the impressions or marks corresponding to some or all of the wounds received by Christ in his trial and crucifixion.

Dr. Coomes, Louisville, Ky., has recorded, in the *Medical Standard*, a case of stigmatisation in a devout Catholic, a female, whom he personally watched along with others appointed to assist him. The first bleeding occurred in June 1891. During attacks of hysterial unconsciousness blood frequently flowed from the right hand, the feet and forehead. After watching her for three hours, "the crusts of the wounds began to be lifted up, and in a few moments the serous portions of the blood began to ooze from beneath the crusts, and slowly run down across the right foot. In a few minutes the blood began to assume a pinkish and then a red colour, until it had the appearance of ordinary blood. There were but a few drops from this foot on this occasion. The left foot has now commenced pouring out serum, which, like that from the right foot, soon became red, and, after a few drops, had issued, the flow ceased." More remarkable stigmata are recorded in this case, but, as the blood was not seen flowing by Dr. Coomes himself, it would not be safe to accept the report, although "no evidences of fraud have been detected, and she has been watched closely during the unconscious state." Dr. Coomes stuck needles again and again into her limbs, dashed her face with water, and tickled her feet, and found complete anæsthesia and absence of reflex action. In this and similar cases it is more than probable that genuine and pretended wounds and hæmorrhages are mixed up together. M. Warlomont, a member of the commission appointed by the Royal Academy of Medicine of Belgium to inquire into the phenomena alleged to occur in the case of Louise Lateau, gave credit to them. The conclusion at which this commission arrived was unanimous—viz., that "The stigmata and ecstasies are real. They can be explained physiologically." The late Mr. Critchett was present at one examination of Louise Lateau, and believed that the phenomena were perfectly genuine.

THE EDITOR.

[*References.*—Dictionnaire de Mystique Chrétienne, art. Extases, Stigmates, &c., Paris, 1858. Maury, Les Mystiques Extatiques et les Stigmatisés, Ann. Médico-Psych., tome i. Jules Parrot, Etude sur la Sueur de Sang et les Hémorragies névropathiques, Paris, 1859. Louise Lateau, de Bois d'Haine, by Dr. F. Lefebvre, Prof. of Pathology in the Louvain University, Physician to the Lunatic Asylums in that town; translated and edited by Rev. J. Spencer Northcote, D.D., London, 1873. Louise Lateau, la Stigmatisée de Bois d'Haine, Warlomont, Bruxelles, 1873. Illustrations of the Influences of the Mind upon the Body, vol. i. pp. 119–126, 292, London, 1884.]

STOLIDITAS, STOLIDITY.—A term meaning stupidity, imbecility; or merely describing the characteristic of the phlegmatic temperament. A synonym of Amentia.

STRAIT-WAISTCOAT.—A short coat of strong material which confines the arms of the violently insane; sometimes without sleeves, and sometimes with long sleeves without openings, which can be tied together behind or before. (Fr. *camisole de force;* Ger. *Zwangsjacke.*)

STRIDOR DENTIUM.—Teeth-grinding. A symptom in certain cerebral diseases. Among the insane it is by far the most frequent in general paralysis.

STRYCHNOMANIA (στρύχνος, nightshade; μανία, madness). An ancient term for the delirium resulting from eating the deadly nightshade. (Fr. *strychnomanie.*)

STULTITIA (*stultus*, foolish). Foolishness. Dulness of the mind. (Fr. *stupidité;* Ger. *Narrheit*). (*See* IDIOCY.)

STUPEMANIA.—A name sometimes applied to mental stupor.

STUPOR (*stupo*, I am stupefied). A state of mental torpor.

STUPOR, ANERGIC.—Term substituted for acute dementia by Dr. Hayes Newington. (*See* STUPOR, MENTAL.)

STUPOR, MENTAL. — **I. Anergic. II. Delusional.**

I. Anergic. (**Syn.** Acute dementia; *Démence aiguë*, Esquirol.) So-called "acute dementia" is seen either as a primary affection following a definite course and ending in death or recovery, or as an accidental and intercurrent symptom in other forms of acute or of long-continued insanity, for instance, in epilepsy, puerperal insanity, ordinary acute mania, or melancholia (especially if accompanied with masturbation), general paralysis, &c. After attacks of acute insanity that do not end in recovery a condition is often found where the patient, though still exhibiting much intelligence, does not regain his normal standard of mind; but this must not be confounded with genuine stupor.

Symptoms.—The patient seems contented to remain in an apathetic condition, taking little interest in his surroundings, making no inquiries about his friends or family, but given up entirely to the mere routine of living and doing as he is told. He may or may not retain a few delusions and hallucinations, and possibly is incoherent and at times uncertain in his disposition, but he will work or remain idle according as he is told, and this condition may last a considerable time without much change, or periodical attacks of excitement or of depression may arise, ending eventually in a pronounced state of real mental stupor. This state is one phase in the course of an attack of acute insanity, but it must not be supposed that an antecedent state of acute excitement or depression is always present. In well-marked cases of acute dementia the symptoms usually come on suddenly, and are essentially negative in character, for the patient seems to be deprived of all manifestations of mental and motor energy. He will stand or sit in the same position for hours without moving, there is a blueness and swelling of the hands and feet (although the thermometer does not invariably show a fall of temperature), slow and feeble circulation, vacant expression, retention (in some cases incontinence) of urine and fæces, complete absence of mental function in the region of will, perception, memory, and often even of consciousness, for the patients as a rule on recovery remember nothing of the condition. The reflex [illegible] involved, for muscular [illegible] cal stimuli is either [illegible] respiratory movements [illegible] extent and frequency, [illegible] to light, sound, taste and [illegible] abolished. In fact there is [illegible] separate the condition from [illegible] death, and the patient is [illegible] dent upon others for his [illegible] There may be either [illegible] everything may be freely [illegible] diminution in the bodily weight [illegible]

Some of the patients are [illegible] will stand or sit in the [illegible] will strongly resist any [illegible] move them or to flex their [illegible] would seem that some [illegible] sciousness is present here, for [illegible] moved forcibly away from a [illegible] make strong efforts to return [illegible] they often appear to [illegible] interference with their fixed [illegible] rigid in some of these resistive [illegible] be the muscular system that [illegible] known the finger-nails driven [illegible] palm of the hand from the [illegible]

A true cataleptic state, on [illegible] hand, is often present, and the [illegible] the patient will retain for some [illegible] position in which they are placed, [illegible] just the appearance of an [illegible] figure. Another symptom [illegible] present is the great susceptibility [illegible] skin to the development of [illegible] shown by drawing the blunt [illegible] pencil lightly along the skin of [illegible] abdomen, or extremities, when a [illegible] immediately follows the [illegible] remains for some time. We have [illegible] in some of these cataleptic states [illegible] power of the extended limbs to [illegible] weight is greater in degree and [illegible] than in ordinary persons. The [illegible] in many respects resembles that [illegible] in hysterical persons by hypnotism. [illegible] dementia may terminate as suddenly [illegible] began, or it may develop into acute [illegible] and the time of duration of the [illegible] state may vary from a few hours to [illegible] months, or even years. This condition [illegible] often confounded with "melancholia [illegible]-ita," from which, however, it is [illegible] guished by the presence in the [illegible] delusions and a greater degree of [illegible] sciousness, whilst the above-[illegible] states of catalepsy and vaso-motor [illegible] tiveness are absent. We have met with profound states of acute dementia [illegible] more frequently among females than males, and in both sexes it is very frequently connected with masturbation or [illegible] genital irritation. Young [illegible] most liable to this form of stupor, [illegible] hereditary taint is frequently present. The pathology is uncertain, but stupor is generally believed to be due to vaso-motor disturbance, and is not connected with organic cerebral lesion, in view of the suddenness of onset and departure of the symptoms and the large percentage of recoveries. All the symptoms point to stagnation in the circulation.

Treatment.—Massage, with regulation of diet and attention to the bowels and bladder, are indicated as the best lines of treatment, and special attention should be devoted to prevent masturbation if possible. The use of the continued current and Turkish baths may be recommended, and we have found cupping over the region of the ovaries very useful in young women, where (as generally happens) menstruation is imperfect or irregular. The form of acute dementia or stupor that is often found as an intercurrent symptom in epilepsy or even in general paralysis calls for no special form of treatment, as it is generally of short duration.

T. Claye Shaw.

II. Delusional * (Fr. *stupidité*).—It is unfortunate that medical psychologists have differed so much in the terms applied to the condition which that of "Mental Stupor" is intended to indicate. There is no doubt a reason for the obscurity and vagueness of definition which have prevailed in reference to it. It arises out of the difficulty of diagnosis. The expression and conduct of the patient may seem to indicate absolute dementia.

Nomenclature.—There are cases in which the ablest alienist is unable to decide whether the mind is what the outward expression would lead us to infer—a complete blank—or the seat of such intense depression and painful delusion as only to simulate dementia. "Mental stupor" may be employed to cover both conditions until it is ascertained which of the two is present. When evidence is forthcoming that a melancholy delusion dominates the mental activity, we may speak of melancholia *cum stupore*, or of mental stupor with delusion, or melancholia attonita. If, on the contrary, we are able to satisfy ourselves that this is not the case, we may speak simply of mental stupor. We prefer this term to acute dementia, which conveys the idea of mental degeneration, thus confounding it with dementia of the genuine type. It has been justly said by Baillarger that acute dementia and *stupidité* are, in the majority of cases, only the highest degree of melancholia *cum stupore*. French alienists agree in rejecting the former term (*démence aiguë*), introduced by Esquirol. No one psychologist has done more to show the true nature of the condition under consideration than Baillarger, but the observer first in the field was Étoc-Demazy, who wrote a thesis on stupor in 1835.

In an article upon this affection which Dr. Hayes Newington contributed to the *Journal of Mental Science* (Oct. 1874), he applied the term anergic stupor if so-called acute dementia is the form assumed, and that of delusional stupor if it is not.

Of one thing there can be no doubt, that the delusional stupor of to-day may be the anergic stupor of to-morrow. In such a case the mental condition has melancholia for its basis.

The writer has, in a paper read before the Psychological Section of the International Medical Congress 1881, given his reasons for believing that there is a kind of auto-hypnotism in those cases in which the dwelling intensely upon an all-absorbing delusion, is followed by mental stupor. A case was reported of a female patient in Bethlem Hospital, in whom the manipulations calculated to awaken a person in the hypnotic sleep restored the patient to normal consciousness of her surroundings and a corresponding healthy expression. Unhappily this lasted only a very short time, but the experiment was very suggestive.

Symptoms.—In the first place, it will clear the road to state, what no one acquainted with the insane will deny, the clinical fact that there are patients who, under intense mental depression with delusions, and possibly, but rarely without, do not speak, eat, dress themselves, but may attend to the calls of nature; do not, in short, respond to the outer world, and would die if left to their own resources. The eyes are closed or only half opened, the facial expression is indicative of depression. There is muscular tension, as shown when one takes hold of the patient's arm; the muscles are felt to contract and may become rigid. In this state it is very difficult to dress and undress a patient. He stands and sits in the same immovable attitude. On recovery, he remembers what has been the predominating thought in his mind and much of what has been addressed to him.

To the above mental affection the names melancholia *cum stupore*, melancholia attonita, and delusional stupor are applied.

* Although it is convenient to recognise two divisions of Mental Stupor, the anergic and the delusional or melancholic, we shall not, under the present section, restrict ourselves to the delusional form of stupor, following in this respect the clinical fact, as the two are observed to occur in the same patient in a large number of cases.

It has been doubted whether "stupor" conveys a correct impression, seeing that we do not connect voluntary resistance with stupor. For this reason some alienists prefer the term melancholia attonita.

Another clinical fact is this: A man may receive a mental shock which paralyses his powers of mind and reduces him to the level of vegetable life. His muscles are passive instead of resistant. He slavers; the nasal mucus collects and trickles down unheeded. Flies crawl over his face without his regarding them; he never speaks, and his existence is only preserved by forcible feeding. His muscles may remain for an indefinite time in a position in which they are placed. The extremities are cold, the hands blue, and apt to have chilblains. He is dirty in his habits. His pupils are generally dilated. On recovery, he has no memory, or a very confused one, of the state from which he has emerged. It is to this condition to which the terms acute dementia, anergic, and apathetic stupor are attached Such are two very different mental states, the one with and the other without conscious depression and delusions, the former being by far the most common.

As we have said, the difficulty lies in the diagnosis.* There may be no symptom distinctly evidencing consciousness of surroundings, and the presence of mental distress and delusions—the condition most frequently and, some would hold, exclusively found in the melancholy form of stupor. A female patient at Bethlem Hospital became markedly cataleptic for at least half an hour at a time, and the muscular resistance was [illegible] slight. There was [illegible] to be fed; she slavered; [illegible] dirty; there was oscillation [illegible] which were of normal size [illegible] eyeballs were usually fixed [illegible] front and occasionally up[illegible] shut and tremulous at times, [illegible] others they were wide open; [illegible] wink if anything was suddenly [illegible] near her eyes; the patellar [illegible] slightly brisk; she did not [illegible] pulled along, when she walked [illegible]cally; she did not speak; she [illegible] dressed. In stupor with delusions it [illegible] said the patient resists, but this [illegible] the case here, and yet, as proved by the patient's statement after recovery, and the proof which test-questions afford of the patient's memory, there had been no [illegible]

Such cases are common; hence the frequent mistake of labelling a case [illegible] of acute dementia, when it is one in reality of melancholia attonita. We are able to give instances in which patients have manifested apathy, silence, immobility, disregard of flies settling on the face, and the saliva dribbling down the chin, and the hands blue and cold, and yet able to give subsequently a coherent account of the delusions under which they were labouring at the time when they were apparently simply stupid. Dr. [illegible] in filling up a form which the writer drew up and distributed a few years ago in reference to mental stupor, added: "Here is a case in which all the symptoms were those of so-called acute dementia, but the case was really one of melancholia cum *stupore*. I cannot find any case in which the initial stage was pure stupor without consciousness, with no depressed state of mind, but which terminated in stupor with depressed feeling and consciousness. I do not think I ever met with such a case, and indeed I am very sceptical that ever such exists. I should prefer to believe that it was melancholic stupor to begin with except I myself had an opportunity of watching the case. It is most difficult from outward symptoms merely to tell real 'anergic' from melancholic stupor. I have seen a case of melancholic stupor end in dementia just as any kind of mental disease may so end."

It must be evident from the foregoing that it is not always possible to differentiate the symptoms belonging respectively to melancholy stupor and anergic stupor or so-called acute dementia. Then, in regard to loss of sensation, it is very certain that a pin introduced into the skin will fail to induce any sign of pain in both conditions. Then again, as to catalepsy,

* Although Dr. Newington has given a table showing the differential symptoms in the two forms of mental stupor, we fear that they will not always enable us to arrive at a correct diagnosis. At the same time, it is well to have them in view. *Anergic:* Invasion very rapid, intellect evidently greatly impaired, memory gone, no sign of emotion, features relaxed, eye vacant and not constantly fixed, volition absent, motor system weak, catalepsy, sensory system and reflexes dull, pupils dilated, extreme emaciation, vascular system profoundly affected, as shown by the pulse being very slow and by cyanosis; tongue clean, or if not it is moist; habits dirty. *Delusional:* Invasion slow, intellect not impaired, memory preserved, features contracted, eyes fixed on one point, usually upwards or downwards, or obstinately closed; presence of volition shown by great stubbornness, motor system little interfered with, patient standing or kneeling from time to time, more ability to bear pain, pupils contracted, nutrition affected *pari passu* with mental state; the disturbance of the vascular system is less marked and comes on later; tongue very dry, furred; refusal of food, constipation; habits rarely dirty. Dr. Newington lays great stress on anergic stupor following acute mania in women only, or at least far more frequently than in men. Heredity is a marked feature in the history of both forms of mental stupor.

we find it present in both states, but it is not likely to occur when there is much resistance.

Although we have taken great pains to show that the more carefully patients are examined in regard to their mental condition when labouring under mental stupor, the more frequently will it be found that some form of delusion was present, we do not deny that delusions may be absent and thought be practically suspended. The probability of a patient having passed into this condition may be suspected if the facial expression is vacant, listless, stupid, mouth often open, the saliva trickling on to the beard or dress, the breath offensive, the pupils dilated, the appetite bad, refusal to take food, evacuations passed involuntarily, skin cold and clammy, hands blue and swollen, pulse very feeble and slow, diminished sensibility, respiration slow and shallow, eyes frequently half closed, the eyeballs turned up, muscular activity slight, sometimes *nil*, patient remaining in the same condition all day, more or less cataleptic, in many instances mute or only repeating a few words, automatic, apathetic, frequently unaware of what is passing around, the mind being more or less a blank.

Such a condition as this may succeed to acute mania: a shock which at once deprives the brain of its power of spontaneous action, or fever, or starvation, or exhausting diseases. It may be inferred that a female patient whom we knew in St. Luke's Hospital, who passed into this condition after acute mania, was free from delusions. There was mutism, mental stupor, and marked catalepsy. She had to be treated as a child, and was fed and dressed. She was dirty in her habits. Again we should be disposed to infer a like mental vacuity in a young man in the same institution, in whom religious depression and delusions appeared to have entirely passed away, and he became taciturn, refused food, and could not dress himself. He stared vacantly about; sometimes standing, sometimes sitting, and in either position as immovable as a stone. No resistance was offered when the writer extended his arms, but there was no catalepsy. He was discharged from the hospital unimproved.

Among the indications of profound stupor we have mentioned the absolute indifference of the patient to flies crawling over the face or to the conjunctiva being touched. This ought to count for something, and yet in a recent case in which this symptom was present it was ascertained that his memory and consciousness were perfectly vivid during his illness. Thus, he remembered seeing a friend, and that he (the patient) would not speak to him as he was suspicious of his intentions. He recollected being pricked in the legs and arms, and that it hurt him excessively, but that he would not show any signs of feeling "through obstinacy." He knew who the attendant was, and he felt that he was kind to him. He said he remembered various occurrences and incidents as well as he would be able to recall events which had happened five months previously at any other period of his life. He was apprehensive of mischief being done to him when he was asleep, for he would wake up with cuts on his fingers and face, and is still of opinion that they were real and that they were done during sleep. He was under the influence of great dread, and the force necessarily used to feed him appeared to him to be done to injure him. He had a reason for sitting still—namely, lest if he walked about there were violent patients who would knock against him or hit him. He recovered.

Dr. Whitwell has shown that the character of the pulse is reflected in the sphygmographic tracing taken by him in cases of mental stupor. "It would at first sight appear that the pulse was exceedingly weak and feeble. . . . . It is certainly small, but is apparently only weak and feeble in that the fluctuations of the vessel are comparatively small, and the variations in its bulk and volume are only within narrow limits and gradual. A sphygmographic tracing shows a typically high tension pulse, in which the cardiac factor is not very active. The line of ascent is short and sometimes somewhat oblique, the latter being masked by its shortness. The apical angle is wide, and the line of descent gradual; the dicrotic wave and aortic notch are usually almost absent, and there is frequently a pre-dicrotic wave present which may tend to blend with the apical angle to form a plateau, probably on account of the feebleness of the cardiac factor. In fact, the tracing indicates a pulse of considerable tension, suggesting difficulty in the peripheral outflow and diminished vigour or power of the ventricular contraction." Dr. Whitwell's tracings during a period in which a patient becomes clearer in mind show quite an opposite condition of the circulation. Even the stage of transition may be shown. We are indebted to him for permission to use the interesting sphygmograms which are appended, and with which he has illustrated a paper in the *Lancet*, Oct. 17, 1891, entitled, "A Study of the Pulse in Stupor" ("Stenotic Dystrophoneurosis")

The descriptions below indicate the patient's state when the tracing was taken.

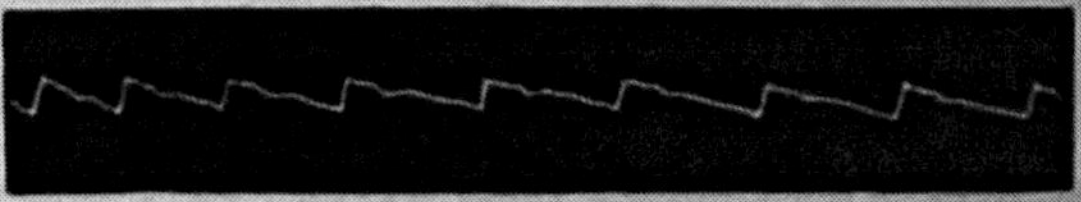

FIG. 1.—Tracing of pulse during stage of stupor, from case of intermittent stupor.

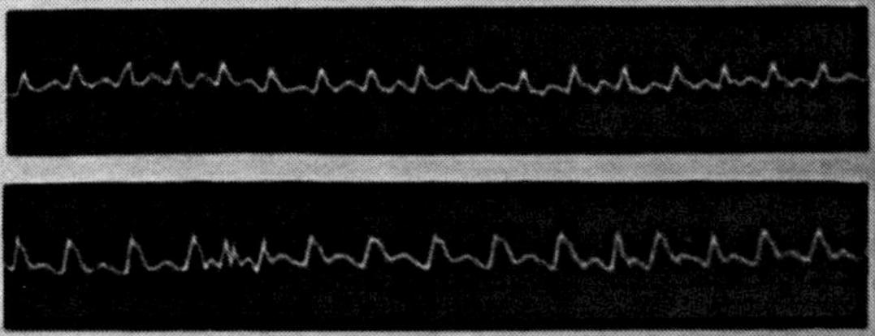

FIGS. 2 AND 3.—Same case under administration of amyl nitrite during stage of stupor.

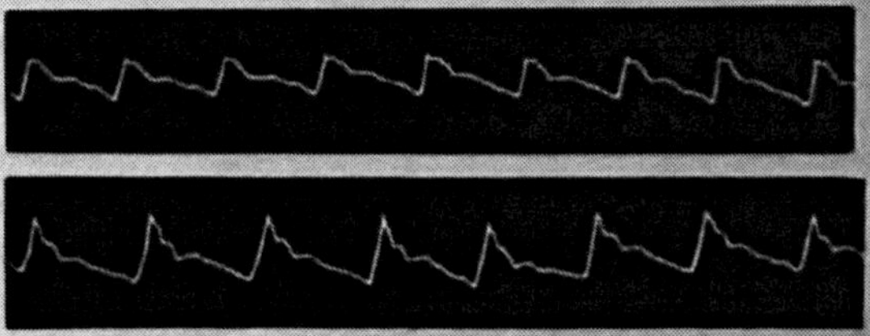

FIGS. 4 AND 5.—Same case during transition stage between stupidity and lucidity.

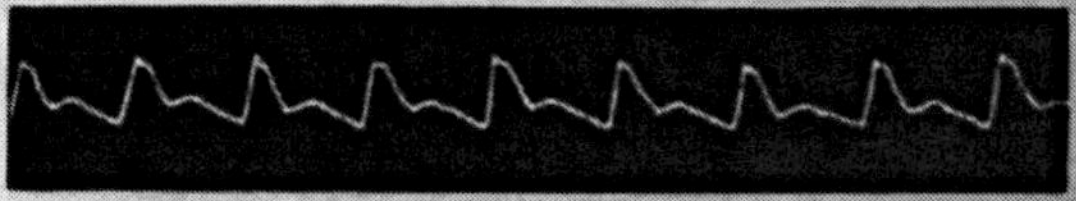

FIG. 6.—Same case during period of lucidity

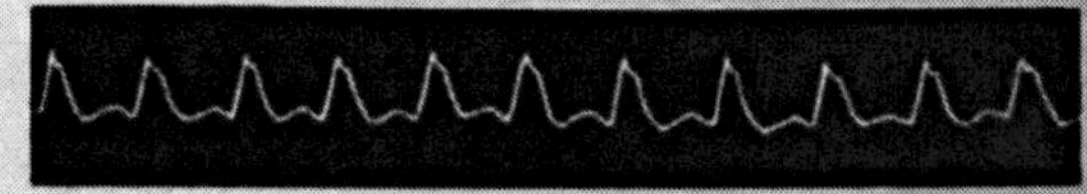

FIG. 7.—Effect of amyl nitrite on pulse during stage of lucidity.

Age.—Usually between twenty and thirty.

Sex.—Young men are especially liable to pass into mental stupor. These cases are generally associated with sexual vice.

Causes.—Any circumstance involving brain exhaustion or strain; shock from fright; loss of relative; sexual excess. Cases of mental stupor following mania, &c., general paralysis, and epileptic attacks, belong to the anergic form.

Circularity.—"By approaching the disease (stupor) from the physical side, Dr. Kahlbaum has made the disorders of motility, and not the form of mental derangement, the essential part of the malady, and has studied rigidity, spasm, choreic movements, and catalepsy, as they occur in the insane, as affections analogous to the occurrence of general paralysis. But I think he carries his views too far, and that as the morbid mental state conditions the motor trouble, it is right to take the former, and not the latter, as the basis of classification; at the same time, it is very important that, in view of the psycho-motor centres, these motor and psychical (as also the sensory) troubles should be brought into relation."*

* From writer's article "Mental Stupor," in the "Transactions of the International Medical Congress, 1881." Subsequent experience has strongly

Pathology.—Brain exhaustion, vaso-motor disturbance, and trophic changes. Using the term mental stupor in its broader sense, cases published by Dr. Whitwell,* in which the cerebral vessels were examined, go to prove that they were diminished in calibre. Cardiac complications favour the theory of arterial stenosis. So does also pallor of the disc in mental stupor, as observed by Dr. Aldridge and Dr. Whitwell. Dr. Wiglesworth thinks that a group of cases can be distinguished, the prominent symptom of which is self-absorption passing into vacuity, with muscular tremors and afterwards rigidity. He regards the pathological basis as a primary inflammatory affection of nerve cells, markedly, but not exclusively, the motor ones, followed by swelling of the cells with displacement of the nucleus. The microscopical appearances of the cortical cells, answering to this description, in two cases of mental stupor, are given by Dr. Wiglesworth, who admits, however, that more observations are necessary.†

In his remarkable thesis on Stupidité, Étoc-Demazy adduces evidence of general cerebral œdema from the post-mortems of patients dying in this mental condition.

Prognosis.—The prognosis of mental stupor with melancholy delusions is not very good. Even in those cases in which the mental cloud is dispersed, serious bodily symptoms are frequently developed. Pulmonary disease insidiously creeps in. Emaciation becomes more and more marked, and the patient succumbs.

Treatment.—In a large number of cases a considerable time will elapse before remedies are likely to take effect. Shower baths have often proved beneficial. The prolonged bath has appeared to be the means of cure when most other remedies have been tried and failed. Nitro-glycerine has been known to remove mental stupor, but with only temporary results so far as we are aware. A moderate form of drill in the form of being placed between two attendants who walk at a good pace is effectual in some instances. Galvanism applied with care to the head may be useful. (*See* Katatonia.) The Editor.

STUPOR VIGILANS (*vigilans*, wakeful). A synonym of Catalepsy.

STUPOROUS INSANITY. (*See* Stupor, Mental.)

STUTTERING. (*See* Stammering.)

confirmed the view here expressed. See, in confirmation, an able article in the *Journal of Mental Science*, April 1892, by Dr. Goodall, Pathologist at the Wakefield County Asylum.

* *Journal of Mental Science*, Oct. 1889.

† See *Journal of Mental Science*, Oct. 1883.

SUB-DELIRIUM.—A low lethargic state complicated with muttering delirium.

SUBJECTIVE CONSCIOUSNESS.—In this mental state, that which occupies the consciousness is something contemplated as the *ego*. "That *objective* force differs in nature from force as we know it *subjectively* is intellectually intelligible, yet to conceive of force in the *non-ego* different from the conception of force in the *ego* is utterly beyond our power" (Spencer). Subjective science is the theory of that which knows.

SUBJECTIVE SENSATIONS.—Sensations caused by internal stimuli, and not due to any external object.

SUCCURSAL ASYLUMS.—Term used (especially in Ireland) for a provincial asylum appropriated to one particular class of lunatics, namely the insane poor who are incurable and tranquil.

SUFFOCATIO HYSTERIA, SUFFOCATIO MULIERUM, SUFFOCATIO UTERINA.—Terms for globus hystericus. (*See* Hysteria.)

SUFFUSIO DIMIDIANS (*suffusio*, an overspreading or clouding; *dimidians*, halving). A symptom in migraine, in which only one-half of the field of vision is perceived by the mind.

SUGGESTION AND HYPNOTISM.—We shall endeavour in this short article to give in a condensed form our views on suggestion and hypnotism.

Definition.—Suggestion in its widest sense may be defined as the act by which an idea is introduced into and accepted by the sensorium. Every idea is transmitted to the brain by a sense organ, but it does not, however, become a suggestion unless it is accepted, and this acceptance often takes place by reason of the tendency to credence inherent in the human mind.

1. The idea may be transmitted directly by the suggested speech to the brain as a *direct suggestion*; or, again, it may be created by the brain in consequence of an impression received—*indirect suggestion*. In the latter case psychical individualism comes into play, so that the same impression may give rise to different suggestions, because each brain-reaction in its own peculiar way transforms the impression differently. The first impression is the germ of the suggestion, and is elaborated by the fertile mental soil.

2. The suggestion having been made, and the idea accepted by the brain, there then follows a centrifugal phenomenon—every suggested idea which has been accepted tends to become an act—*i.e.*, sensation, visual image, movement, action, passion, &c., or in other words, every cere-

bral cell stimulated by an idea stimulates those nerve-fibres which are to realise this idea. This is the law of **ideo-dynamism** as we call it. No one has understood this law better, and illustrated it by more numerous examples, than Dr. Hack Tuke in his "Influence of the Mind on the Body." The idea thus may become a sensation—*e.g.*, the idea of having fleas causes the sensory phenomenon of itching. The idea may become an image—*e.g.*, hallucinations during sleep and when awake. The idea may become a visceral sensation or organic action—*e.g.*, the administration of bread-pills as a purgative, vomiting by a substance believed to be an emetic, &c.; or the idea may become movement or action—*e.g.*, table-turning and the phenomena of thought-reading are based on this fact.

3. In Medicine suggestion may be utilised for **therapeutic purposes**; the brain stimulated by a certain idea tends to realise it as far as possible; it sends additional motor impulses to paralysed muscles; it neutralises painful sensations; it stimulates nerves of secretion; it acts in an inhibitory and dynamogenic manner, thus presiding over all the functions and organs of the body.

4. In order that an idea shall be accepted by the brain and realised by it, it is necessary for **the suggestion to be efficient.** In the normal condition the realisation as well as the cerebral automatism which tend to transform the idea into an act are limited. They are moderated by the higher reasoning faculties of the brain, which constitute the controlling power; reason struggles with the tendency to credence and cerebral automatism. Everything which diminishes the action of the reasoning faculties and weakens the inhibitory control increases the credence and cerebral automatism. Thus, natural sleep, by extinguishing the attention, leaves free play to the imagination, and allows the impressions which arise in the sensorium to become images, and to be accepted as realities. In the waking state credence is increased by religious faith (religious suggestion, miraculous cures), and by faith in medicines or medical practices (cure by fictitious medicines, magnets, metals, electricity, hydrotherapeutics, the tractors of Perkins, massage, the system of Mattei, &c.). The idea of cure suggested by these practices may cause the psychical organ to act and obtain from it the curative effect, not that the sum total of these practices is suggestion, but that suggestion is a factor in every one of them.

Among the means which increase credence and facilitate the transformation of the idea into action, [illegible] hypnotism. Hypno[illegible] adjuvant to suggestion. [illegible]

5. **How shall we [illegible]** Is it, as Braid says, a [illegible] duced by the concentration [illegible] a bright point, and by [illegible] of the mind on one idea? [illegible] jects influenced in this way, [illegible] must be noted, some who are [illegible] their hypnosis, who yet [illegible] memory of everything [illegible] when they were in the hypno[illegible] and in whom we obtain without [illegible] rent sleep all the phenomena [illegible] hypnosis, such as catalepsy, [illegible] and even hallucinations, and [illegible] effects. In those individuals [illegible] susceptible to real hypnotic [illegible] amnesia on waking, the series [illegible] tions, instead of commencing [illegible] sleep, may begin with sensory [illegible] phenomena, or with uninduced [illegible] actions. The sleep may be [illegible] other phenomena, or it may be [illegible] from them. In one word, sleep is [illegible] phenomenon obtained by [illegible] which, although it cannot be pro[illegible] all individuals, if obtained, [illegible] suggestibility, but is not indispen[illegible] the production of the other phe[illegible] hypnosis; sleep is in the same way [illegible] others, a phenomenon of sugges[illegible] It would be best completely to [illegible] the word "hypnotism," and to [illegible] by the term "condition of sug[illegible] If the words hypnotism, hyp[illegible] hypnotic state are to be retained, [illegible] may be defined as a *peculiar [illegible] condition which may be artific[illegible] duced, and which, if brought into [illegible] creases in various degrees the sugges[illegible]* —i.e., *the tendency—to be influenced [illegible] idea which is accepted and realised [illegible] brain.*

6. **How is this Psychical Condition, i.e., Hypnosis—produced?**—All the proceedings of ancient mesmerists and modern hypnotists, the *baquet* of Mesmer, the tree of Puységur, the passes and different manipulations, the staring at a bright object as practised by Braid, the revolving mirror of Luys, &c., may be reduced to one factor—viz., the endeavour to make an impression on the subject, and induce in his sensorium the idea of the phenomenon which we desire to obtain, namely, sleep. The best and simplest means is speech. In very susceptible subjects a simple word is sufficient; in most, however, it must be enforced by gestures, by a firm manner of address, by gentle or by strong insinuation, by the operator fixing the subject's eyes or

closing his eyelids, and by direct command. In hospital practice, where this command is very easy on account of the authority of the physician, it is possible to influence nine subjects out of ten, and to bring almost all,—five out of six—into profound sleep, with amnesia on waking. In private practice, however, success is only obtainable in a smaller proportion of cases; amnesia on re-awaking is produced but in one out of four or five patients operated upon; in most cases, however, we are able after one or more *séances* to produce a variety of the phenomena of suggestibility—viz., motor suggestions, such as catalepsy, paralysis, movements, and various actions; suggestions of sensibility, such as anæsthesia, analgesia, sensations of cold, heat, &c.; suggestions affecting the senses, such as deafness, blindness, anosmia, &c.; sensory images, as hallucinations of the different senses; suggestions of actions, passive obedience, robbery, murder, &c.; post-hypnotic suggestions — *i.e.*, suggestions which are realised a shorter or longer time after waking.

7. **The suggestibility is variable,** and the so-called hypnotic condition comprises various stages. These have been classified as follows by Liébault:—

(*a*) *Somnolency*, difficulty in raising the eyelids; in 1888, 6.06 per cent. of his subjects presented this first stage.

(*b*) *Light sleep*, commencement of catalepsy; the subjects are able to alter the position of their limbs if challenged; 17.48 per cent. of the patients treated presented this stage.

(*c*) The light sleep becomes *deeper*; dulness and catalepsy; ability to execute automatic movements; the subject has no longer sufficient will-power to arrest the suggested automatism; 35.89 per cent. are thus influenced.

(*d*) *Intermediary light sleep*; the subjects are unable to fix their attention on any one but the hypnotist, and can recollect only what has passed between themselves and him; 7.22 per cent. of the patients.

(*e*) *Ordinary somnambulistic sleep*, characterised by complete amnesia on awaking and by hallucinations during sleep; submission to the will of the hypnotist; 24.94 per cent.

(*f*) *Profound somnambulistic sleep*, characterised by amnesia on awaking, and by hypnotic and post-hypnotic hallucinations; absolute submission to the hypnotist; 4.66 per cent.

Our own observations have not led us to observe the exclusive *rapport* between subject and hypnotist in profound sleep noted by Liébault, and we have established the following classification.

(I.) Hypnotic conditions with **persistence of memory.**

(*a*) *Torpor*, somnolence or partial suggestibility (of heat, cold, &c.).

(*b*) *Inability to open the eyes spontaneously.*

(*c*) *Catalepsy* (by suggestion) *with possibility of breaking it.*

(*d*) *Irresistible catalepsy.*

(*e*) *Muscular contractions and analgesia* (by suggestion).

(*f*) *Automatic obedience.*

(II.) Hypnotic conditions **with sleep and amnesia on awaking.**

(*a*) *Amnesia on waking, absence of hallucinations.*

(*b*) *Hallucinations during sleep.*

(*c*) *Hallucinations during sleep, as well as post-hypnotic hallucinations and suggestibility in the awake condition.*

Every one of these stages shares the symptoms of the preceding ones. This classification, however, is purely schematic. Everything is individual, and every subject has his special susceptibility.

We call *artificial somnambulism* that condition of suggestion in which there are active hallucinations.

8. We shall now briefly consider **the different manifestations of hypnosis.** The subject to whom sleep has been suggested rests usually with his eyes closed, the eyelids often tremulously agitated; he is mostly inert, like an ordinary sleeper, except when he is made to act. Respiration and pulse are not altered; if they are, it is due to emotion, and suggestion is able to suppress any phenomena of emotion after one or two sittings. The subject is never unconscious, he hears everything that is said, and even if he is amnesic after waking we may by simple affirmation awake the recollection of everything that has happened during the apparent unconsciousness. The subject can always be made to talk during sleep.

An arm elevated and kept suspended for a few seconds often remains in this position spontaneously. If it does not remain there, it may be brought about by saying, "You are not able to bring it down." This is catalepsy, and is purely suggestive. The subject retains the position which he is made to assume, either because he has not sufficient psychical initiative to change it, or because on account of real or imagined suggestion, he is convinced that he cannot alter it. Some, if challenged, are able to make an appeal to their dulled energy, and to break through the spell, while others are quite unable to do so. The catalepsy may be flabby, waxen or tetanic.

Analgesia and anaesthesia may be spontaneous, due to the fact that the nervous force is concentrated in the brain, and detracted from the periphery. On the other hand, they may not be spontaneous, but may be suggested; they may also be absent. The subjects may be susceptible to illusions—*i.e.*, we may be able to pervert their sensory images—*e.g.*, we may give water the taste of wine. We may also "hallucinate" them—*i.e.*, produce in their brains sensory images of all kinds, visual, auditory, olfactory, gustatory, tactile, visceral, and complex. The hallucinations may be passive, as in ordinary dreams; the subject may be present at the scene which his imagination, prompted thereto by the suggestion, produces, without corporeally taking part in it. The hallucination may be active, spontaneous, or brought about by the suggestion, as in natural somnambulism. The subject, *e.g.*, sees a dog, is frightened, tries to get out of danger, feels himself bitten, gives evidence of pain, puts his hand to the supposed wound, &c. These hallucinations may be more or less vivid as in a dream, and the image may be indistinct or it may be very real. All degrees are possible, according to the impressionability of the subject, and it may be increased by hypnotic training.

A suggestion is *post-hypnotic* when it is suggested during the hypnosis and is realised in the waking condition after a shorter or longer time. Some subjects may realise the suggestion after several months or even after a year.

Negative hallucinations consist in the effacement of existing sensory images from the mind—*e.g.*, the subject on waking does not perceive a certain person; the latter may pinch or prick him or undress him, but he appears unaffected by his presence.

Retro-active hallucinations consist in the creation in the mind of the subject of all kinds of illusory recollections which do not correspond to reality. The subject may be made to believe that he has seen something—*e.g.*, that he passed through a certain street a week ago, and that he has been knocked down and robbed; the image exists in the brain as if the event in question had really happened. Thus, one may produce in the waking condition false witnesses who thoroughly believe what they say.

Amnesia on waking may be the result of the concentration of nervous activity in the sensorium upon the suggested impression during the hypnotic sleep. On waking, this nervous activity is redistributed over the whole [illegible] pression is no longer [illegible] nated by the nervous [illegible] conscious one. In order [illegible] make it once more perce[illegible] sary only to illuminate [illegible] the nervous activity upon [illegible] collection of the impression [illegible] the subject. Thus, we may [illegible] selves that the suggested [illegible] cination is but apparent; [illegible] the subject recollect every[illegible] seen, although in reality he [illegible] thing. The physical and [illegible] the power of perception, but [illegible] tion neutralised all perceptions [illegible] they were produced.

A subject who accomplishes [illegible] action after a long time without [illegible] remembered the suggestion [illegible] interval has only apparently [illegible] collection. This recollection may [illegible] on every occasion when he [illegible] his attention upon himself and [illegible] distracted by his senses, [illegible] neously into the second condition [illegible] sciousness with predominance of [illegible] ginative faculty. When, [illegible] consciousness is normal, when [illegible] to him, and when the nervous [illegible] diffused toward the periphery, [illegible] lection is extinct. After the [illegible] accomplished, he does not [illegible] suggestion of the act; he fully [illegible] what the suggestion has produced [illegible] his own intentional act, because [illegible] have said, the normal and con[illegible] state does not recollect the [illegible] but the second, the concentrated [illegible] nambulistic mental state, does.

(9) The doctrine of suggestion [illegible] from a sociological, historical, [illegible] gical, legal, and therapeutic view, [illegible] large field for contemplation [illegible] does not permit us to enlarge on. [illegible] We must, however, say a word [illegible] about criminal suggestions. It [illegible] averred that suggested crimes [illegible] committed, that the experience of [illegible] but the experience of the laboratory [illegible] somnambulists, it is true, play [illegible] without conviction; as in a natural [illegible] they do not lose the sense of their [illegible] Moreover, the moral sense, either [illegible] or suggested by education, may [illegible] primary suggestion which does not [illegible] contrary suggestions to enter the [illegible] Other somnambulists, however, like [illegible] dreamers, identify themselves with [illegible] *rôle*; their true moral consciousness [illegible] abolished, and they will commit [illegible] overt act. Some conduct themselves like impulsive epileptics; a blind [illegible] impulse leads them to the suggested [illegible]

Others act under the influence of an insane delusion or hallucination—*e.g.*, they will commit murder because they desire revenge or believe it to be their duty. If the moral sense is absent, and if the suggestibility is great, the soil is naturally prepared for insane ideas. An honest man, however, may also commit a crime by suggestion, dragged into it by an impulsive vertigo or guided by an insane idea.

(10) The therapeutical use of suggestion, or **psychotherapeutics**, as it has been well termed by Dr. Hack Tuke, who has so well comprehended its importance, is a most valuable application of suggestion, for which hypnotism is the most efficient adjuvant. Although suggestion may, through the vaso-motor nerves, produce remarkable modifications, as redness, blisters, stigmata, &c., suggestion employed therapeutically is almost exclusively functional in its action. It is of service especially in certain neuroses when there is no organic change, or when the latter is produced by a functional disorder; hysteria, chorea, spasms, tetanus, nervous vomiting, nervous pains, arthralgia, visceralgia, and neuralgia may very often be treated by hypnotic suggestion. Suggestion is often useful in organic diseases when functional disorder accompanies, supervenes upon the lesion, or underlies it, or when the dynamical disorders surpass those of the organic lesion. In this manner it cures sometimes chronic articular pains, and by suppressing the pain and re-establishing the articular movements and the muscular play, it restores the function, and thus also the organ. Suggestion often cures hemianæsthesia, and sometimes even paralysis, of cerebral origin when the seat of the lesion does not make it incurable; it often brings about remarkable improvements in myelitis, ataxy, disseminated sclerosis, &c. It may diminish oppressive sensations in diseases of the chest; it may restore the appetite and favourably influence tubercular affections by modifying the soil affected. Even if it does not cure the disease it may give considerable relief, and it therefore finds its application in all diseases. It is powerless, so far as our experience extends, against mental alienation; there the auto-suggestion is predominant.

Braid made use of hypnotism as a therapeutic agent, but not recognising the *rôle* of verbal suggestion, he proceeded with empirical manipulations. Liébault, of Nancy, first discovered the therapeutical value of suggestion, and applied it in a systematic method of treatment; we ourselves have introduced it into the official *clinique*. To the Nancy school belong the numerous physicians who disseminate in two worlds the benefits of suggestive therapeutics.

H. BERNHEIM.

[*References.*—Bernheim, De la Suggestion et de ses applications à la Thérapeutique, third edition, Paris, 1891; Hypnotisme, Suggestion, Psycho-thérapie, Paris, 1891. Liébeault, Le Sommeil provoqué et les états analogues, Paris, 1889; Thérapeutique suggestive, Paris, 1891. Liégeois, De la Suggestion et du Somnambulisme dans leurs rapports avec la Jurisprudence et la Médicine Légale, Paris, 1889. Beaunis, Le Somnambulisme provoqué, études physiologiques et psychologiques, Paris, 1887. Forel, Der Hypnotismus und seine Handhabung, Stuttgart, 1891. Wetterstrand, Der Hypnotismus und seine Anwendung in der praktischen Medicin, Wien und Leipzig, 1891. Ringier, Erfolge des therapeutischen Hypnotismus in der Landpraxis, Munich, 1891. Moll, Der Hypnotismus, Berlin, 1889. Bérillon, Révue de l'Hypnotisme experimental et thérapeutique, Paris, 1887 à 1892.]

SUICIDE (*sui*, of self; *cædo*, I kill). *Suicidium*. The Abbé Desfontaines has the credit of having introduced this word in the last century.

History.—There has been no period in authentic history in which, so far as we know, there has been immunity from the practice of self-destruction. Further, among the instances which have occurred, there have been many which do not fall under the suspicion of mental disease.

In the history of the *Jews*, of the six cases recorded in the Old Testament that of Abimelech,* shows an attempt at suicide completed by another person. Zimri,† after the murder of the King of Israel discovered that he had a rival in another candidate for the throne, and in consequence destroyed his palace, and himself by fire. The death of Samson by his own action has led to much discussion among the Fathers and other writers, its true character admitting of various interpretations. From any point of view it is a mixed case. The primary object of the act was revenge. In carrying out his intention, he was willing to perish himself. The suicide of Saul‡ is sufficiently simple in its character, and was, so to speak, a natural course to follow in order to save himself from the insults of the Philistine "lest these uncircumcised come and thrust me through and abuse me." The suicide of Saul's armour-bearer was the natural sequel. The last example, that of Ahithophel,§ is as free as the others from mental disorder. We put aside the ingenious explanations given by certain Jewish writers, in order to

* Judges ix. 3, 54; and 2 Sam. xi. 21.

† 1 Kings xvi. 9–18.

‡ 1 Sam. xxxi. 6; 2 Sam. iv. 10; 1 Chron. x. 4, 5.

§ 2 Sam. xvii. 23.

show that the cause of death was mental emotion and not suspension.

The "History of the Jewish War," by Josephus, contains many examples of self-destruction. "Phasælus killed himself; the wife of Pharoras carried poison about her as a provision against the uncertain future, and attempted self-destruction; also Herod the Great made an attempt upon his own life; some hundreds were induced by the pro-suicidal eloquent oration of the Jewish captain, Eleazar, to die by each other's and their own hands, and, finally, the almost equally eloquent anti-suicidal oration of Josephus himself could not dissuade or prevent three or four dozen Jewish captains from willing and compassing death in the same manner."*

The suicide of Judas Iscariot need not detain us. The amount of patristic lore, and of learned but fantastic commentary, which has been expended upon this event, is prodigious.

Greeks and Romans. — The ancient Greeks do not appear to have regarded suicide as a crime. Plato, however, although in his Utopia he does not forbid burial to those who commit suicide, does order that the spot where they are laid should be in a lonely place, unmarked by any stone.† The suicide of Lycurgus, deliberately done, and for a well-intended object, would seem to justify the opinion that the Spartans did not regard suicide with aversion.

The examples of suicide recorded in the classics are numerous, the well-known case of Cato standing prominently out from others of less note. Cicero has spoken of the act as the result of his peculiar character.‡

The self-destruction of Cleombrotus, the Ambraciote, has been, along with that of Cato, charged upon Socrates by some of the Fathers. "If an irresistible eagerness to bathe in the ocean of immortal life seized upon Cleombrotus, after he had contemplated that image of the Blessed which the pencil of Plato, guided by the revealings of Socrates, had sketched on the pages of Phaedo, we must, I presume, conceive him to have been an enthusiastic and religious, rather than a reflective and matured person, whether young or old. He simply had not rightly understood the distinction which Socrates so broadly draws in this very Dialogue between the philosophic death and actual [illegible] should be stated [illegible] the third century B.C. [illegible] act of Cleombrotus as [illegible] for immortality born [illegible] Plato's pages. This, however, [illegible] different position from [illegible] by patristic writers. It [illegible] proved that Socrates and [illegible] opposed to suicide. The [illegible] said of Aristotle. The opposite [illegible] has been maintained in regard [illegible] timents, however, as well as [illegible] philosophers above mentioned.

It would be a serious omission [illegible] refer to the opinions expressed by [illegible]. He held that suicide was an [illegible] under certain circumstances, [illegible] poverty, slavery, grief, in old age [illegible] less disease. Or, again, when [illegible] death was in prospect. Two [illegible] tifications remain, satiety of life [illegible] inability to maintain a position [illegible] ance with the individual's principles [illegible] other Stoic, Marcus Aurelius Antoninus, held that a man should end his [illegible] when his life was no longer in [illegible] with his own conviction. [illegible] old age was a reason for terminating [illegible] before it actually came and weakened [illegible] power to form a reasonable judgment [illegible]

Epictetus has expressed in his [illegible] tation a limited approval of suicide. [illegible] is not, however, very lucid in determining the exact line between causeless, [illegible] therefore criminal, self-murder, and justifiable suicide. By Tacitus, suicide [illegible] regarded as "mors opportuna"—a [illegible] proper and, indeed, meritorious mode of escaping from the sorrows and [illegible] of this life. Pliny the younger [illegible] approved of suicide under certain circumstances. He expressed his surprise that a man of whom he speaks who was old and ill should have chosen to live [illegible] *tamen et vivere volebat.* Epp. lib. [illegible] 18, p. 107 Migault).

With regard to Cicero, his opinions appear to have wavered, and passages may be quoted on either side. In the "De Officiis" occurs a pro-suicidal utterance in connection with the death of Cato. In the "De Senectute," however, the very same act is condemned.†

The same uncertain sound is noticeable in the works of Plutarch. It is said by Migault, whose work is eminently thoughtful, that he did not so much "combat suicide *per se* as suicide à la Zeno, and Chrysippus, and that though he certainly did not approve of the dictum that the

* "Suicide, chiefly in reference to Philosophy, Theology, and Legislation." By H. G. Migault. Heidelberg, 1856, p. 137, fourth section, p. 137.

† "De Legibus," lib. 9.

‡ "De Offic." l. c. 31.

* Migault, *op. cit.*, "Classical Paganism," p. [illegible]

† See the question fully and ably discussed by Migault, *op. cit.*, pp. 108–127.

wise and happy as such ought to die voluntarily, it does not by any means follow that he would have been equally loath to affirm that the over-tried and ill-starred ought not occasionally to do so."*

In respect to Roman law relating to suicides there has been much discussion.

It appears that the clearest notice of ancient punishment for self-destruction among the Romans is contained in Pliny's "Natural History,"† where he writes, "Tarquinius Priscus built the Cloaca by the hands of the people. The labour, however, was, one knew not whether more wearisome or dangerous; and occasionally a Quirite escaped from the tedium of it by suicide. This king now invented a new remedy which had not occurred to anybody before him, and has not occurred to anybody after him. He ordered the corpses of all who died in this manner to be fastened to crosses exposed to the public gaze of the citizens, and at the same time, left to be torn in pieces by wild beasts and birds."‡

Reference should be made here to the remarkable suicidal epidemic among the Milesian virgins who were seized with an irresistible propensity to hang themselves, "all the entreaties and tears of their parents availed just as little as the representations of friends. They, in their suicide, even eluded all attention and cunning of their guards. Thus the evil was considered a divine punishment against which human aid would not be at all able to prevail; but at last a proposal was made by the advice of a clever man, according to which those who hanged themselves should be carried naked across the market-place to the place of burial. This proposition was approved of, and it not only checked the evil, but likewise destroyed in the virgins the desire for death."§

The East.—Among so-called barbaric nations in the East, one feature of suicide was, and is, remarkable, and offers a contrast to the way in which the act was regarded among the Greeks and Romans. This has been well brought out by Migault in the following passage:—"Whereas, the Greek and Roman writers viewed suicide at the utmost as a *human right*, an undoubted privilege, by the using of which the ills and discomforts of the present life might be escaped from, a decorous means of self-deliverance from temporal evils, a deed of philosophical heroism or physical nerve which the Divinity might be presumed to sanction, and Reason be affirmed even to command; suicide on the contrary, assumed, and in part still assumes, under the teaching of sundry barbaric creeds, the developed character of a *religious rite*, a path leading on to greater extra-terrestrial bliss, a deed unto which a sure divine recompense is vouchsafed in a future state of existence, a thing specially well-pleasing and even meritorious according to the estimate of the Godhead, and as such not only permitted and vindicated, but even promulgated and prescribed."*

Zoroaster is cited as asserting that "man is not to compel the soul to emigrate out of the body."

Ariaspes, in the fourth century B.C., took poison in consequence of having understood that he would be executed by his father. The mother of Darius, Sisygambis, when she heard of the death of Alexander, committed suicide. Sutteeism among the Hindoos, and similar practices among the Ethiopians and other peoples, must be regarded as, with few exceptions, practically involuntary suicide. It would be quite beyond our purpose to enter fully into this remarkable development of religious forms of suicide.

The teaching of the Koran is opposed to suicide. "Neither slay yourselves, for God is merciful towards you; and whoever does this maliciously and wickedly, he will surely cast him to be broiled in hell-fire, and this is easy with God."† No proof is forthcoming that the Mohammedans ordered any difference to be made in regard to the funeral rites for those who committed suicide. It is suggested by Migault that the rarity of the deed rendered it unnecessary to make any special law among Mussulmans.

Among Christians.—We believe that the earliest *Christian* law against an attempt to commit suicide was a decree of the Council of Toledo in 693.‡ The punishment consisted of excommunication for two months (duorum mensium spatio, et a catholicorum collegio, et a corpore ac Christi sanguine sacro manebit omnimodo alienus).

At the latter end of the fourteenth century, letters of indulgence were granted by the Parliament of Paris to those who had attempted suicide. The interesting fact is stated that they were on some occasions treated as if possessed (demoniaci), in an

* *Op. cit.*, p. 132.
† Lib. 36, ch. xv. sec. 24.
‡ Migault, *op. cit.*, 173.
§ Plutarch, "De virtutibus mulierum," Opera, tom. vii. p. 22.

* *Op. cit.*, "Barbaric Paganism," p. 4.
† Sale's translation, i. 99.
‡ Mansi, t. xii. p. 71: Concilium Toletanum, xvi. c. 4.

abbey where cases of possession were cared for. It is clear that we have here genuine cases of suicidal melancholia. Migault quotes from Carpentier* the curious passage on which this statement is founded:—"Nostris Demoniacle, Insanus, demens. Lit. remiss. ann. 1384 in Reg. 125. Chartoph. reg. ch. 120: Pierre Nagot a esté le plus du temps, et par especial en temps d'esté, fol et Demoniacle, et s'est plusieurs foys voulu noyer; . . . . et pour cause de ses folies . . . . il fu prins . . . . et porté en une abbaye nommée S. Sever, ... en laquelle abbaye l'on maine les Demoniacles."

Hugh Grotius regarded suicide as a felony, and therefore deserving of severe notice.

Hume, Voltaire, Rousseau, Montesquieu, Montaigne, Gibbon, as also Sir Thomas More in his "Utopia," have defended suicide under special circumstances.

Blackstone† says, "Now the question follows, what punishment can human laws inflict on one who has withdrawn himself from their reach? They can only act upon what he has left behind him, his reputation and fortune. On the former by an ignominious burial in the highway, with a stake driven through his body (and without Christian rites of sepulture); on the latter by a forfeiture of all his goods and chattels to the King."

The Rubric for the Order for the Burial of the Dead was composed in 1661. Accompanying it is the note: "The office ensuing is not to be used for any who die unbaptised or excommunicate, or *have laid violent hands upon themselves.*" On this passage Shepperd remarks that "it must not be considered a new law, but merely as explanatory of the ancient canon law, and of the previous usage in England."

The clown in "Hamlet" assumes that Ophelia will not receive Christian burial on account of committing suicide.

The law in regard to the treatment of the corpse of the suicide was rescinded in the year 1823 (4 Geo. IV. c. 52) having for some years gone into desuetude.

Acts 43 & 44 Vict. c. 41, 45–46 Vict. c. 19, provide that the body of a suicide may be interred either silently, or with any such orderly or Christian religious service at the grave as the person in charge of the body thinks fit.‡

Sir James Fitzjames Stephen says: "Suicide may be [illegible] injurious to society, but [illegible] less degree than murder. [illegible] the person killed we cannot [illegible] injury to survivors is generally [illegible] is a crime which produces [illegible] alarm, and which cannot be [illegible] would, therefore, be better [illegible] regard it as a crime, and to [illegible] any one who attempted to kill [illegible] who assisted any other person [illegible] should be liable to secondary [illegible]ment."*

Frequency.—The formula in [illegible] the increase of suicide has been [illegible] down by Morselli: "In the [illegible] the civilised states of Europe and [illegible] the frequency of suicide shows a [illegible] and uniform increase, so that [illegible] voluntary death since the beginning of the century has increased, and goes on increasing more rapidly than the geometrical augmentation of the population and of the general mortality."†

In view of the erroneous [illegible] which have been drawn from statistics in regard to the increase of insanity, we naturally feel great doubt whether [illegible] allowance has been made for the [illegible] of fallacy which affect the conclusions arrived at, but we append the following:

Table I.,‡ showing the Number of Suicides per 1,000,000 in the different European States, and the Increase or Decrease during certain Terms of Years.

Year.	Country.	Number of Suicides per Million.	Increase per Million.	Term of Years.
1880	Portugal	16	3	5
1880	Spain	19	2	5
1883	Ireland	24	6	5
1878	Russia and Finland	35	1.2 (dec.)	6
1881	Italy	44	7	3
1881	Scotland	48	11	5
1880	Holland	51	Stationary	10
1882	England	74	7	10
1875	Norway	75	33 (dec.)	11
1879	Belgium	90	22	5
1877	Sweden	101	15	5
1880	Bavaria	100	11	5
1877	Austria	144	24	3
1880	Hanover	150	30	5
1877	Prussia	168	34	4
1880	France	216	36	5
1881	Switzerland	240	25	5
1878	Denmark	265	38	5
1878	Saxony	469	170	5

* *Vide* "Glossarium novum ad scriptores medii ævi," s. v., Dæmoniaci.

† "Commentaries on the Laws of England," 1765, book iv. ch. 14.

‡ "Suicide," by W. Wynn Westcott, M.D. London, Deputy Coroner for Central Middlesex, 1885, p. 45.

* Quoted by Westcott, *op. cit.*, p. 49.

† "Suicide," by Henry Morselli, M.D.: International Scientific Series, London, 1881, p. [illegible]

‡ From Westcott, *op. cit.*, p. 60.

We are on safe ground when we take the annual returns of suicides in England and Wales during a certain period, as from 1861 to 1888. Table II. exhibits the increase which has taken place. Taking the first five years (1861–1865) and comparing the frequency of suicide during that period with its frequency during the quinquennium, 1884–1888, we find that there were sixty-five suicides to a million persons living, in the former, and seventy-eight in the latter, term of years, and that the rise was fairly progressive. Again, taking the periods 1861–1870 and 1881–1888, we find the increase per cent. to be as follows:—All ages: persons, 15.2; males, 19.2; females, 8.8.

Table II., showing the Annual Number of Suicides in England and Wales to a Million Persons Living, 1861–1888.

Date.	Male.	Female.	Persons.
1861	100	35	67
1862	97	34	65
1863	97	33	64
1864	98	32	64
1865	99	34	66
1866	91	34	62
1867	91	32	61
1868	105	35	69
1869	109	36	71
1870	106	34	69
1871	99	34	66
1872	97	35	66
1873	99	32	65
1874	104	32	64
1875	101	34	67
1876	111	37	73
1877	109	31	69
1878	107	36	70
1879	123	40	80
1880	120	37	77
1881	116	36	75
1882	113	38	74
1883	111	38	73
1884	117	35	75
1885	114	34	73
1886	125	39	81
1887	122	39	79
1888	124	39	80

Suicide in British India.—Suicide is favoured by the Brahmins. It is on the contrary discouraged by the disciples of Mahomet. It is stated by Dr. Westcott that "the floating British population exhibits a slightly higher ratio than that of the British at home."* We may state on his authority that the laws bearing upon voluntary deaths in British India are enacted by the Indian Penal Code, cap. xvi. ss. 300, 305, 306, and 309. Other regulations will be found in s. 19 of Reg. xix. of 1807; and Nizamut Adawlut Reports, vol. iii. of 1833.

* *Op. cit.*, p. 161.

The same authority estimates the average suicide-rate in India at about 40 per million. The causes of suicide among the natives are mainly four, namely: revenge or accusation, religion, physical suffering, grief, shame, and jealousy. It is stated that women nearly always make a choice of drowning, more particularly in wells. Under the head of religion would of course fall, death by being crushed under the car of Juggernath. Self-immolation (chandi) for the purpose of spiting another person, and making some imaginary charge calculated to turn the neighbours against a person, is said to be still resorted to.

Ætiology of Suicide (predisposing and exciting). **Climate.** — Morselli deduces from the statistics of suicides in Europe that the South (Italy, Spain, and Portugal) gives the minimum proportion, while this seems to rise by degrees as the centre is approached, which is at 50° of latitude. Suicides predominate in the centre of Europe between 47° and 57° of latitude, and 20° and 40° of longitude—a region covering 942,000 square kilomètres. The countries nearest this area have more, those more distant fewer, suicides. The suicidal area, so to speak, is in the temperate zone. It is obvious that it is impossible to isolate the influence of climate from such elements as civilisation, &c., which are concomitants of differing thermal regions. At the same time climate would seem to be a most important factor. Extremes of climate would seem to minimise the tendency to suicide. In Italy the highest averages are in the upper, the lowest in the southern regions.* A similar difference is observed in France, but the fact that Paris is in the north, introduces at once a source of fallacy. Belgium, Switzerland, Austria, and Bavaria present the same relative liability when northern and southern regions are compared. The general conclusion arrived at is that "in the centre of Europe, from the north-east of France to the eastern borders of Germany, a *suicidigenous* area exists, where suicide reaches the maximum of its intensity, and around which it takes a decreasing ratio to the limits of the northern and southern states."†

Telluric Conditions.—It is said that there is an inverse ratio between orography and the frequency of suicide. The highest proportion is alleged to occur in the plain of the Po, and after the valleys of Piedmont, Lombardy, Emilia, and Valicia, comes Latium. The lowest proportion is found in the mountain

* Morselli, *op. cit.*, p. 41.
† *Op. cit.*, p. 50.

regions of Italy. The same holds good in France. In our own country it appears that Scotland and Wales, which to a large extent are mountainous, yield a much lower proportion than the less hilly England. In the region of the Alps there is a minimum of suicides, while in the valleys of the Danube, Bohemia, &c., the proportion of suicide is larger. In Switzerland, the mountainous cantons follow the same rule, and present a contrast in this particular to the valleys of the Rhine, the Aar, and the Rhône. It is only necessary to add, that in Belgium, Sweden, and Norway, the same fact holds good.

Turning from the alleged influence of high and low countries to that of rivers, it seems that the countries where these are on a large scale are those in which the proportion of suicide is high, while in marshy low lands suicides are less common, as in certain provinces in Italy, the Landes in France, Ireland, the districts around the Zuyder Zee, as also in Jutland. Germany presents the same association of suicides with the distribution of large rivers. Further, it is maintained, that the suicidigenous regions are formed by comparatively recent alluvial deposits, as Denmark, Poland, the valley of the Thames, &c. Scotland, Ireland, and Wales, most of Spain and Portugal, are examples of an opposite—that is, an earlier—geological formation, and a lower proportion of suicides. Morselli, to whom we must refer for more detail, asserts, "that the number of suicides always presents a lower average on the chalk and slate soils of the secondary period. Lastly, will be found those few countries on the lime, gneiss, slate and granite rocks of the great Alpine system."*

Interesting as all these statements are, we confess that we accept the conclusions with considerable reserve, first, because the returns of suicide in different countries may differ in their completeness, and therefore may be misleading; and secondly, because the elements of the problem are so exceedingly complex that we are in great danger of referring a maximum amount of suicides to the wrong cause.

Seasons and Months.—As is well known, it was formerly supposed that dark damp weather favoured the occurrence of suicide. It is not surprising that the gloomy month of November in our own country was believed to be a specially obnoxious one in this respect. Statistics in this instance appear to be tolerably free from fallacy, and to allow us to set aside the popular impression, and to prove the association of the maximum amount of suicides with [illegible] Guerry* found that the [illegible] of 85,334 suicides in [illegible] 1835–60 occurred under the [illegible] the minimum under the [illegible]. The order in which suicide [illegible] influenced by the seasons [illegible] Summer, spring, autumn, and [illegible]. This result is based upon large [illegible] data in Europe, and justifies the [illegible] "among the surest and most [illegible]tible results of statistics." The [illegible] Tables given in the work upon which [illegible] the highest authority, we rely, ought to be carefully studied by all who wish to prosecute this important inquiry more thoroughly. One Table is given to show the influence of madness on suicide [illegible] to months, in Italy, France, and [illegible]. "The result agrees with the opinion [illegible] attributes the greater number of [illegible] the spring and summer months to the development of more numerous [illegible] affections. The proportion of [illegible] through madness does not, however, explain entirely the higher ratio of [illegible] *deaths from other causes* during spring and summer; the reason is that the [illegible] change may be brought on either by an inherent suicidal tendency, or by a tendency to madness. It is then to be noted that suicide and madness are not influenced so much by the intense heat of the advanced summer season as by the early spring and summer, which seise upon the organism not yet acclimatised and still under the influence of the cold season. And this also applies to the first cold weather in October and November, when the change from the warm to the cold season is most severely felt by the human constitution, and especially by the nervous system."†

As regards England and Wales [O]‡ no statistics can be obtained. For London, however, they are available, and of great interest. Singular as it may seem, the amount of suicide increases with the increase of daylight. At its minimum in December when the day is shortest, it rises month by month with a slight exception in February, till it reaches its maximum in June, when it falls gradually, with a very slight exception in October, until it

* *Op. cit.*, p. 55.

* Quoted by Morselli, *op. cit.*, p. 62.

† Morselli, *op. cit.*, p. 72.

‡ In this and other instances in which [O] occurs, the statement is Dr. Ogle's, being taken from his valuable paper read before the *Statistical* Society, Feb. 16, 1886, entitled "Suicides in England and Wales, in relation to Age, Sex, Season, and Occupation." His statistics have their own value, and if they differ from those which we give in preceding paragraphs when they refer to the same period and country, the reader will do well to take them as the more correct.

reaches its minimum in the dark days at the end of the year. Even slight exceptions would, Dr. Ogle believes, disappear, were the numbers on a larger scale. Why this greater amount of suicides in the summer than in the winter months is not very easily explained. It is no explanation to say that there is more insanity in the hot than in the cold months. Although there are more admissions to asylums in summer than in winter, it does not follow that the attacks commence in the warm weather. While, however, we do not dispute that this may be the case, we do not find, as might have been expected, that mental disorders are more frequent in hot than in cold climates, a circumstance pointed out by Guislain.

Meteorological Changes and Influence of the Moon.—The number of observations made is limited, and inference must be drawn with caution. We attach so little importance to the observations recorded, bearing on the changes in the barometer in relation to suicide, that we pass them by. As to the lunar influence, a Table is given in Morselli, but only for a single year, in regard to the number of suicides in the different phases of the moon. The proportion per thousand was as follows: New moon, 246.8; first quarter, 255.8; full moon, 238.6; last, 258.8. If this experience is confirmed by more numerous returns it would indicate an increase in suicides in the second and fourth lunar phases, and a decrease in the first and third.

Time of Day.—Of 11,822 suicides which happened in Prussia during four years, 1869–72, the higher proportion per thousand occurs in the night. From other Tables (France and Switzerland) it appears that "the *maximum* occurs from 6 A.M. to 12; at first there is a decrease in the hours P.M., then an increase which falls away from 3 to 6 o'clock, after which the number of suicides continues to diminish regularly in the evening hours until midnight; however, the *minimum* is not reached until the hour preceding the rising of the sun. The daily distribution of suicides is parallel to activity in business, to occupations and work; in short, with the noise which characterises the life of modern society, and not with silence, quiet, and isolation." *

Ethnology.—The influence of race is no doubt a marked factor in the causation of suicide; at the same time it is very difficult to distinguish from the associated geographical conditions, not to mention others which help to determine voluntary death. The annual number of suicides per 1,000,000 of the population is given by Morselli * as follows:

Scandinavia.	
Denmark	127.8
Norway	
Sweden	
Germans of the North.	
Prussia and its Conquests	150
Hamburg	
Ducal Hesse, &c.	
Germans of the South.	
Bavaria	165
Baden	
Würtemberg	
Saxony	
Austria	
German-Swiss, &c.	
Anglo-Saxons.	
England (excluding Wales)	70
United States	
South Australia	
Flemings.	
Netherlands	50
Flemish Province of Belgium, &c.	
Celts.	
Wales	30
Scotland	
Britain	
Ireland	
Celto-Romans.	
France (French Province of Belgium)	11
French-Swiss	
Northern Italy	
Western Romans.	
Spain	27
Peninsular and Lower Italy	
Italian-Swiss	
Eastern Romans.	
Transylvania	50
Roumania	
Slavs of the North-West.	
Russia	42
Bohemia	
Moravia	
Galicia—Buckovina	
Slavs of the South.	
Carniola	30
Croatia and Slavonia	
Dalmatia	
Magyars.	
Hungary	52
Finns and Lapps.	
Finland	40
Norrland	
Russian Baltic Province	
Slavo-Mongols.	
South-East Russia	51

"The peoples with the highest average inhabit the central regions, the chosen zone of the suicide, and after these the other peoples are arranged almost in direct ratio with the ethnical distance which separates them from the Germanic

* Morselli, *op. cit.*, p. 79.

* *Op. cit.*, p. 84.

nations; thus the Germans and the Latins will be found at the two ends of the scale, for although having come forth from the common Indo-Germanic stock, in the descent of European peoples, they will be found from time immemorial at the extremities of their two principal and most distant branches. . . . . The low position in point of numbers held by the English peoples, with regard to suicide, in comparison with the Germanic, whilst the first place in the civilised world as regards power and riches belongs to them without dispute, is astonishing; it is not modern Rome, it is not England, which gives the greater number of suicides. Admitting that in statistics we have to deal with deficiencies and want of exactness, it is not possible that, even if perfectly correct, we should ever have the German averages lower; nevertheless the Anglo-Saxons undoubtedly proceeded from the same stock as the Saxons, Dutch, and Low-Germans. . . . . The divergence between England and the countries where the Celtic or Gaelic race remains most pure, that is to say, Scotland, Ireland, and Wales, will prove the influence of the Germanic element infiltrated, especially in the first of these. And it is not to be wondered at if, under diverse climatic and social conditions, the English colonies in North America, producing a race so distinct from the mother-stock as that of the Yankees, still reveal in the excessive average of suicides so great a difference from their original European brethren."†

Civilisation.—Guided by the statistics which we have given, we must conclude that "madness and suicide are met with the more frequently in proportion as civilisation progresses."* Once more we may point out the effect of civilisation in securing fuller returns than can possibly be the case in uncivilised countries. It is simply impossible to make allowance for this source of error with any degree of certainty. All that we are justified in concluding is the apparent greater liability of the more cultured races of mankind.

Religion.—Jews are shown to be less prone to suicide than Christians. When Protestantism and Roman Catholicism are compared, it appears that those who profess the faith of the former are the most liable to resort to self-destruction. Saxony, Denmark, Scandinavia, and Prussia, are cited by Morselli as presenting an unfavourable contrast to the lower rate of suicide in Italy, Spain, and Portugal. It is stated that in Protestant States the average number of suicides per

* Morselli, *op. cit.*, p. 117.
† *Op. cit.* pp. 83–86.

million is 190, while [illegible] in Catholic States, it [illegible] On the other hand, in [illegible] there is a mixture of [illegible] Christian religion, the average [illegible] suicides per million is 96. [illegible] of Protestantism may partly be [illegible] to its facilitating the development [illegible] intellectual culture; it is the [illegible] countries, and any country with [illegible] inhabitants, who are always [illegible] both in instruction and suicide." [illegible]

Culture.—This brings us to [illegible] element of the complex problem [illegible] the effect of culture. A Table has [illegible] prepared classifying the population [illegible] various countries according to [illegible] and education. The following [illegible] given:* Of four European [illegible] Prussia stands first, both as to [illegible] and suicides. France comes [illegible] in both characteristics. Thirdly, [illegible] and Hungary have about the same number of suicides, although in the [illegible] portion of the uneducated the [illegible] stands in a worse position than [illegible] by about 10 per cent. It is a very [illegible] picture, and one still more highly [illegible] by a more extensive collection of [illegible] for the result establishes the [illegible] rule that suicide occurs in inverse [illegible] ignorance. At the same time we are far from thinking that it is safe to take these statistics as altogether correct guides.

Sex.—The Table referred to in the foregoing section shows a low proportion of female suicides to male suicides. Here, however, it behoves us to remember that sex is itself a complex fact; for example, it includes the relative degree of male and female education as well as the differences, bodily and mental, between the sexes. Morselli confidently states that "in every country the proportion of suicides is one woman to three or four men; as in crime, it is also one in four or five."† This disparity is attributed to the difficulties of existence—the struggle for life which is so much greater among men.

In England and Wales [O], the rate for males during twenty-six years was [illegible] annually per million living, while the rate for females was only 41, or in the proportion of 254 to 100. Indeed, when correction is made for the difference between the age-distribution of males and females, the proportion becomes still more striking, namely, 267 to 100. If the female rate at each age-period is taken as 100, and the male rate reduced to the corresponding figure, the male and female rates diverge more and more widely with the

* Morselli, *op. cit.*, p. 132.
† *Op. cit.*, p. 189.

advance of age, but the regularity of the scale is broken at two periods, namely, in the 15–20 and in the 45–55 years' periods, and in the earlier of these two periods, the female is actually higher than the male rate.

The break in the scale at 45–55 marks the sudden shock given to the female system by the *menopause;* while the exceptional inversion of the male and female rates in the 15–20 years' period marks the conversion of the girl into the woman. Dr. Ogle points out that this period is not only that in which the suicide-rate for females is higher than that for males, but is also the only period in which the general death-rate is higher in the former sex, and is also marked by an exceptionally higher rate of lunacy for females than for males. These three concomitant features of the 15–20 period in regard to suicide, death, and insanity among females are due to puberty, but the tendency to suicide increases with age, so that though a girl and boy are at the same period of age, yet physiologically and pathologically the girl is the elder of the two in sexual maturity and stature.

No doubt, as Dr. Ogle says, the total chance of dying by suicide is much greater than is generally supposed; for 1 out of every 119 young men who reach the age of twenty kills himself.

Tables we have published in the *Journal of Mental Science* (Jan. 1890) show that in this country, from 1861–1888, the result as to the liability of the sexes to suicide may be stated thus: Among equal numbers living of both sexes there were almost exactly three male suicides to one female suicide.

Morality.—Of the various social influences under consideration, that of public morality must not be overlooked, but the tests are in the highest degree illusory. Tables showing the difference in the number of illegitimate children in different countries are altogether untrustworthy tests of comparative international morality. It is apparently well established that where the annual average of suicides undergoes a very marked increase, a corresponding increase of crime occurs. It is a matter of common observation that the murderer frequently endeavours to end his own life. And yet in some countries statistics show that "those that are preeminent in crimes of blood are those where suicide is scarce."* Italy and Spain are examples in point when compared with other European nations. It is certainly almost incredible that where crimes against property predominate, suicides are more frequent than where crimes of blood are frequent.*

* Morselli, *op. cit.*, p. 49.

Depression of Trade.—There is no doubt that agricultural distress increases the number of suicides. Machinery in place of hand-labour has exerted a bad influence in this direction. It has been shown by Morselli that there is no *direct* relation between the cost of bread and the number of suicides, although in twenty-four provinces in Italy, in which wheat rose in price very considerably, suicides increased in number in half these districts—to fifty per cent., remaining stationary in three, and diminishing in nine. On the contrary, in thirty-four provinces, where the price fell considerably, in eighteen of them the number of suicides declined, in three it remained stationary, while lastly, in twelve, there was an increase of suicides. In the year 1869 a favourable condition was enjoyed in Italy, and there was a decided fall in the number of suicides. The same relation between prosperity and fewer acts of self-destruction was observed in 1875, in the same country. Again, if the effect of railways on voluntary deaths be examined into, it would seem that "the States that are most advanced in railway development, are those that generally have the larger averages of suicides." † We are assured that "in France the kilometrical maximum development of railways is in the northern zone, as is the case in Italy, and in these regions the prevalence of suicide corresponds with that of the networks of railways and of their commercial and passenger traffic compared to the population and the geographical superficies." ‡ It must be remembered that this relationship does not necessarily mean that railways *per se* exert an injurious influence on the brain. They may be only one of other indications of modern civilisation.

Political Life.—It is stated that although a predisposing cause of suicide is to be found in the increased individual interest taken by a large number of the people in political life, in great revolutions, as those in Europe, 1848–49, there were fewer suicides throughout the greater part of Europe.‡ Something should be said as to the influence of the prevalent thoughts and speculations of any particular age, but this study is extremely open to erroneous deductions, and definite facts are obtained with difficulty. Two opposite forces may be at work at the same time, and among the same people. For example, in England, the Salvation

* *See* an elaborate Table in Morselli, *op. cit.*, p. 151.

† *Op. cit.*, p. 158. ‡ *Op. cit.*, p. 159.

Army, and a largely increasing body of Agnostics might, and no doubt do, exert their opposite influences on thought at the same epoch.

Density of Population.—It appears impossible to establish any relation between this factor and the number of suicides. Belgium, for example, stands first as regards the number of inhabitants to the square mile, while it is thirty-second in national liability to suicide. It is not necessary to burden the consideration of the causation of suicide with elaborate statistics when the net result fails to show any causal relationship between dense populations and voluntary deaths.

City and Country Life.—The following formula is laid down by Morselli: "The proportion of suicides in all Europe is greater amongst the condensed population of urban centres than amongst the more scattered inhabitants of the country." * This seems opposed to the negative results of the investigation referred to in the last section. Comparisons have been made between the inhabitants of centres of more than 2000 and the rural population. Paris has an unenviable predominance in the scale of capitals in relation to suicide. The researches of Guerry, Lisle, and Legoyt are cited by Morselli as showing that the suicides increase regularly and in every direction in the departments of France, according to their vicinity to the capital. Decaisne states that while there is 1 suicide to 160 deaths in Vienna, 1 in 175 in London, 1 in 712 in New York, there is the large proportion of 1 in 72 in Paris. It appears that as regards London and the provinces, there has always been a larger proportion of suicides in the former. In Berlin the same difference has been observed. In Vienna there is a lower proportion of suicides than in other European capitals. In St. Petersburgh the suicides are very much greater than in the country at large. So in Copenhagen, Stockholm, Brussels, Munich, and Frankfort-on-the-Main, where it stands at a very high rate, and is said to be on the increase.

The influence of [illegible] suicide seems fairly [illegible] large mass of figures wh[illegible] collected together by [illegible] various countries. The [illegible] the foregoing conditions [illegible] occurrence and range of [illegible] but have the effect of [illegible] able caution as to the [illegible] of these causes, seeing that [illegible] inextricably mixed. We [illegible] erred, if at all, in minimising the [illegible] at work in society, from the [illegible] should be led astray by the [illegible] array of figures which are to [illegible] the numerous works which have [illegible] on the subject.

Age.—The tendency to suicide [illegible] in both sexes in direct ratio [illegible] This conclusion has been arrived [illegible] making due allowance for the [illegible] their numbers in the general [illegible] at different ages. According to [illegible] statistics, the stage of life [illegible] ages between twenty-one and [illegible] most favourable to this tendency [illegible] maximum number occurring [illegible] and fifty, but in our own country [illegible] tics show that suicides are most [illegible] between fifty-five and sixty-five [illegible] men and women. As stated by Dr. [illegible] In England and Wales [O], after the tenth year of age, the rate of [illegible] reaches whole numbers, and rises [illegible] until the maximum is reached [illegible] the decennium 55–65, when after [illegible] almost stationary for another decade, the rate falls.

Admissions to asylums show in general a somewhat similar decrease at the more advanced ages. Taking the whole period of life, however, the lunacy-rate reaches its maximum at an earlier period than the suicide-rate, and its decline afterwards is not so regular.

We have given the following table [illegible] the *Journal of Mental Sciences* (Jan. [illegible]) showing the suicides to a million persons living at different ages in England and Wales, 1861–1888:

Table III.—Number of Suicides at Different Ages in England and Wales, 1861–[illegible].

	All Ages.	Under 15	15	20	25	35	45	55	65	75 and upwards.
Persons . .	47,704	261	1858	2887	6914	9000	10,308	9576	5340	1560
Males . . .	35,501	148	875	1797	4915	6735	7813	7669	4306	1243
Females . .	12,203	113	983	1090	1999	2265	2495	1907	1034	317

* Morselli, *op. cit.*, p. 169.

Suicides by children five years of age have been recorded, and it is said even three, but this is difficult to believe. Of 240 suicides committed by children in France, 94 were fifteen years old, 60 were fourteen, 38 were thirteen, 11 were twelve, 16 were eleven, 6 were ten, 4 were nine, 3 were eight, and 8 were seven only. Eighty-one suicides in England and Wales during ten years (1865–74) were committed between ten and fifteen, there being as many as 45 males as against 36 females. Again, in Prussia during the three years 1873–75 8 children terminated their existence under ten years and above five. The antagonism between suicide and crime, as regards age, is shown in one of the Tables prepared by Morselli, who proves that in France during a certain term of years the tendency to suicide was greatest at above seventy in both sexes, while, on the contrary, crime manifested the greatest intensity under twenty-five. The two curves display an inverse parabolic development.*

Celibacy.—Due correction being made for the proportion of married to unmarried persons to the general population, statistical proof is forthcoming of the evil effect of celibacy and widowhood as regards the prevalence of suicide. Sex, however, affects the result, for in Italy, France, and Switzerland there appear to be fewer suicides among the unmarried, while there are more among the married and those in a state of widowhood. The latter condition favours suicide among men more than among women. Celibacy, on the other hand, is not so injurious to women as to men.† It is a melancholy reflection that the unhappy state to which marriage brings a large number of women causes among this class so large a number of violent deaths. It would seem that divorce exercises a more injurious influence on the male than on the female sex. It should be stated that in the case of widows a family has an appreciable effect in lessening the tendency to suicide.

Occupation.—More extended statistics have had the effect of disproving an opinion long entertained of persons residing in agricultural districts as more prone to commit suicide than those who live in towns. We have in the "Manual of Psychological Medicine" endeavoured to expose the old fallacy on this point—the relative liability of rural and urban populations. It has been found in Italy that the highest figures of suicides are associated with those industries which are the least necessary to human existance—*e.g.*, objects of luxury, scientific and musical instruments, fabrication of arms and ammunition, printing, lithographing, and toilet industries. Among such industries as weaving, spinning, building, stone cutting, tailoring, shoemaking, hat manufacturing, &c., there are fewer instances of voluntary death. The proportion rises among those concerned in food, including wine-merchants and beer-sellers.

Among the class devoted to religion in Italy, including nuns, convent maids, and lay sisters, the number of suicides is small. Among those who use their intellectual faculties more severely, journalists, engineers, in short, the literary and scientific classes, there is a distinct increase in the number of suicides. The condition of teachers in Italy appears to be particularly depressing, and, as might be expected, occasions a frequent resort to a violent termination of life as an escape from an unhappy profession. Fortunately, schoolmistresses have a better time of it, and do not follow this course. The commercial classes, including large merchants and bankers, yield a large proportion of suicides. Still greater is the number among the lawyers and doctors.

In England and Wales [O], the death registers during six years (1878–83) exhibit 9000 suicides of males with known occupations. The suicide-rate at each age-period is calculated separately for each occupation, and the rates thus obtained are applied to a standard population, that is, to one with a certain fixed age-distribution. At the bottom of the list are those occupations (the clergy excepted) which entail severe manual labour, and are mostly carried on out of doors by uneducated men. At the top of the list are sedentary occupations, and they comprise a number of callings which lead to intemperance. By far the majority of suicides of servants were among butlers. In the comparatively happy medium is found the great class of shopkeepers. Soldiers may be supposed to enjoy their pre-eminence in self-destruction, chiefly on account of their intemperate habits of life, and partly on account of their being taken from the dregs of the population, not to mention the well-known psychological influence associated with the sight of an instrument of destruction. The high rate among medical men and lawyers is attributed to undue indulgence in the pleasures of the table, and the strain of the nervous system from prolonged mental work. On the whole, suicide is more prevalent among the educated than the uneducated. This is confirmed by its increase in recent years. To some extent higher education

* Morselli, *op. cit.*, p. 226.

† *Op. cit.*, pp. 226, 232.

is only indirectly to blame, since it frequently leads to higher living as well as less exercise, and a less simple and healthy mode of life. Of those among whom the standard of education is not high, nor the amount of healthy exercise small, but who are, notwithstanding, prone to suicide, it is obvious that they are not only an imbibing section of the population, but have had to pass through frightfully hard times. The failures of farmers were, in 1879, suddenly doubled. Taking this and the following year, they were 83 per cent. above the average of four other years (1878, 1881–1883), and it turns out that in 1879 and 1880 suicides among farmers attained their maximum.

In referring to the Annual Report of the Lunacy Commissioners for a comparison of suicide-rate with insanity-rates, in England and Wales, Dr. Ogle observes that while they give the average annual admissions into asylums per 10,000 males, returned in each occupation at the census of 1881, "they unfortunately have taken no account of differences of age-distribution in the different occupations, and consequently the rates given by them are of very little use for purposes of comparison; for the insanity-rates, like the suicide-rates, increase vastly with age, and the age-distribution differs greatly in different professions and industries." "On the whole, there is quite as close a parallelism between the two series of rates as could be fairly expected, seeing on what different principles the two sets of rates have been calculated."

Social Condition.—To a considerable extent the object of this section has been anticipated by the observations made in a previous one. Much stress is laid by Morselli upon the excessive tendency among the military to suicide. The following sentence may be quoted in full:—"Whether this is owing to distance from home and disgust for military life, or to the severity of discipline, this is not the place to discuss, but in the meantime, whenever the psychological conditions of the army are studied, there the heaviest, and we may even say an exceptional, loss may be perceived. And in the comparison which may be made between the soldiers and sailors of different countries, there is such a similarity of data that a still greater value must be attributed to the psychological interpretation of the numbers. The military service is, in fact, everywhere, except in England, regulated by the same rules of conscription, and of the obligation of the citizens, and everywhere the social and material conditions of soldiers are equalised, either by custom and rule, or, which is [illegible] disciplinary orders."*

In 1868 statistics were [illegible] ing that in the north of Germany [illegible] 1 suicide out of 2238 soldiers; [illegible] 1 in 3900; in Saxony 1 in [illegible] Norway, and Prussia had [illegible] Würtemberg 1 in 9748; France [illegible] Sweden and Bavaria 1 in [illegible] and Belgium 1 in 17,800. "From [illegible] to 1871 the mortality by suicide in the English army was 0.379 per thousand of the forces; and, comparing it with [illegible] of men between twenty and [illegible] years of age, which during that [illegible] was 0.107, we find it of more than [illegible] intensity. This intensity, moreover, augmented as time advanced; from [illegible] 1871 it grew from 278 per million to [illegible] the first quinquennial, an average of [illegible] the second, 443), and even reached [illegible] 1869. The tendency then increased with the sending away the troops from Europe [illegible] that in the kingdom (at home) the suicide is 339 per million, but in the English possessions in India it rises to 458. We may suppose that here nostalgia and the [illegible] influence of the climate play a large part."†

Some important observations have been made in regard to the influence of imprisonment on the tendency to suicide. This influence appears to be sufficiently well marked, especially in prisoners [illegible] thirty years of age.

According to returns in Italy, [illegible] guilty of crimes against the person constitute more than half. Naturally, [illegible] prisoners sentenced to long imprisonment most frequently commit self-destruction. Morselli arrives at the conclusion that "solitary confinement produces a greater proportion of suicides than associated imprisonment and the system of [illegible] prisoners." Thus, under the *cellular system* practised in Belgium, Denmark, some prisons in Great Britain, and Italy, the average number of suicides in prison is in the ratio of 1370 per million prisoners; under the *Auburn system*, where practised in Great Britain and Italy, the average is 400; in those prisons where the *mixed system* is adopted, as in Saxony and in some places in Great Britain, the average is [illegible]; and, lastly, where the associated system has been introduced, as in Austria, Hungary, France, Italy, Prussia, and Sweden, the average amounts to 350. Morselli, therefore, disagrees with Baillarger, Moreau, and the French Parliamentary Commission (1875) that "solitary confinement cannot be pronounced injurious to the mind and health of the prisoner."‡

* *Op. cit.* p. 257. † *Op. cit.*, p. [illegible]. ‡ *Op. cit.* p. 264.

Intemperance.—The influence of alcohol or beer in the production of suicide is not disputed. It is stated by Böttcher that 56 per cent. are due to alcoholic excess.* Suicides have risen and fallen in number in Sweden according to the stringency of prohibitory laws as regards drink.

Heredity.—Remarkable examples of hereditary suicide have occurred (pp. 1230, 1231).

Connection of Suicide with Insanity.—It is absolutely impossible to determine the number of suicides due to mental disease. That this number is very large is unquestionable, but it cannot be admitted for a moment that the suicidal act taken alone is any sign of insanity. The customary verdict of juries in cases of suicide—"temporary insanity"—has fostered the idea that voluntary deaths are necessarily committed by madmen. Dr. Westcott made a careful inquiry into the cases of suicide falling under his notice, and has found that in 20 per cent. only was there any proof that the deceased had shown symptoms of mental disease, so far at least as his friends were aware of the fact.

Of male lunatics admitted into asylums in England and Wales, in the course of one year—1887—there were 25.8 per cent. manifesting a *suicidal tendency*, while there was a larger proportion of females—namely, 32 per cent.—which at first sight seems strange in view of the statistics given as regards suicides in the general population. When, however, we take the *actual* deaths from suicide in English asylums during one year (1890) we find there were ten males and four females, showing that inside asylums as well as out of them there are more of the former sex who *commit* suicide.

As to the form of mental disorder of those admitted into asylums with suicidal tendency, in 1887, the great majority (59.6 per cent.) were cases of melancholia, then mania (20 per cent.), and lastly dementia (16 per cent.).

It is unnecessary to pursue this aspect of suicide further, as it is treated by Dr. Savage in the article SUICIDE AND INSANITY (*q.v.*).

Modes of Death.—These vary to some extent according to nationality. Thus in Paris charcoal is largely employed to cause asphyxia. Certain poisons are particularly fashionable in England. In Italy there exists a strong predilection for drowning, and so on. As has been pointed out, the certainty of effect and the minimum amount of pain mainly determine the form of suicide resorted to. With the insane this by no means holds good, for a powerful reason is often found in the delusion under which the patient suffers, for intensifying the suffering in accordance with a morbid fanaticism. The order in which various modes of violent death occurred during ten years (1866–75) was as follows: Hanging, drowning, fire-arms, asphyxia, arms for cutting and stabbings, falls, poison, crushing by railway train. In Italy drowning, together with gunshot wounds, comes first, then we have suspension, falling from heights, wounds by cutting or stabbing, and poisoning being about equal, and lastly charcoal, and crushing under railway trains. In Prussia and Bavaria, there is great uniformity in the preference for suspension, asphyxia being the last on the list. Attention has been drawn to the remarkable regularity which in successive years marks the choice of methods of deaths resorted to by suicides in England. Thus, from 1858 to 1876, the annual average number of suicides per million inhabitants ranged from 66 to 73. Fire-arms were resorted to in an almost uniform proportion every year, varying only from 2 to 5 per million; cutting and stabbing from 11 to 16; poison from 6 to 8; drowning from 10 to 16; hanging from 22 to 30; otherwise from 3 to 7. It is a remarkable fact that a greatly increased preference has been manifested in Europe for death by hanging. It might have been expected that poison and asphyxia by charcoal would have been regarded with more favour, and indeed this has been the case in North America and some other countries.

The order in which the various poisons have been made use of in England during one decennium is as follows: Prussic acid, cyanide of potassium, laudanum, oxalic acid, arsenic, strychnine, the vermin killer, and oil of bitter almonds; whilst in the second and third places occur caustic acids, mercury, preparations of opium and morphia, vegetable narcotics, phosphorus, and salts of copper. Then, in the last place, there are chloral, chloroform, paraffine, and belladona, ammonia, cantharides, salts of lead, zinc and potassium.

In Dr. Ogle's statistics of suicides for England and Wales, strangulation heads the list; then follow drowning and cut-throat. A long way down comes poison; the order of frequency being mainly determined by the comparative facility of access to the means of destruction, although, strange to say, the sailor prefers hanging to drowning. A razor is easily procured, a river or pond is generally near, while a rope is always handy.

Hanging is selected by men, women pre-

* Morselli, *op. cit.*, p. 290.

for drowning, and elect to take poison rather than stab themselves. As might be expected, they rarely shoot themselves, jumping from a height being more common. With men, as age advances, there is an increasing comparative distaste to the use of the gun, poison and drowning, and an increasing preference for the knife and cord.

Morselli emphasises the rareness of violent death by drowning the nearer we approach the north of Europe. "The Slav race is the one which shows less inclination than others to seek death by drowning, not only in Russia, but also in the Slav provinces of Austria-Hungary (Galicia, Buckovina, the military frontiers, and Slavonia). Where the Slavic race mingles with others, as in Transylvania (Slavo-Magyar), or in Bohemia and Moravia (Czech-German), suicide through drowning is somewhat more frequent, still always below that of any other country. Let us note, however, that in later times, even in Austria, suicide by drowning, especially amongst women, is seen to increase. In all the rest of central and northern Europe, death by drowning is chosen in nearly the same number of cases; in Belgium and Ireland, however, it is more frequent than in Germany and Scandinavia. Of the German countries, Saxony and Würtemberg have the greatest decrease of cases by drowning, and in Denmark among Scandinavian countries. In the aggregate of Europe, however, deaths by drowning come after those by hanging, except in the north of Russia. The preference given to drowning in southern climates, and especially in France, Italy, and Spain (of which to tell the truth, we possess only incomplete data), shows how, even in his self-destruction, the suicide adapts himself to the place and season. This is certainly not the only reason of the phenomenon, but there is an undoubted relation between the annual average temperature and the number of deaths by drowning." *

It has been observed that death by suspension and by drowning occur in inverse ratio to one another. In Russia the latter is rare, while four-fifths of the suicides are brought about by hanging. Other members of the Slav race, the Transylvanians and Galicians, manifest the same preference for this mode of death. The Scandinavians also, in the case of Denmark, prefer hanging to other forms of suicide. The Swedes prefer poisoning. Death through the infliction of wounds is highest in our own country. The German, whether at home or abroad, shows a marked choice for [illegible] refer the reader to [illegible] work for a mass of information [illegible] national preferences in regard [illegible] of death chosen.

Doubtless the most remarkable [illegible] of suicides throughout the world is the regularity with which they occur under certain conditions, so that general laws can be deduced from a study of the phenomena, and the extent of violent deaths can be predicated with tolerable accuracy. Those who, like Morselli, refer suicide to the general principle of evolution, regard it as an "effect of the struggle for existence and of human selection." This doctrine of course assumes that it is the weak who are destroyed by their own hands in the struggle for life.

THE EDITOR.

[*References.*—Bareuc, Reflexions sur le Suicide, 1789. Brierre de Boismont, Du Suicide, [illegible]. Bucknill and Tuke, A Manual of Psychological Medicine, fourth edit. 1879. Buckle, H. T., History of Civilisation in England, 1869. [illegible], Appiano, Histoire du Suicide, 1760 and [illegible]. Caro, E., Le Suicide dans ses rapports avec la civilisation, 1856. Casper, J. L., Forensic Medicine, translated from the German, by J. W. [illegible], 1861–5. Casauvieilh, J. B., Du Suicide, [illegible]. Espine, Marc de, Essai analytique de [illegible] Mortuaire Comparée, 1858. Jaccoud, [illegible] Dictionnaire de Médicine, Art. Suicide, [illegible]. Maudsley, Henry, Insanity and Crime, [illegible], Body and Mind, 1873. Mignault, H. G., [illegible] chiefly in reference to Philosophy, Theology, and Legislation, Heidelberg, 1856. Psychological Medicine, Journal of, 1859, 1878, 1879, 1880. [illegible] L. A. J., De l'Homme, 1835, and Essai de [illegible] Morale, 1866. Registrar-General, Reports of, annual. Winslow, Forbes, The Anatomy of Suicide, 1840. Westcott, W. Wynn, Suicide, its History, Literature, Jurisprudence, Causation, and [illegible]tion, London, 1885.]

SUICIDE AND INSANITY.—Suicide may occur in persons who have [illegible] no other sign of insanity. The motive of suicide varies with the education and surroundings of the individual. Suicide is more common in some forms of insanity than in others, but there is hardly a distinct group of cases deserving the term of suicidal mania. Suicide may be accidental or intentional.

In mania and general paralysis of the insane if suicide occur it is generally as the result of accident.

In some cases of slight emotional disorder there may be an intention to pretend to commit suicide which may by accident become effective.

In some neurotic persons, whether the neurosis result from heredity, alcoholism, previous attacks, injuries to the head, or in connection with some bodily ailment such as asthma, gout, &c., slight moral causes may lead to suicide; such cases may be called neurotic suicides, and

* Morselli, *op. cit.*, p. 324.

in those we frequently meet with a history of suicide in other members of the family.

Suicide in insane states may be **accidental** or **intentional.** Intentional suicide may be *impulsive* or *deliberate*.

Impulsive suicide may be
- Neurotic.
- Hysterical.
- Maniacal.
- Alcoholic.
- Epileptic.

Deliberate suicide may depend on
- Egotistical feelings
  - Pain.
  - Worry.
  - Sleeplessness.
  - Ruin.
  - Shame.
  - To avoid persecution, &c.
- Altruistic feelings
  - To save others from suffering.
  - To benefit others.
- or be Indifferent to those
  - As result of "voices."
  - As result of fixed delusion.
  - As result of weak mind.

Suicide in **children** almost always occurs in hereditarily neurotic children in whom suicide may be impulsive or deliberate and is almost always due to some trivial cause. In some, it is accidental.

In **maniacal states** suicide is rarely the result of deliberate purpose. It may result from impulse or in mania of the delirious type, it may follow or depend on hallucinations of the senses, and be due to dread of being injured by some one.

In some slight cases of mania of the emotional or hysterical type there is a tendency to exaggerated mental reflexes, so that the means to commit suicide suddenly suggest the act, such as knives, pistols, trains and heights.

Buoyant feeling in mania or anæsthesia in general paralysis may lead to accidental suicide; thus a patient may believe that he can fly, and jump from a window, or being insensitive to pain may lacerate or burn himself.

Patients who are suffering from **acute alcoholism** often kill themselves, and many who are suffering from secondary depression after alcoholic excess are suicidal; some who having had attacks of insanity following alcoholic excesses commit suicide from dread of a recurrence of ordinary insanity, some suffering from partial weakness of mind due to alcohol commit suicide, while others develop hallucinations of persecution and have sensory hallucinations which drive them to their end.

In **epilepsy** suicide is not frequent but may result from morbid self-consciousness as to the fits; it may occur in the automatic stage of epilepsy, or as the result of uncontrollable impulse.

It is generally accepted as an axiom that no patient suffering from **melancholia** should be trusted. Yet some such patients are much more suicidal than others. The majority of hypochondriacal melancholiacs are not suicidal, though many, like a sea-sick man believe they wish for death. The hypochondriac who is chiefly concerned with his "brain feelings" is rarely suicidal, nor is he who is chiefly concerned with some general bodily feeling such as that of impending death. Patients who believe there is some radical disease of, or obstruction of, the throat or bowels may be suicidal, or they may compass their death by some mutilation which they perform with the idea of giving themselves relief. In some cases in which there are marked waves of mental depression, suicidal impulses may occur at the rise of those waves. In woman, suicidal tendencies do not frequently occur with uterine hypochondriasis, though with disorders of the reproductive system they are very common both in men and in women.

We believe no woman suffering from amenorrhœa and melancholia is free from danger, and no man who believes he is suffering from impotence or spermatorrhœa, or is syphilophobic is trustworthy.

In young people suffering from melancholia the danger is generally due to impulsive acts; after childbirth both homicidal and suicidal impulses often arise; at the climacteric, suicide especially in women, is very common; in unmarried women and in widows there is a great tendency to suicide if melancholia develop.

In young men the fear of spermatorrhœa is potent as a cause. Syphilis, real or imaginary, may also be equally dangerous.

Senile melancholia, especially in men, is highly dangerous. Melancholia related to gout is also generally suicidal.

Simple melancholia of very slight depth is a very common cause of suicide. Melancholia with stupor is more rarely a cause; active melancholia leads to impulsive acts of suicide. Melancholia with persistent hallucinations is also frequently suicidal. With the onset of recurring melancholia and with the entry on convalescence suicidal attempts are common. Pain of body or mind, or sleeplessness may lead to suicide in melancholic patients. The early morning is the period of greatest danger.

Delusional insanity frequently gives rise to suicide. Almost all patients who believe that they are being watched, followed, or spoken about, are likely to be suicidal. The danger is greater in men than in women, and is greater in younger men than in many of middle life.

Delusional insanity associated with ideas of persecution, of jealousy and the like are dangerous.

Simple delusions which have not become organised into delusional insanity may lead to suicide. Thus patients, more especially women who believe they are either injurious to their husbands or children, or that they are in the way, may sacrifice themselves.

Similar are those who seek their death for some religious objects.

Hallucinations of the senses may lead to suicide. Voices may command. Visions may entice. Misery produced by constant occurrence of hallucinations, may act like constant pain.

Suicide occurs in **imbeciles** and occasionally in **idiots**, but in these latter it is usually accidental. In dements and imbeciles it may result from accident or impulse or may be the outcome of some insane train of thought. In such cases a very slight cause may give rise to the suicidal act.

All melancholic patients must be considered suicidal till they are fully known, and as such must be never trusted.

Some risk must be run sooner or later, and it is necessary in curable cases to recognise that the too constant presentation of the idea of distrust to the patient's mind keeps up the morbidly suicidal state. Hence we are inclined to question the free use of suicidal dormitories; they are more preventive than curative.

Most patients who believe themselves to be watched and followed must be treated as suicidal.

Waves of depression occur in many neurotic but otherwise sane people, which often lead to suicide. GEO. H. SAVAGE.

SUICIDE IN RELATION TO LIFE INSURANCE. (*See* LIFE INSURANCE.)

SULPHONAL. (*See* SEDATIVES.)

SUNSTROKE AND INSANITY.—The relationship of sunstroke and insanity has received only a comparatively small amount of attention at the hands of medico-psychologists in this and other countries, and our knowledge of the mental defects and aberrations of intellect, met with as sequelæ of an attack of sunstroke, is as yet ill-defined and unsystematised.

Authors resident in hot climates have concerned themselves largely with the study of the effects of a continued high degree of temperature upon the vital processes of man, and [illegible] to them for our knowledge [illegible] quelæ, such as ardent fever [illegible] lirium, remittent or inte[illegible] complicated with dysenteric [illegible] flammations, congestions, &c.

All observers have experienced the same difficulty in estimating [illegible] effects of the solar rays, and [illegible] culty has arisen not only from the [illegible] of a sufficient number of experiments [illegible] by the common presence of other conditions, such as hot, rarefied, and [illegible] impure air, heat of the body produced [illegible] exercise which is not attended by [illegible] tion, and other conditions too numerous [illegible] mention.

It would be out of place here to [illegible] upon the varieties of sunstroke, [illegible] have been graphically described by Sir Joseph Fayrer, Duncan, Moore, and others, so for the present we purpose to accept the convenient classification of Morehead, who divides the **forms of sunstroke** into two classes—viz.:

(1) **Coup de Soleil—due to direct heat of the sun.**

(2) **Coup de Chaleur—indirectly due to heat and other influences.**

Some writers uphold the view that the direct influence of the sun has probably little or nothing to do with the hyperæmia discovered after death, which they consider to be venous in character, and a secondary phenomenon immediately dependent upon a diminished power of activity of the heart. If this view be correct, the substitution of the term "heat-stroke" for the generic term "sunstroke" would be advantageous, and would convey a more accurate notion as to the actual condition.

On the other hand, the assumption that the direct impingement of the sun's rays upon the head may be attended with an active congestion may possibly be true in some cases, but we do not think this is by any means proved apart from the presence of other important factors.

Dr. Handfield Jones, writing upon functional nervous disorders, remarks that "any man of experience in the manifold disorders of jaded and exhausted nervous systems will recognise at once how close is the resemblance between the results of tropical heat and those produced by the ordinary causes in operation among the struggling multitude in our large towns," and it is with the factors which aid in producing such exhaustion of the nervous system that we have chiefly now to deal.

The relative values of the atmospheric influences, such as heat, humidity, winds, &c., as causes are interesting, but the bodily causes, such as fatigue, bodily habits, excesses—either alcoholic, dietetic, or sexual—and syphilis are the most important, and have an influence specially upon the general vigour of the constitution; and, in rendering a person more or less susceptible to heat, so far predispose him to suffer from it.

Solar heat as an immediate or exciting cause is said to act in two ways, causing (1) **prostration** of the nervous powers and syncope, symptoms of debility, with vertigo, weariness, nausea, and incontinence of urine; or (2) **venalisation of blood**, with absence of perspiration, suppression of urine, and constipation. This latter state, however, is chiefly aided by fatigue, impure air, alcohol, disorders of viscera, and retained secretions; and, further, although the heat of the sun may possibly affect the vaso-motor centre in the medulla oblongata, especially by striking on the unguarded occiput and neck, yet the same symptoms arise when there is no direct influence of the sun upon the person attacked.

The recognition of this fact is important to us, as formerly many cases were not returned in India, but were overlooked, owing to the fact that only those cases occurring after direct exposure to the sun were recorded; and, moreover, when we investigate the previous histories of our cases of insanity this source of error is always open to us.

Undoubtedly, hot climates eventually sap the foundations of life amongst Europeans, and although the hypothesis of acclimatisation—*i.e.*, "that an injurious effect is first produced and then accommodation of the body to the new condition within a limited time," is to a certain extent true, yet the rule does not extend in its application from the individual to the progeny.

It appears that acclimatisation of Europeans in India depends largely upon intermixing by marriage with the natives, otherwise they are apt to degenerate into strumous or nervous types, and fail to reach beyond the third or fourth generation.

The effects of a tropical climate are, so to speak, relative; and beyond the influences of fatigue, over-exertion, overcrowding, bad ventilation, unsuitable dress, retained secretions, unsuitable diets, &c., we have to consider malaria, syphilis, and alcohol, all of which tend to debilitate or contaminate the system, and predispose the individual to the occurrence of sunstroke. From literature, and a limited experience gained by an analysis of fifty-five cases of insanity following sunstroke, we have been led to the belief that India is, perhaps, the country most productive of that affection amongst Europeans, for no less than twenty-three of the cases were said to have occurred there. In eight cases there was a history of malaria, and in five of syphilis, whilst any tendency to alcoholism could only be traced in seven of the fifty-five cases. What the relationship of malaria and syphilis is to sunstroke we are not prepared to say. Undoubtedly syphilis (as first pointed out by Mr. Hutchinson) precedes attacks of sunstroke. Possibly the special and primary syphilitic brain lesions affecting the meninges or vessels, or encephalic nervous substance, may predispose to heat-stroke by weakening the resistive power of the organism and brain, particularly to the effects of heat; but this is mere supposition on our part, and much information is yet wanted before we can assign to syphilis a definite part in the ætiology.

Alcohol especially predisposes to the indirect form of heat-stroke, and, as before stated, is a powerfully co-operating aid to the external and bodily causes, but possibly some observers tend to give this agent too great a prominence as a factor.

With these brief general considerations as to the ætiology, we will now pass on to what is to us the more important part of the subject. The most abiding results of sunstroke are all referable to impaired functional energy of the cerebro-spinal system, and this impairment shows itself either in motor paralysis, sensory paralysis of common or special sensation, hyper- and dysæsthesiæ of the nerves of common and special sensation, in debility, and undue excitability of the emotional centres, and in similar states of the cerebral hemispheres and spinal cord; or more commonly in some nervous defect or perversion consisting in a functional paralysis of one or more of the great nerve centres. In addition to these, the extreme sensitiveness of a patient to the rays of the sun, or to excessive heat ever afterwards, and the effect exercised upon them by alcohol, all point, according to Sir Joseph Fayrer, to an unstable condition of the great vaso-motor centre in the medulla oblongata.

The same author states that undoubtedly an attack of insolation is often attended with meningitis, or cerebral changes, which may destroy life or intellect sooner or later, or permanently compromise the whole health or that of some important function.

The **mental sequelæ** are interesting, and of the syncopal, asphyxial, and hyperpyrexial forms of sunstroke, the two latter appear to be the most important and dangerous.

In many cases the sequelæ may be attributed to the injury which the brain has received during the primary attack, and in the case of the syncopal variety, the temporary loss of nutrition of the brain may result in mental or even physical weakness, which may continue through life.

In infancy heatstroke is certainly a cause of accidental idiocy or imbecility. Dr. Langdon Down states that he has seen a notable number of feeble-minded children, who owe their disaster to sunstroke, while making the passage of the Red Sea and Suez Canal *en route* from India; or from exposure in that country, and he attributes the mental decadence as originating without doubt from the actual exposure to heat. Dr. Shuttleworth has kindly allowed us to copy the records of six cases of imbecility following sunstroke admitted to the Royal Albert Asylum at Lancaster. The parents of idiots and imbeciles are extremely ready to attribute the mental affections of their children to accidental causes; but in these cases the non-existence of hereditary neuroses, the absence of fits and other diseases or accidents likely to have been the cause, as well as the nature, extent, and immediate consequence of the attack of sunstroke, aided us in a great measure in coming to the conclusion that the damage to the mental power was undoubtedly dependent upon sunstroke.

The amount of injury to the mental powers was variable, but all the patients were simple-minded or imbecile, rather than belonging to the lower grades of idiocy.

Sometimes the mental symptoms are found intercurrent with the sopor and coma following the shock, and they may then take the form of delirium or excitement with hallucinations, passing into a condition somewhat similar to that of primary dementia. As a general rule, however, although there may be some trace left of the primary injury to the brain, the progress of the case is more favourable than when the psychosis develops some months, or even years, after the injury. In children, as in adults, the neuroses following sunstroke are somewhat similar to, and have much in common with, the traumatic neuroses. In none of the six cases was there any hereditary, neurotic, or strumous taint, and, moreover, until the period of the actual attacks of sunstroke nothing abnormal or defective had been detected by the parents.

The chief clinical [illegible]

(1) The ordinary [illegible] with absence of bodily [illegible]

(2) The full development [illegible] tively normal dimensions of [illegible] and osseous systems (including [illegible] of the head, jaws, and teeth, [illegible]

(3) The absence of any physical [illegible] or affections of the nervous system [illegible] as paralysis or chorea;

(4) The good use of all the special organs of sense, and absence of [illegible] or hallucinations;

(5) The special affections of speech, either of a temporary character immediately following the attack, or a continued impairment or failure in development of the faculty;

(6) The frequency of the occurrence of fits immediately after the attacks, lasting for a short period but not continued through life;

(7) The limited or perverted morality as seen in various grades, from mere disobedience to propensities peculiar, dangerous, or even homicidal, and sometimes, though rarely, habits of a degraded nature.

(8) The small mental capacity, with failure to improve much by the ordinary educational methods;

(9) The attachments, antipathies, and peculiarities which were in most cases retained through life: their absolute inability to compete with their fellow-beings, and their mental unfitness to aid in their own survival.

Epilepsy is one of the most common of the sequelæ of sunstroke, and occurs in various degrees of severity, from slight epileptiform convulsions to the severest forms of the disease. Maclean, writing upon diseases of tropical climates, states that immense numbers of soldiers were invalided home from India for this affection following sunstroke, but in a large proportion of cases the attacks disappeared before arrival at Netley, particularly in the long voyage round the Cape of Good Hope.

As a rule the disease appeared to be amenable to treatment. The same author also noted a few examples of chorea-like movements of the muscles of the forearm and hands, probably due to nerve irritation.

Dr. Mickle is inclined to the belief that the apoplectiform seizure or the epileptiform *petit mal* of general paralysis has been mistaken for sunstroke. While acknowledging that such an error may possibly occur, our experience has led us to believe that it is more common for the sequelæ of sunstroke to be mistaken for general paralysis.

The frequent occurrence of epilepsy is suggestive, and as in the case of the periodical psychoses, the disorder seems to be a manifestation of an unstable vaso-motor state.

Both idiocy and imbecility may be dependent upon early epilepsy, but the absence of spastic contractures, oculomotor anomalies, deformities and other conditions, together with the absence of progressive mental deterioration associated with the occurrence of the convulsions, is suggestive rather of an acquired psychosis; and further, in cases of epilepsy following upon sunstroke, the mental defect and convulsions appear to be collateral phenomena, both depending upon a common cause, whilst the positive signs of alienism, such as anomalies of character and moral perversions with defective or one-sided development of special faculties, appear to be, in a large measure, different from the progressive deterioration of ordinary idiopathic or hereditary epilepsy.

In adults we have seen the occurrence of episodical attacks somewhat analogous to epilepsy in which there was a periodical attack of depression or excitement, or even conditions closely resembling the epileptiform and apoplectiform attacks of paretic dementia.

Insanity arising from sunstroke is much like that due to traumatism, but as a rule progressive deterioration terminating in dementia is far more common in the latter than in the former. An attack of sunstroke seems to form an acquired predisposition to insanity, and, as in the case of traumatism, the most serious psychoses are developed months or even years after the injury.

Dr. Clouston believes that few Englishmen become insane in hot climates in whom sunstroke is not assigned as the cause, and that that cause gets the credit of far more insanity than it produces. At the Morningside Royal Asylum only twelve cases were admitted in nine years which could be said to have been due to traumatism or sunstroke, being only one-third per cent. of the admissions.

In the case of Bethlem the percentage is much higher, for of 1974 admissions no less than 49 (or 2.6 per cent.) were attributed to sunstroke. Possibly this high percentage may have been due to the admission of large numbers of officers and others who have seen foreign service.

Dr. Mickle believes that sunstroke is not uncommonly a cause of general paralysis among British soldiers in India, and he quotes the authority of Meyer, Victor, Berstens, and others. On careful analysis of the aforesaid forty-nine cases, we have only been able to find one case in which general paralysis really existed, whereas the number that simulated that disease was remarkable. The symptoms in fourteen cases consisted in associated mental and physical defects, which rendered the differential diagnosis one of extreme difficulty. The physical symptoms consisted in tongue tremors, thickness or slurring of speech, pupillar anomalies, altered reflexes (chiefly exaggerated), shaky and interrupted handwriting, tottering or weak gait, loss of control over bladder and rectum, hallucinations, or perversion of all or some of the senses (that of smell least commonly), and mental conditions, such as melancholia or hypochondriasis, but more commonly exaltation, extravagance, excitement, or even acute mania. With such a combination of symptoms the diagnosis of general paralysis appeared to be warrantable, but the cases proved to be deceptive, for after a time the physical signs disappeared, and the patient recovered mentally; or the mental health remained in a weak and permanently impaired condition, as shown by some irrelevancy or inattentiveness; or more commonly by some trace of exaltation or fixed delusions, with a smiling, self-satisfied manner.

Such patients become docile, cheerful, tractable, and industrious, and are perhaps in a condition to resume work, and so they may go on for years, with no motor or special sensory disturbances, and no marked change mentally from year to year.

A very common symptom is cephalalgia, which may occur periodically or persistently, and is probably dependent upon chronic meningitis, with some thickening or opacity of the membrane. Such patients cannot tolerate heat, and a close or heated atmosphere will cause an exacerbation of the sensory symptoms, or even recurrence of the mental disturbance. Alcohol is apt to aggravate the symptoms, and although possibly in some cases it has played a considerable part in the production of the insanity, yet we believe it is far more effective in cases where the brain has been previously rendered weak by sunstroke, for in many cases the primary affection or attack of sunstroke has not been preceded by alcoholic excesses, and, moreover, has not been followed by any immediate mental or motor defect, but it has formed, nevertheless, a predisposition to the disastrous effects of other exciting causes, such as alcohol.

The symptoms arising from locomotor ataxia, various paralyses (either general or circumscribed), epilepsy, senile dementia, and many other conditions may, in some particulars, render the diagnosis difficult, but the greatest difficulty is experienced with such affections as (1) general paralysis; (2) syphilitic disease of the brain and membranes; (3) alcoholic insanity; (4) dementia, with paralysis from local lesions, or circumscribed brain lesions, with dementia and paralysis (from softening, hæmorrhage, embolism, and thrombosis.)

It is not our intention to discuss the differential diagnosis of these affections, for there are few motor, sensory, or psychical elements which can be said to be symptomological of sunstroke.

It is rather by the history, the combination and character of the symptoms, and the subsequent course of the case, that we are able to define a group within which the cases have some common characteristics; and, moreover, the possession of this knowledge may materially guard us in giving our prognosis, and aid in the course of treatment pursued.

General Pathology.—The pathology of the affection is somewhat indefinite. Many writers uphold the view that exposure of the uncovered head to the scorching rays of the sun may give rise to purulent meningitis; but the question may be asked, "Why, when so many people are exposed to the injurious influences, so few suffer from it?" The difficulty in answering this question is increased by the want of a satisfactory physical explanation of the fact.

Obernier has endeavoured to show, by both clinical and experimental observations, that the causes and nature of sunstroke are to be sought in the abnormal increase of temperature in the body; and Liebermeister has further shown that the cerebral symptoms associated with high temperatures are only to a limited degree, if at all, dependent upon cerebral hyperæmia. Sufficient facts are not yet established to justify any decided opinion as to the pathology. Experiments have shown that moderate heat directed upon the cranium causes dilatation of the vessels, and we must conclude that the initial congestion of sunstroke is due in part to heat, and—with due regard to the authority of Liebermeister—there is some probability that on the onset of the symptoms there is some hyperæmia of the pia and brain, or, more accurately speaking, a distension of the whole venous system, and the changes found after death may further assume the existence of a cerebral congestion similar to the congestion found in other organs. Buck is of opinion that a tendency to capillary stasis is induced—the heart labours to overcome the obstruction, and, failing, gives us the syncopal or cardiac variety; or the nervous system, resenting the increased abnormity of the circulation, develops convulsions and coma, as the cerebro-spinal variety of the disease.

Special Pathology.—The post-mortem appearances vary in the different forms of the disease. In ardent fever, serous effusions in the ventricles and between the membranes of the brain have been noted, with turgescence of vessels, and congestion of the pulmonary system. The cause of death is said to be most commonly asphyxia, and not apoplexy, and the most important changes are found in connection with thoracic viscera.

When the medulla is affected accumulation of blood takes place in the right side of the heart and lungs, with secondarily (as a consequence) a want of that fluid duly arterialised in the brain. Roth and Lex state that death in the majority of cases occurs from cardiac paralysis, and only occasionally from cerebral disturbance. Arndt speaks vaguely of a "diffuse encephalitis," as explaining the cerebral symptoms, which often remain after the acute attack; and he points out that during an attack of sunstroke the blood is acid, very rich in urea and white globules, and shows very little tendency to coagulation. Köster and Fox have called attention to the occurrence of hæmorrhages, separation and destruction of the nerve fibres, and extravasation in both vagi and phrenic nerves.

In children, Dr. Shuttleworth has found meningitis, with effusion and traces of old-standing disease of the membranes in one case, and in another the membranes were thickened and somewhat opaque, especially at the vertex.

In the adult we found in one case marked opacity of the arachnoid, with an excess of serous fluid between the convolutions and in the ventricles. The dura mater was apparently normal, and not adherent to the skull-cap. The inner membranes stripped readily, and in one coherent film, leaving the surface of the convolutions intact. The vessels at the base were healthy, and normal in arrangement. There was no marked congestion of the venous system. The convolutions themselves were well formed, and the cortex was of good depth and colour. Striation, however, was ill defined, and there was a considerable amount of œdema of the white substance. On microscopic examination of the cortex cerebri we found a considerable number of spider cells and other evidences of degeneration.

In another case, reported to the Medico-Psychological Association by Dr. R. Percy Smith, the dura mater was found normal, but there was great excess of sub-arachnoid fluid over the surface of the brain, especially at the upper ends of the ascending frontal and parietal convolutions. The pia mater was soft, but peeled readily from the upper surface of the brain, leaving the convolutions intact. The convolutions were somewhat wasted, and the arteries at the base were slightly atheromatous. On section, the grey matter was pale and ill-defined, especially over the whole of the frontal region, and the left lateral ventricle was dilated. The condition of the spinal cord was interesting—the dura mater being distended by fluid in its lower parts, whilst along the cervical and dorsal regions there were numerous hæmorrhagic patches on its outer surface, consisting principally of clotted blood lying in the meshes of thin gelatinous material.

In the lower cervical region the anterior surface of the dura mater was adherent to the posterior surface of the bodies of three cervical vertebræ by old firm adhesions. No compression of the cord or caries of bone could be detected, and the spinal cord itself was firm and healthy, and did not show any signs of degeneration. Köster has described a hyperæmic condition of the brain, and the occurrence of several small ecchymoses under the peri- and subcardium of the left ventricle in a case of death from sunstroke; but he has also described similar results found in the case of a syphilitic woman where excessive increase of temperature could not have been the cause of death; and he further calls attention to the possible occurrence of disturbances of the vaso-motor and respiratory nerve-centres, which must take place in a pronounced form in patients suffering from sunstroke. In the only other case which we have to report the dura mater was found normal, but the veins of the pia mater were deeply congested and full of dark-coloured blood. The inner membranes peeled readily, and left the convolutions intact. There was slight excess of sub-arachnoid fluid, and the white substance of the brain was œdematous; otherwise, beyond considerable injection of the choroid plexus, the brain appeared to be fairly healthy. Both lungs were deeply congested.

THEO. B. HYSLOP.

SURDI-MUTISM. Deaf-mutism (*q.v.*).

SURDITAS VERBALIS (*surditas*, deafness; *verbalis*, pertaining to words). A synonym of Word-deafness.

SURDOMUTITAS (*surdus*, deaf; *mutitas*, dumbness). A synonym of Deaf-mutism.

SURGERY, BRAIN. (*See* TREPHINING.)

SURMENAGE (Fr.). The bodily or mental condition produced by over-exertion or overpressure.

SUSPENDED ANIMATION. (*See* TRANCE.)

SWITZERLAND, Provision for the Insane in.—The care of the insane in Switzerland is, like most other branches of public administration, placed under the supervision of the government of each canton, which is charged with this duty, which forms part of its public health provision. As the resources and needs of different cantons vary greatly, their activity in respect to the relief afforded and to public and private beneficence varies proportionally, and this will explain how it is that several cantons appear more advanced and better equipped than others.

The history of the provision for the insane in the several cantons has not been dissimilar to that of other countries during past centuries. Very little concern was apparently felt regarding those who were not dangerous to society. If dangerous, they were located in the various houses for lepers, which had been established near the large and small towns and boroughs in different parts of the country from the days of the Crusades, houses that were called maladières or maladaires, or "Siechenhäuser" in the German districts. In these houses, situated generally on the confines of those centres in which the necessities of isolation were apparent, there were often to be found congregated all those suffering from disagreeable or dangerous diseases, such as the violent and paralytic insane, &c. At a later date the insane sometimes found refuge in hospitals, where a few rooms or cells were set apart for them, either as a safeguard for the public weal or to afford them, if not special care, at least shelter. The earliest trustworthy date of the construction of a special building for the insane was in 1749, when a building was erected near Berne as an annexe to the exterior hospital, formerly used as a house for lepers. This asylum, to which later two wings were added, still exists, and was the only public establishment in the canton of Berne for the special treatment of the insane under the care of a physician till 1850.

The Bernese Government also had in the ancient convent of Kœnigsfelden (at that time part of the territory of Berne) in Aargau some specially constructed rooms for the reception of lunatics, in connection with the hospital for physical ailments. Zürich and Basle in the same manner set apart accommodation in buildings adjoining the hospitals to receive the more dangerous of the insane of those towns.

In 1810 the first asylum at Lausanne for the Canton Vaud was constructed for seventy patients and joined to the cantonal hospital. In 1838 the Asylum des Vernits for sixty-six patients was erected near Geneva, constructed after plans revised by S. Tuke of York. From the same year date also the laws for the reception and supervision of the insane, the provisional administration of their property, and for the supervision by the State of private asylums.

It was from 1830 to 1840, in consequence of the development of liberal political and administrative ideas in the different cantons of Switzerland, that the lot of the unhappy insane became everywhere ameliorated.

To this end measures were taken at Zürich, Basle, St. Gall, Aargau, Vaud, and, as we have seen, at Geneva and Neufchatel, to improve the organisation of the existing asylums or refuges, and with the special object of affording adequate medical treatment, and several cantons made preparatory studies of plans for the construction of such asylums for the insane.

In consequence of a decision of the Grand Council of the canton of St. Gall, the new hospital and asylum of St. Pirminsberg (St. Gall), erstwhile a convent, but rebuilt and re-arranged for its new destination, was opened in 1847, capable of accommodating one hundred patients. It was situated at an elevation of 826 metres above the level of the sea, 300 metres higher than the valley of the Rhine, and near the baths of Ragatz. Although from a hygienic point of view it offered many advantages, the close proximity of rocky elevations rendered the future enlargement of the asylum difficult, but even these difficulties were overcome when reconstruction became necessary to meet the growing wants of the community, and at the present day the asylum is capable of receiving three hundred patients of both sexes. Large sums were needed for this purpose, and over a million francs have been expended on its reconstruction and renovation. At some distance from the hospital a farm, St. Margarethenberg, has been established for the employment during summer months of a certain number of patients in agricultural labour, especially haymaking.

The State Council of Neufchatel, the insane of which had previously been drafted to the asylums of [illegible]feld (Alsace) and Dôle (France), passed a regulation in 1843 as to the [illegible] of its insane in proper asylums. This legislation enacted that, without [illegible] from the State Council no insane person should be confined for more than [illegible] months in any public or private asylum. Every house is deemed to be a lunatic asylum if several lunatics, or even a single insane person, is placed there and supervised by strangers. For each admission a certificate given by a licensed physician is needed, the date of which is not to be earlier than a fortnight before the actual admission of the patient. In cases when the relatives do not apply for admission of an insane person who is dangerous to the public safety, the State Council interferes on the demand of the local authorities.

A few years later, in 1849 (January 1), the building of a new lunatic asylum (Préfargier) was commenced through the generosity of M. de Meuron, who had it constructed and fitted up entirely at his own expense, and entrusted its working to a committee chosen by the founder and the State Council of the canton. The asylum of Préfargier, which is built from plans prepared by the French architect Philippon and executed by M. Chatelain, is arranged to accommodate from one hundred and twenty to one hundred and thirty patients (male and female) under the managment of a directing physician.

For the reception of private patients a villa has been built accommodating six patients and an assistant physician. The house is under the control of the State Council.

The town of Basle had erected a hospital for its insane in 1834 adjoining the general hospital, capable of accommodating thirty-two patients, while there was additional room for thirty-five to forty incurables. Here it was that, between 1850 and 1860, the director, Dr. Brenner, instituted, for the first time in Switzerland, clinical lectures for the students of the University of Basle.

As this hospital in time became inadequate for the needs of a rapidly increasing population, the canton of Basle passed a legal enactment for the erection of a new building for two hundred and forty patients. This hospital, built on the pavilion system, was inaugurated in the autumn of 1886; each block is destined for a special class of patients. The central building contains the administrative offices and the apartments for a surgical clinic. Two blocks are reserved for quiet patients of both sexes, two for epileptics and the paralytic insane, two for excited patients, and two for private patients of a superior class. The kitchens and wash-houses are in a special building in an extension of the central block. This new establishment meets all the requirements of such special institutions, though it leaves a good deal to be desired, as do all isolated buildings, in regard to the facility for adequate supervision. All these buildings are lighted by gas and heated by steam.

In 1839, the canton of Thurgau inaugurated its asylum for the insane in a section of the cantonal hospital of Münsterlingen, formerly a convent. As this building did not meet the needs of the canton, the former convent of Katharinenthal on the Rhine was fixed upon in 1871 to receive the incurable cases. Münsterlingen, on the borders of the Lake of Constance, can accommodate one hundred and fifty, Katharinenthal two hundred to two hundred and fifty patients of both sexes.

In 1846 the Grand Council of the canton of Berne decided on the erection of a new hospital and asylum for 230 patients of both sexes. This house, called the Waldau, which was built on the rectangular system, with vertical separation of the special divisions, was opened in November 1855. As it had to meet the needs of a population of more than 450,000 it was soon entirely filled, and arrangements had to be made with other hospitals to place in them those of its poor (*assistés*) insane, who could no longer be accommodated in the Waldau, while the authorities have set about the building of a new hospital and asylum at Münsingen, where a large estate has been bought for this purpose. An adjoining estate has afforded the asylum of Waldau the opportunity of usefully and profitably employing its patients.

Clinical lectures have been given here to the students at the University of Berne since 1861.

Waldau, constructed to hold 230 patients, has since been enlarged by several annexes to accommodate the numerous patients belonging to the canton, so that on an average 350 to 360 insane have during the last few years been in residence there.

In 1860 the canton of Soleure opened a new hospital and asylum (the Rosegg) for 150 to 200 patients of both sexes, excellently situated, at 1½ kilometres from the town. The funds for this building have been for several years obtained through annual collections made in the churches.

The canton of Zürich, having in 1814 to 1816, built their first lunatic asylum near the old hospital, used it to the best advantage, while recognising it as but a temporary and inefficient means of relief. But about the year 1860 the suppression of the convent of Rheinau afforded the canton an excellent opportunity to arrange this vast building, which was in excellent condition, for the reception of the incurable insane.

Situated as it was on an island of the Rhine, surrounded by a large, well-cultivated estate of 100 hectares of land, it was enlarged yet more to receive about 600 patients of both sexes.

After having thus amply provided for the most pressing needs, the canton decided on the construction of a new establishment for the reception of curable cases. The estate of Burghölzli, admirably situated at a distance of two miles from the town of Zürich, was chosen for the site of the new building. It was opened in 1870 for 260 patients of both sexes, and the superintendence was entrusted to Prof. Gudden, who shared the calamitous fate of King Louis II. of Bavaria, in 1886.

In 1872 the canton of Aargau inaugurated the new hospital and asylum of Koenigsfelden for 300 patients, by the side of and on the territory of the ancient convent of that name. It was built and arranged chiefly after the plans and directions of its first, and till 1891 only director, M. Schaufelbühl. It is admirably situated at a few minutes' distance from the station of Brugg, on the Aar, between Aarau and Zürich. The buildings of the old cantonal hospital having been abandoned for several years, are still available for the reception of a number of incurables.

In 1873 Bois de Cery was opened near Lausanne for the requirements of the canton of Vaud for 360 patients of both sexes. This building is beautifully situated on an eminence affording a view of Lake Leman, and the greater part of the canton of Vaud to the Jura mountains. Up to the present it still suffices for the needs of the canton, and as it is surrounded by a large tract of land, it affords considerable scope for the manual employment of its patients.

In the same year were established the hospital and asylum of St Urbain, near Langenthal-Olten, in the canton of Lucerne. This vast building, formerly a convent, which was suppressed in 1848, was bought by the Lucerne Government in 1870 with the object of creating an asylum. The immense buildings were found to be admirably adapted for this purpose, while the construction could be accomplished at very little cost. It was opened in November 1873 for 200 patients, but within three years this number was exceeded, so that an addition to the number of beds became necessary. An extensive farm of 120 hectares belonging to the hospital serves to employ with labour the numerous patients drawn from an agricultural district. In furtherance of this object, which gave excellent results in 1881, an agricultural colony has been organised in one of the two farms, containing about 40 hectares.

The pecuniary affairs of this colony have improved notably, and as it is the first that has been organised in Switzerland, it is worthy of record, as the earliest attempt to diminish the cost of maintenance to the State and charitable communities.

Thanks to this diminution of expenses, and to other favourable circumstances of an economic nature, the hospital of St. Urbain has been able to lay aside during the last ten years of administration more than 200,000 francs, while at the same time the terms for the very poor have been considerably reduced. The number of patients has in the last ten years risen to 400.

As the hospital of St. Urbain by reason of its extensive accommodation is more than sufficient for the needs of the canton, the Lucerne Government has entered into an agreement with six neighbouring cantons—namely, Berne, Uri, the two Unterwalden, Zug, and Schaffhausen—for the reception of their poor insane at a low rate.

The last of the hospitals and asylums to be enumerated is that of Marsens, near Bulle, in the canton of Fribourg. It was opened by the authorities of this canton in 1875, and can accommodate 100 patients of both sexes, and is built in separate blocks. Unfortunately, the cost of construction has been so great that, instead of eight, four only of the planned blocks have been built.

Besides these fourteen hospitals and asylums established in Switzerland since 1838, there are two in process of erection for the cantons of Schaffhausen and Grisons, for about 120 beds. The first is under the direction of Dr. Aug. Müller, near Schaffhausen, and the other is situated near Coire.

Some cantons, such as St. Urbain, receive patients under agreements made with an existing hospital, while others again subsidise their pauper insane by providing for their admission into the hospitals of other cantons, as, for example, Glaris, Zug, and Appenzell.

Besides the State provision for the insane, there are large numbers of private asylums or maisons de santé, viz.:—

Münchenbuchsee, at seven miles' distance from Berne, the most important, on account of the number of patients, 100 beds, under the direction of Dr. Glaser.

La Métairie, near Nyon (Vaud), at twenty-two kilometres distance from Geneva, thirty to thirty-five beds, admission to which is placed under the control of the government of Vaud, especially of a council of administration. It is under the direction of Dr. Fetscherin, formerly director of St. Urbain, for persons in easy circumstances; also

Bellevue, at Kreuzlingen, near Constance, for forty to sixty patients, the property of Dr. Binswanger.

Bellevue, near Landeron (Neufchatel), for ten or twelve patients. Proprietress, Madame Scherrer.

Stammheim, near Winterthur, for twelve patients. Proprietor, Dr. Orelli.

Spiez (Marishalden), on the lake of Thun, for twelve patients. Proprietor, Dr. Mutzenberg.

Two special asylums for epileptics have been established for some years near Zürich on the Rütli, with from forty to fifty beds for children of both sexes, and in a new building forty to fifty beds for young girls. The other is at Tschugg, near Cerlier (on the lake of Bienne), canton Berne, for twenty epileptics of both sexes.

In the cantons of Zürich (at Hottingen), of Berne (near Berne), of Basle and Vaud (Etoy, near Aubonne), there exist small philanthropic private asylums for idiots (children). A large number are placed in other asylums for the poor, or in general hospitals or in the poor-houses of the different cantons.

The cantons of Geneva and Neufchatel are the only ones that have established laws for the provision of the insane, while those cantons possessing hospitals have been content with regulations as to the reception and maintenance of the patients in the hospitals and asylums.

The fourteen hospitals and asylums that now exist, with the exception only of those of Geneva and Katharinenthal, are placed under the superintendence of a directing physician, who resides in the house and is responsible for the attendance on and entire management of the patients, as well as for the internal economy of the hospital. He is generally assisted by a second physician and sometimes one or several house pupils. The household management (*l'economie*) is entrusted to a house-steward, aided in some establishments by a farm-steward.

The work of these fourteen hospitals

has become more and more considerable. During the decade ending 1886 these hospitals, constructed to receive about 3300 patients, have admitted 15,927 patients, while 51,105 have undergone treatment in them during this period. The discharges for the same time reached 11,982, of whom 3025 (5.91 per cent. of the number treated) died. Of the admissions, 11.7 per cent. were due to alcoholic influence.

In accordance with the observations of other countries, the number of admissions on the register and of the annual discharges shows a more or less regular increase from year to year, the increase in discharges, however, being proportionately less than that of the admissions, a fact which accounts for the overcrowding that is taking place almost everywhere in asylums. Regular statistics giving the total amount of the work of Swiss asylums for ten years (1877 to 1886) show an annual increase of 2.317 per cent. in the number of resident patients, in that of admissions an increase of 1.23 per cent. per annum, and an increase of 0.942 per annum in the discharges, irrespective of deaths.

The number of insane treated in asylums proportionately to the number of inhabitants has also risen from 1.1133 per thousand of the population in the decade ending 1880 to 1.3378 per thousand in 1886.

A general census of insane persons in the entire territory of the Confederation has only been taken once—in 1870—at the time of the general census. This census placed the number of insane at 7764, which is probably much below the mark, and which in proportion to the population of 2,669,147 inhabitants in 1870 would indicate 1 insane in 343.78, or 2.908 per thousand of the inhabitants.

Besides this general census several cantons have at various times organised others within their boundaries. But these censuses have not sufficiently fulfilled their purpose, seeing that, by the faultiness of organisation and laxity as to proper interrogation, the end proposed was not sufficiently kept in view.

No census of the insane can fulfil its object which does not from the outset distinguish between and include the two large classes of insane, the idiots or cretins, that is to say, those who have suffered from congenital mental derangement, or derangement originating during the first years of life, and those who acquire mental affections during adult life (*e.g.*, the simple mental maladies, curable and incurable, paralytics, epileptics, &c.).

The only cantonal census that has thus distinguished between these forms of mental affection previous to 1880, was that of the canton of Berne, organised in 1871, and based on the results of the federal census of 1870.

The results of this measure were to chronicle the existence of 2804 insane, idiots and cretins, or 5.53 per thousand, or 1 insane for every 180 of the population; in 1870 the census taken in the same canton without distinguishing between these two categories, gave only 2021 insane, or 4.02 per thousand. The most complete census of the insane that has been made in Switzerland was that of the canton of Zürich, taken in December 1888. While the latest and most reliable it furnishes us with certain very startling results, for it indicates 1 insane person to every 103 of the population, or 3261 insane (properly speaking, idiots, cretins, and insane) for 339,014 inhabitants, or 9.610 per thousand.

Of the 3261 insane persons (1542 men, 1719 women) in the canton of Zürich, there are 79.3 per cent. unmarried, 10.5 per cent. married, 6.4 per cent. widowed, 3.8 per cent. divorced; 31.1 per cent. are treated in the public hospitals and asylums, 11.4 per cent. in private asylums, and 41.4 per cent. in their own homes.

Besides these two censuses of real value, others have been promoted for furnishing the cantonal authorities with necessary and important data for the provision for their insane during the years 1830 to 1885: in St. Gall (1836), Soleure (1846), Lucerne (1851 and 1868), Neufchatel (1854), Aargau (1857), Grisons (1874), and Schaffhausen (1885).

Side by side with the census of the insane, statistical researches have been instituted since 1836 in several of the cantons with respect to cretins. Dr. Guggenbühl undertook the establishment of an asylum for the purpose of curing them, or at least ameliorating their condition. He founded this asylum on the Abendberg, near Interlaken, where it existed for ten or twelve years, without, however, bringing about any remarkable results, as was to be expected with a malady that becomes incurable as soon as it has reached a certain developmental stage. But the question, having once been raised, did not remain without fruitful result. Public societies took it up, and there resulted from their investigations a statistical table of the cretins and idiots in Switzerland. From this it has been deduced that there are certain districts which appear more favourable to the development of cretinism than others, and from later censuses, taken especially in the canton of

Berne, it has been found that there at least the number of true cretins has of late sensibly diminished.*

In order to furnish a few more notes on the number of assisted persons in the hospitals and asylums, we mention the following figures:—

In the public asylums of Switzerland there were, under treatment on January 1, 1889, 4214 patients (1986 male, and 2228 female), on December 31, 1889, 4343, or a proportion of 1.48 insane persons treated in the hospitals for every thousand of the entire Swiss population, or if we include the 150 patients treated in the different private asylums, we shall obtain 4500 insane residents, or 1.53 per thousand of the entire population.

In 1885–89, the annual cost of maintenance of these fourteen hospitals and asylums, representing a population of 1,561,686 inhabitants, was 1,782,357 francs, or 1.14 francs for each inhabitant. The different cantons have expended in the construction and fitting up of their hospitals and asylums a round sum of from 14 to 15 million francs.

As the official assistance of the State and the committees cannot fully provide for all the requirements for the amelioration of the lot of the insane, *societies of patronage* have been formed in Switzerland, as in Germany, with the object of—

(1) Combating the prejudices existing in regard to mental maladies;

(2) Looking after the social interests of persons leaving asylums, and thus facilitating their return to society;

(3) Expediting by all useful means or other necessary measures the admission into asylums of all recent cases;

(4) Watching over the moral and material interests of patients while in asylums and during their absence from their homes, and eventually furnishing them with pecuniary assistance.

These societies of patronage having originated in private enterprise and created resources for themselves by annual assessments, as well as by gifts and legacies, soon became of great importance in the domain they had chosen for their field of action. In the nine cantons—Zürich, Berne, Lucerne, Basle (Ville), Appenzell (Rh. ext.), St. Gall, Grisons, Aargau, Thurgau—which reckon such societies among their [illegible] institutions, the number of [illegible] at the end of 1887 was about 13,000, and they possessed at that time a sum of [illegible] francs, part of which was to be [illegible] for the construction of an asylum (Grisons and Appenzell). For the [illegible] needs of one year 32,023 francs were spent by them. It remains only to add that the activity of these societies of patronage grows in importance from year to year, and fulfils its philanthropic purpose with much success.

F. [illegible]

* We must mention here a remarkable work by Dr. H. Bircher (Aargau) on endemic goitre, and its relation to deaf-mutism, and to cretinism, based on numerous observations, and on the material furnished by the examination of military recruits. By his observations he is led even to admit a propagation of the goitre and cretinic degeneration through the influence of water in certain geological formations.

SYDENHAM'S CHOREA.—The ordinary form of chorea, so called to distinguish it from chorea magna, or chorea Germanorum.

SYLLABLE STUMBLING.—A paralytic dysphasia, in which there is difficulty in speaking a word as a whole, although each letter and syllable can be distinctly sounded. It occurs in general paralysis.

SYMBOLISING INSANITY. (See INSANITY, SYMBOLISING; and SYMBOLISM.)

SYMBOLISM.—In some forms of insanity, especially delusional and hallucinational insanity, it is not uncommon for patients to interpret almost everything they see as a sign or symbol of their own feelings and ideas; for instance, that the clock in the room, or the stars in the heavens, bear a special relation to themselves.

SYMPATHETIC INSANITY.—The definition of sympathetic insanity lies in the word itself. It is a disorder of the brain connected with the disease of a more or less distant organ which has no apparent biological relation with the cerebrum. We shall not deal here with the doctrine of sympathies; it will suffice to keep in mind that sympathy is either physiological or abnormal. Sympathetic insanity is a morbid sympathy which has its seat, secondarily, in the brain.

This mental derangement has been known from the most ancient times. Homer mentions it in his "Iliad," and Aristophanes in his Comedies. Hippocrates investigated the relation between mania and irritation of the stomach, and has described the mental disorder connected with menstruation in young women. Aretius, of Cappadocia, places the seat of mania and melancholia in the intestines. Lastly, Galen enunciated his famous theory of humorism, and attributes insanity to the injurious action of the bile.

Galen's views have reigned supreme for centuries, and the fact that insanity originates in the intestines has been admitted by Aëtius, Soranus, Celsus, Oribasius, Alexander of Tralles, Paul of

Ægina, and the Arabian physicians. The schools of Alexandria, Salerno, Cordova, Salamanca, Montpellier and Paris all professed during the Middle Ages the doctrine of humoral pathology, which still had an adherent in the eighteenth century in the person of the famous Boerhaave.

This doctrine was rejected by Stahl, who considered insanity as the result of stasis of the blood, although he attributed to the liver a certain *rôle* in its production.

The doctrine of insanity by sympathy counted in the sixteenth and seventeenth centuries as many adversaries as adherents. Lepois, Willis, and Cullen rejected it, but still at the end of the eighteenth century it was defended by men like Lorry, Tissot, Sauvages, &c.

The enumeration of the different views held up to our own times affords little interest. We must, however, mention the antagonism in Germany between the spiritualistic and somatic schools at the commencement of the nineteenth century. Heinroth and Ideler, on the one hand, declare the preponderant influence of the mind and deny systematically the material origin of insanity, while this view is rejected by Nasse, Friedreich, Amelung, and by Maximilian Jacobi, who was the most vigorous and able adherent of the somatic doctrine, and in fact became the actual founder of the school of sympathetic insanity (B. Ball).

In 1856 and 1857 the Medico-Psychological Society of France held several meetings for the discussion of a thesis of Dr. Loiseau on sympathetic insanity. His work is very complete and carefully written, and is the most important which we possess on this subject. This monograph gave the learned assembly an opportunity for brilliant speeches. "Is there a sympathetic insanity?" About the middle of July 1857 the discussion was closed without any result being arrived at. The adherents of this new morbid state—Archambaut, Belhomme, and Legrand du Saulle—did not succeed in convincing their medical brethren in spite of their eloquence and abundant arguments, and the question was adjourned without having been solved, and in truth it is much more difficult than it might seem to be at first sight.

When one morbid condition appears at the same time as another which affects a more or less distant organ, it is not necessary to see herein sympathy, for it may be merely coincidence, except when their course and constant form prove their causal connection. We repeat that this relation to each other does not always include sympathy. It may exist between two morbid conditions which are parts of the same aggregate of symptoms, and this becomes evident when the clinical study proves clearly a bond between the two phenomena. In other words, a mental disorder may be found to be merely symptomatic after a superficial examination had made it appear to be *psychose par consensus*. This is the case with mental disorders observed in connection with neuroses, with organic central affections, with intoxication, and with a morbid diathesis. Also, as one of the speakers at the debate of 1856 pointed out, the number of sympathetic mental disorders becomes singularly reduced if examined more closely. If we submit them to a severe analysis, we begin altogether to doubt the existence of these disorders as a distinct nosological species.

To give some examples:—

A woman becomes insane during pregnancy, but recovers. Ten years later she has a fresh attack of mental derangement and is believed to be again pregnant; however, a uterine polypus is discovered. The woman undergoes a surgical operation and completely recovers her mental health (G. de Caulbry).

A man has had two attacks of frenzy with an interval of several years; each of these attacks is cured by the expulsion of ascarides (Vogel).

A melancholiac has an hepatic abscess, puncture of which restores physical and mental health.

A girl has become insane in consequence of the suppression of the menses; one morning on getting up she declares that she is quite well. The menses have returned, and with them reason (Esquirol).

A man suffers from cardiac disease; during the exacerbation he suffers from *délire des grandeurs* with hallucinations, while lucidity returns in the intervals (Loiseau).

A phthisical patient notices that the symptoms of his pulmonary affection improve, but at the same time he becomes agitated. Then his sentiments become altered; he becomes suspicious and unsociable (Clouston).

These are some cases from the number of those of sympathetic insanity which are least disputed. Uterine affections, intestinal worms, hepatic suppuration, catamenial disorder, heart disease, and tubercular diathesis—such were the morbid conditions which determined a reaction of the cerebrum. The question is now, of what nature is this reaction?

When our ancestors in medicine invented the hypothesis of sympathy, they had in view two phenomena, physiological or morbid, united by a mysterious link, which the science of their days did not allow them to discover. This gap between the two conditions mentioned was filled up by "sympathy." To-day anatomical and clinical discoveries have cleared up these formerly obscure relations. Chemical analysis and the study of the nervous system account, at least theoretically, for the connection of the two phenomena. Where our ancestors discovered "sympathy," there we see faulty nutrition, intoxication, or cerebral reflex action. We even might say that the term "sympathy" is no longer justified.

Among the examples quoted above there is not one which could not be interpreted clinically. Uterine disorders are specially capable of determining by reflex action profound derangement of the cerebral functions. Nobody doubts that alterations in the nutrition of the brain may be caused by cardiac and hepatic disease and by menstrual disorders. That form of sympathetic insanity which has been the least discussed, and which is connected with helminthiasis, is it sympathetic in the sense understood in former times? Is there no connection between the intestine and the brain? The knowledge we possess of reflex actions compels us to be very reserved on this point. The constant irritation of the mucous membrane causes a profound derangement of the splanchnics, which in its turn radiates towards the cortical cells: such is the theory which is partly proved by facts, since the epilepsy which is so frequently associated with insanity of helminthiac origin, could not be explained without a somatic lesion of the central nervous system.

Lastly, diathesis has such an evidently harmful effect on the nutrition that it is almost impossible to conceive that the brain could be exempt from this influence. To mental disorders in consequence of diathesis is logically due the epithet "symptomatic," which a number of medical men would now desire to apply to all forms of "sympathetic" alienation.

We have thus arrived at an unexpected result: there is no sympathetic insanity.

However, although this term will have to be completely abandoned some day, we must nevertheless recognise the fact that there are certain mental disorders whose course is parallel to that of certain peripheral and visceral diseases, or, in other words, that there are mental derangements whose form, course, and frequent repetitions show complete solidarity with extra-cerebral disorder without allowing us to consider them as parts of the same syndrome. For these forms of disorder we retain in this article, in order to conform with usage, the term "sympathetic insanity."

Heredity favours the formation of such disorders as it does all forms of mental derangement, but it need not be necessarily present. A curious observation which medical men have frequently made is precisely this—the absence of heredity in most cases examined, so that in them the origin of the disorder becomes still more evident.

Do these psychoses possess a constant, well-determined form, and do diseases of one region or of one organ always produce cerebral reactions with a character so invariable that we are enabled to make our diagnosis from them alone? Most observers deny this, and are of opinion that a peripheral disease produces merely a mental disorder, the form of which always varies. We ourselves regard this opinion as too absolute. This is certain, that if in describing an attack of insanity we confine ourselves to stating only an insane conception—*e.g.*, ideas of persecution—we find that this symptom is present in a great number of cases with such monotony that we certainly could not make use of it for the purpose of differential diagnosis; but a mental disorder is composed of complex elements, which we must take into account, and the *ensemble* of which gives the derangement its proper character. The form of the disorder, its mode of appearance, its course, and its duration are valuable indications for its characterisation; utilising these, we might perhaps arrive at better conclusions with regard to the disorders with which we are occupied here. This part of mental science is as yet little advanced, and much remains still to be discovered, but we must not neglect the results already obtained. In England we mention the work of Skae; this great alienist has in his essay on classification sketched with great aptitude most species of mental disorder of a sympathetic nature. We also mention the noteworthy books of Clouston, Maudsley, &c., on insanity connected with phthisis, menstruation, chorea, and neurotic conditions.

Sympathetic insanity may be naturally divided into two categories:

(1) **Insanity produced by functional disorder**, and

(2) **Insanity produced by morbid conditions.**

The disorders of the former class (disorders of puberty, puerperal, menstrual, ovarian, and climacteric insanity) and a certain number of disorders of the latter category (insanity from diathesis, derangement connected with general diseases and with neurotic conditions) will be found in special articles in this Dictionary. We shall therefore limit ourselves to describe summarily some forms of mental alienation which have their origin in visceral and organic affections.

Mental disorders connected with derangements of the *digestive organs* have at all times attracted the attention of the medical world. Hufeland described an abdominal insanity. It is quite true that derangement of almost any abdominal organ may produce mental disorder (Friedreich). It is well known that normal digestion already influences certain individuals intellectually and morally; why should not costiveness or a functional disorder have an influence on the brain? Guislain relates the case of a woman who had auditory and visual hallucinations every time she had constipation.

Lorry, Esquirol, Louyer-Villermay, and Bayle have investigated the intellectual disorders of gastric origin. Esquirol has described after Wichmann, Hesselbach, and Greding *displacement of the transverse colon* as a common cause of alienation. As a matter of fact, this view has been contradicted by Sir William Lawrence, and its value is doubtful.

Hypochondriacal depression, ideas of discouragement with a tendency to suicide, and refusal to take food are the most important of *intestinal psychoses.* Régis has justly recommended washing out the stomach in the case of dyspeptic lunatics.

Mental symptoms in cases of *duodenal catarrh* have been described by Holtorff. The symptoms are those of simple hypochondriasis, but they often border on actual lypemania with morbid exaggeration of the conscience and extreme irritability.

Moral perversion has sometimes been observed. A patient has been known to be very quarrelsome and vicious, who after an evacuation again became sociable.

Although in former times the influence of the *liver* as an ætiological element has been greatly exaggerated, it is nevertheless real and frequent; organic lesions of the liver are, however, rare in the insane (Loiseau). It is different, however, with inflammation of the organ.

Functional alterations of *liver* and *bile-ducts* are a recognised cause of melancholia. Wiedmann and Greding have pointed out the frequency of numerous calculi in the gall-bladder of lunatics. The scientific observations on the *spleen* which we possess, and on the *pancreas*, are neither numerous nor conclusive enough to allow of our drawing conclusions with regard to mental derangement connected with lesions of these organs. The *peritoneum* however seems to have frequently been the cause of mental disorders of a sympathetic nature. We owe the proofs of this latter fact to Bonet, Greding, and S. Pinel. Dr. J. A. Campbell has published a case of sitiophobia, where the post-mortem examination disclosed chronic peritonitis.

Mental disorder, due to *helminthiasis*, is of common occurrence; Esquirol found this to be the case in twenty-four patients among 144, at the Salpêtrière. At the commencement of this century Prost reported numerous cases of helminthiac insanity. This physician even maintains that intestinal worms are one of the most frequent causes of insanity. Esquirol, Ferrus, Frank, and Vogel, have published most interesting observations on cases of this kind. An extensive monograph on this subject has been written by a German physician, Dr. Ernst Vix. This author describes a special symptomatology in connection with helminthiasis—disorders of sensibility of various kinds, perversion of taste, sexual excitement, and a propensity to scatophagia; hemeralopia has been observed in some cases. Of these symptoms, perversion of taste is the most common; it is accompanied by maniacal excitement, and becomes complicated with the refusal of food. We think it is necessary to add various disorders of the nervous system. We have thus observed in some cases palpitations with a tendency to lypothymia. Dr. Vix thinks that helminthiac insanity is more frequent in the female sex than in the male.

Legrand du Saulle quotes numerous examples of insanity caused by irritation due to the presence of *larvæ* in the *frontal sinus.* The form observed was mania frequently complicated with epilepsy.

In spite of Griesinger's scepticism with regard to psychoses of *renal origin*, the latter has been observed by several authors, among whom we mention Savage, Wilks, Scholtz, Petrone, Erlangen. The last-mentioned regards insanity in albuminuria as the first consequence or stage of uræmic intoxication. Without deciding whether this opinion, which holds this form of insanity to be merely symptomatic, be right or wrong, we wish to mention that the principal characteristic of this disorder is maniacal excitement with painful hallucinations, soon followed by a quiet dementia, to which has been given the name of "tranquil stupor." This mental depression must be distinguished from the apoplectic state. The face is calm, the pulse normal. The patient wakes up from his stupor when he is called. Later on other more serious symptoms appear, which hasten the termination.

We know little as yet about mental derangement in *Addison's disease*. Griesinger says that patients affected with it are profoundly depressed. The melancholic form with conditions of anxiety and emotion has been observed by Dr. Rutherford Macphail. The patient whose case is described had attacks of religious exaltation; he refused food, and died in a state of marasmus.

Although *diabetes* is not actually an affection of the kidneys, we shall say a word or two about mental disorders in diabetic patients. Marchal de Calvi was the first to write on this subject in 1864. Later, Legrand du Saulle has given a most characteristic description of diabetes, of the mental symptoms of which he speaks in the following terms: "There is at first an invincible apathy, a complete suspension of the will, or there may be comparative optimism. The patient sees his sexual appetite disappear, and with resignation passes into a condition of impotence. He becomes sleepless and spends his nights in soliloquies without insane conceptions (*sans délire*). At last there appears a morbid excitement, terminating in a desire to sleep, which not being satisfied, causes attempts at suicide."

Lallier makes the interesting remark that thirst and polyuria are frequently absent in insane patients affected with diabetes.

Affections of the *bladder* (cystitis, retention of urine, stone) frequently influence the mental functions, but the disorders thus produced pertain mostly to the moral faculties. In some patients a tendency to suicide is observed.

Psychoses connected with *cardiac affections* frequently present the forms of mania or depression. Mildner asserts that lesions of the aorta produce mania, and those of the mitral valve melancholia. Our opinion is that it is necessary to attach more importance to the remittent course of the mental disorder which may improve at the same time that the cardiac disease becomes modified under treatment. The mania is generally remarkably acute and accompanied by extremely violent acts. Ambitious ideas often appear and make it especially difficult to treat the patient. A patient suffering under these circumstances from melancholia is anxious, he has painful hallucinations and ideas of persecution, and he also shows a tendency to despair, to murder, and to suicide. Some patients are themselves afraid of becoming insane. In all varieties of insanity associated with heart disease there is an irresistible desire to be in motion.

The *cutaneous affections* observed every day in patients in asylums are generally a product of the mental disease in the course of which they appear. They must be regarded as trophic derangements. In a few rare cases, however, a herpetic diathesis is complicated secondarily by intellectual and moral disorders. These forms of mental derangement are, with regard to their symptoms, almost uniform, and follow faithfully the phases of the cutaneous affection, so that their sympathetic nature appears evident. An insane patient had an old eczema on his ears and the nape of the neck, with exacerbations. He attributed this eruption to the sorcery of a priest who had touched his ears with a breviary. This priest continued to cause him sufferings by piercing and burning him at the points which were the seat of the itching. The excitement increased or decreased according to the course of the eczema. Later on ambitious ideas appeared, the patient was a saint and then God himself. Suddenly all the insane conceptions disappeared simultaneously with the appearance of a serious complication; an ulcerous enteritis has by metastasis replaced the eruption. Death occurred in consequence of repeated intestinal hæmorrhage. This example seems to us conclusive. We have ourselves observed several patients with mental disorders in connection with herpetic affections, and we admit, with Guislain, this form of sympathetic insanity, in spite of the objections raised against this view.

Herpetic insanity presents definite characteristics by which it may be recognised. At first there is hypochondriacal excitement, according to the generally remittent course of the eruption, then there are ideas of persecution based on disorders of cutaneous sensibility. One patient feels insects creeping over his skin, another feels himself "ravaged" by a demon, &c. Chronicity sets in and presents as a characteristic form ideas of grandeur with aberration of personality. The patient denies his family, and maintains that he has been changed in his youth; he is a prince, God, &c. This mental symptom, the aberration of personality, may well be pathognomonic of this form of mental disorder.

J. Poya.

SYMPATHETIC NERVOUS SYSTEM, PHYSIOLOGY OF.—Distribution of Sympathetic Nerves.—The physiology of the sympathetic nerve is so dependent on its anatomical distribution, that it is necessary to make a short statement as to the position it occupies in the body. Following mainly Dr. Gaskell's investigation, it is found that the white rami communicantes are formed by an outflow of medullated nerves from both the anterior and the posterior roots of the spinal nerves between the second thoracic and the second lumbar inclusive, which medullated nerves pass not only into their metameric sympathetic (lateral) ganglia, but also form three main streams, upwards into the cervical ganglia, downwards into the lumbar and sacral ganglia, and outwards into the collateral ganglia, passing over the lateral ganglia to form the main portion of the splanchnic nerves and the other rami efferentes. The structure of these visceral nerves is different from that of the first nine spinal nerves. These latter agree in structure with the nerves lying between the second lumbar and the first sacral nerves. But below this point again, the structure of the nerves is the same as that of the thoracic visceral nerves. At the second and third sacral roots arise the pelvic splanchnic nerves, called by other observers the nervi erigentes, that pass directly to the hypogastric plexus without communicating with the lateral ganglia; from this plexus they branch upwards to the inferior mesenteric ganglion (collateral ganglion), and downwards to the distal ganglia of the bladder, uterus, and generative organs.

The upward stream of these visceral nerves is seen in the spinal accessory nerve.

In the spinal cord itself these visceral nerves seem to be formed of two rami, one a ganglionated root in connection with the cells of Clarke's column, the other a non-ganglionated root in connection with the cells of the lateral horn.

The origin of all vaso-motor nerves is to be found in the central nervous system. They pass down from the medulla oblongata, from a spot known as the antero-lateral nucleus of Clarke, run down the cord in lateral tracts, leave the cord by way of the anterior roots of the nerve, and so pass to lateral ganglia, and onwards to the heart and vessels in many directions, some of their non-medullated fibres being reflected back from the lateral ganglia to the membranes and vessels of the cord itself. In their passage through the lateral ganglia, by way of the rami viscerales, they lose their medulla in these ganglia, and pass to their various destinations on the vessels as non-medullated fibres. The blood-vessels of every portion of the head and face receive their vaso-constrictor nerves from the cervical sympathetic. The blood-vessels of all the abdominal organs derive their constrictor nerves by way of the splanchnic nerves, and the corresponding rami efferentes of the upper lumbar ganglia.

The accelerator nerves of the heart leave the spinal cord by the rami viscerales of second, third, and even lower thoracic nerves, pass to the ganglion cardiacum basale, and thence reach the heart directly, or indirectly by way of the inferior cervical ganglion and the annulus of Vieussens. In the lateral ganglia they also lose their medulla.

The nerves that, stimulated, cause peristaltic movements in a large portion of the gastro-intestinal canal, leave the medulla oblongata in the roots of the vagus, lose their medulla in the ganglion of the trunk, and thence run to the intestinal muscles, resembling the vaso-motor nerves in structure and distribution. The lower portion of the intestinal canal is innervated from two sources, one, the thoracic stream of visceral nerves, the other, the pelvic splanchnics above mentioned.

Sympathetic Ganglia.—The ganglia are of four kinds: (1) The ganglia of the posterior roots, root ganglia; (2) The lateral ganglia, the main sympathetic chain; (3) Collateral ganglia, such as semi-lunar, inferior mesenteric; and (4) Terminal ganglia, the ganglia of organs, as of heart, stomach, &c. The root ganglia and the lateral ganglia may be called proximal; the collateral and the terminal ganglia may be called distal.

The functions of these ganglia vary. The root ganglia are probably centres of nutrition, and centres of reflex arcs in a small degree. Gaskell considers the lateral ganglia are only nutritive centres, and not centres of reflex action. Their size alone makes it probable that they possess other functions than that of nutrition of nerves.

Dr. Hale White's investigations seem to show that in the human adult the collateral ganglia hold no specific function. He is inclined to look upon them as degenerate organs in man, like the ganglion of the trunk of the vagus, the pituitary in the pineal bodies, and probably also the medullary portion of the human suprarenal body, derived as it is from the sympathetic system. The terminal ganglia of organs have an automatic function; the secretory nerves of the intestine have the small ganglia of the solar and superior mesenteric plexuses for their centres; the cells of Auerbach's and Meissner's plexuses have an automatic influence on the intestine: the ganglia of the uterus, Fallopian tubes, and of the blood-vessels have an automatic influence upon the organ on which they lie (Hale White).

The vaso-dilator nerves are the inhibitory fibres of the heart, the fibres, with their functions, contained in the chorda tympani and small petrosal nerves, and the nervi erigentes. Anatomically, they differ from vaso-constrictor nerves by not losing their medulla until they reach more terminal ganglia. Their orgin is from the cranio-cervical and the sacral cord.

Double Nerve Supply to Glands, &c.—It is probable that all tissues are connected by efferent nerves of these two kinds. This double supply has been found in the submaxillary, parotid, and lachrymal glands. Thus Michael Foster speaks of two sets of fibres employed in the secretion of saliva, one, cerebro-spinal, vaso-dilator, stimulation of which produces a copious flow of limpid saliva free from mucus, anabolic; the other, sympathetic, vaso-constrictor, coming from the cervical sympathetic; its stimulation giving rise to a secretion rich in organic matter, katabolic.

Influence on the Iris.—There seems to be no need for a dilator muscle of the iris. It cannot be demonstrated in most animals. The sphincter muscle of the iris is supplied by two nerves of opposite character, the one the third nerve that contracts the pupil, the other the sympathetic that inhibits this contraction. The dilatation of the pupil on stimulation of the sympathetic nerve is thus brought about by inhibition of the tonic contraction of the sphincter muscle, if only the radial fibres of the iris possess a sufficient amount of elasticity.

There is no evidence that the same nerve fibre is sometimes capable of acting as a motor nerve, sometimes as a nerve of inhibition.

Influence on the Heart.—"The primary effect of the stimulation of the sympathetic (accelerator) of the heart is an increase both in the rate and strength of the auricular and ventricular contractions; these nerves, therefore, may be justly called motor, because they augment the activity of the cardiac muscle, and that augmentation is followed by exhaustion. Gaskell prefers the term 'katabolic' to motor, because when a muscle is set in action by stimulation of its motor nerve or otherwise, there is a great increase in the destructive changes with subsequent exhaustion. On the other hand, any explanation of inhibition, which is to hold good, must not confine itself merely to the cessation of rhythmical action, but must also explain the diminished contraction and the relaxation of the cardiac muscle. The result of stimulation of these nerves is exactly opposite to that of the sympathetic nerves; there, increased activity followed by exhaustion, symptoms of katabolic action; here, diminished activity followed by repair of function, symptoms of anabolic action." This inhibition can be set in action reflexly by an afferent nerve.

Reflex Action.—It will be seen, in speaking of vascular tone, that reflex action plays an important part. Although the lateral ganglia are nutritive centres rather than reflex, their structure does not prevent the possibility of their acting as reflex centres. But whether or no, a large amount of action of the sympathetic nerve seems to be under reflex influence, the centre of the reflex arc being the medulla oblongata or the spinal cord. Sometimes a sensory nerve is the eisodic nerve, and the sympathetic the exodic; sometimes the relation is reversed. Nor is the perception of a sensory impression necessary. Some impression is made on the peripheral termination of a nerve; the molecular motion it sets up is propagated along the nerve until it reaches a ganglion. In many cases the propagated impulse reaches the ganglion by means of a nerve that is only in close apposition to the actual nerve that is connected with the ganglion. The large quantity of molecular motion thus disengaged discharges itself along another nerve proceeding from the ganglion to a muscle.

Many examples of such a reflex are are themselves illustrations of the part played by the sympathetic in numerous diseases.

Illustrations of Sympathetic Reflex Action.—Thus, facial neuralgia, causing congestion of conjunctiva and lachrymation; salivation occurring in pregnancy; faintness or constipation due to irritation of hepatic or renal calculus; contraction of vessels and arrest of urine, set up by calculus in the kidney; partial cramp of vaso-motors, confined to the extremities of the fingers, seen sometimes in angina pectoris; the effects of cold on the vessels of the extremities, explaining various necroses of the extremities. Perhaps, too, Vulpian's experiment should come under this head, in which, after transverse section of the sciatic nerve, or of the brachial plexus, when the corresponding pulp of the paw of an animal had become quite pale and anæmic, he was able, by slightly rubbing these pulps, to cause a reflex congestion. In mammals, after section of the cord at the mid-dorsal region, sensory excitation of one posterior limb will cause reflex heat-phenomena in the other. Maragliano's observation in fever, testing the variation in the pulse by sealing the forearm in a glass vessel, and taking sphygmographic tracings, irritating the other arm meanwhile by an electrical current, showed the vascular reaction in patients with fever to be generally indicative of constriction, but sometimes of dilatation, and generally more energetic, prompt, and persistent than in the afebrile period. Flux from the intestinal vessels is a sequence of the irritation of some foreign body in the canal, or of the collapse, from perforating ulcer of stomach or intestines. Contraction of cerebral vessels may be caused by the irritation of the proximal end of the divided posterior roots of the sciatic or other spinal nerves. Sciatica may induce saccharine urine, the fourth ventricle being here the centre of the reflex arc. There is the pulse of lead colic. Local dilatation of vessels (paresis of vaso-constrictors), and even evanescent erythema, may result from the action of intense light—*e.g.*, the electric light. Landouzi and Nothnagel have described an angina pectoris vaso-motoria, which they referred to a general arterial spasm, often produced reflexly, especially by exposure to cold, the secretion of milk induced by fœtal movement *in utero*, by the touch of the finger, or of the child's mouth, and the hæmorrhage from a fibrous tumour of the uterus are reflex, or the eisodic nerve may be sensory-sympathetic. From investigations made by Dr. F. Edgeworth, of Bristol, it is seen that large medullated fibres are found in very many of the sympathetic nerves, from the upper dorsal to the third lumbar vertebræ, but in greatest abundance in the uppermost dorsal rami, and in the lower dorsal and upper lumbar. They pass through the ganglion cells of the ganglia on the lateral sympathetic chain, without giving off any branch to them, and they can be traced up to the posterior roots of the spinal nerves, to be connected with cells in the posterior ganglion. It seems therefore certain that these fibres are sensory.

Vascular Tone.—But a chief illustration is the reflex action of the blood upon vascular tone. Goltz says the tone of the arteries is maintained by local centres, situated in their own immediate vicinity; but though such distal ganglia exist, the spinal system is really the centre of the reflex arc, except perhaps for the feeblest impulses. Vascular tone is due to a reflex mechanism, a mechanism brought into action by incessant centripetal excitations, which are probably the blood waves; as regards a vessel the factors of this arc exist—the middle tunic of the vessel, the centripetal nerve fibres in the vascular walls, the bulbo-spinal centre, and the centrifugal vaso-motor nerves.

All the phenomena of reflex congestion and of reflex dilatation of the vessels from any cause are only instances of enfeeblement or abolition, more or less complete, more or less persistent, of the vascular tone.

Influence of Heart on Arteries, and of Arteries on Heart.—The influence of the sympathetic is specially seen in the mutual relationship of the heart and arteries. Let there be from any cause a constriction of most of the small arteries of the body, there is, as a consequence, increase in the arterial tension. The heart strives to overcome this excess of tension, and must employ more energy for this purpose; its contractions become more vigorous, more rapid. This effect is not purely mechanical, but is under the influence of the sympathetic accelerators. Under increased intra-arterial pressure the blood in the ventricle also undergoes at the moment of systole, and of the opening of the sigmoid valves, an excess of tension. This impresses some excitation at the endocardial extremities of the centripetal nerve of the heart; this impression is carried up to the bulb, from which down through the cervical cord is reflected a centrifugal irritation by way of the sympathetic to the intra-cardiac ganglia, and so result increased energy and increased rapidity of the cardiac movements.

Reversing the order of the phenomena, if the left ventricle from any cause be abnormally full of blood, the special impression on the peripheral extremities of the cardiac nerves is carried up by the depressor nerve, a branch of the vagus, to the bulb, and thence by means of dilator nerves a general reflex dilatation of vessels takes place, and especially by way of the splanchnic nerves on the vessels of the mesentery, and the heart is relieved of its pressure; or the dilatation of the abdominal vessels is brought about by inhibition of the vaso-constrictors.

So once again, if an abnormally small amount of blood be in the heart, the reflex action originates from the cardiac nerves, and will react on the vaso-constrictors; the vessels contract, and the blood, receiving an increased *vis a tergo*, flows more abundantly to the heart. Thus the heart may, up to a certain point, play the part of regulator of the vessels, or at least exercise a certain influence on their tone, whilst inversely the vessels rule, up to a certain point, the energy and frequency of the movements of the heart.

Nutrition.—It is probable that the part played by the sympathetic nerve on nutrition is only in so far as the heart's action is kept normal by its influence, and the tone of the vessels preserved. It is certain that section of a nerve supplying the blood-vessels of an area of mucous membrane, or of skin, causes ulceration and destruction of the part. But not only are the phenomena of partial atrophies, of infantile paralysis, of progressive muscular atrophy, constantly met with without any lesion of the sympathetic, except in so far as variations in the blood-supply are concerned, but the peculiar symptoms of progressive hemi-atrophy of the face seem to have little or nothing to do with distinct sympathetic lesion.

Animal Heat.—The influence of the sympathetic on animal heat is exercised: (1) By the vaso-motors of the whole body regulating the amount of blood for combustion in the tissues; (2) By the vaso-motors of the cutaneous vessels partially regulating transpiration from the skin; (3) By the vaso-motors of the lungs, regulating pulmonary transpiration; (4) By the accelerator nerve of the heart ruling not only in part the amount of blood in the tissues, but especially regulating the amount passed through the lungs, and so indirectly the quantity of oxygen assimilated by the blood. The first act, that of heat creation, is the consequence of the chemical phenomena of nutrition. The distribution of the heat created, the variation of it by constriction of vessels, or by restraining chemical action, are among the functions of the sympathetic.

Inflammation.—This nerve plays an important part in inflammation, both by altering vascular tone under reflex irritation, and probably by influencing the molecular (chemical) changes in the vascular walls, changes that favour the migration of leucocytes. For the due understanding of microbic pathology this influence of the sympathetic deserves to be recognised as causing in some cases at least a preliminary condition, without which germ growth would be difficult or impossible. Vaso-motor paresis does not, in the absence of other factors, cause inflammation, but it is an important accessory.

Œdema.—It is on the increased porosity or permeability of the vessel that œdema depends. The endothelium of a vessel is a living tissue with an active metabolism. Whilst even for mechanical dropsy we are compelled to assume a peculiar influence exerted by the wall of the vessel, the latter acquires a still greater importance in other varieties of hydrops. This modification of the vascular endothelium is partly influenced by the condition of the circulating blood, [illegible] by vaso-motor paresis.

General Pathology.—The sympathetic system may be said to possess a very special pathology, but by no means in all cases a recognised pathological anatomy. As a general rule the cells of the semilunar and the superior cervical ganglia are wasted in wasting diseases, but with many exceptions. The most usual lesions are pigmentation, colloid degeneration with proliferation of endothelial cells, and secondary fatty metamorphosis, interstitial hyperplasia leading to atrophy, and sclerosis of nerve elements.

Given a recognisable lesion of a sympathetic ganglion or nerve, certain phenomena are found following this as a consequence. On the other hand, given these same phenomena without a coarse lesion of the sympathetic nerve or ganglion, it is justifiable to say that these depend upon a morbid condition of these structures, even though such a condition cannot be recognised by the usual means of investigation. A ganglion (and we include Clarke's cells under this category) apparently healthy, may be changed in some occult way by the sun's rays, by the circulation of abnormal blood, by what is called "irritation" carried to it from disease in a distant organ, or by emotion. It cannot be doubted that these influences change in some way the equipoise of the ganglion; for, as their result, are seen phenomena precisely corresponding to the effects of coarse experiments upon the sympathetic in animals, and of easily recognised lesion of these organs in man. The starting-point of this irritation is seen, the channels by which the irritation is conveyed, the consequences of the irritative action beyond the ganglion; but the absolute condition of the ganglion itself, in so far as it differs from its state in health, is incapable of being in all cases demonstrated. Moreover, it is a matter of experience that irritations which induce sympathetic phenomena are generally reflex rather than direct.

Effects of Lesion on Cervical Sympathetic.—Section of the cervical sympathetic nerve causes paralysis of, and therefore dilatation, of the vessels of the head and face, with some rise of temperature of the same regions. The pupil is contracted from the inhibitory influence of the sympathetic on the iris being cut off. The contraction of the pupil is due to the unimpeded influence of the third nerve. Not quite so certainly result interference with the secretion of tears, sweat, and saliva, on the affected side, narrowing of the palpebral fissure, and retraction of the eyeball. Myosis may be due to the pressure of a tumour on the cervical sympathetic. It is met with in sclerosis of the medulla oblongata, and in some diseases of the spinal cord, as tabes cervicalis and progressive muscular atrophy.

Exophthalmic Goitre.—Exophthalmic goître is described elsewhere in these pages. It may be allowable to point out the small part played by the sympathetic in the causation of this disease. The phenomena may own a central origin. As a matter of experiment, exophthalmos has been found to be a result of section of the restiform bodies, and therefore may be expected to manifest itself from any destructive lesion of that, if not of other portions, of the medulla oblongata. Lesion also of a portion of the floor of the fourth ventricle would account for any interference with the independent or co-ordinate action of the levator palpebræ, as one portion of the origin of the fourth nerve can be traced into a grey nucleus at the upper part of the floor of the fourth ventricle, close to the origin of the fifth nerve. Lesion too of a small portion of this ventricle on each side of the middle line will include the chief vaso-motor centre of the body, whilst a partial paralysis of the vagus, from lesion of its nucleus, would set free the accelerator nerves of the heart to act without vagus inhibition, and thus induce palpitation.

Headache.—The influence of the sympathetic is sometimes seen in that form of headache that is caused by reflex irritations from the stomach, intestine or uterus.

Migraine.—No morbid condition of the sympathetic will account for the symptoms of migraine, although this nerve is considerably affected. It is closely allied to a nerve storm, described by Dr. Buzzard, affecting the medulla oblongata, in which the nuclei of the fifth nerve, the portio mollis, the vagus, and often the bulbar vaso-motor centre are implicated, associated with tinnitus, neuralgia, vertigo, faintness, and vomiting.

Epilepsy.—The sympathetic takes no part in the causation of epilepsy, except that it is partially responsible for the altered nutrition of the centre or centres from which the local discharge emanates.

Lesion of Nervous Centres. — In lesions of the brain and spinal cord sympathetic phenomena are often found as secondary consequences, or as involved in the causation of inflammation. Probably a paresis of vaso-motors may be one factor in the increased constriction of which, in some cerebral lesions, a high temperature is the manifestation.

Angina Pectoris.—The forms of angina pectoris are various: (1) with spasm of heart, and arterial constriction; (2) a pure neuralgia, which may or may not be associated with disease of the heart or the aorta; (3) a condition of vaso-motor paresis from a central origin, or excited by reflex irritation, or under the influence of emotion. In causation and pathology they are separate diseases, and demand wholly different treatment. The sympathetic takes part in the first form, and is almost wholly responsible for the third.

Diabetes Mellitus. — Diabetes mellitus is discussed elsewhere in these pages. But it may be remarked here that the condition of general arterial pressure and the dilatation of the hepatic artery, and in a less degree of the portal vein, are under the government of the vaso-motor centre, and thus this system of nerves may be associated with diabetes. The connection is almost invariably reflex, and the vaso-motor system generally affects the centre of the reflex arc and the exodic nerve. Dr. Pavy found that injury to the inferior cervical ganglion gave rise to glycosuria.

Neurasthenia.—Neurasthenia is also the subject of a special article. But as to one form of it, Rosenthal sums up the whole nature of the disorder when he says, "L'hystérie n'est qu'une faiblesse de résistance congénitale ou acquise des centres vasomoteurs."

Pigmentation. — Morbid development of pigment, or unusual positions of it, are only abnormalities of a normal condition. The exciting cause may be a diseased state of blood acting directly, as in ague, syphilis, carcinoma, chronic rheumatism, &c., or irritation acting in a reflex manner from a distant organ, and by preference from pelvic or intestinal viscera, or emotion. The irritation, whether direct or reflex, primarily affects the solar plexus, and through it partially paralyses the splenic plexus. The effect of this is first an enlargement of the spleen, and secondly an increase in the formation of pigment. Except in some instances of intense emotional storm, chronicity is an invariable element in pigmentation. For the abnormal deposit of pigment in the skin three factors are necessary: a well-developed papilla, the healthy influence of the sensory nerve, a dilatation of the local vessel. The latter factor is generally induced by a diminution of vascular tone caused by paresis of the vaso-constrictors. This paresis, like the effect on the splenic nerves, can be effected by the direct action of morbid blood, by reflex irritation, and by emotion.

Addison's Disease.—The fact that the symptoms of Addison's disease do not follow the removal of, or other diseases of the supra-renal capsules, seems to be new proof against the possibility of the irritation of bacilli tuberculosi in the supra-renal capsule exciting the phenomena of Addison's disease. But the part played by the sympathetic in the direct causation of Addison's disease is still uncertain.

The variation in the size of the sympathetic ganglia in health is so great that the reported hypertrophy of certain ganglia in acromegaly seems of little importance.

Neuroses of the Extremities.—The dilatation of the vessels of the extremities and the more usual neuroses attended with vaso-constriction and local diminution of temperature depend, the first on paralysis of the vaso-motor of the part affected, and the latter on over-excitation of the vaso-motor centre. In the lesser degrees it is not unusual in this country. In one form or other it is common among the coolies who take service in Natal. The contractile form of the neurosis may determine symmetrical gangrene of the extremities. This seems to be due to chronic spasm, such as might readily be set up in the vessels by prolonged irritation. This condition may easily exist in the vaso-motors that run in the course of the nerves of the extremities, if these nerves are in a state of peripheral neuritis, a fact that has been found in a certain number of cases. It is a true tetanus of the vaso-motors. In one case recorded, in which only the vaso-motor fibres of the arms were affected, a growth was found post-mortem in front of the spine, involving the first dorsal nerve and the sympathetic trunk. This disease is pre-eminently connected with the sympathetic system.

In many other maladies the sympathetic plays an important part by means of its physiological action on circulation, nutrition, secretion, and inflammation. It is thought by some to be the structure specially involved in sea-sickness, and in fatal chorea with great distension of vessels. In diabetes insipidus, in many of the visceral—especially the uterine—neuroses, in purpura hæmorrhagica, in some affections of the skin, this system of nerves, so bound up in the cerebro-spinal centres, takes either a primary or secondary place.

It is certain that anatomical abnormalities of many of the sympathetic ganglia may exist without any corresponding symptoms; and that the sympathetic is constantly in a state of vulnerability, of abnormal excitability to impulses, often from a distant organ, and very frequently affecting it by a reflex mechanism.

E. Long Fox.

[*References.*—Dr. Gaskell, *Journal of Physiology*, vol. vii. Dr. Hale White, *Journal of Physiology*, vols. viii. and x.; Guy's Hospital Reports, vol. xlvi. Dr. Chapin's Fiske Fund Prize Essay. Poincaré, Le Système nerveux périphérique. Dr. Broadbent and Dr. Saundby, On Vascular Tone, Brit. Med. Journ., 1883, vol. ii. Michael Foster, Text-book of Physiology. Eulenburg and Guttman, Sympathetic System of Nerves. Seeligmüller, Lehrbuch der Krankheiten der peripheren Nerven und des Sympathicus. Wunderlich, Das Verhalten der Eigenwärme in Krankheiten. Vulpian, L'Appareil Vasomoteur. Dr. Greenhow, Internat. Med. Congress Reports. Dr. Weir Mitchell and others, American Journal of Science, 1876. E. Long Fox, The Influence of the Sympathetic on Disease, 1885.]

SYMPTOMATIC MANIA. (*See* Mania, Symptomatic.)

SYNALGIA.—By this term Henry de Fromentel ("Les Synalgies et les Synesthésies," Paris, 1888) designates the phenomenon, previously described several times, that by the irritation of some point of the body pain is experienced in another part, often widely separated from the first. He has deduced laws which, as he believes, hold good not for a definite person only but for all who experience synalgias, according to which, for example, an irritation of the skin over the patella produces a synalgia in the hypochondrium of the same side. The undersigned has for many years observed synalgias on himself, but his experience does not confirm the laws given by de Fromentel.

E. Bleuler.

SYNOSTOSIS (*σύν*, with; *ὀστέον*, a bone). The joining together of the bones of the skull. The early or defective closing of the cranium has a great effect on the mental development of the individual. (*See* Idiocy, Pathology of.)

SYPHILIDOMANIA, SYPHILOMANIA (syphilis; *mania*, madness). A form of mental derangement due to syphilis. (Fr. *syphilomanie*; Ger. *Lustseuchenwuth*.)

SYPHILIDOPHOBIA, SYPHILOPHOBIA (syphilis; φόβος, fear). Morbid dread of syphilis. A form of hypochondriasis. In another sense it means fear of giving syphilis to others; an occasional symptom in insanity.

SYPHILIS AND INSANITY, RELATIONSHIPS BETWEEN.—We purpose concisely to consider the possible connections which may exist between syphilis in its different phases and the different forms of mental disorder and disease of the higher nervous organs. We purpose taking the symptoms of syphilis as they are met with at various ages, and also as it affects the different organs of the body, and we shall make as clear as possible the distinction between the moral or intellectual, and the physical or physiological action of the disease in the production of mental disturbance.

We shall point out the effects of acquired and of congenital syphilis, and shall incidentally have to notice that there is no distinct and direct relationship between the severity of the primary diseases and that of the secondary insanity. It is more frequent than not to find that patients who are suffering from neurotic disorders related to syphilis have had but slight constitutional and local syphilitic disease.

It is not, however, correct, in our opinion, to infer from this that the syphilis has been imperfectly treated, and so had developed unchecked in consequence, and that more thorough treatment would certainly have prevented the development of nervous symptoms. In many of the cases in which the nervous symptoms have followed constitutional syphilis treatment has been regularly and continuously applied before the nervous symptoms exhibited themselves, and the continuance of the treatment did not affect the course of the nervous disorder in any way.

Syphilis may produce mental disorder by causing loss or destruction of nerve-tissue, such as organic dementia; it may cause sensory troubles leading to mental disorder; or it may cause disorder of nutrition and function, which may lead to ordinary insanity or epilepsy.

Syphilis does not affect all patients similarly. It is certain that, whatever may be the cause of contagious diseases, the nature of the soil greatly influences the character of the growth. In those who are specially unstable on the nervous side it may be that syphilis and other similar diseases may affect the nervous system most seriously. Our own experience inclines us to believe that syphilis does affect the nervous system of those who by age, habit, or inheritance are nervously weak, and in many such cases it seems to avoid the tissues more affected in others, such as the skin and mucous membrane.

Other questions are involved, and we have to learn under what conditions the cord and what the brain bear the brunt of the disease; how far primarily and how far secondarily these suffer.

A great deal of what has to be said is only to be considered as provisionally true; the fact, however, remains that there are certain relationships between syphilis and nervous disorder, though we cannot fully define them. We are not in a position to show how many of the population suffer from syphilis, and cannot say therefore what proportion of the population who would under any circumstances break down mentally, owe nothing to syphilis as a cause of their disorder. We have, for years, not only asked male patients whether they have had syphilis, but have personally examined them, with the result of sometimes discovering signs of the disease which the patient was himself ignorant of having had. Syphilis may be present in patients whose insanity does not depend upon it, and we know no form of insanity deserving the name of "syphilitic insanity." Syphilis rarely acts as the only cause of insanity; alcoholic or other excesses, strain, injury, or general modes of life act as contributing conditions.

We propose considering the relationships after the following scheme:—

(1) Insane dread of syphilis.

(2) Insane dread of results of syphilis.

(3) Syphilitic fever, delirium, and mania.

(4) Acute syphilis leading to mental decay.

(5) Syphilitic cachexia and dyscrasia, and mental disorder.

(6) Syphilitic neuritis (optic), suspicion, mania.

(7) Syphilitic ulceration, disfigurement and morbid self-consciousness.

(8) Congenital syphilis, cranial, sensory or nerve-tissue defects.

(9) Congenital syphilis, epilepsy, idiocy.

(10) Infantile syphilis, acquired.

(11) Constitutional syphilis, (*a*) vascular or fibrous; (*b*) epilepsy; (*c*) hemiplegia; (*d*) local palsies; (*e*) general paralysis, cerebral, spinal (spastic and tabetic), peripheral.

(12) Locomotor ataxy (*a*) with insane crises, (*b*) with insane interpretation of the ordinary symptoms.

Moral Effects of Syphilis. *Insane Dread of Syphilis.*—This shows itself in several distinct ways. A man contracts syphilis before marriage, and from general causes becomes sleepless and depressed; he may become possessed by the idea that it is all due to the syphilis of the past. He may become truly melancholic, being very sleepless and suicidal.

Or a married man may contract syphilis, and be harassed by the fear of giving it to his wife or to his children.

In the above cases syphilis acts as the idea around which the melancholic feelings group themselves, the whole being but an exaggeration of a real fact.

In other cases the syphilis is the interpretation of morbid feelings without the disease having been contracted. This is true syphilophobia, and is common in young men who usually have been leading unsocial, solitary, and self-conscious lives; they may have been absolutely continent, but more frequently they have indulged in self-abuse. In these cases there is generally complaint of uneasy feelings in the skin which lead to frequently washing themselves; they also often have hallucination of smell, which makes them believe that others can and do detect their syphilitic state. In some the presence of acne adds weight to the delusion, as they believe the eruption to be due to syphilis. Such symptoms are most common in men. They are very rare indeed in young Englishwomen, because they are happily ignorant of the features of the disease. They may occur in women about the menopause, and may lead to false accusations and jealousy of the husband.

We have met with similar ideas in elderly women who almost always had some vaginal or uterine discharge, which seemed to give rise to the notion of syphilitic infection. Elderly widows suffer from disorders of this class. In these cases general treatment and change of air and scene is preferable to too definite specific treatment, though in patients who know they have had the disease we sometimes advise a visit to Aix-la-Chapelle and a complete course of baths and treatment, as this acts beneficially on the general health, and may thus enable the patient to throw off his dread. There is, however, considerable risk in sending such patients abroad without skilled and watchful attendants.

In some cases the dread of syphilis gives rise to ideas of impotence, or at least to unfitness for marriage, and this may be the foundation of melancholia of a very dangerous type.

We saw a strong, vigorous young officer, full of promise in his profession, who was invalided for nervousness and sleeplessness. On arrival in England he was treated for syphilis, which disease he had contracted some years before, and for which he was then carefully treated. Nothing could persuade him that he was not really suffering from syphilis, and that, though attached to a lady suitable to be his wife in every way, he had any prospect of ever being able to marry. His friends could not recognise the danger of his symptoms, and, though they at length obtained an attendant, they would not give him the authority required to control the patient, and the result was his most determined suicide.

To sum up: this class of cases needs patient general treatment; in young cases the termination may be in recovery, but often is dementia. At the [illegible] recovery may take place, but chronic mania with ideas of persecution is more common. In old cases chronic mania or dementia generally result, and apoplexy is not uncommon.

Syphilitic fever may be associated with delirium, and this may form the starting-point of a maniacal attack. We cannot ourselves remember coming across any case quite answering to this, but we have met with some cases which convince us that certain nervously weak people who have worried and drugged themselves into nervous instability may develop [illegible] symptoms out of proportion to their bodily state, and from this further mental disorder may grow.

It is more common, though by no means really common, to meet with *cases in which, with the development of syphilitic disease, general physical and mental weakness is manifested.*

Dr. Wiglesworth recorded one fatal case of this kind at the International Medical Congress at Washington, 1887. We cannot explain the pathology of these cases; they seem to depend on general nutritional disorder rather than on any special vascular or nervous changes, and they therefore deserve to be placed with cases in which the *mental symptoms depend on general cachexia.* It was long supposed that the treatment of syphilis by mercury led to some of the worst cases of constitutional syphilis, and there is no doubt but that serious harm was done by profuse salivation and by too free and too prolonged mercurial treatment. We have met with several cases of constitutional syphilis in which the general health having been seriously affected, the mind has also become disordered; in these cases melancholy of the stuporose form or associated with suspicion were most common. In other cases more or less complete mental weakness was apparent. If the patients with general symptoms be young, there is a fair chance of recovery; but if past middle age, the prognosis is unfavourable. Only general measures are of any avail.

In the course of syphilis local troubles may occur which may give rise to insanity. These may be nervous or nutritional.

Neuritis.—It is not uncommon to meet with optic neuritis in the course of the disease, and we have met this associated with temporary defect of sight, and this caused the patient to be suspicious and violent against those whom he took for his persecutors. Ideas of annoyance, following, poisoning, and the like may arise. Symptoms somewhat like those associated with peripheral neuritis of alcohol or lead may be met with.

The treatment of these cases differs; in some we have had the best results from producing rapid effects from mercurial inunctions or inhalations, while in some the iodides did good, and in others general treatment and the withdrawal of specific treatment led to recovery. The prognosis in these cases depends greatly on the duration of the disease, provided there are no signs of general paralysis; the neuritis and its consequences may pass away.

Nutritional changes may occur depending on local gummata, specific inflammations affecting vessels or the nervous system. As a result of the above there may be disfigurement, and this may give rise to ideas that the patients are pointed at or shunned, or scoffed at, as lepers.

The development of this to an insane degree is slow as a rule, the patient being at first self-conscious and given to solitary occupation. He avoids strangers, and later even shuns his relations. He may take to vices such as drink or masturbation; then develop hallucinations of his senses, which rapidly lead to delusions of persecution. In these cases violence is common, and there is a considerable risk of homicide or suicide.

As these symptoms generally develop before middle life, there is a prospect of amelioration if change and occupation with treatment to counteract the disfigurement are procured.

Congenital Syphilis.—There is a considerable difference of opinion as to the part played by this in the production of idiocy. Medical officers of asylums, such as Drs. Langdon Down, Shuttleworth, Fletcher Beach, only rarely obtain certain evidences of congenital syphilis or specific histories among their patients, but physicians to children's hospitals meet with cases of partial weak-mindedness associated in many instances with this disease.

We believe that congenital syphilis causes death from convulsions and from other diseases, in children who would probably have been mentally defective had they lived, and that many minor nervous disorders occur in such children who are managed at home because they are physically weak, and that these lesser neuroses are seen by out-patient physicians in many patients who die before maturity. But besides this, all physicians connected with idiot asylums recognise that some of their patients are idiotic as the result of congenital syphilis. Dr. Langdon Down puts the proportion as not more than 2 per cent. Dr. Ireland takes no special notice of this as a cause. We have met with several cases in which the correlation was evident. The cases which have come specially under our notice may be classified under three heads: (*a*) those with general defect of development with moral and intellectual want; (*b*) those with sensory defect, and consequent mental want; (*c*) those with epilepsy or paralysis, and consequent epileptic or paralytic idiocy.

The first class is the least definite, and contains children who may be grouped among the various forms of idiots, the only special feature being a distinct history of parental syphilis with evidences of the disease in the patient. We have met such children fairly well formed as to head, but who after early infancy have not developed; they have learnt to walk, but not to talk, and are restless and mischievous, and only to a very small degree educable. They require to be removed from home for the sake of the other children and for special training.

The group (*b*) contains cases in which specific inflammation has caused deafness, or blindness, or both, in early infancy, these defects leading to idiocy by deprivation of sensory stimulation. In some of these cases special education for deaf and dumb and blind fails to develop any really useful mind, and with the growth of sexuality and desire much serious trouble may arise, and the small mental gain effected may be ruined very rapidly. The probable end of these cases is early death from some physical disease such as phthisis.

In group (*c*) we have two divisions, the epileptic and the paralytic; the former frequently begin with convulsive seizures in early infancy, and these fits recurring become habitual and prevent mental development. In some cases the fits cease at some period of life, say about seven or fourteen years of age, but as a rule the mind has been too seriously damaged to recover, and the patient remains a quiet non-epileptic idiot. In the paralytic cases and in some epileptic ones local lesions about the cranium, the membranes, and the brain itself are the cause of the convulsive or paralytic symptoms. As a rule, these paralytic idiots are hopelessly weak, and need asylum care, and they usually live but a short time. In a few cases the general symptoms of congenital syphilis only affect the mind later. Thus, defect of sight or of hearing may act in the same way that disfigurement did in making the patient morbidly solitary, self-conscious, and suspicious; in the end becoming deluded and insane. These cases generally are met with in young women, and the prospect of cure is very slight, most of the patients passing into chronic weak-mindedness or delusional insanity. We have met with one case in which infantile acquired syphilis seemed to be associated with defective mental growth. A young man who bore about him all the marks of acquired syphilis, which was traced clearly to his wet-nurse, broke down soon after adolescence, and suffered from stupor with recurring attacks of excitement, the whole tending to dementia. He belonged to a typically healthy family, and there did not seem to be any probable cause for his malady other than the constitutional syphilis which was manifest, and it seems to us to be likely that it should thus be possible to produce a nervous instability which showed itself at the first critical period of the man's life.

Insanity associated with Constitutional Syphilis.—While studying this group of cases we shall take it for granted that syphilis, when it is considered as constitutional, affects by preference certain tissues, and that nervous and mental disorders will be found to be related to the nature and seat of the diseased process. Fibrous tissues appear to be very liable to syphilitic disease, and we find the periosteum, the pericranium and dura mater liable to thickenings due to syphilis. Vessels also suffer in various degrees from inflammatory changes and the thickenings of their coats; it is doubtful whether the nervous elements in the skull themselves suffer; the syphilitic growths are more common along the superior and central parts, the parts represented by the chief arterial supply. In the spinal cord the posterior part seems to be more liable than the anterior. The symptoms may be due to nutritional changes leading to disorder or to degeneration leading to functional defect. We shall have to refer first to the cases in which the relationship is clear, and after that to some of the cases in which the connection is not so easily established.

Syphilis may give rise to epilepsy, and this epilepsy may lead to mental disorder of the epileptic type. (*See* EPILEPSY.)

Syphilis may give rise to hemiplegia, which again may be followed by dementia.

Syphilis may be followed by local palsies which may be associated with mental disorders.

Syphilis may give rise to pseudo-general paralysis of the insane.

Syphilis may give rise to true general paralysis of the insane, (1) of the *cerebral*; or (2) *spinal*—(*a*) spastic, (*b*) ataxic—type; or (3) of a type beginning with *peripheral* disease.

Syphilis may give rise to epilepsy. If a middle-aged man who has had syphilis has a series of epileptic fits not associated with injury or alcohol, it is probable that syphilis is the cause, and the benefit which follows treatment confirms the diagnosis.

In these cases there is considerable risk of the development of paralytic symptoms, and of dementia, and if these occur the prognosis is unfavourable, as they point to real organic brain injury. It must be remembered that epileptiform fits under the same conditions may point to the development of general paralysis.

Epilepsy may result from local irritative thickening of the membranes, from some local gummatous swelling growing into the surface of the brain, or to some vascular lesion of a specific kind. We believe too that a dynamical change may occur in patients suffering from syphilis which renders them epileptically unstable, like some of the guinea-pigs experimented upon by Brown-Séquard.

In our experience the epilepsy of syphilis tends to stupidity rather than violence, so that it is rare to meet with the regular epileptic maniac whose epilepsy resulted from syphilis. If not cured by treatment the tendency is to local paralysis and to dementia.

Syphilis and Hemiplegia with Dementia.—A very large number of patients are admitted into the general hospitals with hemiplegic systems, and a fair proportion depend on syphilis. Many of these cases recover under treatment, but some remain with permanently contracted limbs and with other motor defects; some, especially of the latter group, are progressively weaker in mind, and become permanent dements. The general history is as follows: A middle-aged patient who has had syphilis a variable number of years before, after some causes of physical or nervous exhaustion, has a fit followed by hemiplegia; there is a partial recovery of power, but the patient has lost all his energy, he is placid and perhaps childish; he may be irritable and emotional; his memory, though at first not much affected, fails apparently from lack of attention; sleep is generally good and appetite large; the bodily weight often increases. This state of mental weakness often remains unchanged for years, and just as such a patient may have a useless and contracted limb which never becomes more palsied, so the mental powers may degrade to a certain point, and there remain stationary.

In some cases the stage of dementia is preceded by mental excitement, so that patients, after a fit, are paralysed and quiet for a time, and then become wild, emotional, and maniacal; this stage may lead to rapid dissolution, or may be replaced by mental weakness similar to the last described. Recurring fits may be present leading to more rapid degeneracy.

Local Paralysis due to Syphilis followed by Insanity.—We believe that it is fully recognised that syphilis has a special, almost characteristic, way of causing isolated local losses of power in which the cranial nerves suffer very frequently, and it is noteworthy that such paralyses may be associated with or followed by various forms of mental disorder. When later discussing the relationship existing between general paralysis of the insane and syphilis we shall have to point out the frequency with which one meets in the last disease with a preceding history of local syphilitic paralysis.

After a cranial nerve-paralysis, or after specific affection of the special senses, treatment may be followed by removal of all the visible symptoms, and yet the patient may slowly from that time exhibit changes in character and habits which tend to eccentricity or insanity. In some of these there is a blunting of the higher moral sense so that low, vulgar, or vicious acts are done quite in opposition to the ordinary habits of the individual; sober men take to drink, and moral men to vice; active men become indolent, truthful ones become untrustworthy, and social men may become morose. At first the changes are nearly always modifications of the finer social adjustments. Patients who have thus begun to degenerate often rapidly go down hill, their powers of resistance as well as their powers of control failing, or temporary improvement may occur.

General Paralysis of the Insane and Syphilitic.—Probably there is no point about which there is more difference of opinion among neurologists than as to the part, if any, played by syphilis in the production of this disease. Those chiefly concerned in the treatment of syphilis have been inclined to think that syphilis is not a frequent cause; while those who have good opportunities of watching the origin of general paralysis of the insane seem to be impressed by the belief that it is a very important factor in the disease. It is noteworthy that among the more educated classes in whom accurate histories can be more readily obtained, a specific history is more frequently met with than among the inhabitants of pauper asylums. Physicians in large consulting practice, and medical officers to asylums for the better classes, as a rule attribute a good deal of importance to syphilis in the production of the disease. General paralysis is most common where syphilis is most common, but this only means that it is a disease most frequently met with in the centres of highly civilised populations. It has been said that syphilis is very common among certain nomadic tribes among whom general paralysis is unknown. We cannot say we trust either of these statements. We believe that at least seventy per cent. of our private cases of general paralysis have clear histories of constitutional syphilis.

We do not look upon general paralysis as necessarily of specific origin, but we consider syphilis is one of its most common causes. We believe it acts in different ways in different persons, and affects different parts of the nervous system, but that its tendency is to start a process of degeneration which ultimately produces the ruin we recognise as general paralysis, and that it may play the sole or only a partial cause.

Syphilis may give Rise to Pseudo- or True General Paralysis.—There is a group of interesting cases in which a history of syphilis is followed in the course of years by symptoms of motor and mental instability. As a rule the symptoms are more physical than mental at the outset, but they vary widely, but generally are diagnosed with assurance of certainty as typical general paralytics; the symptoms run the ordinary course, and may confirm the opinion already formed, but at some period in the development of the symptoms there is a distinct arrest, so that, though permanently damaged, the patient may live for years in a state of restricted intellect. We have met with cases of this kind in which the handwriting and gait were affected to some extent, while the memory was defective and exaggeration of ideas was also well marked, and yet these symptoms remained unchanged for several years. In others, the patients passed into a fat and partly weak-minded state, and there remained for many years, and we have even seen patients who appeared to be in the third and paralytic stage with epileptiform fits, in whom the disease stopped, and the paralysed patient regained a good deal of physical as well as some mental power. In referring to the above cases we must admit that similar arrests of symptoms may occur in other cases of general paralysis than in those depending on syphilis, but in our experience the syphilitic cases provide the more common examples.

In these cases some acute bodily discase or some cause of profuse suppuration may be associated with the amelioration. When referring to these cases we wish to add that the relief is not only temporary, but is in some cases persisting after eight or ten years.

True general paralysis associated with syphilis may be (1) *cerebral* and (2) *spinal* —(*a*) spastic or (*b*) ataxic.

The *cerebral* again divides itself into that of *general* and that of *local* origin.

A certain number of cases begin with progressive loss of power and of self-control, there being a steady loss from the highest and last acquirements to the more organic.

There is nothing to separate these cases from similar ones due to other causes, and the pathology is in no way special. In another group of cases to which allusion has already been made a local syphilitic lesion occurs, and may be recovered from, and yet later a degeneration may arise from the early local lesion.

In our experience it is very common to meet with such a history as the following:—A middle-aged man who has suffered slightly from syphilis years before is exposed to causes of mental and physical exhaustion, and then for the first time has a local cranial nerve defect, the most common being ptosis, external strabismus, and mydriasis. In some cases optic neuritis is present. Energetic treatment is followed by cure of all or most of the local symptoms; the patient returns to work, but sooner or later, generally within two years, irritability and change of disposition, followed by distinct loss of mental power, point to the disease which is making progress. The course of the disease may be either that of excitement or of depression, but dementia with fits is the general end.

We have met with so many of these cases that we cannot but associate the general disease with the evidences of local disease. In some respects the pathology is allied to that of general paralysis following concussion of the brain. As in a ripe pear, general degeneration rapidly follows a slight local injury.

General Paralysis of Syphilitic Origin with (*a*) Spastic Spinal Symptoms. — We recognise a considerable number of cases of this variety of general paralysis with a distinct syphilitic history. Some of the youngest cases of general paralysis which have come under our care belong to this group as well as many of the cases in women. The early symptoms are of the ordinary type, but we believe that in most the pupils will be found rather large and unequal, irregular in outline; the [illegible] is less greasy, and there are [illegible] capillary stigmata over the [illegible] processes, the reflexes are very [illegible] exaggerated, speech is early and [illegible] implicated, and the handwriting is very shaky; the gait is jerky. Though there may be arrest of this disease, in our experience it runs often a rapid course, [illegible] great contraction of limbs and a tendency to bedsores; grinding of the teeth and movements as of swallowing are common; fits may be present, and post-mortem excess of fluid in membranes and lateral ventricles is more common than effusions; there are specially wasted areas, and the pyramidal tracts of the cord are degenerated. It must be remembered that this description in no way differs from general paralysis produced by some other causes, but it has been so frequently met with by us in young specific cases that we believe it should be here recorded.

We believe that the local convolutional waste and the secondary cord degenerations are related and may be found connected with the specific cause.

General Paralysis of Specific Origin with (*b*) Ataxic Symptoms.—Suffice it to say that the mental symptoms may precede the ataxy, may coincide with it, or they may follow the fully developed symptoms.

It is pretty generally accepted in England that locomotor ataxy has very commonly a specific origin. On the Continent, in France especially, this disorder is more commonly considered as allied to the neuroses, but in any case the coincidence of ataxy with syphilis is common.

It is noteworthy that this is more common in men than in women, and that general paralysis with ataxy is also more common with men, that ataxy and ataxic symptoms are rare in women.

There is nothing special in the form of general paralysis with ataxy, but it is noteworthy that in some of these cases there is a marked tendency to remissions or to alternations, so that both ataxy and mental defect pass off in part, or the one develops while the other is in abeyance.

We are sometimes inclined to think that there is a cerebral or intra-cranial ataxy apart from the changes in the spinal cord, and that just as in the spastic general paralysis the degeneration of the cord is secondary, so in ataxic general paralysis the same may be true (*see* Locomotor Ataxy as allied to Neuroses).

General Paralysis of Specific Origin and Peripheral Disease.—At one time a good deal was written about general paralysis "par propagation," and though one recognises local intra-cranial lesions as efficient causes for general paralytic degeneration, and also believes that spinal lesions may lead to the same, it is hard to prove that local peripheral neuritis of a specific or other nature may cause similar changes.

We only suggest the possibility, though we cannot give any cases fully supporting the theory.

Syphilis may lead to uncomplicated locomotor ataxy which may exhibit insane crises or insane interpretation of symptoms (*see* LOCOMOTOR ATAXY AS ALLIED TO NEUROSES). GEO. H. SAVAGE.

SYPHILITIC (HEREDITARY) DISEASE OF THE NERVOUS SYSTEM.—The labours of Hutchinson on certain diseases of the sense organs, especially interstitial keratitis and specific deafness, and their association with a characteristic alteration of the upper median permanent incisors, gave the first great impulse to the study of the subject with which we are concerned in this article.

The subsequent discovery of the frequency of disseminated choroiditis in the subjects of congenital syphilis was a further step in advance. Hydrocephalus was assumed to be present in some syphilitic children on account of the large massive head sometimes found in such children, but the anatomical proof was not forthcoming, and it was generally agreed that in marked contrast with acquired syphilis there was exceedingly little proneness to affection of the central nervous system in the hereditary form. The publication of Heubner's work on syphilitic affections of the cerebral arteries, although it referred only to the acquired disease, gave a fresh impulse to the investigations in morbid anatomy, and within the last fourteen years a great number of examples of disease of the central nervous system in hereditary syphilis, have been described by various observers.

It may, indeed, now be said, in contrast to the early views, that nearly every variety of nervous affection of acquired syphilis has its parallel amongst congenital examples, albeit there are indications of a few broad differences which may be made out as to the relative frequency alike of lesions and symptoms between the two groups.

It is convenient to consider the subject of **hereditary syphilitic disease of the nervous system** from the side of (A) **morbid anatomy**; and (B) **symptomatology.**

The multiplicity of co-existing lesions is often so great that it is difficult to correlate the anatomical and clinical features; but the two sets of observations may be broadly grouped as follows:—

(A) **Morbid Anatomy.**

Lesions of the following tissues: Bones of cranium; membranes (dura mater and pia arachnoid); blood-vessels; brain substance (cortex, ventricles, great ganglia, pons, medulla); cerebral nerves; organs of special sense; associated spinal disease (bones, membranes, cord, spinal nerves).

(B) **Symptomatology.**

(*a*) Convulsions; (*b*) headache and irritability; (*c*) paralysis, aphasia, affections of cranial nerves; (*d*) psychical defects; (*e*) spinal symptoms.

(A) **Morbid Anatomy.** Cranial bones:

(1) *Early Forms.*—The two varieties which have come under our own observation have been (*a*) small definite gummatous infiltrations of the skull bones causing a varying amount of absorption of tissue, and in one case eroding down to the surface of the dura mater (this form we believe to correspond with Parrot's early localised gelatiniform transformation of the skull); (*b*) small areas of caries affecting the inner plate of the bones of the vault, but also in some instances the basis cranii. In connection with both forms exfoliation of small plates of bone may occur.

(2) *Late Forms.*—Localised gummatous infiltrations also occur in the skull in older children, and they may lead to ulceration and some loss of substance; sometimes there occurs a certain amount of localised atrophy without lesion of skin. Thickening is more common. In syphilitic children massive thickening of the bones of the skull has been recognised ever since Mr. Hutchinson drew attention to the prominent frontal present in many of the subjects of interstitial keratitis first described by him. This massive thickening, though most common in the frontal region, tends in older children and young adults to be diffused, and all parts of the skull may show it. Thus, in a case under the care of Dr. Henry Humphreys so marked was the thickening at the base that many of the basal foramina were distinctly narrowed in consequence. There is good reason to believe that this thickening is sometimes slowly progressive over considerable periods. Sections of such bone show great compression of Haversian systems, and the Haversian canals in parts may be almost obliterated.

It must still remain an open question as to the relation between these cases of massive thickening of the skull and the hyperostosis of cranial bones, which are often present in young children. The cranial bosses of soft vascular bone situated around the fontanelle, but extending to a varying degree along the parietals and frontal, were claimed by M. Parrot as syphilitic manifestations. Such masses, which generally become obvious within the first or second year of life, increase to a varying amount, then sometimes undergo absorption and sometimes ossify into spongy lens-shaped osteophytes. These osteophytes may undergo absorption, but not unfrequently result in a light porous form of osseous deposit, and occasionally dense hard bone is the final outcome.

With regard to the *early* cranial bosses, we are now convinced that M. Parrot's view is incorrect. It is true that syphilis and rickets often co-exist, and it is probable that syphilis, as a chronic hindrance to good nutrition, is one amongst other factors of rickets. Thus, the cranial bosses are often present in syphilitic and rickety children, but they occur in children in whom syphilis can be absolutely negatived, and the balance of evidence is in favour of their being rickety manifestations of the skull accompanied by other signs of rickets in the skeleton, but occasionally out of all proportion to changes in the ribs and long bones. The permanent light spongy hyperostosis of skull bones we also believe to be rickety in derivation. But when there is definite massive sclerosis of skull in a child over five years, or in adolescence, we believe the presumption to be in favour of syphilis in addition to rickets.

Asymmetry of the cranium is sometimes found both in rickets and in rickets combined with congenital syphilis. A common form presents flattening of one parietal occipital region with some prominence of the opposite frontal, so that a horizontal tracing of the skull presents a somewhat lozenge-shaped contour.

Craniotabes, by which is meant a form of atrophy commencing in small areas on the inner table and extending through to the outer surface affecting predominantly the postero-lateral regions of the skull, is a condition practically confined to the first eighteen months of life. It is certainly very common in syphilitic children, but it occurs in infants in whom syphilis may be excluded, and the old view, according to which it was considered a manifestation of rickets, is probably the correct one.

The typical hydrocephalic skull, characterised by gaping sutures, large fontanelles, thinning of bones, and more or less spherical contour, is sometimes found in children the subjects of congenital syphilis. It must also be noted that hydrocephalus, only moderate in amount and probably stationary, has also been found post-mortem in some cases where massive thickening of skull bones was present.

Alterations of the nasal bones deserve enumeration, for, although no anatomical proof is forthcoming, it is quite possible that in some cases syphilitic damage to these bones may give the starting-point to meningeal disease. Caries of the nasal bones occurs rarely in congenital syphilis. The commoner conditions are:

(1) Stunted growth, which seems to result from the early interference with nutrition in connection with the prolonged nasal catarrh of the infantile period; and

(2) Chronic periostitis and sclerosis of these bones, leading to thickening.

Dura Mater.—This has been found greatly thickened, assuming an almost cartilaginous consistency in spots. Also hæmorrhage has occurred in connection with pachymeningitis, giving rise to laminæ of fibrine. Inflammatory deposits also have been observed in various stages, and likewise adhesions generally localised, of bone, dura-mater, pia arachnoid, and brain tissue.

The presumption is that in the majority of cases the diseased process begins with an internal periostitis of one or other cranial bone.

In some of the cases (referred to in the previous section) of caries of the inner table the connection with pachymeningitis is obvious. It seems probable (though it cannot be proved) that the initial bone change may in some cases undergo repair so as to leave little obvious sign, whilst the meningeal disease once initiated is slowly progressive.

(3) *Pia Arachnoid.*—All varieties of inflammatory deposit have been found in the pia arachnoid in hereditary syphilis. Thus, patches of green lymph in the meshes of the pia, both on convexity and at anterior and posterior base, have been found in varying amount. Simple acute meningitis is a condition so easily set up in infancy that its presence in a child the subject of hereditary syphilis is not necessarily to be attributed to the syphilitic virus. The more chronic forms show great variety and admit of greater certitude. The simplest form is a milky turbidity, sometimes widely spread and accompanied by brain and nerve changes to be presently described. Another form shows extreme fibroid thickening, and, as we have seen in one infantile case, even a little calcareous change. The fibroid cases may be accompanied, as in Siemerling's remarkable example, by actual gummata situated

in the inflammatory deposit, or, as in one of the earliest recorded examples described by one of us, small arteries may be found in the infiltrated meninges, showing partial thrombosis and Heubner's changes in the inner and middle coat. Traces of old hæmorrhage have also been found in inflammation of the pia as well as in affection of the dura.

(4) *Arteries.*—The characteristic endo-arteritis affecting the inner and middle coats described by Heubner in acquired brain syphilis has been subsequently observed in a considerable number of hereditary cases, and the gratuitous suggestion by a French writer that some of the early examples were really acquired, and not hereditary, scarcely merits consideration.

Not only in the basal arteries, but, as mentioned above, in some of the small arteries on the convexity in the midst of meningeal thickening, similar changes have been found. The small arteries may be diseased when the large ones are healthy, or *vice versâ*, or both may be affected together. They stand out like cords having a milky-looking surface, or may closely resemble dirty white threads. Also in the smaller vessels especially associated with inflammatory deposits peri-arteritis, as well as endo-arteritis, has been demonstrated.

(5) *Brain Proper.*—The most striking and in every way important changes have been found in the cortex. Softening has been occasionally found (Angel Money), but far more frequently hardening. The sclerosis has in our experience occurred in some cases, in small nodular masses, not bigger than split peas, in other cases it has "picked out" convolutions in the same fashion as diffuse glioma but without increase of bulk; but in the majority of examples it has affected large tracts of one or both hemispheres to a varying amount in different regions. Not unfrequently sclerosis has been found associated with a certain amount of atrophy. The narrowing of separate convolutions, the alteration of consistency to that of cartilage, and the very slight alteration of colour towards a brownish pink, are very characteristic features.

The sclerosis may extend for a short depth into the white matter, and in a case aged two years four months, shown to one of us by Dr. Robert Bridges, this condition also affected both optic thalami and part of the roof of the lateral ventricles, But predominantly and often exclusively, sclerosis of congenital syphilis is cortical. Microscopic examination shows an extensive overgrowth of neuroglia and disappearance of nerve cells. Some accompanying alteration of the pia arachnoid is almost invariable, and in not a few cases there is symphysis (as Fournier designates it) between dura, pia arachnoid, and sclerosed cortex. The hypothesis that the initial change is meningitis, and that the fibroid induration and limitation of growth of the cortex are due to the chronic meningitis is a very tempting one. But this hypothesis will not always apply, for in some cases the implication of the pia arachnoid only amounts to a slight opacity. The other hypothesis that the atrophy and fibrosis are the result of deficient blood supply in consequence of associated peri-arteritis and endo-arteritis of the basal or cortical arteries is also attractive, but is inadequate inasmuch as the arterial changes, though frequently present are not constant.

Amongst other lesions of the brain substance may be mentioned a few cases of small hæmorrhages into the white substance and one case of extensive hæmorrhage (Gowers) in a syphilitic boy aged eight years. "The hæmorrhage had apparently commenced in the right ventricular nucleus or outside it, and had burst into the ventricles." There was no visible aneurysm, but there was syphilitic disease of the vertebral and cerebellar arteries.

There have also been recorded a few cases of small yellow indurated foci in different parts of cerebrum and cerebellum (Rochebrune, Chiari, Henoch), which must be regarded as small gummata. Large gummata are exceedingly rare.

Ventricles.—Hydrocephalus has been found in several cases. The effusion has generally in our experience been moderate in amount. The character of the effusion has been recorded in different cases as serous, sanguineous, turbid, or purulent. In the long standing cases the ependyma has been found thickened (*vide* description by Angel Money). There has been often associated meningitis at the posterior base or chronic change in other parts of the brain.

Cerebral Nerves.—Symmetrical gummata have been found by Barlow on the third, fifth, sixth, seventh, and eighth pairs in a boy aged fifteen months old. Microscopic sections showed atrophy of nerve cylinders and infiltration with granulation cells and a very fine stroma. The new growth was less abundant in the interfunicular tissue than in the funiculi themselves. Thickening of the fifth and seventh nerves has been found by Dowse in a girl aged twelve years, the subject of congenital syphilis. Chiari also reports a case in which the right seventh was thickened, and Engelstedt one in which he found the left third nerve diseased, and the muscles supplied by it pale and wasted.

Organs of Special Sense. (1) *Eye.*—Mr. Hutchinson enumerates the following diseases of the eye as occurring in hereditary syphilis: acute iritis, interstitial keratitis, choroiditis and choroido-retinitis, and optic neuritis. For accounts of their morbid anatomy, so far as it has been studied, we refer to the special treatises. We may quote with regard to the microscopic appearances of early choroiditis some observations of Mr. Nettleship. The case on which they were based was a syphilitic infant under the care of Dr. Barlow. The child died just under ten months, and the choroiditis was detected by us at the age of eight months. "The changes in the choroid consist in the presence of small isolated collections of corpuscles in the chorio-capillaris; sections of several of these were found in the part of the choroid which had shown during life little flecks of exudation and none were found elsewhere." "The corpuscles are about as large as pus corpuscles and stain deeply with logwood." "They stand in no evident relation to the blood-vessels, and none of them occur in the deeper part of the choroid." "In all these particulars they differ from tubercle." "The elastic lamina over these deposits is slightly raised and sometimes a little puckered." "In several instances, at the seat of the deposits, a thin layer of flattish cells is present on its inner (retinal) surface immediately beneath the pigment epithelium, but in no sections could any perforation of the lamina be detected." "The epithelium itself appears morbidly adherent." "It may be mentioned that these changes (circumscribed deposits in the chorio-capillaris with a thin layer of flat cells on the retinal surface of the elastic lamina) are precisely similar to what we found in a case of choroiditis from acquired syphilis in which the eye was excised during the progress of the disease."*

(2) *The Ear.*—To the pathological condition underlying the symmetrical deafness first described by Mr. Hutchinson, we have as yet no adequate clue, but it is probably a progressive degeneration of the internal ear or of some part of the auditory nerve.

Associated Spinal Lesions.—In a case under the care of Dr. Bury in which, post-mortem, chronic meningitis with sclerosis of the cortex cerebri and endo-arteritis were found, there was also present distinct sclerosis of the lateral columns and of the internal aspect of the anterior columns. Besides such descending lesions, of which there are a few other cases on record, there are a few examples of independent spinal affections in the hereditary form of the disease. Thus Kahler found, post-mortem, in a syphilitic child, five months old, an area of degeneration in one lateral column which presented atrophy of cells and nerve fibres, a fine reticular growth and vessels with Heubner's change well marked.

Bartels gives details of a remarkable case of a young woman, aged twenty-two, who was the subject of congenital syphilis, and who, amongst other illnesses, suffered from two separate attacks of paraplegia which yielded to anti-syphilitic treatment. When ultimately she died from other causes the vestiges of a caseous, partly softened, gumma were found in front of the articulation between the atlas and the skull, and between the atlas and axis. It was clear that the cord had been somewhat flattened, and that the paraplegia had been caused by compression and myelitis.

In the case of a marasmic syphilitic infant, examined, post-mortem, by Barlow, there was found extensive periostitis of several laminæ of the cervical vertebræ, which it was easy to see might, if the child had survived, have led to cord symptoms. Siemerling, in the case already mentioned, found marked gummatous proliferation of the pia mater all along the spinal cord, tap-shaped processes dipping into the white substance, and the antero-lateral and posterior columns all more or less softened.

Jürgens reports two cases: In one case there was slight pachymeningitis and chronic fibrous arachnitis; in the other case he found a gummatous tumour in the cervical region which involved half of the right lateral column, and also partly invaded the posterior roots.

(B) **Symptomatology.**

(*a*) *Convulsions.* — We have already stated what we believe on post-mortem evidence to be the physical substratum of this symptom in syphilitic children, viz., meningeal and cortical changes varying in degree from extensive sclerosis down to mere opacity of membranes. Although, as in adults, these may be associated with lesions of the calvaria, we have insisted on their frequent occurrence in syphilitic children independently of any true specific disease of the skull. Looking at the subject clinically we now point out the frequency of early convulsions in syphilitic children. Buzzard and Fournier have drawn attention to this, and we have re-

* Path. Trans. xxviii. p. 290.

cords of several family syphilitic groups in which many members have died of early convulsions. The earliest case of convulsions, with subsequent post-mortem verification of extensive meningeal changes, was observed by one of us in a child four months old, but we have notes of several at the age of three months without post-mortem verification, and one of a syphilitic infant who had ten or twelve fits daily from the age of fourteen days to seven months. A great many cases of convulsions have been noted within the first two years of life. As to the character of the fits the early cases have been mostly bilateral with tonic and clonic contractions. In some, laryngismus and carpopedal spasm have been marked (*vide* in this connection observations by Horsley and Semon on cortical origin of laryngismus). In some recurrent attacks of opisthotonos spasms have been observed, followed by persistent head retraction for varying periods, suspected to be due to inflammatory processes at the posterior base. In one infantile case this was proved post-mortem, and what was probably a small softening gumma was found in the neighbourhood.

In one case, aged sixteen months, convulsive seizures occurred, in which the mouth was widely opened and the child became very dusky. No cortical changes of convexity were found, but symmetrical gummata on several cranial nerves. We have seen no case of limited one-sided clonic spasm under the age of twelve months in a syphilitic infant, but we think it is very important to note that syphilitic infants may have bilateral fits and laryngismus within the first year associated with or shortly succeeding the snuffles and rash, and may then have a period of latency for months or years, and subsequently present either one-sided spasm or paralysis.

Examples.—(1) T. Holloway (under care of Drs. Gee and Barlow), snuffles at four weeks, and probably pemphigus. Bilateral fits three or four a month up to one year. Could not sit up till three years, and could not walk till four years. At four years had two right-sided fits within six months.

At six years fell down without convulsion being observed. Paralysed on right side after this, and speech for a time thick and indistinct. Somewhat irritable subsequently. When seen at age of ten years eight months by Dr. Barlow, the child was undergrown and pale, had typical scars at corners of mouth and pegged upper median permanent incisors. The right eye was blind, and there was extensive detachment of retina. The left showed atrophy of disc and old choroiditis. There was some paresis of the right upper and lower limbs, but no spasm, and there was a slight arrest of development (as shown in length and circumference) in right forearm compared with left. There was no evidence of paralysis of any cranial nerve. She heard and understood many things which were said to her, and answered some questions, but could not be trusted in her replies to questions testing common sensation and special sense. There was slight articulatory defect, as of a young child who had not long learned to talk. She was docile, but distinctly retarded in her intellectual development for a child nearly eleven. She died of nephritis, and at the post-mortem her brain showed remarkable sclerosis of both hemispheres, the left being more affected than the right, with marked shrinkage in both transverse and longitudinal measurement. There was also extensive endo-arteritis of all the arteries of the circle of Willis and their branches.

(2) Ada Hare (Barlow). Laryngismus sixteen months old to three years. From three years to seven years free from fits. At seven years had a fit affecting left side of face and left limbs. After this, liable to headaches and to occasional fits.

At eight years and nine months, when seen, had just passed through a series of almost daily fits for period of three months; the left side predominantly affected. She presented characteristic pegged upper median permanent incisors. Intelligence below the average. Could tell her name, but not her age. Had never been able to learn anything at school beyond her letters.

There are, it must be noted, some cases in children and adolescents in which to all intents and purposes we have to do with *idiopathic epilepsy* plus an early specific history or a few characteristic signs, like pegged permanent incisors, interstitial keratitis, choroiditis and specific deafness. There are some cases even in which, as Fournier points out, the only specific element is the family history. The question in these cases may well arise, and indeed has been stated by Dr. Jackson in one of his papers, whether we are justified in considering them as in any true sense syphilitic. The therapeutic test is of some value. We can both of us recall such cases which had not responded to administration of the bromides, but which under grey powder and iodide recovered or markedly improved.

But in a very large number of cases after a shorter or longer interval, fits in a syphilitic child will be replaced or accompanied by other cerebro-spinal symptoms. A very early sign noticed by Bury has been the exaggeration of knee-jerks, but sooner or later one-sided spasm, paresis of one or more limbs, ocular palsy, and progressive mental defect come into evidence.

(*b*) *Headache and Irritability.*—Fournier lays great stress on headache and its increased severity during the night in the affections of the nervous system dependent on congenital syphilis.

In our experience complaints of definite headache in these affections have only been made by adolescents and children over ten years old.

But we have repeatedly observed evidences of great irritability (probably in part dependent on head trouble) in syphilitic infants. It is a matter of every-day experience that syphilitic infants sleep very badly. Phases of continuous screaming have been noticed by us in instances in which subsequently diseased membranes have been proved, and we have also known cycles of one-sided convulsion, paresis, and torpor ushered in by excessive irritability and stiffness of the neck either with the head retracted or held to one side.

Demme records a case of a syphilitic child who had attacks of headache followed by outbursts of rage, then by stupidity, then by diabetes insipidus. In connection with this may be mentioned a case observed by Bury of a syphilitic boy, aged two years, who developed diabetes insipidus, but without any history of headache.

(*c*) *Paralysis.* (1) *Hemiplegia.* — The physical substrata of this symptom in the congenital, as in the acquired, form of syphilis are multiple. Endo-arteritis, with sclerosis and meningeal thickening, is most common in children. Endo-arteritis with softening also occurs, but massive hæmorrhage is rare, and large cerebral gumma is rare.

Clinically, so far as we have seen, hemiplegia has most commonly been preceded by one-sided convulsion, and has been often succeeded at varying intervals by convulsion limited to the paretic side. But it may occur without obvious initial spasm. The patient, without previous warning, may fall down and lose consciousness for a varying period. In other cases there is some prodromal restlessness, irritability, vomiting, or, if the child is old enough, complaint of headache, and then, without loss of consciousness, the patient suddenly loses power down one side of the body and some degree of articulate speech.

Attacks of inherited as well as of acquired syphilitic hemiplegia may be sometimes followed by marked [illegible]. Example: A woman, aged twenty-eight, under the care of Dr. Bury, attended on account of slight speech defect with paresis of right side of face and right upper and lower limbs, and some anæsthesia of the right side. She had scars at the corners of the mouth, deafness, choroiditis, and blindness on the right side; also keratitis and old iritis. The history was that she had had a stroke seven years ago, and was unconscious for nine weeks, and lost her power of speech for twelve months. Five weeks before she attended, she had had another stroke, and had been unconscious for three days.

In many of the initial attacks of hemiplegia paresis of limbs, so far as its gross indications are concerned, clears up to a great extent, and the paresis of the face to a marked extent. The only vestige may be that the child does not use the arm and hand which have been affected quite as freely as those of the opposite limb. But there is a great proneness to subsequent attacks, after which a spastic condition may supervene, and there is a marked liability to supervention of paralysis of the other side of the body, after which one side may be limp and the other spastic, or more commonly both sides more or less spastic. It has been proved post-mortem, in one of our cases, that the paralysis was due to descending degeneration from both sides of the damaged brain of both pyramidal tracts.

(2) *Aphasia.*—In the hemiplegias of children alterations of speech are, as a rule, more transient than in the hemiplegias of adults. Hemiplegia as caused by hereditary syphilis is no exception to this general rule, at all events in the early stage, though at a later period, when extensive degeneration and mental failure have supervened, speech may be lost.

In the following example there were:

(1) Speech defect occurring with a slight attack of right-sided paralysis; and (2) subsequent attack of left-sided partial paralysis, loss of speech with defective control of lips, loss of power of protruding tongue, and difficulty in the first part of deglutition.

Charles Pohlmann, aged 10 years (Barlow), with marked family and infantile history of congenital syphilis, was brought to hospital with the following statement from the mother. Twenty days ago began to suffer from severe headache; ten days ago whilst at dinner found suddenly that he could not ask for what he wanted, made a sound but could not utter such words as bread, milk, &c.; pointed to the objects required; could call his brothers and sisters by name. Speech trouble increased, and four days after onset mother noticed that liquids ran out of his mouth and that he could not hold things properly with his right hand. Has complained of pain in the right leg to-day but was not noticed to drag it. The boy was poorly nourished, had typical pegged upper median incisors, there was a little flattening of the right naso-oral fold when he smiled, and the left corner of the mouth was drawn.

The grip of the right hand was distinctly weaker than that of the left. He used the left hand by preference. There was no alteration of gait. Seemed to understand what was said to him. Pointed to left parietal region in reply to question as to seat of pain. Could only answer "yes" and "no" to questions. Seemed unable to answer questions involving replies other than yes or no.

A few days after admission was able to utter his first name, Charlie, but could not give his surname, and when it was uttered to him he could not repeat it. When asked about his address said "yes" when it was rightly and "no" when wrongly stated. After some hesitation he was induced to write with a pencil. He wrote the letters of his name on dictation, but afterwards when asked to write it without dictation he wrote it with many letters altered. After about four months of mercurial treatment, the slight paresis of the right side of the face and of the right hand had almost disappeared, and the only fault of speech was slight hesitancy, and he was discharged. Six months after the beginning of the first seizure he again complained of headache, and it was found that he could not ask for what he wanted. The day after this, weakness of the left hand appeared. He could lift it up but he could not raise anything in the hand. The speech became worse, he could not put his tongue out and his swallowing became difficult. When re-admitted he apparently understood what was said to him but he could not speak. He was unable to close his left eye or his lips. The left naso-oral ridge was flat when he smiled. When bread was given to him he could not bite it. He could not protrude his tongue and had some difficulty in swallowing; the food seemed to remain in the back of his mouth. He was unable to grasp with the left hand, or supinate with the left wrist. The hand was dropped. The knee jerks were equal; the gait was good. So far as could be ascertained there was no anæsthesia. After a few days he was induced to write his name, which he did with transpositions and omissions of some of the letters, often being unable to get beyond the first two letters. The difficulty in mastication, protrusion of tongue, and in the first part of swallowing very slowly improved. He used to frequently assist the bolus down his throat by pushing it backwards with his finger.

At the end of a fortnight he began to make definite vocal sounds as an attempt at speech—*e.g.*, "hah-ih" represented "Charlie. At the end of a month speech was much improved, the difficulty being chiefly with labials. As he got able to protrude his tongue it deviated slightly to the left. For several months there was defective control over the lips. His writing for some months showed transposition of letters, but at the end of twelve months he wrote a long letter nearly correctly. The left-hand paresis had practically recovered. He was treated with mercurial inunction until the gums became a little spongy.

The pathology of this case is probably endo-arteritis of symmetrical branches of the middle cerebral arteries and degeneration of the cortical centres especially of the third frontal on both sides. The speech defect recovering after the first right-sided hemiplegic attack, but recurring with involvement of lip and tongue movements after the second (left-sided) attack, is remarkably similar to a case of embolic arterial disease recorded by Barlow in which there was symmetrical softening of Broca's convolution, and the convolution corresponding to it on the opposite hemisphere. Pohlmann's case illustrates also several of the points to which we have referred in the earlier part of the section on symptomatology.

Cranial Nerves.—The nerves may be affected apart from disease of the brain and membranes. As we have pointed out in the section on morbid anatomy, they may be affected with gummata and with interstitial neuritis. The nerve affection may be symmetrical, affecting both sides and several pairs, or it may be unilateral, affecting one or more, and remain stationary for long periods. Mr. Nettleship has recorded a case of a syphilitic girl aged fourteen, in whom there existed, along with keratitis and characteristic teeth, paralysis of the third, fifth, and sixth nerves on one side. The condition did not alter during four years. In one of our cases, probably syphilitic, the paralysis of the third nerve had not changed during a period of seven years.

It is noteworthy that separate portions of both the third and fifth nerves may be affected, leaving the other portions intact. Thus ptosis, or loss of the reflex to light, may be the only sign of involvement of the third, and anaesthesia the only sign of involvement of the fifth. Mr. Hutchinson records two cases of ophthalmoplegia externa in congenital syphilis. In one of them it was associated with atrophy of the optic discs.

The comparative immunity of the seventh nerve from syphilitic disease is dwelt upon by Mr. Hutchinson. It is no doubt rare in the acquired form. In hereditary syphilis we have each seen one case in a young infant with concomitant specific rash, &c. In the case before referred to of symmetrical gummata (proved post-mortem), evidence during life of degenerative electrical reactions of the facial was obtained. In another case of a child aged two years and six months, who was profoundly syphilitic, in addition to localised convulsions and other symptoms, there was a persistent one-sided facial palsy of both upper and lower branches, which gave degenerative reactions. In this case it was assumed as probable that there was a separate lesion, gummatous or otherwise, of the facial nerve.

Organs of Special Sense. (*a*) *The Eye.*—For the account of the characteristic signs of the early iritis, interstitial keratitis, and choroiditis of congenital syphilis, we refer to the invaluable researches of Mr. Hutchinson. Concerning choroiditis, the form which is commonest (to quote Mr. Hutchinson) "is characterised by atrophic and pigmented changes, near to the periphery of the fundus." "They are sometimes seen in both eyes, sometimes only in one." "In other cases patches may be seen in all parts of the fundus." "There is yet another form in which no large patches occur, but a great number of small ones, and in which numerous dotted and striated accumulations of pigment are seen in the retina, simulating the condition of retinitis pigmentosa."

We desire to draw attention to the importance of (1) looking for choroiditis in syphilitic infants within the first year of life. We have seen it as small flecks of brownish exudation, without atrophy or massive aggregations of pigment, subsequently verified post mortem, and also as small white rounded areas very like tubercles. (2) In older children (of five or six years, &c.) it is noteworthy what a large extent of choroidal disease may be found in the periphery consistently with moderate vision. The importance of choroiditis disseminata as a diagnostic help cannot be overstated. (3) It seems probable that the atrophy of the disc [illegible] cases of congenital syphilitic [illegible] the nervous system is for the most part due to the participation of the disc in a general choroido-retinitis. We have referred previously to one case of extensive detachment of retina, where probably the starting-point was a choroido-retinitis. (4) Observations are much needed on cases of intra-cranial congenital syphilitic disease, in which papillitis or atrophy of the disc occurs without concomitant choroiditis.

(*b*) *The Ear.*—There is little to be added to Mr. Hutchinson's clinical account given thirty years ago, of the frequently rapid and intractable form of deafness dependent on hereditary syphilis, which comes on mostly between the periods of five years before and five years after puberty, is bilateral, painless, and independent of otorrhoea. In many cases the conduction through the bone becomes lost, which suggests damage to internal ear or nerve, but the pathology of the affection is still unexplained.

Psychical Defects.—We have pointed out in the section on morbid anatomy (1) that the most common brain lesion in cases of hereditary syphilis is a diffuse affection of the cortex, in which certain of the convolutions become hardened and shrunk, and their cells atrophied in consequence of an overgrowth of the neuroglia. (2) That this condition may (*a*) be secondary to a chronic meningitis, itself started by a syphilitic periostitis or occurring independently; or (*b*) occur as a result of a specific endo-arteritis; or (*c*) gradually develop apart from disease either of the vessels or membranes. And we have seen that the symptomatology of brain syphilis in the child is largely made up of phenomena which might be expected to occur during the progress of such cortical changes; the instability of the large nerve cells of the grey matter being expressed clinically by headache, screaming and convulsions, their destruction by paralysis, aphasia, and, as some of the related cases have already indicated, by mental deterioration. Mental impairment, indeed, in our experience, is not exceptional, as writers on insanity have frequently stated, but is one of the prominent features of hereditary syphilitic brain disease. From an analysis of ninety reported examples of brain disturbance in congenital syphilis, we find there are forty, or nearly half, in which some failure of the mental functions is noticed, and we believe that this proportion under- rather than overstates the actual facts.

The clinical type of intra-cranial hereditary syphilis may be stated to be a spastic paresis of the limbs, plus convulsive attacks, and a moderate degree of dementia. In these respects it closely resembles cases of "birth palsy," in which, as a result of meningeal hæmorrhage, certain portions of the cortex are compressed and the convolutions in the affected region become small and indurated; the child is backward or demented, has spastic limbs, and is subject to attacks of epileptiform convulsions.

In both classes—viz., the syphilitic and the "birth palsy" cases—the most pronounced cortical change is to be found in the motor area, that is, in the middle zone of the hemisphere, the fore and hind parts of the cerebrum being comparatively spared. This fact is of interest in connection with the location of mental functions, and gives support to the view that mental processes are not subserved by the frontal lobes alone but probably depend on the healthy action of all portions of the cortex.

The mental disturbance in hereditary syphilis may be considered according to the time of its development under two headings—viz., idiocy and juvenile dementia.

Idiocy. — Congenital deficiency of mind from inherited syphilis is rarer than mental failure coming on in childhood; this may be owing to the number of infants who die from the severity of the cerebral mischief. But we have seen cases of syphilitic children who were truly idiots, that is, whose mental functions have never perfectly developed. Such children may subsequently be seized with eclampsia or other symptoms of brain disease. The idiocy may be the result of a fœtal or an early infantile meningo-encephalitis, or of hydrocephalus.

It is also possible but difficult to establish that a syphilitic taint may weaken nerve elements apart from demonstrable changes, and so lead to idiocy, just as the virus of acquired syphilis predisposes to degeneration of the nerve elements of the posterior columns, and so becomes the chief ætiological factor in locomotor ataxy. Also it must be borne in mind, as Hughlings Jackson pointed out in a case of his own, that syphilis may be grafted on to a brain already imperfect in consequence of insanity in the parents.

Juvenile Dementia.—In the vast majority of cases mental failure comes on in childhood; the child when young is as bright and sharp as other children of the same age, he learns to read and write and cannot in anywise be called backward, then, at an age varying from five to ten his intellect becomes arrested in its development. The parents or teachers notice that he no longer learns his lessons as correctly as formerly, that his memory is failing, that he is less vivacious, takes no interest in his work or his play, and gradually he proceeds to a condition of more or less complete dementia. As a rule, the dementia is preceded and associated with convulsive attacks, hemiplegia or other indications of cerebral mischief. This common variety is illustrated by the following cases:—

(1) Mary A. (Under care of Dr. Bury.) Healthy as a baby till vaccinated, when she became covered with brown spots, also snuffled in the nose—she talked sensibly and played with other children, and had a good memory *till eight years old;* used to learn hymns and sing them, and was fond of music. When about twelve years, had a fit, in which the right side was chiefly drawn up; "she lay for about twenty-four hours partly unconscious, and drew herself up." After the fit the right foot trailed in walking, and then the right side became paralysed. She often had pain in the head—she had two more similar fits before her death; after the third fit she never spoke, that is about nine months before she died. A strong family history of syphilis but none of insanity or other nervous disorder. When fourteen and a half years old, she was lying in bed and quite demented; there was paresis of the right limbs but no marked rigidity. The upper central incisors were pegged, there were old scars at the angles of the mouth, and a characteristic physiognomy. The child was seen again a few months later; she was lying crouched up in bed, her arms and legs rigidly flexed. There was extreme emaciation and advanced dementia. She died a few weeks later, aged fifteen years.

The autopsy revealed thickening of the pia arachnoid, atrophy and sclerosis of the convolutions, and thickening of cerebral arteries. On microscopical examination typical endo-arteritis and atrophy of the pyramidal cells of the cortex (see figures) were conspicuous, and the cord showed a bilateral descending degeneration of both pyramidal tracts.

In the case of Dr. Humphreys already mentioned, similar changes were found post mortem together with hæmorrhagic pachymeningitis and enormous thickening of the skull. The patient was well till three years old, then had a fit in which the right side worked, this being followed by other fits. She was unable to walk at seven years, lost her speech at nine years, and when seen aged eleven, she was a complete idiot. There was spastic paralysis of all the limbs. The eyes showed optic atrophy and choroiditis disseminata, and the teeth were notched and pegged.

(2) Hannah H. Seen in 1882 by Dr. Bury, aged sixteen years, parents dead; the father died of hemiplegia, probably syphilitic. The patient presented typical teeth; signs of old iritis, symmetrical disseminated choroiditis, and symmetrical deafness. She was deaf and had bad sight five years ago, but was then quite sensible. Her mind began to fail when fifteen years old. Now, if left alone patient sits still and does not attempt to do anything, will not offer to get food for herself, is bad tempered, uses very filthy language, but did not do so before her mental failure. She is very frightened at times, tries to catch at something in the air. Is very restless at night, will jump out of bed screaming, but the nurse can soon quiet her. Staggers in walking. This patient was seen again last year, then twenty-four years old, and it is important to observe that her mental condition was not materially worse; she could walk a little, but the lower limbs were somewhat rigid and the knee-jerks exaggerated.

(3) Georgina T. Aged eleven years eleven months, under care of Dr. Barlow. Well marked parental and family history of syphilis. The patient was the result of the sixth pregnacy. Had a rash all over the body when six weeks old with "snuffles," was under medical treatment for eight months. Subsequently got on well up to seven years old. Learnt well at school and was able to do many things which she is now incapable of doing—*e.g.*, she could scrub the steps and hem a handkerchief and put the younger sister to bed. It was noticed that after this time she gradually "went back" in intelligence. Would laugh without reason and for a long time continuously. Her schoolfellows began to call her silly. She became frightened at the least thing. When seen at the age of eleven years eleven months, she was fairly grown and free from signs of visceral disease. She had typical pegged upper median permanent incisors. There were characteristic fissures round the mouth. The nose bridge was good and there was no deafness. She was blind with the left eye, the left pupil was small and immobile to light; under atropine it dilated without revealing any bridles.

Her knee-jerks were exaggerated, and in walking she held her legs rather stiff and carried her head too far forwards. The movements of her hands were good. There was no atrophy.

Mental Condition.—She was irrepressibly cheerful and quite docile. Her memory could not be trusted to carry messages. Her speech was natural, but in answering a question she burst into a meaningless laugh. She could do addition sums. She slept well, and would often desire to go to bed at five o'clock in the afternoon. She had been fond of taking long walks alone but could not be induced to do any housework for more than a few minutes. When seen again eighteen months subsequently her gait was much more spastic, but her mental state had not altered to any extent.

In other cases dementia may exist for a long time without any marked evidence of brain disease, or paralytic defects may not come into relief in consequence of the prominence of mental defects.

And for diagnosis and treatment it is just as important to recognise this fact as we have already pointed out with regard to instances of epilepsy existing alone.

Example:* Annie L., aged fourteen years, came under Dr. Bury's care in February 1882. Strong family history of syphilis. The patient when a baby was one mass of spots, had snuffles, and screamed a great deal. Subsequently was pretty well till her weak state of mind came on about four years ago (ten years old). For the last twelve months her walking has been bad, power to hold her water has been getting less, and her hands and mouth have occasionally twitched. She is a well-nourished girl, has a pleasant face and well-shaped head. There is well-marked disseminated choroiditis, most advanced in the right eye. The corneæ are clear, and the teeth are not typical. The knee-jerks are exaggerated. This and her mental condition are the only indications of disease of the central nervous system.

Mental Condition.—She is easily frightened, cries readily, starts at the least noise, does not speak unless spoken to, then talks of things that happened long ago. She cannot read letters, though she could two years ago, but was never able to read a book. She can name a few common objects, such as a doll, a watch; she calls all coins either a "penny" or a "sovereign;" she has no idea how many fingers she has after she has counted them; she does not notice what is going on around her, does not as a rule indicate her wants in any way, is not vicious, but is timid now, and, when frightened, muscular tremors are noticed.

Variety of Insanity.—There are many degrees of intellectual failure, but not

* This case, cases 1 and 2, and Dr. Humphry's case, are reported in full in the April number of *Brain* for 1883.

many varieties of insanity. In some cases maniacal attacks are recorded, or there are fits of excitement, or the patient is bad tempered and vicious; frequently there is evidence that the patient suffers from hallucinations or illusions. But, as a rule, the cases fall into the class of simple intellectual failure; they are passive, apathetic, deprived of memory, do not understand what is said to them, and lapse into a purely vegetative existence. These cases rarely reach asylums; they are not sufficiently vicious or troublesome, they are apathetic and inoffensive, and are to be found dragging on an existence, aimless and devoid of interest and intelligence, at their own homes or in our union hospitals. We may picture the type as a little child, bright, active, and intelligent, who passes step by step into a state of hopeless dementia, a child whose fondness for play, whose interest in all its surroundings, whose sharp memory and bright intelligence are gradually blotted out by the thick mist which slowly but surely settles down upon and closes in the developing brain, arresting its growth and benumbing or paralysing its highest functions.

If, in conclusion, we contrast brain disease due to hereditary syphilis with that due to acquired syphilis, we find that amentia in association with eclampsia and spastic limbs are to be regarded as typical of hereditary syphilis; hemiplegia, with or without unilateral convulsions, as typical of acquired syphilis in the adult. The morbid anatomy of the former consists mainly of chronic meningitis, endoarteritis, and cortical sclerosis and atrophy; whereas the common lesions in acquired syphilis are gummata and central softening from arterial disease and thrombosis.

Spinal Affections. — We have referred in the section on morbid anatomy to (1) spinal lesions, the result of descending degeneration from cerebral disease; (2) independent lesions in the cord, presumably starting in vascular disease in the cord; (3) lesions of the cord and its membranes, consecutive to damage of the spinal canal, either of the nature of gummata or periostitis.

The above categories probably explain the majority of the cases of spinal affection in congenital syphilis which have recovered completely, or (what is more commonly) have recovered partially with relapses, but in which post-mortem verification has not been obtained.

Thus Dixon Mann has recorded a case of a syphilitic boy aged fifteen, who suffered from lumbar pain, paraplegia with exaggeration of deep and superficial reflexes, paralysis of bladder, and sacral bedsore. Under anti-syphilitic treatment the boy recovered, and Dr. Mann ascribed the condition to a local thrombosis of the vessels of the cord, which had led to softening, and interfered with conductivity for a time, but had not produced actual destruction of tissue.

Dr. Moncorvo has recorded three cases of syphilitic children who presented the clinical features of disseminated sclerosis, and in two of them he observed notable improvement under anti-syphilitic treatment.

Fournier and Laschkewitz have each recorded a case of hyperostosis of vertebræ in congenitally syphilitic subjects, with symptoms pointing to compression myelitis. Under specific treatment rapid diminution of the hyperostosis and of the paraplegia occurred in Fournier's case, and Laschkewitz's case was cured in two months.

With respect to locomotor ataxy, Remak gives details of two cases, one a girl of twelve years and the other a boy of sixteen years, in whom many of the symptoms of this disease were present.

Fournier also describes three cases of ataxy in young people, in whom there was reason to suspect congenital syphilis, though the evidence was not quite conclusive.

We have no post-mortem evidence as yet throwing light on the question as to whether the spinal symptoms depended on definite syphilitic lesions or whether, as in some cases of acquired syphilis, the specific poison may have acted as a powerful predisposing cause.

Spinal Nerves.—Dr. J. A. Ormerod has recorded one remarkable case of a woman aged twenty-three, who was the subject of hereditary syphilis, and who presented a fusiform enlargement on the median nerve, which was attended with paralysis, atrophy and anæsthesia.

Prognosis.—The course of the various nervous manifestations of congenital syphilis is exceedingly varied.

A few lesions appear to go through a cycle and undergo spontaneous and complete subsidence. Others, so far as clinical observation extends, are the outcome of a storm which comes to an end with some irreparable damage done but without tendency to further progress. But of many of the severe manifestations in congenital as well as in acquired syphilis, we may say that they are more commonly scotched than cured.

It is remarkable how promptly active symptoms respond to proper treatment, but post-mortem investigation shows again and again the existence of widespread damage which has not been eradicated, although its active phases may have been controlled.

Examples of spontaneous and sometimes complete subsidence are some cases of interstitial keratitis.

Examples of definite mischief are some of the cases of probable peripheral paralysis of one or more cranial nerve, and some cases of choroiditis disseminata.

An instance of rapidly progressive irreparable mischief is the deafness of hereditary syphilis. Damage to vessels with thrombosis is probably recoverable to a great extent, and the symptoms referable to it show often remarkable and rapid improvement.

The irritability and convulsions dependent on meningeal disease may be controlled, but they are often the harbingers of progressive degeneration, and what may be called the degradation of the functions of both brain and cord. The psychical affections are always to be looked upon as of grave import. For although there may be periods of quiescence yet the ultimate issue tends sooner or later to dementia.

Treatment.—We are of opinion that the paramount lesson of congenital brain syphilis is, that the earliest exanthem stage of the disease should be vigorously treated. The desideratum is not only to get rid of the affections of skin and mucous membrane which will spontaneously subside, but to limit if possible the early damage to tissues which not improbably gives a substratum for later mischief.

We believe that mercurial inunction ought as a rule to be employed in the early stage of the disease. For the later manifestations grey powder is, we believe, the best vehicle of giving mercury internally; but whenever active signs appear mercurial inunction should again be employed. The iodides may be given as intermediate treatment, but we have not found them so well tolerated or so obviously effective in children as mercury.

FIG. 1.

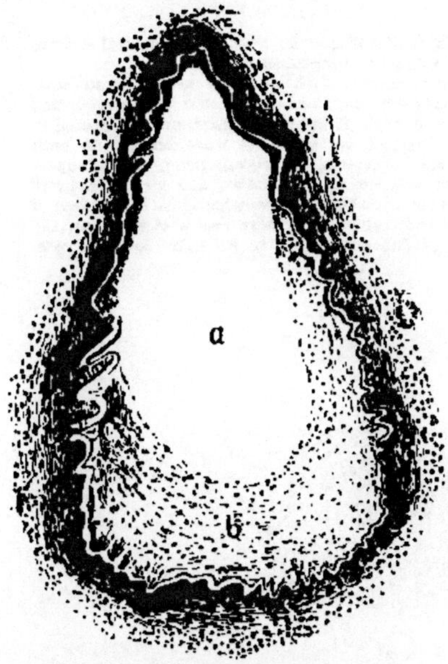

Section of middle cerebral artery from a girl aged fifteen years, the subject of hereditary syphilis and dementia. The letter *a* is placed in the lumen of the vessel, *b* in the middle of a growth, composed of round and fusiform cells, and situated between the endothelium and the fenestrated membrane. (Dr. Bury's case, *Brain*, April 1883, p. 17.)

FIG. 2.

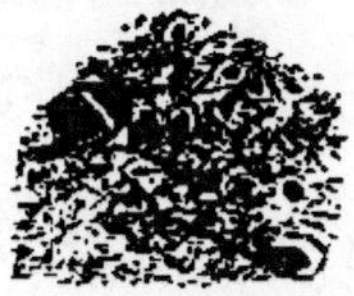

Section of cerebral cortex from upper end of motor region—from the same case as Fig. 1. The drawing shows a group of atrophied pyramidal cells with wide peri-cellular spaces; in many sections of the cortex not a single cell could be found. Sections of the spinal cord showed descending sclerosis of the pyramidal tracts. (Dr. Bury, *Brain*, 1883, p. 16.)

FIG. 4.

FIG. 3.

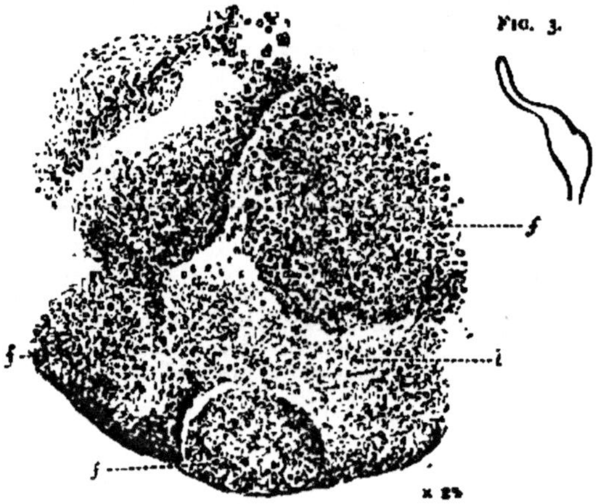

FIG. 3.—Third nerve presenting a fusiform gumma near its superficial origin. From a child aged fifteen months, the subject of congenital syphilis.

FIG. 4.—Section of gumma of motor root of fifth nerve from the same case. *f, f,* funiculi showing destruction of axis cylinders and infiltration with granulation cells, which are most abundant at periphery. *i*, interfunicular tissue infiltrated to less extent with granulation cells. Symmetrical gummata were present on both third nerves, and on the fourth, fifth, sixth, seventh, and eighth pairs at their superficial origin. There was extensive endarteritis of the basilar, and all the arteries forming the circle of Willis. Stellate cicatricial patches were found on the surface of the liver with some subjacent cellular infiltration, and there was a cicatrix on the capsule of the spleen and adhesion of the peritoneum to it. (Dr. Barlow's case, "Path. Trans.," vol. xxviii. p. 291.)

FIG. 5.

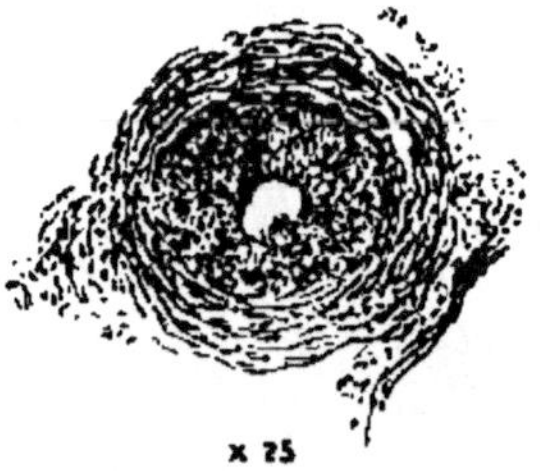

FIG. 5.—Peri-arteritis and endarteritis of arteriole from a syphilitic infant, who died aged ten months. There was extensive chronic meningitis of the convexity, with a few adhesions of bone, dura mater, and pia arachnoid, and one small thin patch of calcification. There was a small area of recent green lymph at the anterior base. In the meningitis of the convexity small arteries could be traced like opaque white threads. These on section showed a gradually narrowing lumen, and for varying distances they were thrombosed. The arteries of the circle of Willis were natural. There were a few spots of superficial softening in the cortex, and the lateral ventricles were slightly enlarged. There was extensive choroiditis in the exudation stage. The meningeal disease probably started when the child was four months old. The choroiditis was first detected when she was eight months old. (Dr. Barlow's case, "Path. Trans.," vol. xxviii. p. 287.)

Fig. 7.

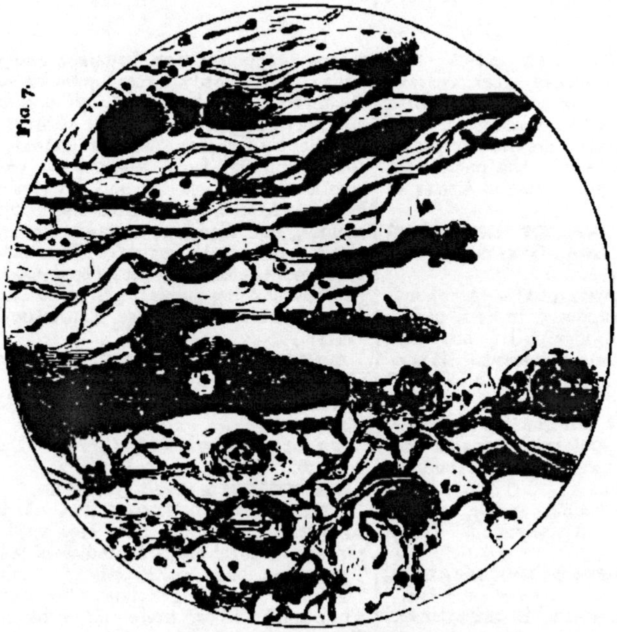

Fig. 6.

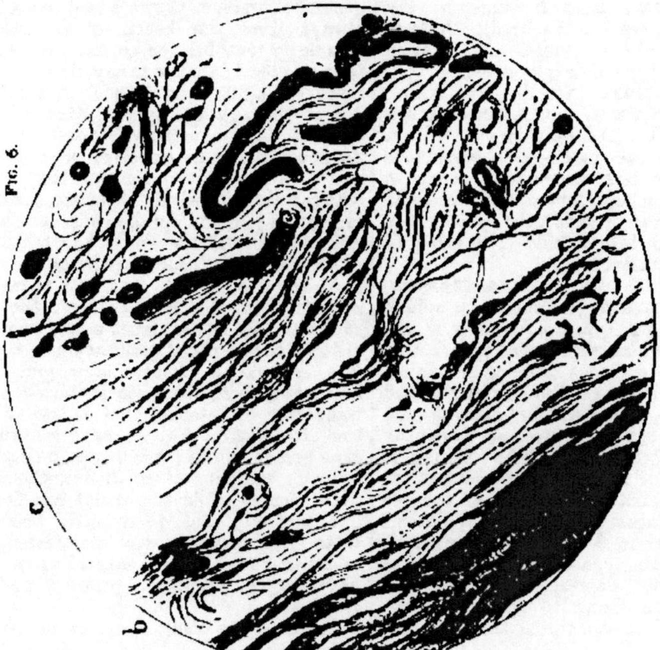

Figs. 6 and 7.—Sections of thick fleshy vascular membrane attached to the internal surface of the dura mater on the right side, from a child aged 11½ years, the subject of hereditary syphilis and dementia, under the care of Dr. Henry Humphreys. The membrane was composed of parallel layers of vessels separated by a little connective tissue. The vessels, chiefly capillaries, had remarkably thick walls. In Fig. 6 *a* represents the dura mater, *b* and *c* the two layers of the false membrane. The thickened vessels in *c* are seen more highly magnified in Fig. 7. In this case the convolutions were exceedingly narrow and wasted, and the brain substance very firm. There was extensive endarteritis. The base of the skull was remarkably thickened. (Dr. Bury, *Brain*, 1883, pp. 13 and 24.)

Thomas Barlow. Judson S. Bury.

SYSTEMATISED MANIA. (*See* Mania, Systematised.)

T

TABES DORSALIS AND INSANITY.—Occasionally tabes dorsalis or locomotor ataxy is complicated with general paralysis of the insane. In other cases of tabes dorsalis, cerebral symptoms sometimes supervene and the patient becomes insane. (*See* LOCOMOTOR ATAXY AS ALLIED TO NEUROSES.)

TABETIC GAIT IN GENERAL PARALYSIS. (*See* GENERAL PARALYSIS.)

TACHE CÉRÉBRALE.—A phenomenon formerly supposed to be a pathognomonic sign of meningitis, but now known to occur in many diseases. It consists in the production of a bright red line by drawing the finger-nail over the skin of the patient, this line lasting longer, appearing earlier, and being broader and deeper-coloured than would be the case in a healthy person.

TACHYPHRASIA (ταχύς, rapid; φράσις, speech). Synonym of Logodiarrhœa (*q.v.*).

TANASIMONOSOPHOBOMANIE. (Fr.) Michéa's term for hypochondriasis.

TANZKRANKHEIT, TANZSUCHT, TANZWUTH. St. Vitus's dance. Chorea.

TAPEINOCEPHALIC (ταπεινός, low or debased; κεφαλή, the head). A term applied to skulls whose conformation shows a low type of development.

TARANTISM. (*See* TARANTULISM.)

TARANTULA, TARENTULA (Taranto, a city of Apulia, where the spiders abounded).—The name of a venomous spider whose bite was said to produce a state of melancholy and stupor which could only be relieved by music, the patient then being excited into a kind of dancing fit called Tarantulism (*q.v.*).

TARANTULISM, TARENTISMUS, TARENTULISM (Tarantula, a spider, originally from Taranto, the city in the vicinity of which venomous spiders were found).—An epidemic dancing mania occurring in Italy in the sixteenth and seventeenth centuries, the dancing and excitement being adopted as a remedy for the bite of the tarantula. Owing to the number of epidemics prevalent at the time, there existed great fear of the bite of the tarantula as causing symptoms ending either in death or permanent injury; accordingly, a bite of any sort induced intense depression. Music and dancing were found to relieve the depression and it was stated that by these means the poison was dispersed and expelled. The remedy induced great nervous excitement, which spread by infection, and very many people became affected by this dancing mania. People danced till they dropped from exhaustion, every emotion seemed excited and suicides occurred. After a time the dancing became annual, but died out towards the end of the seventeenth century. The tarentella were the tunes or songs composed to cure this dancing mania. (Fr. *tarantisme*; Ger. *Tarantismus*). (*See* EPIDEMIC INSANITY.)

TASTE, HALLUCINATIONS OF. (*See* HALLUCINATION.)

TASTE, ILLUSIONS OF. (*See* ILLUSION.)

TAUBSTUMMHEIT (Ger.). Deaf-mutism.

TÄUSCHUNG (Ger.). Illusion.

TEARS, PSYCHOLOGY OF.—Adjectives the most various have been used to express the psychological qualities of tears. They have been called "hot," "cold," "languid," "gushing," "silent," "wearied," "wanton," and we know not what else. They are waves of emotion, and, as a general expression, they are said to spring always from the heart, an expression singularly truthful, for no one ever wept from the head; that is to say, no one ever reasoned himself or herself into tears except through an appeal back to an emotion. There are very few persons who do not under some emotions shed tears, and it is probably quite true that they who can always restrain them are, according to the common opinion, of a hard and unimpressionable nature. The statement often made that insane persons do not shed tears is not all true, but there is some truth in it. We have seen the insane weeping, but we must admit that on visiting the wards of great asylums there is a remarkable absence of weeping in comparison with the noise, irritation, and wandering of intellect that is forced on the attention. Also, we have known a sane person who became insane, owing to a great calamity of grief, overwhelmed with weeping while the sanity remained, but perfectly and persistently tearless when the insanity was manifested, a result that may appear natural when the physiology of weeping is properly understood.

Tears are the result of a nervous storm

in the central nervous system, under which there is such a change in the vascular terminals of the tear-secreting glands that excretion of water from the glands is profuse. Some excretion is always in process in order that the surface of the eye may be laved and cleared of foreign matters which may come in contact with it; but the controlling centre is at a distance. As the muscular power that extends or flexes a finger is at a distance from the part moved, so the excitement to tears is from an irritation in a distant nervous centre, and is removed when the nervous centre is either soothed or exhausted. The persons who weep say that tears afford relief. Nothing is more perfectly true, nothing more clear when the facts are understood. The relief comes, not from the mere escape of tears, which is only a symptom, but from the cessation of the storm in the nervous chain. If the storm be calmed by soothing measures, as when we soothe a child that is weeping from fear, annoyance, or injury, we quiet the nervous centres, upon which the effect ceases. In children the soothing method succeeds, and sometimes it succeeds in adults, although in adults the cessation of tears is more commonly due to actual exhaustion following a period of nervous activity. In grief, the afflicted weep until they can weep no more; then they become calm, or, like children, cry themselves to sleep. Thus tears indicate relief, and show that the nervous system has fallen into the repose of weariness. Persons subjected to many and repeated griefs shed in time fewer tears, and the aged, compared with the younger, are almost tearless. The poor insane patient who ceases to weep becomes griefless; under the continued excitement the grief centre fails or dies. If this were not the case, tears would flow in such a person so long as life lasted. Tears have their value in the life of mankind; they are of value not as tears, although their actual flow gives relief, but as signs that the grief centres are being relieved of their sensibility, and that the nervous organisation is being fitted to bear up against sorrow.

We once crossed the Thames in a boat at Putney with a man eighty-four years of age. He told us: "It is sixty years since I last made this passage in this same place, and then it was to fetch the famous Dr. Hooper" (author of Hooper's "Physician's Vade Mecum") "to see my child Tom lying at death's door with scarlet fever. I was so heart-broken, and cried so terribly, that the men in the ferry-boat, which then plied here, tried to console me. Tom recovered and lived until last year, when he went before me. If he had died of the scarlet fever when he was young, I veritably believe I should have died, too of tears and grief, and yet when he died fifty-nine years later, during all which period he and I had been affectionately attached to each other, I could not shed a tear, nor could I again feel the poignancy of that early grief. I accuse myself of being without feeling, and yet I cannot help it. Can you doctors explain the reason?" We explain it as above, and we think the explanation as accurate in fact as it is clear in theory.

Respecting the nervous excitation which calls forth tears, we have noticed how little it is due to physical pain. It is called forth by fear, by anxiety, by affection, by grief, but not even by pain extending to agony. In the days preceding the use of anæsthetics we have seen patients who were undergoing surgical operations faint; we have heard them cry out and scream until they made the bystanders sick and pale, but they rarely, if ever, shed tears. The parturient woman in the acme of her "great pain and peril" may suffer the extremest physical agony, under which her cries are piercing, but she rarely sheds tears. Indeed, we never recollect seeing the most nervous of her class, under such circumstances, shedding a tear. Strangely, however, during the sleep induced by an anæsthetic like chloroform or ether, we have seen profuse tears, not from suffering, but from some emotional dream induced by the narcotic.

A very slight emotional disturbance will induce the nervous irritation leading to tears in susceptible subjects; and this although the catastrophe has nothing to do, intrinsically, with the person affected. Hence the commotion of tears conjured up in a play. Hamlet, it will be remembered, seizes aptly this point when the player weeps. "What's Hecuba to him, or he to Hecuba?" Of course nothing, yet the player weeps, and maybe the audience weeps with the player. By art another remembrance may be used to call forth tears on the proper occasion. A well-known player was asked how he managed to weep when he willed. He replied, "I call up the remembrance of my dear father, who is dead." On the other hand, anything that produces diversion of mind, when the disturbance is not severe may keep back the outbreak. John Hunter tells us that once when he went to the play to see Mrs. Siddons perform, in a moving exposition of her great powers, he could not join the rest of the house in their tears "because he had forgotten his pocket-handkerchief;" and a friend of my own, an emotional man, told me that at a funeral, where he expected to be overwhelmed with tears, he was completely checked by an absurd reading which the parish clerk gave to a sentence of the service. In these facts there is nothing incompatible, because the more intense the nervous vibrations, the more easy is the diversion of the impulse from one centre to another.

As a rule, the escape, and free escape, of tears relieves the heart and saves the body from the shock of grief. Tears are the natural outlets of emotional tension. But there are exceptions to this rule, and we have more than once seen uncontrollable weeping followed by serious systemic disturbance, affecting principally the heart and circulation. We have known intermittency of the heart induced in this way and assume the most serious character.

Change of scene, mental diversion and outdoor life are the best remedies for the tearful, but an opiate judiciously prescribed is often the sovereign remedy. Other narcotics are injurious. Alcohol, so often resorted to, is fearfully injurious. It disturbs and unbalances the nervous system, keeps up a maudlin and pitiful sentimentality, and sustains the evil. Alcohol is the mother of sorrow. There are other narcotics which are similar in effect, notably chloral; but an opiate given at night-time, under necessity, not only soothes, but controls, and, when prescribed so that the use of it shall not pass into habit, is a divine remedy.

As tears are secreted by glands which lie between their nervous centre and the mucous surface of the eyeball; as they have two functions or duties, one the function of relieving nervous tension, the other of laving the eyeball; so these functions may be called into over-action by internal nervous impulses or vibrations, and by external excitations or what are sometimes called reflex actions. The first is seen in the act of weeping under emotion, the vibration starting in the nervous centres, and extending to the gland from behind, urging it to action; the second is seen in the act of shedding tears from direct irritation of the mucous surface of the eyeball, as when an irritating substance "gets into the eye," and the vibration extends from the mucous surface back to the gland, exciting it to action and causing emotionless tears. In these ways tears afford a good illustration of the mode in which the nervous fibres are capable of conveying to a secreting organ exciting impulses from both sides of a gland lying in their course, and having in connection with it afferent and efferent communications. In both cases the exciting impulse is a vibration; and as when the impulse sets forth from a mere external irritation, as from a particle of dust on the conjunctiva, the effect is in the truest sense mechanical; so, probably, in the case of the emotional irritation, which calls forth tears, the process is as purely mechanical.

In the human animal tears are most easily wrought where the sympathetic nervous system is most developed and most impressionable, and when the three great emotions, fear, grief, and joy, are most active. Hence, women generally are more given to tears than men, and under the peculiar state called hysteria, in which the nervous system is at highest tension, are often seen moved to tears by the three emotions, in turn, during one paroxysm.

B. W. Richardson.

TELESTHESIS (τῆλε, far off; *αἴσθησις* perception). Tact, or perception from remote grounds or circumstances. (Fr. *télaesthèse*; Ger. *Fernfühlen*).

TELEPATHY (τῆλε, afar; *πάθος*, a suffering). The supposed power of one mind to influence or be influenced by another by other channels than those of the senses. Also a synonym of Thought-reading or Thought-transference. (Fr. *télépathie*.)

TEMPER, CHANGE OF.—An early symptom in insanity, especially moral insanity.

TEMPERAMENT (*tempero, I mingle*; Fr. *tempérament*; Ger. *Körperanlage*.)—The theory of temperaments as understood in the present day implies a definite relation between the physical qualities of an individual, such as size and form of body, size and shape of head and face, complexion, colour of hair and eyes, and on the other hand, his mental characteristics, his tastes, disposition, and tendency of conduct, his mode of being affected by external impressions and by disease, and so on.

By this theory individuals are arranged in groups according to their characteristics, and it is claimed that those belonging to any particular group on account of their physical qualities, will be found to resemble one another in their mental and other qualities. These groups, although few in number are so comprehensive that most individuals can be classed in one or other of them, and the name summarising the characteristics belonging to each one of these groups, is the name of the temperament of each member of the group.

The word temperament as met with so frequently in every-day literature and conversation, is unfortunately used in so many varied senses that it is quite incapable of definition, and has, in fact, no distinct meaning. From such sources it would seem that the number of temperaments can be indefinitely multiplied merely by prefixing different adjectives to the word, and the common non-scientific use of the word is therefore of no help whatever in endeavouring to understand the real theory of temperaments.

The word temperament was originally used almost entirely in connection with physical qualities. The earlier physicians had to rely much more on external appearances as an aid to diagnosis than those of the present day have; we find, therefore, that the idea of dividing men into groups according to their general appearance dates from a very early age in medicine. In the writings of Hippocrates, evidence of the conception is frequently met with, and at a somewhat later date the theory was arranged on a scientific basis by Galen, who wrote a work on temperaments which has been translated into Latin by Linacre. Since the time of Galen the theory has been variously modified and extended in detail from time to time, but the basis of his teaching has been the basis of all teaching and writings on the subject from his time to the present.

Galen describes nine different varieties of temperament; there were four simple uncomplicated temperaments, the dry, the moist, the hot and the cold: then there were four temperaments formed by mixtures of these qualities, the hot and moist, the hot and dry, the cold and moist, and the cold and dry, which from their descriptions appear to correspond to the later sanguine, bilious, phlegmatic and melancholic temperaments respectively. Finally there was a ninth temperament named the "balanced" in which no quality was in excess, but the individual's characteristics were so arranged and evenly balanced that he was perfect. It served as a basis from which to describe the others.

The names used later on, sanguine, bilious, &c., were derived from the humoral pathology. It was supposed that a person's temperament depended on the presence in his system of an excess of one of the humours, or of a preponderating influence of the organ concerned in the production of that humour. Four main temperaments were described therefore, according as the heart and blood, the liver and bile, the spleen and black bile (the spleen being then supposed to secrete black bile) or the brain, pituitary body and phlegm were more influential in determining the qualities of the individual; the names were respectively: Sanguine, bilious or choleric, atrabilious or melancholic, and pituitous, lymphatic or phlegmatic.

Since these early times the number of temperaments described has remained as a rule at four. Some authors since it has been known that the spleen does not secrete black bile, and that black bile is bile in another form, have dropped the melancholic temperament, considering it to be a mixture of the others; some have added another, the nervous temperament, and so have kept the numbers at four, and others have added the nervous and dropped the bilious and melancholic temperaments. The main temperaments, like Galen's balanced temperament, are used as types, for it is obvious that very few individuals correspond exactly to the typical description; a person is said to have one or other of the temperaments according as his characteristics most closely correspond to the description of the ideal of that one.

The names and descriptions of the divisions have been so often re-arranged that it is difficult to find two authors agreeing altogether in detail, but the four main temperaments described below have definite characters and are those usually described; the melancholic, according to this classification, being properly a mixture of the bilious and the nervous.

(1) **The Sanguine Temperament.**—Individuals of this temperament vary in height but are oftener short, and usually not stout until later on in life, when they have a tendency in that direction. The head and bones are small, features well defined, nose rather short, and lips of medium thickness, not thin; neck short. Complexion fair and bright, often ruddy, hair reddish and plentiful in early life, eyes blue. Mentally persons of this temperament are characterised by great susceptibility to external impressions and to the feelings of pleasure or pain attached to these impressions; their mental movements are rapid but shallow, they are impulsive, emotional and excitable, easily provoked and as easily forgetting. They lack persistence and have bad memories. They have often powerful imaginations and clever thoughts. The sanguine temperament is useful in preventing narrowness of mind, and in initiating new ideas, but is not suitable to an older age than that of childhood, and lacks the steadiness necessary in life. The diseases said to be especially common in those of this temperament are diseases of the circulatory system and heart, hæmorrhages and acute inflammations. Illnesses in these individuals, including insanity, generally run an acute course.

(2) **The Nervous Temperament.**—In persons of this temperament the figure is slight but often tall. The head is small and narrow, the forehead being proportionately large. The features are small and sharply cut, the nose and chin pointed and the lips thin. The skin is dark and dull, the complexion sallow, the hair is usually brown and the eyes dark or grey. They are restless and active; speech rapid. Mentally their activity is great, but they are characterised by too much changeability. They think readily, but have bad memories; suffer much from emotions of hope and fear, but easily get over them afterwards. They imagine well and are much influenced by their environment. They have tender feelings, but can forget easily; very susceptible to sensations. They seem to be particularly liable to insanity, especially mania, and to diseases of the nervous system.

(3) **The Bilious or Choleric Temperament.**—Individuals of this temperament are usually short and thickly built, and even if tall they are correspondingly big. The head is large and square; features large and not well defined, nose outspread, mouth wide, skin rough and hairy. Complexion, hair and eyes dark in colour. Voice rough. Movements clumsy but strong. Mentally they are capable of much exertion; they are not impulsive, but steady in thought and judgment; memory good; speech deliberate but decided; they make up their minds about anything and stick to it. They are passionate and jealous, and do not forget an injury; their feelings are not easily excited, but are strong when roused. Affection strong. They are perhaps less liable to disease than those of any other temperament, but are said to be more frequently affected with the symptoms usually included under the heading, "lithic acid diathesis." There is no particular form of insanity assigned to individuals of this temperament, but they are possibly more liable to general paralysis or mania than the other forms. The question of the connection between temperament and insanity has never been adequately gone into.

(4) **The Phlegmatic or Lymphatic Temperament.**—Men of this type are, as a rule, thick set, short-necked, bulky individuals with want of proportion in their build. The head is not large, the features are not well defined. The hair is light or sandy and often thin, the eyebrows light. The complexion is colourless and pasty, the eyes have a washed-out appearance, often greyish in colour. The skin is unhealthy looking; speech is slow and movements sluggish. Mentally, individuals with this temperament have good judgment, but are slow; common sense fairly good and memory good; not emotional; heavy and plodding; feelings persistent, thought not powerful. Much lack of energy. Persons of this temperament are liable to chronic, strumous diseases, and to chronic catarrhs. In them disease runs a slow, atypical course. They are liable to dementia rather than to other forms of mental affection.

Since the commencement of the idea the theory of temperaments has been variously applied, sometimes fancifully, sometimes with a firm basis of fact. Among the common modes of application are the following:—Each age of man, childhood, youth, middle age and old age has a particular temperament assigned to it, the sanguine, bilious, melancholic, and phlegmatic respectively; a particular temperament has been supposed to prevail at each season, the sanguine in spring, and the bilious, melancholic and phlegmatic in summer, autumn and winter respectively. Nations and races have also had a particular temperament ascribed to each of them. More important from a medical point of view are the following:—Climate is supposed to influence temperament, to be a predisposing cause to certain diseases in persons of particular temperaments, and to affect persons differently according to their temperament. Men of different temperaments are also said to be liable to different diseases, to different classes of diseases, and to be differently affected by the same disease; and if an individual becomes insane, the form the insanity takes is said to depend partly on his temperament, as mentioned in the description of the different varieties.

In the time of the humoral pathology it was supposed that the organ and humour concerned in the formation of an individual's temperament were especially prone to disease, and we occasionally find some sort of evidence of this in the present day.

It must be confessed that the theory of temperament is not of much use in medicine at present, as far as diagnosis and treatment are concerned. In the earlier days of medicine when fewer means of diagnosis, such as the thermometer, stethoscope, and other instruments, were known, the patient's appearance was of more value as an indication for treatment. However, even without any special knowledge of a theory of temperament, no thoughtful practitioner in the present day prescribes for a patient without involuntarily reminding himself that the same drug may affect two persons in quite a different way, and he judges what its effect may be very much by the physical and mental qualities of the individual. It is also a matter of ordinary experience that the course of the same disease may be quite different in two different people, and the treatment is varied accordingly. Moreover, even now, certain diseases are occasionally associated with particular physical appearances, for instance, in examining a case of diabetes, we almost invariably look to see if the hair is of a reddish colour.

Granted that the theory of temperaments as above given proved, it is clear that a knowledge of it can be made useful in prophylactic medicine. If people of a certain temperament are liable to certain diseases, or if diseases run particular courses, according to the temperaments of the patients affected, the causes of the diseases can be avoided in the former cases, and in the latter we can treat accordingly. If it be known that certain climates are dangerous to individuals of any one temperament, they can be advised either to remove from the dangerous place or to be on their guard against the affections to which they are liable. In the case of insanity also, if it be true that men of particular temperaments are liable to corresponding particular forms of madness, one can know what to expect and provide accordingly; moreover the treatment of that and any other disease must be adapted to the temperament of the patient, if it is clear that the way in which the disease affects the individual, and the sort of treatment the disease is amenable to in his case, depends on his temperament.

It has been said that in the inheritance of physical qualities, corresponding mental characteristics and liability to disease are also inherited; the recording of the temperament of the parent, might, if this be the case, influence the bringing up and career of the child.

WILLIAM GEO. WILLOUGHBY.

TEMPERATURE IN PERIPHERAL NERVES.—The conditions of temperature in the trunks of peripheral nerves may be considered under two heads: First, as to the question whether any heat is evolved when a nervous impulse travels along a nerve trunk; and secondly, as to the question whether any heat is given off from a nerve during the process of dying.

(1) The question as to **whether heat is set free during the passage of a nervous impulse** was attacked as long ago as 1848 by Helmholtz.* This observer worked with a thermopile, and using the sciatic nerves of a frog failed to find any evidence of heat being evolved from a nerve during the passage of a nervous impulse. His instrument was sensitive to one-thousandth of a degree Centigrade.

Heidenhein* repeated these experiments with a similar result. On the other hand Oehl† and Valentin,‡ employing much the same method, obtained evidence pointing to the production of heat in a nerve trunk during the passage of a nervous impulse. Schiff§ experimenting with a thermopile on the nerves of warm-blooded animals such as cats, rabbits and white rats obtained a similar positive result.

The invention of an instrument for measuring with extreme delicacy any variation in temperature by Callendar‖ provided the writer with a very reliable method for re-investigating this question. The electrical resistance thermometer depends on the principal that the electric resistance of a metal wire varies approximately as its temperature. If the temperature of the metal wire be altered, its resistance to the passage of a constant current can be observed by means of a galvanometer. By those means very small variations of temperature can be calculated. The degree of sensibility which it was usually found convenient to work with was one five-thousandth of a degree Centigrade. In this research ¶ the sciatic nerves of frogs were used, and taking pains to eliminate all sources of error it was found that there was no evidence of any heat being evolved from a nerve trunk when a nervous impulse was generated in the nerve.

The fact that no heat can be detected by an instrument so delicate as to show variations of one five-thousandth of a degree Centigrade, or less if desired, is of interest in comparing the activity of muscle with that of nerve. In the case of muscle, energy when liberated appears as work done, and as heat liberated in the proportions varying under different conditions; whereas in the case of a nerve trunk there is no evidence of the energy of a nervous impulse appearing in any form but that of the impulse.

(2) **As to the Production of Heat in a Nerve during the Process of Dying.**—Using Callendar's electrical resistance

* Müller's *Archiv f. Anat. u. Physiolog.*, 1848, s. 158.

* *Studien d. Physiolog. Institut zu Breslau*, iv. s. 250, 1868.

† *Gaz. Med. de Paris*, p. 225, 1866.

‡ *Archiv f. Patholog. Anat.*, xxviii. s. 1, 1863.

§ *Arch. d. Physiolog. Normal et Patholog.*, p. 157, 1869.

‖ *Phil. Trans.*, 1887, A., p. 161.

¶ *Journal of Physiology*, p. 208, 1890.

thermometer the writer found that if the thermal condition of a nerve trunk be continuously observed it will be found that—due precautions being taken—heat is evolved from the nerve as it loses its irritability and dies.

The technique of the experiment cannot be gone into here, but it is enough to state that the vitality of the nerve can be estimated by the amount and existence of the natural nerve current. The natural nerve current disappears on the death of the nerve, and so forms a criterion of its vitality. Experiment goes to show (1) that a nerve in dying evolves heat, and (2) that this evolution of heat corresponds roughly with the intensity of the natural nerve current; this relation is not, however, absolutely constant.

Humphry Davy Rolleston.

Temperature of the Body in Insanity, and the Use of the Thermometer in its Treatment.—The older authors frequently attributed the more acute varieties of insanity to "inflammation" of the brain, and Bayle in his first account of general paralysis in 1822 called it an inflammation of the membranes. But no scientific observations were made on the temperature of the body in any form of insanity until after the clinical thermometer was brought into use by Wunderlich, and his results had been published in his classical work. Dr. Saunders, of the Devon Asylum, was the first to use the instrument in asylum practice, and to publish in 1865 a general estimate of its future importance, with a case of general paralysis, in which, after a congestive attack, the temperature as tested by the thermometer was shown to be 106°. In 1867 we made a series of observations on the temperature of the body in the insane, as tested by the thermometer in 305 patients in the Carlisle Asylum, the results being compared with observations on forty sane persons living under the same conditions. The chief results obtained, which have not been upset by any subsequent observations, were the following:—The average temperature of the body is higher in the insane than in the sane. It is highest in general paralysis, falling gradually in the following mental diseases: viz., acute mania, epileptic insanity, melancholia, simple mania, and dementia. Subsequent observations have shown us that puerperal insanity has a higher average temperature than even general paralysis, there being a large number of cases of the former disease—23 per cent. of the whole number—with a temperature over 100°, some of them even reaching 106°. Dementia is the only form of insanity the average temperature of which is below that of health. The great characteristic of every form of insanity is that the difference between the night and day temperatures is less than that of health, and this is owing to the rising of the night temperature and not to the lowering of the morning temperature. In general paralysis the night temperature is nearly always higher than the morning temperature, if a sufficient number of observations are taken in all the stages of the disease in any case. The night temperature of every form of insanity is higher than that of health. The greatest differences of temperature are found in puerperal insanity, general paralysis, epileptic insanity, and acute mania in different cases. Increased mental exaltation and excitement to any great extent always raised the temperature from 1° to 5.8° in different cases. In *folie circulaire* there is a different temperature for the depressed, the sane, and the elevated periods, the last being the highest by 2.2° in some cases. The congestive attacks of general paralysis are almost always accompanied or followed by a rise in temperature, this commonly passing over 100°. We once had a case in which it reached before death 107.4°. A continuous and marked rise in the average temperature in any case commonly shows acute brain excitement or advancing cerebral disease. The average frequency of the pulse in insanity corresponds with the mean temperature, but the rises in the evening temperature have no necessary corresponding rises in the evening pulse. The differences in the temperature between the insane and the sane are actually not great in amount, on the average being under 1° when a large number of cases are taken. Though this difference seems small yet it is very significant and very important. It indicates how profoundly the brain action is affected in insanity, the changes extending not only to the mental functions but to the thermic centres. These differences of temperature are partly explained by the recent observations of Roy and Sherrington and others as to the vaso-motor centres of the brain being situated in the cortex; each functional area thus includes such a centre for itself, through the action of which, with that of the cortical cells, there results an automatic arrangement through which those areas receive an increased supply of blood and produce increased heat when active, and have a diminished supply with a lessened temperature when functionally at rest. Many observers have demonstrated by the use of delicate surface thermometers that functional activity in individual brain areas causes increased temperature there.

We have found a few cases of very low and very high "neurotic" temperatures among the insane, that were quite exceptional and apart from general experience. Bechterew found that the insane generally have not the same resistive power as the sane against low temperatures, their bodies losing heat more rapidly when subjected to great cold.

Many observers in this country, in France, Germany, Italy, and America, have since made observations on the temperature in the insane, especially in general paralysis. Among those may be mentioned Macleod, Mickle, Turner, Bechterew, and Croemer, and their results confirm generally our observations in 1867.

To any one engaged in practice in the department of mental diseases the thermometer is of the greatest service. It is useful and often essential, (1) in the differential diagnosis of those diseases from the continued fevers, inflammation of the nervous centres, traumatism, and from other diseases; (2) in the diagnosis of many acute brain affections, accidents, and bodily diseases among the insane; and (3), in the treatment of most cases of acute mental disease. Before deciding to send any patient to an asylum we think the temperature should always be taken. We have known cases of the delirium of typhus and typhoid fevers, scarlet fever, meningitis, septicæmia, uræmic delirium, cerebro-spinal meningitis, drunkenness, and opium poisoning sent to asylums as labouring under technical insanity, and some of the cases were so sent by able and experienced men in our profession. The use of the thermometer would in most of these cases have averted such mistakes. Then, every medical man with experience among the insane knows how in certain cases bodily disorders of every kind may occur without any complaint on the part of the patient. The sensory anæsthesia and reflex dulness that so often accompany acute and chronic insanity, together with the disturbed reasoning, will often abolish or inhibit the pain of acute pleurisy or peritonitis, will stop the cough of pneumonia and phthisis, and prevent a maniacal patient with broken ribs or serious internal injuries from complaining or saying that anything is wrong. We have to think, and feel and reason for the patient, and come to conclusions from his objective signs alone. The thermometer helps us greatly to do this, for its indications are absolute so far as they go. We think it a safe rule that whenever the temperature of any insane patient is found to be above 99.5°, a careful physical examination should be made to discover bodily disease or injury; not that such a temperature is that may not be caused by cortical brain excitement. We have known a purely maniacal and neurotic temperature of 104° to occur in a case that was not a general paralytic, had no organic brain disease, and was not a puerperal case.

It is in the third department mentioned however—viz., the ordinary diagnosis, prognosis, and treatment of mental diseases, that we would say the regular use of the thermometer was most important of all. We do not consider the clinical history of any case of insanity complete except the morning and evening temperatures have been taken several times in the course and different stages of the disease. The difference between the morning and evening temperature, and that between one stage and another may be very slight, but yet may be very important. We always estimate that in psychiatry a difference of a degree of temperature may have as equal significance with two or three degrees in fevers and inflammations. If the temperature of a maniacal, melancholic, or general paralytic patient is found to have risen from 98.4° to 99.4°, it will in most cases be as important an indication for diagnosis and treatment in a case of insanity, as an increase of three degrees in a case of fever or inflammation. In melancholia neurotic rises of temperature over 100° are uncommon, and only occur in the very acutely excited and some stuporous cases. Such cases are commonly serious. In mania the temperature often rises above 100° from the cortical excitement alone. We have seen it rise from 98.5° to 103° in two hours, and fall again to normal in the next five hours, though that is uncommon. In acute mania, especially of the delirious type, a temperature about 100° is not necessarily alarming, but when it keeps day by day over 100° it is more serious. In the melancholic variety of stupor the temperature of the body is often half a degree or even more over the normal. In the "anergic" variety ("acute dementia") it is commonly lowered, but in a few cases the heat of the body and cavities is slightly raised, while the extremities may be as low as 94° or 95°. In puerperal insanity the use of the thermometer is essential to diagnose septic conditions, metritis, peritonitis, pelvic inflammation and abscesses; and, apart from these complications, to show how the case is progressing. The cases with the highest temperatures are always those where there is greatest risk of death.

We have found large doses of quinine have immediate effects in reducing the temperature and benefiting the patient in these puerperal cases and in others also, while the reduction by antipyrin seemed to be accompanied by lowered vital energy. We have seen puerperal cases recover, whose temperature had been over 105°. In phthisical insanity most valuable indications are given by the thermometer. In rheumatic insanity the temperature rises and falls as in articular rheumatism, and should be watched in the same way. In epileptic insanity an ordinary fit or series of fits, or even an access of epileptic mania seldom raises the temperature much and then only for a short time. The thermometer is of great use in the acuter varieties of alcoholic insanity, and after alcoholic convulsions, the temperature being often found then to be increased. It is in general paralysis that the temperature has been most studied, both in this country and abroad. Its indications have given rise to very different conclusions, Blandford saying that the disease must be essentially an inflammatory process because it is high, and Turner coming to an opposite opinion. Mickle's careful investigations agree in the main with ours. All agree that in the acuter stages of the disease the temperature is high, and that it is increased in the evening, that before, during and after congestive attacks it rises to a truly febrile stage, commonly over 101°, sometimes even to 107°, and that for a certain time in the second stage of the disease when there is hebetude, fattening, and muscular torpor, the temperature may fall below the normal. We pointed out in 1868 how valuable a means of diagnosis between the congestive attacks of general paralysis, of locomotor ataxia, and of other cerebral organic disease and ordinary epilepsy, we had in the thermometer, and also that by it we could frequently detect organic brain disease. The regular use of the thermometer has unquestionably marked a distinct advance in psychiatry, and it seems probable that its extended use with more delicate instruments will still further help the mental physician and benefit the insane. T. S. Clouston.

[*References.* — Wunderlich, Das Verhalten der Eigenwärme in Krankheiten, Trans. by Woodman, New Syd. Soc. Saunders, Report of the Devon Asylum, 1865. Clouston, Journ. Ment. Sci., April 1868. Mickle, Journ. Ment. Sci., April 1872; Macleod, Lancet, Nov. 19, 1870. Croemer, Zeitsch. für Psychiatrie, 1879. Turner, Journ. Ment. Sci., 1889. Voisin, Traité de la Paralysie Générale des Aliénés, 1879.]

TEMPERATURE OF THE HEAD, NORMAL.—Sect. I.—In studying the temperature of the head, under the circumstances which concern us in this article, we have only to do with the central nervous mass, and with the tissues lying between it and the exterior. We can go still further, and make our limit interiorly the cerebrum.

Now there is no question that the brain has the highest temperature of any organ in the body except the liver. But in man we cannot examine the temperature of the brain by any direct process. We are consequently forced to examine it from the skin of the head. The question, therefore, which at once arises is this: Can the temperature of the brain make itself felt on the exterior surface through the intervening tissues?

Transmission of Heat from Brain to Skin.—Contrary to former belief, none of the animal tissues can come under the designation of *really bad conductors* of heat. Bone, brain-tissue (white or grey), skin, liver-tissue, kidney-tissue, all conduct more or less readily. Even fat, whether in the solid, semi-solid, or semi-liquid condition, is not nearly so bad a conductor as has been supposed.

Thus, for a difference of temperature of 0.1° C. (0.18° F.) between the two sides of pieces 10 mm. (0.39 inch) thick, the following are the average percentages of conduction:—

Bone (compact tissue) . . .	77·77
Bone (spongy tissue) . . .	89.78
Bone (compact spongy) . .	74·74
Brain (grey and white tissue) .	85.00
Muscle (parallel to fibres) . .	82.73
Muscle (across fibres) . .	76.50
Liver	93.00
Kidney (cortical substance) . .	97.70
Kidney (medullary substance) .	91.95
Fat (solid)	50.00
Fat (semi-solid) . . .	40.00
Fat (semi-liquid)	36.00

But the conductivity of skin remains to be considered. In earlier observations, experimenting on 3 mm. (0.118 inch) of the scalp of sheep, the writer came to the conclusion that, through this thickness, the average transmission was only 67.5 per cent. Later experiments have shown that through *10 mm.* the conduction is 70 per cent. As this thickness could not be obtained naturally, pieces of skin were laid one upon another, and pressed closely together. This method is decidedly adverse to the power of conductivity of the tissue, so it may safely be assumed that 70 per cent. is below the mark.

Now, taking the compact spongy tissue of bone as an example, a change of temperature of 0.1° C. (0.18° F.) on one side of a piece 10 mm. (0.39 inch) in thickness would cause a change of temperature on the opposite side of 0.07474° C. (0.1345° F.).

It is therefore evident that, so far as conductivity is concerned, there is not the slightest difficulty in detecting changes of temperature on the surface of the brain—and even deeper, brain tissue being itself so good a conductor—by examinations made on the outer surface of the skin. It follows inevitably that the temperature of the brain is always influencing the temperature of the exterior of the head. The real difficulty is in locating on the skin thermal points of the cerebral surface. The conduction of heat not being *rectilinear*, the part of the cerebral surface directly underlying a given point of the skin may not affect in the greatest degree the temperature of that particular point, but the temperature of some other point more or less distant; simply because the easiest path of transmission is to this latter point.

We now pass to the examination of the temperature of the skin of the head taken in detail.

SECT. II.—**Divisions of the Head.**—It is necessary, at the outset, to pick out and to define, as far as possible, certain points of the skin in which the examinations are to be made. Different observers have done this in different ways. Our method was as follows: First, the surface was divided into three main portions, called respectively, *anterior*, *middle*, and *posterior regions*. The anterior region was thus formed: A line was drawn across the top of the head between the angles made by the frontal and zygomatic processes of the malar bones of the two sides, this line touching the fronto-parietal suture on the longitudinal median line. All the portion of the head in front of this line was included in the anterior region. The middle region was bounded in front by the line just described; its posterior boundary was formed by a line drawn parallel to the last line, between the mastoid processes of the two sides. The posterior region included the portion of the head lying behind the posterior boundary of the middle region. The longitudinal median line of the head divided each of the three regions into right and left symmetrical halves. Each region was subdivided by horizontal and perpendicular lines forming smaller spaces. These spaces varied in their measurements; a fair average would be about 20 mm. (0.787 inch) vertically by about 16 mm. (0.63 inch) horizontally. In the anterior region there were on each side 27 of these spaces, in the middle region 34, and in the posterior region 27, making a total of 88 on each side of the head.

Commencing with the anterior region, we will compare symmetrically [illegible] spaces of the two sides.

Now the first thing of importance that is found in such a comparison, when thoroughly carried out, is this:—*In none of the subdivisions of this region is the temperature uniformly higher on one side than on the other; on the contrary, in every space it may be higher on the right side or on the left side, in turn.*

We must, therefore, seek on which side, in the majority of cases, the higher temperature is found. Now, of the twenty-seven spaces eighteen are in favour of the right side, and nine are in favour of the left side. But, still further, equality of temperature is found in sixteen spaces. The number of comparisons of each pair of spaces was 100, making a total for the whole region of 2700 observations. Of these 2700 cases, 1343 are in favour of the right side, 1137 are in favour of the left side, and 220 show equality of temperature. The percentages of these results are as follows:—In favour of the right side 49.74, in favour of the left side 42.111, in favour of equality 8.149. If we take alone the cases in which either the right side or the left side predominates, thus leaving out the cases of equality of temperature, we have 54.153 per cent. in favour of the right side, and 45.847 per cent. in favour of the left side. But, if we take the averages of all the proportionate numbers of times in which each side is superior in temperature to the other, we find that the left side has the greater average; the mean for the left side being 75.069 per cent. while the mean for the right side is 68.117 per cent., that is to say, in the spaces in which the left side has the larger number of cases of higher temperature the average majority is greater than the average majority found in the spaces in which the right side has the larger number of cases of higher temperature.

The part of the region in which the spaces are situated which show a majority in favour of the left side is roughly bounded by the longitudinal median line, on the inside; by a line drawn upward from the external angular process, on the outside; and by a horizontal line touching the upper border of the frontal eminence.

We next proceed to consider the **thermometric values of the differences of temperature between the two sides.** It is found that the mean difference of temperature is not far from the same, whether the right side or the left be the warmer. Thus the mean difference of temperature in favour of the right side is 0.255° C. (0.459° F.); and the mean difference in favour of the left side is 0.241° C. (0.434° F.) The greatest difference noted was 0.461° C. (0.83° F.) and was in favour of the left side; the smallest difference noted was 0.076° C. (0.137° F.), and was in favour of the right side.

Coming, in the next place, to the middle region, we have, as before stated, 34 spaces on each side to compare. We find here, as in the anterior region, that every space may be of higher temperature on either the right side or on the left side, in turn. Seeking for the side of the head on which the majority of cases of superiority of temperature occurs, we find that seventeen spaces are in favour of each side, the two sides being thus equal in this respect. Fifteen spaces show equality of temperature. The number of comparisons of each pair of spaces was, as in the case of the anterior region, 100, making a total of 3400 observations. Of this number, 1637 are in favour of the right side, 1956 are in favour of the left side, and 107 show equality of temperature. The following are the percentages of these figures:—In favour of right side 48.147, in favour of left side 48.706, in favour of equality 3.147. Omitting the cases of neutrality, we have: For right side 49.714 per cent.; and for left side 50.289 per cent. The mean percentage in favour of the right side in the seventeen spaces which, in the majority of cases, are of a higher temperature on this side is 65.634, and the corresponding percentage in favour of the left side is 66.852.

With regard to the position of the different spaces showing majorities in favour of one side or the other, it may be stated in a general way, that, in the case of the left side, they cover a part of the region extending downward from the longitudinal median line for about 92 mm. (3.6 inches), taken on a line passing through the external auditory meatus, and forward from the posterior boundary of the region to within about 16 mm. (0.63 inch) of the anterior boundary. Below and in front of this tract, the right side predominates, with one signal and important exception, which exists in a spot lying just back of the angle formed by the frontal and zygomatic processes of the malar bone, where the higher temperature is in favour of the left side by a decided majority.

Taking the thermometric differences observed in the middle region, we find that the mean difference of temperature in favour of the right side is 0.0589° C. (0.106° F.); and the mean difference in favour of the left side is 0.1103° C. (0.198° F.) The greatest difference of temperature noted was 0.264° C. (0.475° F.), and was in favour of the left side; the smallest difference noted was 0.016° C. (0.028° F.), and was in favour of the right side.

We will now examine the last of the regions—the posterior. We have twenty-seven spaces on each side to compare. We find in this region, as in the anterior and middle regions, every space sometimes warmer on one side, and sometimes warmer on the other. In eleven spaces the average superiority of temperature is on the right side; and in sixteen spaces it is on the left side. In eleven spaces equality of temperature is found. Of the 2700 comparisons—100 on each pair of spaces as before—1191 are in favour of the right side, 1429 are in favour of the left side, and 80 show equality of temperature. The percentages of these results are as follows:—For right side 44.112, for left side 52.926, for equality 2.962. If we leave out the cases of equality of temperature, we have:—For right side 44.458 per cent., and for left side 54.542 per cent. The mean percentage in favour of the right side, in the eleven spaces which show superiority of temperature on this side, is 66.449; and the mean percentage in favour of the left side, in the sixteen spaces which show left superiority of temperature, is 69.102.

It is almost impossible, even approximately, to designate, without the aid of a diagram—and a far more detailed account of the method of measuring spaces than has been given in this article—the position of the spaces of this region which are in favour of the right and left sides respectively. The best that can be done is to try to point out the position of the eleven spaces which are in favour of the right side. Start from a point about 20 mm. (0.78 inch) distant horizontally from the occipital protuberance, and draw a line upward, parallel to the longitudinal median line, for a distance of about 63 mm. (2.48 inches); then from the summit of this line draw another line horizontally to the anterior boundary of the region (posterior boundary of the middle region); in the tract thus enclosed will be found the eleven spaces in question.

With regard to the thermometric differences of temperature found in this region, the mean difference in favour of the right side is 0.186° C. (0.334° F.); and the mean difference in favour of the left side is 0.066° C. (0.118° F.) The greatest difference was 0.386° C. (0.694° F.), and was in favour of the right side; the smallest difference was 0.008° C. (0.0144° F.), and was in favour of the left side.

Having considered the relative temperatures of symmetrically situated spaces of the two sides of the head, we must next look at the **relative temperatures of spaces on one and the same side, in the same and in different regions.** This part of our subject will be summarily dealt with, as its investigation, in any degree approaching detail, would lead into complications fit only for a special experimental essay. First, all the comparisons must be condensed into comparisons of the three regions taken in their totalities. Second, the results on the two sides of the head are best taken together, as the error in so doing is of slight importance. Acting on these conditions, we have the following values for the three regions:—In favour of anterior region, 34.344 per cent.; in favour of middle region, 33.8 per cent.; in favour of posterior region, 31.856 per cent.

We have finally to deal with the **absolute thermometric values of the three regions.** The following figures give the average temperatures of both sides of the head taken together:—Anterior region, 33.824° C. (92.883° F.); middle region, 33.785° C. (92.093° F.); posterior region, 33.505° C. (92.309° F.) These figures represent the results of observations made under strictly experimental conditions; but, taking individuals at random, they may not always hold good. A temperature of 36.1° C. (96.98° F.) is of common occurrence in the anterior and middle regions, and 35° C. (95° F.) may be found in the posterior region.

SECT. III. — **Effect of Intellectual Work.**—Nearly every one of the eighty-eight spaces on each side of the head has been examined with regard to the effect on its temperature of intellectual work; and every space thus examined has shown a rise of temperature following the mental exertion. The rise of temperature under these circumstances would, therefore, seem to be universal, and not confined to any particular locality. Different kinds of mental work were employed, but, whatever the nature of the work, it was always found necessary that it should present some difficulty in its accomplishment, or should decidedly excite the interest. But although the whole of the surface is thus affected, yet certain parts appear to have their temperatures raised more readily and in a higher degree than others, and this, too, no matter what kind of work is done. The parts in question may be said, in a general way, to lie over a tract of the surface of the brain formed by the posterior portions of the 1st and 2nd frontal, and the anterior ascending parietal (4th frontal) convolutions; and, possibly—crossing the fissure of Rolando—the anterior portion of the posterior ascending parietal (ascending parietal) convolution.

With regard to the thermometric value of the rises of temperature observed, the following are the averages for the three regions:—Anterior region, 0.034° C. (0.0612° F.); middle region, 0.0375° C. (0.0675° F.); posterior region, 0.0296° C. (0.0533° F.). Higher rises, however, frequently occur, such as 0.085° C. (0.153° F.) in the anterior region; 0.092° C. (0.1656° F.) in the middle region; and 0.044° C. (0.0792° F.) in the posterior region.

We have next to examine the comparative effect of intellectual work on the two sides of the head. The general result of experiments made on this point is as follows: 66.346 per cent. of the observations show that the rise of temperature is higher on the left side; 19.231 per cent. are in favour of the right side; and 14.423 per cent. show that the rise is equal on the two sides.

The thermometric differences may be thus briefly stated:—Average for left side, 0.00439° C. (0.007092° F.); average for right side, 0.00234° C. (0.00421° F.). Here also, as in the case of the comparison of spaces on one and the same side, the rises of temperature may be much greater than the averages just given; they may, in fact, be nearly doubled.

Effect of Emotional Activity.—It is exceedingly difficult to bring emotional conditions of the mind under experimental control. Only one class of these conditions has been found available for the purpose. It is that condition of mind which is induced in many persons by the reading or recitation of poetry or prose of an emotional character. Such reading or recitation may be either aloud or to one's self. Moreover, listening to the reading or recitation of another person may produce the same effect. When the mental condition in question is thoroughly established, the writer has never failed to find a rise of temperature. Like intellectual work, emotional activity produces a rise of temperature in all parts of the surface; also the portion of the head which appears to be most affected in intellectual work, seems to be most affected during the emotional condition.

The following are the average rises of temperature in the three regions:—Anterior region, 0.0385° C. (0.0693° F.); middle region, 0.041° C. (0.0738° F.); posterior region, 0.036° C. (0.0648° F.). Rises of temperature of 0.1° C. (0.18° F.), and even 0.2° C. (0.36° F.), are not, however, uncommon in the anterior and middle regions.

Although the investigation of such an emotion as anger—or, in a milder form, vexation—cannot easily or safely be made the object of a deliberate experiment, yet, in a number of instances, the writer has had the unexpected opportunity of witnessing, in the course of experiments having other objects in view, the effect of this state of mind. The result has been a marked and rapid rise of temperature—0.3° C. (0.54° F.), and 0.4° C. (0.72° F.)—but its position with reference to particular parts, and its comparative effect on the two sides of the head have never been satisfactorily determined.

We come, lastly, to consider *the comparative effect of emotional activity on the two sides of the head.* The following is the general result of comparing symmetrically situated spaces:—The rise of temperature is higher on the left side in 60.416 per cent. of the observations; 21.528 per cent. are in favour of the right side; and in the remaining 18.056 per cent. the temperature rises equally on the two sides.

The average thermometric differences of rise of temperature are as follows:—Left side, 0.0059° C. (0.0106° F.); right side, 0.00495° C. (0.0089° F.).

J. S. LOMBARD.

[*References.*—J. S. Lombard: Regional Temperature of the Head, 1879, and Experimental Researches on the Temperature of the Head, 1881. Proceedings of Royal Society, Nov. 17, 1881, pp. 173–198; and Jan. 7, 1886, pp. 1–6; also unpublished experiments. H. C. Boyer, Archives de Neurologie, 1880, fasc. 1er. Boeck et Verhoogen, Circulation Cérébrale (Inst. Solvay, Bruxelles, 1890). Dorta, Sur la Température Cérébrale, &c, Genève, 1889.]

TEMPORARY INSANITY.—A name applied to short outbreaks of insanity; its most common use is as a jury's verdict in suicide. (*See* MANIA TRANSITORIA.)

TEMULENCE (*temulentus*, drunken). A term generally used as synonymous with drunkenness. It is sometimes used to describe any state in disease resembling drunkenness.

TENTIGO VENEREA (*tentum*, the penis). A synonym of Nymphomania.

TENTIGO VERETRI.—A synonym of Satyriasis.

TERRORS, NIGHT. (*See* NIGHT TERRORS.)

TESTAMENTARY CAPACITY IN MENTAL DISEASE.—There are three well-marked stages in the history of the law of testamentary capacity in mental disease: (1) From the earliest recorded decisions to 1848, each case of disputed testamentary capacity was determined upon its own merits; (2) from 1848 to 1870, the doctrine promulgated by Lord Brougham in *Waring* v. *Waring* (6 Moo. P. C. 341, *et seq.*), that the least degree of insanity would vitiate a will made under its influence, prevailed; (3) since the judgment of Lord Chief Justice Cockburn in *Banks* v. *Goodfellow* (1870; L. R. 5 Q. B. 549)* the Courts have recurred to the earlier and sounder criterion—was the capacity adequate to the act? It will be convenient to trace the historical development of our law of testamentary capacity before we attempt to ennunciate its leading doctrines, or to illustrate their practical appreciation, at the present day.

(1) One of the earliest and most satisfactory definitions of testamentary capacity in mental disease proceeded from the Star Chamber. In *Combe's Case* (Moor. 759, 4 Burn's E. L. 61; 3 Jac. I.) it was argued by the judges in that famous tribunal "that sane memory for the making of a will is not at all times when the party can speak 'yes' or 'no,' or had life in him, nor when he can answer to anything with sense; but he ought to be of judgment to discern and to be of perfect memory; otherwise the will is void" (*cf. Winchester's Case*, 6 Co. 23 *a*. Trin. 41 Eliz. K. B.). In the beginning of the reign of Charles I., *Herbert* v. *Lowns* (1 Ch. Rep. 24, 3 Car. I.) carried the doctrine of *Combe's Case* a little further. "To a disposing memory it is necessary there be an understanding judgment, fit to direct an estate." In the time of Charles II. we find a will made by "a sickly child, newly *pubes*, and without the knowledge of his curators . . . . in the absolute favour of the nurse under whose care he had been," reduced as inofficious (Nisbet's Doubts, temp. Car. II. 207). *Dew* v. *Clark* (1826, 3 Add. 79–209, and Add. 123 *et seq.*) is the next case of importance in the history of the definition of testamentary capacity The facts were these: Ely Stott died November 18, 1821, leaving a widow and a daughter by his first wife. The amount of his personal estate was nearly £40,000. By his will, dated May 26, 1818, Stott gave to his daughter, to whom he had conceived a violent and irrational aversion, a life interest only in a comparatively small portion of his property. It was held by Sir John Nichol that this unfounded antipathy had prevented the testator from properly appreciating his daughter's claims upon him, and that the will must be pronounced against. In *Harwood* v. *Baker* (1840, 3 Moo. P. C. 282) the criteria of testamentary capacity are

* An interesting discussion upon this case before the Medico-Psychological Association in 1881, will be found reported in the *Journal of Mental Science*, No. cxix. new series, No. 83, pp. 471–4.

stated by Erskine, J., in the following terms: "In order to constitute a sound disposing mind, a testator must not only be able to understand that he is by his will giving the whole of his property to one object of his regard, ... but he must also have capacity to comprehend the extent of his property and the nature of the claims of others whom by his will he is excluding from all participation in that property. The protection of the law is in no cases more needed than it is in those where the mind has been too much enfeebled to comprehend more objects than one, and more especially" (which was the case in *Harwood* v. *Baker*) "when that one object may be so forced upon the attention of the invalid as to shut out all others that might require consideration" (*ubi supra* at p. 290). With the exception of one or two points of detail, mainly suggested by recent American decisions, the language of Erskine, J., is a complete and accurate statement of the modern law of testamentary capacity. (*Cf.* also *Gillespie* v. *Gillespie*, Fac. Dec. February 11, 1817; *Durling* v. *Loveland*, 1839, 2 Curt. 225; *Durnell* v. *Corfield*, 1844, 1 Rob. E. R. 51.)

But the period under consideration enriched our law, not only with an exhaustive definition of testamentary capacity, but also with a philosophic analysis of "lucid interval" and "insane delusion," and a clear statement of their legal consequences.

Thus, in *ex parte Holyland* (1805, 11 Ves. 10) Lord Chancellor Eldon, dissenting from a dictum of Lord Thurlow, declared that complete restoration to previous mental vigour is not necessary to the existence of a lucid interval: while in *Towart* v. *Sellars* (1817, 5 Dow, p. 56) it was impliedly held that the question for consideration in such cases was, Has the testator recovered, not a sound, but a disposing mind? The modern definition of "insane delusion" also belongs to this period. In *Mudway* v. *Croft* (1843, 3 Curt. 671) the following passage from Dr. Ray's "Medical Jurisprudence" (p. 131) is expressly adopted: "It is the departure from the natural and healthy character, temper, and habits which constitutes a symptom of insanity, and in judging of a man's sanity it is consequently as essential to know what his habitual manifestations were as what his present symptoms are." The interest of this quotation, thus incorporated into the law of England, lies in the fact that it does away with all rigid objective standards, provides that each case shall be tried on its own merits, and assigns to a man's mental constitution and history their proper place in an inquiry into his testamentary [illegible]. (*Cf. Chambers* v. *Yatman*, [illegible] 448.)

The medico-legal relations of lucid intervals, insane delusions, and insanity generally were clearly formulated in our early case-law. Insanity was held to be *primâ facie* evidence of testamentary incapacity. (*Cf. Hall* v. *Warren*, [illegible] Sir W. Grant, M.R., 1804; *In re* [illegible], 1837, 1 Curt. 594; and *Snook* v. [illegible], 1848, per Lord Langdale, M.R., 11 [illegible] 105.) It was not, however, conclusive (*Rodd* v. *Lewis*, 1755, 2 Cas. temp. Lee, 176), and the presumption arising from an inquisition *de lunatico inquirendo*, or from residence in an asylum, might be rebutted by proof of a lucid interval, or that the insanity or delusions were irrelevant or immaterial. *Cartwright* v. *Cartwright* (1793–95, 1 Phillim. 90, 122) is an instructive instance. A., a patient in an asylum, made a will in which she left practically her whole fortune to her nieces. The circumstances under which the will was executed were as follows: On August 14, 1775, A. was supplied with pen, ink, and paper by Dr. Battie, the superintendent of the asylum, to quiet and gratify her, though he considered her at the time quite incapable of making a will. Her attendants retired, but watched her. She was so agitated and furious that they were fearful she would attempt some mischief to herself. At first she wrote upon several pieces of paper, and got up in a wild and furious manner, and tore the same, and threw them in the fire; and, after walking up and down the room many times in a wild and disordered manner, muttering and speaking to herself, she wrote the paper which was the will in question. Probate was granted upon the grounds that (*a*) the will was originated and executed by the testatrix, and (*b*) the provisions were "wisely and orderly framed." This decision has frequently been cited in support of the contention that the law at one time made the instrument in dispute the best, if not the sole, criterion of the capacity to execute it. But it is doubtful whether Sir William Wynne intended to lay down any such rule (*cf. Chambers* v. *Yatman*, 2 Curt. 415, 447), and, if he did, it has long since been distinctly repudiated (*Brogden* v. *Brown*, 1825, 2 Add. 441). Other authorities of the same character as *Cartwright* v. *Cartwright* are *Clarke* v. *Lear* (Mar. 1791), *Coghlan* v. *Coghlan*, of which the date is not recorded.

Laing v. *Bruce*, a Scotch case (1838, 1 Dunlop, 59), may be consulted as an illustration of an insane delusion which was held insufficient to suspend testamentary capacity. A., the testatrix, was under delusions, which were intermittent and considered trifling by her friends, about her money matters. It was decided that her capacity to *revoke* a will was not destroyed.

(2) For more than twenty years, a doctrine, or perhaps we should rather call it a dictum, of Lord Brougham's perplexed English judges in administering the law testamentary, viz.: In *Waring* v. *Waring* (1840, 6 Moo. P. C. *et seq.*) an elderly lady, excessively penurious and eccentric, very irritable and quarrelsome, had disinherited her brother under an insane delusion that he had joined the Roman Catholics, towards whom she entertained a strong aversion. In accordance with the decision of Sir John Nicholl in *Dew* v. *Clark* the facts of which have already been stated, and, it may be added, in strict obedience to the existing law, the testatrix's will was set aside. But Lord Brougham, in giving judgment, went out of his way to criticise the popular definition of *monomania*, declared that the mind, being one and indivisible, if unsound upon a single subject, could not be really sound upon other subjects, and impliedly held that a person partially insane was incompetent to make a will. In *Smith* v. *Tebbitt* (1867, 1 P. and D. 401), Lord Penzance, then Sir J. P. Wilde, construed Lord Brougham's language in this sense, and said: "If disease be once shown to exist in the mind of the testator, it matters not that the disease be discoverable only when the mind is addressed to a certain subject, to the exclusion of all others, the testator must be pronounced incapable. . . . . The same result follows though the particular subjects upon which the disease is manifested have no connection whatever with the testamentary disposition before the Court."

Now, with reference to these propositions, it must be observed (1) that they are not established by the earlier cases to which we have referred, and (2) that both in *Waring* v. *Waring* and *Smith* v. *Tebbitt* the presence of insane delusions, distinctly operating upon the mind of the testator, reduces any metaphysical discussion of the degree of mental disease which destroys testamentary capacity to the proportions of an *obiter dictum*. Lord Brougham in the one case, and Sir J. P. Wilde in the other, had to decide, not whether a monomaniac is incapable in law of making a will, but whether a particular will made under the influence of insane delusion was valid. The testatrix in *Waring* v. *Waring* disinherited her brother under an erroneous and insane belief that he had become a Roman Catholic. The testatrix in *Smith* v. *Tebbitt* thought that her sister, to whose prejudice the will in dispute was made, was a child of the devil, for whom the deity had reserved the hottest place in hell. These cases clearly fall within the *ratio decidendi* of *Dew* v. *Clark*, and neither called for, nor gave judicial authority to, any deliverance upon the legal consequences of monomania in general.

(3) Lord Chief Justice Cockburn in *Banks* v. *Goodfellow* (1870, L. R. 5 Q. B. 549), and Sir James Hannen in *Boughton* v. *Knight* (1873, 3 P. and D. 64), have re-established the earlier and sounder criterion—"was the capacity adequate to the act?" (*Cf. Blewitt* v. *Blewitt*, 1833, per Sir J. Nicoll, 4 Hagg. E. R. 410; and *Morison* v. *Maclean's Trustees*, 1862, 24 Dunlop 265; per Lord Justice Clerk Inglis, at p. 631.)

In *Banks* v. *Goodfellow*, A. had made a will in favour of B., his niece, who had lived with him for many years, and to whom he had always expressed an intention to leave his property. At the time of executing this will A. was under a delusion that C., to whom he had borne a violent hatred, and who was actually dead, was still alive. C. had no claim whatever upon A. It was left to the jury to say whether A. had made that will, uninfluenced by his delusions. The jury found in favour of the will, and probate was granted, the Court of Queen's Bench refusing to reverse the finding of the jury. "It is essential," said the Lord Chief Justice Cockburn, "to the exercise of the powers of making a will that the testator shall understand the nature of the act and its effects; shall understand the extent of the property of which he is disposing; shall be able to comprehend and appreciate the claims to which he ought to give effect; and with a view to the latter object that no disorder of the mind shall poison the affections, pervert his sense of right, or prevent the exercise of his natural faculties, that no insane delusion shall influence his will in disposing of his property, and bring about a disposal of it which if the mind had been sound would not have been made. Here then we have the measure of the degree of mental power which should be insisted on. If the human instincts and affections of the moral sense become perverted by mental disease, if insane suspicion or aversion take the place of natural affection, if reason and judgment are lost, and the mind becomes a prey to insane delusions calculated to interfere with and disturb its functions, it is obvious that the condition of testamentary power fails, and that a will made under such circumstances ought not to stand." In a later passage, the Lord Chief Justice said: "No doubt, when the fact that a testator has been subject to any insane delusion is established, a will should be regarded with great distrust, and every presumption should, in the first instance, be made against it. Where insane delusion has ever been shown to have existed, it may be difficult to say whether the mental disorder may not possibly have extended beyond the particular form or instance in which it has manifested itself. It may be equally difficult to say how far the delusion may not have influenced the testator in the particular disposal of his property. And the presumption against a will made under such circumstances becomes additionally strong when the will is, to use the term of the civilians, an inofficious one, that is to say, one in which natural affection and the claims of near relationship have been disregarded."

In *Boughton* v. *Knight*, Sir James Hannen laid down the law of testamentary capacity to the jury in language which sounds like an echo from *Harwood* v. *Butler* (see *ante*). "There must be a memory to recall the several persons who may be fitting objects of the testator's bounty, and to comprehend their relationship to himself, and their claim upon him. . . . . A sound mind does not mean a perfectly balanced mind, free from all influence of prejudice, passion, or pride. The law does not say that a man is incapacitated from making his will if he proposes to make a disposition of this property moved by capricious, frivolous, or even bad motives. . . . Eccentricities as they are commonly called of manner, of habit, of life, of amusements, of dress and so on must be disregarded. But there is a limit beyond which one feels that it ceases to be a question of harsh unreasonable judgment of character, and that the repulsion which a parent exhibits towards one or more of his children, must proceed from some mental defect in himself" (*cf. The Hopper Will Case*, 33 N. Y. 619; *Smee* v. *Smee* 1879, 5 P. D. 84). In concluding this part of our subject, we propose to contrast very shortly the development of English with that of American testamentary law. Both started from the same point. Both have reached the same goal. In the United States, as in England, testamentary capacity was originally, and is now, treated as a question of fact. Even in the intermediate, or as we might perhaps not improperly call it the metaphysical period, the laws of England and America had the same postulate—viz., the difficulty of determining where sanity ended and insanity began. But from this postulate the English and American Courts drew widely different conclusions. According to Lord Brougham and Lord Penzance, mental disease was so subtle and intangible that no legal tribunal could with safety undertake to define its degrees, and the only prudent course was to hold any degree of insanity fatal to civil capacity. American lawyers, on the other hand, seem at one time to have inclined to the view that the proper inference from the common postulate was that the mere possession of understanding was enough to create testamentary power. The case of *Alice Lispenard* (26 Wendell 255) went furthest in this direction. The mental characteristics of the testatrix were these: she was washed and dressed like a child even when thirty-five years of age; her head wagged from side to side; she dribbled at the mouth; had sudden fits of anger, so that she would strike children; would sit for hours in front of a window, and continue in that position even after the shutters were closed, &c. The rule of testamentary capacity adopted in this case was that in pronouncing upon the validity of a will, the Courts will not measure the understanding of the testator, but if he have any reason at all, and be not an absolute idiot, totally deprived of reason, he is the lawful disposer of his own property, and his will stands as a reason for his actions. Senator Verplanck, in delivering the judgment of the Supreme Court in this case said: "To establish any standard of intellect or information beyond the possession of reason in its lowest degree, as in itself essential to legal capacity, would create endless uncertainty, difficulty, and litigation; would shake the security of property, and wrest from the aged and infirm that authority over their earnings or savings which is often their best security against injury and neglect. If you throw aside the old common law test of capacity, then proofs of wild speculations or extravagant and peculiar opinions, or of the forgetfulness or the prejudices of old age, might be sufficient to shake the fairest conveyance or impeach the most equitable will. The law therefore in fixing the standard of positive legal competency has taken a low standard of capacity; but it is a clear and definite one, and therefore wise and safe; it holds . . . . that weak minds differ from strong ones only in the extent and power of their faculties: but unless they betray a total loss of understanding, or idiocy, or delusion, they cannot properly be considered unsound." These observations were somewhat qualified by other parts of the judgment, but they are sufficiently strong to show the tendency of the American Courts at that time. The doctrine suggested in the *Lispenard* trial was, however, repudiated in the famous *Parish Will Case* (*Delafield* v. *Parish*, 1862, 25 N. Y. 9), in which it was laid down that the testator must have sufficient capacity to comprehend perfectly the condition of his property, his relations to the persons who were, or should, or might, have been the objects of his bounty, and the scope and bearing of the provisions of his will: he must have sufficient active memory to collect in his mind without prompting the particulars or elements of the business to be transacted, and to hold them in his mind a sufficient length of time to perceive at least their active relations to each other, and to be able to form some rational judgment in relation to them (*Converse* v. *Converse*, per Redfield, J. 21 Verm. R. *Blanchard* v. *Nestle*, 3 Denio 37).

The leading doctrines in the modern law of testamentary capacity in mental disease may be shortly stated in the form of propositions.

I. A testator must be able at the time when he makes his will both to recall, and to keep clearly before his mind (*a*) the nature and extent of his property, and (*b*) the persons who have claims upon his bounty; and his judgment and will must be sufficiently unclouded and free to enable him to determine the relative strength of these claims.

II. An insane person can make a valid will if (*a*) *in spite of his insanity* he has a disposing memory, judgment and will as defined above, or (*b*) he is enjoying what is called a *lucid interval* at the date of its execution.

The case of *Banks* v. *Goodfellow*, already noted, is an illustration of a delusion which was foreign to the subject-matter, and did not therefore affect the validity of a will. A curious rider might, however, be added to the doctrine established by that case. Suppose that A. makes a will disinheriting B., C., and D., to whom he had no insane dislike, and who had strong claims upon his bounty. At the time of executing this will, the name of E., towards whom A. had a violent and insane hatred, but who had no claims whatever upon him, had been mentioned to A., and had rendered him incapable of estimating the comparative claims of B., C., and D. The delusion in such a case would be foreign to the subject-matter of the will, but there can be little doubt that it would destroy for the time the capacity of the testator. (*Cf. Creagh* v. *Blood*, 2 J. & La Touche, Irish, per Sir Edward Sugden, L.Ch. at p. 515.)

A fortiori, testamentary capacity is not destroyed by a delusion which quickens the testator's faculties. *Jenkins* v. *Morris* (1880, 14 Ch. D. 674), a decision upon the contract of a lunatic, is a case in point. A. leased a farm to B. At the date of the lease A. laboured under the delusion that the farm was impregnated with sulphur and was anxious to get rid of it for this reason. Rational letters written by A. in reference to the lease were put in evidence, and it was proved that, in spite of his delusion, he was a shrewd man of business. The lease was held valid.

III. A lucid interval is not necessarily a complete restoration to mental vigour previously enjoyed; nor is it merely the cessation or suppression of the symptoms of insanity (*Dyce Sombre* v. *Prinseps*, 1856, per Sir John Dodson, 1 Deane, at p. 110); it is the recovery of testamentary "memory, judgment and will."

IV. An insane delusion is not merely an unfounded though colourable suspicion, nor even a belief which no rational person would have entertained; it is a persistent and incorrigible belief that things are real, which exist only in the imagination of the patient, and which no rational person can conceive that the patient when sane would have believed.

V. Neither subsequent suicide nor supervening insanity will be reflected back upon previous eccentricity so as to invalidate a will. (*Cf. Hoby* v. *Hoby*, 1828, per Sir John Nichol, 1 Hagg. 146; *aliter* in the case of previous insanity, *Symes* v. *Green*, 1859, 1 S. & T. 401.)

VI. Affective or moral insanity does not generally destroy testamentary capacity.

Frere v. *Peacocke* (1846, 1 Rob. E. R. 442, per Sir H. Jenner Fust, at p. 456) appears to be the chief, if not the sole, authority for this proposition. A., the validity of whose will was in question, took an irrational pleasure in hearing of the sufferings of others, rubbing his hands, grinning and otherwise manifesting his gratification at evil tidings. Probate of the will was granted. There can, however, be little doubt that insanity of character, if sufficient to unhinge the disposing mind, would destroy testamentary capacity.

VII. Upon the executor who propounds a will rests the burden of proving (*a*) testamentary capacity, (*b*) knowledge and approval of its contents, and (*c*) due execution.

The reason for this rule cannot be better stated than it was in an American case, *Crowninshield* v. *Crowninshield* (2 Gray

526). "The hair-at-law rests securely upon the statutes of descent and distribution until some legal act has been done by which his rights under those statutes are lost or impaired."

A testatrix gave instructions for her will, which was prepared in accordance therewith. At the time of execution, the testatrix merely recollected that she had given those instructions, but believed that the will which she was executing accurately embodied them. Sir James Hannen held that the will was valid. (*Parker* v. *Felgate*, 1883, 8 P. D. 171, 173, 174.) If the testatrix had merely authorised her solicitor to make a will, and had she said, "I do not know what you have put down, but I am quite ready to execute it," the will would be invalid. (*Hastilow* v. *Stobie*, 1865, 1 P. & D. 64, overruling dicta of Sir Creswell Creswell in (*a*) *Middlehurst* v. *Johnson*, 1860, 30 L. J. Prob. 14; and (*b*) *Cunliffe* v. *Cross*, 1863, 3 S. & T. 36.

VIII. *Primâ facie*, an executor is justified in propounding his testator's will, and if the facts within his knowledge at the time he does so tend to show eccentricity merely on the part of the testator, and he is totally ignorant at the time of the circumstances and conduct which afterwards induce a jury to find that the testator was insane at the date of the will, he will, *on the principle that the testator's conduct was the cause of litigation*, be entitled to receive his costs out of the estate, although the will be pronounced against. (*Cf. Boughton* v. *Knight*, 1873, per Sir James Hannen, 3 P. & D. pp. 77–80; and *Smee* v. *Smee*, 1875, 5 P. & D. at p. 90.)

A. WOOD RENTON.

TETANOID EPILEPSY. — A name given by Pritchard to those epileptic fits in which there is only one form of spasm, the tonic. The patient falls unconscious, is rigid for a few moments and then recovers.

TETANUS HYDROPHOBICUS (τέτανος, a state of tension; hydrophobia, *q.v.*). A form of pharyngeal spasm at every act of deglutition, simulating the muscular spasms of hydrophobia. Rose has described a variety as occurring after injury to the pneumogastric and other cranial nerves.

THANATOPHOBIA (θάνατος, death; φόβος, fear). A morbid fear of death. (Fr. and Ger. *Thanatophobie*.)

THEFT IN GENERAL PARALYSIS, &c. (*See* GENERAL PARALYSIS, and KLEPTOMANIA.)

THELYGONIA (θῆλυς, female; γονία, race or offspring). A term very loosely used for nymphomania, properly employed for female offspring or the procreation of female children.

THEOMANIA (θεός, God; μανία, madness). Religious madness. The form of mental disease in which patients believe themselves to be the Deity, or to be inspired to proclaim his will infallibly to mankind. Under one variety of monomania, Esquirol placed "those who believe themselves gods, profess to be in communication with Heaven, and believe they have a celestial mission. They proclaim themselves to be prophets or soothsayers. Such are theomaniacs. . . . The *melancholia enthusiastica* of Paulus Ægineta belongs to the same variety" ("Mal. Ment." ii. p. [illegible]). (*See* RELIGIOUS INSANITY.) (Fr. *théomanie*; Ger. *der religiöse Wahnsinn*.)

THERAPEUTICS.—The reader is referred to the observations on the treatment of the various forms of mental disorder made under their several heads by the contributors of these articles. He is also referred to the following articles: BATHS; DIET; ELECTRICITY; FEEDING (FORCIBLE) OF THE INSANE; NEUROSIS, FUNCTIONAL (MASSAGE); PREVENTION OF INSANITY; SEDATIVES.

A few remarks may, however, be offered here which may serve to assist the student and general practitioner.

The first question which the mental physician asks is, whether there is a distinctly abnormal condition of the bodily organs the removal of which will favour the disordered brain functions—the proximate cause of the attack of insanity. It was to this point that Max Jacobi directed all his endeavours from the moment a patient was placed under his care. If he carried his somatic doctrines too far it remains true that the leading idea of medical treatment must centre in this doctrine. So long as a disordered liver disturbs the healthy action of the mind, so long as a disorder of the colon occasions melancholia, so long as suppressed gout causes the patient to regard himself as a miserable sinner; in short, so long as any of the viscera are the seat of disease, and the physician disregards such disorder of the bodily organs, he clearly fails to fulfil the first indication of treatment. Were it necessary, many illustrations could be given of the importance of ascertaining in the first instance the condition of other organs of the body than the brain—instances in which the removal of disease in a distant organ has been followed by rapid mental recovery, but it may suffice to refer to the action of emmenagogues in relieving some cases of insanity.

Although hellebore has been extolled in addition to the time-honoured remedies for amenorrhoea, there can be no doubt that the most effectual drug is the permanganate of potash in doses of 2 or 3 grs. three times a day. That larger doses may be advantageously employed is shown by the effect produced by some patients having taken in mischief the whole contents of the pill-box amounting to at least 30 grs., but with the desired effect. We should, however, not feel justified in prescribing such large doses. This treatment should be accompanied by

Counter-irritation. — Following the well-known aphorism that active disease in one organ or part of the body is incompatible with disease in another, medical men have endeavoured, not without a certain amount of success, to set up inflammation or irritation of the skin in order to divert the morbid action of the central organ to the periphery. The remarkable recoveries from insanity following upon a carbuncle in the neck have led to the employment of setons or blisters on the skin. It must be admitted that beneficial results do not follow so frequently from artificial as spontaneous inflammation. At the same time the imitation of nature in this respect is not unfrequently followed by satisfactory results. Counter-irritation is therefore one mode of treatment which it is the duty of the mental physician to employ whenever it seems indicated.

Depressant Treatment.—(1) *Depletion* is rarely justifiable. The lancet so much in favour as a remedy in former days under the mistaken idea that inflammation of the brain or its membranes caused the symptoms of insanity cannot be said to be within the range of practical mental therapeutics. We hesitate to attribute the change which has taken place in the treatment of the insane altogether to an alteration in the sthenic character of disease. Certain it is that the indiscriminate bleeding which was practised up to the early part of this century and even later, was injurious. It would be pleasant to think that the profuse depletion practised by the estimable Rush, was justified by the more robust type of the constitution in his day, but the reaction which set in against it was not, so far as we are aware, based upon this convenient theory, but upon the mischief it had done. That there are cases in which the local abstraction of blood, as by leeches behind the ear, may be of service is no doubt true, and of course intercurrent disorders may require topical bleeding, as for example the application of leeches in amenorrhœa.

(2) *Antimony* is not a depressant which is justifiable save in the rarest instances; yet not only was it employed a century ago in almost all cases of maniacal excitement but in much more recent times it has to our knowledge been the sheet-anchor in at least one public asylum. When we speak of the non-employment of this drug, we do not exclude its use in very small doses in combination with morphia. In fact, although very rarely resorting to it even in this form, we have seen valuable results from its exhibition in cases of mania where morphia was prejudicial without, but useful with, tartrate of antimony. The combination of a grain of morphia with one-eighth of a grain of tartar emetic was for many years a favourite remedy at the York Retreat. Dr. Bucknill found that the benefit to be derived from antimony did not occur in those cases in which it produced nausea, but that on the contrary it bore a close relation to the tolerance the patient had for it, and that the results were most satisfactory with those patients labouring under acute mania and of strong constitution in whom there was little general disturbance of the health.

(3) *Purgatives.*—Although the old-fashioned administration of purgatives was excessive there can be no doubt that occasionally they are useful, and no form is better than a pill containing calomel 1 gr., aq. ext. aloes 2 grs., pil. col. co. 2 grs.; to be taken twice a week at bedtime. By this means the action of the liver is sufficiently excited in cases of mental depression in which it is sluggish. Mercurials may be said to be uncalled for, except as an occasional alterative and purgative, and as an anti-syphilitic remedy. Their abuse in former days is well known. There is no encouragement for their employment in the early stage of general paralysis, where one might have expected it to be beneficial.

Tonics and Stimulants.—(a) *Tonics.*—The indications for the use of tonics in mental disorder are the same as those in disease accompanied with weakness in non-mental affections. Cases of anæmia obviously call for the exhibition of iron. Amongst tonics we may enumerate the following as specially valuable: Iron, arsenic, phosphorus, quinine, strychnia. A good form of tonic is Easton's syrup, which combines several of these bodies. (For the action of quinine *vide* article.)

(b) *Stimulants.*—The use of stimulants to procure sleep in cases of maniacal insomnia has been already referred to. The form of mental disorder in which they are imperatively called for is that of acute delirious mania (*q.v.*). In some instances of melancholia, rum and milk may be given to the patient if he wakes early with great depression, but in the majority of cases, food, especially Brand's extract of meat, is better than any stimulant.

Narcotic Treatment.—(*a*) *Opiates* have unquestionably a highly important place in the treatment of mental disorders. When to use and when to refrain from using opium is indeed one of the most difficult and delicate problems for the mental physician to solve. Monstrous doses have been administered, but such a practice is reprehensible. That opium in increasing doses within moderate limits may be advantageously employed in acute mania is supported by considerable evidence. In melancholia again, it may be allowed that opium exerts a calmative and in the end a curative influence, but that it fails in many instances where previous experience indicates its use is but too certain. It is of great importance to remember that the use of opiates for either mania or melancholia requires careful attention to the dietary in use at the same time. A plentiful supply of food, and in some cases stimulants, will ensure a success of this treatment when it would otherwise entirely fail; and if the appetite is decidedly interfered with by opium, the objection to its use may be so great as to counter-indicate its administration.

(*b*) *Hypodermic injections of morphia*, commencing with as small a dose as one-tenth of a grain of morphia on account of possible idiosyncrasies, may be employed with great benefit. It has been administered in enormous, and we think dangerous, doses by Aug. Voisin in some cases of melancholia, the maximum dose having been fifteen grains. We should not care to go beyond two grains, and then only after cautiously raising the dose. Vomiting is likely to occur from the use of large doses, or if this does not happen, the special symptoms of opium poisoning may alarm the physician.

The hypodermic injection of remedies has during the last few years greatly advanced, and has certainly not always been accompanied by the care which is desirable.

(*c*) *Hyoscyamus* retains its high position as a hypnotic in the treatment of the insane. One or two drachms of the tincture may be given at bedtime, or a considerably larger dose. It is generally better to combine it with other drugs, as the bromides or choral.

The hypodermic injection of hyoscyamine and hyoscine needs great caution, and the effect of these drugs should be carefully watched. It is allowable to use it in institutions in cases in which it would be unsafe to employ it when the patient is subsequently left in the hands of non-medical persons.

Sedatives, as choral, paraldehyde, the bromides, sulphonal, &c.

Chloral is justly regarded with more or less apprehension, but although frequently abused, it has its place. We cannot commend the large doses which have been given in some asylums, and that some ninety pounds were given by the late Dr. Gray, of Utica Asylum, to 600 patients in the course of eighteen months, would find no justification at the present day, when we know its injurious as well as beneficial effects. The excuse for its employment is the less now that we have a drug like sulphonal, which, in the large majority of cases, exerts the desired influence in the insomnia of the insane, the dose being from fifteen to forty grains. In some cases a drachm is well borne by the patient. Paraldehyde in doses of one or two drachms, repeated if necessary, is undoubtedly a valuable addition to our hypnotics in the treatment of the insane.

Cannabis Indica.—This drug has been very frequently employed to induce sleep or to allay maniacal excitement. We have, however, found the effect somewhat uncertainly beneficial in consequence of the special action of the drug becoming complicated with the mental symptoms. Effects may follow the administration of a moderate dose, which are in the first instance alarming, but are not likely to be of a serious nature, and will probably disappear on the administration of a stimulant. The tincture (B.P.) may be given in doses of from ten to twenty minims.

Bromide of potassium and *bromide of ammonium* retain a high position in asylum practice, apart from epilepsy, although a note of warning in regard to their deteriorating influence when too long continued has not been wanting.

The whole subject of hypnotics and sedatives is fully considered in the article (*q.v.*) by Drs. Ringer and Sainsbury.

Baths.—Their use in various forms is described by Dr. Duckworth Williams in a special article (*q.v.*). It is needless to point out the cruel use which may be made of the cold water douche, as we do not believe that it is ever so used in England, nor, we trust, at the present day, on the Continent, where many years ago we witnessed its abuse. That it should have been resorted to in order to force a patient to give up a delusion is not perhaps surprising, considering the multitude of means employed to frighten the insane out of their delusions. We only mention the practice here to reprobate it.

Electricity.—The reader is referred to Professor Arndt's article on this remedy in mental disorders.

Feeding.—The extreme importance of supplying not merely an ample diet for the insane, but an exceptionally large amount in the exhaustion so frequently associated with acute mania, must be here insisted upon in the strongest possible manner. We refer the reader to the article on acute delirious mania. The stimulus which Dr. Clouston has given to the copious use of nutritious food has been of the greatest value. Again, the enforcement of some form of nourishment, as beef tea, &c., on waking in the morning, in cases of melancholia, must be emphasised. Attention to this one point will often render sedatives unnecessary.

We conclude this article by singling out the treatment of one form of mental disorder—mania—on account of its importance and the necessity for instant treatment. It is contributed by Dr. Conolly Norman as supplementary to his article on mania.

"The diet requires careful regulation. It must be always borne in mind that with great mental excitement there is apt to be combined digestive trouble and a tendency to exhaustion. The food should generally be of a light and nutritious nature. The state of the tongue and so forth will indicate more exactly what is desirable in each case. In severe cases there is often refusal of food from inattention or mere excitement. This is a symptom which must on no account be neglected, otherwise the patient's strength will run down rapidly and dangerously. Artificial feeding should therefore, in severe cases, be adopted early. Concentrated predigested foods, with the addition of alcohol, are indicated.

To procure sleep is of the first importance in the treatment of acute mania. The induction of rest by day is often followed by sleep at night, but in the majority of cases insomnia is a very troublesome symptom. Regulated exercise in the open air when the patient's strength permits it, is invaluable in this respect. Two hours' steady walking out of doors seems to produce more healthy weariness and disposition to sleep than a whole day spent in aimless motor excitement. But in many cases, especially the more severe, this is out of the question. Packing in the wet sheet is often of great service. The prolonged warm bath is sometimes useful. A tepid bath at bedtime, or a cold bath followed by a thorough rubbing, will sometimes act well. Of drugs, the best are morphia, sulphonal, and paraldehyde. Methylal is useful in alcoholic cases. Morphia is not indicated in mild cases. In very severe cases where there is an urgent need of sleep, it should be used in full doses, guarded with ether or alcohol. Sulphonal is generally remarkably safe. Its prolonged use is no doubt somewhat depressing. Paraldehyde requires the dose to be constantly increased. Chloral is sometimes useful, but its depressing effect on the heart must be carefully watched, and it must be remembered that if it fails to produce sleep it is likely to increase excitement. The "chloral habit" also is very easily and rapidly formed. Something may be hoped from hypnotism in mild cases, especially of a recurrent type.

Of calmatives, as distinct from soporifics, the most valuable is probably digitalis. Sulphonal in small repeated doses is certainly effectual in producing temporary sleep in some cases. The bromides are chiefly useful in cases in which there is marked sexual excitement. Their indiscriminate use has undoubtedly done much harm, and they share with the opium preparations the evil credit of having turned many acute maniacs into chronic dements, at least prematurely.

Of late years hyoscine has attained some reputation in the treatment of excitement. It is a drug which requires to be used with great caution. Apart from its mere depressing action it appears distinctly to have a specific effect in diminishing motor restlessness. Its chief virtue, however, seems to be owing to the decided 'shock' which results from its administration. It may occur that in exceptionally favourable circumstances the interruption to the morbid current thus effected may be followed by permanent improvement, but the experience of most of those who have used this drug has been disappointing." * THE EDITOR.

THERMO-ANÆSTHESIA (θερμός, warm; ἀναισθησία, want of sensation). The loss of perception of heat and cold by the skin and mucous membranes. This may vary in degree from absolute inability of perception to the loss of recognition of slight differences in temperature; it may accompany ordinary sensory anæsthesia or exist apart from it, or there may be a perversion of the sensations, cold applications giving a sensation of warmth and *vice versâ*; or electrical stimulation may give rise to the sensation of cold or heat. Its pathology is still obscure, but it usually occurs in lesions of the cord involving the lateral columns.

THINGS. — In psychology "things" are opposed to sensations. Sensations are modes of the brain being affected, while "things" are the results of mental synthesis of sensations; each "thing"

* The general or moral treatment of mania is given under TREATMENT.

implies sensations and uniting energy of mind.

THLAPSIS DEPRESSIO (θλάω, I break). Depression, melancholy.

THOUGHT. (*See* CONSCIOUSNESS; PHILOSOPHY OF MIND, p. 37.)

THOUGHT-READING, THOUGHT-TRANSFERENCE.—The fictitious power claimed by some of being able to read the thoughts of others by personal contact. The phenomena are due to the practised art of muscle-reading; that is to say, that the operator can divine by the muscular movements of the person who is the subject of experiment the direction in which his thoughts tend. It is an interesting instance of the mind acting on the body during intense mental concentration, the corresponding involuntary movements being appreciated by another.

THYMOPATHIA (θυμός, the mind; πάθος, an affection). Term for mental affection or derangement. (Fr. and Ger. *Thymopathie*.)

THYROID GLAND IN RELATION TO MENTAL DISEASE.—The Committee of the Clinical Society of London, nominated December 14, 1883, to investigate the subject of myxœdema (Dr. Ord, Chairman), arrived at these conclusions amongst others: That clinical and pathological observations, respectively, indicate in a decisive way, that the one condition common to all cases is destructive change of the thyroid gland; that the most common form of destructive change of the thyroid gland consists in the substitution of a delicate fibrous tissue for the proper glandular structure; that interstitial development of fibrous tissue is also observed very frequently in the skin, and with much less frequency in the viscera; the appearances presented by this tissue being suggestive of an irritative or inflammatory process; that pathological observation, while showing cause for the changes in the skin during life, for the falling off of the hair and the loss of the teeth, for the increased bulk of the body, as due to the excess of subcutaneous fat, affords no explanation of the affections of speech, movement, sensation, consciousness, and intellect, which form a large part of the symptoms of the disease; that the full analysis of the results of the removal of the thyroid gland in man demonstrates, in an important proportion of the cases, the fact of the subsequent development of symptoms exactly corresponding with those of myxœdema; that in no inconsiderable number of cases the operation has not been known to have been followed by such symptoms, the apparent immunity being, in many cases, probably due to the presence and subsequent development of accessory thyroid glands, or to accidentally incomplete removal or to insufficiently long observation of the patient after operation; that myxœdema, as observed in adults, is practically the same disease as that named sporadic cretinism when affecting children; that it is probably identical with cachexia strumapriva and that a very close affinity exists between myxœdema and endemic cretinism; that while these several conditions appear in the man to depend on, or to be associated with, destruction or loss of the function of the thyroid gland, the ultimate cause of such destruction or loss is at present not evident.* (*See* CRETINISM and MYXŒDEMA.)

TICKLISHNESS, AND THE PHENOMENA OF TICKLING.—The several forms of special irritability exhibited by the peripheral endings of sensory nerves known as ticklishness, seem to have attracted the attention of some of the older writers on physiology, and Scaliger proposed to class "titillation" as a sixth and separate sense. Although no modern observers have followed up this view, there can be no question that the general phenomena of ticklishness are distinct and characteristic enough to be differentiated from those of ordinary sensation and of the peripheral irritability which gives rise to afferent impulses necessary for reflex action.

Ticklishness becomes of interest to the student of psychology because it appears to be something superadded to the simple capability for receiving stimuli suitable for provoking unconscious reflex results observable among some of the lowest organisms, and yet falls short of the more definite sensory impressions which enable the higher centres to judge of the nature and properties of external objects.

It is distinctly an appeal to consciousness, but at the same time one of an elementary and primitive order. As such it appears to be one of the simplest developments of mechanical and automatic nervous processes in the direction of the complex functioning of the higher centres which comes within the scope of psychology.

In several ways does tickling differ from ordinary sensation. In the first place it almost invariably involves and accompanies an impulse to movement of the usual reflex character. But this conscious impulse, though at times strong, is not of the same emphatic nature as that which gives rise to actual pain. Indeed, it may,

* Supplement to vol. xxi. of the Clinical Society's Transactions.

and often does, lead to muscular contractions beyond the control of the will without producing any consciousness of pain whatever. Again, we find that the parts where tactile sensation, which enables us to determine the character of external objects by contact, is most acute, such as the tips of the fingers or of the tongue, are scarcely at all sensitive to titillation. That sensitiveness to tickling is not locally coincident with sensitiveness to pain is evident, since those parts of the body where pain is caused by a slight degree of violence such as the upper part of the tip of the nose, are far from being the most ticklish.

In endeavouring to classify the various phenomena of ticklishness for the purposes of more detailed study, we find, as is so frequently the case with regard to natural phenomena, that no sharp and rigid partition lines can be drawn.

A convenient classification may be attempted by dividing the nerves concerned into (1) those close to the surface, and (2) those more deeply situated.

(1) The *superficial* irritability or ticklishness responds in nearly all cases to very slight stimuli. It is commonly but not always associated with the nerves supplying the minute hairs which cover the skin of the body and of the extremities, with the exceptions of the palms and soles, and the last joint of the digits. These sensitive hairs are especially abundant in such situations as the orifices of the ear and nostril.

The ticklishness associated with hair may be again subdivided in accordance with its subjective characters into (*a*) that which is distinctly distasteful, and (*b*) that which is rather agreeable than otherwise. The former appears to have to do with warning intimations of the presence of parasites and other noxious insects. There can be no doubt that the struggle for existence between man and the minute parasites which prey upon him has been a very sharp one in the past, so that we might reasonably expect to find traces of it in his structure and habits. Even in modern times in some parts of the world where cleanliness is neglected, and other circumstances favour the increase of vermin, there is still a conflict of clashing interests of this nature which is quite keen enough to leave a permanent impress on the race through the action of the laws of natural selection.

The small hairs on the integument, while they are probably the remains of a thick natural coat which formerly harboured the enemy, may now be regarded as so many minute sentinels which instantly notify an invasion, and by the irritation caused by the movements of an insect among them, induce us to rid ourselves of its presence before it becomes a source of danger to comfort and health.

The agreeable sensations which accompany a light touch as of a hand stroking the hirsute surface of the skin may be owing to several causes. In some instances the sensations are probably connected with the sexual appetite, and may be the vestigial relics of the caresses of courtship referable to some out-of-date methods of making love. We find that in some animals local titillation of the skin, although in parts remote from the reproductive organs, plainly acts indirectly upon them as a stimulus. Thus Harvey records that by stroking the back of a favourite parrot (which he had possessed for years, and supposed to be a male), he not only gave the bird gratification—which was the sole intention of the illustrious physiologist—but also caused it to reveal its sex by laying an egg.

The pleasure derived from caresses may often be due to obscure association of sexual feelings, even although, owing to the many complications of the primary instinct due to the cultivation of the higher faculties and changed habits of life, both individual and social, it might be scarcely recognisable as such. In short, the beaten track of an old reflex may remain open, although its original purpose is a thing of the remote past. There are without doubt certain vestigial reflexes of this and parallel kinds still occasionally manifest which are legacies of an earlier state of development, but which may even yet be of serious import in stimulating or directing the bodily and mental energies (*see* Reflex Action).

Doubtless another reason why caresses of the nature of gentle titillation are pleasurable may be attributed to the beneficial effect in previous ages of the assiduous care bestowed by the parent upon the offspring, and by the several animals of a troop upon one another, which conduced to cleanliness and freedom from parasites, and therefore to physical well-being. If the conflict with parasitic enemies were ever as severe as seems to have been the case, a group of animals which habitually and systematically freed themselves and one another from a common foe, as we constantly see monkeys do, would be more healthy, and therefore more likely to survive in times of stress than another group the members of which were too stupid or indifferent to act in this manner. It is obvious also that if an animal found such services immediately pleasurable, it would be the more ready to submit to them, and would derive corresponding benefit.

Another and distinct form of superficial sensitiveness to tickling appears to be closely associated with certain reflexes partially under the control of the will. This is found where the small hairs are absent, in connection with the smooth skin of the palms and soles, and mucous surfaces, such as the palate and fauces, the interior of the nose, conjunctivæ, glans penis, and other parts.

In these situations appropriate stimulation provokes certain movements and other reflex phenomena. As a rule, the sensation produced when the part is slightly tickled is subjectively unpleasant unless associated with these movements, and becomes intolerable if the irritation is increased. The special form of ticklishness here displayed appears to find its *raison d'être* in provoking and coercing the higher centres to cease from all inhibitory action, and to allow the reflex mechanism free play. Every one who will try the experiment of tickling his palate or the soles of his feet, and at the same time endeavouring by an effort of will to restrain all movements, will experience the strength of this prompting sensation of tension and discomfort. The ticklishness of the palm and sole seems to be to a great extent vestigial, and probably originally had to do with conditions of life now obsolete (*see* REFLEX ACTION).

(2) We now come to the ticklishness which apparently is attributable to a special function of nerves more deeply situated, since it is not called forth by a light touch on the skin, but is generally most manifested when stimulation is of such a character as to affect the deeper structures.

This form is what is most generally spoken of as "ticklishness" in popular parlance, and to the physiologist it is very interesting from the remarkable and uniform series of phenomena which accompany it. It is plainly an altogether different thing from the superficial forms already dealt with, since light touches on the integument, even where the small hairs are most abundant and sensitive, do not produce the results following stimulation, for which this form of ticklishness is especially noteworthy. Certain regions of the body, such as the axillæ, and contiguous parts, the flanks, lower ribs, &c., are most ready to respond to appropriate provocation. Children, as soon as they become active, are more sensitive than adults. It is observable that the accompanying sensation is at first distinctly pleasurable, and one may say that there is an actual appetite for this kind of nerve irritation, since a child will invite its playmate to tickle it. But after a few moments, especially if stimulation has been at all vigorous, a reverse feeling is exhibited. The proceeding becomes distasteful, and the child will writhe and twist about to avoid it. Yet the moment it is desisted from the child will again, by gesture, attitude, and speech, invite its repetition, and again as before, after a certain point, show its distaste by movements of avoidance. The muscular results of this reflex stimulation may be slight and controllable by a moderate inhibitory effort, or they may be violent and convulsive, and totally beyond the power of the subject to check them. The movements also are invariably accompanied with laughter, generally of an uncontrolled, open-mouthed, and spasmodic character.

To any physiologist who seeks to discover the reason for these and similar obscure facts concerning the bodily functions and attributes by an appeal to evolutionary laws, it is evident that such pronounced and noteworthy phenomena as the above, following a like cause in all cases and universally prevalent, cannot be explained on any other ground than that they either are, or have been, of some definite utility. For it appears to be a law that whenever any salient characteristic is observable and is universally distributed among the members of a species, it must either be of undoubted use in the life economy at the present time, or must in the past have played an important part in preserving the race from extinction, or in furthering its more perfect development and adaptability to environment.

Now, since no present probable useful office can be discovered for this curious appetite and the extraordinary phenomena which accompany the act of tickling, it seems more than likely that we have here one of those strange vestigial reflexes which were of vital importance in the remote past. What the utility can have been is an interesting and obscure problem, and one which seems well worthy of the attention of competent observers. The close and invariable association of laughter with this form of tickling gives some promise that the solving of the question at issue will throw light on the curious and important psychological problems respecting the origin and primary basis of laughter and the sense of the ludicrous.

LOUIS ROBINSON.

TIC NON DOULOUREUX (Charcot). A hysterical affection of the face usually one-sided, characterised by frequently repeated spontaneous paroxysms of twitching of the facial muscles, and hemi-anæsthesia of the same side of the face. Though as a rule spontaneous, the paroxysms are occasionally brought on by stimuli, as in a case of Charcot's where energetic spasm occurred on exposure of the eye on the same side of the face.

TIGRETIER, TEGRETIER. — A psychopathy of hysterical origin first described by Nathaniel Pearce ("The Life and Adventures of Nathaniel Pearce," London, 1831, i. 290) occurring among the native women of Abyssinia. The subjects became imbued with a religious emotionalism in which delusions of demoniacal possession giving rise to paroxysms of excitement were prominent. Courbon (*Progrès Médical*, 1884, 39, 774), while denying the truth of Pearce's account, remarks that severe forms of hysteria are common among the women of Abyssinia and that they find expression in strange mental delusions (Hirsch).

TINNITUS AURIUM (*tinnitus*, a ringing or tinkling; *auris*, the ear). The humming or other noises heard in the ear and not due to external sounds. It gives rise to illusions of hearing in the insane.

TITUBATION (*titubo*, I stagger). A staggering gait, sometimes dependent on disease of the nervous system. (Fr. *titubation*; Ger. *Wanken*.)

TOBACCO, Effect of, on the Nervous System.—The influence of tobacco on the nervous system, and on the production of cerebral nervous disorders, must be attributed to the two substances, nicotine and pyridine, which are contained in tobacco, and which belong to the strongest poisons. Nicotine might be compared to hydrocyanic acid. Different sorts of tobacco contain different quantities of these substances. Cigars from Havanna contain two per cent. of nicotine.

Physiological Action of Nicotine.—Nicotine produces in cold-blooded animals restlessness, rapid disturbance of consciousness, clonic spasms, loss of reflexes and arrest of respiration, and lastly death. In small warm-blooded animals a very small dose causes death in a few seconds with symptoms of paralysis. Large warm-blooded animals after a full dose fall down dead without any convulsions; small doses cause tonic and clonic spasms, which return at intervals, and afterwards death through inspiratory tetanus or paralysis. In man, doses from 0.001 to 0.003 grammes are poisonous, and cause headache, vertigo, somnolency, indistinctness of vision and hearing, general weakness with fainting, difficulty of breathing, a sense of cold, vomiting and lastly tremor and spasms in the extremities. All these symptoms are direct nervous symptoms, and are not due to any change in the blood. In very minute doses nicotine stimulates the brain and nerves (thus favourably influencing mental work, and promoting peristaltic action of the intestines). It is striking how soon the system becomes accustomed to this dangerous poison.

Physiological Action of Pyridine.—Excitement of the medulla oblongata with violent spasms of the whole body, and excitement of the spinal cord and of the intra-muscular nerve terminations with rapid paralysis.

There are two ways in which these poisonous substances may be brought into the human body: (1) by inhaling the dust of tobacco in cigar and tobacco manufactories; (2) by smoking or by taking snuff. The nicotine being soluble in water is absorbed from the aqueous smoke of the tobacco and is mixed with the saliva and the inhaled air of the smoker.

Of disorders among the labourers in tobacco manufactories we know congestion of the brain, several forms of neurosis, præcordial oppression, palpitation, anæmia, general weakness and insomnia; we also sometimes find very severe cases of anæmia with weakness of the muscles of the lower extremities, and with dragging gait. Another symptom is spasm of the muscles of the forearm, the cause of which is undoubtedly intoxication, because other labourers who exert their hands and arms much more than labourers in the tobacco factories, never suffer from these spasms.

As diseases of smokers must be considered: — (1) chronic hyperæmia (catarrh) of the pharynx and stomach, with all its consequences; (2) diseases of the brain, spinal cord and nerves; (3) disease of the sensory nerves. We have to deal with the latter two conditions only. It is an undoubted fact that the abuse of tobacco may produce elementary and complicated mental disorders with anxiety, illusions or hallucinations of vision, and depression. Some authors (Jolly, Simon, Krafft-Ebing) attribute to the tobacco a *rôle* in the ætiology of general paralysis. Other symptoms of the brain affection are: insomnia, vertigo, loss of memory and severe headache. If the spinal cord is affected we find a compound of symptoms which are so similar to locomotor ataxy that they may easily be confounded: lancinating pains in the legs, paræsthesia, ataxic gait, Romberg's symptom, disorder of the intestines and bladder, and loss of sexual appetite. It is of importance for the differential diagnosis, that the knee-jerk is not absent. Among the symptoms of disorder of the nervous system we find neuralgia and spasms in various nerve tracts; also disorders of sensibility in the form of hyperæsthesia, hyperæsthesia, and paræsthesia of the skin, and muscular tremor. Allorythmia of the heart and cardio-stenosis (angina pectoris) must also be reckoned among these symptoms, because nicotine influences the automatic ganglia of the heart. Of great importance are the disorders of the sensory nerves, among which we find temporary hyperæsthesia of the acoustic and optic nerve; a characteristic symptom is also amblyopia, which is always bilateral. The papillæ appear at first normal but afterwards slightly discoloured in the macular half. The cause of the visual derangement is a well-defined paracentral scotoma, which includes the fovea centralis, and extends from here in an oval form as far as or even beyond the yellow spot. Inside this scotoma, white appears as grey, red as dark, and green as grey; the acuteness of vision decreases to one-third, one-sixth or even one-thirtieth of that of normal vision. The periphery of the visual field is normal. This amblyopia never passes over into amaurosis. Closely related to this amblyopia produced by tobacco is alcoholic amblyopia. The abuse of tobacco mostly going hand in hand with that of alcohol, it is often difficult to decide which of the two is the actual cause. Amblyopia caused by tobacco was first observed in 1835 by Mackenzie, and accurately described in 1864 by Hutchinson.

All the morbid phenomena caused by the abuse of tobacco appear the earlier if the proportion of nicotine in tobacco is greater. The **prognosis** is favourable, if we succeed in preventing the further ingestion of the poison, that is to say, if the patient abstains from smoking. This statement includes the most important point of the treatment, which in addition should be tonic (quinine, iron, strychnine, hydro-therapeutics.) Relapses very easily occur after renewed smoking.

The Europeans learned the use of tobacco from the American Indians; Columbus and his successors found them smoking. Tobacco is said to be an Indian word, whilst the word nicotine is derived from Jean Nicot, who was in 1560 French ambassador at Lisbon, and promoted the importation of tobacco. About the middle of the seventeenth century the use of tobacco had become general; many people began to protest against it, and most Sovereigns attempted to prohibit it. James I. himself wrote a work against it: "Misocapnus (καπνός, smoke), [illegible] Tabaci lusus regius," which appeared in 1603 in London. A. [illegible]

TOBSUCHT (Ger.). Mania.

TODTENSCHLUMMER (Ger.). Trance or catalepsy.

TOLL (Ger.). Mad, furious, [illegible] raging or delirious.

TOLLHEIT, TOLLKRANKHEIT, TOLLSINNIGKEIT, TOLLSUCHT (Ger.). Various terms denoting maniacal fury, madness, insanity.

TOLLWUTH (Ger.). A term applied to acute mania, also hydrophobia.

TOM O'BEDLAMS.—A race of mendicants who levied charity on the plea of insanity. The Bethlem Hospital was made to accommodate six lunatics; but in the year 1644 the number admitted was forty-four, and applications were so numerous that many inmates were dismissed half cured. These used to wander about as vagrants, chanting mad songs, and dressed in fantastic clothing to excite pity. Under cover of these harmless "innocents" a set of sturdy rogues appeared called Abram men who shammed lunacy, and committed great depredations. (*See* ABRAM MAN.)

> "With a sigh like a Tom o' Bedlam."
>
> *King Lear.*

TONOPSYCHAGOGIA (τόνος, vigour, strength; ψυχή, the mind; ἄγω, I do or act). Term denoting the act of inducing proper tone to the mind. (Fr. and Ger. *Tonopsychagogia.*)

TORPEDO (*torpeo*, I am numbed). Narcosis or numbness.

TORPEFACTIO UNIVERSALIS.—Torpidity of the whole body.

TORPID (*torpeo*, I am numbed). Incapable of exertion. Benumbed.

TORPIDITAS (*torpeo*, I am numbed). Incapability of exertion. Numbness.

TORPOR (*torpeo*, I am numbed). Deficient sensation, numbness, torpidity. (Fr. *torpeur.*)

TORPOR, MENTAL.—A term applied to the slowness of feeling or action, the mental numbness and lack of response characteristic of pronounced melancholia, especially its stuporous form.

TORT IN LUNACY.—A tort may be defined, with sufficient accuracy for the present purpose, as a wrong independent of contract.

The authorities bearing upon the liability of a lunatic in tort are both ancient and meagre, but the following points have been settled:

(1) If a lunatic commit an assault he is liable in *trespass*. In the case of *Weaver* v. *Ward* (Hob. 134, Pasch. 14 Jac.) it was said that "if a lunatic hurt a man

he shall be liable to trespass, though if he kill a man it is not felony."

The meaning of this statement appears to be that a degree of unsoundness of mind which would offer a complete defence to a charge of murder is no answer to a civil action for assault. The reason assigned for the rule is, that "wherever one person receives an injury from the voluntary act of another, this is a trespass, although there were no design to injure" (Bac. Abr. Trespass, G. I.). It would be out of place to comment here upon the absurdity of applying the word "voluntary" to the act of a lunatic. Probably the true explanation is that the lunatic was capable of paying damages, which it was the object of the action to obtain (*cf.* Hobart, Rep. 181).

(2) In *Cross* v. *Andrews* (Cro. Eliz. 622) it was decided that "if an innkeeper be so distempered that he is *non sanæ memoriæ*, and a guest, knowing thereof, inns there, when his goods are stole, an action upon the case lies against the inkeeper; for if the defendant will keep an inn he ought at his peril to keep safely his guests' goods, and if he be sick his servants ought carefully to look to them." (*Cf. Mason* v. *Keeling*, arg. 12 Mod. 332, Mich. 11 Will. 3; *Ridler* v. *Ridler*, Abr. Eq. Cas. 279, Mich. 1729; *Haycraft* v. *Creasy*, 2 East 104.)

(3) In *Mordaunt* v. *Mordaunt* (39 L. J. P. & M. 57), it was said in argument that a lunatic is liable to an action for false representation, and Kelly, C.B., added, "and also for a libel," but without citing any authority for the assertion.

It appears, therefore, to be the law that a lunatic is liable for torts; but there can be little doubt that in England, as in America (*cf. Dickenson* v. *Barber*, 9 Mass. 225), the mental state of a defendant would very properly be considered by the jury in awarding damages.

A. Wood Renton.

TOUCH, HALLUCINATION OF. (*See* Hallucination.)

TOUCH, ILLUSION OF. (*See* Illusion.)

TOUCH, INSANITY OF. (*See* Délire du Toucher; Doubt, Insanity of.)

TOXIC IDIOCY. (*See* Idiocy, Toxic.)

TOXIC INSANITY. (*See* Insanity, (Toxic; and Pathology.)

TOXIPHOBIA. — Many people are under the impression that some person or persons desire to poison them. Such a suspicion may occasionally have some justification, but in the vast majority of cases it is groundless. In a paper published in the *Dublin Journal of Medical Science*, for February 1876, we have stated that we are constantly consulted by persons who aver that they are being poisoned, or that attempts to poison them are being made. So common is this apprehension of poison that we regard it as a well-defined form of monomania, and propose to term it *Toxiphobia*. In our paper we give an account of sixty-three cases of toxiphobia, of which we have taken notes. The persons who consulted us belonged to all classes of society, not excepting the very lowest, and they did not embrace, with two exceptions, recognised lunatics. Some of them were persons discharging important official and professional functions. The sixty-three cases did not include any in which there was a reasonable suspicion of poison. The following is a rough classification of the sixty-one cases: Eight men imagined that women were administering love potions or philters to them, but no woman made a similar complaint. Twelve men felt certain that their wives were trying to get rid of them by means of poison, whilst nine women were equally satisfied that their husbands were animated by a similar desire. Three female and two male domestics alleged that fellow-servants were attempting their lives by poison. One man and four women believed that their families were endeavouring to poison them. Two persons stated that certain of their relatives had been made away with by means of slow poison in order that their property might pass into the hands of the poisoners. In eight cases persons alleged that the people with whom they lodged invariably tried to poison them in order to get hold of their effects. A Petty Sessions clerk thought that the disappointed candidates for the office to which he had recently been appointed were, through a revengeful feeling, trying to murder him. A gentleman believed that an unsuccessful rival in a love-affair had bribed the servants of the former to poison him. The wife of a labourer in gas works insisted that a female of her husband's acquaintance sought to poison her so that she might marry her husband. A person who supposed himself an important witness for the plaintiff in a long-pending Chancery suit, lived in continual apprehension of being murdered by emissaries of the defendant. He was constantly changing his lodgings, cooked his own food, would not use milk or other articles into which poison could be readily introduced, but nevertheless seems to have plied his business (that of an attorney's clerk) intelligently and creditably. The wife of a barrister believed that her husband was anxious to get rid of her in order that he might marry a younger woman. She asserted that he was in the habit of pressing her to drink wine, which to her seemed always to possess a peculiar flavour; the wine, however, when examined, was found devoid of peculiar flavour, or of toxic qualities. This lady entertained her suspicions for many years, but kept them to herself, until she divulged them to her analyst. It would appear that her mental aberration was not suspected by her friends or relatives. Another woman who suspected that her husband was poisoning her slowly, succeeded, by false representations, one of which was that poison had been detected in her food, in persuading her relatives to share her opinion. In this case, the husband and wife were separated. Subsequent events proved his innocence; but though the toxiphobiac's relatives recanted their opinion of her husband's conduct, she did not, and refused to return to him. This lady was clever, agreeable, and on every point, save one, apparently perfectly sane.

The Petty Sessions clerk above referred to had some whimsical notions relative to what he termed the attempts to *get the poison into* him. He produced a nightcap and shirt, which he said were charged with some subtle poison, for when he used them they made his "skin creep," and produced a pain like the sting of a nettle. He believed that his persecutors came at night and blew into his room through the window (if open), through the keyhole, and even down the chimney, a white powder, which, when inhaled, caused irritation of the lungs, followed by "weakness." This man did his duty properly, and no doubt no one suspected that he was a monomaniac. Some toxiphobiacs constantly bring articles for analysis, and seem satisfied when informed that they are free from poison. On the other hand, they are sometimes incredulous when informed of the negative result of the analysis. A young gentleman formed the idea that a young woman, who had matrimonial designs upon him, was in the habit of drugging his food. He always expressed doubt when informed that nothing could be detected in the articles which he suspected. On one occasion, however, some fine shreds of tobacco were found in some tea which he produced for analysis, but when taxed with having put the tobacco in himself, he confessed that he had done so with the view of testing whether analysis was capable of discovering minute traces of foreign articles in food.

CHARLES CAMERON.

TRACHELISMUS, or **TRACHELIASMUS** (τραχηλίζω, I bend back the neck). A bending back of the neck. This name was proposed by M. Hall to designate the first symptoms of epilepsy, believed to be contraction of the muscles of the neck with consequent distension of the veins, causing cerebral congestion. (Fr. *trachélisme.*)

TRACTION. (*See* PERKINISM.)

TRACTORATION. — Same as Perkinism.

TRACTORS.—The metallic rods used in Perkinism.

TRADE-MARKS, insane persons may apply for (Patents Act, 1883, s. 99, quoted *supra* under PATENTEES, INSANE).

TRANCE.—Under Lethargy (*q.v.*) and Ecstasy (*q.v.*) we have described and defined the condition which is present in trance. The French words *léthargie* and *extase* are terms synonymous with trance. According to Parrot, *léthargie* occupies a position between coma-vigil and carus, but it is very certain that the distinction between all these terms is far from definite. It has been pointed out in the article on Ecstasy that Prichard employed the term in precisely the same sense as that of trance. At the same time there may be a condition of prolonged semi-unconsciousness, partaking of the character of profound sleep which characterises trance, without there being that mental attitude and significant facial expression which we associate with genuine ecstasy. When this mental state is present the compound term "ecstatic trance" is expressive. Two cases of a striking character are recorded in this work (p. 525).

Alcoholic trance has been described by Dr. T. D. Crothers in its relation to criminal cases, of which he has recorded several well-marked examples. His conclusions may be briefly summarised. In inebriety, a state of trance may arise, in which the condition of the brain involves the suspension of all memory and consciousness of acts and words, the individual going automatically about, with little or no indication of his actual state. The higher brain centres are in abeyance as in spontaneous or artificial somnambulism. This condition may last for several days or only for a few moments. Crime may be committed without motive or apparent plan, but when carefully studied the details and methods of execution will be imperfect. After this condition has passed away there is no remembrance of what has occurred. This condition cannot be successfully simulated. A person labouring under alcoholic trance is for the time being a dangerous and irresponsible madman, who should not be punished as a criminal, but should be confined in an asylum.*

A striking case of trance or lethargy has been recorded by Dr. Clark, Medical Superintendent of the Kingston Lunatic Asylum, Ontario.

We give a condensed report of the case. Having heard of a female patient who had been in a trance for years, all efforts to arouse her being without results, he visited her and found a thin old woman in bed, about sixty-nine, apparently fast asleep. Respirations were irregular, and varied from 24 to 44 per minute. The pulse quickened and rose from about 80 to 120. The eyes were half closed, and the woman appeared to be oblivious to everything that was going on. Both her father and mother had suffered from insanity. The patient married when very young, although she had the character of being peculiar; she had a family, and three years after the birth of her last child her disposition changed, and she became untruthful, whimsical, and easily worried. There is a history of fits, probably hystero-epileptic in character. In 1862 the woman fell into a state of trance which lasted for seven years or more. The condition was one of almost continual sleep, the patient occasionally waking up for a few minutes and conversing rationally. She was informed of the death of a particular friend, and the announcement aroused her, but her return to normal health was very gradual. For another period of seven years of wakefulness, she interested herself in her daily affairs. She seemed astonished to find people and places changed. About thirteen years before Dr. Clarke's visit she gradually passed into the trance state in which he saw her. When examined in 1890 by Professor T. Mills and Dr. Clarke, there was marked rigidity of the right knee and leg—*e.g.*, the patellar reflexes were absent. The left foot was drawn as if the tendo Achilles was contracted, the right foot being drawn down, but not in such a marked manner as the left. Tickling the soles of the feet did not cause any reaction. Orbicular reflexes were brisk, but it was noticed that flies crawling over the face did not excite them; the pupils reacted to light. Bread was put into her mouth, but remained there without any effort being made to swallow.

On October 9, 1890, she was placed under Dr. Clarke's care. Efforts were made to arouse her, but without avail. Her friends stated that she had been in this state of trance for more than eleven years. She remained in this condition until February 1891, when she died; during these four months she was closely watched, and until the last week of her life gave little indication that she had the slightest knowledge of the fact that she lived. Her temperature was almost always sub-normal, sometimes falling to 95 degrees. She was very clean in her personal habits. The amount of urine passed was very small, and the bowels were seldom moved. It was possible to arouse her for a few moments, to the extent of making her open her eyes, but she gave no indication of consciousness. The facial expression was almost death-like. Early in February 1891, a marked change took place, diarrhœa developed and the woman evidently suffered pain. On the 4th, she was undoubtedly awake, and in the evening spoke in a hoarse whisper asking for a sour drink. This was the second time of speaking in the course of thirteen years. On the following day she fell asleep again. In the afternoon she again awoke, and fed herself, and in the evening spoke naturally. On the 7th Dr. Clarke found her lying on the floor; she could not speak. On the 16th of February she steadily grew worse, and died on the 26th. On examining her brain after death it weighed 35 ozs., and presented a perfectly healthy appearance; there were no adhesions with one slight exception; the ventricles were free from disease. No microscopical examination was made. There were *ante-mortem* clots in the longitudinal and lateral sinuses, the clots in the lateral sinuses being particularly well organised. Heart weighed 3¾ oz.; walls of right auricle and ventricle unusually thin; valves normal; walls of left ventricle hypertrophied. Ascending aorta dilated into a fusiform aneurism, capacity about twice that of normal. No atheroma and no pressure effects noticed, abdominal aorta atheromatous; *ante-mortem* clots in abundance. Apex of right lung a mass of tubercle; in fact, tubercles were found scattered throughout the whole lungs, and in the apex a small cavity existed; hypostatic congestion marked. In the left lung a few tubercles were found, and there was some hypostatic congestion; nutmeg liver. The stomach was large, and about two inches from the pyloric orifice was a constricted portion, which was undoubtedly not the result of inflammatory action, but the natural shape of the viscus, suggestive of a rudimentary second stomach. The intestines

* See reprint of paper read by Dr. Crothers, editor of the *Journal of Inebriety*, before the International Congress of Medico-Legal Science, held in New York, June 1889.

were small, adhesions everywhere, and there were several constricted portions, without there being complete stricture, and above the constrictions there was much distension. The kidneys were small.

The value of this case of trance, which certainly did not present any indication of ecstasy, is greatly enhanced by the report of the autopsy. (*See* SLEEP, p. 1173.) THE EDITOR.

[A highly instructive case of "Suspended Animation" or Trance was reported by the late Mr. Dunn (London) and was examined by Dr. Todd at his request (*Lancet*, Nov. 15 and 29, 1845). See Prof. Gairdner's case, *Lancet*, Dec. 1883].

TRANSFERENCE.—The act of carrying thoughts from one person to another, applied to so-called mind-reading or thought-reading. It is also used in hypnotism to denote the passage of suggestions from the operator to the subject. Charcot has employed the word to indicate the change from one part of the body to another of certain phenomena of hysteria, such as anæsthesia, by the action of certain agents, such as blisters, faradism, or magnets and metals. The transfer is seldom lasting, and the so-called agents undoubtedly act suggestively to the patient. Sensitiveness to certain metals by certain individuals has been described by Burg, Dumontpallier, and others, but these evidently act in the same manner.

TRANSITORY INSANITY. — Attacks of insanity are frequently of short duration and in a general sense may be called transitory, that is, passing away (*transitus*) quickly, but the term is used in a more definite and technical sense, and especially is this the case with transitory mania (*q.v.*). Attacks of mental depression sometimes come and go in the same day, and are frequently associated with intestinal derangement.

TRANSITORY MANIA (Mania Transitoria), OR FRENZY (*Transitorische Tobsucht*). — We understand by transitory mania that kind of acute frenzy (*Tobsucht*) which, developing suddenly and rapidly, soon reaches its climax under symptoms of severe active cerebral hyperæmia, of ungovernable spontaneous motor impulses, and of violent anger with complete absence of consciousness. The paroxysm does not change in intensity, and, after a comparatively short time, mostly not more than twelve hours, the attack subsides, after a profound sleep of several hours, without leaving any recollection of the events during the paroxysm and without leaving behind any pathological change of the brain or mental defect. The attack does not seem to be at all connected with previous mental derangement or with any discoverable heredity; lasting, more or less violently, a shorter or longer time, it usually disappears without medical aid and terminates in complete recovery. It does not leave behind any somatic or psychical changes, nor does it injure mental integrity, and, as a rule, it never returns. The form of mental alienation, equally important from a forensic and clinical point of view, is not a sudden attack of ordinary mania with a rapid course, but it is a special form of mental disorder with an ætiology, pathogenesis, and course of its own. It is closely related to ordinary mania, but its character and symptoms distinguish it typically from all other maniacal forms, so that it has a just claim to a place in the science of mental disorders as a psychosis *sui generis*.

In most cases it was formerly considered to be an acute maniacal phenomenon, as is sufficiently indicated by the terms which are still in use: mania transitoria (acuta, acutissima); mania brevis, ephemera, furiosa; mania subita acutissima, mania ferox, furor maniacus, raptus maniacus, &c.

Transitory frenzy (*Tobsucht*) has nothing in common with mania (*manie*), but it bears unmistakably the fundamental character of frenzy. We ourselves lay special stress on calling it *transitory frenzy*, from purely scientific reasons, as well as because all the most important arguments against the existence of the disorder in question have been taken from the incorrect term, transitory "mania."

The symptoms of transitory mania originate from a certain somatic basis; as in all other psychoses, it would be impossible to explain them from a purely psychological point of view. It is certain that we know the clinical picture only, not the deeper anatomico-pathological reasons and the minute morbid changes which temporarily take place in the brain; but from the fact that the disorder is always accompanied by an unmistakable cerebral hyperæmia we may safely conclude that the morbid mental and somatic phenomena are caused by an irritation of the central nervous system. We know that the brain does not alone influence and originate mental acts, and that there are mental disorders which do not directly originate in the central nervous system, but that many somatic factors, especially disorders of circulation, may by their influence on the cerebrum produce deuteropathic mental derangement. In such cases the psychosis has not, as we have pointed out, a direct origin in the central nervous organ, but an extra-cerebral factor (the circulation) determines in a predisposed brain to an outbreak of some mental disorder. In transitory mania the blood flowing into, but not being able to flow out of, the cranial cavity, causes, in consequence of the vascular dilatation, a condition of extreme cerebral irritation, which, extending over all the sensory and motor tracts, produces mental excitement, a temporary aberration and a wild motor discharge, which disappear as soon as normal circulation is restored. Compared with other psychoses, in which we are unable to guess during life or even to find after death the slightest material change, transitory mania gives us at least a clue to its somatic origin, and shows us pretty clearly the cause of the pathological changes which temporarily take place in the brain. The theory is accepted by Emminghaus that the symptoms of mania as a whole have their origin in congestion. A most ardent representative of this vaso-motor theory is Professor Meynert, and the circumstance that attacks of frenzy may appear in conditions of anæmia (in consequence of hyperæmia in some parts of the brain) does not constitute an objection to the theory. We certainly believe that, as a rule, the typical *mania transitoria is produced by hyperæmia of the cortex of the anterior lobes of the brain.* This view is supported, not only by the well-known results of post-mortem examination in pure frenzy, as well as in *dementia paralytica* with symptoms of frenzy (Simon), but also by the fact that even the most scrupulous physical examination of individuals labouring under typical transitory mania yields a perfectly negative result.

This fact, however, does not at all exclude the view that hyperæmia in consequence of somatic changes may cause transitory mania.

Transitory mania is produced by the co-operation of predisposing and occasional causes. The latter sometimes, the former rarely, may be proved to be present; not unfrequently, however, it is impossible to state at all the actual causes, and to find out among the various influences which reciprocally act upon each other which was first and which was last.

The reason that the ætiology and pathogenesis of transitory mania are much less known than we should desire, lies, not so much in the difficulty of the subject, as in the circumstance that the disorder in question is comparatively much more rarely the object of medical treatment than any other psychosis. There not being any prodromic stage the alienist is not present at its outbreak. Moreover, the disorder takes such a rapid course that the physician, if he is not altogether too late on account of its short duration, is only able to observe the paroxysm on the *stadium decrementi*, and has to confine himself to the observation of symptoms. In most cases the patient and his antecedents are completely unknown to him, and, instead of any history, he has nothing but the scarce and unreliable *data* of the patient and his relatives, so that he is unable to write a thorough and objective history of the case and to find with anything like scientific certainty the ætiology of the derangement.

The ætiological factor, however, does not merely lie in external influences, as all occasional factors have been proved to be only of comprehensive and individual value; the external factor *may*, but *does not necessarily*, lead to transitory mania.

Any constitutional abnormality which influences the circulation, and thus creates a tendency to active hyperæmia and habitual congestion of the head, predisposes an individual to transitory mania. Intercurrent secondary diseases exercise a predisposing influence only when they act quantitatively upon the circulation of the blood and produce cerebral hyperæmia.

In addition to these, we have to consider as a predisposing factor anything which tends to decrease the power of cerebral resistance against hyperæmia, produced by occasional causes, and to increase cerebral excitability—*e.g.*, any weakness or exhaustion of the nervous system. Such an irritable weakness may be acquired by excessive physical and mental work, especially nightwork, by a fast life, by long-continued or frequently repeated excitement, as grief or distress, and by passions of any kind which impede nutrition, consume vital energy, and do not allow the brain to rest from its condition of irritation; also by insomnia, by former attacks of mental derangement, by acute diseases of the central nervous system during infancy or later (inflammation or concussion of the brain), by injury to the head, by typhoid and intermittent fever, and by former or existing nervous diseases—in short, by any condition entailing physical and mental exhaustion.

Heredity does not seem to have any appreciable influence on the pathogenesis of transitory mania; it is certainly not a *conditio sine quâ non.* We have not been able to prove it in any cases which have come under our observation. Of much greater importance, however, is the sex, men being much more predisposed to the disorder, while women are so only during puberty. The reason for this does not seem to lie in the difference between the male and female organism, but rather in the difference of their relative social position, and in the habits of life of the female sex, where all those influences which serve to diminish the power of cerebral resistance are mostly absent, as overwork and all kinds of excess, which in the male sex so frequently prepare the soil for transitory mania. This is not extraordinary, for the female sex is, in consequence of the conditions mentioned, protected to a considerable extent against some other forms of psychosis, as—*e.g.*, progressive paralytic dementia.

With regard to special individual predisposition, military men seem to be specially liable; we must, however, take into consideration that in no other class of people are the circumstances mentioned above so frequently present.

With regard to age, we may safely say that transitory mania only occurs in persons between about twenty and sixty years. In children we know of only one case; in old people we have not heard of any case at all.

Climate and nationality do not seem to be in any way connected with predisposition; neither is any special formation of the cranium, nor any special stages of life or phases of development, which, like puberty, menstruation, pregnancy, and lactation, so frequently predispose to mental disorder.

For the production of transitory mania it is necessary that, in addition to the predisposition of the central nervous system, there should be present an exciting cause, an external influence. The less the predisposition, the stronger must it be. The disorder in question being based on active cerebral hyperæmia, it is evident that any condition must be considered an occasional cause which influences the circulation and tends to produce a determination of blood to the brain, such as *strong drinks, mental excitement, physical and mental overwork, rapid change of temperature, indigestion and gastric disorders,* and *poisoning with carbon monoxide.* In addition to these, there are also other more distant ætiological elements, like sexual excitement, bad ventilation, stimulants, &c., whilst climate and especially the season of the year may be of some influence. In any case, transitory mania, like all other psychoses, does not develop from a single cause, but is produced by a complication of causes.

Transitory mania or frenzy differs from ordinary frenzy as well as from all other mental disorders, by the absolute absence of any prodromic symptoms which usually precede all other psychoses. Without any special somatic disorders or mental abnormalities having been present, there is suddenly an outbreak of extreme motor excitement, loss of consciousness, and a paroxysm of the wildest anger.

If there are any prodromic signs at all they are more of a somatic than psychical nature—*e.g.*, flushing of the face, intense headache and sense of pressure and hammering in the head, a sense of discomfort, palpitation, asthma, vertigo, perspiration on the forehead, tinnitus aurium, and chromatopsia.

The principal characteristic of transitory mania is the spontaneous and ungovernable intense excitement produced by the cerebral irritation and the morbidly exaggerated motor impulse, which, however, does not consist as in other and milder forms of frenzy, of a more or less harmless restlessness, but in a wild paroxysm with a blind desire of destruction. The excitement extends with great intensity over the whole of the motor sphere, so that not single muscles but the whole muscular system is under its influence. All the wild motor discharges are without any purpose and object.

We have specially to remark that the cerebral excitement discharges itself also through the organ of speech, so that every idea is at once expressed either by words, or by inarticulate cries, screams, and shouts.

In transitory mania there is no connection with the external world, so that external events are either not at all appreciated, or they are misunderstood and misinterpreted in a subjective sense. The formation of ideas is here exactly the same as in acute delirium in certain conditions of fever and intoxication, when the formation of ideas corresponds to the motor impulse, and the brain produces with an enormous rapidity, but without any logic and without association, a multitude of contradictory ideas, which do not become fixed, and disappear as rapidly as they came.

An attack of transitory mania is always accompanied by an outbreak of anger and rage, which, like all affections originating in a pathological soil, is specially energetic and ungovernable, and is nourished by the false apperception of the external world and even by the outrages committed by the patient himself in this condition.

Some somatic symptoms, accompanying the condition in question, are, pressure and a sense of heat in the head, lively and sparkling eyes, which protrude from the orbits, redness of the conjunctiva, a threatening or staring look, dilatation or irregularity of pupils, redness of the face and contraction of the facial muscles, grimaces, foul tongue, increased salivary secretion, exaggerated and irregular respiration, rapid heart beat and pulse (from 100 to 120), fulness of the vessels, high temperature, painful sensations in the contracted muscles, and, lastly, absence of urinary secretion and intestinal movements.

There may also be various forms of cephalalgia, spasm of the pharynx, burning pains in the epigastrium, asthmatic or gastric troubles, nausea and muscular tremor. Symptoms of paralysis, however, never occur.

Transitory mania is the only psychosis which finds its termination in sleep. As rapidly and suddenly as the attack came, so suddenly it also disappears. The tremendous excitement and irritation of the nervous system and the exaggerated muscular effort are naturally followed by a reaction in the form of absolute exhaustion and a desire for rest. All symptoms calm down, and profound uninterrupted sleep ensues, during which the pulse sinks to its normal condition.

We quite agree with the words of Emminghaus that we have here a process, in which the whole energy accumulated in the cerebral cortex is rapidly used up, and the cells having become exhausted and unexcitable in consequence of energetic discharges, during a profound sleep all the energy consumed during the excitement is renewed.

The amnesia following the disorder is specially intense. Emminghaus explains it thus: that during the attack but little internal work is done by the cortical cells, which at once discharge themselves, so that afterwards peripheral influences and their central effects are unable to awaken any recollection of the time of the attack, the perceptive and apperceptive function of the cells acted much too feebly at the time. Recollection generally reaches as far as the moment of the outbreak, and perhaps includes darkness before the eyes, &c., but then completely ceases.

There are, however, many varieties in the characteristic symptoms of transitory mania, such cases being called imperfect cases. One of the most frequent abnormalities is that the disorder does not take the usual course of one single attack of uniform intensity terminating in a profound, uninterrupted sleep, but is resolved into a series of short attacks interrupted by intervals of exhaustion and comparative rest. Neither is the termination of the attack in sleep always the same. Sleep is *never* absent, but its duration varies (from two to sixteen hours), and it also may be very slight and often interrupted.

Another abnormality of transitory mania is, that its duration may be very much protracted, there being cases in which the attack lasted several days.

Lastly, the paroxysm may be slight, amnesia may be incomplete, and a mental defect may remain behind.

It will now be necessary to state the difference between transitory mania and allied psychoses, of which we mention:

(1) Ordinary raving mania;
(2) Periodical frenzy;
(3) Raptus melancholicus;
(4) Raptus epilepticus;
(5) Conditions of transitory neuralgic dysthymia;
(6) Pathological anger;
(7) Other transitory disorders of consciousness in general, and, in particular, during a half-awake condition (*Schlaftrunkenheit*).*

As sub-species of transitory frenzy we mention:

(1) Transitory mania produced by alcohol (mania, or ferocitas ebriosa; mania a potu).

(2) Transitory mania during confinement (mania a partu; or, mania puerperalis transitoria), which has been described by Krafft-Ebing as well as by ourselves (*loc. cit.*).

With regard to **therapeutics**, we may briefly say that the treatment of transitory mania can only be symptomatic.

It would be impossible to administer any medicines during the paroxysm, and afterwards we must trust to the *vis medicatrix naturæ*. The patient must be isolated, and anything that might irritate him, carefully avoided. He must be kept away from bright light or loud noise, and he must be allowed to divest himself of his clothing if it molests him. We have tried the usual treatment of cold baths, hypodermic injection of morphia, &c., but only with very moderate success. *Transitory mania will take its own course, and cannot be cut short by any remedies.* It is, however, impossible to generalise, and the physician will have to take into consideration the individuality of his patient.

As the term "transitory" mania implies, the disorder terminates in recovery, so that there can be no question as to the results of post-mortem examinations. It is not impossible that death might occur,

* Our space does not allow us to describe the differences minutely, but we refer the reader to our treatise on transitory mania (pp. 71–119).

not through the attack itself, but by a secondary disease, and even if in such a case the autopsy should not reveal any signs of hyperæmia, it does not follow that the latter was not present, because, as Emminghaus says, any signs of cortical congestion may disappear after or even during the agony of death. We also cannot believe that dilatation of the cortical vessels, or hæmorrhage into the cortical substance, will be found, as it occurs in severe forms of frenzy, for our opinion is that death can only occur in some rare cases if the attack extends to centres important to life, and even then scarcely any pathological changes would be found. Death might occur in consequence of the bursting of a miliary aneurism through the hyperæmia which causes the attack, but we must remember that the occurrence of miliary aneurism in the cortical vessels is extremely rare.

With regard to the **medico-legal aspect** of the question we remark:

How the motor and mental excitement expend themselves depends mainly on accidental external circumstances and the surroundings of the patient. If the latter are unfavourable it may happen that during the paroxysm the patient commits acts which make him liable to be punished by law, especially if the antecedents of the patient are such as to indicate that he might be capable of committing them. Thus it may happen that persons, in consequence of there being trace of prior mental disorder, and the deed being in accord with their mental history, are convicted, although innocent, and perhaps even condemned to death.

Therefore transitory mania, and especially those forms of it connected with alcohol and parturition, are of great forensic importance. It is a condition of unconsciousness which excludes free will, and makes the individual irresponsible while the condition lasts, because there is no possibility of free choice *pro* or *contra*; in addition to this the motives for the deed are merely organic and lie in the morbid motor excitement and the pathological frenzy. The patient, driven by the morbid impulse, could not help acting as he did.

Although in some cases the intellect may be less deranged and consciousness less obscured, and the patient may seem to have a certain method in his doings, we must bear in mind that the association of certain ideas takes place mechanically and as a matter of habit, so that nevertheless the patient was not master of himself and his actions, and was unable to avoid doing what he did. The wrong he did was not intentional, but was [illegible] by powers over which nobody [illegible] control. Therefore an individual, [illegible] doing wrong, under such [illegible] is not punishable.

OTTO VON SCHWARTZER.

[*References.*—R. von Krafft-Ebing, Die Lehre von der Mania transitoria, 1865; Die [illegible] schen Störungen des Selbstbewusstseins, [illegible]. Otto von Schwartzer, Die transitorische [illegible], eine klinisch-forensische Studie, 1880. [illegible], Fall v. M. tr., Irrenfreund, 1871, vii. Von Krafft, Fall v. M. tr., Allg. Zeitschrift f. Psych., [illegible], xxviii. Braun, M. tr., Allg. Z. f. Psych., [illegible], xxv. Cook, M. tr., Philad. Med. and Surgical Reporter, 1873, xxviii. Van Holsbeek, De la Folie subite, passagère au point de vue médico-légale, Bullet. de l'Académie de Méd. de Belg., [illegible], 1869. Lotz, Fall v. Melanch. tr., Allg. Z. f. Psych., xxv., 1860. Hofmann, Fall von M. tr., [illegible] des Med. Doctoren Coll., 1879, 20, ii. [illegible], Jour. Psych., Annal. Méd. Psych., 1871. [illegible], 23, ii., 1868, Fall v. tr. furrib. Delir. [illegible], Mania acutiss., Allg. Z. f. Psych., xxiii. Von Krafft, Ueber eine Form d. Rausches welche als Manie verläuft, D. Z. f. Staatsarzneikunde, [illegible], xxvii. Ettmüller, Cas. Viertelj. f. g. M., [illegible]. Bonnet, Cas. Annal. méd. Psychol., 1874–5. [illegible], Cas. Friedreich's Blätter, 1867–5. Otto von Schwartzer, Bewusstlosigkeitszustände, [illegible]. Lehrbücher der gericht. Psychopath. und [illegible]. Von Büchner, Balfour Browne, [illegible], [illegible], Casper-Liman, von Krafft, Maudsley, Arndt, [illegible], Meynert, Griesinger, Lombroso, Leidesdorf, Krapelin, Tardieu, Savage, Liman, [illegible] Geisteszustände, 1869. Lombroso e [illegible], [illegible] med. l. 1874. Motet, Zurech. d. [illegible]. [illegible] Hôpitaux, 1870. Tuke, F., Beurth. d. [illegible] v. Gericht. British Med. Journ., 1875. v. [illegible], Sulla procedura nei giudizii cr. e civ. p. [illegible] l'alienazione mentale, Napoli, 1870. Laycock, D. gericht. Beurth. Geistesgestörter Med. Times and Gaz. 1867, x.–xi. Eastwood, Medico-legal Uncertainties, Journal of Mental Science, 1869, &c. Und die einschlägigen Arbeiten, von Adamkiewicz, Brierre de Boismont, Schlager, Lippe, Mendel, Emminghaus, Carrara, Tyler, Russell Reynolds, Everett, Legrand du Saulle, Verga, Jacoby, Livi, Browne, [illegible], Meschede, Zulé, Mosing, Hagen, Lombroso, [illegible], Laurent, Nicolson, Telman, Erlenmeyer, [illegible], Scrzcaka, Bonnet and Bulard, Otto, [illegible], [illegible].]

TRANSITORY MELANCHOLIA. (*See* MELANCHOLIA TRANSITORIA.)

TRAUMATIC FACTOR IN MENTAL DISEASE, THE. — Under the above head may rightly be included all injuries produced by external violence affecting the nervous system, so as to become factors in the production of mental disorder or defect; and it is narrow and unscientific to limit the scope of the subject to direct injury of the head. And, contrary to the classification of many, we do not include insolation under the head of traumatic injury. The clinical similarity of some examples of the two does not justify us in huddling all cases from injury and from insolation promiscuously together. Nor do we deal with the surgical aspects of the subject.

From the shock of a blow, several events

may follow, perhaps successively. As a primary effect, there may be jar, shake, violent vibration of the brain, or brain and cord; and this—when occurring in concussion—chiefly through the medium of the excessive commotion and propulsion of the cerebro-spinal fluid, dashed to and fro by the external impact, as shown by Duret. The practical result is more or less suspension of fewer or more of the functions of the brain, or brain and cord. Next, there may follow the molecular alteration and the perversions of function manifested as ordinary psycho-neuroses; or as traumatic neurosis, or neurasthenia, or hysteria; and, finally, there may be sub-acute or chronic organic disease of the brain, and sometimes of other parts of the nervous system.

In the later and more typical cases a neurosis is first engendered, and on this basis the resulting insanity or deterioration of mind is formed by further nervous and mental reductions.

If cranial, the original injury may chiefly affect the bony structure, or the brain itself, or the intra-cranial blood-vessels.

Even in some of the, clinically, so-called functional cases, the brain may really have undergone some fine material damage; and, in them, paralysis of ordinary type affecting the limbs on the side the same as the cranial hurt is very suggestive of damage to the opposite cerebral hemisphere by counterstroke.

The morbid conditions arising from the incidence of external force, and constituting a factor in the production of mental disease, may either be **immediate**, or be **secondary**, and more or less remote. The **immediate** morbid conditions may be concussion of the brain (molecular perturbation); or bruise, crush, or rupture of its substance; or hæmorrhage into it, or into the sub-dural, sub-arachnoid and ventricular spaces; or vaso-motor results of damage to brain, cord, or sympathetic. Compression of brain may come from effused blood, inflammatory products, or depressed bone. Local anæmia or œdema of brain may quickly follow some of these conditions.

The **secondary** conditions following injury, and promoting mental disease, may be slow nutritive alteration of brain, acute or chronic inflammation, and exudation, suppuration, sclerosis, secondary degeneration, and the destructive changes following hæmorrhage, softening, inflammation or ischæmia of brain. Even tumour of the brain may arise out of injury, and in its turn influence the production of mental disease.

As a factor of mental disease, injury may act either as a predisponent or as an excitant. Nervous and mental abnormalities may promptly follow injury, and then disappear; but may leave behind them, either some impress—manifest or latent—which inclines to the production of mental disorder; or else some progressive organic change, which ends in a similarly disastrous effect on mind. On the contrary, the mental symptoms may spring from the moment of injury, or merely separated therefrom by a short interval characterised only by slight indications of impending nervous and mental failure or perversion.

The operation of the traumatic factor is thus seen to be in some cases slow, slight, and simply predisposing; or it may lead to the production of neurasthenia or of hysteria, or of both—or of a traumatic neurosis not always quite the same—and, on the basis of any of these, to an established morbid psychosis of traumatic origin; or it may be expressed either in primary coarse, or else fine, subtle, brain-damage, and secondary organic and often destructive brain disease. Or this operation of the traumatic factor may merely be to precipitate, and somewhat modify, an already partially prepared or nascent insanity; or it may be the direct excitant of an insanity formed and ready equipped to spring forth on the stroke.

The traumatic factor frequently is cooperative with other factors in the production of mental disease; its action modifies, and is modified by theirs; and the cases often have mixed features as the result.

The *age* of the patient has some influence on the type of insanity of traumatic origin, which, indeed, evinces a tendency to take the forms of insanity most frequent at the same particular stage in life.

The tendency to the production of insanity by injury is increased in neurotic subjects; in those of the insane diathesis; in the irritable, wayward, sensitive, impulsive; in the syphilitic, or those deteriorated by other disease, or by mental overwork, anxiety, insomnia or privation; and in those given to alcoholic or sexual excesses.

The **prognosis** is extremely unfavourable in the organic cases. But a number of the functional cases recover. Severe mental symptoms, immediately following the injury, may clear up well; those beginning late, and slowly progressive, present an unfavourable forecast; so does convulsion, tending to become habitual; and so do cases of the paranoiac type.

After cessation of the immediate effects

of the blow, there is ordinarily an interval—often long—before the onset of supervenient mental disease. In this interval, some deviations from the normal are usually manifest. Frequently, there is a change in character and disposition. Unusual impatience, irascibility, overbearing domineering urgency, outbursts of rage, or moody taciturnity and suspicion, may be evinced, or an uneasy nervous state; downcast sadness and hypochondriacal notions enthral the subject; nightmare and painful dreams break the rest. Partial or general failure of memory and of mind may come; or fatigue on the slightest mental exertion or strain of attention; or a dazed, bewildered, confused state of mind. Addiction to alcohol and coition are apt to be manifested; and, in the traumatic neurotic state now existent, the effects of sexual indulgence, drink, narcotics, extreme heat, physical exertion, mental overwork, agitation or anxiety, are easily produced and unusually severe. Gradually deepening, these conditions may form the prodromic stage of the supervenient psychosis; or, now, there may be great disquietude, tremor, headache, suicidal and homicidal impulses, insomnia, and possibly an expansive phase. Pain in the head may be general, or chiefly at the site of old injury, or radiating thence, and associated with cranial tenderness or numbness, &c. As to the special senses, there may be the most various *sensorial* (*a*) failure and loss; or (*b*) morbid over-acuteness; or (*c*) perversion. Early or late, may be paresis, paralysis, spasm, convulsion, tremor, chorea, ataxia, contracture, vertigo.

The symptoms and course of the mental disease vary, partly with the many varieties of situation, kind, extent, and severity of the brain-injury, and of every accompanying, primary, or secondary functional cerebral impairment; and partly with the particular nervous and mental tendencies of the individual.

The Traumatic Factor at Different Stages of Life.—External violence may affect the *embryo* or *fœtus in utero*. The grave effects—upon the development of the young—of injury of the germ-layers of the embryo of lower animals prepares us for the possibility of something analogous in the human being. And striking examples are forthcoming in which severe physical shocks, sustained by the pregnant mother, and partially conveyed to the womb, have wrought disaster to the nervous and mental development of the coming child; as in the case of pregnant women, in besieged towns, subjected to the violent shocks, vibration and tumultuous commotion of the modern bombardment.

In being born, also, the infant is liable to sustain cranial and cerebral injury, hurtful to its future mental state. So, in *difficult child-birth* the depression of vitality, the prolonged asphyxial state to which the infant may be exposed, the ecchymosis, hæmorrhage, or contusion, the brain may suffer in the expulsive efforts, or from distortion, depression, or even fracture of the skull bones—all may strike at the very foundations of the integrity of the nascent mind. Even the intervention of the *forceps* does not always avert the disaster, and their unskilful use has to answer for many an indented skull, damaged brain, and maimed intellect. And these ill-results of difficult labour occur chiefly in civilised luxurious races, with their bigger child-heads, and more fragile delicate women.

In *infancy* and *childhood* the risks of brain-injury are freely, and often needlessly, incurred. At these stages of life, injury to the skull and brain is apt to be the starting-point of idiocy, imbecility, convulsion, choreiform or athetosis movements, hemiplegia, contracture, talipes, wasted limbs; irritable, quarrelsome temper, proneness to aggressive tendencies, violence, impulsive excitement, destructiveness and automatism; these latter symptoms, in some cases, immediately of epileptoid origin. The tendency is to progressive mental failure, fatuity, and death. The necropsies present traces of old meningeal hæmorrhage, destructive local lesion, or local atrophy, of the cerebral cortex; or, often, wasting of one cerebral hemisphere only, or chiefly, and more extreme in some parts of it than in others.

After incurring head-injuries, some children take convulsions, as the predominant symptom; these convulsions tend to become inveterate; and the subjects perhaps grow up exhibiting mental fluctuations, irritability, violence, occasional delusions, mental automatism, and irregularly progressive dementia, much as in the epileptic. Eventually dying, they may show some wasting of the brain, with developmental irregularity of gyri and sulci. And they, like the last cases, may present cranial bone-changes following the injury.

In *youth*, as an outcome of injury, may be cases like those described for childhood; or quasi-maniacal attacks of excitement may occur with mischievous, violent, destructive tendencies, the attacks often being either recurrent or sub-continuous;—or there may be moral insanity, ideo-impulsive insanity, hebephrenia, and a variety of paranoia.

In the *adult*, and especially following *cranial* injury, we have chiefly found four great groups of mental disorder:—

(1) One consisting of the ordinary forms (even if modified) of functional mental perversions of the more simple type (psycho-neuroses);

(2) A second, constituted of paranoia and its immediate congeners;

(3) A third, comprising mental and other symptoms dependent on severe traumatic organic brain-disease and alteration, whether due to secondary morbid processes, or to these as well as to primary damage of the brain;

(4) And the fourth, consisting of functional neuroses of certain types, with mental symptoms. They may also be incidentally present in the other groups.

The second and third groups comprise the cases more fully and characteristically of traumatic nature.

Special Semeiography and Necroscopy in the Adult.—(1) The **first** great group, then, consists of functional mental disorders, modified it may be, but in a general way of the ordinary type of psycho-neuroses. And it is only necessary to mention them briefly. According to our observation the traumatic cases practically consist of:—

(*a*) Examples of a kind of cerebro-mental automatism;—consciousness becoming greatly obscured for a considerable space of time, or more briefly and recurrently, although the individual affected moves about amongst his fellows, perhaps attracts no special notice, perhaps makes long journeys, and for a time lives a life of which he retains no recollection, or perhaps unconsciously commits himself by various acts—*e.g.*, larcenies.

(*b*) Modified symptoms—*i.e.*, varieties, of stuporous insanity may occur.

(*c*) Acute hallucinatory insanity with unsystemised delusions is not infrequent. The hallucinations are chiefly of sight and hearing, are of import hostile to the sufferer, and the delusions are such as those of being derided, of mockery, of accusations as to moral or legal wrongdoing, of impending disaster, of annoyance, persecution, evil design or conspiracy against the patient. Emotional dejection and lack of control may culminate in *raptus*, with explosive violence directed against self or others.

(*d*) Melancholic depression forms the last sub-group to name here, and may present the symptoms of simple melancholia, with suicidal attempts; or delusions of wickedness or uselessness, vivid hallucinations with harmonising delusions, chiefly of depressive kind, morbid fears, and in some a failure of memory.

(2) The **second** great group contains paranoia and its immediate congeners. Injury in early life may assist in forming a natural bent to paranoia. Unsystemised delusional insanity, with hallucinations coming at first, may, or may not, gradually be replaced by the systemisation of established paranoia. In this group there may also be symptoms of organic brain or cord disease, of traumatic origin.

Some traumatic subjects become moody, unsociable, impatient, ill-tempered, irritable, and gradually may pass into a state of acute excitement, with suicidal attempts or homicidal assaults, and perhaps convulsions. These acute symptoms may pass off, and leave a suspicious, resentful, embittered, morose, surly, taciturn state, with delusions of conspiracy against the subject. Or a period of early excitement may give place to a chronic, depressed, hypochondriacal, persecutory, aggressive, dangerous, often homicidal state, with suspiciousness, irascibility, and paroxysmal transports of fury, sometimes on a convulsive (epileptoid) basis. Expansive symptoms may commingle with these. The end is usually dementia and death. Or, after the change of character already described as often preceding psychoses of traumatic origin, there may be marked headache, insomnia, irascibility, suspiciousness, suicidal or homicidal impulses, or assaults under delusions of identity, failure of memory, or its recurrent obscuration in connection with convulsions.

Persecutory and hypochondriacal delusions are frequent. Those of poisoning of, or conjugal infidelity to, the subject, if present, mark, in some examples at least, a complication of the traumatic factor by the alcoholic.

In many cases are dissolute excesses of various forms, brutality to spouse, children or friends, moral perversity, and eventually, perhaps, still graver outrages, violent brutal impulses, and occasional outbursts of acute mental excitement.

The course is long and changeful in clinical aspect and in degree of severity. Frequent as symptoms are insomnia, headache, vertigo, local pareses; various sensory and sensorial anomalies which may consist of perversion, or of morbid increase, diminution or loss, of sensibility.

(3) The **third** great group is a large one, including, *inter alia*, "organic" dementia, which sometimes is of the senile form —*i.e.*, senile dementia, precipitated and

modified by injury;—focal brain-lesions often with epileptoid states; diffuse brain disease, including general paralysis. Long, or considerably, after severe skull fracture, may come epileptiform seizures, of either the graver or milder type, or both, which increase in frequency, and are associated with violence and mental automatism similar to those so often manifest in epileptic mental disorder, and with progressive incoherence, mental confusion and dementia. Turning movements may occur, or tonic spasm, or spasmodic twitches, or local paralyses; hemiparesis or hemiplegia may be partial or general on the side affected, and either persistent, and augmented for the time being, after the convulsive seizures, or only appearing then and temporarily. Partly in dependence on these seizures, the mental state fluctuates from the noisy, restless, incoherent, to the oppressed, inert or semi-comatose. Similarly related to the convulsive attacks, and similarly fluctuating, are the most varied disorders and defects of speech, comprising many examples from all of the great orders of speech affections, namely, those of intellection, those of diction, and those of articulation. Vision, or other of the special senses, may fail or cease.

At the necropsy, are changes in the bone at the site of the old fracture, with bony bosses on the inner surface, local chronic pachymeningitis, perhaps cohesion of dura, pia and brain cortex; or cortical atrophy, and various old destructive or indurative lesions of the cortex beneath the seat of cranial injury; sequelæ of old sub-dural hæmorrhage, and of the usual type, or of old sub-arachnoid or pial hæmorrhage, the latter appearing partly as atrophic degenerate portions of the cortex. As evidence of counter-stroke at the time of the original injury—and situate at the opposite pole of the cranial sphere—may be the traces of bruise or crush of the cortex, or traces of meningeal hæmorrhage, or of local, acute, or chronic meningitis — *e.g.*, old adhesion-bands, and meningeal thickening, and areas of adhesion and decortication, chiefly affecting the base of the brain. Atrophy, more obvious in the grey than in the white, has befallen the cerebral hemisphere chiefly affected; and the ventricular ependyma is often granulated.

In some traumatic cases, with marked meningeal thickening and opacity, cerebral atrophy, pallor, and fine changes, chiefly, and irregularly distributed, in one hemisphere—is gradual dementia, and sometimes a mild expansive state reminding one of general paralysis.

Conditions, at least resembling general paralysis, may also come gradually some months after severe cranial injury. Preceded by strangeness of manner, emotional depression, severe cranial pain, hallucinations and delusions—come physical symptoms as of general paralysis, mental failure with large ideas (although of some fixity) completing the resemblance. But under active treatment such cases may vastly improve for years, eventually deteriorating, however, on the lines of dementia, spastic paraparesis, and various speech affections. At the necropsy, are slight brain wasting, some chronic meningeal thickening and opacity, slightly increased dural adhesions to the calvaria, the traces of old hæmorrhage into the sub-dural space; and degeneration of the pyramidal tracts of the spinal cord.

In these last two sub-groups we have cases at least closely allied to general paralysis, or forming the links between it and some other organic brain diseases, or perhaps to be taken as modified varieties of general paralysis itself. And there are other cases holding a somewhat analogous position, but the limits of space will scarcely permit us to more than mention them.

Such are cases *with* (*a*) indistinctly or moderately marked signs as of general paralysis in speech, face and tongue, &c., *and, besides, either with* (*b*) suicidal attempt and slightly dangerous tendencies, emotional dejection, delusions of melancholic and hypochondriacal type; hallucinations and delusions as to hostility against him, annoyance and persecution; severe cranial pain, and some symptoms of hystero-neurasthenia; *or else with* (*b*) severe cranial pain, emotional depression, weeping, or excitement under delusions, and especially under vivid hallucinations, as to hostility towards him, his persecution in various ways, his condemnation and impending death; *or else with* (*b*) a dazed confused state of mind, hallucinations, and some self-satisfaction. In the last case, the considerable clearing up of these symptoms links it with a sub-group, there is not space to describe, in which the mental and physical symptoms follow quickly or comparatively soon after the injury, simulate general paralysis of the expansive and excited, or of the depressed type; but soon clear up or vastly meliorate.

We next take unquestionable cases of general paralysis of the insane.

Traumatic General Paralysis.—In some examples at least, one cerebral hemisphere is much more affected than the other by adhesion and decortication, and by a greater extent, degree and duration of the other conditions of the cerebral lesion of general paralysis, including secondary wasting, sometimes slight and moderately diffuse induration, and in some a state of lesion partially like that of the demented convulsive cases described at the beginning of this third great group. In some there are old meningitic thickening and adhesion bands, and cerebro-meningeal cohesions, about the base of the brain and the anterior portion of the mesial surface of the cerebral hemispheres. The optic nerves are often involved, and secondary descending systematic spinal degenerations are frequent.

Other cases follow much more closely the usual general paralytic type of distribution of the cerebral lesions, and of their respective degrees in different parts.

The patients may be dangerous, inclined to violence, and perhaps suicidal or homicidal in paroxysms of excitement. Hallucinatory voices are apt to threaten, or pronounce danger or harm to the subject. The earlier symptoms may subside and leave some self-satisfaction in possession. But expansive symptoms may be prominent in phases, or throughout, while before and with them is the fundamental failure of mind. And now and then come paralytic seizures, with mental dulness, oppression, and increase of the impairment of speech and writing. In many cases there is severe pain in the head, especially in the earlier stages. Increased tendon reflexes and cloni are often found in the later stages, also hemiparesis, and contractured limbs—chiefly on the more paretic side.

Some examples are marked by the relative predominance, or striking nature, of such symptoms as excitement, noisy raving, violence, destructiveness, in the earlier stages; vivid hallucinations of hearing and of other special senses; often a long precedent change of character and disposition; irritability of temper, readiness to outbursts of anger and aggressiveness. Also, frequent recurring apoplectiform and epileptiform seizures with (left) hemiplegia, increased knee jerks, and ankle-cloni. In these the brain-lesions and wasting are often chiefly of the *right* cerebral hemisphere.

Or the clinical aspect may be different, presenting mental depression and symptoms of hypochondriacal or melancholic type, or other delusions of hostility, poisoning and persecution; perhaps vivid and terrifying hallucinations and illusions of special sense, besides quarrelsomeness, irritable morose ill-temper, hatefulness, urgent and protracted cursing, reviling or threatening language, (right-side) epileptiform seizures with post-convulsive recurring (dextral) hemiplegia, and increased embarrassment of speech, delusional refusal of food, obstinate constipation. Here the adhesion and decortication and other lesions, as well as the atrophy, sometimes at least, predominate in the *left* cerebral hemisphere.

(4) The **fourth** great group comprises many examples of traumatic neurosis which is engendered with especial facility if there is already a neurasthenic or hysteric basis, but which may be produced independently of the pre-existence of these; and which, on the other hand, may become manifest as, or may occasion, traumatic neurasthenia, and then, on this basis, hysteria. Elements of mental perversion or failure are present. Here come a considerable number of the examples of so-called "railway-brain," or "railway spine," "spinal concussion," "functional," "ideal," "psychical," paralyses, &c., accompanied by psychic change, occasioned by injury. The injury may be slight. Cases with definite organic lesions and symptoms are here excluded from this group, although often attended, also, by similar symptoms.

The overt psychosis is closely preceded by symptoms such as loss of memory of the time immediately following the accident, and perhaps of that immediately preceding it; back pains from sacrum to nape, headache, malaise, uneasy disquietude, insomnia.

The morbid psychosis established, there are melancholy—often of hypochondriacal type with great irritability—sadness, indifference to friends and family, distress, oppression, sombre feeling rising into fear and culminating perhaps in seizures of terror or in suicidal attempts; despair, often with præcordial pain, oppression and palpitation; variable, fickle and tumultuous emotional changes; vivid and terrifying recollections and dreams of the accident or injury. Frequent, are self-study as to symptoms, and concentration of mind upon them, irascibility, anxiety, inclination to delusive notions about being annoyed, vague, torpid, confused, easily fatigued mental action, rapid fatigue in attention and confusion in the exercise of reading, silence, slow replies, limitation of volition, hallucinations, insomnia, failure or loss of memory—general, or partial, or severe; often many hysteric symptoms; and a host of sensorial, sensory, motor, vaso-motor and trophic symptoms, on which there is not space to dwell.

WM. JULIUS MICKLE.

TRAUMATIC IDIOCY (*see* IDIOCY, TRAUMATIC), **TRAUMATIC INSANITY, TRAUMATIC EPILEPSY, TRAUMATIC HYSTERIA** (τραῦμα, a wound). Idiocy, insanity, epilepsy, and hysteria following injury.

TRAUMATISM AND INSANITY.—Under this term may be comprised those cases of mental disorder in which either the immediately exciting cause is traumatic, or in which the symptoms are directly referable to a traumatic origin. Cases in which the actual declaration of an impending mania was due to some injury are not classed under this heading. It may be pointed out that so large is the proportion of cases in which there is absence of heredity that they may not unequally be divided into two great classes, in one of which there is heredity and in the other not. It is with the latter that this article chiefly deals. The traumatism may be of every variety, and the disorder appears to be but little influenced by the degree of its severity. The subject as a whole will be discussed under three heads:—(1) **Insanity following head injuries**; (2) **following other kinds of injuries**; (3) **following surgical operations.**

In all these varieties the onset may be either acute or chronic—*i.e.*, it may date practically from the injury, or may occur after an indefinite period of quiescence. In the acute or direct form the insanity would seem to be but the morbid development of disturbances which, showing first as traumatic fever, next pass on to delirium, and then, progressively as it were, into some form of insanity. Nothing is commoner in hospitals than to see delirium tremens, produced by a slight accident, occur in an intemperate person. True delirium tremens however is much more often diagnosed than actually seen; and the different varieties of delirium met with in alcoholic patients require to be much more carefully distinguished from each other than has hitherto been the case. The vast majority of these patients recover wholly from their mental disturbance, but in a certain small proportion, even though with total absence, as far as can be ascertained, of heredity, the psychosis persists for a greater or less length of time, and in patients who are prematurely old or broken down may pass on into chronic dementia. Cases of traumatic insanity following the delirium of drink are only more frequent than those following the delirium of the specific fevers or pneumonia in that intemperance is the commonest of vices in adults. In the treatment of all these cases, the great object to keep in view is [illegible]. So long as abundance of food is taken and digested the case is hopeful, but with refusal or inability to take food rapid wasting sets in and death frequently follows, sometimes occurring with extreme suddenness.

(1) **Head injuries are especially prone to** be followed by traumatic insanity. There are no cases in which it is less possible to predict the amount of mental damage likely to become permanent. The most severe cerebral lesions may result in complete mental recovery, while very slight disturbances ofttimes lead to the gravest results. Strangely enough cerebral injuries in which the patient has remained for days or weeks in a state of coma are little likely to be followed by any form of insanity. Loss of memory or some one or more functional impairments rather than any general psychosis, will probably constitute the permanent lesions. Yet this is far from being an absolute rule. In a case under the writer's care a patient remained for some weeks in a state of insensibility, with occasional explosions of violence. Recovery slowly ensued; but great irritability of temper developed. Some years after the original accident he had an attack of acute mania. In such a case, however, the symptoms might most properly be regarded as dating from the traumatism, and persisting throughout, though with intervals of improvement. Amnesia and aphasia may occur; if recovery takes place from these conditions it is usually gradual, though sometimes sudden.

The principal psychoses occurring at a late stage are associated with traumatic epilepsy. In these instances distinct pathological changes will be found, such as ostitis of the skull or pachymeningitis. The period of quiescence may extend over several years. The nature of the pathological lesion will determine its duration. No cases of insanity offer more hopeful prospect of relief by operation, especially of course when the starting-point of the epilepsy can be sharply localised in the cerebral cortex. There is a close relation in ætiology between these cases and the reflex insanity to be presently mentioned. Insanity in any form may follow this traumatic epilepsy as it may ordinary epilepsy. Of the other psychoses due to cerebral lesion, and not associated with epilepsy, the forms are manifold, so that it is impossible to say with truth that one is more apt to occur than another, and no general rules can therefore be laid down either for treatment or prognosis. But whatever the form, it will always be wise and will often be profitable to search for some reflex cause. If such be diagnosed the treatment resolves itself into one of surgical possibilities. If no operative measure can benefit the results of the traumatism, each instance must be considered and treated apart from its traumatic origin. There is, however, in all, broadly speaking, an intolerance of alcohol. A glass of wine or beer may induce an irritable explosion, and suffice to turn these patients from apparently sane beings into irresponsible criminals. One of the best tests of complete recovery from head injuries is the absence of any vertigo in stooping or looking down from a small height. The existence of any amount of glycosuria is an unfavourable symptom. A large proportion of the cases tend, according to Lasègue, to general paralysis and dementia.

(2) With regard to the **other injuries** insanity is an extremely rare but still an occasional sequel. These psychoses may be considered with those following surgical operations, for the main features of both are similar. It is desirable, however, to mention at once the reflex psychoses occasionally met with. These are usually connected with the presence of a foreign body, an adherent cicatrix involving a nerve or such like cause, and manifest themselves as attacks of delirium, markedly periodic in their occurrence. Thus a case has been described by Wendt in which the auriculo-temporal nerve was involved in a scar, and the irritation gave rise to periodic attacks of an epileptic nature. Brown-Séquard has mentioned an instance in which the presence of a foreign body in the foot set up similar disturbance. The treatment of such psychoses is obvious and satisfactory. Such occurrences indicate the necessity of considering every case of mania from a surgical as well as from a medical point of view.

(3) As a rare sequel of **surgical operations** insanity occurs. Less closely allied to traumatic insanity than might at first be supposed, though possessing some features in common, it is of even greater importance, for the probability of its occurrence might contra-indicate operation. Up to the present, however, so few cases have been recorded that it is wiser to note facts than to draw conclusions. It is eminently desirable that every instance should be made known, and the complication will probably then be found far more common than at present suspected. This variety of insanity presents certain features: (1) It is especially prone to occur with complete absence of heredity and even in individuals free from any neurotic taint; (2) there is always a period of quiescence after the operation, usually from three to eight days; the longest period known to the writer was eight weeks; (3) the onset of the insanity *per se* appears to exercise no injurious influence on the progress of the wound; (4) when the mania is acute and the operation has been grave in degree rather than in accidental complications, death may follow, though the wound progresses normally.

In the less remarkable variety there is either heredity or a neurotic tendency. The writer is of opinion that when the latter takes the hysterical form the patient is less likely to have any grave mental disturbance after operation. The hysterically disposed are in fact good subjects; a somewhat remarkable fact. In those who are eccentric rather than insane, operations will not infrequently be followed by transitory mania of no gravity. If the psychosis is influenced by, or originates in, any surgical malady, the removal of this is likely to improve the mental condition. Thus, hallucinations of smell have been known to cease after ovariotomy performed on a girl who was insane, and other surgical operations performed on the insane have met with success as good as in persons of normal mental stability.

It seems unquestionable that mania may be set up by an anæsthetic in persons free from any predisposition to insanity. No anæsthetic known appears free from this possible risk. Here the cause is toxic not traumatic. Insanity, however, of this variety, follows directly on the administration of the anæsthetic and persists. There is no quiescent period. The patient really never recovers from the loss of consciousness into which for weeks or months the anæsthetic had plunged him. But when complete recovery from the anæsthesia has taken place, and the mind fully reverts to and remains in its normal condition for a varying period, the anæsthetic cannot be held accountable. Moreover, insanity has followed operation when no anæsthetic was employed, and mental disturbance has been observed to follow wounds before anæsthetics were even invented. Again, the drugs often used in surgical dressings, such as carbolic acid, or iodoform, might be thought the true factors. Or the morphia, so often employed in after-treatment, or the traumatic fever in the manner already described, might evoke the disturbance. All these possibilities must be admitted, but still cases of insanity occur after surgical operation when no one of these agents has been used. In a perfectly aseptic operation there is often no pain whatever, and no traumatic fever. Seeing, however, that one form of puerperal insanity is associated with a septic condition, it is possible that failure to maintain asepsis during the after-treatment may predispose.

The writer has not been able to trace clearly any such connection in any instance. When a wound unites by first intention, there can be no appreciable absorption of any drug such as iodoform or carbolic acid, and insanity has followed abdominal operations, such as herniotomy and ovariotomy, in which no cavity was washed out by any drug, and in which the union was perfect. The emotional state, induced by the anticipation of an operation, may be a predisposing factor. It is extremely difficult to estimate the degree of this mental condition, but, none the less, an endeavour should always be made to do so. We have here to judge, not by the mental symptoms shown beforehand, but by the degree of control the patient is exercising in order to subdue them. Relaxation of the mental tension, when the subject of anticipation is over, may be very great, and will seem all the greater, if the mental condition has not previously been taken into account. A certain degree of mental excitement, if not undue in amount, is not unfavourable. Those who have neither hope nor fear are not the best subjects for operations.

Coincidently with the mania the wound may progress in a perfectly normal manner, but the temperature will commonly be raised, so that the chart does not give a true picture of the surgical aspect of the case. Should mental disorder follow surgical operation, it would be desirable to substitute other dressings for those in use, to abstain from employing iodoform, belladonna, eserine, or any such drugs which have been known to set up delirium. The urine should be examined, for renal disturbance, such as might be produced by carbolic acid, might have given rise to the insanity. Should any anæsthetic be required during the after-treatment, it would be wise to employ one different from that originally given. There is no reason why an anæsthetic, if necessary, should be withheld. Chloroform is, speaking generally, the best to employ in persons actually insane.

This insanity may occur at any period of life. The youngest case in the writer's knowledge was a boy ten years old, who after excision of the knee-joint suffered from sub-acute mania, with melancholia and delusions running a [illegible] course and followed by recovery. The [illegible] was a woman aged sixty-five, who was [illegible] with chronic mania after an amputation, and drifted on into dementia, which promised to be incurable.

With regard to prognosis the present state of our knowledge does not warrant us in speaking very decidedly. In the majority of cases, where the mania is of moderately acute type and the wound does well, complete recovery follows. In patients whose constitution is broken down by alcoholism, renal disease, or such like, the mental disorder is likely to persist and prove incurable, though the wound may recover slowly. When the operation has been a grave one, such as ovariotomy or lithotomy, death will often ensue, if the attack of mania is acute, even though the wound progresses perfectly. Several cases, however, of acute mania following amputation of the thigh, have ended in recovery. It follows, therefore, that the mental and the surgical aspect of the case must be to a great extent considered apart; the mental being the more important of the two. Throughout, however, the possibility of the insanity being of the reflex kind already mentioned, must be kept in view, especially if the attacks are periodic. In many cases the hair will be found to become coarse and stiff, and the return of the normal condition in this respect is a favourable indication that recovery is commencing. If a wound has become aseptic, it would be proper to adopt any further surgical procedure that might be thought necessary to improve the condition in this respect. For example, if an excision of the knee-joint had failed and the wound had become septic, amputation might be resorted to, and would be more likely to benefit than injure the mental condition. (*See* TRAUMATIC FACTOR IN MENTAL DISEASE.)

CLINTON T. DENT.

TREATMENT (GENERAL).—General or moral treatment is conveniently separated from the medicinal, although in practice they are so intimately connected.

We shall consider in this article, rest in bed, occupation, exercise and amusements, schools, appeals to reason, seclusion, mechanical restraint.

Rest in Bed.—Rest has been, there can be little doubt, too much neglected in the treatment of the insane, notably in melancholia, and mischief has been done in some instances by forcing the patient to take exercise or to amuse himself. Especially does this hold true in those cases of mental depression which are the result of family trouble, and poverty, loss of memory and the power of application in consequence of over-study and other forms of mental strain in the first instance. The brain craves repose, and it is worse than useless to attempt to restore its exhausted energies and tone by the excitement of the theatre or the concert, however useful these may be at another stage of the disorder. We are not aware that any physician at the head of an asylum has carried out this mode of treatment more effectively than Dr. Rayner, the late superintendent of the Hanwell Asylum (Male Department) where the writer has known cases markedly benefited by it. In a paper read at the International Medical Congress, Berlin, 1890, Dr. Neisser (Leubus) advocated this treatment.

Occupation, Exercise and Amusements.—Important as under some circumstances is the complete rest of mind and body, it is no less important to distract the attention of patients from themselves by various forms of amusement and by daily exercise in the open air.

If idleness is a curse to the sane, it is the parent of mischief and *ennui* to the insane, and especially to the pubescent and adolescent cases. The lives of the idle insane are miserable and without interest: their morbid fancies riot unchecked, while evil habits, quarrelling and destructiveness are all encouraged by the absence of any definite amusement or occupation. Walks, games, and entertainments must be encouraged, but these may not afford a sufficient object, and should be supplemented by some useful occupation or they are apt to pall. The insane are idle from various causes—from apathy, incapability of sustained attention, mental pre-occupation from delusions, and it may sometimes be said from perverse laziness. Employment, Nature's universal law of health, alike for body and mind, is specially beneficial to the insane, seeing that it displaces insane ideas by new and healthy thoughts, revives the familiar habits of daily activity, restores self-respect by showing the patient that he is good for something, while it promotes the general bodily health. Out-door employment is no doubt the best, and the garden and farm are invaluable means of treatment. All kinds of workshops are needful for amateurs as well as for artisans. Painting and printing also furnish interesting occupation. We have found the latter of great utility in concentrating the attention. The kitchen and laundry are the workshops for female patients of the humbler grades, while the employments of the higher class are mainly those to which they are accustomed at their own homes. Nursing their fellow patients is a valuable occupation for both sexes, so far as it can be safely introduced. Drilling is very useful, especially for the class referred to by Dr. Shuttleworth in his article, IDIOTS AND IMBECILES (*q.v.*). For those who are incapable of better employment, even their whims should be taken advantage of to encourage employment, for the immediate object is not the value of the labour but the benefit of the patient. The latter and the general health should determine the nature and duration of the work. Great risks must often be run in the employment of patients in placing tools and lethal weapons in their hands. This risk is inevitable before the patient can be allowed to return to the outer world and it is a risk which the public scarcely appreciate.

Employment will be encouraged and fostered by a healthy tone of activity pervading the whole asylum, by praise, extra privileges, and in certain cases by small money payments. If inexcusable idleness may sometimes be met by deprivation of privileges, this must never have reference to food.* Insanity is as a rule of an asthenic type, and those who labour under it require ample support, the idlers not excepted.

One thing must never be forgotten, that occupation and amusements are sovereign remedies for the destructive habits of many patients. Pent-up nervous energy must have vent, and if it does not find relief in occupation of some kind, or in games, it will assuredly be discharged upon animate or inanimate objects, often involving great destruction of clothing. Doubtless the greater recognition of this fact would frequently make all the difference in the amount of violent excitement in an asylum, and so prevent, in many cases, the resort to seclusion and to mechanical restraint.

Farm labour, a most useful resource in our county asylums, and a universally recognised mode of employment, may, it is granted, be carried too far, but the evil arising from excess of work is small indeed compared with the far greater evil of an idle objectless life.

However easy it may be to introduce occupation in asylums for the poor, this is by no means the case in institutions for the insane of the educated class. A few years ago an American asylum physician requested us to take him to Bethlem Hospital for the special

* It would seem needless to say that nothing can ever justify the punishment of the insane for refusing to work, yet such a course has been advocated within a recent period.

purpose of ascertaining the various ways in which the male patients were occupied, as he had found it extremely difficult to secure this desirable result. He soon became aware that precisely the same difficulty was experienced in this hospital, notwithstanding the strongest conviction that occupation is of the utmost utility. Some of the patients were at that time engaged in bringing out a manuscript journal, *The Bethlehem Star*,* which excited considerable interest, and diverted the minds of many from morbid self-inspection. Again, a few patients were occupied in drawing or painting. Many were reading books and newspapers. At the same time there were no means of healthy outdoor occupation in addition to games of skill. On the other hand, for the female patients, the American visitor saw no lack of work, in sewing, needlework, &c., in addition to the musical practice on the piano. Amusements are no doubt more readily introduced than definite occupation. There are games of chance and skill—chess, draughts, billiards, and then there are the periodical concerts and private theatricals. Out of doors there are raquets, tennis, and croquet, cricket, football, and skittles. Lectures, the magic lantern, and recitations, have their place, and are greatly appreciated by some patients. Nowhere have we seen them so systematically carried out as in some asylums in the United States.†

Schools in Asylums.—The most successful and continuous endeavour to occupy a certain number of patients in an asylum by means of imparting school knowledge was carried on at the Richmond Asylum, Dublin, by the late Dr. Lalor, into the working of which we carefully inquired some years ago. It has always appeared to us that asylum chaplains might do very good service by superintending this mode of occupying the time and attention of patients, but unfortunately the number who take any interest in the subject is quite insignificant. Surely the gloomy monotony which is apt to creep into these institutions would be greatly lessened, if not prevented, by systematic instruction imparted in an able and interesting manner, and by the more frequent use of musical instruments. One great advantage of united tuition is, that it brings a number of patients together, and subjects them to a certain amount of wholesome rivalry. It excites whatever desire to excel may remain in the breast of a lunatic, rouses sluggish faculties, and stimulates laudable emulation. The attention is diverted for at least some hours from the delusions under which the patient labours, and is concentrated upon other subjects. It seems, indeed, impossible that the occupation and diversion of the mind which a school (including music, singing, &c.) provides, can be other than beneficial. The immediate effect in causing actual recovery may not be apparent, and Dr. Lalor did not pretend that such was the case, but we are satisfied that an excited patient not unfrequently becomes tranquil after being brought into the class. It may even avert, or at least postpone, the period when a patient threatened with fatuity, sinks into hopeless dementia. As regards incurable cases, upon which educational efforts may seem, at first sight, entirely thrown away, we must think that vicious habits are in many instances broken, and the direction of the thoughts turned, for a time at least, into a healthier channel. We believe that more has been done in asylums to induce the Greek scholar to read his Homer, the German scholar his Goethe, and to encourage the artist and musician to interest themselves in the pursuits they followed before they entered the asylum, than to *teach* those who are more or less ignorant. In short, more has been attempted among private patients than among the pauper class. And it is to this point—the introduction of well qualified, and therefore well paid, schoolmasters and mistresses into some county asylums—that we are anxious to attract fresh attention.* The head inspector of national schools (Ireland) stated, ten years after the Dublin school had been in operation, that "the experiment of bringing lunatics under regular instruction has been attended in this place with great success."

* This Journal first appeared in 1875, expired in seven weeks after a delicate and critical state of health, and was resuscitated in 1879, but soon came to an untimely end. In 1880 it returned to life, only to expire after a brief career. In 1889 a new journal appeared, *Under the Dome*, which for a considerable time was a success, and lasted nearly a year. We are glad to add that it is now resumed, and is for the first time printed, the editor being the medical superintendent, Dr. Percy Smith. At the Edinburgh Royal Asylum, the *Morningside Mirror*, and at the Montrose Royal Asylum the *Sunnyside Chronicle* have long flourished.

† At the British Medical Association Meeting 1883, Dr. Yellowlees brought forward in the Psychology Section the subject of occupation in asylums, but unfortunately it was an extemporary address and has not appeared in print. The Editor is glad to find from the rough notes with which the speaker has kindly favoured him, that the remarks he has made are in full accordance with the sentiments of the superintendent of the Gartnavel Asylum.

* See article on the Richmond Asylum School (Dublin), in the *Journal of Mental Science*, Oct. 1875.

It may be added, that long ago Dr. Brigham instituted winter classes in the State Lunatic Asylum, near Utica (N.Y.), and that Dr. Pliny Earle actively encouraged the introduction of schools into asylums. The late Dr. Kirkbride (Philadelphia) informed us that he considered a well-organised school would be valuable in any large hospital for the insane, as at least an useful occupation of the mind. Instead of having a schoolroom he employed the "companions" of patients to encourge them in reading and conversation every day.

In Scotland Dr. W. A. F. Browne formed classes in the Dumfries Asylum. In these classes drawing was taught, and the patients were instructed in Greek and Latin.

Appeals to Reason.—It has been laid down over and over again that it is of no use to attempt to argue an insane man out of his delusions. As a general rule this is no doubt true, but it may be too broadly stated and too invariably acted upon. The rule may hold good at one stage and be no longer applicable at another. It will be always open to the objector to the employment of reason in all cases to say that it only succeeds when the patient would have recovered without having resorted to this mode of moral treatment—one form of legitimate rationalism. We can only set against this facile objection, that we have known instances in which success followed the appeal to reason when other means have failed and there was no indication of recovery. Thus, the patient who believes that her husband has been killed by an imaginary plot, will sometimes recover her senses when she really sees him. At any rate it is certainly a duty to make the experiment of bringing actual facts to bear upon the delusion under which the patient labours. Instances to the point will be found recorded in the *Journal of Mental Science* (Oct. 1886), in a paper read before the Annual Meeting of the Medico-Psychological Association, by Dr. Savage. M. Parant has written an able defence of this mode of treating the insane.

It is an abrupt transition from rational methods of treatment to pass to seclusion and mechanical restraint.

Seclusion.—That many of the objections which apply to mechanical restraint apply also to seclusion must be admitted. That it may be terribly abused is very certain; at the same time its use was one of the means by which Dr. Conolly felt himself enabled to dispense with restraint of the mechanical kind. His model of a padded room was before him, as he lectured at the Hanwell Asylum on the substitutes for restraint, and at the end of the course of his lectures he presented the writer with it as a memorial of the importance he attached to seclusion used in moderation. When M. Battelle, of Paris, insisted on the impossibility of introducing non-restraint into the Paris asylums, his reply was that one of the important if not essential means of introducing it—the placing an excited patient in a padded chamber—was not resorted to. Even at the present day it is rare to see a padded room in use in foreign asylums. In our own country there are superintendents who never resort to seclusion and have no padded room. We cannot but think, that if Conolly attached too much importance to this mode of treating certain patients, the other extreme, of regarding the padded room as never useful, is a very questionable position to take.

Mechanical Restraint. — The most prominent feature of the reformed method of treatment of the insane has unquestionably been the reduction of the amount of personal restraint. When the first blow was struck at the barbarous treatment of lunatics a century ago, the chains were removed from the limbs of the patients for whose safety, or the safety of those around them, they were employed. Under the old system the employment, amusement, and rational treatment of the insane were almost out of court—they seemed absurd. In the course of time, the milder forms of restraint which had been substituted for iron fetters were deemed not only unnecessary, but absolutely cruel. That it was possible to conduct an asylum without them was proved by Gardiner Hill, Charlesworth, and, above all, by John Conolly. But it was not sufficient to prove that it was possible to do without any mechanical restraint, it was also necessary to show that it was distinctly better for the patient, under all circumstances. The scientific physician had to show that medical and moral treatment sufficed to either remove the disorder which led to the resort to restraint, or to combat successfully the outbreaks of violence to which the insane are liable. He found it difficult to do this. By the employment of a number of attendants he was indeed able to coerce the most violent patients in an asylum. In some instances, however, he was doubtful whether this prolonged physical struggle was not as irritating to the patient as the strait-waistcoat; whether the flesh and blood which contested for mastery did not excite more resentment in the breast of the patient than the unconscious garment to which the patient could not attribute personal animosity. It was also felt that a physician ought not to be called upon to bind himself in the treatment of his patients to pursue or to eschew any one form of treatment.

It has thus come to pass that the whole question of mechanical restraint has been re-discussed in these latter days, and there has been undoubtedly a certain reaction against the iron rule to which the superintendents of asylums had been subjected since the triumph of Conollyism. Reactions mark the history of medicine no less than that of nations in their religion and politics. They are sanctioned by an experience of the disadvantages as well as the advantages which flow from the extreme position originally taken. A more moderate one would have been better in the first instance, but then all reforms are themselves reactionary protests against some abuse, and it would seem almost impossible to start such a movement without an amount of enthusiasm which is apt to override a strictly logical and scientific demand. The dread of the return to evil ways from which there has been an escape, naturally induces good men to shut their eyes to the value of some practices which have been swept away along with those of a highly objectionable character. In the present instance, it may well be that an excellent man, penetrated by an intense admiration of what had already been achieved in the amelioration of the condition of the insane, and with the fervent desire to extend it, went too far in his iconoclastic fervour, and like the English Puritans under Cromwell destroyed some things which might have been usefully retained, and proclaimed as a dogma admitting of no exception (unless surgical), that which involved a difference of degree rather than of kind. Thus, whether a violent patient should be held down by the strong hands of attendants, or secured in bed by certain appliances, involved a question of the kind of material employed and not a principle, seeing that both practices were examples of restraint. It was so, at any rate in those cases in which the one form of restraint was substituted for the other, for it would be falling into a grave error, and doing a great injustice to Conollyism, to assume that there were no other alternatives. It is the legitimate boast of those who abolished the strait-waistcoat that, to a very large extent, suitable moral and medical treatment humanised the maniac, and that occupation, exercise, amusements and humanity, were the true substitutes of the mechanical restraint which was so rampant half a century ago. We are most anxious to [illegible] this injustice to a movement for which we feel so much sympathy and to which the insane are so much indebted. It is only against the fanaticism which makes a fetish of the non-restraint system, that we ought to protest. We have lived to see the day, at one time little expected, when the Legislature has passed an Act which among other things recognises restraint and lays down regulations in regard to it. The Lunacy Board has from time to time admitted the necessity of some form of bodily restraint.

The occasions in which mechanical restraint is employed by those who occasionally use it are as follows:

(1) Cases of intense desire in patients to take away their own life. In some patients the consciousness of loss of control is accompanied by the demand to be restrained from self-injury. A voluntary patient was admitted at Bethlem Hospital with self-applied mechanical restraints.

(2) Cases of self-mutilation other than from suicidal impulse, namely, from the influence of delusion to mutilate.

(3) Some cases of self-abuse in which during an acute stage it becomes necessary to save the patient from the consequence of his own acts.

(4) Surgical cases in which the patient would interfere with the necessary treatment of wounds, &c.

(5) Some cases of extreme violence involving danger to others.

(6) Cases of intense and ceaseless restlessness threatening fatal exhaustion.

We conclude this, as well as the allied article on THERAPEUTICS (*q.v.*), with a special reference to the treatment of mania, by the writer of the article on that form of insanity. It is, as already intimated, supplementary to Dr. Conolly Norman's article.

"In no branch of lunacy practice has more advance been made of recent years than in the treatment of the maniacal condition. Violent purgation and free depletion, which were once esteemed panaceas, on the supposition that the affection was symptomatic of sthenic inflammation, are now as obsolete as the swing-chairs and surprise baths of a somewhat earlier period, methods which no doubt rested on the implicit assumption that excitement is the indication of a moral and not a physical aberration. More recently the practical difficulties which attend the management of mania were too often met by the prolonged use of seclusion and by the stupefying effects of calmatives and narcotics. The dangers attendant upon the indiscriminate use of both these methods are now at length fully recognised by alienist physicians.

The first great indication in dealing with a case of mania is to procure rest. In the majority of cases this can undoubtedly be best effected by means of treatment in an asylum. Mild cases may be treated under special circumstances in a private house, or better in a general hospital.

The primary object is to separate the patient as thoroughly as possible from his old surroundings. Only in this way can we obtain for the brain such relative rest as that organ is capable of enjoying. There must be not merely a cessation of business worries, but a freedom from the bustle and anxiety of ordinary domestic life. The over-acuteness of sensibility, characteristic of the maniac, renders him liable to excitement from the most trivial sources of irritation. Our aim must be as far as is possible to free him from all care, to shut him off from all objects with which he has formed, or is likely to form, morbid mental associations. We find from experience that the sight of home surroundings perpetually recalls home cares and duties, and that the enormous mass of associations connecting the patient with relations and immediate friends renders it difficult for him to procure mental tranquillity in their midst. For this reason it is generally essential to isolate the sufferer. It is also true that friends are often not judicious in their treatment of the maniac, and that to play the part of nurse to a relative in a state of mental excitement is such an entire reversal of the ordinary relations of life (not to say such a mental and physical strain) that it is quite out of most people's power. Isolation may then be carried out in a private house, seldom in the patient's own residence, or in a hospital, provided there is abundant attendance and medical care, and if the structural arrangements are suitable, provided that the case be a mild one. Severe cases (*i.e.*, cases in which excitement is very high, or in which the general physical symptoms are serious) are best treated in an institution devoted to the care of the insane.

Rest in bed is the best treatment for a large number of early cases, and should be adopted in all cases where the general strength is markedly failing. It should be accompanied by careful watching. It is the experience of the writer that a large number of cases of mania, whether primary or recurrent, can be cut short by rest in bed with careful nursing and the utmost quiet possible.

Akin to the treatment by rest in bed is the question of seclusion. This is a mode of dealing with maniacal disturbance which has been unduly discredited by having been long abused. It is, nevertheless, of the greatest value when carefully carried out. Undoubtedly there are many cases in which seclusion brings comfort to the patient, and for the time an immediate alleviation of his urgent symptoms. It should therefore be unhesitatingly adopted with the object above indicated, of procuring rest. It should never be carried out except under the strictest medical control. It should never be resorted to merely to give relief to attendants or to promote the tranquillity of the wards. Care must be taken that the secluded patient does not develop habits of masturbation, dirtiness, or destructiveness. Tendencies this way must be regarded as indications unfavourable to seclusion or as signs that it has been too much prolonged. The room must be kept at a genial temperature, and it must be seen that the patient is warmly clad, particularly in winter, and in the case of persons who are exhausting themselves by continuous excitement. It may be necessary to provide clothes of some strong material, wool-lined, and locked at the back.

With convalescence or the passage into a more or less chronic condition, care should be taken to provide employment for the sufferer. Occupation, of course, of a non-exciting kind, is an agent of the utmost value whether in preparing patients for a return to the world or in steadying and tranquillising those whose recovery will never be so complete as to enable them to regain their place in society.

Mania is perhaps that form of mental disturbance which most severely tries the capabilities of those who are in immediate charge of the patient. Nowhere are patience and tact more requisite. Nowhere is discipline, tempered with sympathy, more valuable. Kindness, good humour, and readiness of resource on the part of attendants will often render tractable a patient otherwise intractable, while, on the contrary, inconsiderate language and the injudicious exercise of authority produce irritation and disturbance. This element of personal influence, so hard to reckon up, is yet of inestimable value. The general rules for the treatment of all forms of insanity have here a special application, and must be ever in the mind of any one who would successfully treat maniacal conditions." THE EDITOR.

TREMENS. Trembling. (*See* DELIRIUM TREMENS.)

TREMOR (*tremor*, a trembling).—**Definition.**—Tremor may be defined as a fine or coarse clonic spasm of regular or irregular distribution and of limited range, occurring either as the physiological expression of certain nerve states, or as a symptom of certain pathological conditions.

No one can study cases of general paralysis, hysteria, &c., without having his attention forcibly directed to muscular tremor, its diagnostic import, and the different forms which it assumes. It is absolutely necessary, however, to bear in mind that tremor may arise in the course of other disorders altogether free from mental disorder; hence the importance of endeavouring to differentiate as far as possible between tremors arising from different causes. To the superficial observer one tremor does not differ from another in character, but further observation will show that distinctions exist and must be recognised.

For the purposes of description the subject may be considered (1) **physiologically**, when it may be (*a*) of purely *physical* origin (as in shiverings and rigors), or (*b*) of *mental* derivation (as in grief, anger, fear, &c.); (2) **clinically**, as a symptom (*a*) of certain toxic conditions (such as poisoning by alcohol, lead, mercury, and arsenic, or in the abuse of alcohol, opium, chloral, tobacco, arsenic, tea, and coffee), (*b*) of certain neuroses (such as general paralytic conditions, paralysis agitans, chorea, insular sclerosis, general paralysis of the insane, exophthalmic goitre, hysteria, cerebral tumours, &c.), or (*c*) as evidence of exhaustion whether muscular or nervous (such as febrile deliriums, general asthenic states, &c.); and lastly, we have to investigate it (3) as a **hereditary** affection, and (4) as occurring in the **aged** apart from muscular weakness or nervous degeneration. It may thus represent the spasmodic hyper-activity of nerve cells in health, or be the exponent of the exhaustion or deterioration of nerve cells in disease. In dealing with these varieties of tremor, we shall reserve a fuller description for such forms as occur in diseases allied to insanity.

The induction of tremor by cold is a *physical* phenomenon due in all probability to the stimulation of the sensory cutaneous nerve-endings, whereby an irritation of the cerebral motor centres is engendered, these being further incited to action by the temporary cerebral hyperæmia which follows the action of cold on the skin. Its indications are a rapid, at times tumultuous, movement of the muscles of mastication (chattering) and the arms, the trembling extending later on to the head and trunk, and last of all affecting the lower extremities. Its peculiarities are the irregularity of the tremor, which is now of small now of wide range, the horizontal tremor of the head, and [illegible] the approach of the clonic contractions to a tonic spasm in the trunk muscles. The fingers individually show little or no tremor, the spasms being confined to the larger limb and trunk muscles and the muscles of mastication. In rigors due to other causes, such as irritation of mucous tracts, puriform accumulations, or at the commencement of symptomatic or idiopathic fevers, the cause and expression of the tremor are exactly the same. The *mental* causes of tremor will be found to lie in those agitated states wherein the patient gives vent to an emotional overflow of grief, anger, fear, &c. Here the tremors are usually excessive in degree, and last only so long as the mental perturbation is extreme; there is usually tremor of the outstretched arms and hands mostly in a perpendicular direction, and in excessive states of terror there is tremor of the lower jaw, while emotional and twitching fibrillation of the lips and tremor of the flexor and extensor muscles of the legs are not uncommon. The tremor here appears to be due to a loss of that controlling power of the motor centres subserving the muscular tonicity by the exercise of such emotional states, and this loss of tone control is further illustrated by the occurrence of sphincteric relaxation during great fear or excitement.

In disease tremor is of frequent occurrence, and we may consider it systematically according to the above classification.

In *toxic states* the tremor may be the outcome of an acute or chronic action of a drug.

Alcohol.—In the sub-acute form of delirium tremens, the tremor occurs early in the affection, is present only on movement, and is fibrillar, irregular, and wide in range, affecting usually the superficial strata of muscles of the upper extremities, the face and tongue, being frequently associated with occasional twitchings of the trunk muscles. In the acute form the tremors are much more pronounced, and the oscillatory movements are not limited to the superficial but extend to the deeper muscular planes, so that the tremors assume a more general type, and may become so extensive as to be transformed into clonic convulsions simulating epileptiform seizures. In the chronic forms of alcoholism the tremor ranges from slight fibrillar oscillations on exertion, and after drinking bouts, to the permanent extensive tremors of all the superficial muscles of the arms, face, neck, and even the trunk.

The tremor as one of the earliest signs of alcoholic excess may be limited to the fingers, or affect the hands, forearms, arms and lips as well. In the hands there is fine individual, generally vertical, fibrillation of the fingers, which is most marked when the patient is told to extend the hand and separate the fingers; that affecting the forearms is also vertical, fine and irregular, the individual clonic spasms varying in degree, while when the neck muscles are affected the tremor is most evident during speech, and in the erect posture. The levator anguli oris and alæ nasi show marked tremor in old drunkards (Pieters), and the tremor of the lips, at first slight, increases with continuance of alcoholic excesses until it becomes so marked as to distinctly affect the speech, to which the tongue tremor also lends the quavering and stuttering characteristic of alcoholic ingestion. All these tremors are exaggerated on movement, and as the system becomes more and more impregnated with the poison, so the groups of muscles sharing in the tremor increase in number, while the tremor itself grows in severity. The diagnosis between chronic alcoholism and general paralysis by means of the tremor alone is difficult and well-nigh impossible. It is mainly through the association of other symptoms that the distinction between these affections can be drawn.

Mercury.—The tremors of mercurial poisoning, popularly known as "metallic tremors" and "the trembles," are very distinctive; they commence in the face and tongue, then proceed to the hands and arms, coming on gradually and being increased by excitement or emotion (Gowers); they may exist for years without causing much inconvenience, but when they become aggravated through the continued exposure to mercurial influence, they extend to all parts of the muscular system, involving the extremities, the head and neck, the facial muscles, the tongue, muscles of deglutition and the trunk muscles, as well as the muscles of respiration. The degree of tremor increases on movement, so that ultimately walking becomes jerky or choreic, and the patient makes involuntary grimaces, while the speech is indistinct, stammering, and tremulous. The tremor at first ceases on lying down, and in the absence of voluntary effort, but in the later stages is constant though lessened on rest. There is no nystagmus. When constant it resembles paralysis agitans, but differs in that it affects the muscles of the head and neck, is much more marked on movement, and that there is no fixity or rigidity of feature, or festination. The tremor is less wide and less irregular than in disseminated sclerosis, where there is also marked nystagmus. From general paralysis it is to be diagnosed by the excess of the tremor and the presence of stomatitis; from plumbism by the blue line on the gums and the special palsy in the latter.

Lead.—The tremor in plumbism is not very frequent in its occurrence; it may be fine as in the senile variety, but it may also resemble that of paralysis agitans, though the increase on movement distinguishes it from that affection; it is also slower, wider, and more irregular in its distribution; it may, as pointed out by Gowers, affect chiefly the flexors of the elbow and wrist, and the supinator longus —the muscles which escape paralysis. The lips and tongue may also be implicated, and if there is no paralysis, the distinction between it and the tremor of mercury poisoning is difficult.

Opium and Chloral.—The tremor found in chronic poisoning from these drugs offers no special characteristics, being merely the expression of an enfeebled exhausted muscular system coupled with anæmia, and the fibrillar oscillations are therefore like those of asthenia. The loss of co-ordinative power which follows the abuse of chloral may in a measure assist in the production of the tremor.

Arsenic.—The tremor in the chronic abuse of this drug, as well as in slow poisoning by its means, closely approximates to the alcoholic variety. In other cases it simulates that of lead, especially when extensor palsy co-exists. In many cases, however, it is not due to any specific action of the drug itself, but is a consequence of the muscular degeneration.

Tea and Coffee.—Max Kohn has described a sensory disturbance which he designates the delirium tremens of coffee, in which there is delirium with abnormalities of the sensory functions and tremor. Tea taken in excessive quantities causes similar disturbances, and acting as these agents do by stimulating the cutaneous sensibility, and causing excitement of the motor functions even in small quantities, the phenomena they induce when taken in large quantities are easily explainable. The tremors offer no special characteristics.

Coming now to tremor as a symptom of certain *neuroses*, we have to consider its occurrence in various paralytic conditions.

In **hemiplegia**, the condition known as post-hemiplegic chorea is sometimes, but rarely, met with, and consists of a somewhat irregular, minute, fibrillary quivering, usually limited to the arm affected, and best seen in those forms of hemiplegia (*e.g.*, the infantile) in which recovery is taking place; it is also seen occasionally in cases of muscular atrophy, in certain forms and stages of cerebral and cerebellar disease, such as tumours, softening, &c., and in locomotor ataxy. Another form of tremor, not choreic in character, being more rhythmical and limited, is to be met with in paralysed limbs. *Athetosis* is a slow mobile spasm of intermittent type, uninfluenced by repose, and inco-ordinate in its nature; it is limited as a rule to the fingers and wrists, to the feet and toes, though occasionally it has been observed in the face and eyelids.

Paralysis agitans affords us a typical illustration of rhythmical tremor. It varies in range from a minute continuous fibrillation to a severe oscillation, and as its amplitude increases its rate lessens, diminishing from about 7 to 4.8 contractions per second. In the early stages of the affection the tremor is fine, increasing in range as the malady progresses; it is continuous during rest, and at first it can be controlled for a very short period by a strong effort of will; in the early stage, too, the fibrillation may not be apparent during rest. Its other peculiarities are, the horizontal tremor of the arms, the significant attitude of the hand, the thumb oscillating against the index finger forming the so-called pill-rolling movement, the bent attitude, the fixed and vacant facial expression, and the unsteady festinating gait. There is a slight increase in amplitude of range of the tremor on movement, but this is by no means so marked as in insular sclerosis or the toxic forms of tremor. The groups of muscles affected are mainly those of the hand and fingers and of the wrist, while those of the upper arm are less, and those of the shoulder least concerned in the tremor. This, as above mentioned, is generally horizontal, but it may be lateral or antero-posterior in direction, occasionally supinatory and pronatory movements predominate. In some few cases the shoulder muscles are mainly affected, the degree of muscular implication diminishing downwards instead of upwards. In the lower extremities the intensity of tremor diminishes from below upwards. The trunk muscles are occasionally affected, but the head is generally free from tremor, such oscillations as are to be observed being due to the tremor of the arms. The tremors of paralysis agitans and disseminated sclerosis are slow oscillations as distinguished from the tremors of alcoholism, general paralysis, exophthalmic goitre and mercurial poisoning, which are far more rapid. The speech presents the peculiarity observed in the gait; there is, as it were, an articulatory festination, a tendency to run words into one another.

Chorea. — Though the purposeless movements of chorea are not strictly to be included among tremors, they, save for their amplitude, partake of the nature of irregular tremor of extremely wide range and slow action. It was this consideration that led Duchenne at first to regard cases of insular sclerosis as instances of chorea in which the irregular oscillations had increased in rapidity while diminishing in amplitude. It will not be necessary for us here to enter on the characteristics of choreic and choreiform movements and habit spasm—they will be found described in other parts of this work.

Insular Sclerosis.—The tremor peculiar to this affection presents certain peculiarities; in the first place it occurs only on attempted movement, it is jerky, extremely irregular and increased by effort, emotion, and attention directed to the movement. The tongue shows tremors of a jerky inco-ordinate character when protruded, but the facial muscular action is generally calm. Ocular muscular tremor or nystagmus is common. Articulation has been called "syllabic," staccato or scanning, with a tendency to clip the ends of words. The tremor in the early stages is limited to the hands, but later on the legs share in the spasms, inducing a peculiar gait which has originated another name for the malady — spastic paraplegia.

General Paralysis. — The muscular tremors in a typical case of general paralysis are frequently indicative of the hyper-emotional mental condition and the lack of controlling power. In the earliest stages there is to be noted an irregular loss of restraining power, an inability to gauge correctly the amount of force necessary to be expended in carying out fine movements, hence the smile becomes a quivering expanded grin, the tongue is projected with a jerk with coarse fibrillar tremors when kept out for a while, and the hands and arms are moved through wider ranges than necessary for the accomplishment of actions. Later on the muscular tremors grow more prominent and assume a fibrillar type, becoming associated with the earlier ataxy; the tongue when protruded exhibits a fine rippling tremor, irregular, and at times spasmodic; the lips show twitchings, wave-like fibrillations, jelly-like but unrhythmic oscillations on exertion, like those of a person in a state of intoxication and who is on the verge of tears; there is tremor of the head on movement, and the facial muscles show a spasmodic tremulation as soon as they are called into action, now on one side, now on another, or on both; the occipito-frontalis, zygomatici and levatores labii twitch and quiver, while at rest the face is quiescent and lacks life and expression. The hands show rhythmic twichings, especially in the small palmar muscles, while convulsive spasm of the wrist and elbow muscles, or of the muscles of the thigh and arm, are not uncommon. All these involuntary movements are mainly to be noted during voluntary action or on passive movement, and may become so extreme as to involve both sides of the body in a quivering convulsive tremor. The hand when extended also trembles, generally with slight dashes and jerks of inco-ordination. The speech demonstrates not only the muscular tremor and inco-ordination, but also the deteriorating mental state. With the former only can we concern ourselves here, referring the reader for a detailed description of the latter to the article on General Paralysis. The hesitating, slurring, slovenly articulation with its quivering tremulous dwelling on vowels and its blurring of consonants, the shuffling, stumbling and sliding over dentals, and the stuttering repetition of labials and gutturals, all indicate the unsteadiness and insubordination of the articulatory muscles during speech. The handwriting, too, is a mirror of the mental and bodily retrogression, the shaky, imperfectly-formed letters, the inco-ordinate jerkings and unexpected dashes, the blots and smears, are all indications of the muscular incompetency, while the elision of letters, the re-duplications, misspelt words and the running of words into one another denote the mental imperfection. As the disease advances, the groups of muscles implicated become larger, and the tremors grow coarser and of larger amplitude, the speech becomes mumbling, shaky, quivering, stammering, and very indistinct, the fibrillations become spasmodic upheavals of muscular masses, the power of voluntary movement gradually grows less, and the patient slowly becomes more and more enfeebled, sinking into a helpless incapacity, the facial muscles being the last to retain a vestige of the familiar tremors of the early stages.

Exophthalmic Goitre.—The tremor is fine, rapid, regular or irregular, and occurs only on movement. At times the fibrillation may be so regular as to resemble paralysis agitans, and again it may be so irregular as to simulate chorea. It may be general or partial, and has been known to be unilateral when the goitre and exophthalmos were also unilateral (Gowers). Marie has noted that in the regular form the tremor is more rapid than in paralysis agitans.

Hysteria.—Tremor may occur in this affection either as a fine irregular oscillation, increased or only present during movement, or it may be coarse and rhythmical, continuing during rest, and being influenced by voluntary movement. In whatever form it may be present it varies greatly not only in rate but also in amplitude, and is nearly always associated with those motor disturbances known as hysterical paralysis and contractures, when in all probability it is but an expression of the weakness of the affected muscles, since it is usually only after maintained muscular effort that the tremor commences. It is by no means constant, being present at one time and easily evoked, and absent at another. When present, attention directed to the limb, or handling it, increases the tremor. The coarse form may consist of a rapid rhythmical oscillation of the head or hands, and in the legs the tremor may be brought about by attempts to straighten the contracted joints. Emotion necessarily increases the tremor, and there may be isolated tremors of a group of muscles of one side of the face, &c., but these are rare. Hysterical chorea may here be mentioned, an imitative representation of chorea minor, coloured by hysteria. (*See* Hysteria.)

Convulsive Tremor, a name given by Prichard to the condition known as myoclonus multiplex, is characterised by shock-like jerkings of the trunk and larger limb muscles, and it may vary from very slight to extremely intense clonic contractions. They may be constant, or cease during sleep, or occur only in paroxysms. Gowers regards the affection as allied to senile chorea. (*See* Convulsive Tremor.)

Acute disease inducing muscular weakness brings about in consequence a fine form of tremor, which occurs only on movement and is but an expression of the imperfect response to highly energised cortical centres (as in the delirium of fevers, acute mania), or of the easily fatigued muscular fibre conjoined with the action of an exhausted nerve cell (as in convalescence from severe illness, the prostration of starvation, &c.). In old standing heart affections slight muscular tremors are to be met with, and especially tremor of the head and hands on exertion.

The pulsatile jerking of the extremities in heart disease must not be mistaken for a rhythmic tremor.

Old age presents us with a peculiar form of tremor; we are not speaking of the tremor due to muscular weakness, but an extremely fine regular and rapid oscillation which at first occurs only during muscular exertion, ceasing entirely during rest and sleep. It is earliest observed in the arms and hands, the neck muscles being affected later on. After some time it occurs both during rest and on exertion, and presents so close an analogy to paralysis agitans (except that the other signs of the affection, the peculiar gait, the fixed look, and the affected speech, are absent) that it has been regarded as a modified form of that disease. It is especially to be noted in the writing, a typical example of which is furnished by Fig. I. in the article on Handwriting (*q.v.*).

Another form of tremor, apparently independent of disease, but in all probability due to **hereditary nervous weakness**, has been described by Gowers and others. It is usually fine in range, sometimes irregular and unequal in degree of movement, and there is no concomitant muscular weakness or rigidity, which distinguishes it from the tremor of paralysis agitans. It occurs in young or middle-aged persons, is capable of being controlled by the will, so that it does not show itself in the writing, and occasionally it ceases during rest. The hands and neck muscles are those mainly affected, but the face and tongue may also share in the tremor, such cases being frequently mistaken for early general paralysis. Emotional states, especially if severe or long-continued, have been assigned as the direct cause, while an inherited neurotic disposition, either from gross nervous lesion or functional nervous disorder, has been found in most cases.

Diagnosis.—This is involved and has been anticipated in the description of the several varieties of tremor. It would be extremely difficult in some cases, did not the affections in which they severally occur present other symptomatic evidences of distinction, and it is merely for the purpose of description and not for differentiation that they have been thus grouped. The broader forms of tremor are certainly distinctive, though even in these, unless great caution is exercised, errors of diagnosis may be made. The handwriting illustrating varieties of tremor will be found in a separate article. (*See* HANDWRITING OF THE INSANE.)

J. F. G. PIETERSEN.

[*References.*—Gowers, Diseases of the Nervous System. Quain, Dictionary of Medicine. Charcot, Diseases of the Nervous System, Syd. Soc., 1889. Bristowe, Theory and Practice of Medicine. Roberts, The Theory and Practice of Medicine. Finlayson, Clinical Manual. Bevan Lewis, Text-book of Mental Disease, London, 1889. Bucknill and Tuke, Psychological Medicine. Savage, Insanity. Clouston, Mental Disease, London, 1887.]

TREPHINING.—Those conditions of mental disease in which surgical interference has been employed for relief or cure are those of (**I.**) injury to the brain and skull, (**II.**) general paralysis, (**III.**) imbecility when resulting from microcephaly, hydrocephalus, &c., (**IV.**) hallucinations (cerebral sensory disorders), and (**V.**) chronic epilepsy. In the following brief statements reference will not be made to details of surgical technique, since these are all contained in well-known text-books of operative surgery and monographs on the surgical treatment of diseases of the central nervous system, it being sufficient to remark in passing, that no operative interference is justifiable without conformity with the Listerian principle of asepsis and antisepsis. Further, to profitably discuss the application of operative measures to the above-stated disease states, allusion will first be made to the pathological condition which it is desired to relieve, and then will follow a discussion of the treatment which it is suggested should be at present adopted. Finally, no space will be occupied in discussing the question of risk to life, except where specially prominent (*see* **III.**), since the condition of all these cases is one of hopeless incapacity and death, unrelieved if surgery can do nothing for them. For this reason the mortality percentage, after such operations, although extremely small, is of no scientific value or interest to the community.

The difficult question of estimating the value of the results of such treatment is considered last.

I. Injury to the Brain and the Skull.—*Pathology.*—Cases in which various forms of insanity have followed severe injury to the brain or skull are commonly spoken of as cases of traumatic insanity, a very unfortunate expression. The first and most complete account of cases in which surgical treatment was resorted to for the direct purpose of relieving the mental condition are those recorded by Skae and others, later by Bacon, Hartmann, and Talcott (*see also* Mickle). In all these cases there was a direct injury to the head, resulting in the production of a localised lesion in the skull and a cicatrix. The cortex of the brain consequently was damaged in each instance, and further, adhesions necessarily formed between the dura mater, bone, and brain. The disorders of function caused by these structural conditions were in three cases mania, in two cases morose depression and delusions. The predominance of mania is of course in accord with the observations of Krafft-Ebing in regard to symptoms in chronic epilepsy. In each case the injured bone was removed, consequent upon which recovery commenced and was obtained in each of the recorded instances; one case being observed for four years and another six years.

Operative Procedure. — The surgical treatment of these cases has hitherto been limited to the removal of the injured bone, and apparently with remarkably good results; in fact, the latter are so good as almost to suggest that unfavourable cases have not been published, were it not for the results of operating for chronic epilepsy (*q.v.*). In each instance the improvement in the patient commenced from the time of the operation, so that the relation of cause and effect is well marked in such cases.

In accordance with the experience of the last-mentioned condition it would certainly seem that the reparation of the seat of mischief should not be confined to removing the bone, but also that the operation should be extended to the dura mater and excision of the affected cortex, since this is usually the starting-point, sooner or later, of epileptic convulsions.

In any case there can be no doubt that early operation should be resorted to in all cases of obvious traumatic lesion and in which mental disease has developed.

II. General Paralysis.—*Pathology.*—The condition known as general paralysis is still a *terra incognita* so far as the early stages of the disease-changes in the central nervous system are concerned. It is assumed by some that there is, concurrently with the degenerative changes in the brain, an increase of the intracranial tension, and evidence of the same in the shape of increased pressure under which the cerebro-spinal fluid escapes when the dura is punctured, is stated to have been observed during the operation of trephining. It has further been assumed that this pressure prevents the proper emptying of the peri-vascular lymphatics and consequently induces secondary degenerative changes. It cannot be conceded that these statements concerning the pathology of the disease have been established, though there has doubtless been observed an apparent excess of cerebro-spinal fluid. The degenerative changes are of themselves of a nature that could not be expected to improve as a result of operation, if they are, as is generally considered, primary in the development of the condition.

Operative Procedure.—Claye Shaw and Batty Tuke have respectively operated upon these cases or caused them to be operated upon. In each case simple trephining with puncture and partial excision of the dura mater was performed. In Claye Shaw's first case there was unquestionably considerable improvement, the patient becoming coherent and having no delusions, the speech remaining unaltered. Seven months after the operation the patient died after the onset of convulsions which had commenced only twelve days previously. In the second case in which there was in addition the symptom of great pain in the head, similar treatment also produced so much change as to enable the patient to be discharged. He was subsequently readmitted six months later and died three months afterwards from convulsions. These two cases commence the epoch of trephining for the deliberate relief of general paralysis, and as the result of empirical treatment must be regarded as noteworthy. The propriety of the more general employment of operation will be discussed directly, but it must be admitted that Claye Shaw's results are gratifying in view of the hopeless nature of the disease. It was proposed by Shaw and also by Batty Tuke to keep the drainage wound open so as to prolong the escape of the cerebro-spinal fluid. There would be no difficulty in doing this, and in view of the considerations expressed above it would be quite justifiable. In Batty Tuke's case the patient relapsed in a few days from the mental amelioration, but did not again suffer from headache. The general adoption of this procedure has been disputed by Adam, Revington, and Percy Smith on the ground that the improvement may have been due to spontaneous remission of the disease and on account of the want of exact knowledge of the conditions which the operation is supposed to relieve. The cases in which it would seem that this empirical treatment is likely to be at all successful in palliating the disease are, as has been previously suggested by Claye Shaw, those in which there is notable pain in the head and convulsions. Finally he thinks that operative treatment should be undertaken during the early stages of changes in speech.

To sum up: Since the operation in itself cannot be considered dangerous and since the condition is universally regarded as fatal, and further, since simple trephining can unquestionably relieve the pain when that is present. it might be tried purely empirically.

III. Imbecility (Microcephaly, &c.). —*Pathology.*—Since Lannelongue's well-known communication on the advisability of opening the skull in cases of microcephaly, that treatment has been freely adopted in those patients in whom it was reasonable to assume that there was either defective development of the extensible bony envelope of the brain, or pathological increase of the intra-cranial tension with no corresponding compensation on the part of the growth of the skull. Putting aside such states as cannot be shown to satisfy either of these two conditions, we are left to consider the propriety of surgical interference in cases of microcephaly and hydrocephalus. While speaking on the question of pathology it is perhaps hardly necessary to do more here than allude to the necessity of excluding in any given case the possibility of the particular condition under observation being due, either in part or in the main, to that very obscure but commonly spoken of class of cases in which encephalitis is considered to have occurred in early life and to have been the starting-point of the mental degradation (*cf.* Strümpell, &c.). To return to the cases of (1) *Microcephaly* and (2) *Hydrocephalus*: the former of which must be considered at some length.

(1) *Microcephaly.* — This is not the place to introduce the academic discussion (Broca and Virchow) as to whether the brain condition or skull condition in microcephaly (*q.v.*) is more strictly primary. It is sufficient to remark that in microcephaly a ready distinction may be drawn between the cases according as they are of greater or less severity. Thus, as regards the *cranium*, in the former case, the fontanelles close within the first few months of birth, synostosis of the sutures occurs, and hyperostosis of their margins, while the bone subsequently increases in thickness, but not or only very slightly in superficial area. In the less severe cases the fontanelles do not close so early. Synostosis may be confined to one suture producing plagiocephaly, or only to parts of sutures; the bones of the cranium extend, but very slowly, and individual bones may cease growing after the first year or two of extra-uterine life. As regards the brain in a certain proportion of the former cases, the arrangement of the cortical mantle has been found to be primarily defective and no direct evidence of intra-cranial tension present. In the remainder there is an obvious crowding of the elements of the encephalon and apparently an inhibited tendency of development. In the latter cases (the less severe), and in which the cerebral development has, as suggested, proceeded further, the defect, so far as the brain is concerned, is that due to want of space. Next, as regards other structural conditions observed in microcephalic idiocy, these may be summed up as consisting of arrest of development of the other parts of the body, and in addition of anomalies of development. Coming next to disorders of function, in the worst cases there is great difficulty in procuring the education of simple acts necessary to life—*e.g.*, swallowing. There is at first contracture of usually all the limbs, and, if this passes off and normal movements are not established, the condition becomes one of flaccid paralysis. Finally a severe form of functional disturbance not infrequently present is that of convulsions.

Operative Procedure.—The operation for the relief of microcephaly so far has been designed towards cutting away the synostosed sutures, thus giving room as well as allowing for the natural distension of the bony capsule. The technique of the operation has been variously described, and performed. We believe that the best—*i.e.*, the least disturbing—is the following. The plan must include the performance of the operation piecemeal, since we believe we have shown that a danger to life in the shape of hyperpyrexia may thus be avoided, and it goes without saying that, similarly, shock is much excluded thereby. The first operation consists of a simple incision—*i.e.*, one about 4 centimetres long, parallel with and close to the middle line. A disc of bone averaging 1 to 1.5 centimetres is removed, the wound is closed, and treated in the ordinary way. On subsequent occasions further portions are removed as follows: Parallel incisions are made with a small saw, in the skull one centimetre apart, and continued for 4 to 6 centimetres, according to the condition of the patient. In this manner long strips of bone are removed along the lines of the sutures, so as to free one-half of the parietes of the skull from the middle line. If this be insufficient, as evidenced by the after-condition of the patient (*vide infra*), the other side may be similarly operated upon. The procedure thus described is not the usual one, nor that which is employed by several surgeons at the present time, some preferring to cut away the bone by pushing forceps between the dura and the bone, and so conveniently dividing the latter. While believing that this may be utilised in later operations we cannot help feeling that at the commencement, at any rate, it is a source of danger. The wound ought invariably to heal in a few days by the first intention.

Results of the Operation. — Lannelongue in his second communication, recounting the general results of operation in twenty-five cases, considered that he had thereby obtained permanent improvement in the mental condition, that education before impossible became easy, and in cases where pain was obviously present that it appeared to be relieved. From our own observations, which are confirmatory of those made by the American surgeons, but especially Keen's, the first effect of the operation is to produce noteworthy amelioration of the mental symptoms. If the patient were restless before, he is afterwards unquestionably quieter, does not scream or have apparent attacks of pain as before the operation, and is more amenable. As regards changes in the other disturbances of function referred to, contracture diminishes, and use of the hands and prehension commence. It learns to swallow and to eat. Even in partial operations we have noticed this improvement to continue for six months where the operation was undertaken within the first year of life. It remains now to consider whether the improvement is permanent or whether it will relapse, and finally whether it is possible to obtain it in individuals who have arrived at the fourth or fifth year. Of the latter case, a single experience of our own shows that, as Maunoury found, when only a partial operation is performed, the condition becomes stationary, or may relapse into its former condition three to six months later. At the present time it is impossible to speak definitely on this matter until the after-examination of cases shall have extended over several years. As regards the influence of age in deciding upon the performance of the operation it is obviously most advisable to treat the case as early as possible—*i.e.*, three months after birth. There can be little doubt, on the other hand, that the operation is not promising after the eighth or ninth year on account of the growth of the skull (Merkel). It would be advisable therefore to propose if possible a limit of age after the passing of which it is unlikely that any improvement would result from surgical interference.

(2) *Hydrocephalus.*—Its pathology and treatment need no examination here, it being sufficient to state that relief by operation is called for.

IV. Operative Interference for Hallucinations.—Burckhardt has proposed to remove, in cases of very definite hallucination, the special sense receptive centre which can be determined to be the seat of disturbance, or at least to divide the communicating channels between such centres. He has excised with this object in view portions chiefly of the verbal auditory sense centre. From his carefully published cases it is clear that (1) the hallucinations were diminished, and the mental state improved; (2) the cases were not cured.

Further evidence however is required before this procedure can be generally adopted.

V. Effects of Surgical Treatment in cases of Chronic Epilepsy. — *Pathology.* — Any reference to surgical treatment of cases in which mental deficiency or aberration is present would be incomplete without brief mention of the results of operating in cases of chronic epilepsy, as to the changes produced in the intellect. The mental deficiency, which is so characteristic of chronic epilepsy, is commonly attributed to two distinct causes: (*a*) the cerebral exhaustion produced by the fits; (*b*) the interference with the cerebral functions generally by the action of the original epileptogenic lesion. The operations undertaken for the treatment of chronic epilepsy have hitherto been performed in cases where either there has been a cicatrix involving the bone, &c., or where the focal lesion has been sought for and excised.

The epilepsy in some of these cases has not been cured, but in all those carefully reported there has been observed for a period very shortly after the operation a distinct improvement in the mental state. The patient becomes brighter, takes an intelligent interest, is more careful and attentive, and more receptive of instruction. As just stated, this has been noted even where the fits have not been arrested. The improvement cannot therefore be invariably attributed to the abolition of the exhausting attacks, but it must be due to the removal of some factor by the operation.

It has been surmised that the changes in the conditions of intra-cranial pressure which are induced by the opening of the skull is the source of this improvement. At present, however, it is impossible to satisfactorily explain the causation of the alteration. VICTOR HORSLEY.

TRISTEMANIA, TRISTIMANIA. Synonyms of Melancholia. (Fr. *tristemanie.*)

TRISTITIA (*tristis*, sad). A synonym of Melancholy as distinguished from melancholia (tristemania).

TROMOMANIA (τρομέω, I tremble; μανία, madness). A synonym of Delirium Tremens.

TROPHONEUROSIS (τροφή, nourishment; νεῦρον, a nerve). Atrophy of a part from interference with the nervous influence connected with its nutrition.

TRÜBSINN (Ger.). Melancholia. (Fr. *trophoneuroses*.)

TRUGBILD (Ger.). An illusion.

TRUNKSUCHT (Ger.). Habitual drunkenness, dipsomania (*q.v.*).

TROPHIC LESIONS IN THE INSANE. (*See* BEDSORES; HÆMATOMA AURIS, &c.)

TRUSTS (LAW OF) IN RELATION TO LUNACY.—The Trustee Acts 1850–1852 enable the proper Court

(1) To divest a trustee (or mortgagee) who is lunatic or of unsound mind of property vested in him;

(2) To appoint a new trustee in place of a trustee who has become lunatic or of unsound mind;

(3) To appoint a new trustee where a person in whom a power of appointment is vested becomes of unsound mind.

The most recent work on this subject is Williams's "Petitions in Chancery and Lunacy," to which the reader is referred.

A. WOOD RENTON.

TUBERCULOSIS. (*See* PHTHISICAL INSANITY.)

TUMOURS ON THE BRAIN AND INSANITY. (*See* PATHOLOGY.)

TUMULTUS SERMONIS.—An irregular or stuttering manner of reading.

TURBATIONES ANIMI (*turbatio*, a disturbance; *animus*, the mind). Mental affections.

TURKEY and Egypt.—It appears that in 1560 an asylum called the Suleimanié was founded at Constantinople. It was erected by Sultan Suleiman near the Mosque and the Tib-Khané, or School of Medicine.*

The original name for asylums in Turkey was Dar-ul-Shifá. Subsequently they were termed Timar-Khané, or nursing establishments. Since 1873 the Turks have called them Timar-Khané (Homes for Invalids). In Mr. Burdett's recent work it is stated that after the cholera of 1873 all patients till then confined in the Suleimanié asylum were transferred to the Toptaschi building at Scutari, and there they remain. It is maintained by the prefecture of Constantinople. In it are confined men and women belonging not only to the Ottoman Empire but other nationalities. In March 1884 there were 492 patients, of whom 441 were Musselmans, 35 [illegible] Jews.

The description given of the former state of the Scutari asylum is deplorable in the extreme, the patients being chained by the neck to their cells, while wild beasts were kept in the same place. Even in 1884 in the civil hospital at [illegible], insane patients were very badly treated, two were chained by the neck to the floor of the passage leading from the door of the hospital to the wards of the patients; another was chained to the floor at the entrance to one of the rooms occupied by the ordinary patients; while another was secured in the same manner to the flooring of a cell in the court-yard. Mr. Burdett, from whose laborious work these particulars are taken, states that all the chains were long, massive and heavy, and attached to the neck by thick strong iron rings. A fifth was hypochondriacal, but was not chained. It is added that the shrieks and howlings of the others were heard throughout that quarter of [illegible] and greatly disturbed the inhabitants, and there seems no reason to suppose that the terrible condition of the inmates of the hospital has been ameliorated.

Dr. J. H. Davidson, the medical superintendent of the County Asylum, Cheshire, communicated to the *Journal of Mental Science*, April 1875, an interesting account of a visit to the asylum at Constantinople (Toptaschi in Scutari), under the charge of the visiting physician, Dr. Mongeri. There were two medical assistants, a surgical assistant and a dispenser. There were 300 males and 74 female patients in the asylum at the time of Dr. Davidson's visit. The disparity of the sexes is due to a religious scruple as to not placing females in a lunatic asylum. Some lunatics ramble about the streets without clothing, and are regarded with veneration. All the inmates of the institution, Mussulmans or Christians, rich or poor, must be dressed in the asylum uniform. The costume, it seems, resembles that worn by the dervishes. Acts of insubordination at the time of the medical visit are immediately suppressed by a shower bath, given in the presence of a numerous staff in order to overawe the patient. There are preserved in the asylum the chains, collars and *fallacca*, in use in former times. These are replaced by the camisole, which is, however, stated to be rarely used. Reil's belt is sometimes resorted to. The prolonged bath for ten or twelve hours is frequently employed, as is also the Turkish bath. There is little or no employment for the patients. Dr. Davidson states that Dr. Mongeri has reformed the

* "Hospitals and Asylums of the World," by Henry C. Burdett, 1891, vol. i. p. 58.

asylum: "He had many difficulties and prejudices to contend with, but these have, in a great measure been happily overcome by his unflagging energy and indomitable perseverance, and the patients now confined in the Timar-Khané experience a judicious and humane treatment."

Egypt.—The asylum at Cairo has from time to time been described by English visitors. In 1877 it was visited by Dr. Urquhart, and by Mr. W. S. Tuke in 1878. In 1888 Dr. F. M. Sandwith described its condition.*

They agreed in regard to its miserable condition. Mr. Tuke spoke of the dirt and squalor which at once struck any one familiar with an English county asylum. The impression received by him was most unfavourable. At the Coptic Church of St. George, at Old Cairo, the visitor is shown a pillar to which a chain is attached. To this pillar a person labouring under acute mania is fastened for three days without food—a procedure which is regarded as almost a certain cure of the malady."

Dr. Urquhart wrote: "The whole place is so utterly beyond the ken of civilisation, that it remains as hideous a blot on the earth's surface as is to be found even in the Dark Continent." †

Dr. Sandwith states that the patients were removed in 1880 from the asylum, or more correctly, warehouse, to the remains of a palace in the suburbs of Cairo. In 1884 the chiefs of the department which controls the asylum and hospitals retired, and a native pasha and Dr. Sandwith succeeded them. He found "240 men and 60 women clothed in rags, sitting all day long upon their beds, without exercise and without occupation. Any men who had the reputation of having been dangerous were made to wear chains similar to those used in Egypt for hard labour convicts. These chains are six feet long, are fastened by a key round both ankles, and weigh 5½ lbs. On the ground floor with stone pavement, were the dormitories—some excellent rooms on the first floor being unused; and in a secluded corner of the ground floor, on the maleside, were four dark, barred dungeons, each provided with a central hole leading direct into a cesspool beneath. In the walls and floors of these dungeons were fixed iron rings for fastening the ankles, and either the waist or the wrists of the unfortunate patient; while under him was placed a wooden plank, with a red leather cushion for his head fastened to it. . . . . But perhaps the worst things noted were the latrines. These were triangular holes in the flooring, communicating directly, by means of a shaft inside the wall, with the numerous rectangular cesspool passages, which honeycombed the old palace and its grounds. The smell from these latrines, even when kept externally clean, could be traced for several yards. . . . . There were no official visitors to the asylum, strangers were refused admission, and patients' friends could rarely obtain entrance. The attendants were effete and useless men and women drafted from the general native hospital." Dr. Sandwith proceeds: "I had already had the pleasure of striking the chains off all prisoners, treated in the twenty-three hospitals under the control of the Sanitary Department, and I now removed all chains from the asylum. . . . . As a substitute we provided camisoles made in Cairo, after the pattern of some kindly sent to me by Dr. Savage. I may mention here that these were very seldom required, but when used for acute mania, they answered the purpose admirably. . . . . The patients were induced to employ themselves in the kitchen, &c., and in six months the male airing yard had become a flourishing garden. Good bath rooms were provided. The drainage was attended to. In short the whole place was transformed. As is well known, the most common cause of insanity in Egypt is smoking Indian hemp. Religious excitement is another cause, but it is often difficult to distinguish between cause and effect. The asylum generally contains two or three Mussulman fanatics who believe themselves prophets. One patient believed himself to be the great Mahdi from the Soudan. Another patient, a chronic melancholiac, had been an officer in Arabi's army. Dr. Sandwith notes with satisfaction how the attendants control their patients with good-humoured chaff. He has never seen anything like unkind treatment. A very small number of the lunatic population are sent to the asylum because the native retains his relative at home as a religious duty. The word employed for an insane person is magzoob (struck by the wrath), or *magnoon* (the victim of ginua or madness.) Alcohol, Indian hemp, and domestic trouble are the chief causes of insanity among women. Dr. Sandwith makes the observation, that general paralysis appears to be unknown to the cereal-eating natives, although they frequently have syphilis, and indulge in great excesses. It is occasionally met with among well-to-do Orientals in good circumstances, "who eat meat freely, use their brains more than their hands, and are not strict tee-

* *Journal of Mental Science*, Jan. 1889, p. 473.
† *Ibid.* April 1879, p. 48.

totallers." He has found among the Cairo insane, several with trembling of the lips and tongue, without other symptoms, while others with ideas of grandeur turn out to be haschisch cases. The Editor.

TURKISH BATHS. (*See* Baths.)

"TURN OF LIFE," AND INSANITY. (*See* Climacteric Insanity.)

TWINS, INSANITY IN (Fr. *folie gémellaire*). — The extraordinary resemblances that exist between twins when they have attained the adult age have long attracted attention, and if in some cases there is absolutely no likeness, and in others the likeness is no more striking than might be expected in children of the same parents, and necessarily akin to one another in character and organisation, we are, on the other hand, compelled to recognise that there is so close a resemblance between some twins, either intellectually, as regards the physiognomy and the expression of the face, or in respect to states of health and disease, that it seems almost to amount to identity.

It is not only in external likeness that these resemblances exist; it is also, and especially, in the intimate organisation of the nervous system, and in the physiological consequences that result.

The same disease has sometimes been known to occur in twins, almost at the same moment, and following the same course—a proof of the close relationship between the two natures. When the disease in question is a mental aberration the proof acquires a greater force, and leads naturally to the conclusion that the cerebral organisation of the two individuals must have the deepest analogy.

Some few cases of insanity of twins have been placed upon record. By this is meant the mental aberration, developed almost simultaneously in both twins, exhibiting the same kind of delirium, and outside of the usual conditions of occurrence of communicated insanity, or *folie à deux*. As a matter of fact twins may, like any other members of an insane family, become the subjects of mental derangement one after the other, and manifest the same symptoms of perturbation of the intelligence.

But by insanity of twins is to be especially understood, the mental derangement developed in conditions peculiar to twins, and characterised by the three following peculiarities:

(1) **Simultaneity of occurrence;**

(2) **Parallelism of insane conceptions and of other psychological disturbances;**

(3) **Spontaneity of the delirium in each of the individuals affected.**

These three characteristics may be found in the highest degree in the following cases:

Case I.—*Acute Mania with Predominance of Mystical Ideas, and Multiple Hallucinations occurring almost simultaneously in Twin Sisters.*

(*a*) *Family History.*—The father was a sober, healthy man, a gendarme, he married early, and had six children, four girls and two boys. All the children had been healthy up to the date of the commencement of this observation. The father died at the age of fifty-two of sudden apoplexy, without ever having presented cerebral symptoms, or intellectual disturbances.

The mother's history is wanting. She died in childbed at an early age.

The twins, left orphans at five years of age, were brought up together in Lorraine until they were fourteen. They had always presented the closest physical resemblance, so much that it is not easy to distinguish one from the other. They are both tall, of robust constitution, and of sanguine temperament. They have a fresh colour, high cheekbones, round faces, brown hair and eyes.

With respect to character, Louise is more serious, and even sadder than Laure, who has always been of a gay disposition. Louise, however, has always lived a hard life, and since her husband's illness, besides the unhappiness that it had caused her, she has undergone frequent privations, sometimes even wanting for food.

The two sisters have always been united by the most tender affection; their education has been the same, and it is worth while noting that exaggerated devotion formed no part of their training. This is an important point, inasmuch as the delusions in both are essentially of a mystical nature.

From the age of fourteen their existences become separate. They are both twenty-nine years old at the present time. Louise came at once to Paris; Laure remained in the country for some years. Louise married in Paris when she was twenty-one. She has a delicate child seven years old.

Existence for this woman, in business as a greengrocer, has been a long struggle. Her husband fell seriously ill, with albuminuria, three years ago. During the whole of this time the wife has tended her husband devotedly, but without neglecting the interests of her little business. On the evening of the 16th of November 1883, a priest was called to administer the last sacraments to the husband.

The wife dismissed him because she did

not like the look of his face. This may have been the beginning of mental disturbance. At any rate, in the course of the night, the insanity broke out in all its intensity. She threw herself on her husband's neck, kissed him, and exclaimed, "Jean is cured, I see the good God." From this moment she became more and more agitated; she went to the window to sing hymns, broke the panes of glass, insulted those present, and struck the doctor who was standing at the patient's bedside. The police having arrived to remove her, she rushed down into the street upon seeing them, and tried to prevent them entering the house, crying: "I am death, you shall not pass." It must be said that for six days she had been watching her husband, almost without eating. She had never exceeded the bounds of moderation in the use of alcoholic beverages.

Upon removal to the Prefecture (Central Police Station) she exhibited all the symptoms of maniacal agitation, giving way to an unceasing loquacity, stating that she was the Virgin Mary, and that she could resuscitate the dead. Insomnia absolute.

During this time a new complication occurs in this domestic drama. Laure, the twin sister of Louise, is seized with a fit of mental aberration almost at the same moment.

Called to the bedside of her brother-in-law, she had already watched there one night, when Louise, in her presence, had suddenly become insane. Two days later the man had died, and Laure had been to the funeral. At her brother-in-law's grave she had begun to talk nonsense, and no sooner had she been conducted home than an attack of furious delirium broke out. Four days after the fit of insanity that had necessitated the removal of her sister, she was taken to the Asile Ste.-Anne, under the care of Dr. Bouchereau. The following are the separate histories of these two patients:

(*b*) *Case of Louise.*—Removed to the *Clinique*. Louise was admitted on November 17, 1883. Treatment, chloral 4 grammes (one drachm). Prolonged bath.

The day after admission the patient is calmer, she asks for news of her husband; and has no longer any delusions.

The 9th of December she is still calm. She is told with the greatest caution of the death of her husband, and appears very resigned.

On December 11, as she appeared quite restored to reason, she was taken to see her sister. She was kind and affectionate to Laure, who is still in full maniacal delirium. Towards the end of the visit, Louise became excited; she would not leave her sister, and it was with some difficulty that she was conducted back to her ward. The rest of the day she talked nonsense, and was unreasonable.

December 14.—The patient is seized with irresistible impulses. She throws herself on those who come near, bites the attendants, and kicks them.

At the same time she appears to have hallucinations of hearing. She hears accusations to which she replies by the acknowledgment of an imaginary guilt.

December 21.—Appearance of menses; agitation increasingly violent. She strikes an attendant; placed in a separate room, she removes a panel of the door. She refuses food, spits out her medicine, passes the night without sleep. Treatment: Prolonged baths, bromide of potassium, chloral, &c.

The agitation did not cease for a moment until January 2, when there was an interval of calm, but on the 4th of January, the symptoms returned in all their intensity.

January 12.—Hallucinations of sight. Thinks she sees her husband running about in his nightdress, calls him by his name, says she is a bee, that she has a great deal of work to do. Does not cease for a minute to sing and shout, and to knock against the walls of the cell.

January 17.—Shouted and jumped all the day. At dinner-time she escaped from the attendants and rushed into the garden, round which she ran three times, allowing herself afterwards to be reconducted to her cell.

January 19.—Still excited. Throws herself against the walls; sees trees upon which are birds, calls them, and tries to catch them.

The agitation continues until Feb. 5. At this date she is feverish and obliged to remain in bed. Milk diet—saline purgative, which operated. The patient began to grow calmer from this time, asked if her family inquired after her, and wanted to go and nurse her sick husband. Not being allowed to do so, she exclaimed, "I am here for the remainder of my life." Sleep is fairly good.

February 24.—Return of agitation; patient breaks everything, tears her clothes, loses her sleep. This, with few intermissions, is her condition until the end of March.

April 3.—She is calmer; saw her brother-in-law for a quarter of an hour, and talked with him in the parlour. Appeared gay and contented.

April 6.—The patient was shown to the

class at the Clinic; her sister was also brought in, and the meeting was most affectionate, but after a few minutes they became agitated and were removed.

Louise was excited until the 21st of the month, when she became relatively calm.

May 3.—The patient still calm; works and sleeps well; she eats gluttonously, her appetite being insatiable. The affective sense is much blunted. She makes no inquiries about her child, and remains indifferent to her position, except that she claims her liberty on the ground that she has been here long enough, and finds it tiresome.

June 7.—The patient is calm, and she no longer appears insane. She manifests, however, an unnatural indifference to her position, only expressing from time to time a fear of a return of the agitation. "It seems to me," she says, "as if it were going to return."

(c) *Case of Laure.*—This patient was admitted under the care of Dr. Bouchereau on November 27, 1883, in a state of violent maniacal excitement. She broke the windows, banged the doors, and declaimed in an incoherent manner, mystical and ambitious ideas being predominant. She is the Virgin Mary, the Queen of France, &c. She crosses herself frequently, goes on her knees, lifts up her arms and turns her face upwards in the attitude of prayer.

During the following weeks the excitement continues, her movements are sudden and her acts purposeless. She has sudden fits of agitation, threatening, biting, striking, throwing herself upon the attendants, and committing other acts of impulsive violence. She gives way to insults and bad language, and often sings for hours together. Occasionally she undresses herself. She always goes barefooted, refusing to wear anything on the feet. At times she throws herself at full length in her cell and pronounces an incoherent monologue, or else she will be found upon her knees praying. She often sees the Saviour, the saints and angels. Sometimes, however, it is, on the contrary, serpents that appear. She has several times repeated that it is sought to make her swallow poison.

She often breaks out into sudden and prolonged fits of laughter. Her appetite is generally good. Insomnia is almost absolute. She talks, sings, and makes a noise at night.

The maniacal excitement and impulsive phenomena remained about the same until the middle of February. From this date her acts became less disorderly, and although still more or less excitable, she was no longer violent, [illegible] at sewing: the incoherence of [illegible] unchanged. There were all kinds of hallucinations—strange noises and [illegible] visions. Sometimes the sky would open, and she would see the doctors who spoke and made signs to her. Sometimes she saw women hanged, or cut up in pieces. From time to time she had genital hallucinations.

March 20.—The patient is calmer and occupies herself more than before, but there is still the same incoherence of ideas. She often laughs without being able to assign a reason.

April 1.—Her attitude is better. The patient is civil and works fairly well. She exhibits real pleasure when she receives a visit from her husband or children.

From time to time she has a slight agitation with shrieks and cries, but these last only a few minutes, and are not frequent.

April 6.—She is brought into the presence of her sister in the lecture-theatre of the Clinic, and the two patients reciprocally exciting one another have to be separated.

May 4.—Laure is fairly calm, her memory is good, and she remembers some facts in connection with her admission to St. Anne. She is, however, far from being completely cured; her attitude is often singular, and her ideas incoherent or confused. She imagines that she is being "worked;" she feels a weight in the abdomen and uterus, and disagreeable sensations in other parts of the body; she will not, however, explain more fully as *we know better than herself what is the cause of it.*

She believes that she is descended from an illustrious family, perhaps even from a royal one. She knows that the heavens and earth belong to her because the devil has crowned her.

It is more particularly in the intermediary condition, between sleep and waking, and chiefly in the morning that she has visions. She sees children, and quarters of the moon descending from heaven. Three days ago she saw a big man with a big woman in a complete state of nudity.

She appears to be greatly concerned about her twin sister, for whom she has always had the warmest affection. She is constantly asking to be discharged, as her presence is necessary at home, her husband being obliged in her absence to place the till in the hands of a stranger.

Menstruation is regular, lasting last time about three days. There is some anæmia, a soft systolic murmur at the base, and a continuous musical *bruit* in the two carotids.

May 11.—Examined again from a psychological point of view. The patient persists in her delusions. She has visions particularly towards the morning; she believes that she is queen, having been crowned by the devil and another person; she also believes that she is a spirit. She says that her father is dead; he was the Wandering Jew.

To recapitulate: these twin sisters, very alike both morally and physically, were both seized with delirium accompanied by maniacal excitement, hallucinations of the sight and of other senses, ambitious and mystical ideas, and general intellectual disturbance. The symptoms broke out under circumstances in which each had been painfully shocked, but without its being possible to explain the coincidence by contagion.

Louise had been separated from her sister as soon as the delirium commenced. It is evident that the delirium, which occurred at four days' interval in the two sisters, must be attributed to one and the same cause, that is, to the same moral traumatism. And it is only by the most intimate resemblance of cerebral organisation that we can explain so striking a parallelism of symptoms under the influence of this cause.

Cases like the preceding are not common, but several authentic observations of the kind have been recorded. The following are sufficiently conclusive to be worth quoting:

CASE II.—"*Délire de Persécution*" *occurring simultaneously in Twin Brothers*.*—I have, at the present time in my wards, says Moreau de Tours, two brothers, twins, affected with monomania. Their mother was mad. A maternal aunt is at the Salpêtrière. Their eldest sister has a son, nineteen years old, remarkable for his intelligence and for a singular aptitude for mathematics. For the last two years this young man has by himself done all the bookkeeping of one of the most important houses in Paris. When he was four or five years old it was noticed that the whole of the left side of the body was much less developed than the right. The same want of symmetry exists at the present time, and is sufficiently evident to attract attention.

The twins resemble one another physically to such a degree that they might easily be taken one for the other. Morally, the likeness is no less complete, and presents the most remarkable peculiarities.

* Moreau de Tours. "La Psychologie Morbide," pp. 139 (note) and 172.

For instance, the dominant ideas are the same. Both believe that they are the objects of imaginary persecutions, the same enemies have sworn their ruin, and they adopt the same means to this end. Both of them have hallucinations of hearing. Unhappy and morose they never speak a word to anybody, and answer with reluctance such questions as are addressed to them. They always keep alone, and never speak to one another.

A very curious fact has been observed over and over again by the attendants, and also by ourselves. From time to time, at irregular intervals of two, three or more months by the spontaneous effect of the disease, and without any appreciable cause, a marked change occurs in the state of the two brothers.

Both of them come out of their stupor and habitual prostration at the same period, and sometimes the same day. They utter the same complaints and come of their own accord to beg the doctor to restore them to liberty. We have known this to occur, strange as it may appear, even when they were separated by several miles: the one being at Bicêtre, the other at Ste.-Anne. The closest parallelism is here seen, bringing the twin brothers into sympathy as to one and the same mental disorder, both suffering from the monomania of persecution. They presented the paradoxical phenomenon, which has previously been noted in other cases, of manifesting at the same day, and at the same hour, recurrences and transformations of their delirium. Lastly, there existed, as we have seen, hereditary antecedents pointing without doubt to mental disease in the family. The importance of this fact will be seen further on.

A most remarkable case of the same kind was recorded by Dr. Baume in the *Annales Médico-psychologiques* for 1863, which is as follows:—

CASE III.—*Singular Case of Insanity. Suicide of Twin Brothers. Strange Coincidences.* — Mental pathology gives rise to the most inexplicable problems, but the following case, says the author, has appeared to me peculiarly strange.

Two brothers, twins, fifty years of age, Martin and François, worked as contractors on the railway from Quimper to Châteaulin.

Martin had given signs, five years previously, of temporary mental alienation, and two months ago he had experienced a relapse, but of short duration. His family declare that there is no hereditary predisposition.

Towards the 15th of January (the present month) the brothers were robbed of three hundred francs, the money having been removed from a trunk in which they placed their common savings. During the night of the 23rd, François, who lodged at Quimper, and Martin who resided with his children at the Lorette (five miles from Quimper), dreamt at the same hour, three o'clock in the morning, the same thing, and both awoke suddenly crying out, "*I have him; I've got the thief; they are hurting my brother!*" giving way to the same extravagances, and manifesting their great agitation by dancing and jumping on the floor. Martin seized upon his grandson, whom he took for the thief, and would have strangled him had he not been prevented by his children. This agitation became gradually worse; he complained of violent headache, declaring that he was lost. On the 24th it was with great difficulty that he was persuaded to remain at home, and towards four in the afternoon he went out, followed closely by his son. He kept along the side of the river Steir, uttering incoherent sentences, and attempted to drown himself. He was only prevented by the energetic interference of his son. The police, upon the warrant of the neighbouring mayor, brought him to the asylum at seven in the evening, Martin, then insane, being in the greatest state of agitation.

Whilst Martin had reached at the outset the extreme limits of acute insanity, his twin brother, François, promptly enough calmed on the morning of the 24th, passed the day in seeking after the perpetrator of the robbery. Towards six o'clock in the evening it so happened that he encountered his brother, just as he was struggling with the gendarmes, who were taking him to the asylum. He exclaimed: "Oh, my God! my brother is lost! if they take him for the thief they will murder him!" After gesticulating wildly he proceeded to the Lorette, to the ambulance of the railway works, complained of violent pains in the head, and said it was all over with him, using some of the same incoherent expressions as his brother. He requested to be attended to, which was done. He soon said he felt better, and left under the pretence of business, going and drowning himself at the very same place where his brother had unsuccessfully attempted to do the same thing some hours before. He was recovered from the water but did not survive.

Martin, admitted into the asylum on the evening of the 24th, died suddenly on the morning of the 27th. During this period of time there was no lucid interval, and the first two nights were passed in a state of extreme agitation, the patient thinking that he was God, the emperor, &c.

On the 26th, after a bath of several hours' duration, with cold affusions on the head, he was somewhat calm; but at ten P.M. the excitement returned with renewed violence. He dashed his head several times against the wall, and also attacked the attendants. Finally, the overseer of the section had just got him back to bed in the same state of excitement, when without any apparent cause he expired in our presence. The strongest restoratives had been used to no effect.

At the post-mortem examination, thirty-eight hours after death, we found a venous hæmorrhage between the two layers of the arachnoid, over the posterior half of the encephalon. There were about four hundred grammes of dark fluid blood mixed with soft granular clots. The hæmorrhage due to the excitement of the patient and his attempts to dash out his brains against the walls, had probably occurred but a few moments before the fatal issue.

So died these twins. Their mental aberration, due to the same cause, manifested the same peculiarities, and after breaking out at the same time would have ended by the same kind of suicide, at the same spot, had not one of the brothers been prevented from executing his impulse by circumstances independent of his will.

The *Journal of Mental Science* contains three cases of the same kind.

Dr. Savage* relates two, and it is worthy of note that in each instance there was a condition of profound lypemania.

The third was observed by Dr. Clifford Gill. Twin sisters, twenty years of age, and bearing the greatest resemblance to one another both physically and morally, became insane almost simultaneously. A most remarkable parallelism, both physiological and pathological, had previously existed. On one occasion one of the sisters being at Scarborough, and the other at York, the latter suffering from headache and biliousness, said to her mother that her sister was suffering in the same way, and the supposition turned out to be quite correct. One of the sisters manifests symptoms of maniacal excitement with a predominance of erotic ideas; the other has attacks of mania with hallucinations, and a predominance of religious delusions. In both cases the mental symptoms are intermittent.

Dr. Flintoff Mickle, in the same journal, relates the case of twin sisters, who, like the preceding, showed the greatest resemblance both morally and physically.

* *Journal of Mental Science*, January 1883.

The symptoms are exactly the same in each subject, being those of melancholia of the religious type. Both imagine that they are damned, have a tendency to suicide, and suffer from hallucinations of the sight. But whilst one became insane for the first time at the age of twenty-nine, the other, who went to America after her marriage, instead of remaining like her sister in England, did not lose her reason until twelve years later. This makes it all the more remarkable that her delusions should be identical with those of her sister, and that their religious terrors should be expressed in the same terms.

Cases such as the above are not frequent in medical literature, but it is probable that they would be more so if the twins were not separated from one another in most instances when the insanity has occurred.*

As the interest of the observations resides chiefly in the parallelism between the two subjects, it is evident that most cases of the kind fail to be recorded. It is probable, however, that, once the attention of alienists is drawn to the question, cases will become more numerous—so much so as to no longer be exceptional.

As it is, some interesting conclusions may be deduced from the documents that we possess.

If insanity in twins were only to be looked upon as a natural curiosity, and worthy of record in the chapter of *casus rariores*, it would be of little interest to science, but such is certainly not the case.

It must first be observed that the likeness between twins may vary extremely in degree. Sometimes it exists in the most striking manner; in most instances it is much less, and in some twins there is as much difference as in the ordinary children of the same family.

Now, in all the cases of insanity of twins that we have collected, the closest physical and moral resemblance has always been noted. Not only have the features been alike, but the intellectual and moral dispositions have also coincided in a remarkable degree. The nature of the delirium has been essentially the same, and with the exception of Dr. F. Mickle's case, the date of the first symptoms was the same, so that it is rational to see in these intellectual disturbances the evidence of a deep analogy in the cerebral organisation and the physiological function.

* See a very interesting case reported by Dr. McDowall (Morpeth) in the *Journal of Mental Science*, July 1884, with portraits showing the most marked resemblance.—Ed.

Sometimes, as in the case of Moreau de Tours, the attacks occur at the same time in both patients, and are separated by intervals of remission common to both.

Some of these patients have a family history of insanity, but others are entirely free from any hereditary taint of the kind. There exists then an intellectual and moral affinity, extending beyond the ordinary limits of consanguinity.

Nothing is, of course, more common than the same kind of insanity in different children of the same parents constituting a family, but at the root of these morbid manifestations we generally find heredity, and we cannot wonder at different branches of the same tree bearing the same fruit.

Twins are brothers with a closer tie. Born at the same time, conceived under identical circumstances, they have experienced the same influences during the whole period of gestation, and in some, if not in all cases, there has resulted a striking resemblance of cerebral organisation and of physical health. Such can be the only possible origin of these pathological symptoms which, breaking out at the same moment, follow an absolutely identical course, characterised by the same phases and same observations.

Some accessory points complete the likeness, and confirm these conclusions. The affection and proverbial sympathy existing between twins are developed to the highest degree in the subjects of these pathological observations; their influence upon one another morally is not beneficial; nearly always, in the course of their illness, the contact of the two individuals has been most harmful to both.

In these phenomena may be seen a still more convincing proof of the profound likeness of the two organisations, which react with such a deep intensity upon one another.

To sum up in a word our conclusions, we may say that heredity dominates the whole question, and that insanity in twins is but the highest and most striking manifestation of this force, which kneads living matter at its will, and reigns through the whole series of organised beings. B. Ball.

TYPHOID FEVER. (*See* Fever, Enteric; Post-Febrile Insanity.)

TYPHOID STATE.—A name given to the symptoms characteristic of the late stages of typhoid and typhus fever, but which occur also in other diseases. The patient lies on his back, unable to move himself, in a state of low muttering delirium, subsultus, the pulse feeble, and the mouth and lips covered with sordes.

TYPHOMANIA (τῦφος, stupor; μανία, madness). Hippocrates employed the word τυφομανία to denote a state of stupefaction in which the patient is suddenly deprived of his senses as if thunderstruck, in which sense, according to Hippocrates, it may have been immediately derived from τυφέω or τυφώς, a whirlwind). A state of lethargy complicated with low muttering delirium. The term has been also applied to acute mania running a rapid course and attended by exhaustion. Dr. Luther Bell first described it in 1844; hence it is called Bell's disease. (Fr. *typhomanie.*) (*See* ACUTE DELIRIOUS MANIA.)

TYRIASIS.—A term meaning, among other things, satyriasis.

U

UNCONSCIOUS CEREBRATION.—That activity of intellect and mental modification which goes on without the consciousness of the subject. It is analogous to the automatic unconscious movement of the limbs from habit, as, for instance, the movement of the legs in going upstairs. A frequently occurring example of unconscious cerebration is the following:—Occasionally during conversation one forgets a name or a phrase, which baffles all attempts at recollection at the time, but when the subject has been dropped, and the mind is engaged with something else, the name or phrase will spontaneously recur.

We have under AUTOMATISM referred to the very early enunciation by Laycock of the reflex action of the brain, and the later adoption of a similar, although not altogether identical, doctrine by Dr. Carpenter, under the designation of unconscious cerebration. It should be added that Griesinger, at a somewhat later period than Laycock, but prior to Carpenter, recognised psychical reflex action in an article contributed to the *Archiv für Physiolog. Heilkund*, entitled "Ueber psychische Reflexactionen, mit einem Blick auf das Wesen der psychischen Krankheiten."

The following are Dr. Laycock's earliest contributions to the subject:—*The Edinburgh Medical and Surgical Journal*, July 1838; "Treatise on the Nervous Diseases of Women," 1840; Paper read before the British Association for the Advancement of Science, 1844, published in the *British and Foreign Medical Review*, January 1845, entitled, "On the Reflex Function of the Brain." Laycock always referred to the original views of Unzer and Prochaska, who appear to have recognised, although dimly, the reflex action of the ganglia at the base of the brain.

Reflex action of the cerebrum might presumably occur with or without consciousness. The point to which Carpenter specially directed attention was its unconscious action. His views were first enunciated in the fourth edition of "Human Physiology," 1852. He maintained that while "the extension of the doctrine of reflex action to the brain was first advocated by Dr. Laycock," he had not clearly stated that such action might be unconscious. He, however, accepted Dr. Laycock's statement that he had fully intended to convey that idea. He regards unconscious cerebration as synonymous with the "Mental Latency" of Sir William Hamilton.*

UNCONSCIOUS KINÆSTHETIC IMPRESSIONS (κινέω, I move; αἴσθησις, sensation; kinæsthesis, meaning therefore sense of movement). Unconscious kinæsthetic impressions are those impressions pertaining to our sense of movement which, though at first necessary, can from habit be dispensed with, as far as consciousness of their existence is concerned, in the guidance of our actions.

UNCONSCIOUSNESS.—The antithesis of consciousness (*q.v.*).

UNCONTROLLABLE IMPULSES.—In most mental diseases self-control is lost, but in some forms the loss of power of self-control is the main feature of the case. The commoner impulses are towards suicide, homicide, destruction, stealing, drinking and immorality. (*See* DESTRUCTIVE AND IMPULSIVE ACTS.)

UNDUE INFLUENCE.—It is necessary, in considering the law of undue influence, to draw a clear distinction between gifts *inter vivos* and testamentary dispositions.

(1) **Undue Influence in Procuring Gifts Inter Vivos.**—Here there are two groups of cases.

(*a*) The first group consists of those cases in which there has been some unfair and improper conduct, some coercion from outside, some over-reaching, some form of cheating, and generally, though not always, some personal advantage obtained

* "Principles of Mental Physiology," 1874, pp. 515–543.

by a donee placed in some close and confidential relation to the donor.* *Lyon* v. *Home*† may be taken as an illustration. A., a widow, aged 75, within a few days after first seeing B., who claimed to be a "spiritual medium," was induced from her belief that she was fulfilling the wishes of her deceased husband, *conveyed to her through the medium of B.*, to adopt him as her son, and transfer £24,000 to him; to make her will in his favour; afterwards to give him a further sum of £6000; and also to settle upon him, subject to her life interest, the reversion of £30,000—these gifts being made without consideration and without power of revocation. Giffard, V.C., decided that the gifts were fraudulent and void.

(*b*) The second group consists of cases where the relations between the donor and the donee have at, or shortly before, the execution of the gift been such as to raise a presumption that the donee had influence over the donor. In such cases the Court throws upon the donee the burden of proving that he has not abused his position, and that the gift made to him has not been brought about by any undue influence upon his part. In this class of cases it has been considered necessary to show that the donor had independent advice, and was removed from the influence of the donee when the gift to him was made. This proposition may best be illustrated by a few cases. In *Huguenin* v. *Baseley* (1807, 14 Ves. Jun. 273), a voluntary settlement by a widow upon a clergyman, who had not only acquired considerable spiritual influence over her, but was entrusted by her with the management of her property, was set aside. The *ratio decidendi* in this and similar cases appears to have been that a confidential relation being proved to exist between the donor and the donee, the Court will presume that it continued up to and at the time of the gift, unless this inference is *clearly disproved by the donee*. It seems, however, that this statement of the law must be taken with the following qualification. "When a gift is made to a person standing in a confidential relation to the donor, the Court will not set the gift aside *if of a small amount* simply on the ground that the donor had no independent advice. In such a case some proof of the exercise of the influence of the donee must be given. . . . But if the gift is so large as not to be reasonably accounted for on the ground of friendship, relationship, charity, or other ordinary motives on which ordinary men act, the burden is upon the donee to support the gift" (per Lindley, L.J., in *Allcard* v. *Skinner*, *ubi sup.* at p. 185; *cf. Rhodes* v. *Bate*, L. R. 1 Ch. 258).

In *Bainbrigge* v. *Browne* (1881, 18 Ch. D. 188), it was held by Fry, J., that, when a deed conferring a benefit on a father is executed by a child who is not emancipated from the father's control, if the deed is subsequently impeached by the child, the *onus* is on the father to show that the child had independent advice, and that he executed the deed with full knowledge of its contents, and with a free intention of giving the father the benefit conferred by it. If this *onus* be not discharged the deed will be set aside.

The case which has carried the doctrine under consideration to the furthest extent is *Allcard* v. *Skinner* (1887, 36 Ch. D. 144–193).

In 1868, A. was introduced by N., her spiritual director and confessor, to S., the lady superior of a sisterhood, and became an associate of the sisterhood. N. was one of the founders, and also the spiritual director and confessor, of the sisterhood, which was an association of ladies who devoted themselves to good works. In 1871, A. having passed through the grades of postulant and novice, became a professed member of the sisterhood, and bound herself to observe (*inter alia*) the rules of poverty, chastity, and obedience by which the sisterhood was regulated, and which were made known to her when she became an associate. These rules were drawn up by N. The rule of poverty required the member to give up all her property either to her relatives, or to the poor, or to the sisterhood itself; but the forms in the schedule to the rule were in favour of the sisterhood, and provided that property made over to the lady superior should be held by her in trust for the general purposes of the sisterhood. The rule of obedience required the member to regard the voice of her superior as the voice of God. The rules also enjoined that no sister should seek the advice of any extern without the superior's leave. A., within a few days after becoming a member, made a will bequeathing all her property to S., and in 1872 and 1874, handed over and transferred to S. several large sums of money and railway stock. In May 1879, A. left the sisterhood, and immediately revoked her will, but made no demand for the return of her property till 1885, when she commenced an action against S. for that purpose, on the ground that she had

* Per Lindley, L.J., in *Allcard* v. *Skinner*, 1887, 36 Ch. D. at p. 181.

† 1868, L. R. 6 Eq. 655, 682. Mr. Hume Williams's book on "Unsoundness of Mind" contains an amusing and instructive account of this and similar cases.

disposed of her property while acting under the paramount and undue influence of S., and without any independent and separate advice. It was held by the Court of Appeal that although A. had voluntarily, and while she had independent advice, entered the sisterhood with the intention of devoting her fortune to it, yet as, at the time when she made the gifts she was subject to the influence of S. and N., and to the rules of the sisterhood, she would have been entitled on leaving the sisterhood to claim restitution of such part of her property as was still in the hands of S.,* if her own delay and acquiescence since leaving the sisterhood had not barred her claim.†

"The equitable title of the donee," said Lindley, L.J., "is imperfect by reason of the influence inevitably resulting from her position, and which influence experience has taught the Courts to regard as undue. Whatever doubt I might have had on this point, if there had been no rule against consulting externs, that rule in judgment turns the scale against the defendant. In the face of that rule the gifts to the sisterhood cannot be supported in the absence of proof that the plaintiff could have obtained independent advice if she wished for it, and that she knew she would have been allowed to obtain such advice if she had desired to do so. I doubt whether the gifts could have been supported if such proof had been given, unless there was also proof that she was free to act on the advice which might be given to her. But the rule itself is so oppressive and so easily abused that any person subject to it is in my opinion brought within the class of those whom it is the duty of the Court to protect from possible imposition. The gifts cannot be supported without proof of more freedom in fact than the plaintiff can be supposed to have actually enjoyed."‡

(2) **Undue Influence in Procuring Testamentary Dispositions.**—Here a very different rule of law prevails. In the case of gifts or other transactions *inter vivos* it is considered by the courts of equity that the influence arising from natural or professional relationships, if exerted by those who possess it to obtain a benefit for themselves, is an undue influence. Gifts or contracts brought about by it are, therefore, set aside, unless *the party benefited by it can show affirmatively** that the other party to the transaction was placed in such a position as would enable him to form an absolutely free and unfettered judgment. Upon the other hand, the natural influence of the parent or guardian over the child, or the husband over the wife, or the attorney over the client, may lawfully be exerted to obtain a legacy so long as the testator thoroughly understands what he is doing, and is a free agent.

The mere existence, therefore, of a relationship which renders "undue influence" possible will not invalidate a testament in favour of the person who is in a position to exercise such influence. There must be proof that he did exercise it.

In *Parfitt* v. *Lawless* (*ubi supra*) the plaintiff, a Roman Catholic priest, had resided with the testatrix and her husband many years as chaplain, and for a part of the time as confessor. He was confessor at the time when the will in dispute was made. There was no evidence that the plaintiff had interfered in the making of such will, or had procured or brought about by coercion or spiritual dominion, a gift which it contained of the residuary estate to himself. It was held by Lord Penzance that there was no evidence to go to a jury upon an issue of undue influence.

In *Parker* v. *Duncan* (1890, *Law Times* May 10), the will of a female pauper was propounded by the Chairman of the Board of Guardians of the Union in which she resided. The property consisted wholly of policies of insurance upon the life of the deceased, and these the testatrix disposed of absolutely to the plaintiff. It was shown that the plaintiff had himself taken the alleged instructions for the will and had got it prepared by his own solicitor, whom he refused to allow to see the testatrix. Of the attesting witnesses, one was a friend of the plaintiff's, the other was a nurse in the workhouse infirmary

* It was admitted on the appeal that as regards money given by A. to S., and applied by the latter to the charitable purposes which A. and S. were equally anxious to promote, there was no equitable claim to restitution.

† Cotton, L.J., dissented from the opinion of the majority of the Court, and held that A.'s claim was not barred by her delay.

‡ *Ubi sup.*, pp. 184, 185.

* The reason of this rule appears to be that in cases of gifts and contracts there is a transaction in which the person benefited at least takes part; in calling upon him to explain the part he took and the circumstances that brought about the gift or obligation, the Court is plainly requiring of him an explanation within his knowledge. But in the case of a legacy under a will, the legatee may have, and in point of fact, generally has, no part in or even knowledge of the act; and to cast upon him, on the bare proof of the legacy and his relation to the testator, the burden of showing how the thing came about, and under what influence or with what motives the legacy was made, or what advice the testator had, would be to cast a duty on him which in many, if not most, cases he could not possibly discharge (per Lord Penzance, *Parfitt* v. *Lawless*, 1872, 2 P. & D. 469).

in which the testatrix had died. The will was declared to be invalid.

The mere fact that in making his will a testator was influenced by immoral considerations does not amount to "undue influence" so long as the dispositions of the will express the wishes of the testator (*Wingrove* v. *Wingrove*, 1886, 11 P. D, 81).

As to "undue influence" in procuring marriage, *see* MARRIAGE, *supra*.

A. WOOD RENTON.

UNEMPFINDLICHKEIT (Ger.). Defect or absence of sensibility. Dysæsthesia, anæsthesia; apathy.

UNITED STATES. (*See* AMERICA, PROVISION FOR INSANE IN.)

UNPARDONABLE SIN.—A common delusion of patients suffering from melancholia, especially in connection with religion, is that they have committed the unpardonable sin mentioned in the Bible. The opinion as to what the sin is varies with different patients, but it is generally connected with blaspheming against the Holy Ghost as they are led to infer from the Bible; or else connected with sexual acts. It seems that the idea of impossibility of forgiveness, and the idea that the patient alone has committed it, make the "unpardonable sin" a favourite delusion.

UNSEEN AGENCY, MONOMANIA OF. (*See* MONOMANIA OF UNSEEN AGENCY, and MONOMANIA.)

UNSINNIG (Ger.). Mad, irrational.

UNSINNIGKEIT (Ger.). Madness, insanity.

UNSOUND MIND. (*See* NON COMPOS MENTIS.)

UNSOUNDNESS OF MIND. (*See* DEFINITION.)

UNTERSCHEIDUNGSZEIT. — Perception-time.

UNWORTHINESS.—A common delusion in religious melancholia.

URANOMANIA (*οὐρανός*, heaven; *μανία*, madness). Monomania involving the idea of a divine or celestial origin or connection; a species of megalomania.

URGENCY CERTIFICATES. (*See* CERTIFICATES, MEDICAL.)

URINARY BLADDER, Influence of the Mind on the.—The influence of pyschic activity in promoting contraction of the bladder, resulting in more or less urgent desire to micturate, is well known. The emotion of fear produces an especially strong and often immediate effect on the bladder as well as sometimes on the bowels; this fact has not escaped the observation of Rembrandt, who, in his picture of the youthful Ganymede in the clutches of the eagle, represents the child as both crying and urinating. Intellectual activity produces a slighter degree of vesical contraction. Mental suspense has a well-marked continuous action in causing contraction of the bladder; this action is familiar to public speakers, to students awaiting examination, to criminals expecting execution. (Such action is frequently combined with stimulation of the kidneys; thus Casanova in his instructive *Mémoires* refers to the excessive flow of urine he experienced on the evening of the day he was imprisoned at Venice.)

The immediate reaction of the bladder to external stimulus has been experienced by most persons on putting the hands into cold water; even the sight of the cold bath is sufficient in some individuals to produce the desire for micturition. Any suggestion in the normal condition of the idea of micturition is often sufficient to produce contraction of the bladder, and the usual accompanying sensations; in this way children and young girls, the hypochondriacal, hysterical, and nervous persons generally, frequently experience spasmodic contractions of the bladder, which are liable to become habitual; such contractions may become a constant source of trouble and anxiety to the individual affected by them. The bladder may also be influenced by suggestions received during the hypnotic state; Binet and Féré, Moll and others have in this way caused subjects to urinate one or more times on awakening from the hypnotic condition. In various morbid nervous conditions the bladder may be affected; thus, in attacks of *petit mal* the central nervous convulsion may not uncommonly terminate in a powerful vesical contraction. Trousseau's magistrate, who unconsciously urinated in a corner of the council-chamber, is well known. Dr. Colman* mentions the case of "a respectable girl, twenty years old, who came under observation recently. She had attended the hospital for twelve months for ordinary epileptic fits, and frequent attacks of *petit mal*, consisting chiefly of sudden desire to pass urine. Usually the sensation had been transient, and she had been able to retain control over her bladder. On a recent occasion, however, when she was at a public entertainment, the attack of *petit mal* was of longer duration than formerly, and while in the unconscious condition she deliberately lifted her clothes and began to void urine in public; and it was with the greatest difficulty that her friends prevented the authorities from handing her over to the police."

While such facts as these here briefly

* "Post-Epileptic Unconscious Automatic Actions," *Lancet*, July 5, 1890.

summarised have long been open to observation, it is only within recent years that accurate and precise demonstration has been brought forward as to the delicate character of the reactions of the bladder to psychic stimuli. To Mosso and Pellacani, by their classical and decisive investigations on the human subject in 1882, is due the credit of demonstrating that contractions of the bladder result directly from the irritation of any sensory nerve; and also that all conditions of the organism which raise the blood-pressure and excite the respiratory centres, produce an immediate and measurable effect upon the bladder. Some preliminary experiments with dogs, by means of the plethysmograph, showed that a caress or an affectionate look produced an immediate contraction of the bladder. Several series of observations were then made with young girls about the age of twenty. A catheter, connected with a tube leading to a plethysmograph, was inserted into the bladder, the subject lying quietly on her back with her legs slightly open and raised. On lightly touching the back of the first subject's hand with the finger a notable contraction of the bladder was at once registered. On winding up the instrument which turns the registering cylinder in connection with the plethysmograph there was another less marked and less rapid contraction; while the bladder was dilating after this contraction Mosso addressed a trivial remark to the girl, a trifling contraction at once occurred and was repeated when she spoke in reply; it was ascertained that these contractions were not due to the abdominal movements of respiration. Some experiments were then made on a very intelligent girl as to the effect of the psychic representation of pain in producing contraction of the bladder. On saying, "Now I am pinching you," but without pinching, there was immediately a manifest contraction, without respiratory change. When the girl spoke there was a still stronger contraction, and this was repeated when a pleasantry was addressed to her. "These phenomena may be considered as the most delicate examples of reflex movement which are produced in the organism, and they correspond to what we have already remarked in animals." On another girl similar experiments were carried out to show the effects of mental exertion. On making some unimportant remark to her there was a trifling contraction; when the object of the experiment was explained, by telling her that she would have to multiply figures to see what would happen in her bladder, there was a more powerful contraction; she was then asked how many eggs it took to make seven dozen. During eight or nine respirations the question produced no effect, then contraction slowly began, and when she had found the answer the bladder slowly dilated to its original volume. "From these experiments which we have repeated on a large number of persons, it must be concluded that every psychic event and every mental effort is accompanied by a contraction of the bladder."

It was found that every influence which contracted the blood-vessels contracted also the bladder, and shortly afterwards Pellacani made some allied investigations as to the effect of drugs in producing vesical contractions.* He found that alcohol and coffee, active agents on the heart, vessels and nervous system, also influence the bladder walls. "For alcohol we have observed a short period of dilatation, followed by a longer period of progressive augmentation of tonus, particularly when the person is in a state of intoxication. The action of coffee on the bladder of man is much prompter than that of alcohol." Gallic acid produces powerful contraction of the bladder by its astringent action on the vessels. Pilocarpine produces very powerful and rapid contraction.

François-Franck and Pitres took up this question so far as animals are concerned, and declared their results at the Collège de France in 1884–5. They experimented on dogs, and observed simultaneously the curves of arterial pressure and of pressure in the bladder. They found that the bladder frequently contracted before the manometer indicated any vascular contraction; that the bladder contraction usually ended before the vascular; and that not seldom, under the influence of feeble cerebral excitation, there was an energetic vesical contraction independently of all vaso-motor contraction. Their experiments, they concluded, fully confirmed the results reached by Mosso and Pellacani.

There is, therefore, no doubt that "the bladder," in Mosso's words, "is an æsthesiometer more certain than the blood pressure, and not inferior even to the iris."

HAVELOCK ELLIS.

[*References.*—Mosso et Pellacani, Sur les Fonctions de la Vessie, Archives Italiennes de Biologie, tome I, 1882. Article, Encéphale (Physiologie), in Dictionnaire encyclopédique des Sciences Médicales. D. Hack Tuke, Influence of the Mind upon the Body, vol. ii. pp. 61–62.]

URINE. Physical Characters.—Normal urine is a fully clear fluid, of an

* "Archives Italiennes de Biologie," tome ii. 1882.

amber or light pale yellow colour, of sp. gr. 1020, reaction slightly acid and with a well-known peculiar odour.

Quantity varies according to temperature, amount of liquid taken, action of the skin and other causes, but it is usually stated to range under our ordinary life conditions between 1000 and 1500 cubic centimetres per day.* There are differences between the urine secreted at different hours. The minimum is secreted between two to four A.M., and the maximum between two and four P.M. (Weigelin), but these differences are not important for our purpose. The amount is *diminished* by profuse sweating, diarrhœa, thirst, non-nitrogenous food, diminution of the blood pressure, and in some diseases of the kidneys. In severe maniacal attacks the decrease appears to have an inverse relation to the rapidity of development and the intensity of the paroxysm, for in milder cases it is not nearly so great (Addison). Lombroso made observations in cases of mania, epilepsy, idiots, and laments, and found that the quantity was less than usual. Rabow† found the quantity diminished in melancholiacs. With advancing dementia the quantity diminishes as well as the absolute amount of urea and chlorides.

It is *increased* by copious drinking, by increase of the general blood pressure, or of the pressure within the area of the renal artery. The passage of a large amount of soluble substances (urea, salts and sugar) into the urine, a large amount of nitrogenous food, and by various drugs. Nervous excitement in hysteria and like conditions is apt to be followed by polyuria. In states of mental anxiety or suspense, the amount is sometimes increased, but this must be distinguished from mere frequency of micturition. We may have polyuria, without the presence of sugar in the urine, following injury to a certain part of the floor of the fourth ventricle (Cl. Bernard). Ebstein‡ collected a series of cases in which polyuria was developed in connection with or in consequence of primary disease of the brain. The occurrence of polyuria in epileptics is frequent. After each fit, in addition to the increased quantity of urine passed, it is richer in chlorides and more deficient in urea than a corresponding volume taken from the total quantity passed in twenty-four hours. When the fits occur at greater intervals, the quantity excreted in twenty-four hours is usually markedly reduced after each one. The quantity of urea is, as a rule, not great, and occasionally there is an increase of xanthin (Rabow). In general paralysis in the earlier stages there is an increase in the quantity of urine, but as dementia advances the quantity lessens (Rabow). In the melancholic first stage, however, Mendel estimated that the quantity of urine is lessened.

* Vogel reckons a centimetre for each kilo of body weight.

† *Archiv f. Psych. und Nervenkr.*, Bd. vii. Heft 1.

‡ *Deutsch. Archiv für Klinische Med.*, Bd. xi. 1873.

The specific gravity varies considerably under different mental conditions. Merson* estimated that in general paralysis the *mean* specific gravity did not materially differ from that of health, and that the absolute quantity of urine, though slightly below that of health, was, in truth, slightly in excess of the latter, if estimated according to body weight. The most concentrated urine is excreted at night. Sutherland and Rigby† stated that the specific gravity in mania and melancholia ranges most usually between 1021 and 1030 in the former, and frequently exceeds 1030 in the latter, whereas in dementia it is usually found to be between 1011 and 1020. Sediments of one sort or another occur in almost every case of mania and melancholia, especially the latter; in dementia not so frequently. It may be stated generally that in periods of excitement the relative amount of solids is increased, but that during periods of freedom from excitement, both in mania and melancholia, there is a diminution. In dementia, considering the large amount of food consumed, this diminution may be considered as an evidence of slow chemical change. Lombroso found the specific gravity diminished in melancholia, almost normal in mania, and increased in dementia previous to an attack of excitement. He also states that urea, chloride of sodium, and phosphoric acid are diminished in maniacs and melancholics during their periods of freedom from excitement. Rabow found the specific gravity increased in melancholia, urea diminished and chloride reduced to a minimum. In advancing paralysis with dementia the specific gravity appears to be increased, and a turbidity due to urates is common.

In polyuria, due to mental states or other nervous conditions, the urine is very dilute and copious, while the specific gravity may be as low as 1001. The mean specific gravity of the urine of 248 cases admitted to Bethlem and estimated within a week of their admission was acute mania (66 cases), 1026; melancholia (68 cases), 1025; partial dementia and delusional

* "West Riding Asylum Reports," vol. iv. p. 63.

† *Lancet*, vol. ii. 1845, p. 241.

(54 cases), 1020; general paralysis of the insane (60 cases), 1021.

The **colour** of the urine depends largely upon the colouring matters in it, and upon variations in the amount of water. In the sudden polyuria occurring after an attack of hysteria, it may be as clear as water. The urine passed after an epileptic fit is sometimes remarkably clear owing to the tendency to increase of the water. In mania and melancholia during the acute periods the prevailing colour of the urine is high; in dementia it is light.

The **reaction** is usually acid, and this is markedly so where there is excitement or prolonged muscular exertion. Sutherland and Rigby found it to be acid in at least 80 per cent. of the maniacal and melancholic cases, but in dementia the proportion was much smaller, viz., 63.54 per cent. A twenty-four hours' collection of urine is normally acid, but if portions of the twenty-four hour urine be examined as it is secreted, certain portions are normally slightly alkaline or neutral; for instance, the urine secreted after a meal is often alkaline, the accepted explanation being that hydrochloric and other acids are poured out into the stomach for the purposes of digestion, hence a temporary increased alkalinity of the fluids within the circulatory system and the separation of a greater proportion of base than acid through the kidneys, so also the ingestion of a purely vegetable diet renders the urine alkaline, as is ever the case with the herbivoræ; on the other hand the urine of the carnivoræ has a high degree of acidity, and people who consume much animal food secrete urine the acidity of which is greater than that of persons eating less meat.

The cause of the normal acidity used to be referred to acid phosphate of soda, but the more correct view is to consider it due to loose combinations of organic acids and salts; for instance, if the ordinary sodic phosphate, Na_2HPO_4, which has an alkaline reaction, be dissolved with an equivalent weight of hippuric acid (142 : 179) a strongly acid re-acting fluid is obtained which may be considered with equal justness either a solution of acid phosphate of soda and hippurate of soda, or a solution of neutral sodic phosphate and free hippuric acid. Similar reactions are obtained from the union of uric acid with the alkaline phosphates; in other words the acid reaction of the urine mainly depends upon loose combinations between the uric and hippuric acids and the alkaline phosphates. The acid reaction given by the urine of the aforementioned cases admitted to Bethlem was in mania 83 per cent.; dementia and delusional, 88.3 per cent.; general paralysis, 90 per cent.; melancholia, 99 per cent. (This estimate is open to objection, for in many instances the specimens obtained did not represent the amount passed during the twenty-four hours.)

The constituents of the urine to be studied mainly divide themselves into six divisions.

(1) **Nitrogenised Bodies of the Nature of Urea:** Urea, uric acid, allantoin, ammonia, oxaluric acid, xanthin, guanin, kreatin, kreatinine, sulphocyanic acid.

(2) **Fatty Nitrogen Free Bodies:** Fatty acids of the series $C_2H_2O_2$, oxalic acid, lactic acid, glycero-phosphoric acid.

(3) **Carbohydrates:** Inosite, gum.

(4) **Aromatic Substances:** Hippuric acid, the ether-sulphates of phenol, cresol, pyrocatechin, indoxyl, scatoxyl and others.

(5) **Mineral Constituents:** Chlorides of sodium and potassium, sodic phosphate, phosphates of calcium and magnesium, calcic carbonate, potassium sulphate, and others.

(6) **Colouring Matters.**

In disease there are also albumins, grape and milk sugar, bile acids and bile colouring matters, methæmoglobin, hæmatoporphyrin, oxymandelic acid, leucin, tyrosin, cholesterin, fat, cystin. A great number of medicinal agents are also separated, changed, or unchanged, by the urine. We shall not refer further to the 6th section.

(1) **Urea and Allied Bodies.** *Urea*, $CO(NH_2)_2$.—Since more than half the nitrogen excreted by the kidneys is in the form of urea, its excess or diminution is a measure of nitrogen changes in the body; in order therefore to appreciate, or even to detect, deviations from normal elimination, it is first necessary to understand fully the variations according to body weight, age, sex, food, rest, or exertion, which may be considered normal. In the outset it may be premised that ordinary clinical determinations of urea excretion, so many of which are to be found published in clinical literature, have but a restricted value; this is epecially true of those which are unaccompanied with exact details of diet. Quite independent of all other circumstances, the urea excretion varies much according as nitrogen is taken into the body in large or small quantities. For example: the same individual,* other conditions being similar, excreted (during twenty-four hours) the following quantities of urea on different diets:

* O. V. Franque, "Dissert." Wurzburg. 1855.

Purely animal food . .	51–92 grms.	
Mixed food, animal and vegetable	36–38	,,
Vegetable food . . .	24–28	,,
Nitrogen free food . .	16	,,

In the adult male the urea is estimated by Vogel to be from .37 to .60 gramme per kilo of body weight; a smaller number than this represents the female excretion. The greatest urea excretion is to be found in men who are undergoing excessive exertion with a full animal diet. Under ordinary conditions of adult life, with gentle daily exercise, and in a state of health, there is approximately nitrogenous equilibrium, that is, the output of nitrogen is equal to the intake. During a few days there may be some nitrogen storage, but this is followed by an increased excretion, sooner or later. On the other hand, severe muscular exertion considerably increases nitrogenous excretion, and then if a period of rest should follow there is nitrogen storage; for example, in a prolonged period of mania with excessive activity, followed by a lull, one would expect the nitrogen stores in the body to be drawn upon considerably, and the nitrogenous output to considerably exceed the nitrogenous intake, while in the lull, there would be more or less quiescence, and in consequence there should be theoretically nitrogen storage; but whether this is so or not, information from an accurate research is much needed. Oppenheim * has shown that the increased urea excretion on exertion is in part due to the dyspnœa which accompanies such exertion.

Dr. Campbell Clark found a diminution of urea in some degree in all his cases of puerperal insanity, although in one case only was that diminution at all striking. If at any time, however, there was a tendency to increase, that increase was in proportion to the degree of sleeplessness and mania in the case.

Excretion of Urea under Abnormal Conditions.—All fever is accompanied by a loss of nitrogenous balance; the nitrogen stores are attacked, and a greater excretion of urea follows than can be accounted for by the food given. In diabetes there is also increased excretion of urea and loss of nitrogenous balance. In all diseases accompanied by dyspnœa there is loss of nitrogenous balance, the output being greater than the intake. In progressive pernicious anæmia, leucæmia, scurvy, hyperæmia of the kidneys, and in phosphorous poisoning, there is increase in the excretion of urea. Many drugs also increase urea elimination. It is also stated that breathing in compressed air, or any artificial rise of temperature, has the same result.

* Pflüger, *Archiv f. Phys.* Bd. xxiii.

Lessened Urea Excretion.—At the end of acute fevers, when the temperature goes down and convalescence commences, there is generally some nitrogen storage, which is necessary to replace the nitrogen lost during the fever. In most maladies of the kidney and liver there is decreased urea excretion, the diseased organs are not capable of carrying on their functions properly, and if the diminished excretion passes a certain limit the condition known as uræmia arises. In gouty conditions of the body the urea output is, as a rule, smaller than in health. Rabow * found in a case of melancholia a daily excretion of urea from 6 to 20 grammes, but when the same person recovered the excretion rose from 9.9 to 20 grammes. In mania he found in one case an excretion of 14.59 grammes as a daily average during a period of excitement, and 23.5 grammes during a period of quiet; but no details as to diet are given. It therefore may well be that during the excitable period but little food was taken, and during the quiet period much taken; if such were the case the nitrogenous output may have been greater in relation to the intake in the first (excitable) period than in the second (quiet) period. Johnson Smyth † has found in thirty cases of secondary dementia a remarkable decrease of urea, as compared with healthy men living on the same diet. Addison ‡ investigated sixteen cases of mania, and his summary of these cases is as follows:

(1) Quantity diminished;
(2) Specific gravity high;
(3) Intensely acid;
(4) Sodic chloride less during mania than in convalescence;
(5) Diminution of urea;
(6) Phosphoric acid less during states of mental excitement;
(7) Sulphates in eleven cases greater in convalescence than during the attack.

Mania (Averages).

	During Attack.	During Convalescence.
Quantity . . .	664.6 c.c.	1584 c.c.
Specific gravity	1025	1016 ,,
	grammes.	grammes.
Urea	21.25	30.80
Sodium chloride	2.33	3.88
PO_4	1.43	1.98
SO_3	1.39	1.49

* *Archiv f. Psych. u. Nervenkr.*, Bd. vii.
† *Journ. Ment. Sci.*, vol. xxxvi. p. 517.
‡ *Ibid.*, vol. xi. p. 262.

In this otherwise careful research there are no exact data as to the composition of the food.

In **general paralysis**, there is some discrepancy of opinion, Addison found less urea excreted than in health. Merson,* on the other hand, considered the daily average showed an increase. Sander† found the excretion to be small in general paralysis. Rabow found relatively more urea in the first stage and with the advance of dementia a diminution in the amount. In the melancholic first stage the urea is less increased as a rule. In dementia, and especially where the vitality is low, all observers agree that the urea is diminished below the normal standard.

In cases of **hysteria** and **catalepsy**, Strubing‡ found during the seizures a diminution of urea. The most recent researches on the amount of urea excreted by general paralytics are those made by Dr. John Turner,§ and Dr. W. Johnson Smyth.‖ Turner's cases were all on a diet which it is computed was equivalent to 12.2 grammes of nitrogen and 342 grammes of carbon. The number of cases in which it was possible to collect complete samples of the urine for twenty-four hours was 61, and the mean daily quantity of urea excreted by these was 24.5 grammes. In eighteen cases in the first stage of the malady the mean was 24.7 grammes, maximum 33.4; minimum 18.2. In thirty-five cases in the second stage, the mean was 24.6 grammes; maximum 42.0, minimum 13.4. In eight cases in the third stage the mean was 23.6 grammes; maximum 34.0; minimum 15.6. He therefore concludes that there is a real diminution of urea excretion among general paralytics. Smyth's cases were ten in number, and the observations were continued for seven days. The observations seem to have been made with especial care and the results compared with those obtained from two healthy men living on the same diet.

The mean results are as follows:

	Two healthy men.		Mean of ten cases of general paralysis.
Total amount of urine	1356 c.c.	...	1578 c.c.
	grammes.		grammes.
Total solids per day .	37.8	...	47.0
Urea, per day . . .	23.2	...	26.0
Uric acid	0.9	...	3.1
Phosphoric acid . .	1.2	...	1.6

* "West Riding Asylum Reports."

† Griesinger, "Mental Pathology and Therapeutics" (New Syd. Soc. Transl.), 1867.

‡ *Deutsch. Arch. f. Klin. Med.*, 1880, Bd. xxvii. p. 125.

§ *Journ. Ment. Sci.*, Oct. 1889.

‖ *Ibid.*, Oct. 1890.

These observations do not agree with Turner's, for the urea is not diminished but rather increased. The quantity of urine, the total solids, and especially the uric acid also, all show a considerable increase.

In an analysis of the urine in three cases of epilepsy, Gibson* found the average twenty-four hours' secretion of water a little above, of urea, chloride of sodium and phosphoric acid below the normal amount. The nightly average of water and NaCl was less than the daily; of urea equal; of phosphoric acid greater. No constant change in the urine of the fit nights, but a tendency to increase of water, urea and chloride of sodium. There was also increase of all the constituents in the hours following fits. With regard to other maladies: In osteomalacia,† in lepra, pemphigus,‡ impetigo,§ in chronic rheumatism, and generally in chronic anæmic diseases, a lessened excretion of urea has been observed.

Uric Acid.—A. B. Garrod‖ considers that a man excretes one part of uric acid per 120,000 parts of body weight; hence a man weighing 56.5 kilos would excrete normally 0.47 grammes during the twenty-four hours. Thudichum puts it at 0.5 gramme, and Neubauer and Vogel, in saying that the excretion varies between 0.2 and 1.0 gramme, also put the mean daily excretion for persons of standard weight at 0.5 gramme. The eating of a highly nitrogenous diet raises the excretion of uric acid; under these circumstances, Ranke found as much as 2.1 grammes, the urea itself being much increased. Ranke considered that gentle bodily movements diminished the excretion, and excessive movements raised it. It is, indeed, doubtful whether muscular activity has much to do with increase or diminution of uric acid. The old idea also, that sugar produces an excess of uric acid, is pretty nigh exploded, for direct experiment has shown no increase so long as the digestion is not affected, even when large quantities of sugar have been consumed. The general consensus of opinion at present is that the varying quantities of uric acid depend in the main upon individual peculiarity.

Since uric acid closely follows urea, in all the cases previously mentioned in which urea has been found in excess or the reverse, uric acid will also be found in excess of normal or below normal. Thus an increase has been noted in pyrexia, in

* Roy. Med. Chirurg. Soc., 1867.

† Schmuziger and Leube, Peters, *Med. Wochenschrift*, 1882, p. 361.

‡ Kaposi, "Kantkrankheiten," p. 481.

§ Beneke, *Arch. f. Wiss. Heilkunde*, Bd. ii. 36.

‖ "Proc. Roy. Soc.," vol. xl. pp. 484, 485.

which there is an increase in the number of respirations, especially in croupous pneumonia. Scheube found the greatest amount of uric acid the day following the highest fever. Ranke, Virchow, Mosler, Salkowski, Pettenkofer, and Voit, with others, have found in leucæmia a great increase of uric acid. In one case recorded by Bartels it is said to have reached the quantity of 4.2 grammes in the twenty-four hours. In splenic anæmia uric acid has also been found abnormal in quantity. Coignard* in a case of dyspepsia found as much as 1.38 gramme of uric acid excreted within the twenty-four hours. The researches of Garrod have shown that in gout there is a decreased kidney elimination, while there is a normal or possibly increased secretion of uric acid in the tissues. The uric acid is decreased in diabetes, in anæmia, in many affections of the kidney, and in some other diseases. The influence of mental states and diseases upon the secretion of uric acid is very little known, Johnson Smyth found that uric acid was increased in mental diseases generally, the increase being greatest in general paralysis, epilepsy and melancholia; on the other hand, uric acidæmia is said to give rise to a variety of disorders of the nervous system. In his Croonian Lectures (1874) upon functional derangements of the liver, Murchison associated with lithæmia aching pains in the limbs and lassitude, pain in the shoulder, hepatic neuralgia, severe cramps in legs, &c., headache, vertigo and temporary dimness of sight, convulsions, paralysis, noises in the ears, sleeplessness, depression of spirits, irritability of temper, cerebral symptoms and the typhoid state. Haig† found that "when the urine excreted during a headache is carefully separated from that before the headache began, or after it left off, an excess of uric acid relative to urea is always found (say the relation of 1 to 20 or 1 to 25). Before the headache begins there is often a relation of 1 to 40—i.e., diminished uric acid, and after it ends the same. If we have a mixture of before or after with the headache urine, the excess in one direction may balance that in the other, and the result comes out near 1 to 33, or normal." The same author found that in epilepsy, just as in migraine, "the excretion of uric acid is greatly diminished before the attack—that is, mental exaltation corresponds to a minus excretion of uric acid and headache, an epileptic fit or mental depression corresponds to a plus excretion, which is, to some extent, the result of the previous minus excretion (retention)." Migraine, or the headache of uric acidæmia, is looked upon as a local vascular effect of uric acid. "Epilepsy resembles migraine in the mental brightness and well-being, with scanty excretion of uric acid, which may precede both, in the excessive excretion of uric acid and mental depression which may accompany both, and in the subnormal temperature which is often found in both." Hysteria is also regarded as one of the mental effects of uric acid, and as a variety or mixed condition between ordinary epilepsy and simple mental depression. Haig does not, however, agree with Broadbent that the high arterial tension is "probably the most important factor in the secretion of the pale and watery urine which accompanies an hysterical attack," but states that, as a matter of fact, "during the high arterial tension and contraction of arterioles and capillaries in the attack, the urine is scanty and of high specific gravity, containing much uric acid; and it is only when the tension falls and the capillaries are relaxed at the end of the attack that it becomes pale and watery. Further, he believes that the unconsciousness which follows epileptic fits will last a long or short time according as the uric acid which occasioned them is slowly or quickly driven out of the blood, and that the stupor is not really due to exhaustion of the nerve-centres any more than the heavy, languid, and sleepy feeling so often met with in the morning hours during the plus excretion of uric acid, is due to want of sleep in the previous night. The same author has noticed the presence, absence, or alteration in amount, of certain forms of tremor in a fairly constant relation with the amount of uric acid in the blood. He also ascribes uric acidæmia as being an important factor in the production of some forms of aphasia, vertigo, and insomnia.

Allantoin and *oxaluric acid* are both bodies which occur rarely, if at all, in human urine; whilst *xanthin*, *guanin*, *kreatin*, *kreatinin*, *sulphocyanic acid*, &c., are, for our purposes, comparatively unimportant.

(2) **Oxalic acid** ($C_2H_2O_4+2H_2O$), in the form of oxalate of lime, is found in the urine in variable quantity; sometimes it is absent. Its presence is evidently rather due to the nature of the food eaten than to special decompositions within the organism. Oxalate of lime is also found in the intestinal contents, but the urine is the only secretion in which it is found normally. Oxalate of lime is a very insoluble salt; it occurs whenever a solution

* *Jahresb. f. Thierchem.*, 1880, p. 247.

† *Brain*, part i. 1891.

of oxalic acid or of a soluble oxalate is mixed with an aqueous solution of a soluble lime salt. The precipitate may be amorphous or it may be in a crystalline form, such as dumb-bells, octahedra, or sometimes as four-sided prisms, rarely as spheroids. The crystals are insoluble in acetic, soluble in hydrochloric, acid. Hence, to find readily oxalate of lime crystals in a urinary sediment, it is well to treat the sediment with acetic acid, which will dissolve phosphates and leave oxalate of lime and uric acid sediments undissolved. The reason why so insoluble a salt as lime oxalate can exist in solution in the urine was discovered by Neubauer, who found that it was soluble in a solution of acid phosphate of soda. If to a solution of hydrosodic phosphate a few drops of chloride of lime are added and followed by a solution of ammonic oxalate, no precipitate occurs; but if sufficient soda solution is added to neutralise the acid phosphate, then down comes the lime oxalate. A similar change takes place in the urine on standing; the acid phosphate of soda and the sodic urate interact, first forming acid urate of soda, and little by little the acid phosphate of soda disappears from the urine, and the oxalate falls slowly down, the slow deposit being most favourable for the production of crystalline forms. A similar, perhaps identical, process takes place occasionally in the bladder, and then there is a formation of urinary calculus.

At one time it was supposed that a particular disease known as oxaluria existed, but, although it may be that in one human body more oxalic acid is excreted through the kidneys than another, there is great doubt whether as a distinct malady oxaluria exists. Beneke stated that under continued depressing mental influences oxalic acid crystals appeared in the urine constantly and in very large numbers, and at the same time the quantity of lithic acid became increased, while no change had taken place in the manner of living.

Glycero-phosphoric Acid. — Since the brain and nervous system are so largely made up of combinations of glycero-phosphoric acid united with complex albuminoids, it is only reasonable to imagine it possible that, if there should be any actual loss by wasting of the nervous tissues, there would be an excretion of phosphorus, either in the form of phosphoric acid or of glycero-phosphoric acid, the latter being the more probable. Although there have been many estimations of total phosphates in the urine of persons affected with general paralysis and other brain diseases, and although there is a widespread belief that phosphates are generally increased in these maladies, the researches hitherto have been far from satisfactory because the all-important factor has been usually neglected of careful previous estimation of the intake in the food of phosphates. This remark does not, however, apply with the same force to glycero-phosphoric acid, which has been ascertained to be excreted in such small quantities in health that, in order to estimate it, 10 litres of the normal urine require to be operated upon. Hence, if found in sufficient quantity to weigh when operating upon a quarter or half a litre of urine, we may, in our present state of knowledge, consider such a quantity pathological.

A series of researches on the excretion of glycero-phosphoric acid in the urine of the insane would be of the highest value, and it is strange that it has not been more often undertaken. The most important work in this direction of late years has been done by Dr. E. Birt, at the West Riding Asylum, Wakefield, and his results published in *Brain* (October 1886). In 1884 Zuelzer* maintained that "from the nervous tissue when in a state of lowered irritability the delivery of material is augmented, and that it is lessened in conditions of exalted irritability. Further, that each of these series of conditions is, in respect to the tissue change, differentiated by urinary qualities peculiar to it, and of such kind that, in depressed conditions (traumatic or pathological destructive brain lesions, chloroform, ether, morphia, narcosis, &c.), the phosphoric and glycerin phosphoric acids of the urine are increased; whereas excited conditions (as induced by strychnia, phosphorus, alcohol in small doses) are attended by a diminished amount of those products in the urine." According to Zuelzer†, the normal gravimetric proportion of the P_2O_5 to the N in the twenty-four hours' urine of the adult, is 18 or 20 to 100. In blood, the mean proportion is as 4 to 100; in muscle, 15 to 100; in brain and other nervous organs which contain the greatest amount of lecithin, 45 to 100. Lépine and Eymonnet‡ estimated the normal amount of glycerin phosphoric acid in grammes at 0.25 to 100 N, or about 1 per cent. of the total P_2O_5. They also noted "an increase in the renal excretion of the phosphorus compounds — parti-

* "Untersuch. über die Semeiologie des Harn," s. 57. u. ff. (quoted from Birt).

† Birt, *Brain*, Oct. 1886.

‡ *Comptes Rendus des Séances de l'Acad. des Sciences*, t. xcviii. 1884, No. 4, p. 239, *vide* Birt.

cularly the glycerin phosphoric acid—as a result of gross cerebral lesions, epilepsy, and use of chloral or bromides. Thus, in a case of hæmorrhage into the external capsule and outer part of the lenticular nucleus, the urine excreted during the first six hours contained per litre."

N		P_2O_5		R
2.5	...	0.54*	...	21.6
0.0268	...	1.07		

"Forty-eight hours later, the proportion was normal." In one case of general paralysis of two years' duration in which there was exaltation, Birt found a large absolute quantity of the glycerin phosphoric acid, then during a period of stupor an increased elimination of the inorganically combined P_2O_5. In two other cases there existed a notable discharge of glycerin phosphoric acid in connection with the occurrence of paralytic motor phenomena, which contrasted strongly with the absence of that compound when the patients had regained their normal state. Birt says, "One does not constantly find an excretion of glycerin phosphoric acid following the convulsive attacks of general paralysis." Similarly in epilepsies, even when an enormous series of fits rapidly proceeds to a fatal issue.

Lépine and Jacquin † "found the proportion of the P_2O_5 to the N much below normal on the days between the fits, once as low as 8.6 per cent. In those patients the proportion notably increased immediately after a fit, the rise being absolute, and chiefly due to an increase of the earthy phosphates. An augmentation of the earthy phosphates was also noted when the patients had merely experienced sensations of a fit being imminent, or had undergone an attack of vertigo." In a case of recurrent mania, Birt found the ratio of P_2O_5 to the N was constantly lower when excitement was absent. "No organically combined P_2O_5 was found while the mental affection ran its usual course. As soon, however, as a depressed condition became established (partial collapse from peritonitis, so far induced by morphia), a large elimination of glycerin phosphoric acid occurred." In a case of severe melancholia, there was excess of discharge of glycerin phosphoric acid when the disturbance of cerebral function was greatest.

(3) **Carbohydrates.**—Inosite, gum.

(4) **The Aromatic Substances.**—Hippuric acid. The ether sulphates of phenol, cresol, pyrocatechin, indoxyl, scatoxyl and others, are comparatively unimportant.

(5) **Mineral Constituents.**—These depend mainly upon the food; it is pretty certain that soluble salts of the alkalies and the alkaline earths, and in fact all salts which enter the circulation, are excreted by the kidneys, but most of the earthy phosphates in wheat meal, and all the silica, and most of the iron, are excreted by the bowel.

Dr. Adam Addison found that the quantities of chloride of sodium, phosphoric and sulphuric acids, excreted during the course of a maniacal paroxysm, occurring in acute mania, epilepsy, general paralysis, melancholia or dementia, are less than the amounts excreted in an equal time during health. In chronic melancholia the quantities of chloride of sodium, phosphoric and sulphuric acids are reduced below the mean, and sometimes the minimum of health. In idiocy, dementia (paralytic and common), the urea, chloride of sodium and sulphuric acid range above and below the normal mean of health; in some cases the amount of phosphoric acid is greater than the mean according to weight, but in the majority of cases it ranges between the minimum and mean found in healthy adult men. Sutherland and Rigby found crystals of triple phosphates in dementia at the rate of 25 per cent.; crystals of oxalate of lime were seen in every fourth case of melancholia, or at the rate of 25 per cent. In mania the proportion was 17.85, and in dementia only 2.08 per cent. Mendel* estimated that the quantity of phosphoric acid excreted by the kidneys under the influence of brain disease, and compared proportionately to the other solid principles of urine, varies considerably from 2.49 to 3.93 per cent. The substance is excreted in greater quantity at night than during the day. In the chronic maladies of the encephalon there is a decrease in the absolute quantity of phosphoric acid excreted every day, as well as the relative quantity in connection with the other solid principles of urine. In cases of maniacal excitement there is an increase in the absolute and relative quantity of the substance. Increase in the quantity is also observed during attacks of epilepsy and apoplexy, and after the administration of chloral and bromide

* In Birt's paper the quantities found by analogies are expressed in grammes, or parts of a gramme. Where two series of figures are given, under the heading P_2O_5, the first indicates the phosphoric acid in combination with alkalies or alkaline earths, the second the glycerin phosphoric acid. The numbers under R denote the gravimetric ratio of the respective P_2O_5 to 100 N.

† *Revue Mensuelle de Méd. et de Chir.*, tome iii. 1879, Nos. 9 et 12, quoted from Birt.

* *Archiv für Psychiatrie*, Bd. iii. Heft 3.

of potassium. The decrease of the substance in chronic cases of brain disease must be attributed generally to diminution of muscular activity, dependent on the protracted course of the disease. In other cases it may be ascribed to the general weakness or exhaustion of the nervous system, the result of imperfect assimilation. Bence Jones has endeavoured to show that a distinction between inflammation of the brain and delirium tremens is to be found in the increased amount of phosphoric acid (alkaline and earthy phophates) in the urine of patients with inflammation of the brain. This test is of little practical value, for the sources of phosphoric acid in the urine are so numerous that it would require the evidence of a vast number of analyses to convince one that inflammation of brain tissue would so much increase the amount of phosphoric acid in the urine that this fact alone would suffice for the diagnosis between an inflamed and non-inflammatory condition of the brain. In delirium tremens Bence Jones found excess of urea, sulphates and albumen.

In puerperal insanity Dr. Campbell Clark found chlorides were scarcely traceable, being so low as 0.36 grammes in twenty-four hours; for fourteen hours of day urine the minimum was 0.09 gramme, and for ten hours of night urine 0.24 gramme. He concludes that "the deficiency of chlorides may be partially, but insufficiently accounted for, by (*a*) the anorexia and atonic dyspepsia; (*b*) saline deficiency in the food administered; (*c*) sluggish digestion, owing to artificial, instead of natural, alimentation; (*d*) the pyrexia, which must in these cases be regarded as only of moderate import; (*e*) moisture of the skin." He also considers that "it is exceedingly probable that in some way yet to be ascertained chlorides accumulate in the system, and have some pathological significance in this disease, which we know not. The loss to urine and mucous secretions have three possible explanations: (*a*) Chlorine starvation; (*b*) chlorine infiltration of tissues; (*c*) chlorinæmia. Campbell Clark found a decrease in the quantity of phosphoric acid in puerperal insanity, being as low as 0.2 gramme in twenty-four hours, the minima being 0.07 for day urine, and 0.25 gramme for night urine, and he considers that the quality rather than the quantity of mental excitement is more likely to account for the changes in the excretion of the phosphoric acid.

Albumen.—Rabenau* has several times observed the occurrence of albumen in many cases of paralysis at some time or another. Richter*, however, states that this constituent is not frequently present, and, if it is, is not connected with the cerebral disease. In epileptics, quantitative and qualitative changes occur. Formerly it was repeatedly stated that sugar and albumen occur immediately after the fits. The sugar question is now settled, since all recent works on this subject agree that urine passed after the epileptic attacks is free from it. On the contrary in regard to albumen, Huppert† found that a certain amount is found after every attack. Rabow found albumen in eight, but no sugar in the urine of ten, epileptic lunatics immediately after the fits. Sometimes the reaction was so slow and feeble that it might have been easily overlooked. Huppert arrived at the conclusion that albumen appears in the urine after every well-marked fit of epilepsy. It is not found in urine which is passed just before or during a paroxysm. It continues to be present in urine passed from three to eight hours after a fit. The more severe the fit the more abundant the albumen. Mere cases of epileptic vertigo may be quite unattended by this phenomenon unless the attacks follow one another rapidly. The amount excreted is never large; there may be sufficient, however, to form the ordinary flocculi with heat and nitric acid, but often there is only a white cloudiness or mere opalescence, especially after mild epileptic fits. The largest quantity of albumen is found in the first urine passed after the fit, and the greatest average amount in those patients who have long suffered from severe attacks. Such urine is remarkable for its clearness and increased quantity; its specific gravity generally ranges from 1012 to 1020. In severer forms of epilepsy there are sometimes hyaline cylinders and (in males) spermatozoa in the urine. The cylinders are found in the first or second urine after the fit, but they do not remain present so long as the albumen does.

The spermatozoa also occur in the first urine after severe attacks, and in about a tenth of the cases exist in such numbers that the conclusion is inevitable that a definite though slight ejaculation of semen is coincident with the fit. It probably is due to a direct nerve irritation, that is, one which bears the same relation to the central nervous centres as the convulsions do. A true seminal emission is not a phenomenon of epilepsy in Dr. Huppert's experience. Red blood corpuscles are seldom present in the urine after epileptic

* *Archiv von Psych. und Nervenkr.*, Bd. iv. p. 787.

* *Archiv von Psych. und Nervenkr.*, Bd. vi.

† Virchow's *Archiv*, Bd. lix.

attacks, or their number if present is so small that they can be considered of no significance. Even where there were subconjunctival petechiæ, Dr. Huppert could not find an increase of red blood cells in the urine even with the most careful microscopic examination; while blood cells on the other hand are almost always present. This absence of red corpuscles points to the arteries as the source of albumen in epilepsy. Since Liebermeister, Cohnheim and Hering have shown that nervous congestion, even without rupture of bloodvessels, is always accompanied with an abundance of red corpuscles in the urine as soon as albuminuria commences. While the urine of patients with progressive paralysis of the insane, after epileptiform or apoplectiform attacks, agrees with that of epileptics in containing albumen and hyaline casts, it differs from the latter in containing red blood corpuscles in some quantity either isolated from one another or in groups of six to twelve of each.

Fürstner* found albumen in the urine of those labouring under delirium tremens, and that the quantity of albumen was proportioned to the intensity of the delirium. Albumen is sometimes found in the urine of habitual drinkers.

The same author considers that albumen is far from being a constant symptom of epileptic fits; a transitory reaction of albumen is often found, but not always. In three cases of status epilepticus which ended fatally, no trace of albumen could be found. Rabenau found albumen to be present more commonly in paralytic insanity than in any other cerebral disease, and thinks it independent of alteration of the kidneys. De Witt found albuminuria after the convulsions of general paralysis, while König, Richter, and Mendel, on the other hand, usually found it absent.

Dr. Campbell Clark† found albumen was present in 9 out of 23 cases of puerperal insanity; the precipitate was usually slight.

Sugar. (*See* DIABETES.)—Sugar in the urine has been found in several cerebral diseases and cerebral lesions, in which there were no evident pathological changes in other organs. Recklinghausen‡ found melituria in the case of a tumour of the fourth ventricle; Dompeling§ in a tumour of the medulla; Giovanni‖ in sclerosis of the right cerebellum; Zenker¶ in disease

* *Archiv*, Bd. vi. Heft 3.

† *Journ. Ment. Sci.* Oct. 1887 and Jan. 1888.

‡ Virchow's *Archiv*, Bd. xxx. s. 360. 1864.

§ Ref. *Centralbl. für die med. Wissenschaft*, 1869, s. 144.

‖ *Jahresbericht*, 1876, Bd. ii. s. 269.

¶ "Ueber die Natur. Vors. in Speyer," 1861.

of the fourth ventricle: Mosler* in a case of softening of the nucleus dentatus in the cerebellum. Diabetes coincided with a case described by Mosler,† in which there was a new formation in the fourth ventricle, with a case of tubercle in both hemispheres described by Roberts,‡ with chronic inflammatory changes in one of the calamus scriptorius (Lancereaux) with cysticercus in the brain (Frerichs)§ with encephalitis of the fourth ventricle and its surroundings (Pribram)‖ with carcinoma of the glandula pituitaria (Massot).¶

Gooden** found that there was sugar in many cases of epilepsy, paralysis, and chorea, but that this disappeared as symptoms were relieved by treatment. Ordinarily there was no diuresis; urine often turbid and ammoniacal.

Glycuronic acid, $C_6H_{10}O_7$, also reduces copper. Glycuronic acid when pure is in the form of white amorphous granules, its anhydride forms fine colourless acicular crystals. In urine it is in combination with urea, probably as uroglycuronic acid. It rotates a ray of polarised light 35° to the right. It is doubtful whether glycuronic acid is present in normal urine, but its presence has been ascertained as a result of taking certain drugs—*e.g.*, brombenzol, †† nitro-benzol,‡‡ quinine derivatives,§§ phenol, benzol and indol.‖‖ According to Ashdown,¶¶ the best way is to ferment the urine after the manner of Salkowski, and thus, after having destroyed the sugar, to see whether it reduces copper, if it does, glycuronic acid is probably present. Salkowski's method of fermentation is to simply fill a tube very similar in shape to the ureometer of Doremus, with the urine, and put a little mercury in the bend; a little good yeast is passed up by means of a curved pipette, and the urine kept for a number of hours at a fermentation temperature.***

* *Deutsch. Arch. f. klin. Med.*, Bd. xv. s. 229, 1875.

† Virchow's *Archiv*, Bd. xliii. s. 225.

‡ *Arch. gén.* 1866, tom. ii.

§ *Charité Annalen*, Bd. ii. 1877, s. 653.

‖ *Prager Vierteljahrschrift*, 1871, Bd. cxii. s. 28.

¶ *Lyon Méd.*, 1872.

** *Lancet*, 1854, p. 656.

†† *Zeitschrift f. physiol. Chemie*, 1879, Bd. iii. p. 156; 1881, Bd. v. p. 309. Jaffé, *Ber. d. Deutschen Gesell.*, Bd. xii. p. 306.

‡‡ *Centr. f. Med. Wissen.*, 1875, No. iv.

§§ *Zeitsch. f. Physiol. Chemie*, 1880, Bd. iv. p. 296.

‖‖ Baumann, *Archiv f. ges. Physiol.*, 1876, Bd. xiii. p. 299; *Zeitsch. f. Physiol. Chem.*, 1877, Bd. i. p. 68.

¶¶ "Laboratory Reports, Royal College of Physicians, Edinburgh," vol. ii.

*** On the reduction of copper solution by kreatinine, *see ante*.

Examples of Urine Analysis. — The following few analyses of urine are added as examples of the possibility of determining quantitatively several of the organic principles in the collection of twenty-four hours' renal secretion.*

Mania.—*Acute Mania with Refusal of Food.* — Female, height about 5 feet; weight, 8st. 8 lbs.=54.45 kilos. *Food consumed:* Bread, 2.5 ozs.; tea, 1 pint; milk, 2 ozs.; sweetened arrowroot, 1 pint (made by thickening milk with arrowroot). Analysis of the urine of twenty-four hours Nov. 4-5, 1889: Quantity, 770 c.c.; reaction, slightly acid; specific gravity, 1007; sugar and albumen, absent. Total solids, 13.04 grms.; ash, 2.42 grms.; volatilised chlorine calculated as NaCl, 1.6 grm.; organic solids, 9.02 grms. SO_3 as mineral sulphate, .60; uric acid, not estimated; hippuric acid, .03; kreatinine, .05; nitrogen by soda lime, 3.39 grms. (=7.26 grms. urea).

Melancholia.—Female patient, height 5 feet 2 inches; weight, 6st. 12lb.=43.5 kilos. *Food consumed:* Bread, 14 ozs.; butter, 1 oz.; tea, 2 pints; milk, 2 ozs.; potatoes, 5 ozs.; meat, 3 ozs.; 3 ozs. of a pudding made of rice and milk; water, 8 ozs. Analysis of the urine of twenty-four hours Nov. 4-5, 1889: Quantity, 1688 c.c.; reaction, slightly acid; specific gravity, 1010; sugar and albumen, absent. Total solids, 32.72 grms.; ash, 7.76 grms.; volatilised chlorine calculated as NaCl, 9.32 grms.; total organic solids, 15.64 grms. SO_3 as mineral sulphate, .31; ether sulphate, .06; organic sulphur, .05; hippuric acid, not estimated; kreatinine, .053; nitrogen by hypobromite=4.91 equal to 10.51 urea; nitrogen by soda lime=5.57 equal to 11.93; phosphoric acid, not estimated.

General Paralysis.—J. A., male, aged 43, height 5 feet 7 inches; weight, 12st. 13 lbs.=77.6 kilos; patient in the first stage of general paralysis; a complete collection of twenty-four hours Nov. 4-5, 1889. *Food consumed:* Tea, 1.5 pint with sugar and milk (milk 3 ozs.); cocoa, 1.5 pint; water, 1 pint; bread, 16 ozs.; butter, 1 oz.; potatoes, 13 ozs.; meat pie, 17 ozs. (contains about 6 ozs. meat, 1.5 ozs. haricot beans, also flour and suet). Composition of the urine: Total quantity, 2475 c.c.; reaction, slightly acid; specific gravity, 10124. Total solids, 67.32 grms.; ash, 20.54 grms.; volatilised NaCl, 16.43 grms. Mineral sulphate, 2.40; ether sulphate, 0.30; organic sulphur, 0.14; chlorine, 14.89; uric acid, 0.03 (?); phosphoric acid, 2.16; kreatinine, .113; nitrogen by soda lime, 10.08 = urea 21 grms.

A. Wynter Blyth.
Theo. B. Hyslop.

* The cases were patients in the Berrywood Asylum, under the care of Dr. Greene, to whom we are indebted for the opportunity of making these analyses.

UTERINE DISORDERS AND INSANITY.—We may first point out the influences of disordered functions of the sexual organs not depending upon serious organic change. One of the most obvious of these is what is best described as dysmenorrhœa from obstruction that is caused by mechanical impediment to the natural flow of the menses. Stenosis or contraction of the os externum uteri is the most obvious impediment. With or without this, may exist acute flexion of the neck of the uterus. When this condition exists the normal hyperæmia of menstruation culminates in intense congestion. Hyperæmia often entails hyperplasia. Acute pains due to tension of the swollen tissues and spasmodic contraction follow; and the sympathetic and reflected action upon the ganglionic, spinal and cerebral centres is often greater than can be borne.

With or without dysmenorrhœa, another trying condition is menorrhagia. The loss of blood entails alteration in the quality of the blood. The nervous centres are ill-nourished, and therefore prone to morbid action.

It is important to form a definite and rational idea of the terms hysteria and neurosis. Too often they are mere words used to conceal ignorance. This is an *asylum ignorantiæ* which ought to be closed. Hysteria is not an independent entity. It is a symptom. If we cannot trace the symptoms and its cause, commonly underlying disorder of the sexual system, the rational course is to infer that our skill is deficient, and not to bow down before an idol of the imagination. This is certain, that, in many cases, hysteria is the forerunner of insanity. This also is certain, as the result of large clinical experience, that hysteria is cured by removing the causes of dysmenorrhœa. Our case-books teem with cases of syncope, loss of memory, epilepsy, perversion of senses, hallucinations, associated with dysmenorrhœa, many of which were relieved or cured by removing the cause of the dysmenorrhœa.* The study of the influence of diseased ovaries opens another field of inquiry. Négrier affirmed that the influence of the ovaries and the activity of their function is in direct proportion to their volume. This is difficult to

* This subject is discussed with some fulness in the Lumleian Lectures on the Convulsive Diseases of Women, before the Royal College of Physicians, 1874.

prove. But when we pass to diseased ovaries we are on more certain ground. Marked increase of size is presumptive evidence of disease. Négrier relates a remarkable case of mutilation and suicide at the last day of menstruation in which the ovaries were much above the normal size.

There may be an acquired neurotic diathesis, the relic of disease in childhood, as chorea. In our Lumleian Lectures we specially illustrated this point, adducing cases of malarious infection, from which the subjects had apparently recovered. When menstruation or pregnancy supervened the latent disease was evoked, and ague fits recurred. We have noted similar examples in which epilepsy and chorea, apparently cured, returned under the stress of menstruation or pregnancy.

The connection between amenorrhœa, chloro-anæmia and nervous disorders is deserving of careful study. Trousseau said that chlorosis was essentially a nervous disease. Certainly we have seen reason to conclude that in some cases nervous disturbances have preceded the chlorosis. More frequently what is called anæmia with amenorrhœa is the antecedent condition. The arrested function is commonly associated with disorder or perversion of the intestines or hæmogenetic functions. And this cannot last long without entailing weakness or perversion of the nervous functions. The word anæmia conveys a very imperfect idea of the state of the blood. Toxæmia with spanæmia would express the state more nearly. The blood becomes not only deficient in red globules, but it becomes contaminated by the absorption and retention of matters that ought to be excreted.

If we examine the neuroses that attend morbid conditions of the uterus and ovaries we obtain striking evidence of causation. A frequent state is displacement of these organs, not necessarily diseased in tissue. The most common is retroflexion or retroversion, with or without prolapsus of the uterus. These can hardly exist without entailing some disorder of menstruation, and this is enough to disturb the nervous equilibrium. But in addition to this, the displaced organ presses upon other organs, as the bowel and bladder, impeding their functions, and especially it presses upon the sacral plexus, and so causes constant irritation of the lower segment of the spinal cord, a part of the nervous system, as we have seen, more highly organised than it is in the male. So-called sympathetic, reflex, or diastaltic phenomena are frequent. In not a few instances these minor nervous disorders culminate in melancholia and mania. We have the histories of cases in which the subjects had been insane for long periods, with no sign of amendment until they came under our care. We discovered pronounced retroflexion with hyperplasia of the uterus. This being corrected by surgical treatment rapid recovery ensued. In one most striking case, the subject returned to her home, bore twins, and has since been in perfect physical and mental health. Dr. Bennington brought before the British Gynæcological Society* a case equally remarkable. Dr. C. E. Louis Mayer† in a memoir on the relations of the morbid conditions of the sexual organs and psychoses, relates some instructive cases. Schroeder van der Kolk relates the case of a profoundly melancholic woman who suffered from prolapsus uteri, in whom the melancholia used to disappear directly the uterus was restored. Fleming mentions two similar cases, in which the melancholia was cured by the use of a pessary, in one of them returning whenever the pessary was removed. "In one instance," says Maudsley, "I saw severe melancholia of two years' duration disappear after the cure of prolapsus uteri." This case was, we think, treated by us. Dr. Arbuckle, of the West Riding Asylum, communicated to us (1882) a most interesting case of inversion of the uterus which he reduced after our method, after many attempts by other plans had failed. The inversion had lasted a year. She was very anæmic, emaciated, with mind enfeebled. She got perfectly well after the restoration of the uterus. It is probable that inversion of the uterus entails pressure upon the ovaries and disturbance of their function. Griesinger says he has observed very successful cases of recovery from hysterical insanity by means of local treatment of the genital organs after all other means had failed.

Examples of nervous disorder have been observed in connection with displacement of the ovaries. Occasionally one ovary sinks down in Douglas' pouch getting below the level of the uterus. Severe nervous symptoms follow, and have been relieved by maintaining the ovary in its proper place, or by removing it. Trouble is especially liable to occur when the ovary is enlarged to the size of an orange or even less. In such a case removal by operation is clearly indicated.

The influence of disease of the ovaries is not less remarkable. Physiology points

* *Brit. Gyn. Journ.*

† *Verhandlungen der Gesellschaft für Geburtsh.* 1869.

to the ovary as the ruling organ in woman, "Propter ovaria mulier est quod est." Accordingly we might expect that the disease of this organ would cause most disturbance of the nervous system. Evidence bearing upon this conjecture has been growing of late years. But it has long been foreshadowed. Thus Icard* relates that Professor Coste had brought together in the Musée de France a fine collection of uteruses and ovaries taken from women of all ages who had committed suicide during menstruation.

The following history is doubly instructive. Boyer relates the case of a lady who, during her first pregnancy, became insane. Ten years later the mental alienation having returned it was concluded that she was pregnant. Boyer removed a polypus from the uterus and she quickly recovered. This is an illustration amongst many of the analogies between ordinary gestation, and the carrying an intra-uterine tumour.

There is one form of insanity which is of extreme importance in its medico-legal aspects. Dr. Skae refers to cases of cancerous disease of the uterus and rectum accompanied by the delusion of violation. But this form of sexual hallucination is not always associated with recognisable disease of the sexual organs, nor even with other indications of mental disorder. It is this feature which makes the subjects of sexual hallucination the more dangerous. I have been consulted in several cases of false charges of rape or seduction of this kind. It is often difficult to differentiate depravity from disease. (*See* CLIMACTERIC INSANITY; MENSTRUATION; OVARIOTOMY.) R. BARNES.

* "La femme pendant la période menstruelle," *Etude de Psychologie morbide et de Médecine légale.* 1890.

UTERINE DISPLACEMENTS AND HYSTERIA.—The derivation of the word hysteria indicates the connection that existed in the minds of ancient medical men between the womb and the disease hysteria. The symptoms of slight uterine displacements such as anteversion and anteflexion, and retroversion and retroflexion are so indefinite, if they exist at all, that it seems very fanciful to connect the hysterical state with the supposed displacements. (*See* CLIMACTERIC INSANITY; HYSTERIA; MENSTRUATION AND INSANITY; PATHOLOGY; and UTERINE DISORDERS AND INSANITY.)

V

VAGABUNDENWAHNSINN (Ger.). Insanity with special tendency to travel or wander about from place to place.

VALENTINSKRANKHEIT (Ger.). A term used for epilepsy.

VAMPIRISM.—The belief in vampirism was the result of a mixture of ignorant superstition and actual sensory hallucination. It was believed that the bodies of the dead left their graves by night and returned to their old haunts—on these occasions they sucked the blood of men, women, and children in large quantities. According to Dom Calmet, "On dit que le vampire a une espèce de faim qui le porte à manger le linge qu'il trouve autour de lui dans son cercueil. Ce rédivive sorti de son tombeau, ou un démon sous sa figure, va la nuit embrasser et serrer violemment ses proches ou ses amis, et leur suce le sang au point de les affaiblir, de les exténuer et d'entraîner leur mort. Cette persécution ne s'arrête pas à une seule personne; elle s'étend jusqu'à la dernière personne de la famille, à moins qu'on n'en interrompe le cours en coupant la tête ou en ouvrant le cœur du revenant, dont on trouve le cadavre dans son cercueil, mou, flexible, enflé et rubicond, quoiqu'il soit mort depuis longtemps."

The naturalist, Tournefort, in his "Voyage de Levant," gives a remarkable account of what he witnessed in the island of Micon, in 1701. He and his companions saw the corpse of an islander exhumed whose supposed return to life and nightly prowling about in search of blood, had rendered him an object of dread. Everybody, he says, had lost their heads. The higher class were as much carried away as the uneducated. "It was a genuine disorder of the brain, as dangerous as mania and hydrophobia. Families left their houses and went to the outside of the town to pass the night there."

It was a common thing in countries where vampires were credited, to open the grave of the suspected vampire and burn the corpse. If the body was less decomposed than might have been expected, a confirmation of the superstition was obtained. Many persons died from the fear created by the belief of having been visited and attacked by vampires.

Calmeil records the case of a female patient in an asylum who laboured under the delusion that she was visited at night by a vampire.

In the morning she was free from any fear or painful sensations; when she retired to rest and wished to sleep, a naked figure appeared and sitting upon her chest sucked blood from her breast. She consequently endeavoured to keep awake and besought the attendants to prevent her from falling asleep. Sometimes the same spectre prowled about her bed, and she redoubled her exertions to put the vampire to flight by blowing loudly at him and shaking the curtains. Visual and tactual hallucinations were clearly the cause of her delusion. Her physical health was robust.

French alienists call those who accuse themselves of having sucked blood from others, *vampires actifs*. THE EDITOR.

[*References.*—Dom Calmet, Traité sur les apparitions, les esprits, &c., tome ii. p. 88. Calmeil, De la Folie considérée sous le point de vue pathologique, philosophique, historique et judiciaire, 1845, tome ii. p. 425.]

VAPEURS (Fr.). Hysteria or hypochondriasis.

VAPORES UTERINI. (From the ancient idea that vapours arose from the uterus and passed into the brain.) Hysteria.

VAPOURISH.—Hypochondriacal or hysterical.

VAPOURS.—Popular term for hypochondriasis, or hysteria.

VECORDIA. (Lat. *vecordia.*) Idiocy. Insanity.

VEITSTANZ (Ger.). A term used either for chorea major or tarantism.

VENEREAL DISEASES AND INSANITY.—Venereal diseases are often the causes of insanity, and influence the delusions and other symptoms of insanity. (*See* SYPHILIS AND INSANITY; and SYPHILOPHOBIA.)

VERATRUM OR HELLEBORE.—The celebrated remedy for madness among the ancients. We have already cited the story of Melampus and his cure of the daughters of Prœtus. What was the hellebore to the use of which tradition refers the success of Melampus and others?

The term hellebore—derived by some from *ἑλεῖν*, to slay, and *βορά*, food—was formerly supposed to be the same species as our black hellebore or Christmas rose, designated *melampodium* in old pharmacopœias. Tournefort and Bellonius, however, who found the true hellebore of antiquity—the *ἐλλέβορος μέλας* of Dioscorides — growing abundantly in Asprospezzia (the ancient Anticyra) and Mount Olympus, pointed out that it was a different species.* Black hellebore does not contain veratria, differing in this from white hellebore, a plant of an entirely different order. It is no longer officinal. Woodville says of the hellebore which was found in Anticyra, and which he considers to be a species of *Helleborus niger*, though differing from it in having a large branched stem, that Tournefort tried the effect of simple doses of the extract with the result that violent spasms and convulsions were induced. It is very probable that the ancients used both black and white hellebore. Stevenson and Churchill† in their work already referred to, state that Mayern administered from two to three grains of the extract of the root of white hellebore, *H. albus vulgaris*, *Veratrum album* (Die Weisse Nieswurzel) which grows in Greece as well as the black hellebore, with considerable advantage in maniacal cases, and that Greding employed it in twenty-eight instances of mania and melancholia, of which five recovered, some were relieved, while others derived no benefit. It was formerly officinal, constituting the *Vinum Veratri*, 1851.

We may add that Sowerby‡ in his "Botany" says: that both *H. viridis* and *H. fœtidus* (the only *British* hellebores) have been often used instead of the true ancient or Greek *Helleborus officinalis* or *H. niger orientalis*§ of Sibthorp.

Gilbert Burnett, once Professor of Botany, King's College, London, observes that Tournefort was correct in supposing the *H. niger orientalis* of Dr. Sibthorp to be the hellebore of the ancients "as he found it in the island of Anticyra." As it may not be easily procured, he regards *H. viridis* as the safest substitute for it, though less active and as more nearly allied to the ancient Greek plant than *H. fœtidus*.

Pliny's references to hellebore in his "Natural History" are of much interest. "It is the black hellebore which is known as the melampodium. It purges, while the white hellebore acts as an emetic.‖ In former days hellebore was regarded with horror, but more recently the use of it has become so familiar that numbers of studious men are in the habit of taking it for the purpose of sharpening the intellectual powers required by their literary investigations. Carniadis, for instance,

* See Stevenson's and Churchill's "Medical Botany," vol. i.; and Woodville's "Botany," vol. ii. p. 276.

† Vol. iii. p. cxxxvi.

‡ "Botany," vol. i. p. 58.

§ *σκαρφή* of the Modern Greek; *sopkme* of the Turks.

‖ He adds that the difference between them applies, according to most writers, to the root only.

made use of hellebore when about to answer the treatises of Zeno; Drusus, too, among us the most famous of all the tribunes of the people, and whom in particular the public rising from their seats greeted with loud applause—to whom also the patricians imputed the Marsic war—is well known to have been cured of epilepsy in the island of Anticyra; a place in which it was taken with more safety than elsewhere from the fact of Sesamoïdes being combined with it. In Italy the name given to it is *Veratrum*.

"The ancients used to select those roots the rinds of which were the most fleshy from an idea that the pith extracted therefrom was of a more refined nature. This substance they covered with wet sponges and when it began to swell used to split it longitudinally with a needle, which done, the filaments were dried in the shade for future use. At the present day, however, the fibres of the root with the thickest rinds are selected and given to the patient just as they are. The best hellebore is that which has an acrid, burning taste, and when broken emits a sort of dust.

"Black hellebore is administered for the cure of paralysis, insanity, dropsy—provided there is no fever, chronic gout and diseases of the joints; it has the effect, too, of carrying off the bilious secretion and morbid humours by stools. It is given also in water as a gentle aperient, the proportion being one drachm at the very utmost, and four oboli for a moderate dose."*

One of the disputed treatises of Hippocrates is on hellebore. We find no mention in it of its employment in mental disorders.

The correspondence between Hippocrates and Democritus makes, however, a distinct reference to its use in this disease. The latter says: "I am persuaded that if to me you should give hellebore to drink, as to the insane, it would be right that the insane should escape it, and according to your art you would have blamed it as being itself the cause of madness. For hellebore, when given to the sane pours darkness over the mind, but for the insane it is very profitable."† Whether this was written by Democritus, or not, the production is unquestionably very ancient and, as such, of great interest. In favour of its genuineness, it may be mentioned that no one disputes Hippocrates having visited Abdera, the residence of the philosopher, and that he was on familiar terms with him.

As will be seen from the foregoing, much confusion has arisen in regard to the varieties of hellebore used in ancient and modern times, and we fear that in spite of the attempts which have been made to elucidate the subject, some obscurity still remains. THE EDITOR.

* Bohn's trans., vol. v. p. 99.

† Works of Hippocrates, Frankfort edit. 17

VERBAL AMNESIA.—A synonym of Amnesic Aphasia. (*See* APHASIA; POST-EPILEPTIC INSANITY.

VERBIGERATION. — **Definition.** — A psychopathic symptom first exactly described and appreciated in its clinical aspect by Kahlbaum, finds its external expression in the frequent repetition, either spoken (in which case it is done in a wearisome monotone) or written, of one and the same word or sentence, or of one and the same sound.

Diagnosis.—It is necessary also that the cause of the phenomenon should *not* be a *psychic* one, and to distinguish whether this is so or not is in many cases difficult, but, nevertheless, *monotonous utterances of insane persons* which appear to simulate verbigeration, may in most instances be differentiated from genuine verbigeration by an eliminative diagnosis. We have to point out primarily that such distinctions, which seem, at first, to puzzle the observer, are not uncommon in mental science, if we call to mind the fact that every alienist has to distinguish abnormal euphoria, as seen in a maniac or general paralytic, from the sense of well-being of a paranoiac; or the depression of a melancholiac from the degree of mental exhaustion which approximates closely to melancholic depression, and from the depression due to delusions, which is but an analogue of the depression of normal mental life. In all the mental phenomena evinced by the insane, the observer must grasp the difficulty he has to encounter, whether such are the immediate primary consequences of a pathological process or whether they represent secondary symptoms, induced by a psychic evolution from some primary mental affection by the influence of association of ideas. An example will illustrate this. Melancholia is an immediate primary production of certain morbid conditions, even as micromania, which represents a different clinical symptom of that affection. But the expectation of punishment and hanging is a mental process resulting from an association of ideas, and corresponding to the normal experience of the individual, and is therefore a *secondary* symptom—not verbigeration. This division of mental phenomena into primary, immediate and direct, and secondary, mediate and indirect, is of great importance. Without it mental science will never be kept free from romance and become an exact medical science.

Symptoms.—We now return from these prefatory remarks, which should help us to take a correct clinical view of the subject, to verbigeration itself. The first quality we have to attribute to the symptom of verbigeration is, that it is a *primary* or direct pathological phenomenon. It originates without any process of consciousness, and is as little or only in the same degree subject to will-power as the flight of ideas is. We shall later on show that there is likewise a certain relationship between the mode of origination of verbigeration and that of the genesis of the flight of ideas, in so far as we have to regard two factors as co-operating for the production of either symptom.

Verbigeration is an abnormal and unnecessary repetition of words. It can only take place when the normal flow of ideas is deranged, and the repetition is uncontrollable (this, however, does not imply that the individual himself feels it to be so). From this unconscious compulsion we derive another descriptive characteristic of verbigeration—viz., that for its reproduction we have to apply the form of *direct oratio*. If there is a reproduction in *oblique oratio*, it loses its peculiar character. A female patient, who constantly stationed herself at the main gate of the asylum, used to call out all the day long to every passer-by, whether physician, attendant, or fellow-patient, "Please, my golden doctor do give me the keys." For the sake of experiment we once gave her the keys, but she nevertheless remained unchanged in her attitude with the keys in her hand, saying in the same tone as before, "Please, my golden doctor, do give me the keys." It is clear that an entry in a journal such as this, "The patient constantly stations herself at the door, *wants* to get home, and *asks* for the keys," would be incorrect. In reality, all one can state is that the patient repeats in a verbigerating monotone the sentence, "Please, do give me the keys." It is also clear that from this aspect the diagnosis of the case becomes quite different, for there is no delusion causing it.

We have selected the above example, although it does not exhibit a good development of the symptom in question, because it serves to explain why the symptom of verbigeration is so often disregarded or misinterpreted, for we believe that the—one might almost say—instinctive tendency of the observer naturally leads him to the endeavour to find out the subject-matter of the ideas of the patient from his utterances, and in consequence those slight anomalies which lie in the sphere of imagination and speech, are easily overlooked. Verbigeration as a symptom, is not rare, and nearly always occurs combined with other derangments of the *motor* sphere. At other times we find verbigeration alternating with complete taciturnity (so-called mutism) in the same subject. The voluntary motility in the locomotor apparatus seems in most patients also greatly affected; they show conditions of rigid immobility and cataleptic flexibility (*see* KATATONIA). This combination of psychomotor phenomena is so frequent, that Kahlbaum has called verbigeration a pathognomonic symptom of katatonia. Verbigeration, however, also occurs in epileptics (in the post-convulsive stage), as well as in the course of general paralysis. In association with the latter, the whole clinical picture is generally a peculiar one, in so far as other conditions of motor inhibition, peculiar to katatonia, may be also developed (mental stupor).

After what we have said in our introductory remarks, it is not difficult to distinguish the verbal repetitions produced by persons insane in other ways from genuine verbigeration. If persons with hallucinatory ideas give vent to their anger under the influence of continual molestation, in always the same stereotyped bad language, if melancholiacs always reiterate the same lamentations and self-accusations, or if persons with religious paranoia always repeat the same formulæ, these and all other analogous phenomena are *psychologically* induced, they are indirect *secondary* symptoms. Their peculiar qualities are not lost by reproduction in *obliqua oratio*. We have to mention here that weak-minded individuals and children will often repeat the same phrases to wearisomeness, but this is primarily so different from verbigeration that we do not deem it necessary to add remarks as to the differential diagnosis. We find the same in idiots, imbeciles, hebephrenics, and in cases of terminal dementia and functional psychoses as well as in general paralysis. In the last named, loss of memory is of great moment, as supporting the development of the phenomenon. In the rare cases of extreme general amnesia, such as is described as occurring in heavy drinkers, phenomena, similar in their external manifestations, have been observed.

The theory of the ætiology of verbigeration has not yet been clearly formulated. Kahlbaum referred the contradistinctive phenomena of verbigeration and mutism occurring in one and the same individual to a condition of alternating clonic and tonic spasm of the cerebral apparatus of speech. But, according to our view, this furnishes us only with a clever picture, but no physiological explanation whatever. On the other hand it seems thoroughly justifiable to look for a common pathological source of verbigeration and mutism. Those who would draw a parallel between verbigeration and recurring compulsory ideas, and refer verbigeration to a condition of recurrent irritation in the speech centre, have not taken into consideration the incontestable clinical fact of the coincedent occurrence of verbigeration and mutism; this comparison, moreover, would leave unexplained the phenomenon of which we have not yet made mention, that in verbigeration the words are forcibly enunciated *in an extremely strained manner and with evident difficulty*. We are therefore inclined to the supposition that two factors co-operate in the production of this symptom: first, that there exists in the *speech* centre, as well as in the other parts of the sphere of voluntary motion, a state of inhibition in which a pathological factor is assumed to influence the psychical part of that apparatus. One phenomenon of this state of more or less general inhibition, is the psychomotor inability of speech or mutism. If now a stimulus of sufficient strength influence the speech centre, the inhibition may perhaps be broken through. The effort necessary for this is seen in mimetic co-movements, and in the forced tone with which the words are communicated. Later on, this state of general inhibition will result in the inability to replace by new ideas the ideas first put into action in thought and speech. If, then, this state of irritation becomes permanent, the patient will not be able to rid himself of the first words or sound, and will be compelled to repeat them, the consequence being the origination of verbigeration.

With regard to **prognosis**, verbigeration is a symptom of some importance. Generally it occurs in the middle of a state of stupor (*see* KATATONIA), and then we are unable to draw any conclusion with regard to its further progress. Sometimes it precedes that condition, and then associates itself with a peculiar pathos (pathetic verbigeration), which, if it develops from a state of depression, is a reliable indication that a condition of general motor inhibition or mental stupor is coming on.

With regard to the treatment of this symptom nothing is as yet known.

CLEMENS NEISSER.

VERFOLGUNGSWAHN, [illegible] (Ger.). Delusions of persecution. A general term for insanity of persecution.

VERGIFTUNGSIRRESEIN (Ger.). Insanity due to toxic agents such as alcohol, lead, &c.

VERRÜCKTHEIT.—Syn., French Folie systematisée progressive (Régis); psychose systematisée progressive (Garnier); délire chronique (Magnan).

Putting aside for a moment the cloud of verbiage with which this term has been enshrouded, and the hopeless confusion in which specialists have contrived to leave it, we simply define it as a mental condition, the essential and constitutional characteristic of which is a systematised delusion or group of delusions persistently held. It is almost always primary and constitutional, and not consecutive to other mental disorders.

Under PARANOIA we have given the definition, symptoms, course, and prognosis of this form of mental disorder, but there remain a few points to which it may be well to refer under this heading. Judging from recent German psychological literature, the term appears to be less in use than formerly, while that of paranoia is more in favour. Profs. Wille and Meynert, while admitting a primary mental affection (*primäre Verrücktheit*), corresponding, from the standpoint of nomenclature, to mania or melancholia—*i.e.*, truly primary and without mental weakness, affirm that there are many cases in which it is difficult to determine, in the early stage, whether they belong to primary *Verrücktheit*, or to melancholia. Meynert maintains that the former is more frequent in his experience than the latter. Some years ago this assertion would have been regarded as impossible, for the majority of German psychologists were unwilling to accept this classification, although it had been for long maintained by certain French alienists, and they maintained that there was no such thing as *Verrücktheit*, as a primary psychosis, but that it was always secondary—i.e., consecutive to a state of melancholia or mania, and a symptom or result of enfeeblement of the mental faculties. Having regard to the French synonym already given, M. Magnan believes that there are two forms of systematised insanity: (1) *folie systematisée progressive*, always developed in distinct periods, and (2) *folie systematisée des dégénérés*, which is irregular in its course and atypical in character. M. Ball, on the other hand, does not admit that the latter constitutes a separate form of mental disorder, holding that the former is itself, as the term "progressive" implies, destined to degenerate. According to M. Régis, "both views are to a certain extent correct; it is right to admit that there exists a typical systematised insanity, characterised by a uniform development in three periods, the most important of which is that met with among the degenerated." He also points out that the Italian school of psychologists have anticipated the French in the discussion of this subject and that "they include all systematised insanities under the genus 'paranoia,' which they divide into two distinct forms—degenerative, and psycho-neurotic" (see p. 887 of this Dictionary). If this grouping is in accordance with the division proposed by the French, it is even more complete; the Italian alienists maintain, in short, that systematised is always consecutive to generalised insanity, of which it forms a more advanced stage; when it is primary in the patient himself, it has succeeded a generalised insanity in the *ancestor;* when it is secondary, the transformation from generalised to specialised insanity has taken place in the *same* individual.* M. Régis' definition of *folie systematisée progressive* (paranoia primaria) is more lucid than that frequently given—namely, a chronic, distinct form of insanity without disturbance of the general mental functions, characterised by hallucinations, especially of hearing, the mental affection tending to become systematised and terminating in a transformation of the personality. It forms an integral part of the individual. Patients have indeed received the germ of the disease at birth, but this is developed under the influence of the slightest cause—*e.g.*, want, domestic trouble, &c. It is more frequent among women and the unmarried. It especially attacks gloomy, defiant, proud and misanthropic characters. We cannot follow in detail M. Régis' description of the several stages or forms of progressive systematised insanity, but may state that he embraces under the term, (1) a stage of subjective analysis or hypochondriacal insanity; (2) a stage of insane development, which includes (*a*) persecution-mania, treated of in this Dictionary in a special article by M. Paraut; (*b*) religious insanity, and another subdivision (*c*) characterised by eroticism, jealousy, and political schemes; (3) stage of complete transformation, marked by exaltation, or megalomania, finally ending, it may be, in dementia.

A very similar classification is given under the head of paranoia, or primary Verrücktheit, in the new edition of Griesinger, edited by Dr. Levinstein-Schlegel, and may be regarded therefore as reflecting German as well as French opinion, so far at least as they are represented by their alienists.

It appears, however, to the writer that clinical observation scarcely justifies the belief in so definite and invariable a scheme as that here laid down, very fascinating as it certainly is. Thus, to mention no other instance, we are satisfied that cases of persecution-mania occur not unfrequently quite apart from this alleged order of mental events. That it may be found as one stage of so-called *Verrücktheit* he does not deny, but he claims for it an independent existence also.

The essentially chronic character of this form of mental disease has been insisted upon, although it is true that some alienists have admitted an acute form of paranoia (*paranoia acuta*), but this view seems to us to militate altogether against the really systematised character of the disorder and to confound it with a state of temporary delusion from which we have always supposed it was the intention of those who have introduced the term to differentiate it.

THE EDITOR.

[*References.*—Griesinger, Patholgie u. Therapie der psychischen Krankheiten für Ärzte und Studirende, 2nd ed. 1861. Idem, 5th ed., edited by Dr. W. Levinstein Schlegel, Berlin, 1892. Arndt, Lehrbuch der Psychiatrie für Ärzte und Studirende, 1883. Sander, Ueber eine specielle Form der primären Verrücktheit, Griesinger's Archiv, 1868, Bd. i. Heft 2. Snell, Die Ueberschätzungsideen der Paranoia, Jahres-Versammlung in Hannover, 1889. Schüle, Klinische Psychiatrie, 1886. Krafft-Ebing, Lehrbuch der Psychiatrie. Salgó (Weiss), Compendium der Psychiatrie, 1889. Meynert, Klin. Vorlesungen, p. 140. Kraepelin, Psychiatrie, 2nd ed. Neisser, Ueber die originäre Verrücktheit, Archiv für Psych., Bd. i. Heft 2. Werner, Ueber die Psychiatrische Nomenclatur, Verrücktheit und Wahnsinn.]

VERSTANDESKRANKHEIT (Ger.). Mental disease.

VERSTANDESSTÖRUNG; VERSTANDESVERWIRRUNG (Ger.). Derangement of intellect.

VERTIGO (*verto*, I turn around). Dizziness with fear of falling; giddiness; swimming of the head. (Fr. *vertige;* Ger. *Schwindelsucht.*)

VERTIGO, EPILEPTIC. (*See* EPILEPTIC VERTIGO; EPILEPSY.)

VERWIRRTHEIT. — **Syn.** Confusional insanity.

Definition.—This term is applied to confused mental conditions in several forms of insanity. Sometimes it is applied to the incoherent condition present in acute delirious mania; at other times

* "Manuel pratique de Médecine mentale," par le Dr. E. Régis (with a preface by Prof. Ball), 2nd edit., Paris, 1892.

it is employed to describe a mild phase of ordinary mania. It is also used to describe some sub-acute states of paralysis. More frequently it is employed to characterise mental confusion with hallucinations (*hallucinatorische Verrücktheit*). It is said that hallucinations in this condition are generally auditory and less frequently visual; voices are heard of a threatening character. From this may arise depression and attempts at suicide. A patient recently admitted into Bethlem Hospital (before admission, he himself complained to us of mental confusion) said he could not understand what had happened to him; he was unable to concentrate his thoughts; felt impelled to commit motiveless acts, and to injure those around him without any feeling of malice. He was also suicidal. He had no delusions, strictly speaking, and his case could not be placed under acute mania; his general condition was one to which the term in question would be applied by some German alienists, but we should rather regard it as an early stage of impulsive and suicidal insanity. In not a few cases of persons charged with the commission of criminal acts there exists a real mental confusion, apart from epilepsy, which may be confounded with feigning insanity.

Esquirol did not distinguish confusional insanity from actual dementia (*démence*). Ideler (1838) considered that confusional insanity and dementia differed only in degree, and held that although it might be a primary mental affection, it was far more frequently the secondary result of other forms of insanity.*

The term was employed by Griesinger to represent mental confusion without actual dementia on the one hand, or any specialised delusion on the other.

We have spoken of mental confusion in connection with paralysis. Meynert applies it to certain states with aphasia and amnesia.

Chronic confusional states have been clearly described by Fürstner (1876) who distinguishes confusional insanity with hallucinations from acute mania and acute primary *Verrücktheit* or paranoia (with which Westphal appears to confound it), while according to him the transition to stupor is very characteristic.

Too much importance is attached to the term when it is made use of in the sense of a primary and distinct form of insanity, and English alienists for this reason rarely employ the term confusional insanity, although, of course, they frequently speak of confusional mental states when they occur as symptomatic of various forms of mental disease. The same opinion is held by Jolly, the successor to Westphal at the Charité, Berlin.

Wille, on the other hand, has treated *Verwirrtheit* as a distinct disorder, and describes its causation, course, symptoms, diagnosis, prognosis, and treatment.

With regard to **differential diagnosis**, he distinguishes it from transitory mania, mental epilepsy (*epileptisches Æquivalent*), and post-epileptic insanity, from acute mania, melancholia agitata, acute paranoia, primary dementia, and some stages of general paralysis. It can hardly be confounded with transitory mania; the history of the case should serve to prevent a mistake in diagnosis between confusional insanity, epilepsy, and acute mania.

With regard to so-called acute paranoia, there is wanting the essential symptom of systematised delusions. As regards primary dementia, there is no doubt a very strong resemblance in the main symptoms when it occurs in a mild form, but when it is well pronounced, it ought to be readily distinguished from confusional insanity, when the term is correctly used. The course of the two forms of disorder would serve to distinguish them, seeing that primary dementia (more correctly "anergic stupor") either passes into genuine incurable dementia or ends in recovery, while confusional insanity recurs in the same form—*i.e.*, without passing into either of the terminations just mentioned.

Some statistics show that confusional insanity, understood as a distinct affection, is followed by recovery in a large number of cases (according to Krafft-Ebing as many as 70 per cent.); on the other hand, Meynert and Wille do not give such favourable results, the proportion of recoveries not exceeding 46 per cent.

Treatment.—This must obviously be directed towards strengthening the system generally by means of generous diet, probably stimulants, and if, as is frequently the case, insomnia is present, by sedatives and hypnotics—*e.g.*, paraldehyde, sulphonal, or the bromides. If the mental condition has arisen from overwork, complete mental rest is obviously indicated, or if it is associated with masturbation, the treatment recommended in the article thereon (*q.v.*) must be adopted. (*See* MANIA HALLUCINATORIA.)

THE EDITOR.

[*References.* — Schüle, Klinische Psychiatrie, 1886. Wille, Die Lehre von der Verwirrtheit, in Archiv für Psychiatrie, Bd. xix. Krafft-Ebing, Lehrbuch der Psychiatrie. Griesinger, Die Pathologie und Therapie der psychischen Krankheiten. Kraepelin, Psychiatrie, 1887.]

* *Cf.* Wille in *Archiv für Psychiatrie*, Bd. xix. Heft 2, to which paper we are indebted for several of the statements in this article.

VERWORRENHEIT (Ger.). A term employed to express a higher degree of confusional insanity than *Verwirrtheit* (*q.v.*).

VESANIA (*ve*, a privative particle, *sanus*, sound). Madness, fury or rage, unsoundness of mind. *Vesaniæ* — the name of an order in Cullen's nosology and the eighth class of Sauvages in his "Nosologia Methodica," of 1763. (Fr. *vésanie*; Ger. *Wahnsinn*.)

VÉSANIQUES (Fr.). Individuals who present a perfectly characteristic abnormal mental condition, but whose insanity is not connected with obvious material lesions. They have nearly the same chance of life as that of other men (Ball).

VETERNOMANIA (*veternus*, lethargy; *μανία*, madness). The same as Typhomania. (Fr. *véternomanie*.)

VETERNOSITAS (*veternus*, aged—old people being somnolent). Comavigil.

VETERNUS.—Lethargy.

VIGILANCE (*vigilo*, I watch). Insomnia.

VIGILATIO, VIGILIA (*vigilo*, I watch). Morbid loss of sleep.

VIGILIÆ NIMIÆ.—Morbid loss of sleep.

VIS MENTALIS.—Mental power. A term for the power proper to the brain, in distinction from **Vis Nervosa**, or the power peculiar to the rest of the nervous system. (Fr. *la force mentale*.)

VISCERAL HYPOCHONDRIASIS, VISCERAL MELANCHOLIA.—Common delusions in melancholia and common morbid fears in hypochondriasis are those connected with the abdominal organs, such as fears of or delusions of intestinal obstruction. (*See* HYPOCHONDRIASIS, and MELANCHOLIA.)

VISCERAL INSANITY. (*See* SYMPATHETIC INSANITY.)

VISION, FUNCTIONAL DISTURBANCES OF. (*See* HALLUCINATIONS, and ILLUSION.)

VISIONARY. — Visionary means a person who is in the habit of seeing spectres, which are classed as subjective, because no one else can see them at the same time. The word is sometimes also used to designate a person of a fanciful and credulous turn of mind. Many people have experienced visual hallucinations at some period of their lives, generally in a condition of nervous strain or bad health; but it is only when such visions occur frequently, or their communications seem to have a definite import, or connected purpose, that they begin to interest others. Of such kind are the phantoms of the dead, spirits bearing messages from the unseen world, angels, or demons. Some treat all such apparitions as entire delusions, mere symptoms of brain or nervous disease; others consider that occasional revelations take place from the unseen world either by the exercise of faculties inherent in man, but only brought into action under very unusual conditions, or by some divine or spiritual power exercised by beings who wish to enter into communication with living men. On examining a series of narratives of ghosts and other phantoms, we soon perceive that they collectively support no particular description of the world beyond the grave, but reflect the prejudices, ignorance and credulity of the ghost-seer. We have a Greek who sees the shade of a drowned mariner mourning that he cannot cross the river Styx till his body is buried; or the phantom of an unbaptised child who bewails the misery it is suffering from having died before the rite necessary to salvation; or a Mussulman who sees in the jungles, or the desert, the green mantle of the Iman Ali mounted on his charger; or a Hindoo ghost who complains that low caste men have polluted his tomb. These stories are sometimes strangely well attested, but never more firmly than the narratives of witchcraft, which within less than two hundred years formed the subject of judicial inquiries under which thousands of innocent people were condemned to death. It is certain that some of these unfortunates really fancied that they had communion with evil spirits. Visions are not unfrequently accompanied by voices, or sometimes voices alone are heard. Probably auditory hallucinations are commoner than visual ones.

One of the earliest visionaries of which we have record was Epimenides of Crete, an epic poet, who lived in the days of Solon. He was reputed to have the power of leaving his body and conversing as a spirit with spirits. Religious visionaries were very common during the Middle Ages. Many of them were female devotees who, through severe penances, seclusion, and spiritual exercises, had rendered their nervous system at once weak and excitable, thus becoming liable to hysteria and religious ecstasies. Amongst the most noted of female visionaries were St. Theresa, St. Hildegarde, and Joan of Arc. Coming to our own century, we have Catherine Emmerich, a German nun, and Frederika Hauffé, the seeress of Prevorst, whose manifestations are described by Dr. Justinus Kerner.

The Catholic Church admitted that men might see good or bad spirits. If the seer had visions of saints or angels, and his revelations were agreeable to the faith, they canonised him; if he were visited by demons, they exorcised him; if he set himself against the Pope, they burned him, as they did Savonarola. Sometimes they took advantage of the morbid zeal of a missionary to send him on dangerous missions, as they did to Marcello Mastrilli. He was the son of the Marquis of San Marzano, and at an early age took religious vows. While in a church at Naples a workman let fall from a great height a hammer, which struck Mastrilli on the head, causing compression of the brain. During his illness and convalescence he had several visions of St. Francis Xavier, who held in one hand a bell, in the other a taper, telling him to choose. Mastrilli made his way to Goa, where he opened the tomb of Xavier, and put between the fingers of the dead Saint a paper saying that he was his servant, and would follow his example. The Father Mastrilli then went as a missionary to the Philippine Islands, where he committed a number of pious extravagances. With great difficulty he got landed in Japan at the height of the persecution, in the hopes of converting the Siogun Dayfusama. He was seized and beheaded after undergoing many cruel tortures (1637).

Visionaries were common in the fervent state of feeling at the rise of the Reformation, and during the prolonged contest with Catholicism. Luther was himself, at least during his residence at the Wartzburg, subject to visual and auditory hallucinations, which he attributed to the persecution of devils. During the struggles of the Puritans in England, and the Presbyterians in Scotland, against the Stuarts, the claim to have inspirations and visions was often made, and sometimes gained great influence with heated devotees. Emanuel Swedenborg may be said to be the prince of visionaries, and there is still a considerable sect who accept his revelations; those who reject them have no choice but to regard him as the subject of delusional insanity.

Even in our own day many claim to have communication with the souls of the departed, but the old credulous and uncritical spirit now generally shelters itself under quasi-scientific forms. We have the spiritualists especially strong in the United States, who boast of a stray scientific man among their number. Allied with them is a host of magnetisers, clairvoyants, mediums, and spirit-rappers, who claim to establish a regular commerce with the world of souls, and will tell the whereabouts of lost lovers and stray dogs. These doctrinaires have a large occult literature of periodicals and books, a key to which may be found in the "Journal du Magnétisme." Many of these persons still preserve sufficient mental balance to manage their own worldly affairs, and not unduly to interfere with those of others. What may be said to be common to most of them is a longing or groping towards the unseen world, a decided taste for the wonderful, a disposition to read symbols in nature, or to find mystic meanings in Scripture, with a condition of the nervous system passing from heightened sensibility into actual disease, sometimes manifested by hallucinations of the senses, motor spasms, and a tendency to chimerical ideas and strange conduct.

WILLIAM W. IRELAND.

[*References.*—History of the Supernatural, by W. Howitt, London, 1863. Ennemoser's History of Magic. Le Estasi Umane da Paolo Mantegazza, Milan, 1887. Through the Ivory Gate: Studies in History and Psychology, Edinburgh, 1889, by W. W. Ireland, containing accounts of Swedenborg, W. Blake, and G. Malagrida.

VISUAL HALLUCINATIONS. (*See* HALLUCINATIONS.)

VISUAL MEMORY.*—Memory by means of mental imagery; objects and their attributes being seen "in the mind's eye." Mr. Galton found by means of a series of questions addressed to various individuals that the faculty of memory by mental imagery occurs to a varying extent in almost every person, especially in non-scientific people. As a sex women possess the faculty to a greater extent than men do. He came to the conclusion that "an over-ready perception of sharp mental pictures is antagonistic to the acquirement of habits of highly generalised and abstract thought;" that the highest minds are those in which the power is subordinated for use when necessary. From the replies to his questions by one hundred men, at least half of whom were distinguished in intellectual work, Galton found that the power of mental imagery varied from that of those who could "see" the image "brilliant, distinct, and never blotchy," to that of those who had merely a general, vague, uncertain "idea," and some could recollect the objects yet never "see" them at all "in their mind's eye." The intermediate answers were nearer to the replies of those possessing the highest powers, than to those whose powers were zero. One out of every sixteen spoke of their mental imagery as being clear and

* The Editor is indebted to Mr. Galton for permission to use the diagrams in this article, and to Messrs. Macmillan, the publishers of *Nature*, for the blocks from which they are printed.

bright. The replies as to colour representation showed a smaller power of *complete* mental imagery. There was a larger percentage of those whose power was *nil*. Instances of unusually powerful mental imagery are common. Some artists have painted from a mental image; chess players, as is well known, can sometimes play games blindfolded, and have more than one game going on at the time; musicians have occasionally mental images of their music, and some speakers have images of their manuscript. Sharp sight is not necessarily accompanied by clear visual memory, nor are the visualising and identifying powers necessarily combined; some persons can combine in one perception more than can in reality be seen at one time by the two eyes. As a rule images do not become stronger by dwelling on them; the first mental image usually remains unalterable, even though the need of its correction be afterwards recognised. The visualising faculty being a natural gift has a tendency to be inherited; some young children possess it strongly. It can be developed by practice. As a nation the French possess it in a high degree.

Mr. Galton could find no closer relation between high visualising power and the intellectual faculties than between verbal memory and those same faculties. In some professions the power is of great help, especially, for example, in that of an inventive mechanician.

To imaginative people numerals almost invariably appear in the form of mental imagery. In some cases the reproduction almost amounts to hallucination. Galton found, in connection with this mental imagery of numerals, that in almost one in thirty adult males, and one in fifteen females, an invariable "*form*" appeared whenever a numeral was thought of, in which each numeral had its proper place. "*Forms*" of this kind are of various shapes and outline in different individuals, and in *Nature** and elsewhere Mr. Galton gives various diagrams of these "*forms*."

(1) One form is that contributed by Mr. George Bidder, Q.C., the son of the well-known "calculating boy." As already intimated, heredity is frequently observed. His account is as follows:—

"One of the most curious peculiarities in my own case, is the arrangement of the arithmetical numerals. I have sketched them to the best of my ability (Fig. 1.) Every number (at least within the first thousand, and afterwards thousands take

FIG. 1.

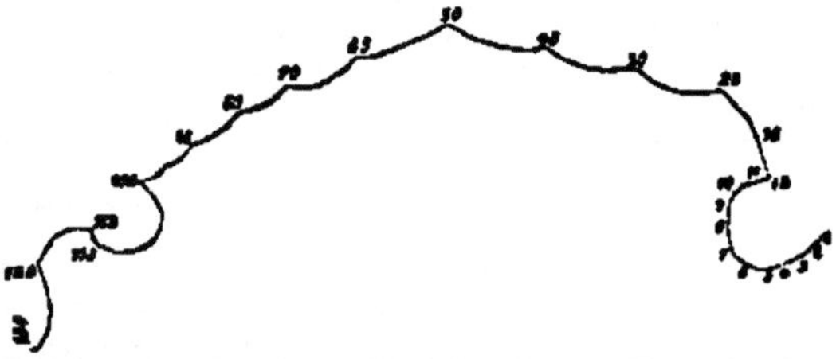

the place of units) is always thought of by me in its own definite place in the series, where it has, if I may say so, a home and an individuality. I should, however, qualify this by saying that when I am multiplying together two large numbers, my mind is engrossed in the operation, and the idea of locality in the series for the moment sinks out of prominence. You will observe that the first part of the diagram roughly follows the arrangement of figures on a clock-face, and I am inclined to think that may have been in part the unconscious source of it, but I have always been utterly at a loss to account for the abrupt change at 10 and again at 12."

Mr. Galton suggests that this is due to the wrench given to the mental picture of the clock-dial in order to make its duodecimal arrangements conform to the decimal system.

(2) Another correspondent thus describes his own visualised numerals:—

"The representation I carry in my

FIG. 2.

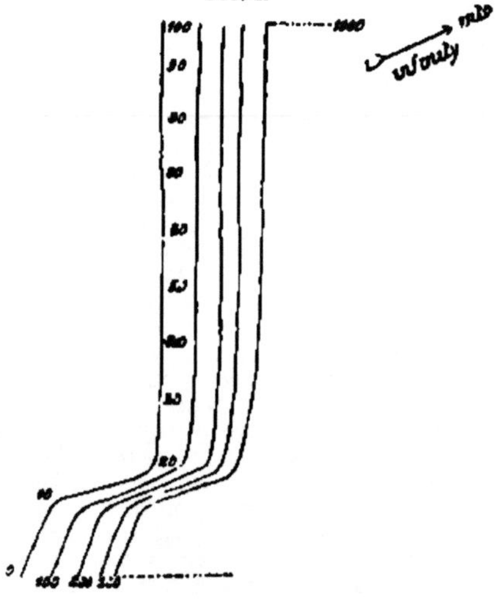

* Jan. 15, 1880.

mind of the numerical series is quite distinct to me, so much so that I cannot think of any number but I at once see it (as it were) in its peculiar place in the diagram. My remembrance of dates is also nearly entirely dependent on a clear mental vision of their *loci* in the diagram. This, as nearly as I can draw it, is reproduced in Fig. 2.

"It is only approximately correct (if the term 'correct' be at all applicable). The numbers seem to approach more closely as I ascend from 10 to 20, 30, 40, &c. The lines embracing a hundred numbers also seem to approach as I go on to 400, 500, to 1000. Beyond 1000 I have only the sense of an infinite line in the direction of the arrow, losing itself in darkness towards the millions. Any special number of thousands returns in my mind to its position in the parallel lines from 1 to 1000. The diagram was present in my mind from early childhood; I remember that I learnt the multiplication table by reference to it, at the age of seven or eight. I need hardly say that the impression is not that of perfectly straight lines; I have therefore used no ruler in drawing it."

(3) The next example (Fig. 3) is thus described by the contributor:—

"From the very first I have seen numerals up to nearly 200 range themselves always in a particular manner, and in thinking of a number it always takes its place in the figure. The more attention I give to the properties of numbers and their interpretations, the less I am troubled with this clumsy framework for them, but it is indelible in my mind's eye even when for a long time less consciously so. The higher numbers are to me quite abstract and unconnected with a shape. This rough and untidy production is the best I can do towards representing what I see. There was a little difficulty in the performance, because it is only by catching oneself at unawares, so to speak, that one is quite sure that what one sees is not affected by temporary imagination. But it does not seem much like, chiefly because the mental picture never seems *on* the flat, but *in* a thick, dark grey atmosphere deepening in certain parts, especially where 1 emerges, and about 20. How I get from 100 to 120 I hardly know, though if I could require these figures a few times without thinking of them on purpose, I

FIG. 3.

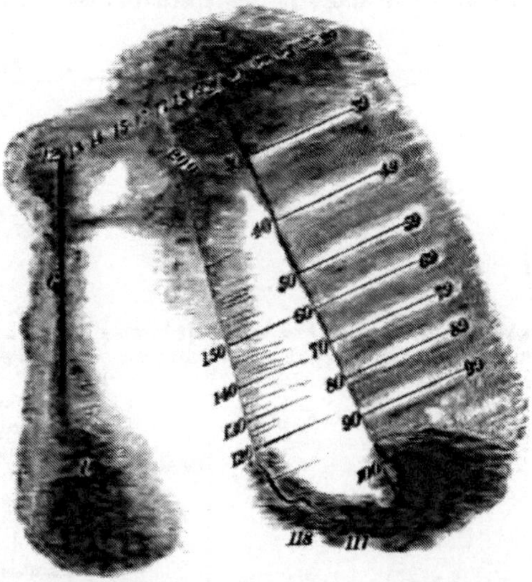

should soon notice. About 200 I lose all framework. I do not see the actual figures very distinctly, but what there is of them is distinguished from the dark by a thin whitish tracing. It is the place they take and the shape they make collectively which is invariable. Nothing more definitely takes its place than a person's age. The person is usually there so long as his age is in mind."

(4) A lady thus writes:—

"Figures present themselves to me in lines (as in the annexed diagram). They

FIG. 4.

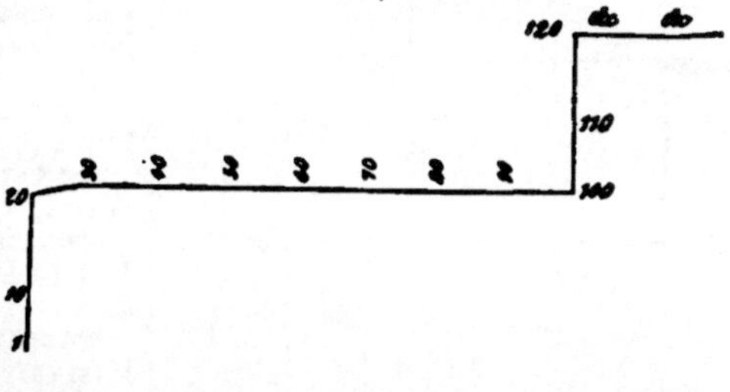

are about a quarter of an inch in length, and of ordinary type. They are black on a white ground. 200 generally takes the place of 100 and obliterates it. There is no light or shade, and the picture is invariable."

(5) A sister of this lady contributes another diagram representing her visualising experience:—

"Figures always stand out distinctly in Arabic numerals; they are black on a white ground, of this size [the specimen

FIG. 5.

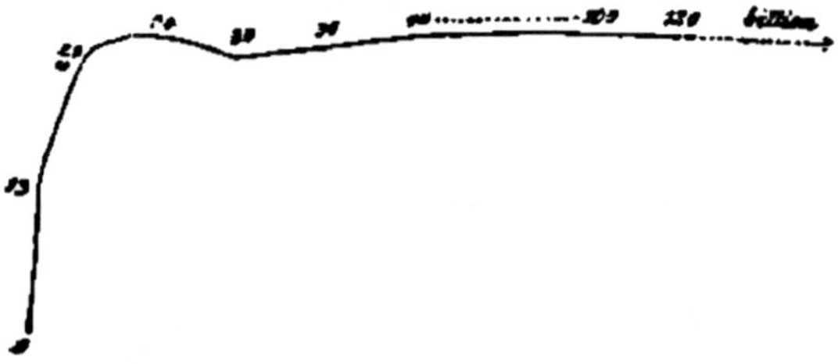

was clear and round, and in rather large ordinary handwriting], but the numeral 19 is smaller than the rest."

FIG. 6.

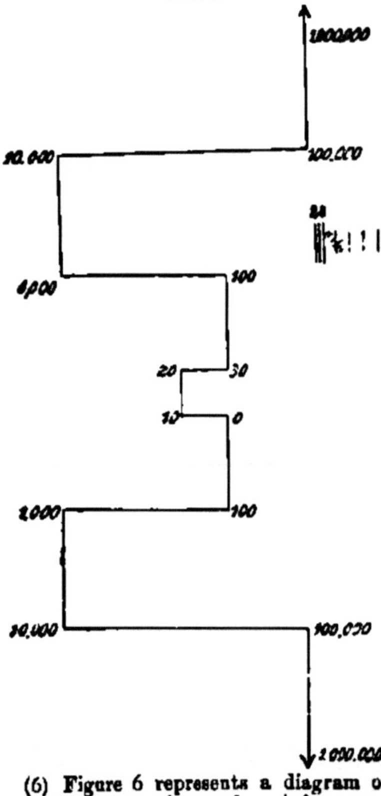

(6) Figure 6 represents a diagram of visualised numerals seen by a lady.

"The accompanying figure lies in a vertical plane, and is the picture seen in counting. The zero point never moves; it is *in* my mind; it is that point of space known as "here," while all other points are outside, or "there." When I was a child the zero point began the curve; now it is a fixed point in an infinite circle. . . . . I have had the curious bending from 0 to 30 as long as I can remember, and imagine each bend must mark a stage in early calculation. It is absent from the negative side of the scale, which has been added since childhood."

(7) The last diagram representing visualised numerals is thus described by Mr. Galton's correspondent:—

"As far as 12 the numerals appear to be concealed in black shadow; from 12 to 20 is illuminated space, in which I can distinguish no divisions. This I cannot illustrate, because it is simply dark and light *space*, but with a tolerably sharp line of division at 12. From 20 to 100 the numerals present themselves as follows, but less distinctly."

FIG. 7.

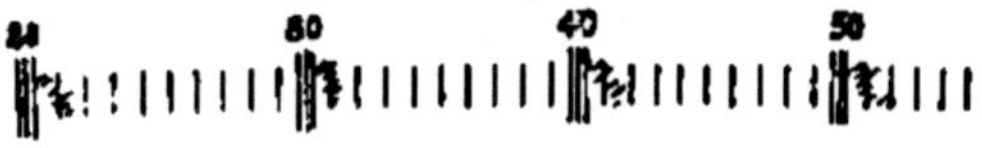

W. G. WILLOUGHBY.

[*References.*—F. Galton, Visualised Numerals, Journ. of Anthropolog. Instit., 1880; Nature, Jan. 15, 1880; Human Faculty, 1883.]

VITUS'S DANCE, ST., AND INSANITY. (*See* CHOREA AND INSANITY; SAINT VITUS'S DANCE.)

VOIX DE POLICHINELLE; or, **PUNCH'S VOICE.**—A bell-like tone of voice occasionally noticed, as in a case of Morel's, just before and during a periodical outbreak of violent homicidal mania.

VOLITION. (*See* PHILOSOPHY OF MIND, p. 40.)

VOLITIONAL INSANITY. (*See* INSANITY, VOLITIONAL.)

VOLUNTARY BOARDERS. (*See* LAW OF LUNACY; SCOTTISH LUNACY LAW, &c.)

VOMITING, HYSTERICAL. (*See* HYSTERIA, MOTOR DISTURBANCES IN, p. 622, and DIGESTIVE APPARATUS IN, p. 636.)

VOX ABSCISSA. (*See* APHONIA, HYSTERICAL.)

W

WAHLZEIT (Ger.). Will time.

WAHN (Ger.). A delusion.

WAHNBILD (Ger.). An illusion.

WAHNIDEE (Ger.). An insane idea, a delusion.

WAHNMUTH; WAHNSINN; WAHNSINNIGKEIT; WAHNWITZ (Ger.). Various terms for insanity or madness.

WAHNSINN.—This term was defined by Griesinger as comprising "states of exaltation characterised by assertive, expansive emotions (*affirmativer, expansiver Affect*), associated with persistent excessive self-estimation (*anhaltende Selbstüberschätzung*) and extravagant fixed delusions (*ausschweifende und fixe Wahnvorstellungen*), which arise therefrom."* The New Sydenham Society's translation, by Drs. Lockhart Robertson and James Rutherford (1867), renders *Wahnsinn* monomania. As stated by Griesinger, Heinroth included almost all the mental symptoms of this form of disorder under the term "ecstasis paranoica," and Jessen under *Schwärmerei*, and partly under *Aberwitz*. Griesinger's *Wahnsinn* does not correspond to Jacobi's *Wahnsinn*, as the latter psychologist comprised under this term melancholia with delusions. Most French alienists term these conditions, "monomanie (aigue) d'ambition, d'orgueil, de vanité," and also adopt Rush's term, amenomania. Great stress was laid by Griesinger upon recognising a distinct form of exaltation apart from the megalomania of the first stage of general paralysis, in which recovery frequently follows without any symptoms of paralysis. It should be stated that the recent edition of Griesinger's work (1892), edited and greatly altered in form and substance by Dr. Levinstein-Schlegel, does not treat *Wahnsinn* as a separate form of insanity, as Griesinger himself did, and only refers to it incidentally in the chapter on *Paranoësien*.

When the burning question of the definition of "Verrücktheit" was discussed at the Congress at Hamburg, in 1876, Westphal proposed a certain classification of the primary forms of this systematised mental disorder, but Hertz shortly afterwards opposed Westphal's proposal, and adopted the term *Wahnsinn* instead of *Verrücktheit*. He maintained that it was undesirable to eliminate the former term from psychological nomenclature, because "Verrücktheit" does not signify the acute primary and curable form, and also because it does not express the essential element of the disorder, which begins and ends with delusion (*Wahn*). Again, *Wahnsinn* is an old recognised term. Although we have already treated of *Verrücktheit* in a separate article, it is necessary for the complete understanding of the term at the head of our present article to refer freely to the history of the word in consequence of its relation to *Wahnsinn*. It must be understood that *Verrücktheit* in colloquial German means only insanity, without any differentiation. In 1845 Griesinger first used the expression in the sense of an incurable secondary mental affection, more especially marked by delusions of persecution and of grandeur; he qualified the term by the addition of the word "partial," which corresponds to the *délire partiel* of French alienists. He recognised also an *allgemeine Verrücktheit*, that is, a general confusion of ideas passing into actual dementia. Prior to Hertz, Snell, in 1865, applied the term *Wahnsinn* to a mental condition answering to that of Griesinger's *Verrücktheit*. It closely resembles the monomania of Esquirol. Griesinger himself subsequently modified his original view in the sense of the contention of Snell, Hertz, and also Nasse, all of whom regarded the subject from the same point of view.

Schüle adopts the term *Wahnsinn*, and divides it into acute and chronic. He subdivides further into (1) systematised acute primary insanity, (2) chronic systematised depressive insanity, (3) chronic systematised expansive insanity.

At the annual meeting of German medical psychologists in 1889, Dr. Werner introduced a discussion on the various terms now under consideration, and rejected them all in favour of the term "paranoia," which, as we have seen, is adopted by Dr. Levenstein-Schleger. Adopting this all-embracing term, he gives the following subdivisions of what formerly would have been called *Wahnsinn*: (*a*) acute primary, (*b*) chronic primary, (*c*) acute hallucinatory (*e.g.*, Krafft-Ebing's *Wahnsinn* from inanition), (*d*) chronic hallucinatory, and (*e*) secondary paranoia, following other forms of insanity.

* "Die Pathologie und Therapie der psychischen Krankheiten," von Dr. W. Griesinger. Stuttgart, 1861.

As reflecting German medical opinion it is important to note that those who took part in the debate which followed, expressed their concurrence with Werner in adopting the term *paranoia* to the exclusion of *Wahnsinn*, *Verrücktheit*, and *Verwirrtheit*, with the exception of Kirn and Kraepelin, who maintained that this course would confound together curable *Wahnsinn*, and incurable *Verrücktheit*. To this Mendel replied that prognosis should not be made the basis of classification.

We are quite in accord with Werner and the new German school in the clean sweep they would make of these disastrous terms, to which we gladly add that of katatonia. They deserve a decent burial—nay, to be buried with psychological honours, and a salute from every medical association in Europe devoted to psychiatry. How long the substituted term paranoia will maintain its present proud position we dare not undertake to prophesy. (*See* PARANOIA.)

THE EDITOR.

[*References*.—Griesinger, Die Pathologie und Therapie des psychischen Krankheiten, 1861. Krafft-Ebing, Lehrbuch der Psychiatrie, 1883. Schüle, Klinische Psychiatrie, Specielle Pathologie und Therapie der Geisteskrankheiten, 1886. Archives de Neurologie, 1890, No. lvii. p. 418. Dr. Willibald Levinstein-Schlegel's Griesinger, 1892, vol. i. p. 388, *et seq.*]

WAHNSINNIG; WAHNSÜCHTIG (Ger.). Mad, maniacal, insane.

WAHNSINNIGER (Ger.). A lunatic.

WAHNVORSTELLUNG (Ger.). A hallucination.

WAISTCOAT, STRAIT.—Formerly a favourite means of restraining violent lunatics. (*See* TREATMENT, and STRAIT WAISTCOAT.)

WAKEFULNESS. A common symptom in the insane. (*See* INSOMNIA.)

WARNINGS.—The popular term for the aura of epilepsy.

WASSERWUTH (Ger.). A form of insanity in which the patient seeks to commit suicide by drowning.

WEAKNESS OF MIND. (*See* IMBECILITY, and DEMENTIA.)

WEANING AND INSANITY. (*See* LACTATIONAL INSANITY, and PUERPERAL INSANITY.)

WEIGHT OF BRAIN.—Dr. Crochley Clapham has given in his article (p. 164) the main results of investigations into the weight of the brain in the sane and the insane. We add to his bibliographical references the following: Sims, "Med.-Chir. Trans." 1835, vol. xix; Clendinning, "Recherches sur l'Encéphale," 1886, "Traité de la folie" 1841; "Med.-Chir. Trans." 1838, vol. xxi.; Goodsir, "Edin. Med. Surg. Journ." 1845, vol. lxiii.; Peacock, "Monthly Journ. of Med. Science," vol. vii. (N. S. i.) 1847; "Edin. Monthly Journ." Oct. 1854 (with Dr. Reid); "Path. Trans." 1859, vol. x. and vol. xii., 1860–61; "Memoirs of Anthrop. Soc. of London," vol. i. 1865; Skae, "Ann. Rep. Roy. Edin. Asylum for 1854, Appendix;" Bucknill, "Path. of Insanity," Brit. and For. Med.-Chir. Rev. 1855, vol. xv.; Bucknill and Tuke, "Psych. Med." 1862, p. 419; Boyd, "Phil. Trans." 1861, vol. cli.; "Brit. and For. Med.-Chir. Rev." Jan. 1865; "Journ. of Ment. Sci." Jan. 1865, vol. x.; Broca, "Sur le volume et la form du cerveau," Bull. de la Soc. d'Anthrop. 1861, t. iii.; John Marshall, "Phil. Trans." 1864, vol. cliv.; "Anthropol. Rev." 1863, vol. i.; Thurnam, "Journ. of Ment. Sci." 1866; "Wagner, das Hirngewicht der Menschen," 1870; A. Mercier (Zürich), "Journ. of Ment. Sci." Appendix, 1891.

Dr. Thurnam gives as the average weight of the brain in 1030 English, Scotch, and Germans as 47.7 ozs. average. The same for women is given as 42.7 ozs. With regard to the weight of insane brains, he gives the average weight of the brain in 257 men at the Wilts Asylum as 46.2, while the average weight of the brain in 213 women was 41 ozs.

After the brain of Cuvier, which weighed 64.5 ozs. comes that of Dr. Abercrombie (Edin.) 63; next Spurzheim, 55.06; then Dirichlet, the celebrated mathematician, 53.6; Daniel Webster, 53.5; Lord Chancellor Campbell, 53.5; Dr. Chalmers, 53; Gauss, 52.6; Dupuytren, surgeon, 50.7; Whewell, 49; Tiedemann, 44.2. The average of ten distinguished men between fifty and seventy years of age amounted to 54.7 oz. (Thurnam *op. cit.* p. 32.)

THE EDITOR.

WERWOLF; or, WERE-WOLF (A.S. *wer*, a man; and wolf). A superstition, at one time common to almost all Europe, and which still lingers in Brittany, Limousin and Auvergne, existed that an animal, sometimes under the form of a wolf followed by dogs, sometimes as a white dog, sometimes as a black goat, and occasionally in an invisible form, prowled about, carrying off and devouring children; its skin was said to be bullet-proof, unless the bullet had been blessed in a chapel dedicated to St. Hubert. In the fifteenth century a council of theologians convoked by the Emperor Sigismund gravely declared that the were-wolf was a reality. The French equivalent *loupgarou* is probably a corruption of *loupwer-ou* or *war-ou*, the *ou* being for *orc*, an ogre. (For classical allusions, *see* LYCANTHROPY.) Herodotus also describes the

Neuri as sorcerers who had the power of assuming once a year the shape of wolves. Pliny relates that one of the family of Antæus was chosen annually by lot to be transformed into a wolf, in which shape he continued for nine years. St. Patrick, we are told, converted Vereticus, King of Wales, into a wolf. Giraldus Cambrensis tells us (Opera, vol. v. p. 119) that Irishmen can be changed into wolves. Nennius asserts that the "descendants of wolves are still in Ossory," and re-transform themselves into wolves when they bite ("Wonders of Erin," xiv.; Brewer, "Phrase and Fable").

WET-BRAIN.—Excessive serosity of brain and membranes, seen in general paralysis, &c.

WET-PACK. (*See* BATHS.)

WHISPERING. (*See* APHONIA, HYSTERICAL.)

WHYTT'S DISEASE. — A name given, in compliment to Dr. R. Whytt, of Edinburgh, to hydrocephalus.

WILL. (*See* PHILOSOPHY OF MIND, p. 40.)

WILL, Disorders of.—The study of the disorders of the will is very obscure, and can only be brought forward as an attempt. If we were only to state facts, the task would be easy, but if we try to penetrate into their reasons and causes, we soon enter the region of hypothesis. We shall not go into the inextricable problem of free-will, which dominates the whole subject, because we think that we may safely leave it alone as being purely speculative. Indeed, whether we are thorough fatalists, or enthusiastic believers in free-will, we cannot deny that there is a moment when these two hostile theses find a ground of reconciliation — the moment, when a voluntary act commences, in other words, when a certain psychological mechanism comes into play. Whatever the antecedents of a voluntary act are, whether it results from the freewill, as some maintain, or whether it is the result of a rigid connection of cause and effect, as others suppose, we must admit, that the voluntary act exists as a fact, and that from a practical standpoint at least, its antecedents and causes are but of secondary importance. We will commence our subject at the exact moment when the voluntary act begins. Thus defined, the mechanism of a voluntary act requires three essential factors:—

(1) A previous decision, a choice (free or not);

(2) The activity of certain images or motor intuitions;

(3) The usual movements effected by the different parts of our body.

We generally consider the beginning and the end only, and neglect the intermediate phase, that of the motor image. This is a great mistake, because, if we do not take it into account, we cannot understand the disorders of the will. We are too much inclined to believe that it is sufficient to will in order to be able to carry out our ideas. It is, however, sufficient to reflect upon the matter in order to see that every one of our voluntary actions, even the simplest, must be *learnt*. To take a glass of water and to swallow it, is an operation very difficult and often impossible for a little child. For a voluntary action to be safely executed it is necessary that the movements required for it be inscribed in our brain in consequence of trials and former experiences. These motor residua (potential movements) constitute what has aptly been called a *motorium commune*, without which our volitions and desires would never be realised.

The will, regarded as the power to govern ourselves and to co-ordinate our actions with one purpose in view, is far from possessing all the power which many authors attribute to it. A rapid glance at its lesions will furnish the proof of this. We shall divide the disorders of the will into two groups: (1) Those cases which result in a want of impulse, and (2) those which result in a want of inhibition.

(1) **Aboulia** may be regarded as the type of the disorders of the will, caused by want of impulse. The patients have the latent will, but they are unable to bring it into action. One of the earliest observations of this kind is due to Esquirol; it is that of a distinguished and eloquent magistrate who was perfectly well aware of his sad position. "If they spoke to him about travelling or about looking after his business, he would answer: 'I know that I ought to do it, but also that I cannot do it; your advice is very good, and I wish I could follow it, but give me will, give me that will which decides and executes. It is quite certain that I have a will only in order not to will.'" All observations of aboulia are but varieties of one and the same type. The condition of depression may advance into complete torpor. During the last influenza epidemic, which raged in France, a great number of cases of aboulia occurred. A distinguished literary gentleman, well known by his activity, confessed to us that he had been for several days in a condition of complete aboulia. The most simple volitional actions (taking a journal from a table, or writing his signature) could not be realised and seemed to him an enormous effort.

This condition seems to be the result not of a weakening of the motor centres but of the stimulation they receive. There exists in all aboulic patients a comparative insensibility, a general depression of the affective and emotive life, and thus the active life finds itself deprived of its mainspring.

With aboulia we may connect certain morbid conditions often met with in the degenerated, such as insanity of doubt (*folie du doute, Grübelsucht*) and agoraphobia. The hesitation and impotence of will are extreme. Cordes (*Archiv für Psychiatrie*, iii.) who suffered himself from agoraphobia, and was able to study it in himself, regards it as a functional paralysis, which indicates certain alterations in the motor centres. The primitive cause is, according to him, "a paresic exhaustion of the motor nervous system of that part of the brain which presides not only over locomotion, but also over the muscular sense."

Lastly, we have to mention the psychical paralyses (paralyses from ideas) which have first been studied by Russell Reynolds, and of which a certain number of cases have since become known; they may even be artificially produced in hypnotised individuals. The patient's mind becomes gradually possessed by the fixed idea that one of his limbs is paralysed, and he becomes unable to move it. It appears that this imaginary paralysis is due to a condition of temporary inertia of the motor images which are indispensable for the carrying out of an intended movement; for to imagine a movement is already the commencement of this movement, and to think a movement impossible is to inhibit the motor images from rising, or at least from attaining such an intensity as to bring about the movement.

(2) **Impulses.**—The alterations of the will which we have just mentioned, represent different degrees of non-acting; they are forms of inertia. In the second group, which comprises the phenomena known as *irresistible impulses*, great activity is displayed either with or without the will. The power of control is still reduced to impotency, but in all cases of this group the inhibition or arrest fail. The will, in fact, is the power not only to do something, but also to leave something undone; it not only produces impulse, but also inhibition. The power of inhibition seems to represent a superior degree in the evolution of the will: in the child the impulsive form reigns at first exclusively, and according to Preyer it is only about the tenth month that inhibition shows itself in the very humble form of voluntary arrest of the natural evacuations. We have also to remark, that like all the higher forms of mental activity, the inhibitory will-power has but an unstable and precarious existence: the commencement of drunkenness, somnolentia, even simple fatigue are sufficient to render us unable to control our reflexes. It must also be noted how difficult voluntary attention is to most people, and how few are capable of it for any length of time; therefore attention on one subject can only be maintained by a constant act of inhibition. The intimate mechanism of inhibition is unfortunately very little known, in spite of the researches of several distinguished physiologists, and the obscurity which reigns over this question in physiology prevents any attempt to explain the psychological mechanism.

However this may be, inhibition exists as a fact in our normal life, and it disappears in cases of irresistible impulse. It is necessary to draw attention to the fact that the transition from the sane condition to the pathological forms is almost imperceptible. Even people who are completely sane have their brains traversed by foolish abnormal impulses, but these sudden and unusual conditions do not pass into action, because they are bound down by a contrary force. In other cases there are *bizarre* actions, which escape the controlling power of the will (tics, whims, &c.), and are in themselves neither reprehensible nor dangerous, or there are also simple volitions—still restrained, however—of more serious actions (to bite or to strike). Such is the case of an amateur artist, who, finding himself in a museum before some valuable picture, felt the instinctive desire to tear the canvas.

We find a further stage of impulse in those patients who, alone or with the help of another person, strive against the attack of some violent proclivity and succeed in mastering it. Lastly, in its highest degree, the impulse is completely irresistible; it has the blind and unconscious power of an instinct, and the will as well as the inhibitory power is annihilated. The symptoms of this species (robbery, incendiarism, suicide, homicide, &c.) have been so often studied that it will suffice to have mentioned them here.

The will is therefore not an imperative entity, reigning in a world of its own, and distinguishing itself by its actions, but it is the last expression of an hierarchical co-ordination of tendencies, and as every movement or group of movements is represented in the nervous centres, it is clear that with the paralysis of each single group, one element of co-ordination disappears. Dissolution of the will is absence of co-ordination, which terminates in an independent, irregular and anarchical action. Moreover, we may ask, whether in certain human beings (not to speak of idiots and individuals labouring under dementia) the will has ever constituted itself, so that we might speak in such cases not of disease of the will, but of congenital atrophy. A great number of hysterical patients seem to belong to this class; their prodigious instability, their caprices, which incessantly appear, keep them in a permanent condition of disequilibration and of moral ataxy. There is a constitutional impotency of the will; it is unable to develop because the conditions necessary to its existence are wanting.

Annihilation of the will shows itself also in most hypnotised individuals, and this is due to the exclusive predominance of the idea or action suggested by the operator, who, occupying the place of the conscience, does not allow of any consideration or of any choice. Several authenticated cases, however, of obstinate resistance, have been reported; some subjects do not accept suggestions on certain points, and preserve during the hypnosis that power of personal reaction which is the foundation-stone of the will.

TH. RIBOT.

WILLENLOSIGKEIT. (*See* ABOULOMANIA, or ABULIA.)

WILLS. (*See* TESTAMENTARY CAPACITY.)

WINE-MADNESS. (*See* OINOMANIA.)

WIT.—The wit in mania is sometimes better than in the same person when healthy, due probably to the rapid association of ideas common in mania (Savage).

WITCHCRAFT.—Speaking with historical exactitude, the subject of witchcraft is a psycho-pathological phenomenon which includes numerous forms of the mental alienation of the early and middle ages. Demonomania, theomania, lycanthropy, choreomania, vampirism, and hysterical anomalies, are all examples of the various developments of witchcraft. In this article, however, we shall more particularly study demonolatria, or the morbid subjection and subordination of the subject to the devil, and devil-worship. The transition from demonolatria to lycanthropy, choreomania, or hysterical insanity, is easy of comprehension, but we will discuss these separate manifestations apart.

Those mentioned in the New Testament as being possessed of the devil, or afflicted with a malignant spirit, do not come under the same category as the voluntary and wicked devil-worshippers. Until the twelfth and thirteenth centuries the possessed were pitied, and were even considered as inspired, so long as they did not devote body and soul to the demon's service, or use him as their instrument. Later on, demon-worshippers and those afflicted with evil spirits were looked upon as one class; the bewitched and witches were also similarly regarded, while even the later representatives of the prophets and magicians, who, under the supposed influence of good spirits, had been favourably regarded in former times, came to be accused of the practice of witchery and were called heretics, so that they fell under the ban and persecution of the Church.

Demonolatria or witchcraft considered psychologically, especially under lycanthropic colouring, tends oftenest to forms of melancholia, of melancholia with delusions, and a confused personal identity, or even its abolition. That witchcraft may generally be considered as a form of melancholia, a morbid mental affection due to the influence of those times, with loss of personality, delusions of guilty conscience, morbid self-accusations, and a desire for expiation, is proved in fact by the confessions of the supposed witches and sorcerers at their trials. We find that those who in the estimation of others were really witches, or believed themselves such, not only confessed all their evil deeds, but complicated their trials with confessions that even to their judges seemed exaggerated and impossible, accusing themselves of horrible and unnatural crimes, such as the wholesale murder of hundreds of children, and other deeds that could not be proved. We must therefore regard demonolatria in the light of an insane delusion of guilt, an active melancholia with a morbid craving after self-accusation, self-humiliation, and an uncontrollable impulse to pretend to have committed the most absurd and nefarious crimes. We do not wish to convey the impression that all were instances of melancholia, but certainly a goodly proportion evinced melancholic tendencies, while others were maniacal, paranoic, epileptic, or hysterical subjects. Demonolatric witchcraft has always been a more or less complex form of psychosis, even as melancholia itself frequently is; it reflects all the tendencies of those times modified by the influence of Christianity. It might almost be said that the mythology of the early people with its gods of good and evil, but still always gods, precociously foreshadowed the absolute monotheism which admits of only one God, that of good, while evil not having its gods in the Christian doctrine, declared itself anachronistically in the actions of these unfortunate beings. Their belief was not an absurd improbable outcome of isolated minds, such as that of those voluntarily practising witchcraft, for their excited imagination was the result of the admixture of the new Christian religion with the blind and mistaken beliefs of their ancestors. The practice of witchcraft, even when newly disguised under the influence of Christianity, was, as we find it in the earliest times, anything but Christian in its aspects, being in fact twin sister to polytheism. Indeed, the two principles of good and evil are to be found in all the religions brought from Asia in times much anterior to Græco-Roman civilisation, as well as in the Jewish, Chaldean, Indian, and Egyptian traditions. The Greeks also, in their *εὐδαιμόναι* and *κακοδαιμόναι*, possessed geniuses of good and evil, and the *manes* of Rome were but the *κακοδαιμόναι* of the Greeks. The satyrs, sylvans, and fauns, were, like the Greek centaurs, so many witches who were nevertheless respected as part of that ancient polytheistic religion which tolerated all divinities, when the people of one country sometimes, through superstitious fear, even sacrificed to the gods of a neighbouring State, though such were not officially included in their religion. That which the poor witches of Christian lands merely fancied that they had done, all those horrors of the witch-revels (sabbat) that their diseased imaginations could suggest, was openly performed by the Greeks and Romans in the excesses of their Bacchanalian, lycean, and lupercalian feasts. It is certain that the nebulous legends of German mythology, which came to us fresh from their Asiatic origin, and which had to bear a severe shock in their encounter with Christianity—when the gods of the Greeks and Romans were already overturned, and the Christian religion raised on their ruins after some centuries of strife—had a strong influence on the development of that witchcraft which flourished in subsequent times, and reached its acme at the commencement of intellectual and scientific progress. Magic must not be confounded with witchcraft, as Bodin remarks, for magic is of Persian origin, signifying the divine and natural sciences. Under the Romans, magicians were punished only when it was believed that they caused death by poison or other means.

From the Laws of Moses, published fifteen hundred years before Christ, it is seen (says Bodin) that Chaldea, Egypt, and Palestine, were infested with witches. Indeed, Asia Minor, Greece and Italy, then only half populated, were equally troubled. God's anger was turned against the land of Canaan, not for the idolatrous and other misdeeds common to all peoples of those times, but on account of the abominable witchcrafts and sorceries that were then practised (Deuteronomy xviii.). After the Trojan war, which occurred 200 years after the Law of God, we have all the cruel witchery of Medea, the transformation of Circe and Proteus, and the Thessalian sorceries. From these facts it may be deduced that the belief in witches need not have been introduced by the German invasion, although the latter may subsequently have exercised an influence on the common Greek and Roman fables that were dying out amongst the people.

We will not attempt to describe at any length the acts of the witches or the horrors of their midnight meetings. In their revels lycanthropy and demonolatria are fused together. The grossest crimes and most barbarous cruelties were practised at their orgies, which were presided over by some representative of their common deity, the devil; infants were sacrificed, and their flesh, after having been boiled with toads, serpents, and the like, was made into an ointment, which was reputed to possess bewitching and mysterious qualities. Sometimes, to render the ceremony more sacrilegious and impious, the presiding sorcerer repeated an infernal mock mass, uttering the most fearful blasphemies over the consecrated wafer, which was subsequently mixed with their powders and unguents to render the profanation more diabolical. At the end of the ceremonies great banquets were eaten, in which infants' flesh was a prominent dish, after which the witches returned to their ordinary occupations quietly, and without leaving any trace of their revels.

Towards the end of the sixteenth century a medical explanation was given by some of this ecstatic state, and of its auditory visual and sensory hallucinations. Houllier declared the bewitched to be simply suffering from a form of melancholia, and that the supposed influences by evil spirits were simply sensory hallucinations. Even in the third and fourth centuries it was believed that the appearance of flying witches was purely imaginary, and due to an ecstatic state or a melancholic phantasm. The fact, however, that in Norway, Livonia, and Germany, where there were more converts, there were also more witches than in the southern countries, tended to maintain an error which already had largely taken root in religious fanaticism. In the first centuries of the Christian era, witchcraft was tolerated among the French, Germans, Goths, Lombards, and Saxons, and it was only in the fifth century that the French began by the Salic laws to punish witches, but their punishments were only slight, except when serious crimes were committed, a fine being imposed on those who attended the witches' revels. As yet the devil did not appear in witchcraft, and it is only in the eighth and ninth centuries that he was supposed to be present at their festivities, and the Church then began to take serious notice of these practices. In the ninth century we find mention made of a trial for witchcraft in Spain, but the condemnation of witches to the stake in any considerable numbers only began in the thirteenth century; the number of victims increased in the fourteenth, and reached its greatest height in the sixteenth century, from which time such punishment gradually died out, but in the eighteenth century was still in vogue. The institution of the Inquisition in 1183 by Pope Innocent III. marked the commencement of a perfect epidemic of trials and torturings of those who were accused of witchcraft; the arbitrary proceedings of the inquisitors who, to satisfy their private revenge, gratify their cupidity, or place out of power those whom they feared, condemned both the innocent and guilty to the flames, further raised popular indignation against the practices in which these unfortunate beings were supposed to indulge. Many of the trials reveal the fact that perfectly sane persons were made to suffer in common with those poor hallucinated melancholiacs who were but too ready to confess to diabolical practices. The so-called witches of those times may conveniently be classified into two groups, (1) those with visions or hallucinations of the senses who were affected with mental depression, and (2) those who actually infested the country killing men and boys, and hiding in the woods with lycanthropic impulses. We can hardly consider these as similar to the howlers and jumpers of later years, in that their affection was not a truly epidemic one; they are rather examples of cynanthropia with demoniacal colouring. Such cases under the interpretation of those times may be considered as appertaining to witchcraft. About 1436 in Switzerland there arose a class of men living in Vaud who worshipped the devil and ate human flesh; they infested the country about Berne and Lausanne; unbaptised infants were specially prized by them for their hideous practices, and the real acts committed by them under the influence of a morbid impulse were mixed up with hallucinations to which they freely confessed at their trials. One witch declared that at their meetings they made ointments and unguents of infants' flesh with which the novices were anointed when they were initiated into their horrible mysteries. In England, in Leicester, in 1340, a like epidemic of demoniacal and impulsive character occurred, while Knyghton speaks of another epidemic of impulsive and demoniacal cynanthropia, which broke out in this country in 1355. Witch trials and witch executions became so common after the famous Bull of Pope Innocent VIII. ("Summis desiderantes affectibus"), of December 5, 1484, issued at the request of two fanatics named Heinrich Institor and Jacob Sprenger, who had published a treatise, (The "Malleus Maleficarum") systematising the whole doctrine of witchcraft, and laying down a regular form of trial, that it has been estimated* that as many as nine thousand (?) persons suffered death subsequently to that edict. Through the spread of civilisation and the reformed religion, and not the barbarous cruelties of the Church, witchcraft gradually died out among the European nations towards the end of the seventeenth century, after having existed for over three hundred years.

A. Tamburini.
S. Tonnini.

WOD (Saxon). Insane.

WODNES (Saxon). Insanity, madness.

WOLF-MADNESS. — An occasional delusion in the insane is, that a patient considers himself changed into an animal. When this occurs with regard to a wolf, it has been called wolf-madness. (*See* Lycanthropy.)

WOODNESS (Saxon, *woed*). Madness. (Used by Spenser.)

WORD-BLINDNESS.—The state of mind of a patient to whom the sight of a word, previously understood, conveys no idea of its meaning. He may at the same time perfectly understand the spoken word. There is almost always some organic cerebral lesion. (*See* Mind-blindness.)

WORD-CLIPPING.—A symptom in general paralysis of the insane (*q.v.*).

WORD-DEAFNESS. — The state of mind of a patient to whom the sound of a word, previously understood, conveys no idea of its meaning. The sight of it may still convey the idea, and the rest of the patient's mental power may be

* Sprenger, "Life of Mohammed."

perfectly sound. The cause is usually an organic cerebral lesion. (*See* MIND-DEAFNESS, and POST-APOPLECTIC INSANITY.)

WORKHOUSES. — Though workhouses or poorhouses in some form are of rather ancient date, and since the reign of Elizabeth have been recognised parochial institutions, it was not until the year 1834, and the adoption of the Poor Law Amendment Act, William IV., c. 76, that they came into any special relation with the care and treatment of the insane, though doubtless large numbers of the insane poor were detained in the older workhouses.

From a much earlier date than 1834 considerable attention had been given to the condition of the insane. Several reports of committees of the House of Commons before this date had disclosed by abundant evidence that on the whole the condition and treatment of the insane of every class, and not the poor only, were far from satisfactory.

The observations of Pinel in France, and the valuable experience of such institutions as the Retreat at York and some other asylums of a similar character had shown by actual experience how much the comfort and well-being of this class of sufferers might be improved and their recovery facilitated by a more humane and rational treatment than that hitherto adopted. In this way the public mind had become prepared to accept and to enforce if possible a new departure in all that belonged to the care and treatment of the insane. Many active and philanthropic minds combined to give effect to these new principles of treatment. Nevertheless abuses lingered, and long after 1834 much remained to be done. By the influence of the Poor Law Commissioners appointed under the Act of 1834, larger and better workhouses began to be erected, and a more strict oversight was maintained over the administration of the Poor Law than had ever existed before. The visits of the inspectors appointed by the Commissioners disclosed many evils, and much deplorable neglect in the care of the insane poor in workhouses as well as with those boarded out or maintained in their own homes. Notwithstanding these disclosures the condition of the insane poor detained in workhouses remained in the main very unsatisfactory for many years after the passing of the Poor Law Amendment Act.

The paucity of asylum accommodation, the unwillingness of guardians to increase the expenditure, to say nothing of the fact that for many years the chief object in the minds both of the central and the local authorities was the suppression of voluntary pauperism, diverted special attention from the insane. To these various causes may be assigned the explanation of that neglect which undoubtedly existed. Abundant evidence that such neglect was common is disclosed in the second Report, 1836, of the Poor Law Commissioners. At this time, much of the neglect was of a gross and scandalous character. That the condition of the insane poor detained in workhouses remained unsatisfactory after a quarter of a century of Poor Law Administration may be gathered from a Report of the Commissioners in Lunacy in 1859 appended to their twelfth annual report. This Report was made after an inspection of the great majority if not the whole of the workhouses in England and Wales.

Since the date of that Report there has been on the whole a steady improvement in the arrangements made for the care and custody and proper selection of such insane persons as seem fit to be detained in workhouses.

The periodical visits of the Commissioners in Lunacy, and the inspectors appointed by the Poor Law Board (now the Local Government Board), combined with the good example set by many Boards of Guardians, have done much to elevate the character of the great majority of workhouses, probably of all. Many have made special provision in wards set apart for the insane with properly trained attendants.

The battle with voluntary pauperism having been won, the authorities discovered that there existed a vast number of impotent poor, whose impotence arose through no fault of their own; this view being recognised, increased and increasing attention has of late years been paid to ameliorate the condition of this class, of which improvement, increased accommodation and comfort, with better nursing and supervision of the insane inmates form no small part. That the improvement has been general and satisfactory may be inferred from the forty-third report of the Commissioners in Lunacy, in which they say of workhouses, "We are able to give on the whole a fairly satisfactory report of the arrangements and provisions made in these institutions for the patients who reside in them." The Report further says that 11,259 insane persons were resident in these workhouses on January 1, 1891. This number is probably double the number resident in these institutions at the time when the Commissioners in their annual report gave such an unfavourable account of their treatment and condition.

It may not be out of place here briefly

to refer to the legislation affecting paupers (including the insane, and their reception and treatment in workhouses.

By the 8 & 9 of George IV. c. 40, justices might require overseers to furnish lists of insane poor when mentioned, and their condition certified by a medical practitioner.

By the 4 & 5 William IV. c. 76, sec. 45, 1834, no dangerous lunatic shall be kept in any workhouse for a longer period than fourteen days. This provision was no doubt violated for many years, no definition of the word dangerous being given.

By the 8 & 9 Vict. c. 100, sec. 3, Commissioners are directed to visit and examine the insane inmates of workhouses at least once in each year. By the 16 & 17 Vict. these powers are much enlarged.

By the 16 & 17 Vict., pauper lunatics, not in any asylum, but residing at their own homes, are to be visited and their condition reported on once in each quarter by the district poor-law medical officer. For this a fee is paid. The medical officer of the workhouse is to make a like return as regards the insane inmates of the workhouse, but without fee. By the 25 & 26 Vict. c. 3, sec. 20, the form of the list as regards the workhouse is altered, and the medical officer is required in each case to say whether it is a fit one to remain in the workhouse or not, how the patient is employed—if restrained or not—and whether the accommodation therein is or is not sufficient.

By the 25 & 26 Vict. c. 3, sec. 20, no person being a lunatic, or alleged lunatic, shall be detained in any workhouse for more than fourteen days, unless the medical officer of the workhouse shall certify in writing that he or she is a proper person to be detained, and that the accommodation is sufficient.

By the 16 & 17 Vict. sec. 67, the relieving officer is bound after receiving notice that a pauper residing within his district is insane, within three days to have him taken before a justice with a view to his removal to an asylum. This is modified by the 48 & 49 Vict., which authorises the relieving-officer to remove such person to the workhouse in the first instance, where he may be further detained provided the medical officer of the workhouse shall certify in writing that he or she is a fit person to be so detained. This might be done without the intervention of a magistrate.

By the Lunacy Act of 1890, these provisions are modified. The relieving-officer or constable may still remove an insane person to the workhouse, where he may be detained for three days, at the expiration of which time he must be taken before a magistrate, who may, if he thinks fit, remit the case to the workhouse. For the permanent detention of an insane pauper in any workhouse, the magistrate must have the certificate of the medical officer of the workhouse (for which no fee is paid), and an independent medical certificate saying the case is a suitable one to be so detained. This is to be confirmed at the end of fourteen days by the certificate of the medical officer of the workhouse. This magisterial order is only in force for fourteen days, unless the medical officer shall certify that it is a proper case to be detained, in which case the magistrate's order becomes of continuing force.

Such are the provisions now in force as regards the detention of insane persons in workhouses. It will be seen from this brief retrospect, that, stage by stage, the legislature has shown an increasing desire to protect the liberty and promote the protection of the insane pauper. This contrasts favourably with the neglect of the early part of the century.

Future legislation, will, in all probability tend more and more to assimilate workhouses in all that relates to the insane poor with asylums, to the great advantage of the insane pauper and the ratepayer. The Commissioners will probably reserve for themselves some power to define the sort of cases which each workhouse is fit to retain; it is obvious that one workhouse may differ widely from another in this respect. The Commissioners in Lunacy have absolute power to discharge any insane inmate of a workhouse, or to direct his removal to an asylum.

A brief consideration of the mental condition of a large proportion of the cases which come under the observation of the medical officers of every large workhouse will be useful and will enable us to deduce some reasons why a much greater use might be made of our workhouses than has hitherto been done in the care and at least preliminary custody of large groups of the insane.

(1) Large numbers of men and women in every stage of dementia—arising from the numerous forms of gross brain disease. Paralysis, softening of the brain so-called—the dementia stages of epilepsy—the dementia due to alcoholic and syphilitic poisoning, and lastly every form of senile decay.

(2) Imbecility in every stage, from simple weak-mindedness to idiocy. Many of these cases are aggravated in their aspect on admission by drink, want of food, fatigue, and general privation. Large

numbers improve under the influence of warmth, rest, and wholesome food. This includes numerous imbecile and epileptic children of all ages.

(3) Cases of dementia following acute mania or melancholia, for the most part, persons discharged from asylums.

(4) Cases of acute excitement of a maniacal character due to alcohol. A small proportion of cases of active insanity, mania and melancholia.

No one familiar with the condition of a large proportion of persons admitted into workhouses, especially those situated near large centres of population, can fail to observe the inevitable difficulty of dealing with this class with strict adhesion to the letter of the law. The mental conditions, for the most part transitory, set up by drink and want, are well calculated to mislead an officer zealous for a strict adhesion to legal requirements — hence the period of probation allowed under the Act of 1890 becomes most valuable. It would have been well and of great advantage had the period of detention under the order of the relieving-officer, who for the most part acts on medical advice, been extended from three days to seven and the medical officers been bound to certify in every case. In this way the somewhat hasty manner in which doubtful cases have to be dealt with would have been to a great extent avoided, and asylums would have been less likely to be burdened with a class of cases, needing but rest and good food, than they are under the hasty action now in force. Patients in the independent class are never sent to an asylum on such brief notice, but in the great majority of cases abundant time is taken to form a correct medical opinion as to the nature and prospects of the case. This period of probation is as necessary in the case of the indigent poor as it is amongst the self-maintaining class.

The continued increase in the number of rate-supported asylums, the constant extension of others, and the steady increase in the population detained in them is likely under the influence of the representative bodies who now have the management of these institutions to lead to some inquiry as to how far it may be possible to reduce the cost of pauper lunacy.

A very superficial inspection of every large pauper asylum is enough to satisfy a skilled observer that there must be hundreds of persons retained in these asylums who do not require the special organisation of an asylum for their safe custody and care, or cure. The cost of the erection of an asylum is of necessity great, and its maintenance a heavy burden on the ratepayers. Whilst a wise philanthropy and Christian sympathy alike require that the sick and afflicted should receive all needful care and comfort, they fail to see why this should be given in needless excess to one group of cases only, long after all hope of cure has passed away.

The victims of cancer, rheumatism, phthisis, and a host of other disabling diseases and infirmities seem to be as deserving of and to require as much comfort as, if not more than, a hopeless imbecile or a chronic dement. The experience of numerous workhouses has abundantly shown that the wants of this class of insane persons may be well and cheaply met in a well-managed workhouse. It seems most probable that in the near future some effort will be made to more largely utilise our workhouses or other economically conducted institutions as a relief to the overburdened asylums than has hitherto been done.

No one who is familiar with the legislation affecting the insane during the present century can fail to be satisfied that it has on the whole been dictated by prudence and benevolence, and that it has surrounded an afflicted class with safeguards and comforts which do credit to our liberality and Christian charity. The asylums erected and managed for the sole benefit of the insane poor are amongst the noblest institutions of any age or country. In recent legislation there is not wanting evidence to show that in the desire to maintain the liberty of the subject, the fact that insanity is a disease requiring to be met by all the aid which medical science can bring to bear upon it, has been somewhat forgotten. There need far more care and far more discretion in dealing with the cases of mental disturbance which come under the cognisance of the Poor Law authorities. There seems a prospect that an immense burden will be cast upon pauper asylum management in mere details of administration; and that the exercise of medical skill in the treatment of this disease is likely to be replaced by constant and wearing attention to minute and numberless legal details. The cause of medical science and its full and free application to the habits of the insane cannot fail to starve under too minute legal restrictions which serve only to hamper that freedom of action without which the full benefit to be derived from treatment is impossible. The tendency of the legal mind in its anxiety to protect the liberty of the subject is to forget the fact that insanity is a sickness as little amenable to legal dicta as fever or consumption. S. W. North.

WUD (Scotch). Mad.

X

XANTHOPSIA (ξανθος, greenish yellow; ὄψις, vision). Yellow vision, a subjective visual disturbance due to the ingestion of certain drugs—*e.g.*, santonin. The disturbance is evidently central, as no staining of the ocular media has been observed, and the retina betrays only a slight hyperæmia. There is first an exaggerated appreciation of the violet spectral rays, but ultimately the reflection of light from white objects is tinged yellow; with this there is a diminished, or even abolished, appreciation of the violet rays of the spectrum. Lassitude and mental depression are accompaniments of this condition, and if the drug has been taken in large quantities, tetanic spasms and coma may result. This visual phenomenon is said to occur in patients suffering from jaundice, but if so it is rare, at least in a highly marked form.

XENELASIA (ξενηλασία, from ξένος, a stranger; ἐλαύνω, I expel or banish). There was a law among the ancient Spartans thus named, by which strangers of doubtful reputation or morality, were excluded from their society for fear of corrupting the youth and contaminating them with foreign vices. It was essentially a law for the prevention of criminal contagion.

Y

YOUNG-HELMHOLTZ THEORY.—A theory brought forward by Young and elaborated by Helmholtz to account for the quality of visual colour sensations. According to it there are three fundamental colour tones, by admixture of which all colours are formed. These colour tones are green, red, and violet. It is then assumed that in every part of the retina susceptible to colour three kinds of nervous elements exist, each corresponding to one of the above three sensations of colour. Every colour sensation is therefore a complex affair whose character is determined by the relative intensities of excitation of the three. (Ladd.)

YOUTH, INSANITY IN. (*See* DEVELOPMENTAL INSANITIES.)

Z

ZELOTYPIA (ζῆλος, emulation; τύπος, impress or type). A morbidly passionate zeal in mental or bodily exertion. (Fr. *zélotypie.*)

ZITTERWAHNSINN (Ger.). Delirium tremens.

ZOANTHROPIA (ζῶον, an animal; ἄνθρωπος, a man). A melancholy madness with fixed ideas. It is a general name for those forms of insanity where a man imagines himself an animal. (*See* CYNANTHROPIA; LYCANTHROPIA, &c.) (Fr. *zoanthropie.*)

ZOANTHROPIC MELANCHOLIA. (*See* MELANCHOLIA ZOANTHROPICA; CYNANTHROPIA; LYCANTHROPIA.)

ZOARA, ZOARE.—Insomnia.

ZOÖMAGNETISM (ζῶον, an animal; magnetism). Animal magnetism.

ZOÖPSYCHOLOGIA (ζῶον, an animal; ψυχή, the mind or soul; λόγος, a discourse). The doctrine of the existence of the mind in animals. (Fr. *zöopsychologie*; Ger. *Thierseelenkunde.*)

ZORNWUTH (Ger.). Maniacal fury, frenzy.

ZWANGSBEWEGUNGEN (Ger.). Compelled movements.

ZWANGSJACKE, ZWANGSWAMMS.—Strait-jacket.

ZWANGSVORSTELLUNGEN (Ger.). Imperative ideas.

APPENDIX.

BRAIN, ANATOMY OF.—The accompanying figure (borrowed by kind permission of Dr. Gowers from his "Diseases of the Nervous System," vol. ii.) is inserted here to illustrate the description given on page 168 of the motor and sensory types of the cerebral cortex.

The drawings were made from frozen sections of the fresh brain stained by Bevan Lewis's method with aniline blue black. The motor type is five-laminated, and is taken from the ascending frontal convolution; the sensory type shows six layers, and is taken from the first annectant gyrus. The method of staining brings out the connective tissue and nerve-cells with their nuclei and nervous processes so long as these are uncovered by myelin. In the superficial layer, therefore, we see merely the neuroglia cells. The layer of fibres arranged parallel to the surface, and the felted layer underneath it, may be demonstrated either by Exner's osmic acid method or by Weigert's or Friedmann's hæmotoxylin method.

The small pyramid layer is slightly thicker than the superficial layer. Its cells are closely compacted, and they are surrounded by a fine network of medullated fibres, which is not shown. The third layer of large pyramids is rather more than twice the thickness of the small pyramid layer, and is broader in the motor than in the sensory area. The cells are further apart from each other than are the small pyramids. They normally contain near their nucleus yellowish brown granular pigment, in greater or less quantity. Besides their apical and basal processes, lateral processes arise from these and from the body of the cell, and pass outward, dividing dichotomously, and forming a felt-work loose in the outer, close in the inner (Baillarger's outer stripe), part of the lamina. The fibres throughout the lamina begin to be arranged in bundles directed radially.

The ganglion-celled layer in the five-laminated type shows the mixed character of its large and small irregular multipolar cells. The "giant" cells of Betz, or motor cells of Lewis, are seen in the motor type (left hand); but are absent from the sensory type (right-hand section). In this layer

FIG. 1.

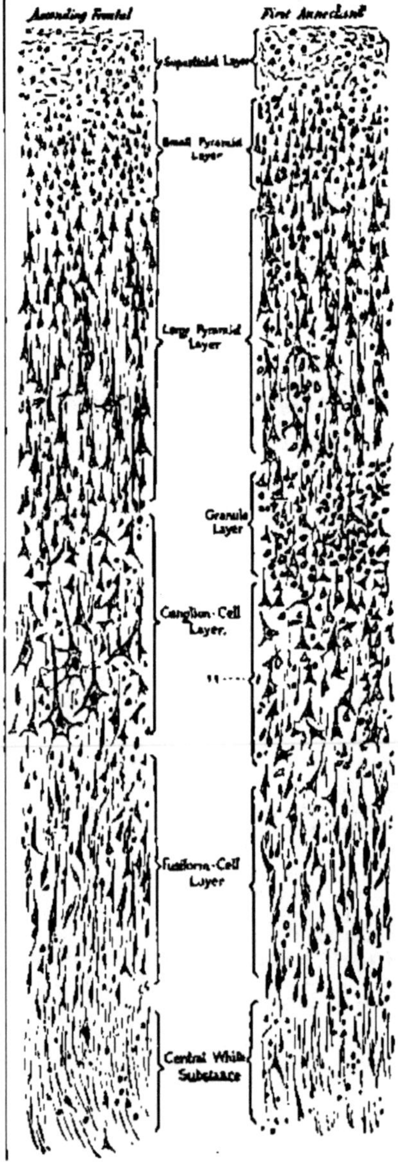

the nerve-fibres are arranged in bundles radiating outwards. Between the bundles in the outer part of the lamina the nerve-fibres form an open meshwork. In the inner portion they are closely compacted so as to form a stripe visible to the naked eye (Baillarger's inner stripe). The ganglion-celled layer is, in the motor region, not sharply separated from the large pyramid layer; but in the sensory region the granule layer lies between them. In the occipital lobe the ganglion-cell layer is very small, and is almost entirely replaced by the granule layer. In the frontal lobe the granule layer is present, but not so well developed as it is behind the motor region.

The fusiform layer presents much the same appearance in both motor and sensory regions. Its cells are separated by bundles of fibres passing into the white matter of the centrum ovale.

The structure of the cornu Ammonis differs materially from either of the above types, but it is not possible to describe it in the space allotted to anatomy.

Fig. 2 shows very clearly the cells of the third cortical layer of the ascending frontal convolution. We are indebted to the late medical superintendent of the Wakefield Asylum, Dr. Herbert Major, for the drawing. ALEX. BRUCE.

FIG. 2.

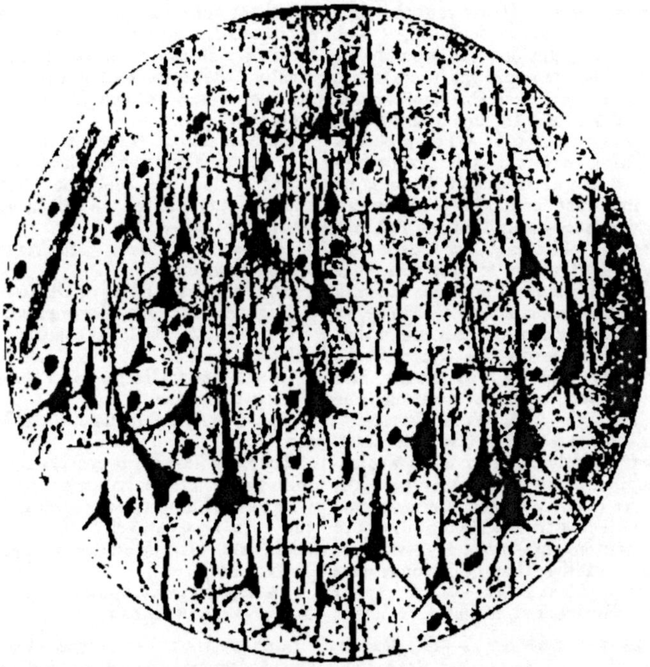

Third cortical layer of ascending frontal convolution. × 200.
H. C. M. ad nat. del.

CONTRACTS OF LUNATICS.—The judgment of Lord Esher, M.R., in *The Imperial Loan Company* v. *Stone* (1892, 8 Times L. R. 408), adds an important rider to, if indeed it does not materially modify, the doctrine laid down in *Moulton* v. *Camroux* (18 L. J. Ex. 68). The facts were as follow: The plaintiffs sued to recover the balance due upon a promissory note signed by the defendant as surety. The defendant pleaded that when he signed the note he was—*as the plaintiffs well knew*—of unsound mind, and incapable of understanding what he was doing. The action was tried before Mr. Justice Denman and a jury. The jury found that the defendant was not of sane mind, but could not agree as to whether or not the plaintiffs were aware of the fact. Thereupon Mr. Justice Denman entered judgment for the defendant, being of opinion that the onus lay *upon the plaintiffs* to show that they did not know that the defendant was of unsound mind. This decision was, however, reversed by the Court of Appeal, and the judgment of Lord Esher contained the following remarkable passages: "If one went through all the cases," said his lordship, "and endeavoured to point out the grounds on which they rest, one would get into a maze. The time has come when this Court must lay down the rule. In my opinion the result of the cases is this: When a person enters into a contract and afterwards alleges that he was insane at the time he entered into the contract—I mean an ordinary contract—and that he did not know what he was doing, and proves that this was so by the law of England, that contract is as binding upon him in every respect, *whether executed or executory*, as if he were sane, unless he can prove that at the time he made the contract the plaintiff knew that he was insane, and so insane as not to know what he was about." A. WOOD RENTON.

GALL-STONES IN THE INSANE.—At the Quarterly Meeting of the Medico-Psychological Association, May 19, 1892, Dr. Beadles (Colney Hatch Asylum) read a paper with this title. He found, out of fifty consecutive post-mortems performed on female lunatics, that gall-stones were present in eighteen cases—*i.e.*, thirty-six per cent. He does not, however, maintain that insanity is a cause of their occurrence. Other factors have to be considered. On inquiry he was not able to find that gall-stones are at all frequent among male lunatics. Among the cases above mentioned there was not, as might perhaps have been anticipated, a larger proportion of melancholiacs. It must be remembered that among the sane gall-stones are much more frequent in the female than the male sex.*

INEBRIATE RETREATS.—The extent to which institutions have been established under the Inebriates Acts, 1879, 1888, is very limited, as will be seen from the following:—

Dalrymple House, Rickmansworth, Hertfordshire.

St. Veronica's Retreat, Chiswick.

High Shot House, Twickenham.

Old Park Hall, Walsall, Staffordshire.

Tower House Retreat and Sanatorium, Westgate-on-Sea, Kent.

The Grove, Fallowfield, near Manchester.

They are licensed to receive 100 persons, but there are only about 60 inmates. Compulsory powers are required to render the "Inebriates Act," 1888, a success. (*See* HABITUAL DRUNKARDS, LEGISLATION AFFECTING.)

IRRSINN.—Idiopathic, constitutional and organic psychosis.

RULES IN LUNACY.—The *Rules in Lunacy*, 1892, came into operation on March 1, 1892, and from that date the rules of 1890 and the orders of March 5 and of August 1891 are annulled.† The rules of 1892 are in the main a consolidation of the old rules (*see* CHANCERY LUNATICS). The following provisions and forms are new:

The Masters.

10. The masters may make orders as regards administration and management, and they may direct by whom and in what manner the costs of any proceedings are to be paid. **Masters to make orders.**

11. Any person affected by any order, decision, or certificate of a master may appeal therefrom to the judge without a fresh summons, upon giving notice of appeal within eight days from the date of the order, decision, or certificate complained of, or such further time as may be allowed by the judge or master. The notice of appeal shall be given to the persons, if any, interested in supporting the order, decision, or certificate, and a copy thereof shall, within the aforesaid period of eight days, be left at the masters' office, and the masters shall thereupon bring the matter before the judge. **Appeal from orders of Masters. Forms 2, 3.**

14. The masters shall inquire into the circumstances of any delay in the conduct of proceedings before them or in proceeding upon their orders, certificates, and directions, and for that purpose may call before them all parties concerned, and may certify accordingly where it seems to them expedient. **Masters to inquire into delay.**

54. In any case, where, pending the appointment of a person to exercise in relation to the property of a person of unsound mind not so found by inquisition any of the powers of a committee of the estate, it appears to the masters desirable, that temporary provision should be made for the expenses of the maintenance, or other necessary purposes or requirements of the lunatic, or any member of his family, out of any cash or available **Temporary provision for maintenance.**

* See *Journal of Mental Science*, July 1892.

† And see Lunacy Act of 1891 (54 & 55 Vict. c. 65).

securities belonging to him in the hands of his bankers or of any other person, the masters shall be at liberty by certificate to authorise such banker or other person to pay to the person to be named in such certificate such sum as they certify to be proper, and may by such certificate give any directions as to the proper application thereof by that person, who shall be accountable for the same as the masters direct.

Provisions as to lunatics so found by inquisition to apply.

55. In all cases not otherwise herein specially provided for, the provisions of these rules relating to lunatics so found by inquisition and the other general provisions of these rules shall apply to applications relating to the property of persons of unsound mind not so found by inquisition, except that the certificate referred to in Rule 32 shall not be made, and that the masters may make orders appointing persons to exercise, in relation to the property of persons of unsound mind not so found by inquisition, the powers of a committee of the estate.

Applications as to Persons mentioned in s. 116 (1) (d) of the Lunacy Act, 1890, not being lunatic.

Applications as to persons incapable through disease or age of managing their affairs. Forms 10, 11.

56. The provisions of these rules as to persons of unsound mind not so found by inquisition shall apply to applications respecting the property of any person who though not a lunatic is through mental infirmity arising from disease or age incapable of managing his affairs.

Masters to keep a register of Committees and Receivers.

74. The masters shall keep a book or books, in which shall be made, in respect of every committee, receiver, or other person liable to account, entries showing in a tabular form the following particulars, that is to say:—

(1) The title of the matter.
(2) The names of the committees, receivers, or other persons liable to account.
(3) The date fixed for the delivery of accounts or of affidavits in lieu of accounts.
(4) The date in each successive year when the accounts or affidavits are delivered into the master's office.
(5) The date in each successive year when the accounts are passed.
(6) The balance or sum, if any, in each successive year directed to be paid into Court by the committee, receiver, or other person liable to account.
(7) The date fixed for the last-mentioned payment.
(8) The date of the actual payment into Court.
(9) The dates of all orders made in the particular matter, and also such other particulars as the Lord Chancellor may from time to time by writing direct.

Master to inform Committees of person of allowance for maintenance.

106. The masters shall inform the committees of the person upon their appointment of the annual amount allowed for the maintenance of the lunatic, or shall supply them with a copy of the scheme for maintenance, where a scheme has been provided.

Committee of person to report to Visitors as to expenditure.

107. Each committee of the person of a lunatic shall annually or from time to time and as often as may be required of him render to the board of visitors an accurate statement in writing of the various sums expended by him, the better to enable the visitors to ascertain and report whether the lunatic is being suitably maintained and whether any additional comforts can be provided for him. The visitors may dispense wholly or partially with the requirements of this rule if in any case they think it desirable so to do.

Committee of person to report to Visitors as to health of lunatic.

108. Each committee of the person of a lunatic shall half-yearly make a report to the board of visitors as to the mental and bodily health of the lunatic. If there is a medical attendant of the lunatic such medical attendant shall either countersign the report of the committee, or shall make a separate report which shall accompany that of the committee to be forwarded direct to the board of visitors.

Power to Visitors to summon Committee of person.

109. The board may summon the committee of the person of the lunatic to attend before them and to give such information in his possession relating to the lunatic as they may require.

129. The following fees shall be payable in respect of proceedings under the Lunacy Acts, 1890 and 1891:— Fees.

In addition to the old fees on certificates and attendances, and the fee of £2 on every order, the following fees, where the clear annual income of the person to whose property the order relates amounts to £100 and upwards:

	£	s.	d.
(a) On an order authorising a particular lease an amount equal to one-fourth the stamp duty payable on the lease;			
(b) On an order authorising a sum of money to be raised by mortgage or charge for every £100 or fraction of £100 of the amount to be raised	0	2	0
(c) On an order approving or authorising a contract for sale of any property for every £100 or fraction of £100 of the amount of the purchase money	0	2	0
(d) On an order authorising a sale by auction where the reserve price is fixed or approved by the masters for every £100 or fraction of £100 of the amount of the reserve price	0	2	0
(e) On an order conferring a general authority to sell or grant leases	10	0	0

Provided that the fees payable under the heads *a*, *b*, *c*, and *d*, shall not exceed £10.

Provided also that the fees payable under the heads *a*, *b*, *c*, *d*, and *e* shall not be payable upon any order made while percentage is payable upon the income of the person to whose property the order relates.

THE SCHEDULE

Referred to in the Foregoing Rules.

Form 1.

Title of Proceedings.

(*a*) Application as to alleged lunatic:—In lunacy: In the matter of *A.B.*, a person alleged to be of unsound mind.

(*b*) Application as to lunatic so found by inquisition:—In lunacy: In the matter of *A.B.*, a person of unsound mind.

(*c*) Application as to lunatic not so found by inquisition:—In lunacy: In the matter of *A.B.*, a person of unsound mind not so found by inquisition.

(*d*) Application in lunacy and in the Chancery Division:—In lunacy and in the High Court of Justice, Chancery Division: In the matter of *A.B.*, a person of unsound mind (*or as the case may be*).

(*e*) Application as to person through mental infirmity arising through disease or age incapable of managing his affairs: In the matter of *A.B.*, and in the matter of the Acts 53 Vict. c. 5, and 54 & 55 Vict. c. 65.

(*f*) Application for vesting order:—In lunacy: In the matter of the trusts of an indenture dated the and made between and . In the matter of *A.B.*, a person of unsound mind (*or as the case may be*), and in the matter of the Lunacy Acts, 1890 and 1891.

Form 2.

Notice of Appeal from an Order of a Master.

[*Insert the Title of the Proceedings.*]

Take notice that of desires to appeal to the judge from the order of the master made in this matter, dated the [*if part only is appealed from add:* so far as it directs that].

And that he intends to ask that the said order may be discharged [*or* varied] and that it may be ordered that

Dated the day of

(Signed)

To , Solicitors for

and to Messrs.

his solicitors.

FORM 3.

NOTICE OF APPEAL FROM A CERTIFICATE OF A MASTER.

[*Insert the Title of the Proceedings.*]

Take notice that of intends to appeal from the certificate of the master made in this matter, dated the

And that he intends to ask that the said certificate may be varied as follows: [*state the variation*].

And that such consequential directions may be given or corrections and alterations made in the said certificate as may be necessary.

Dated the day of .

(Signed)

To , Solicitors for

and to Messrs.

his Solicitors.

FORM 10.

NOTICE TO PERSON THROUGH MENTAL INFIRMITY ARISING FROM DISEASE OR AGE INCAPABLE OF MANAGING HIS AFFAIRS.

Mr. *A.B.*,

Take notice that a summons, of which a copy is within written, was on the day of issued by me (*or* by *C.D.* of), and that in pursuance thereof, orders may be made on the ground that you are, through mental infirmity arising from disease [*or* age], incapable of managing your affairs, for the purpose (*state the purpose*)—*e.g.*, of rendering your property, or the income thereof, available for the maintenance or benefit of yourself [*or* of yourself and your family, *or* for carrying on your trade or business], and that if you intend to object to such orders being made notice of such objection must be signed by you and attested by a solicitor, and filed at Room No. at the Royal Courts of Justice, London, within seven clear days after your receipt of this notice.

Dated the day of .

(Signed) *C.D.*,

(or) *X.Y.*,

Solicitor.

FORM 11.

NOTICE OF OBJECTION BY PERSON THROUGH MENTAL INFIRMITY ARISING FROM DISEASE OR AGE INCAPABLE OF MANAGING HIS AFFAIRS.

I, *A.B.*, of , having been served with a notice of a summons for an order respecting my property under the Acts 53 Vict. c. 5. and 54 & 55 Vict. c. 65, hereby give notice of my intention to object to such order being made.

Dated the day of .

A.B.

Witness,

M.N.,

Solicitor.

A. WOOD RENTON.

SYNONYMS.—Although in the body of the work under the various forms of mental disease we have given the corresponding terms in use in the German and French languages, it will assist the reader to have the most important placed before him in a tabular form.

English.	Latin.	French.	German.
Idiocy.	Amentia.	Idiotisme.	Idiotie. Blödsinnigkeit (angeborene).
Imbecility.	Mentis imbecillitas innata.	Imbécillité.	Imbecillität. Schwachsinn (angeborener).
Cretinism.	Cretinismus.	Crétinisme.	Kretinismus.
Mania.	Mania.	Manie.	Manie. Tobsucht.
Acute delirious mania.	Delirium acutum.	Manie suraigue. Délire aigue.	Acutes delirium. Delirium acutum.
Melancholia.	Melancholia.	Mélancolie. Lypémanie.	Melancholie. Schwermuth.
Mental stupor.	Stupor.	Stupeur or stupidité.	Stupor.
(*a*) Anergic.		Stupeur simple, sans délire ou passive.	Apathischer Stupor. Anergetischer Stupor.
(*b*) Delusional.	Melancholia cum stupore. Melancholia attonita.	Mélancolie avec stupeur.	Attonität. Status attonitus. Katatonia.
Delusional insanity. Intellectual monomania.	—	Conception délirante. Idée fixe. Folie systematisée progressive. Psychose systematisée progressive. Délire chronique. Paranoia.	Wahnvorstellung. Wahnsinn. Fixe Idee. Verrücktheit. Paranoia.
Imperative ideas. Obsession.	Obsessio.	Impulsions obsédantes. Obsessions intellectuelles.	Zwangsvorstellungen.
Dementia.	Dementia acquisita.	Démence.	Blödsinn (erworbener).
General paralysis of the insane.	Insanorum paralysis generalis.	Paralysie des aliénés. Paralysie générale.	Allgemeine progressive Paralyse. Paralyse der Irren.
Moral insanity.	Mania sine delirio.	Folie raisonnante. Folie lucide raisonnante. Monomanie affective. Manie des actes.	Das moralische Irresein.
Hypochondriasis.	Hypochondriasis.	Hypochondrie.	Hypochondrie.
Hysterical insanity.	Insania hysterica.	Folie hystérique.	Hysterisches Irresein.
Epileptic insanity.	Epilepticorum insania.	Délire épileptique.	Epileptisches Irresein.
Puerperal insanity.	Puerperarum insania.	Folie puerpérale.	Puerperales Irresein.
Insanity of puberty.	Pubescentium insania.	Hypochondrie des jeunes.	Pubertätsirresein.
Climacteric insanity.	Insania climactorica.	Aliénation climactérique.	Klimakterisches Irresein.
Senile insanity.	Insania senilis.	Démence sénile.	Seniles Irresein.
Toxic insanity.	Insania toxica.	Délire toxique.	Irresein in Folge von Intoxication.
Delirium tremens.	Delirium tremens.	Delirium tremens.	Delirium tremens. Säuferwahnsinn.
Religious insanity.	Mania religiosa.	Folie religieuse. Délire mystique.	Religiöser Wahnsinn. Mania religiosa.
Erotic insanity.	Erotomania.	Délire érotique.	Liebeswahnsinn. Erotomanie.
Persecution mania.	—	Délire de persécution. Maladie de Lasègue.	Verfolgungswahn.
Traumatic insanity.	Insania traumatica.	Délire traumatique.	Traumatisches Irresein.
Communicated insanity. Double insanity.	—	Folie à deux. Folie simultanée. Folie imposée.	Inducirtes Irresein.
Syphilitic insanity.	—	Folie syphilitique.	Luetisches Irresein.
Circular insanity.	—	Folie circulaire. Folie à double forme.	Circuläres Irresein. Cyklisches Irresein.
Confusional insanity.	—	—	Verwirrtheit.

BIBLIOGRAPHY.

In compiling the following Bibliography, illustrative of the history of the literature of insanity, the writer has been fully aware of the difficulties of the task. In the first place, it could not have been accomplished at all, without the generous co-operation of those who were interested in the subject and who rendered valuable assistance. In the second place, it was necessary to keep it within the limits imposed by the general scheme of the Dictionary. The Bibliography, therefore, is confined to works written in the English language, and does not include what has appeared in journals devoted to this special subject. But, although this broad rule was laid down as fundamental, it will be found that certain important reprints and articles are named; and a Catalogue of the psychiatric periodicals of the world is appended.

The reader will find references attached to the articles in the body of the Dictionary, which will in some measure remedy the inevitable omissions for which the writer craves indulgence.

To those in search of further information it may be stated that references and authorities will be found in these valuable works:—

Bibliotheca Britannica, a general index to British and Foreign Literature, by Dr. R. Watt, 4 vols. 4to, Edin. 1824. The first and second volumes give authors; the second and third give subjects.

Also the *Index Catalogue* of the library of the Surgeon General's Office of the United States Army. Published under the superintendence of Dr. J. S. Billings, during the last decade. Vol. vi. contains "Insanity," with very full references to periodical literature.

Besides the British Museum, there are various medical *Libraries* of the first importance. The library of the Faculty of Physicians and Surgeons in Glasgow is specially rich in old works, and a very complete Catalogue is published by Alexander Duncan, B.A., London, librarian of the Faculty; 4to, Glasgow, 1885. It is preceded by an index of subjects.

The Library of the Royal College of Surgeons, England; and the Library of the Royal College of Physicians, Edinburgh, are now in the process of being catalogued under authors and subjects. Both libraries are worthy of the distinguished corporations to which they belong.

The *Medical Digest* by Dr. Neale is indispensable in searching for information regarding what has been written during the last fifty years.

The *Journal of Mental Science*, which has been published regularly since 1853, contains many valuable papers, reviews and very complete references (Index Medico-Psychologicus, &c.) to the current literature of insanity. As a detailed index to the contents is now being prepared by Dr. Rayner, in addition to that by Dr. Blandford (published in 1879), the stores of information contained in the Journal will be much more accessible.

The periodical published for the Neurological Society of London, *Brain*; and also *Mind*, which is described as a Quarterly Review of Psychology and Philosophy, are the other English magazines in this sphere.

The quarterly *Bulletin* of the Société de la Médecine Mentale of Belgium is valuable in indicating the current course of continental work; while for standard information regarding foreign bibliography, these works may be named:—"Versuch einer Literärgeschichte der Pathologie und Therapie der psychischen Krankheiten," by Dr. J. B. Friedreich, 1830; "Leçons Orales sur les Phrénopathies," by Dr. J. Guislain (2nd ed. by Dr. Ingels), 1880; "Dictionnaire encyclopédique des Sciences Médicales," publié par Dechambre, 1864-78.

There is no mention of *Asylum Reports* in this Bibliography. They are published annually by nearly all the institutions of this country. Sometimes, but of late more rarely, they have included scientific expositions on diet, and kindred subjects. The recent tendency, however, is to reserve scientific discussions for scientific journals; and to deal with the events of the asylum year from a popular or domestic point of view. The laborious statistics appended to these reports still await resurrection and orderly arrangement.

The *Reports* of the Commissioners in Lunacy for England, Scotland, and Ireland are published annually, and are documents of the first importance. A general index to these Blue Books would be valuable, but too lengthy for insertion here.

Certain of the Reports of the Committees of Lunacy of the British Colonies and of the United States are useful discussions on the present condition of asylums and the insane.

For instance the fifth Report (1887) of the Pennsylvania Committee is an ample volume profusely illustrated with plans. These works are so numerous, however, that only a few of the more important are named in this Bibliography.

The English literature of insanity assumes a specialised form about the end of the eighteenth century, and it will be observed that public interest in the subject varies much from time to time. Although there is a sprinkling of books from the end of the sixteenth century onwards, it is really since the beginning of the century that the bulk of the literature increases.

The general treatises of a few authors who dealt with insanity in some special way, are named here, but the ordinary routine authorities in medicine need not be cited. It is unnecessary to print the names of Hippocrates, Aretaeus and Galen in this connection.

The plan of the Bibliography is chronological. Under each year are placed the names of the authors in alphabetical order, with the titles of their works.

It is to be noted that, unless otherwise stated, all the works named have been published in London, and that the size is octavo.

The following contractions are used :—

B. M. J.—British Medical Journal.
D. M. J.—Dublin Medical Journal.
E. M. J.—Edinburgh Medical Journal.
G. M. J.—Glasgow Medical Journal.
Ill.—Illustrated.
L.—The Lancet.
M. T. & G.—Medical Times and Gazette.
N. D.—No date of publication given.
N. P.—No place of publication given.
P.—Pamphlet under 100 pages.
P. P.—Privately printed.
Trans.—Translation.

Other contractions are self-explanatory.

1584.—Scot, Reginald.—The discoverie of witchcraft wherein the lewde dealing of witches and witchmongers is notablie detected, &c. &c.

1586. Bright, T.—A treatise of melancholie, containing the causes thereof—with the phisicke, care and spirituall consollation for such as have thereto adjoyned an afflicted conscience. (Also 1613.) 12mo.

1621. Burton, R.—The Anatomy of Melancholy.

1640. Ferrand, J.—Erotomania, ΕΡΩΤΟΜΑΝΙΑ, or a treatise discoursing of the essence, causes, symptoms, prognosticks, and cure of love, or erotique melancholy. (Trans. fr. French by Ed. Chilmead.) Oxford.

1648. Donne, John.—ΒΙΑΘΑΝΑΤΟΣ ; a declaration of that paradoxe or thesis, that selfe homicide is not so naturally sinne that it may never be otherwise, &c. 4to.

1649. Bulwer, J.—Pathomyotomi ; or a dissection of the muscles of the affections of the mind.

1662. Helmont, J. B. Van.—Oriatrike, or physic refined. Fol.

1666. Harvey, G.—Morbus Anglicus, or the anatomy of consumption with discourses on melancholy and madness caused by love.

1682. Willis, Thomas.—Opera omnia. 4to. Amst.

1689. Harvey, G.—The art of curing diseases by expectation ; with remarks on a supposed great case of Apoplectick Fits. 32mo.

1695. Ridley, H.—The anatomy of the brain, containing its mechanism and physiology together with some new discoveries and corrections of ancient and modern authors, upon that subject. To which is annexed a particular account of animal functions and muscular motion. The whole illustrated with sculptures after life. Illus.

1700. Brydall, John (of Lincoln's Inn).—Non Compos Mentis ; or the law relating to natural fools, mad folks, and lunatick persons.

Herwig, H. M.—The art of curing sympathetically or magnetically proved to be most true, with a discourse concerning the cure of madness, and an appendix to prove the reality of sympathy. (Trans. fr. Latin.) 12mo.

1705. Fallowes, T.—Ἡ *κρατιστη των μελαγχολων των και μαινομενων ιατρεια* ; or the best method for the cure of lunatics. With some account of the incomparable Oleum Cephalicum used in the same.

1711. Mandeville, B. De.—A treatise of the hypochondriack and hysterick passions.

1717. Blakeway, R.—An essay towards the cure of melancholy.

1722. Anon.—A description of Bedlam with an account of its present inhabitants both male and female. To which is subjoined an essay upon the nature causes and cure of madness.

1723. Perry, Charles.—On the causes and nature of madness. As also the natures and properties of opium and volatiles considered in a remonstrance to Dr. Herm. Lufneu, on his behaviour touching a late case. To which is added a postscript. P.

1725. Blackmore, R.—Treatise of the spleen and vapours, or hypochondriacal and hysterical affections. With three discourses on the nature and cure of the cholick, melancholy and palsies.

1729. Robinson, N.—A new system of the spleen, vapours and hypochondriacal melancholy, wherein all the decays of the nerves and lowness of the spirits are mechanically accounted for ; to which is subjoined a discourse on the nature, cause, and cure of melancholy, madness and lunacy.

1730. MANDEVILLE, B.—A treatise of the hypochondriack and hysterick diseases. In three dialogues. 2nd ed.

1733. CHEYNE, G.—The English malady or treatise of nervous disease of all kinds. (5th ed. 1735.)

1742. CHEYNE, G.—The natural method of cureing the diseases of the body, and the disorders of the mind depending on the body. Pt. 1. General reflections on the œconomy of nature in animal life. Pt. 2. The means and methods for preserving life and faculties. Pt. 3. Reflections on nature and cure of chronical distempers.

1746. FRINGS, P.—A treatise on Phrensy. (Trans. fr. Latin.)

MANNINGHAM, SIR R.—The symptoms, nature, causes and cure of the febricula or nervous or hysteric fever, vapours, hypo, or spleen.

1748. MEAD, R.—A treatise concerning the influence of the sun and moon upon human bodies, and the diseases thereby produced. (Trans. from Latin by T. Stack.)

1755. BILLINGS, P.—Folly predominant, with a dissertation on the impossibility of curing lunatics in Bedlam.

MEAD, T.—Medica Sacra; or a commentary on the most remarkable diseases mentioned in the Holy Scriptures. (Trans. by T. Stack.)

1758. BATTIE, W.—A treatise on madness. 4to.

HALLER, A. VON.—Medical Cases.

MONRO, J.—Remarks on Dr. Battie's treatise on madness. 16mo.

1765. WHYTT, R.—(1) Observations on the dropsy in the brain, experiments with opium, lime water, and the effects of blisters. (2) Observations on the nature, causes and cure of those disorders which have been commonly called nervous, hypochondriac or hysteric. To which are prefixed some remarks on the sympathy of nerves. Edin. (Also 1768.)

1774. BRUCKSHAW, S.—One more proof of the iniquitous abuse of private madhouses.

1776. WILSON, A.—Nature and origin of hysteria.

1777. POMME, P.—On hysterical and hypochondriacal disease. (Trans.)

1779. ROBINSON, N.—On the spleen, vapours and hypochondriack melancholy.

1780. FAWCETT, B.—Observations on the causes and cure of melancholy, especially of that which is commonly called religious melancholy. Shrewsbury.

1782. ARNOLD, T.—Observations on the nature, kinds, causes and prevention of insanity. 2 vols. Leicester. (2nd ed. Lond. 1806.)

1783. ANON.—An historical account of the origin, progress, and present state of Bethlem Hospital. 4to.

MONRO, A. (2)—Observations on the structure and functions of the nervous system. Ill. Fol. Edin.

1787. PERFECT, W.—Methods of cure in some cases of insanity, epilepsy, &c. Rochester.

PERFECT, W.—Select cases in the different species of insanity, lunacy or madness, with the modes of practice as adopted in the treatment of each. Rochester.

1788. FALCONER, W.—Influence of the passions upon disorders of the body.

ROWLEY, W.—Treatise on female nervous, hysterical, hypochondriacal, convulsive diseases, apoplexy and palsy, with thoughts on madness, suicide, &c.

1789. FAULKNER, B.—Observations on the general and improper treatment of insanity, with a plan for the more speedy and effectual recovery of insane persons. P.

HARPER, AND.—A treatise on the real cause and cure of insanity, in which the nature and distinctions of this disease are fully explained, and the treatment established on new principles. P.

LAVATER, J. C.—Essays on physiognomy. (Trans.) 3 vols.

1791. BRANDRETH, JOS.—On the use of large doses of opium in insanity. (Med. Com.)

PERFECT, W.—A remarkable case of madness, with the diet and medicines.

1792. FERRIAR, J.—Medical histories and reflections. 3 vols. Warrington, 1792-8; also Lond., 1810-13.

FOTHERGILL, A.—On the effects of hyoscyamus or henbane in certain cases of insanity.

PARGETER, W.—Observations on maniacal disorders. Reading.

1796. ANDERSON, A.—On chronic mania. New York.

BELCHER, W.—Address to humanity; containing a letter to Dr. Munro, a receipt to make a lunatic, and seize his estate; and a sketch of a true smiling hyœna.

1798. CRICHTON, A.—An enquiry into the nature and origin of mental derangement, comprehending a concise system of the physiology and pathology of the human mind. 2 vols.

HASLAM, J.—Observations on insanity, with practical remarks on the disease, and an account of the morbid appearances on dissection.

HASLAM, J.—Observations on madness and melancholy, including practical remarks on those diseases, together with cases, and an account of morbid appearances on dissection. (2nd ed. Lond. 1809.)

1800. JOHNSTONE, J.—Medical jurisprudence: on madness, with strictures on hereditary insanity.

1801. PERFECT, W.—Annals of insanity.

1802. BEDDOES, T.—Essays on some of the disorders commonly called nervous. Part II. containing observations on insanity. Bristol.

1804. Brown, J.—Works, edited by W. Cullen Brown.

Cox, J. M.—Practical observations on insanity; in which some suggestions are offered towards an improved mode of treating diseases of the mind, and some rules proposed which it is hoped may lead to a more humane and successful method of cure, with remarks on medical jurisprudence as connected with diseased intellect. (2nd ed. 1806; 3rd ed. 1813.)

Rowley, W. A.—Treatise on madness and suicide; with the modes of determining with precision mental affections from a legal point of view, and containing objections to vomiting opium and other malpractices. (3rd ed. 1813.)

Trotter, T.—An essay, medical, philosophical and chemical, on drunkenness.

1805. Bakewell, S. G.—The domestic guide in cases of insanity. Stafford.

1806. Anon.—A short letter to a noble Lord on the present state of lunatic asylums of Great Britain. P. Edin.

Pinel, P.—Treatise on insanity. (Trans.) Sheffield.

1807. Duncan, Andrew (attributed to).—Address to the public respecting the establishment of a lunatic asylum in Edin. 4to. Edin.

Highmore, N.—Treatise on the law of idiocy and lunacy.

Report.—Parliamentary Committee.

Stark, W. (architect).—Remarks on public hospitals for the cure of mental derangement. (Glasg. 1810.) 4to. Edin.

Trotter, T.—A view of the nervous temperament; a practical inquiry into the increasing prevalence, preventive treatment of those diseases, &c.

1809. Duncan, A.—Observations on the architecture of hospitals for lunatics. Edin.

1810. Black, W.—A dissertation on insanity, extracted from between two and three hundred cases in Bedlam, with tables. (2nd ed. 1811.)

Crowther, Bryan.—The Rabies Piratica, its history, symptoms, and cure; also the Furor Hippocraticus, or Graecomania, with its treatment.

Halloran, W. S.—An enquiry into the causes producing the extraordinary addition to the number of the insane. Cork.

Haslam, J.—Illustrations of madness.

1811. Beck, T. R.—On Insanity. New York.

Crowe, A. M.—A letter to Dr. R. D. Willis.

Crowther, B.—Practical remarks on insanity, to which is added a commentary on the dissection of the brains of maniacs, with some account of diseases incident to the insane.

Parkinson, J.—Observations on the Act for regulating madhouses, and a correction of the statements of the case of Benjamin Elliot, convicted of illegally confining Mary Daintree, with remarks addressed to the friends of insane persons. P.

Tuke, S.—On the state of the insane poor. (Philanthropist.) Lond.

Tuke, S.—On the treatment of those labouring under insanity, drawn from the experience of the Retreat. Phil.

1812. Collinson, G. D.—A treatise on the law concerning idiots, lunatics, and other persons *non compotes mentis*. 2 vols.

Duncan, A.—On the progress and present state of the Edinburgh Lunatic Asylum. Edin.

Paul, Sir G. O.—Observations on the subject of lunatic asylums. Gloucester.

Rush, Benjamin.—Medical inquiries and observations. Vol. 2 contains, influence of physical causes on the moral faculty; also articles upon diseases of the mind. Phil. (5th ed. 1835.)

1813. Sutton, T.—On delirium tremens.

Tuke, Samuel.—Description of the Retreat, an Institution near York for insane persons of the Society of Friends, containing an account of the origin and progress, the modes of treatment, and a statement of cases.

1814. Adams, J.—Treatise on the supposed hereditary properties of disease, with notes, particularly on madness and scrofula.

Anon.—A new governor of the asylum. A vindication of Mr. Higgins from the charges of "Corrector." York.

Atkinson, Mr. (late Apothecary to the York Asylum).—Retaliation; or hints to some of the governors of the asylum, York.

"Corrector."—A few remarks on Mr. Higgins' publication. York.

Higgins, G.—A letter from Mr. Higgins to Earl Fitzwilliam, on the subject of the abuses of the York Asylum. York.

Hill, G. N.—An essay on the prevention and cure of insanity, with observations on the rules for the detection of pretenders to madness.

1815. Adams, J.—Hereditary peculiarities of the human race, with notes on gout, scrofula, and madness, and on the goitres and cretins of the Alps and Pyrenees.

Bakewell, S. G.—Letter on mental derangement. Stafford.

Eddy, T.—Hints for introducing an improved mode of treating the insane in the asylum, &c. P. New York.

Ellis, Sir W. C.—A letter to Thomas Thompson, Esq., M.P., containing considerations on the necessity of proper places being provided by the Legislature for the reception of all insane persons, &c. Hull.

Forster, T.—Sketch of the new anatomy of the brain, with its relation to insanity.

Gray, Jona.—A history of the York Lunatic Asylum, containing the minutes of the evidence on the cases of abuse lately inquired into by a committee, addressed to Wm. Wilberforce, Esq. York.

LUCETT, J.—An exposition of the reasons which have prevented the process for relieving and curing idiocy and lunacy, and every species of insanity from having been further extended, with an appendix of attested cases, and extracts from the reports of the committee, consisting of their Royal Highnesses the Dukes of Kent and Sussex, and several noblemen and gentlemen.

MARSHALL, R.—The morbid anatomy of the brain in mania and hydrophobia, with the pathology of these two diseases, and a sketch of the author's life, by S. Sawrey.

SPURZHEIM, S. E.—Physiognomical system, by Drs. Gall and Spurzheim. (2nd ed.) Lond.

TUKE, S.—Practical hints on the construction and economy of pauper lunatic asylums: including instructions to the architects who offered plans for the Wakefield Asylum. Ill. 4to and 8vo. York.

1816. ANON.—Observations on the laws relating to private asylums, and particularly on a Bill for their alteration, which passed the House of Commons in the year 1813.

BETHLEM.—Observations of physician and apothecary upon evidence. Lond.

BETHLEM.—Observations by the governors of Bethlem Hospital on a report by the Commissioners in Lunacy. N. D.

HALLIDAY, SIR A.—A letter to Lord Binning, containing some remarks on the state of lunatic asylums in Scotland. P. Edin.

REID, J.—Essays on hypochondriacal and other nervous affections. (3rd ed. 1823.)

REPORT of, and evidence taken before the Select Committee of the House of Commons, to consider of provision being made for the better regulation of madhouses in England. (8vo, 1815.) Fol.

ROGERS, J. W.—A statement of the cruelties, abuses and frauds which are practised in madhouses. 2nd ed.

UPTON, J.—A letter upon the treatment and dismissal of the late medical officer of Bridewell and Bethlem.

1817. BURROWS, G. M.—Cursory remarks on a Bill, now in the House of Peers, for regulating of madhouses, with observations on the defects of the present system.

CAPPE, CATHERINE.—On the desirableness and the utility of ladies visiting the female wards of hospitals and lunatic asylums. P. York.

FORSTER, TH.—Observation on the casual and periodical influence of peculiar states of the atmosphere on human health and disease, particularly insanity. With a table of reference to authors.

FORSTER, TH.—Observations on the phenomena of insanity, being a supplement to the above. P.

HASLAM, J.—Considerations on the moral management of insane persons. P.

HASLAM, J.—Medical jurisprudence as it relates to insanity according to the law of England.

MAYO, T.—Remarks on insanity. Founded on the practice of John Mayo, M.D., and tending to illustrate the physical symptoms and treatment of that disease.

PARKMAN, C.—On the management of lunatics, with illustrations of insanity. Boston.

REPORT.—Select Committee on Lunatic Poor, Ireland.

RETURNS by Clergy of Scotland as to Lunatics.

SPURZHEIM, S. E.—Observations on the deranged manifestations of the mind, or insanity. (Also 1835.)

1818. DUNCAN, A.—A Letter to His Majesty's Sheriffs-Depute in Scotland, recommending the establishment of four national asylums for the reception of criminal and pauper lunatics. P.

HALLORAN, W. S.—Practical observations on the causes and cure of insanity. Cork.

HASLAM, J.—A Letter to the Governors of Bethlem Hospital, containing an account of their management of that institution for 20 years, elucidated by original letters and documents, with a correct narrative of the confinement of James Norris, &c.

1819. COOPER, T.—Tracts on Medical Jurisprudence. Including Haslam's treatise on insanity: with a preface, notes and a digest of the Laws relating to Insanity and Nuisances, &c. Phil.

HASLAM, J.—On sound mind; contribution to the natural history and physiology of the human intellect.

WADD, W.—On the malformations and diseases of the head. Ill. 4to.

1820. BURROWS, G. M.—An inquiry into certain errors relative to insanity.

1822. PRICHARD, J. C.—A treatise on diseases of the nervous system. Part I. [no more published]. Convulsive and maniacal affections.

1823. HASLAM, J.—A letter to the Right Hon. the Lord Chancellor on the nature and interpretation of unsoundness of mind and imbecility of intellect. P.

WILLIS, F.—A treatise on mental derangement (Gulston Lect. for 1822).

1824. WILDE, R. H.—Conjectures and researches concerning the love madness and imprisonment of Torquato Tasso, 2 vols. 12mo. New York.

1825. MORISON, SIR A.—Outlines of lectures on mental diseases. Ill. (2nd ed. 1826.)

1826. HOOPER, R.—The morbid anatomy of the human brain, being illustrations of the most frequent and important organic diseases to which that viscus is subject. Fol.

MILL.—Account of morbid appearances on dissection in various disorders of the brain.

1827. CULLEN, W.—The works of William Cullen (contain chapters on insanity). 2 vols. Edin.

KNIGHT, P. S.—Observations on the causes, symptoms and treatment of derangement of the mind, founded on an extensive moral and medical practice in the treatment of lunatics. Together with the particulars of the sensations and ideas of a gentleman during his mental alienation, written by himself during his convalescence. Ill.

SYER, J.—A dissertation on the features and treatment of insanity. Containing a retrospect of the most important modern theories on the subject, &c.

1828. ABERCROMBIE, J.—Pathological and practical researches on diseases of the brain and spinal cord.

ANON.—A few observations on the Bill now in progress through Parliament to regulate the cure and treatment of insane persons.

BURROWS, G. M.—Commentaries on the causes, form, symptoms and treatment, moral and medical, of insanity.

CHARLESWORTH, E. P.—Remarks on the treatment of the insane and the management of lunatic asylums; being the substance of a return from the Lincoln Lunatic Asylum to the circular of His Majesty's Secretary of State. [With a plan.] P.

COMBE, G.—The constitution of man considered in relation to external objects. 16mo. Edin.

CONOLLY, J.—Introductory Lecture, University of London.

HALLIDAY, SIR A.—A general view of the present state of lunatics and lunatic asylums.

J. W. (late a keeper at a lunatic asylum). —Practical observations on insanity and the treatment of the insane, addressed particularly to those who have relatives or friends afflicted with mental derangement. Also hints on making the study of mental disorders a necessary adjunct to medical education.

MORISON, SIR A.—Cases of mental disease, with observations on the medical treatment, for the use of students.

1829. HALLIDAY, SIR A.—A letter to Lord Robert Seymour, with a report of the number of lunatics and idiots in England and Wales. P.

PRICHARD, J. C.—A review of the doctrine of a vital principle, with observations on the instrumentality of the brain and nervous system on the operation of the mind.

RICHARDS.—On nervous disorders.

1830. CONOLLY, J.—An inquiry concerning the indications of insanity, with suggestions for the better protection and care of the insane.

CROWTHER, C.—Some observations respecting the management of the pauper lunatic asylum at Wakefield. P. Wakefield.

FARR, W.—On the statistics of English lunatic asylums, and the reform of their public management. P.

HASLAM, J.—Letter to metropolitan commissioners in lunacy. P.

NEWNHAM, W.—Essay on superstition, being an inquiry into the effects of physical influences on the mind, in the production of dreams, visions, ghosts and supernatural appearances.

PALMER, W.—An enquiry as to the expediency of a county asylum for pauper lunatics. Exeter.

REPORT.—Minutes of evidence taken by the committee appointed to enquire into the charge preferred against Dr. Wright, apothecary and superintendent of Bethlem Hospital.

TATE, G.—A treatise on hysteria.

TREVELYAN, A.—The insanity of mankind. P. Edin.

UWINS, D.—Remarks on nervous and mental disorder with special reference to recent investigations on insanity. P.

WYMAN, R.—A discourse on mental philosophy as connected with mental disorders. Boston.

1831. COMBE, A.—Observations on mental derangement, being an application of the principles of phrenology, and the elucidation of the causes, symptoms, nature and treatment of insanity. 12mo. Edin. (Also 1834, &c.)

DUNNE, CHARLES.—Brand's lunacy case, a full report of this most interesting and extraordinary investigation.

NIMMO, W.—Illustrations of the theory of mental derangement. Glasgow.

1832. ALISON, SIR A.—The Criminal Law of Scotland. 2 vols.

SEYMOUR, E. J.—Observations on the medical treatment of insanity.

WINSLOW, F.—Suggestions for an improved treatment of mental derangement. P.

1833. ALLEN, M.—Essay on the classification of the insane. Ill.

ALLEN, M.—Cases of insanity with medical, moral, and philosophical observations on them.

ALLEN, M.—Observations on the Lunatic Act, entitled an Act for the better cure and protection of insane persons in England, including views and general information on the moral and medical treatment of insanity. N. D.

AYRE, J.—Researches on dropsy in the brain, chest and abdomen.

BAKEWELL, S. G.—Essay on insanity. (2nd ed. 1836.) Edin. P.

BROUSSAIS, F. J. V.—On irritation and insanity, a work wherein the relations of the physical with the moral conditions of man are established on the basis of a physiological medium. To which are added two tracts on materialism and an outline of the association of ideas. (Trans. by T. Cooper.)

ESQUIROL, J. E. D.—Observations on the illusions of the insane, and on the medico-legal question of their confinement. (Trans.) P.

FARREN.—Essays on the varieties in mania exhibited by the characters of Hamlet, Ophelia, Lear and Edgar.

FLETCHER, R.—Sketches from the case-book, to illustrate the influence of the mind on the body, with the treatment of some of the more important nervous disturbances which arise from this influence.

HALFORD, SIR H.—Essays and orations. 12mo. 2nd ed. Ill.

MADDEN, R. R.—The infirmities of genius.

PRICHARD, J. C.—A treatise on insanity. From the Encyclopædia of Practical Medicine. 12mo.

SHELFORD, L.—Practical treatise on the law concerning lunatics.

UWINS, D.—A treatise on those disorders of the brain and nervous system which are usually considered and called mental.

1834. ANON.—Reasons for establishing and further encouragement of St. Luke's Hospital for lunatics. 4to.

MAYO, T.—Clinical facts and reflections, also remarks on the impunity of murder in some cases of presumed insanity. (Also 1847.)

MAYO, T.—An essay on the relation of the theory of morals to insanity. P.

1835. GALL, F. J.—On the origin of the moral qualities and intellectual faculties of man and the conditions of their manifestations. (Trans. by W. Lewis.) 6 vols. Boston.

NEVILLE, W. B.—On insanity, its nature, causes, and cure.

PHILIP, A. P. W.—A treatise on the more obscure affections of the brain.

PRICHARD, J. C.—A treatise on insanity and other disorders affecting the mind.

1837. BARLOW, H. C.—A dissertation on the causes and effects of disease, considered in reference to the moral constitution of man. Edin.

BROWNE, W. A. F.—What asylums were, are, and ought to be. Lectures delivered before the Managers of the Montrose Royal Lunatic Asylum. Edin.

COLQUHOUN, L.—Report of proceedings under a brieve of idiotry. 2nd ed. Edin.

FARR, W.—Statistics of insanity.

HILL, R. G.—Total abolition of personal restraint in the treatment of the insane; a lecture on the management of lunatic asylums.

1838. CROWTHER, C.—Observations on the management of madhouses, illustrated by occurrences in the West Riding and Middlesex Asylums.

ELLIS, SIR W. C.—A treatise on the nature, symptoms, causes and treatment of insanity, with practical observations on lunatic asylums, and a description of the Pauper Lunatic Asylum for the county of Middlesex at Hanwell, with a detailed account of its management.

MAYO, T.—Elements of the pathology of the human mind. 12mo.

MOSELEY, W. W.—Eleven chapters on nervous or mental complaints, and on two great discoveries, by which hundreds have been, and all may be cured with as much certainty as water quenches thirst, or bark cures ague.

STOCK.—A practical treatise on the law of non compotes mentis, or persons of unsound minds.

WALKER, A.—Intermarriage. (2nd ed. 1841.)

1839. ANON.—Documents and dates of modern discoveries in the nervous system.

BURGESS, THOMAS H.—The physiology or mechanism of blushing: illustrative of the influence of mental emotion on the capillary circulation, with a general view of the sympathies, and the organic relations of those structures with which they seem to be connected.

COOKE, W.—Mind and emotions in relation to health and disease.

EARLE, PLINY.—A visit to thirteen asylums for the insane in Europe; to which are added a brief notice of similar institutions in transatlantic countries; and an essay on the causes, duration, termination and moral treatment of insanity, with copious statistics. (Also Phil. 1845.)

HILL, R. G.—On the management of lunatic asylums, and the total abolition of personal restraint, with statistical tables.

HOLLAND, SIR H.—Medical notes and reflections.

MILLINGEN, J. G.—Aphorisms on the treatment and management of the insane, with considerations on public and private lunatic asylums, pointing out the errors in the present system. 12mo. (2nd ed. 1842.)

PERCY, JOHN.—An experimental enquiry concerning the presence of alcohol in the ventricles of the brain. Nottingham.

RAY, I.—A treatise on the medical jurisprudence of insanity.

1840. BLAKE, A.—A practical essay on delirium tremens. 2nd edit. revised.

LAYCOCK, T.—Treatise on the nervous diseases of women; comprising an enquiry into the nature, causes and treatment of spinal and hysterical disorders.

MORISON, SIR A.—The physiognomy of mental diseases.

PAGAN, J. M.—The medical jurisprudence of insanity.

PERCEVAL, J.—A narrative of the treatment experienced by a gentleman during a state of mental derangement, designed to explain the causes and nature of insanity.

REVIEW.—Organisation and management of lunatic asylums. (B. and F. Med. Chir. Rev.)

WINSLOW, F.—The anatomy of suicide.

1841. ANON.—On the want of remedial treatment for the poor of unsound mind in England, and on the proposal to confine them in wards of workhouses.

BINGHAM, N.—Observations on the religious delusions of insane persons, etc.

COOKSON, W. D.—Treatment of the insane in the Lincoln Lunatic Asylum. P.

FARR, W.—Report upon the mortality of lunatics. (J. Stat. Soc. and L.)

HEYWOOD, T. — The want of remedial treatment for the poor of unsound mind.

JACOBI, M.— Construction and management of hospitals for the insane. (Trans.) (Introd. by S. Tuke.)

NEWELL, SARAH.—Facts connected with the treatment of insanity in St. Luke's Hospital, with letters on the subject. P.

PATERNOSTER, R.—The madhouse system.

POOLE, R. — Memoranda regarding the Royal Lunatic Asylum, Infirmary and Dispensary of Montrose.

1842. ELLIOTSON, J.—Numerous cases of surgical operations without pain in the mesmeric state, &c.

GUTHRIE, G. J.—Injuries of the head affecting the brain. 4to.

LAYCOCK, T.—On lunar influence. L.

PRICHARD, J. C.—On the different forms of insanity in relation to jurisprudence. 12mo.

WEBSTER, JOHN.—Observations on the admission of medical pupils to the wards of Bethlem Hospital for the purpose of studying mental diseases. 3rd ed. P.

WINSLOW, F.—On the preservation of the health of body and mind.

1843. BARLOW, REV. J.—Man's power over himself to prevent or control insanity. 12mo.

CHEYNE, J.—Essays on partial derangement of the mind in supposed connection with religion. Dublin.

DAVEY, J. G.—Medico-legal Reflections, &c. (case of McNaghten for the murder of Drummond). P.

DE VITRE, E. D.—Observations on the necessity of an extended legislative protection to persons of unsound mind. P.

GAVIN, HECTOR.—Feigned insanity.

RUMBALL, J. Q.—Letter to the Lord Chancellor upon insanity.

SAMPSON, M. B.—Criminal jurisprudence considered in relation to cerebral organisation. (2nd ed. enlarged 1855.)

SEARLE, H.—A treatise on the tonic system of treating affections of the stomach and brain.

STARK, J.—Letter to Sir Robert Peel on the responsibility of monomaniacs for the crime of murder. P. Edin.

WINSLOW, F.—The plea of insanity in criminal cases. 12mo.

1844. ACLAND, H. W.—Feigned insanity, how most usually simulated and how detected. (P. P.) 12mo.

A MATRON.—A letter to Lord Ashley on the general government of lunatic asylums. P.

GRANTHAM, J.—Facts and observations in medicine and surgery (including insanity).

HECKER, J. F. C.—Epidemics of the middle ages. (Syd. Soc. Trans.)

MORISON, T. C. — On the distinction between crime and insanity. (Prize essay.)

MORRIS, B. R.—On the proximate cause of insanity. P.

MORRIS, B. R.—Observations on the construction of hospitals for the insane.

REPORT of the Metropolitan Commissioners in Lunacy to the Lord Chancellor.

SHEPPARD, J.—Observations on the proximate cause of insanity, being an attempt to prove that insanity is dependent on a morbid condition of the blood. 12mo.

WIGAN, A. L.—A new view of insanity. The duality of the mind proved by the structure, functions and diseases of the brain, and by the phenomena of mental derangement, and shown to be essential to moral responsibility. With an appendix (1) on the influence of religion on insanity; (2) conjectures on the nature of mental operations; (3) on the management of lunatic asylums.

WIGAN, A. L.—A few more words on the duality of the mind and on some of its corollaries. P. P. P. N. D.

1845. COSTELLO, W. B.—A letter to Lord Ashley on the reform of private lunatic asylums. P.

ESQUIROL, J. E. D.—A treatise on insanity. (Trans. and abridgment of Des Maladies Mentales. Paris, 1838). Phil.

NEWNHAM, W.—Human magnetism, its claims to dispassionate enquiry, being an attempt to show the utility of its application for the relief of human suffering.

STEWARD, J. B.—Practical notes on insanity.

THURNAM, J.—Observations and essays on the statistics of insanity; an enquiry into the causes influencing the results of treatment in establishments for the insane, to which are added statistics of the Retreat, near York.

WILLIAMS, JOSEPH.—An essay on the use of narcotics and other remedial agents calculated to produce sleep in the treatment of insanity. (Prize essay.) P. (Also 1848.)

WINSLOW, F.—An Act (8 & 9 Vict.) for the regulation of the care and treatment of lunatics, with notes. 12mo.

1846. GALT, J. M.—Treatment of insanity. New York.

HOOD, SIR W. C.—Statistics of insanity. (Also 1855 and 1860.)

MOORE, G.—The use of the body in relation to the mind.

NOBLE, D.—The brain and its physiology.

TWINING, W.—On cretinism.

WINSLOW, F.—On the incubation of insanity. (2nd ed. 1854.)

1847. CONOLLY, J. — Construction and government of lunatic asylums.

CONOLLY, JOHN. — Letter to Benjamin

Rotch, Esqre. On the plan and government of the additional lunatic asylum for the county of Middlesex, about to be erected at Colney Hatch. P.

FEUCHTERSLEBEN, BARON E. VON.—Principles of Medical Psychology. (Trans.).

LABATT, S. B.—An essay on the use and abuse of restraint in the management of the insane, with copious notes. P. Dublin.

MILLINGEN, J. G. — Mind and matter, illustrated by considerations on hereditary insanity and the influence of temperament in the development of the passions.

ROBERTSON, C. A. LOCKHART.—The consciousness of right and wrong, a just test of the plea of partial insanity in criminal cases. Edin.

ROBERTSON, C. A. LOCKHART.—Notes on the application of the trephine to the treatment of insanity, the result of injury to the head. P. Edin.

SCOTT, W. R.—Education of idiots.

SEYMOUR, E. J.—Thoughts on the nature and treatment of several severe diseases of the human body. Vol. I. only published, includes insanity.

1848. BURNETT, C. M.—Insanity tested by science and shown to be a disease rarely connected with permanent organic lesion of the brain; and on that account far more susceptible of cure than has hitherto been supposed.

BURROWS, G.—On the disorders of the cerebral circulation and the connection between affections of brain and disease of heart.

DENDY, W. C. — Cerebral diseases of children.

GRAHAM, T. S.—Observations on disorders of the mind and nerves in which their causes and moral treatment are particularly considered.

MAYO, T. — Outlines of medical proof. P.

REPORT. — The evidence taken on the inquiry into the management of the Fishponds private lunatic asylum, Bristol.

ROBERTSON, C. A. LOCKHART.—A report on the recent progress of psychological medicine and mental pathology.

WILLIAMS, J.—Insanity, its causes, prevention and cure; including apoplexy, epilepsy, and congestion of the brain. (2nd ed. 1852.)

WINN, J. M. — A critical treatise on the general paralysis of the insane.

1849. MAYO, T.—Sequel to "Outlines of medical proof." P.

OGILVIE, G. M.—A few remarks on the provision made for the insane in India, with suggestions for its extension and improvement, without encroaching on the public treasury.

WINGETT, W. S.—The defects of the lunacy law; a vindication in the decision in the case of Nottidge *v.* Ripley. P. Dundee.

1850. ANON.—Familiar views of lunacy and lunatic life, with hints on the care and management of those who are afflicted with temporary or permanent derangement. By a late medical superintendent of an asylum for the insane.

DAVEY, J. G.—Contributions to mental pathology, and on the past and present state of the insane in Ceylon.

ESSAYS on subjects connected with insanity read before the society for improving the condition of the insane.

GRANT.—Short notes in reply to Dr. Davey's work, entitled, "Contributions to mental pathology."

HAINS, A.—Trial case of alleged insanity.

JARVIS, E. — On insanity of the sexes. Louisville.

MONRO, H.—Remarks on insanity: its nature and treatment.

PRICHARD, J. C.—A medical man obtains a will from a sick lady during the absence of her husband.

ROBERTSON, C. A. LOCKHART.—An essay on the moral management of insanity (Society for improving the condition of the insane).

ROBERTSON, C. A. LOCKHART. — An essay on the improvements made by the moderns in the medical treatment of mental diseases (Society for improving the condition of the insane).

SEATON, J.—Practical observations and suggestions on the treatment of mental affections. 8vo.

TREVELYAN, A.—The insanity of mankind. P. Edin.

1851. ANON.—A letter to the right honourable the Committee of the House of Lords, relating to Chancery lunatics.

BADELEY, J. C. — On the reciprocal agencies of mind and matter, and on insanity (Lumleian Lectures).

BUCKNILL, J. C. — An enquiry into the classification and treatment of criminal lunatics; a letter addressed to Samuel Trehawke Kekewich, Esq. P.

LEY, W. — A letter to Dr. Williams on criminal lunatics. P. Oxford.

MONRO, H.—Articles on reform in private asylums, and on improving the condition of the insane. (2nd ed. 1852.)

SYMONDS, J. A. (elder).—Sleep and dreams. (Two lectures.) 8vo. London and Bristol. P. 2nd ed.

WHITEHEAD, J.—On the transmission from parent to offspring, of some forms of disease, and of morbid taints and tendencies. (2nd ed. 1857.)

WOOD, W. — Remarks on the plea of insanity, with statistics of the probable duration of life in the insane. (2nd ed. 1852.)

1852. BUCKNILL, J. C. — The law and theory of insanity. P.

BURNETT, C. M.—Crime and insanity: their causes, connections and consequences.

COOK, W.—Mind and the emotions, considered in relation to health, disease and religion.

CUMMING, W. F. — Notes on lunatic asylums in Germany, and other parts of Europe.

DICKSON, T.—Asylums for the insane. Observations on the importance of establishing public hospitals for the insane of the middle and higher classes, with a brief exposition of the nature of insanity. P. (2nd ed. 1855.) Edin.

FEUCHTERSLEBEN, BARON E. VON.—The dietetics of the soul.

HOLLAND, SIR H. — Chapters on mental physiology (founded chiefly on chapters contained in "Medical notes and reflections" by the same author). (2nd ed. enlarged, 1858.)

SWAN, J.—The brain in relation to the mind.

VEITCH.—Essays on mental derangement.

WILLIAMS, J.—The lunacy question; or the lunatic benefitted and protected, with an enquiry into public and private asylums. 2nd ed.

1853. AITKEN.—Specific gravity of the brain. (G. M. J.)

ANDERSON, W. J.—Hysterical and nervous affections in women. 12mo.

BURNETT, C. M.—What shall we do with the criminal lunatics? A letter to Lord St. Leonards. P.

CARTER, R. B.—Pathology and treatment of hysteria.

DAVEY, J. G.—On the nature and proximate cause of insanity.

DUNCAN, J. F.—Popular errors on the subject of insanity examined and exposed. 12mo. Dublin.

GALT, J. M.—Essays on asylums for persons of unsound mind. Richmond, U.S.A.

NOBLE, D.—Elements of psychological medicine; an introduction to the practical study of insanity for students and junior practitioners. (2nd ed. 1855.)

SEATON, J. — The present state of psychological medicine, with suggestions for improving the laws relating to the care and treatment of lunatics. P.

1854. ADLER, G. J.—Letters of a lunatic. New York.

BUCKNILL, J. C.—The law and theory of insanity. (B. and F. Med.-Chir. Rev.)

BUCKNILL, J. C.—Unsoundness of mind in relation to criminal acts. (The first Sugden prize essay.) 12mo. (2nd ed. 1857.)

DIAMOND, H. W.—Physiognomy of insanity; a series of photographic portraits from the life, with brief medical notes. P. 4to.

HOOD, SIR W. C.—Suggestions for the future provision for criminal lunatics.

HUXLEY, J. E.—History and description of the Kent Asylum.

KNAGGS, S.—Unsoundness of mind considered in relation to the question of responsibility for criminal acts.

LINDSAY, W. L.—Histology of the blood in the insane. P.

MAYO, TH.—Medical testimony and evidence in cases of lunacy (Croon. Lect. for 1853); with an essay on the condition of mental soundness. 12mo.

MADDOCK, A. B.—Practical observations on nervous and mental disorders.

PEDDIE, A.—The pathology of delirium tremens and its treatment. Edin.

PRICHARD, T.—Statement of cases treated at Abington Abbey Asylum, Northampton.

PETERS, J. C.—A treatise on nervous derangement or mental disorders, based upon the clinical experience of T. J. Rückerts. New York.

TODD, R. B.—Clinical lectures on paralysis, disease of the brain and other affections of the nervous system.

TUKE, D. HACK.—The asylums of Holland: their past and present condition. (Journ. Psych. Medicine.)

WINSLOW, F.—Lettsomian lectures on insanity.

1855. BLACKIE, G.—Cretins and cretinism. Edin.

BRODIE, SIR B.—Psychological inquiries.

BUCKNILL, J. C.—Medical testimony and evidence in cases of insanity. P.

BUCKNILL, J. C.—Pathology of insanity. (B. and F. Med.-Chir. Rev.)

CARTER, R. B.—On the influence of education and training in preventing diseases of the nervous system. 12mo.

DUNN, ROBERT.—A case of suspension of the mental faculties, of the powers of speech, and special senses, with the exception of sight and touch, continuing for many months.

FALRET, J. P.—Clinical lectures on mental medicine, delivered at the Salpêtrière. Part I. General symptomatology. (Ed. J. H. Blount.)

HOLLAND, SIR H. — Medical notes and reflections. (Also 1839 and 1840.) 3rd ed.

LEECH, JOHN.—The iniquity and impolicy of confining drunkards as lunatics. A more equitable remedy suggested. With postscript and appendix containing startling hints to genuine Britons who value civil and religious liberty. P. Glasgow.

LINDSAY, W. LAUDER.—Chemico-microscopical character of the blood in the insane. Ill. P.

LINDSAY, W. L.—The histology of the blood of the insane. Ill.

LINDSAY, W. L.—Treatment of the insane. P. Edin.

REPORT of the Irish Commissioners inquiring into the erection of District Lunatic Asylums in Ireland. (Also 1859.)

REYNOLDS, J. RUSSELL.—Diagnosis of diseases of the brain and spinal cord.

TUKE, D. HACK. — William Tuke, the Founder of the York Retreat. (Journ. Psych. Medicine.)

TUKE, D. HACK.—On the progressive changes which have taken place since the time of Pinel in the moral management of the insane, and the various contrivances which have been adopted instead of mechanical restraint. (Prize essay.)

WILSON, C.—The pathology of drunkenness. Edin.

WINN, J. M.—Treatment of puerperal mania.

WINSLOW, F.—The case of Luigi Buranelli medico-legally considered. P.

1856. ABBOTT, J. — The handbook of idiocy, &c.

ANON.—Flemish interiors. (Author of "A glance behind the Grilles.")

ANON.—The education of the imbecile and the improvement of the invalid youth.

CONOLLY, J.—The treatment of the insane without mechanical restraints.

LAVATER, J. C.—Essays on physiognomy. (Trans.) N. D.

LAYCOCK, T.—The principles and methods of medical observation and research, with copious nosologies and indexes of fevers and of constitutional, cutaneous, nervous and mental diseases. (2nd ed. 1864.) Edin.

LINDSAY, W. LAUDER.—Scottish Lunacy Commission. P. Edin.

MAYO, TH.—Supplement to the Croonian lectures. Medical testimony and evidence in cases of lunacy (Greensmith's case). 12mo. P.

MIGAULT, H. G.—Eight historical dissertations on suicide.

MORISON, SIR A.—Lectures on insanity. Edin.

SNAPE, C.—A letter to the committee of visitors of the Surrey Lunatic Asylum in reference to the case of D. Dolley, deceased. P.

WILLIAMS, CALEB.—Observations on the criminal responsibility of the insane (Cases of Hill and Dove.)

WILLIAMS, J. W. HUME.—On unsoundness of mind. (2nd ed. 1858, v. 1890.)

1857. HILL, R. G.—Concise history of the entire abolition of mechanical restraint in the treatment of the insane, and the introduction of the non-restraint system.

LINDSAY, W. LAUDER.—Our lunatic asylums. P.

MADDOCK, A. B.—Practical observations on mental and nervous disorders, illustrated with cases. 2nd ed.

MOSELEY, G.—On mental disorders, their nature, cause and treatment.

REPORT by Commissioners appointed to enquire into the state of lunatic asylums in Scotland, and the existing law in reference to lunatics and lunatic asylums in that part of the United Kingdom.

SOLLY, S.—The human brain, its structure, physiology and diseases.

TWEEDIE, A. C.—Mesmerism and its realities further proved by illustrations of its curative power in disease, as well as by its development of some extraordinary magnetic phenomena in the human body. P. Edin.

WATSON, J. — The Parrish Will Case, critically examined in reference to the mental competency of Mr. H. Parrish to execute the codicils appended to his will. New York.

WEBSTER, JOHN.—Notes on Belgian lunatic asylums, including the insane colony at Gheel.

WILKINSON, J. J. G.—The homœopathic principle applied to insanity: a proposal to treat lunacy by spiritualism. P.

1858. BANKS, J. T.—On nervous diseases and nervousness, lapsing into melancholia and insanity.

BUCKNILL, J. C.—A manual of psychological medicine, containing the lunacy laws, the nosology, statistics, description, diagnosis, pathology, and treatment of insanity. With an appendix of cases. Ill. (With Dr. Hack Tuke.)

BURGESS, J.—The medical and legal relations of madness—showing a cellular theory of mind and of nerve force, and also vegetative vital force.

COPLAND, JAMES.—A dictionary of practical medicine. 3 vols. London.

DUNN, ROBERT.—An essay on physiological psychology.

GULL, SIR W.—Abscess of the brain (P. P.)

HOWE, S. G.—On the causes of idiocy.

JAMIESON, R.—A discourse on the physiology of the phrenical action of the cerebrum. (Diagrams.) P. Aberdeen.

MULOCH, T.—British lunatic asylums, public and private; with an appendix relating to Dr. Pathman, Lady Lytton Bulwer, and Mrs. Turner. P. 12mo.

NOBLE, D.—The human mind in its relations with the brain and nervous system

PARRISH, JOSEPH.—The mind unveiled; a brief history of twenty-two imbecile children. 12mo. Phil.

PEDDIE, A.—The necessity of some legalised arrangements for the treatment of dipsomania, or the drinking insanity.

ROBINSON, G.—The circulation of the blood (including the peculiarities of the cerebral circulation, and their connection with the phenomena of epilepsy and apoplexy).

SKAE, D.—On dipsomania. E.M.J.

TUKE, D. HACK.—A manual of psychological medicine, containing the lunacy laws, the nosology, statistics, description, diagnosis, pathology and treatment of insanity. With an appendix of cases. Ill. (With Dr. Bucknill.)

1859. ARLIDGE, J. T.—On the state of lunacy, and the legal provision for the insane.

AUSTIN, T. J.—A practical account of general paralysis.

BOISMONT, BRIERRE DE.—Hallucinations. (Trans.)

BUCKNILL, J. C.—Psychology of Shakespeare. London and Exeter.

CONOLLY, J. — The physiognomy of insanity; thirteen papers by Dr. Conolly, illustrated by photography by Dr. Diamond. (M. T. & G.)

DIAMOND, H. W.—The physiognomy of insanity; thirteen papers by Dr. Conolly, illustrated by photography by Dr. Diamond. (M. T. & G.)

GASKELL, S.—On the want of a better provision for the middle and labouring classes when attacked or threatened with insanity. (Trans. Soc. Sci. Assoc.)

MACNISH. R.—The anatomy of drunkenness.

REPORT of Irish Commissioners inquiring into the erection of District Lunatic Asylums in Ireland. (Also 1855.)

ROBINSON, G.—On the prevention and treatment of mental disorders.

SCHROEDER VAN DER KOLK.—Spinal cord and epilepsy. (Trans.).

SEYMOUR, E. J.—A letter on the laws which regulate private lunatic asylums in England, with observations on the law of interdiction in France.

WINSLOW, F.—On softening of the brain.

1860. ALDIS, C. J. B.—The power of individuals to prevent melancholy in themselves. A lecture. P.

ANON.—Philosophy of insanity. Glasgow.

BUCKNILL, J. C.—The medical knowledge of Shakespeare. London and Exeter.

BUSHMAN, J. S.—Religious revivals in relation to nervous and mental diseases. P.

COMBE, A.—The principles of physiology applied to the preservation of health and to the improvement of mental and physical education. (Edited and adapted by Sir J. Coxe.) Ill. Edin.

DOWN, J. LANGDON.—On lead poisoning. (M. T. & G.)

HOOD, C.—On the condition of the blood in mania. P.

HOOD, SIR W. C.—Criminal lunatics; a letter to the Chairman of the Commissioners in Lunacy. P.

LALOR, JOSEPH.—Observations on the offices of resident and visiting physicians of district lunatic asylums in Ireland. P. Dublin.

LAYCOCK, T.—Mind and brain; or the correlations of consciousness and organisation. (2 vols.) (2nd ed. 1868.) Edin.

MARCET, W.—Chronic alcoholic intoxication; with an enquiry into the influence of the abuse of alcohol as a predisposing cause of disease. (2nd ed. 1862.) 12mo.

TUKE, HARRINGTON.—Private lunatic asylums as contrasted with other residences for the insane. (L.).

WINSLOW, F.—On obscure diseases of the brain and mind. Disorders of the mind and their incipient symptoms, pathology, diagnosis, treatment, and prophylaxis. (3rd ed. 1863.)

1861. CHRISTISON, SIR R.—On some of the medico-legal relations of the habit of intemperance. (Lecture conversazione Roy. Coll. of Surgeons, 1858). P. Edin.

DOWN, J. LANGDON.—Account of a case of idiocy in which the corpus callosum and fornix were imperfectly formed and the septum lucidum and commissura were absent. (Trans. Med. Chir. Soc.).

FAIRLESS, J.—Suggestions concerning the construction of asylums for the insane, illustrated by a series of plans. P. Edin.

GASKELL, S.—A plea for establishing and regulating houses for the reception of patients convalescent from, or afflicted with, incipient symptoms of insanity. (Trans. Soc. Science Cong.)

LAYCOCK, T.—The scientific place and principles of medical psychology, an introductory address.

MCCORMAC, HENRY.—Metanoia, a plea for the insane.

MILLAR, J.—Hints on insanity. London. (2nd ed. 1868.)

PEACOCK, T. B.—On the weight and specific gravity of the brain. (Trans. Path. Soc.)

REYNOLDS, J. RUSSELL.—On epilepsy, its symptoms, treatment and relation to other convulsive diseases.

RITCHIE, R. P.—An inquiry into a frequent cause of insanity in young men.

SMITH, J. IRVINE.—Report of proceedings under brieve of cognition on James Sinclair Lockhart, Esq., of Castlehill and Cambusnethan at Edinburgh, 1860. (P. P.) Ill. Glasgow.

SHAFTESBURY, EARL OF.—Speech at the Freemasons' Hall, on behalf of a benevolent asylum for the insane of the middle classes (especially those of limited means). P.

SKAE, D.—The legal relations of insanity. Edin. P.

WATSON-WEMYSS, A.—On legislation and provision for the care of the insane. P. Edin.

WATSON-WEMYSS, A.—Remarks on the county asylums for pauper lunatics, with a sketch for a plan for these. P. Edin.

1862. BLAKE, J. A.—Defects in the moral treatment of insanity in the public asylums of Ireland, with suggestions for their remedy.

DOWN, J. LANGDON.—On the condition of the mouth in idiocy. (L.)

GAIRDNER, W. T.—On delirium tremens (in author's "Clinical Medicine").

JARVIS, E.—Employment for patients in British lunatic asylums. Dorchester, U.S.A.

LAYCOCK, T.—The antagonism of law and medicine in insanity and its consequences; an introductory lecture. P. Edin.

LAYCOCK, T.—Practical notes on the diagnosis, prognosis and treatment in cases of delirium tremens. P. Edin.

MANIFOLD.—On delirium tremens. (M. T. & G.)

MCCORMAC, H.—On the management of asylums for the insane. (Dub. Med. Press.)

MITCHELL, SIR A.—On various superstitions in the North-West Highlands, and

Islands of Scotland, especially in relation to lunacy. P. 4to. Edin.
NEEDHAM, F.—On the necessity for legislation in reference to habitual drunkards. P.
SIDNEY, REV. E.—Earlswood and its inmates. (A lecture.)
YELLOWLEES, D.—Homicidal mania, a biography. (E. M. J.)

1863. ADDISON, A.—On the pathological anatomy of the brain in insanity.
BIRD, R.—Drink-craving, an outline. P.
CLARKE, J. LOCKHART.—Notes of researches on the intimate structure of the brain. (Pro. Roy. Soc.)
CONOLLY, J.—A study of Hamlet. P.
DUNCAN, J. F.—Cases of syphilitic insanity and epilepsy. P. Dublin.
DUNN, R.—Medical psychology, comprising a brief exposition of the leading phenomena of the mental states; and of the nervous apparatus through which they are manifested, with a view to the better understanding and elucidation of the mental phenomena or symptoms of disease. P.
NIGHTINGALE, FLORENCE.—Notes on hospitals. Ill. 4to.
SKAE, D.—The classification of the various forms of insanity on a rational and practical basis.

1864. ANON. (? Dr. Black of Chesterfield.)—A voice from Derby to Bedlam. P.
ANSTIE, F. A.—Stimulants and narcotics; their mutual relations.
BROWNE, W. A. F.—The moral treatment of the insane.
BYRNE, T. E. D.—Lunacy and law, together with hints on the treatment of idiots. P.
CHAPMAN, J.—A new method of treating disease through the agency of the nervous system, by means of cold and heat. P.
FRY, D. P.—The Lunacy Acts (England). (2nd ed. 1877.)
MCLEOD, K.—On fatty degeneration in insanity. (Trans. North. and Durham Med. Society.)
MARSHALL, JOHN.—On the brain of a bushwoman, and on the brains of two idiots of European descent. (Phil. Trans.)
MAUDSLEY, H.—Insanity and crime: a medico-legal commentary on the case of George Victor Townley. (With Dr. Lockhart Robertson.) P.
MITCHELL, SIR A.—The insane in private dwellings. Edin.
REPORT.—Case of George Victor Townley.
ROBERTSON, CH. LOCKHART.—Insanity and crime; a medico-legal commentary on the case of George Victor Townley (with Dr. Maudsley). P.
SCOTT, CHARLES (advocate).—The convict Bryce, being a letter to the Secretary of State. P. Edin.
WILLIAMSON, W.—Thoughts on insanity and its causes, and on the management of the insane. 2nd ed. P.

1865. BLACK, C.—The insanity of George Victor Townley. P.
BLAKE, J.—The moral treatment of insanity, and suggestions for the appointment of a Royal Commission to report on the best system. P.
BOYD, ROBERT.—Notes of a visit to some of the Northern and Midland County asylums. P. Wells.
DUNCAN, J. F.—Personal responsibility of the insane. P. Dublin.
FOX, F. & C.—A report on the past and present state of Brislington House private asylum for the insane.
LINDSAY, W. LAUDER.—On temporary insanity. P. Edin.
MITCHELL, SIR A.—Blood relationship in marriage in its influence upon the offspring. P. Edin.
STANLEY, W. S.—Thoughts on the mind and its derangements, with hints to the friends of patients. P. Dublin.
TAYLOR, A. S.—The principles and practice of medical jurisprudence. Ill.
TUKE, J. BATTY.—On the statistics of puerperal insanity as observed in the Royal Edinburgh Asylum. (E. M. J.)
WILLIAMS, S. W. D.—On the efficacy of bromide of potassium in epilepsy, and certain psychical affections. P.
WISE, THOMAS A.—Observations on the claims of infirm and imbecile children on public attention. P. Cork.

1866. ALTHAUS, J.—On epilepsy, hysteria and ataxy.
BLANDFORD, G. F.—Lectures on insanity. (M. T. & G.)
BROWN, I. BAKER.—On the curability of certain forms of insanity, epilepsy, catalepsy and hysteria in females. P.
DOWN, J. LANGDON.—An account of a second case of idiocy, in which the corpus callosum was defective. (Trans. Roy. Med. and Chir. Soc. London.)
DOWN, J. LANGDON.—Marriages of consanguinity in relation to degeneration of race. (Lond. Hosp. Rep.)
DOWN, J. LANGDON.—Observations on an ethnic classification of idiots. (Lond. Hosp. Rep.)
DUNCAN, P. W.—A manual for the classification, training, and education of the feeble-minded, imbecile, and idiotic. (With Mr. Millard.)
HAMMOND, W. A.—Insanity in its medico-legal relations; opinion relative to testamentary capacity of J. C. Johnstone. P. New York.
HOVELL, D. B.—Medicine and psychology.
MACGREGOR.—Notes on twenty asylums in England and Scotland visited during July and August, 1866. Glasgow.
MADDEN, T. M.—On insanity and the criminal responsibility of the insane P. Dub.
MILLARD, W.—A manual for the classification, training, and education of the feeble-minded, imbecile, and idiotic (with Dr. P. W. Duncan.)
MURRAY, W.—A treatise on emotional

disorders of the sympathetic system of nerves.
SANKEY, W. H. O.—Lectures on mental diseases. (3rd ed. 1884.)
SEGUIN, E. — Idiocy and its treatment, by the physiological method (edited by E. C. S.). New York.
1866-70. RUSSELL.—Chorea and insanity. (M. T. and G.)
1867. BUCKNILL, J. C.—The Mad folk of Shakespeare (being 2nd ed. of "Psychology of Shakespeare." See 1859 and 1860.)
DOWN, J. LANGDON.—On idiocy and its relation to tuberculosis. (L.)
REID, J.—On the symptoms, causes and treatment of puerperal insanity.
TUKE, J. BATTY.—Cases illustrative of the insanity of pregnancy, puerperal insanity, and insanity of lactation. (E. M. J.)
WEMYSS, A. WATSON.—Remarks on the Lunacy Acts for Scotland and district pauper lunatic asylums. P. Edin.
WINSLOW, F.—On uncontrollable drunkenness, considered as a form of mental disorder, with suggestions for its treatment, and the organisation of sanatoria for dipsomaniacs. P.
1868. ALLBUTT, T. CLIFFORD.—On the state of the optic nerves and retina, as seen in the insane. P.
ANSTIE, F. A. — Hypochondriasis. (Reynolds' Medicine, vol. ii.)
BEAMAN.—On epilepsy. 12mo.
GRAY, J. P.—Insanity and its relations to medicine. P. Utica. U.S.A.
JACKSON, J. HUGHLINGS.—Study of convulsion. (Trans. St. Andrews' Med. Grad. Assoc.)
JACKSON, J. HUGHLINGS.—Cases of disease of the nervous system in patients the subjects of inherited syphilis. (Trans. St. Andrews' Med. Grad. Assoc.)
JACKSON, J. HUGHLINGS.—Physiology and pathology of chorea (E. M. J.)
LINDSAY, W. LAUDER. — Typhomania. (E. M. J.)
MANNING, F. N. — Report on lunatic asylums to the Government of New South Wales (with plans, &c.). Sydney.
MAUDSLEY, H.—Physiology and pathology of mind. (2nd ed. 1868: 3rd and 4th ed. *vide infra*.)
MORRIS, J. — Irritability: popular and practical sketches of common morbid states and conditions bordering on disease: with hints for management, alleviation and cure.
PRICHARD, T.—Report of cases of insanity treated at Abington Abbey, Northampton, 1862-67, with an inquiry into the causes of the increase of insanity, and observations on English asylums. P. Northampton.
THOMAS, M.—Notes of thirteen cases of delirium tremens. P. Edin.
TUKE, J. BATTY.—Objections to the cottage system of treatment for lunatics as it now exists, and suggestions for its improvement and elaboration. (E. M. J.)
1869. ALLBUTT, T. CLIFFORD.—On a case of cerebral disease in a syphilitic patient.
CLARK, SIR JAMES, BART.—Memoir of Dr. Conolly, comprising a sketch of the treatment of the insane in Europe and America.
CLOUSTON, T. S.—On the use of hypnotics, sedatives and motor depressants in the treatment of mental diseases. (Amer. Journ. Med. Sciences.)
DAVEY, J. G.—The insane poor in Middlesex.
DOWN, J. LANGDON.—A case of an asymmetrically developed brain. (Trans. Path. Soc.)
DOWN, J. LANGDON.—A case of arrested development. (Trans. Path. Soc.)
DOWN, J. LANGDON.—A case of microcephalism. (Trans. Path. Soc.)
DUNCAN, GEORGE.—The various theories of the relation of mind and brain reviewed.
ELAM, C.—A physician's problems. [Degenerations, moral and criminal epidemics, illusions, &c.]
GALTON, F.—Hereditary genius, an inquiry into its laws and consequences.
GUY, W. A.—Insanity and crime; and on the plea of insanity in criminal cases. (Stat. Soc. Journ.)
HOWDEN, J. C.—Granular degeneration of nerve-cells in insanity. (L.)
JACKSON, J. HUGHLINGS. — Disease of both lobes of the cerebellum. (Medical Mirror.)
LAYCOCK, T.—The theory of delirium tremens. (L.)
LINDSAY, W. LAUDER.—Insanity in British emigrants of the middle and upper ranks. (E. M. J.)
LINDSAY, W. LAUDER.—Suggestions for the proper supervision of the insane in the British Colonies. (Brit. and For. Med.-Chir. Rev.)
MARCET, W.—An experimental inquiry into the action of alcohol on the nervous system. (M. T. and G.)
REPORT of the Committee on Intemperance for the lower House of Convocation of the province of Canterbury.
RUTHERFORD, W.—On the morbid appearances met with in the brains of 30 insane persons. (With Dr. Batty Tuke.) (E. M. J.)
SCHROEDER VAN DER KOLK.—The pathology and therapeutics of mental diseases. (Trans.)
SHETTLE, R. C.—A brief paper on the pathology of insanity. P. Reading.
TUKE, J. BATTY.—On the morbid appearances met with in the brains of 30 persons. (With Professor Rutherford.) (E. M. J.)
WINN, J. M.—Nature and treatment of hereditary diseases. P.
1870. ANON.—The treatment of lunacy, a reply to the *Lancet*, Jan. 22, 1870. By Medico-Psychologicus.
BACON, G. MACKENZIE.—On the writing of the insane. P.

CLOUSTON, T. S.—The use of the thermometer in the diagnosis and treatment of insanity. (B. M. J.)

CLOUSTON, T. S.—Observations and experiments on the effects of opium, bromide of potassium and cannabis Indica in insanity. (Fothergillian Prize Essay.) (Med.-Chir. Rev.)

CLOUSTON, T. S. — The use of chloral in affections of the nervous system. (B. M. J.)

HILL, R. G.—Lunacy, its past and present.

JONES, C. HANDFIELD. — On delirium tremens. (M. T. & G.)

JONES, C. HANDFIELD. — On functional nervous disorders.

LINDSAY, W. LAUDER.—American hospitals for the insane contrasted with those of Britain. (E. M. J.)

LINDSAY, W. LAUDER.—Causes of insanity in arctic countries. (B. & F. Med.-Chir. Rev.)

LINDSAY, W. LAUDER.—Illustrations of pathology and morbid anatomy in the insane. (E. M. J.)

LINDSAY, W. LAUDER. — Legislation for inebriates. (E. M. J.)

LINDSAY, W. LAUDER.—Mollities ossium in relation to fractures among the insane. (E. M. J.)

MAUDSLEY, H.—Body and mind (*see* 1873).

SEGUIN, E.—New facts and remarks concerning idiocy. New York.

1871. ALLBUTT, T. CLIFFORD.—On the use of the ophthalmoscope in diseases of the nervous system, &c. Ill.

ANON.—Behind the bars. Boston.

ANON.—Our lunacy system. (B. M. J.)

BLANDFORD, G. F. — Insanity and its treatment. (4th ed. 1892.) Edin.

BROWNE, SIR JAMES CRICHTON.—Chloral hydrate, its inconvenience and danger. (L.)

BROWNE, SIR JAMES CRICHTON.—Clinical lecture on mental and cerebral diseases. Leeds.

BROWNE, J. H. BALFOUR.—The medical jurisprudence of insanity. (Another ed., San Francisco, 1875).

DAVIS, A. J.—Mental disorders, or diseases of the brain and nerves, developing the origin and philosophy of mania, insanity, and crime. Boston, U.S.A.

GRAY, J. P.—Insanity, its dependence on physical disease. Utica, U.S.A.

GREENE, R.—On bromide of potassium; and on nitrite of amyl. (Sussex Asyl. Rep.)

HAMMOND, W. A.—A treatise on diseases of the nervous system. 1st ed. New York.

HAWKES, J.—On the general management of public lunatic asylums in England and Wales. P.

LINDSAY, W. LAUDER.—Gheel in the north. (B. & F. Med.-Chir. Rev.)

LINDSAY, W. LAUDER.—Physiology and pathology of mind in the lower animals. P. Edin.

LINDSAY, W. LAUDER.—Insanity in the lower animals. (B. & F. Med.-Chir. Rev.)

MADDEN.—On puerperal mania.

NEEDHAM, F.—Brain exhaustion. P.

PARRISH, T.—The classification and treatment of inebriates. New York.

RAY.—A treatise on the medical jurisprudence of insanity. 5th ed.

REPORT on spiritualism. (London Dialectical Society.)

REYNOLDS, J. RUSSELL.—On the scientific value of the legal tests of insanity.

ROBERTSON, C. A. LOCKHART. — The alleged increase of lunacy.

ROBERTSON, A.—Observations on aphasia. (G. M. J.)

WICKHAM, R. H. B.—Visits to some licensed asylums at Balfron. (E. M. J.)

WILKINS, E. T.—Insanity and insane asylums. Ill. (Rep. to State of California.)

WOOD, W. D.—Hamlet from a psychological point of view.

1872. BRETT, W.—The sources and rules of life, or how to prevent insanity in individuals, and revolutionary madness in nations. P. N. P.

BROWNE, SIR JAMES CRICHTON.—Conium in the treatment of acute mania. (L.)

BROWNE, SIR JAMES CRICHTON.—Cranial injuries and mental diseases.

BROWNE, SIR JAMES CRICHTON.—Lectures on mental and cerebral diseases. Leeds.

BROWNE, SIR JAMES CRICHTON.—Simple melancholia.

BROWNE, J. H. BALFOUR.—Handbook of law and lunacy; or the medical practitioner's complete guide in all matters relating to lunacy practice. (In conjunction with Dr. Sabben.)

CARNEGIE, D.—The licensing laws of Sweden. (Glasg. Phil. Soc.)

CLOUSTON, T. S.—What cases should be sent to asylums? and when? (B. M. J.)

COXE, SIR JAMES.—On the causes of insanity, and the means of checking its growth, being the Presidential address delivered to the Medico-Psychological Association. Edin.

DAVEY, J. G.—On dipsomania. P.

DOWN, J. LANGDON. — On the relation of teeth and mouth to mental development. (Trans. Odont. Soc.)

ELAM, C.—On cerebria and other diseases of the brain.

ELMER, J.—The practice in lunacy under commissions and inquisitions, with notes of recent cases and recent decisions. An appendix containing forms and costs of proceedings, the statutes and general orders. 5th ed.

FISHER, T. W.—Plain talk about insanity, its causes, forms, symptoms and the treatment of mental diseases. With remarks on hospitals and asylums, and the medico-legal aspect of insanity. Boston, U.S.A.

GREENE, R.—Cases illustrative of the treatment of mania. Note on hydrate of chloral. (Sussex Asyl. Rep.)

LINDSAY, W. LAUDER.—Colonial Lunacy Boards. (E. M. J.)

MITCHELL, S. WEIR.—Injuries of nerves and their consequences.
REPORT from the select committee on habitual drunkards, together with the proceedings of the committee and minutes of evidence. (B. B.)
REVIEW.—The Quarterly Review on drink, the vice and the disease.
SABBEN, J. T. — Handbook of law and lunacy. (With Mr. Balfour Browne.)
SMITH, C.—On mental capacity in relation to insanity, crime and modern society. P.
THOMSON, J. B.—Criminal lunacy in Scotland from 1846 to 1870, both inclusive. (E. M. J.)
TROUSSEAU, A.—Lectures on clinical medicine. (Trans.)
TUKE, D. HACK.—Illustrations of the influence of the mind on the body in health and disease. (2nd ed. 1884.)
TUKE, J. BATTY.—On a case of hypertrophy of the right cerebral hemisphere with co-existent atrophy of the left side of the body. (Jour. Anat. & Phys.)
1873. BROWNE, SIR JAMES CRICHTON. — Hysterical mania and senile insanity.
BROWNE, J. H. BALFOUR.—Responsibilty and disease: an essay. P. 16mo.
CAMPBELL, J. A.—Feeding *versus* fasting. (B. M. J.)
ECKER, A.—The convolutions of the human brain. (Trans.) Ill.
GULL, SIR W.—On a cretinoid state supervening in adult life in women. (Clin. Soc. Trans.)
JACKSON, J. HUGHLINGS.—Clinical and physiological researches on the nervous system. (No. 1, the localisation of movements in the brain.)
LIVEING, E.—On megrim, sick headache, and some allied disorders: a contribution to the pathology of nerve storms.
MAUDSLEY, H.—Body and mind; an inquiry into their connection and mutual influence, specially in reference to mental disorders. Gulst. Lectures (1st ed. 1870), 2nd ed. enlarged and revised, to which are added psychological essays.
NEWINGTON, H. H. — Mania à potu. (E. M. J.)
RAY, J.—Contributions to mental pathology. Boston, U.S.A.
SHEPPARD, E.—Lectures on madness in its medical, legal, and social aspects.
SKAE, D. — Morisonian lectures on insanity.
SUTHERLAND, H.—The histology of the blood of the insane. (Trans. Med.-Chir. Soc.)
TUKE, J. BATTY.—On the morbid histology of the brain and spinal cord as observed in the insane. (B. and F. Med.-Chir. Rev.)
YELLOWLEES, D.—Asylum notes. Edin.
1874. BROWNE, SIR JAMES CRICHTON.—Epileptic hemiplegia. (L.)
BUCKNILL, J. C.—The law of murder in its medical aspects.
DAY, H.—Brain injuries. Stafford. P.
DICKSON, J. T.—The science and practice of medicine in relation to mind, the pathology of the nerve centres, and the jurisprudence of insanity.
FOX, E. LONG.—The pathological anatomy of the nerve centres. Ill.
GREENE, R.—Pleuritic effusion with acute mania. (Pract.)
MAUDSLEY, H.—Responsibility in mental disease. (4th ed. 1880.)
MICKLE, W. J.—Morphia in the treatment of insanity. (B. M. J.)
MICKLE, W. J.—Potassic bromide in syphilitic insanity. (Pract.)
NEEDHAM, F.—Insanity in relation to society. P.
REPORT.—First Report of the Lunacy Law Reform Association.
WINSLOW, F. L. S.—Manual of lunacy, a handbook relating to the legal care and treatment of the insane.
YELLOWLEES, D.—Insanity and intemperance. (B. M. J.)
YELLOWLEES, D.—The criminal responsibility of the insane. (Soc. Science Cong. Glasg.)
1875. ALLEN, N.—State medicine in relation to insanity. Boston, U.S.A.
FOX, E. LONG.—The influence of the sympathetic on disease. Ill.
GRABHAM, G. W.—Remarks on the origin, varieties and terminations of idiocy. Ill. P.
HUTH, A. H.—Marriage of near kin.
JACKSON, J. HUGHLINGS.—Nervous symptoms in cases of congenital syphilis. (Journ. Ment. Sci.)
LINDSAY, W. LAUDER.—Tables regarding superannuation of officers and servants of British hospitals for the insane.
LINDSAY, W. L.—Tables regarding superannuation of officers and servants of British hospitals for the insane.
MICKLE, W. J.—Lesions of both corpora striata. Recovery from paralysis. (B. M. J.)
RIBOT, TH.—Heredity, a psychological study of its phenomena, laws, causes and consequences. 2nd ed.
ROBERTSON, A.—On the unilateral phenomena of mental and nervous diseases. (G. M. J.)
SAVAGE, G. H.—Insanity of childbirth. (Guy's Hosp. Rep.)
SAVAGE, G. H.—Overwork as related to insanity. (L.)
SHUTTLEWORTH, G. E.—The training of idiots. (B. M. J.)
SHUTTLEWORTH, G. E.—Two cases of microcephalic idiocy. (B. M. J.)
SUTHERLAND, H.—On the artificial feeding of the insane.
TUKE, J. BATTY. — Morisonian lectures on insanity for 1874. (Edin.)
WYNTER, A.—Borderlands of insanity.
YEATS, W. — Remarks on the present method adopted for the disposal and treatment of the subjects of mental disease. (E. M. J.)

1876. BROWNE, SIR JAMES CRICHTON.—The antagonism of medicine.
BROWNE, SIR JAMES CRICHTON. — West Riding Asylum Medical Reports. 6 vols., 1871-6. Edited by Sir J. Crichton Browne.
BUCKNILL, J. C.—Psychological medicine in America. (M. T. & G.)
BUCKNILL, J. C.—Notes on asylums for the insane in America.
CLOUSTON, T. S.—Disorders of speech in insanity. (E. M. J.)
DOWN, J. LANGDON.—On the education and training of the feeble in mind.
DOWN, J. LANGDON.—The obstetrical aspects of idiocy. (Trans. Obstet. Soc.).
FERRIER, D.—Functions of the brain. Ill.
HAMMOND, W. A.—A treatise on diseases of the nervous system. 6th ed. New York.
JAMIESON, R.—The increase of mental disease. P.
LEWIS, W. BEVAN.—Thermal changes in epilepsy and the epileptic status. (M. T. & G.)
MANN, E.C.—Insanity : its etiology, pathology, diagnosis and treatment, with cases. New York.
MAUDSLEY, H. — Physiology of mind. 3rd ed.
REPORT.—Propositions and resolutions of the Association of Medical Superintendents of American institutions for the insane. Phil., U.S.A.
SAVAGE, G. H.—Cases of insanity relieved by acute disease. (Pract.)
SAVAGE, G. H.—Consideration of cures in insanity. (Guy's Hosp. Rep.)
SKAE, W.—Classification of mental diseases. P. Edin.
WEST RIDING ASYLUM Medical Reports, *vide* Sir J. Crichton Browne, *supra*.
WILBUR, H. B.—Governmental supervision in the management of the insane. Syracuse, U.S.A.
1877. ALLBUTT, T. CLIFFORD. — Mental anxiety as a cause of granular kidney.
BUCKNILL, J. C.—The law of insanity. (Lumleian Lectures.)
BUCKNILL, J. C. — Notes on asylums for the insane in America.
BUCKNILL, J. C.—The priest and physician. (Meeting of Brit. Med. Assoc. at Manchester.)
CAMPBELL, HUGH.—A treatise on nervous exhaustion and the diseases induced by it, with observations on the nervous constitution, hereditary and acquired; and on the origin and nature of nervous force and animal electricity. 16mo. 14th ed.
CARPENTER, W. B.—Principles of mental physiology, with their application to the training and discipline of the mind and the study of its morbid conditions. 4th ed. Ill.
CLOUSTON, T. S.—An asylum or hospital home. Massachusetts, U.S.A.
CURWEN, J.—Address on mental disorders. Phil., U.S.A.
EARLE, PLINY.—The curability of insanity. P. Utica, U.S.A.
FOLSOM, C. F.—Notes on the early management of disease of the mind. European and American progress, modern methods, &c., in the treatment of insanity. Boston, U.S.A.
GLEN, ALEXANDER, Barrister-at-Law.—The statutes relating to lunacy, comprising the law relating to pauper lunatic hospitals and licensed houses, inquisitions in lunacy and criminal lunatics. 2nd ed. (The first edition was by John Frederick Archbold, barrister-at-law.)
GRANVILLE, J. MORTIMER.—The care and cure of the insane; being a Report of the "Lancet" Commission on lunatic asylums in 1875-77. 2 vols.
GRIESINGER, W.—Mental pathology and therapeutics. (Trans.)
IRELAND, W. W.—Idiocy and imbecility. Ill.
LEWES, G. H.—Physical basis of mind.
LEWIS, W. BEVAN.—Relationship of nerve cells of cortex to lymphatic system of the brain. Ill. (Proc. Roy. Soc.)
MAGNAN, V.—On alcoholism : the various forms of alcoholic delirium and their treatment. (Trans. by W. S. Greenfield.)
MICKLE, W. J.—Syphilis in the insane (B. and F. Med.-Chir. Rev.)
PARRISH, J.—An open letter to Dr. Bucknill (on inebriety). P. New Jersey, U.S.A.
ROBERTSON, A.—On medico-psychological evidence and the plea of insanity in courts of law. (G. M. J.)
SAVAGE, G. H.—Heredity in mental diseases. (Guy's Hosp. Rep.)
WILBUR, H. B.—Report on the management of the insane in Great Britain. 2nd ed. P. Albany, U.S.A.
WINSLOW, F. L. S.—Spiritualistic madness.
1878. BAIN, A.—Mind and body. 6th ed.
BEACH, FLETCHER. — On the diagnosis and treatment of idiocy, with remarks on prognosis. (L.)
BUCKNILL, J. C.—Habitual drunkenness, and insane drunkards.
CLARKE, E. H.—Visions, a study of false sight. Boston, U.S.A.
COXE, SIR JAMES.—Lunacy in its relations to the State, a commentary on the evidence taken by the committee of the House of Commons on Lunacy Law in the session of 1877. P.
CURWEN, J.—Report on the care of the insane. Phil., U.S.A.
FERRIER, D. — Localisation of cerebral disease. (Gulst. Lect.) Ill.
GRAY, J. P. — Mental hygiene. Utica, U.S.A.
HAMILTON, A. M.—Nervous diseases, their description and treatment.
HAWKINS, REV. H.—Friendly talk with a new patient. Visiting day at the asylum. Work in the wards, by asylum attendants. P.

JOLLY, F.—Hysteria. (Ziemssen's cyclopædia.)

LALOR, J.—On the use of education and training in the treatment of the insane in public lunatic asylums. P. Dublin.

LEVINSTEIN, E.—Morbid craving for morphia. (Trans.)

LEWIS, W. BEVAN.—Cortical examination of motor area of brain. (Proc. Roy. Soc.) Ill.

LINDSAY, W. LAUDER.—The protection bed and its uses. (E. M. J.)

LINDSAY, W. LAUDER.—Theory and practice of non-restraint. (E. M. J.)

MICKLE, W. J.—Cheyne Stokes' respiration in mental disease. (B. M. J.)

ORD, W. M.—On myxœdema. Med. Chir. Trans.

ROBERTSON, A.—On insanity. (In Finlayson's Clinical Manual.)

SAVAGE, G. H.—Treatment of insanity, especially by drugs. (Guy's Hosp. Rep.)

TUKE, D. HACK.—Broadmoor, the State asylum for insane criminals in England. (Trans. Congrès Internat. de Médecine Mentale.)

TUKE, D. HACK.—Insanity in ancient and modern life, with chapters on its prevention.

TUKE, D. HACK.—On the best method of tabulating the causes of mental alienation. (Trans. Congrès Internat. de Médecine Mentale tenu à Paris.)

WELDON, MRS. GEORGINA.—The history of my orphanage ; or the outpourings of an alleged lunatic. P.

WILKS, S.—Lectures on diseases of the nervous system.

1879. ANSTIE, F. A.—Art. "Alcoholism" in Reynolds's System of Medicine (vol. ii.).

BLANDFORD, G. FIELDING.—General index to the first 24 vols. of the Journ. of Ment. Science.

BUCKNILL, J. C.—A manual of psychological medicine. containing the lunacy laws, the nosology, statistics, description, diagnosis, pathology, and treatment of insanity. With an appendix of cases. Ill. (With Dr. Hack Tuke.) 4th ed.

CALDERWOOD, H.—The relation of mind and brain. Ill.

CAMPBELL, J. A.—On the treatment of excitement by sedatives or otherwise. P.

CHANNING, W.—Buildings for insane criminals. Boston. P.

CLOUSTON, T. S.—The study of mental disease: introductory lecture delivered in the University of Edinburgh on the institution of the lectureship on mental diseases. P.

JACKSON, J. HUGHLINGS.—Articles "Convulsion" and "Apoplexy": Reynolds's System of Medicine (vol. ii.).

LEWES, G. H.—Problems of life and mind.

LINDSAY, W. L.—Mind in the lower animals in health and disease. 2 vols.

LINDSAY, W. L.—Rib fracture in English asylums. (Amer. Journ. of Insanity.)

MCCLINTOCK, A. H.—Remarks on the semeiology of chronic alcoholism. (L.)

MAUDSLEY, H.—Art. "Insanity" in Reynolds's System of Medicine (vol. ii.).

MAUDSLEY, H.—Pathology of mind. 3rd ed.

PETITION.—Criminals in lunatic asylums; a petition to the House of Lords by asylum officials. (L.)

ROBERTSON, A.—On some of the pathological and physiological relations of brain, and higher nerve functions. (Presidential address, Glasg. Path. and Clin. Soc.)

SAVAGE, G. H.—Some uncured cases of insanity. (Guy's Hosp. Rep.)

SIBBALD, J.—Insanity in its public aspect. Edin.

TUKE, D. HACK.—A manual of psychological medicine, containing the lunacy laws, the nosology, statistics, description, diagnosis, pathology and treatment of insanity. With an appendix of cases. (With Dr. Bucknill.) 4th ed.

TUKE, D. HACK.—Historical sketch of the medico-psychological association. Introductory to Dr. Blandford's index to Journ. of Ment. Science.

WOOD, W.—Insanity and the lunacy law. P.

1880. BALFOUR, W. G.—Remarks on private lunatic asylums, a reply to Dr. Bucknill. (B. M. J.)

BASTIAN, H. C.—The brain as an organ of mind. Ill.

BEARD, G. M.—Nervous exhaustion. New York.

BRYCE, P.—The mind, and how to preserve it. N. P. P.

BUCKNILL, J. C.—On the care of the insane and their legal control.

CAMPBELL, J. A.—Insanity, its treatment and prevention. (The presidential address of the Border Counties Branch of the Brit. Med. Assoc.) P.

CLOUSTON, T. S.—Puberty and adolescence medico-psychologically considered. (E. M. J.)

CROTHERS, J. D.—Clinical studies of inebriety. (Med. and Surg. Reporter.) Phil., U.S.A.

HEIDENHAIN, R.—Animal magnetism. Physiological observations. (Trans. by Dr. Wooldridge.)

JACKSON, J. HUGHLINGS.—Optic neuritis. (Ophth. Soc. Trans.)

KIRKBRIDE, T.—On the construction, organisation, and general arrangements of hospitals for the insane, with some remarks on insanity and its treatment. 2nd ed. Ill. Phil., U.S.A.

MAUDSLEY, H.—Responsibility in mental disease. 4th ed.

SPENCER, HERBERT.—Works—specially the principles of psychology.

SUTHERLAND, H.—Alcoholism in private practice. (B. M. J.)

TUKE, D. HACK.—The Cagots. (Journ. of the Anthropological Institute.)

TUKE, HARRINGTON. — Address on the lunacy laws. (Med. Soc. of Lond.) (L.)
TUKE, J. BATTY.—Asylums with unclosed doors. (B. M. J.)
WILBUR, H. B.—A glance at the past and present condition of the insane. P.
WINN, J. M.—The collapse of scientific atheism. P.
ZIEMSSEN, H. V.—Cyclopædia of practical medicine. (Trans.) (Contains diseases of the nervous system.) 17 vols.

1881. BEACH, FLETCHER.—The morphological and histological aspects of microcephalic and cretinoid idiocy. (Int. Med. Cong. Lond.)
BENEDIKT, M.—Anatomical studies upon brains of criminals. (Trans.) New York.
BUCKNILL, J. C.—The late Lord Chief Justice of England (Cockburn) *re* lunacy. P.
CAMPBELL, J. A.—Note on the absence of beer in an asylum dietary. P.
CLOUSTON, T. S.—The teaching of psychiatric medicine. (Int. Med. Cong. Lond.)
DOWSE, STRETCH.—Syphilis of the brain and spinal cord. 2nd ed.
FRASER, W.—On the recent increase in pauper lunacy. P. Edin.
GUY, W. A.—The factors of the unsound mind, with special reference to the plea of insanity in criminal cases, and the amendment of the law.
LOMBARD, J. S.—Experimental researches on the temperature of the head.
LUYS, J.—Brain and its functions. Ill. (Trans.) 2nd ed.
MICKLE, W. J.—General paralysis of the insane, correlative to locomotor ataxia. (L.)
MICKLE, W. J.—Insanity with malarial anæmia and cachexia. (Pract.)
MICKLE, W. J.—Morphia in melancholia. (Pract.)
MITCHELL, S. WEIR.—Lectures on diseases of the nervous system, especially in women.
RAYNER, H.—Gout and insanity. (Trans. Int. Med. Cong. Lond.)
ROBERTSON, A.—On percussion of the skull. (Trans. Int. Med. Cong. Lond.)
ROBERTSON, A.—On unilateral hallucinations and their relation to cerebral localisation. (Trans. Int. Med. Cong. Lond.)
SAVAGE, G. H.—Exophthalmic goitre and mental disorder. (Guy's Hosp. Rep.)
SHEPPARD, S. — Lunacy law reform. (L.)
SHUTTLEWORTH, G. E.—Some of the cranial characteristics of idiocy. (Trans. Int. Med. Cong. Lond.)
SULLY, J. — Illusions: A psychological study.
THOMSON, D. G.—Treatment of the insane in private houses. (L.)
TUKE, D. HACK.—Mental stupor. (Trans. Int. Med. Cong. London.)
TUKE, J. BATTY.—On insanity and hysteria. (Encyclopædia Britannica.)
WARD, H. O.—The first requisites in the physician and nurse for the cure of insanity. P. Phil., U.S.A.
WEATHERLY, L. A.—The domestic treatment of the insane. (Pract.)
WILBUR, H. B.—Chemical restraint in the management of the insane. New York.
WINSLOW, F. L. S.—Fasting and feeding psychologically considered. L.
YELLOWLEES, D.—On disorders of the mind. (Glasgow Health Lectures.)

1882. ALTHAUS, J.—On failure of brain power.
ANDREWS, J. B.—Insanity (Wood's Domestic Medicine, vol. ii.).
ANON.—Only a twelvemonth, or the county asylum. Belfast.
BATEMAN.—The idiot, his place in creation, and his claims on society.
BEACH, FLETCHER.—Types of imbecility. (M. T. and G.)
BLANDFORD, G. F. — Art. "Insanity" (Quain's Dictionary of Medicine).
BUCKNILL, J. C.—The responsibility of Guiteau. P.
CAMPBELL, J. A.—Notes of three abdominal cases of interest. P.
CAMPBELL, J. A.—The necessity for careful physical as well as mental examination prior to sending patients to asylums. P.
CAPPIE, JAMES. — Causation of sleep. (1st ed. 1872.) 2nd ed. Edin.
CLOUSTON, T. S.—Female education from a medical point of view. Edin.
COBBOLD, C. S. W.—Art. "Hæmatoma auris" (Quain's Dictionary of Medicine).
DRAPER, J.—The responsibility of the insane in asylums. P. American.
HAMILTON, A. M.—Idiocy and nervous diseases of adult life. (Wood's Domestic Medicine, vol. ii.)
LEWIS, W. BEVAN.—The human brain: histological and coarse methods of research. A manual for students and asylum medical officers. Ill.
MICKLE, W. J.—Localization of the cerebral centres of the cerebral cortex. (M. T. and G.)
MICKLE, W. J.—Meningeal tuberculosis of the cerebral convexity. (M. T. and G.)
OSLER, W.—On the brains of criminals, with a description of the brains of two murderers. P.
RIBOT, T.—Diseases of memory. (Trans.)
SAVAGE, G. H.—Exophthalmic goitre with mental disorder. (Guy's Hosp. Rep.)
SAVAGE, G. H. — Hypochondriasis and hypochondriacal insanity. (Guy's Hosp. Rep.
SIBBALD, J. — Art. "Insanity" (Quain's Dictionary of Medicine).
STEARNS, H. P.—Insanity: its causes and prevention. New York.
TUKE, J. BATTY.—Art. "Morbid Histology" (Quain's Dictionary of Medicine). (With Dr. Saundby.)
TUKE, J. BATTY.—Notes on the anatomy of the pia mater. (E. M. J.)

TUKE, D. HACK.—Chapters in the history of the insane in the British Isles. Ill.

URQUHART, A. R.—Home treatment of insanity. (Trans. Perth Med. Assoc.)

WEATHERLY, L. A.—Care and treatment of the insane in private dwellings. 12mo.

WORCESTER, S.—Insanity and its treatment. Lectures on the treatment of insanity and kindred nervous disorders. New York and Phil.

1883. ALLEN, N.—The prevention of insanity. Boston. P.

BROWNE, SIR JAMES CRICHTON.—Education and the nervous system. (In the Book of Health, ed. by M. Morris.)

CAMPBELL, J. A.—Four years' treatment of insanity at Garland's Asylum, with remarks. P.

CHARCOT, J. M.—Lectures on the localisation of cerebral and spinal diseases. (Trans. W. B. Hadden.)

GALTON, F. — Enquiries into human faculty and its development.

HAMILTON, A. M.—Manual of medical jurisprudence, with special reference to diseases and injuries of the nervous system.

HAMMOND, W. A.—Treatise on insanity in its medical relations.

LOWE, LOUISA.—The bastilles of England, or the lunacy laws at work. Vol. I. (no more published.)

MANN, E. C.—A manual of psychological medicine and allied nervous diseases.

MAUDSLEY, H.—Body and will: an essay concerning will in its metaphysical, physiological and pathological aspects.

MICKLE, W. J.—General paralysis from cranial injury. (M. T. & G.)

MICKLE, W. J.—Tubercular pericarditis in insanity. (L.)

MORSELLI, H.—Suicide. (Trans. 2nd ed.)

MOUAT, F. J.—Hospital construction and management. (With Mr. Snell.) Ill. Fol.

OPPERT, F.—Hospitals, infirmaries, and dispensaries. Ill.

PARRISH, J.—Alcoholic inebriety from a medical standpoint. Phil., U.S.A.

ROMANES, G.—Mental evolution in animals.

ROSS, J.—Diseases of the nervous system. 2nd ed. 2 vols.

SNELL, H. S.—Hospital construction and management. (With Mr. Mouat.) Ill. Fol.

STEPHEN, SIR JAMES FITZJAMES.—A history of the criminal law of England. 3 vols.

SUTHERLAND, H.—Lectures on insanity. (M. T. and G.)

TUKE, D HACK.—Hypnotism, especially in relation to the mental condition present. (Bull. de la Société de Médecine Mentale de Belgique.)

WINSLOW, F. L. S.—Hand-book of attendants of the insane. 2nd ed.

1884. ALLBUTT, T. CLIFFORD. — On visceral neuroses.

BEACH, FLETCHER.—Facts concerning idiocy and imbecility. (Health Exh. Lit., vol. xii.)

BROWNE, SIR J. CRICHTON.—Report to the Education Department upon the alleged overpressure of work in public elementary schools. (Blue Book.) Fol.

BUCKNILL, J. C.—The abolition of private asylums. (Nineteenth Century.)

BUCKNILL, J. C.—The relation of madness to crime. (Lect. at London Institute.)

FOLSOM, C. F. (with the assistance of Hollis R. Bailey, attorney and counsellor-at-law). Abstract of the statutes of the United States, and of the several States and territories, relating to the custody of the insane. Phil., U.S.A.

HARRISON, GEORGE L.—Legislation on insanity, a collection of all the lunacy laws of the states and territories of the United States to the year 1883 inclusive; also the laws of England on insanity; legislation in Canada on private houses; and important portions of the lunacy laws of Germany, France, &c. Phil., U.S.A.

JACKSON, J. HUGHLINGS.—Croonian lectures on evolution and dissolutions of the nervous system. (Brit. Med. Journ.)

KERR, NORMAN.—On inebriety. P.

MADDEN, T. M.—On insanity and nervous disorders peculiar to women in some of their medical and medico-legal aspects. Dublin.

MOULD, G. W.—The management of the insane. (Lectures.) 12mo. Manchester.

SANKEY, W. H. O.—Lectures on mental diseases. 2nd ed.

SAVAGE, G. H.—Insanity and allied neuroses. (3rd ed. 1891.)

SAVAGE, G. H.—Some modes of treatment of insanity as a functional disorder. (Guy's Hosp. Rep.)

SEGUIN, E.—Opera minora. New York.

SHUTTLEWORTH, G. E.—The health and physical development of idiots. (Health Exh. Lit., vol. xii.)

STRAHAN, S. A. K.—Hepatic abscesses, secondary abscesses in brain. (M. T. and G.)

STRAHAN, S. A. K. — Morphia habitués, their treatment. (L.)

STRAHAN, S. A. K.—Nocturnal insanity. (L.)

STRAHAN, S. A. K.—Tumours of the cerebellum and phenomena associated therewith. (B. M. J.)

STEWART, T. GRAINGER.—An introduction to the studies of diseases of the nervous system. Ill. Edin.

THUDICHUM.—A treatise on the chemical constitution of the brain.

TUCKER, G. A.—The Gheel Colony. P. Birmingham.

TUKE, D. HACK.—Illustrations of the influence of the mind on the body in health and disease. 2 vols. 2nd ed.

TUKE, D. HACK.—Sleep-walking and hypnotism.

YELLOWLEES, D.—Lunacy and pauperism. P. Glasg.

1885. CAMPBELL, J. A.—Treatment of maniacal excitement. P.

CAMPBELL, C. MCIVOR.—Handbook for the instruction of attendants on the insane. With Drs. Clark, Turnbull and Urquhart.

CLARK, A. CAMPBELL.—Handbook for the instruction of attendants on the insane. With Drs. Campbell, Turnbull and Urquhart.

CLOUSTON, T. S.—The position of the medical profession in England in regard to certificates of mental unsoundness and civil incapacity. (E. M. J.)

FOTHERGILL, J. M.—The will power, its range and action.

FOX, E. LONG.—Influence of the sympathetic on disease.

GAIRDNER, W. T.—Insanity: modern views as to its nature and treatment. (Morisonian Lectures, 1879.) P. Glasg.

GOWERS, W. R.—Lectures on the diagnosis of diseases of the brain.

IRELAND, W. W.—The blot upon the brain. Ill. Edin.

MEYNERT, T.—Psychiatry, a clinical treatise on diseases of the fore-brain. (Trans.) New York.

MICKLE, W. J.—Feeding by rectum in insanity. (Pract.)

MITCHELL, S. WEIR.—Diseases of the nervous system. 2nd ed.

PAGE, H. W.—Injuries to the spine and spinal cord.

PAYNE, C. G.—My experience in a madhouse. (Pall Mall Gazette.)

TITCOMBE, SARAH E.—Mind cure on a material basis. Boston, U.S.A.

TUKE, D. HACK.—The insane in the United States and Canada.

TURNBULL, A. R.—Handbook for the instruction of attendants on the insane. (With Drs. Clark, Campbell and Urquhart.)

URQUHART, A. R.—Handbook for the instruction of attendants on the insane. (With Drs. Clark, Campbell and Turnbull.)

WARNER, F.—Physical expression, its modes and principles.

WESTCOTT, W. WYNN.—Suicide, a social science essay.

1886. CLOUSTON, T. S.—The relationship of bodily and mental pain. (B. M. J.)

CREIGHTON, C.—Unconscious memory in disease.

EAST, E.—The private treatment of the insane as single patients. P.

FOLSOM, C. F.—Mental diseases. (American system of medicine.) Boston, U.S.A.

HARRIS, R.—Before trial: What should be done by client, solicitor and counsel, from a barrister's point of view; together with a treatise on the defence of insanity. P.

MACLEOD, M.D.—On puerperal insanity. (B. M. J.)

MAUDSLEY, H.—Natural causes and supernatural seemings. (2nd ed. 1887.)

MICKLE, W. J.—General paralysis of the insane. 2nd ed., enlarged.

MOSELEY, G.—Mental affections and nervous disorders of recent origin or long-standing. Their causes are now successfully treated by a special method. P.

RENTON, A. WOOD.—Monomanie sans délire. "the irresistible criminal impulse theory." Edin.

SAVAGE, G. H.—Evolution of mental disorders. (Guy's Hosp. Rep.)

SHUTTLEWORTH, G. E.—Clinical lecture on idiocy and imbecility. (B. M. J.)

SIBBALD, JOHN.—On work and rest health lecture. 16mo. Edin.

SUTHERLAND, H.—The premonitory symptoms of insanity. B. M. J.

1887. BEACH, FLETCHER.—Idiocy and imbecility due to inherited syphilis. (Trans. Washington Int. Med. Cong.)

BEACH, FLETCHER.—Lecture on the influence of hereditary predisposition on the production of imbecility. (B. M. J.)

BLANDFORD, G. F.—Address on the treatment of insane patients. (Trans. Washington Internat. Med. Cong.)

BLYTH, A. WYNTER.—On poisons. L.

BUTLER, V. S.—The curability of insanity and the individualized treatment of the insane. 12mo. New York.

CLARK, A. CAMPBELL.—Experimental dietetics in lunacy practice. (E. M. J.)

COMBE, A.—Observations on mental derangement. Abridged and edited by Sir Arthur Mitchell. Edin.

DOWN, J. LANGDON.—On the mental affections of childhood and youth. (Letts. Lect. 1887.)

EVEREST, L. F.—The defence of insanity in criminal cases. P.

GRANGER, W. D.—How to care for the insane. New York.

HAWKINS, REV. H.—An address to asylum attendants—off duty and invalided. 16mo. Lond.

HAWKINS, REV. H.—Made whole. An address on leaving an asylum.

LUDD, G. T.—Elements of physiological psychology: a treatise on the activities and nature of the mind from the physical and experimental point of view.

MAUDSLEY, H.—Natural causes and supernatural seemings. 2nd ed.

MILLS, C. K.—The nursing and care of the nervous and insane. Edin.

SAVAGE, G H.—Insanity following the use of anæsthetics. (B. M. J.)

SAVAGE, G. H.—Mental symptoms with locomotor ataxia. (B. M. J.)

SHAFTESBURY, EARL OF.—The life and work of the seventh Earl of Shaftesbury, by E. Hodder. 3 vols.

STEWART.—Our temperaments, their study and their teaching.

SUCKLING, C. W.—Diagnosis of diseases of the brain, spinal cord and nerves.

SUCKLING, C. W.—The brain and its troubles: hints to brain workers. P. Birmingham.

TUCKER, G. A.—Lunacy in many lands. Ill. Sydney.

TUKE, D. HACK.—On the various modes of providing for the insane and idiots in the United States and Great Britain; and on the *rapprochement* between American and British alienists in regard to the employment of mechanical restraint. (Trans. Ninth Internat. Medical Congress, held at Washington.)

WARNER, F.—The children: how to study them. (Lectures.)

WARNER, F.—Three lectures on the anatomy of movement; a treatise on action of nerve centres and modes of growth.

WOOD, H. C.—Nervous diseases and their diagnosis; a treatise upon the phenomena produced by diseases of the nervous system with special reference to the recognition of their causes. Phil. U.S.A.

ZIEGLER, S.—A textbook of pathological anatomy and pathogenesis. 3 vols. (Trans. by D. McAlister.) 2nd ed.

1888. BRAMWELL, BYROM.—Intra-cranial tumours. Ill. Edin.

BROWNE, SIR JAMES CRICHTON.—Responsibility and disease. (Lect. Coll. of State Med.)

CAMPBELL, J. A. — Note on the order of admission of lunatics to asylums. P.

CLOUSTON, T. S.—Science and self-control. P. Edin.

FÉRÉ, CH.—Assistance of the insane in private dwellings in Scotland. (Trans.) P. Glasg.

FINLAY, D. — Clinical observations on epileptic insanity. Glasg.

JACKSON, J. HUGHLINGS.—On the diagnosis and treatment of diseases of the brain. (B. M. J.)

KERR, NORMAN.—Inebriety: its ætiology, pathology, treatment and jurisprudence.

KINKEAD, R. J.—Insanity, inebriety and crime. P. Dublin.

MERCIER, C. A.—The nervous system and the mind: a treatise on the dynamics of the human organism.

MICKLE, W. J.—Insanity in relation to cardiac and aortic disease and to phthisis. (Guls. Lect.)

RANNEY, A. L.—On nervous diseases. Phil., U.S.A.

REPORT of a committee of the Clinical Society of London on myxœdema. (Clin. Soc. Trans.)

SAVAGE, G. H.—Homicidal mania. (Fortnightly Review.)

SAVAGE, G. H.—Syphilis and its relation to insanity. (Trans. Int. Med. Cong.)

TUKE, D. HACK.—Folie à deux. (Brain.)

TUKE, D. HACK.—Hallucinations and the subjective sensations of the sane. (Brain.)

TUKE, J. BATTY. — On open doors. (B. M. J.)

1889. ALEXANDER, W.—The treatment of epilepsy. Edin.

ANDERSON, T. MCCALL. — On syphilitic affections of the nervous system: their diagnosis and treatment.

ARMSTRONG, W.—Lunacy legislation in the Australian colonies. Melbourne.

BANCROFT, J. P.—Separate provision for the recent, the curable, and the appreciative insane. (Rep.) Concord, U.S.A.

BROWNE, SIR JAMES CRICHTON. — The hygienic uses of imagination. (Address in psychology—Leeds meeting of British Medical Association.) (B. M. J.)

BULLEN, F. ST. JOHN. — A review of methods for the exact registration of coarse changes in the brains of the insane.

CHAPIN, JOHN.—Address on the history of American asylums.

CHARCOT, J. M.—Lectures on diseases of the nervous system. (Trans.)

CLOUSTON, T. S.—Diseased cravings and paralysed control. (E. M. J.)

EADE, SIR PETER.—Chorea and insanity. (B. M. J.)

GAIRDNER, W. T. — The physician as naturalist. Glasgow.

GREENE, R.—Care and cure of the insane. (Universal Review.)

GREENE, R.—Hygiene of asylums for the insane. (Trans. Hastings Sanit. Cong.)

IRELAND, W. W.—Through the ivory gate: studies in psychology and history. Edin.

JACKSON, J. HUGHLINGS.—On lead poisoning. (B. M. J.)

KINKHEAD, R. J.—Irish medical practitioner's guide. Dublin.

KRAFFT-EBING, R. VON. — An experimental study in the domain of hypnotism. (Trans.) New York.

LETCHWORTH, W. P.—The insane in foreign countries. Ill.

LEWIS, W. BEVAN.—A textbook of mental diseases, with special reference to the pathological aspects of insanity. Ill.

SAVAGE, G. H.—Pathology of chronic alcoholism. (Trans. Path. Soc.)

SAVAGE, G. H.—Handwriting in insanity. (Ill. Med. News.)

SAVAGE, G. H.—Septic puerperal insanity. (Med. Soc. Trans.)

SPITZKA, E. C.—Insanity, its classification, diagnosis and treatment. New York.

STEWART, JAMES.—Treatment of inebriety in the higher and educated classes. P.

SUCKLING, C. W.—Syphilis of the nervous system. (Birm. Med. Rev.)

TUCKEY, C. L.—Psycho-therapeutics or treatment by sleep and suggestion.

TUKE, J. BATTY.—Lunatics as patients, not prisoners. (Nineteenth Century.)

TUKE, D. HACK.—The past and present provision for the insane poor in Yorkshire, with suggestions for the future provision for this class.

1890. ANON. — Mad doctors; by one of them. P.

BARNES. — On the correlations of the

sexual functions and mental disorders of women. (Brit. Gynæcological Soc.)
BEARD, G. M.—Nervous exhaustion (neurasthenia), its symptoms, nature, sequences and treatment. (Ed. by Dr. Rockwell.)
BRISTOWE, J. S.—Art. on Insanity; Treatise on the theory and practice of medicine. (1st ed. 1876.) (7th ed.)
BROWN-SÉQUARD.—Have we two brains or one? (Forum.)
BROWNE, SIR J. CRICHTON.—Responsibility and disease.
BRUSHFIELD, T. N.—Some practical notes on the symptoms, treatment, and medicolegal aspects of insanity. P. (P. P.) Edin.
CAMPBELL, HARRY.—Flushing and morbid blushing, their pathology and treatment. Ill.
COWLES, E.—Training schools of the future: Rep. of Nat. Conf. of Charities at Baltimore.
ELKINS, F. A.—A case of homicidal and suicidal insanity. Ill. Edin.
ELKINS, F. A.—Report on an epidemic of influenza (140 cases) at Royal Edinburgh Asylum. (With Dr. G. M. Robertson.) P.
ELLIS, HAVELOCK.—The criminal.
FOLSOM, C. F.—Insomnia, disorders of sleep.
FRASER, A.—A guide to operations on the brain. (Plates 42, atlas.) Large fol.
FRY, D. P.—The lunacy laws: containing the statutes relating to private lunatics, pauper lunatics, criminal lunatics, commissioners of lunacy, public and private asylums, and the commissioners in lunacy; with an introductory commentary, notes to the statutes, &c. (Ed. by G. F. Chambers.) 3rd ed. (See also 1864.)
JACKSON, J. HUGHLINGS.—Lumleian lectures on convulsive seizures. (B. M. J.)
MANTEGAZZA, P.—Physiognomy and expression. (Trans.)
MERCIER, C. A.—Sanity and insanity.
MOLL, A.—Hypnotism. (Trans.)
NEEDHAM, F.—Thirty years of lunacy. (Presidential address, Psychological Section, Brit. Med. Assoc.)
OBERSTEINER, H.—Anatomy of central nervous organs in health and disease. (Trans). Ill.
POPE, H. M. R.—Law and practice of lunacy. (Ed. by Boome and Fowke.)
REPORT of committee appointed by the medico-psychological association to enquire into the question of the systematic training of nurses and attendants on the insane.
ROBERTSON, G. M.—Report on an epidemic of influenza (140 cases) at Royal Edinburgh Asylum. (With Dr. Elkins.)
STARR, M. A.—Familiar forms of nervous disease. New York.
STREET, C.—Lunacy Act of 1890. P. Edin.
SUCKLING, C. W.—On the treatment of disease of the nervous system.
TIFFANY, F.—Life of Dorothea Lynde Dix. Ill. Boston, U.S.A.
TUKE, J. BATTY.—The surgical treatment of intra-cranial pressure. (B. M. J.)
WARNER, F.—A course of lectures on the growth and means of training the mental faculty.
WILLIAMS, J. W. HUME.—Unsoundness of mind in its legal and medical considerations. (*Vide* 1856.)

1891. BEACH, FLETCHER.—Psychological medicine in John Hunter's time, and the progress it has since made. (Hunterian Oration.)
BERNHEIM, H.—Suggestive therapeutics: a treatise on the nature and uses of hypnotism. (Trans.) Edin.
BRAMWELL, BYROM.—Atlas of clinical medicine (includes mental diseases). Edin.
BROWNE, SIR JAMES CRICHTON.—On old age. (Introductory lecture, Victoria University, Leeds.) (L.)
BURDETT, H. C.—Hospitals and asylums of the world, their origin, history, construction, administration, management and legislation. Ill. 2 vols.
CAMPBELL, HARRY.—Differences in the nervous organisation of man and woman, physiological and pathological. Ill.
CAMPBELL, J. A.—The utilisation of county hospitals and asylums for teaching purposes. P.
CARLSEN, J.—Statistical investigations concerning the imbeciles in Denmark, 1888–9.
CLOUSTON, T. S.—The neuroses of development. (Morisonian lectures for 1890.) Ill. Edin.
ELKINS, F. A.—On a case of phosphorus poisoning, the mental symptoms and pathological appearances. (With Dr. J. Middlemass.)
FELKIN, R. W.—Hypnotism; or, psychotherapeutics. Edin.
GREENE, R.—Construction and arrangement of asylums. (7th Int. Cong. Hyg.)
GREENE, R.—Hospitals for the insane, and clinical instruction in asylums. P.
HORSLEY, V.—On craniectomy in microcephaly. (B. M. J.)
KERR, NORMAN.—Inebriety and criminal responsibility.
KERR, NORMAN.—Should hypnotism have a recognised place in ordinary therapeutics? P.
PAGE.—Railway injuries.
REPORT of committee of the Medico-psychological Association, to formulate propositions as to the care and treatment of the insane.
REPORT, Charity Organisation Society, on the feeble-minded, epileptic, deformed and crippled.
ROBERTSON, A.—On insanity. (In Finlayson's Clinical Manual.) 3rd ed. Glasg.
SAVAGE, G. H.—Insanity and allied neuroses, practical and clinical. 3rd ed. Ill.
SAVAGE, G. H.—The warnings of general paralysis of the insane. (B. M. J.)

SAVAGE, G. H.—Post-graduate lectures. (M. P. & G.)

SAVAGE, G. H.—Glycosuria, diabetes and insanity. (Med. Soc. Trans.)

STRAHAN, S. A. K. — Consanguineous marriages. (Westminster Rev.)

STRAHAN, S. A. K.—Instinctive Criminality: its true character and rational treatment. P.

TUKE, J. BATTY.—A plea for the scientific study of insanity. (B. M. J.)

TUKE, D. HACK.—Prichard and Symonds in especial relation to mental science, with chapters on moral insanity. Ill.

WALMSLEY, F. H.—The desirableness of throwing open our asylums for the post-graduate study of insanity. P.

WARNER, F.—Report on 50,000 children in schools. (Charity Organisation Society.)

WEATHERLY, L. A. — The supernatural. (With Mr. Maskelyne).

WEISMAN, A.—Essays on heredity and kindred biological problems. Vol. I. 2nd ed. (Trans.)

1892. BLANDFORD, G. F.—Insanity and its treatment, lectures on the treatment, medical and legal, of insane patients. 4th ed. (See 1871.) Lond. and Edin.

CAMPBELL, J. A.—On pneumonia in asylums. (L.)

CAMPBELL, J. A.—A case of tumour of the brain, the result of an apoplexy. (With Dr. J. Coats.)

CLOUSTON, T. S. — Clinical lectures on mental diseases. (1st ed. 1883.) Ill. 3rd ed.

ELKINS, F. A.—Concerning the kinsmen and friends of insane patients. P. Edin.

HERTEL, DR. — Overpressure in High Schools in Denmark. (Introd. by Sir J. Crichton Browne.)

HOWDEN, J.—Pathological index for use in hospitals and asylums. P.

SAVAGE, G. H.—Influenza and neuroses. (Trans. Med. Soc.)

SHAW, J.—Epitome of mental diseases, with the existing regulations as to single patients.

STRAHAN, S. A. K. — Marriage and disease. A study of heredity and the more important family degenerations.

TUKE, J. BATTY.—The surgical treatment of intra-cranial pressure. (B. M. J.)

TUKE, D. HACK.—Dictionary of Psychological Medicine. Ill. 2 vols.

TUKE, D. HACK.—Retrospective glance at the early history of the Retreat, York; its objects and influence. Ill.

WALMSLEY, F. H.—Outlines of insanity.

A. R. URQUHART.

PSYCHOLOGICAL SOCIETIES.

Societies for the Study of Psychological Medicine have been established in various countries. Some of them publish journals, a list of which will be found in the Bibliography incorporated with this work. The following societies are all interested in psychiatry, more or less directly :—

England.—Medico-Psychological Association of Great Britain and Ireland. (*See* Article.) It may be added to the article that nearly 200 now hold the certificate of proficiency in psychological medicine. The examination of attendants has been only lately opened to those engaged in nursing the insane, yet there are nearly 300 who have been trained, and who have successfully passed the examinations. The Report of a Committee, adopted at the annual meeting of 1891, formulates propositions as to the care and treatment of the insane, and sets forth the current opinion of the members at the present time.—The Neurological Society of London, founded in 1886. This Society now numbers about 150 members ; the meetings are held in London. The organ of the Society is "Brain, a Journal of Neurology."—The Psychological Research Society. (*See* Article.)

France.—Société Médico-Psychologique de Paris. Founded in 1852, and named a Society of public utility by a decree of December 11, 1867. This Association gives four prizes for the best work in psychiatry. — Société de Psychologie physiologique: founded in 1885; meets monthly in Paris.—Société de Hypnotisme.—Société Médico-légale de France.

Belgium.—Société de Médecine mentale de Belgique; founded in 1869: meetings held four times a year.

Holland.—Nederlandsche Vereeniging voor Psychiatrie; founded in 1871 ; two meetings are held annually.

Germany.—Gesellschaft für Psychiatrie und Nervenkrankheiten. This Society meets eight times a year in Berlin, and numbers about 180 members.—Psychiatrie Verein ; meetings in Berlin three times yearly, with 130 members.—Verein deutscher Irrenärzte ; one meeting annually, with about 360 members.—Psychiatrischer Verein der Rheinprovinz; about 60 members ; two meetings annually in Bonn.—Östdeutscher irrenärztlicher Verein ; about 50 members ; two meetings annually in Breslau.—Verein südwestdeutscher Neurologen und Irrenärzte ; one annual meeting in Baden-Baden, with about 60 members.—Verein der Irrenärzte Niedersachsens und Westphalens ; one yearly meeting in Hanover.

Austria.—Wiener Verein für Psychiatrie.

Italy.—Societá Freniatrica Italiana, Milan.

Spain.—Academia Frenopatica.

America. — The Association of Medical Superintendents of American Institutions for the Insane. This association was founded in 1844, and holds meetings annually. A noteworthy utterance of opinion in reference to the treatment of the insane was published by this Society in 1876, under the title of "Propositions and Resolutions." — The Medico-Legal Society of New York, founded in 1883, is supported by the professions of law and medicine, and now numbers many members.—The National Association for the Insane, and the Prevention of Insanity, Philadelphia. — The New England Psychological Association.

A. R. U.

PSYCHOLOGICAL LITERATURE.

Asylum Magazines.

Great Britain:—Bethlem Royal Hospital: The Bethlehem Star (1875-1879), Under the Dome (1889-1892); Dumfries Royal Asylum: The New Moon, or Crichton Royal Institution Literary Register (1844); Edinburgh Royal Asylum: The Morningside Mirror (1845); Perth Royal Asylum: Excelsior (1857); York Asylum, Bootham: The York Star (1857); Church Stretton Asylum: Loose Leaves (occasional); Glasgow Royal Asylum: The Chronicles of the Cloister, The Gartnavel Gazette. (A few numbers.)

America:—The Retreat Gazette, Hartford, Conn. (A few numbers.) The Asylum Journal, Brattleboro', Vt. (1842-6); The Opal, Utica (1851-61); The Meteor, Tuskaloosa, Ala. (1872-6); The Friend, Harrisburg, Pa. (Two years.)

Periodical Literature. —: Allgemeine Zeitschrift für Psychiatrie und psychisch-gerichtliche Medicin, herausgegeben von Deutschlands Irrenärzten, Ed. Laehr and others, 1844 (Berlin); Alienist and Neurologist, Ed. C. H. Hughes, quarterly, 1880 (St. Louis); American Journal of Insanity, Ed. Med. Off. of New York State Lunatic Asylum, quarterly, 1844 (Utica); American Journal of Neurology and Psychiatry, Ed. by Drs. McBride, Gray, and Spitzka, quarterly, 1882-5 (New York); American Journal of Psychology, Ed. Stanley Hall, quarterly (Mass.); Annales Médico-Psychologiques, Journal de l'aliénation mentale et de la Médecine légale des Aliénés, Ed. Ritti and others, every two months, 1843 (Paris); L'Anomalo, Gazzetino antropologico, psichiatrico, medico-legale con pagina di letteratura dei folli ed appendice varia del medico generico, monthly, Ed. Dr. Angelo Zuccarelli (Naples); Archiv der deutschen Gesellschaft für Psychiatrie und Gerichtliche Psychologie, Ed. Erlenmeyer and others, 1858-66 also 1872 (Neuwied); Archiv für Psychologie, für Aerzte und Juristen, Ed. Friedrich, 1834 only, afterwards as Blätter für Psychiatrie, 1837-8 (Erlangen); Archiv für Psychologie und Nervenkrankheiten, Ed. Grashey, von Krafft-Ebing, Pelman, Schuchardt, Schüle. 1868 (Berlin); Archiv psichiatrii, neurologii, i sudebnoi psichopatologii, Ed. Kovalewski, quarterly, 1883 (Charcov); Archiv sudebnoi Meditsini, quarterly, 1869-71 (St. Petersburg); Archives de Neurologie, revue des Maladies nerveuses et mentales, Ed. Charcot, every two months, 1880 (Paris); Archivio di psichiatria scienze penali ed antropologia criminale, per servire allo studio dell' uomo alienato e delinquente, Ed. Prof. Lombroso, quarterly, 1880 (Turin and Rome); Archivio Italiana per le malattie nervose e più particolarmente per le alienazioni mentali organo della Società Freniatrica Italiano, Ed. Dr. Andrea Verga e Serafino Biffi, 1863 (Milan); Beiträge zur experimentellen Psychologie von Hugo Münsterberg (Mohr, Freiburg); Brain—a journal of neurology, Ed. by Dr. de Watteville, for the Neurological Society of London, quarterly, 1878 (London); Bulletin de la Société de Médecine Mentale de Belgique, Ed. Dr. J. Morel, quarterly, 1873 (Ghent); Bulletins de la Société de Psychologie Physiologique, President, Prof. Charcot (Paris); Centralblatt für Nervenheilkunde und Psychiatrie für die gesammte Neurologie in Wissenschaft und Praxis mit besonderer Berücksichtigung der Degenerations-anthropologie, Ed. Erlenmeyer, monthly, 1877-1878, Coblenz. Centralbl. f. Nervenheilkunde, &c., Ed. Kurella. L'encéphale, Journal des Maladies mentales et nerveuses, Ed. Prof. Ball and others, quarterly, 1881 (Paris); Friedreich's Blätter für gerichtliche Medicin und Sanitäts-Polizei, Ed. v. Hecker, fortnightly, 1863 (Nürnberg); Giornale di Neuropatologie, Ed. Dr. Vizioli, fortnightly, 1882 (Naples); Der Irrenfreund Psychiatrische Monatsschrifte für praktische Aerzte, Ed. Brosius, monthly, 1859 (Heilbronn); Jahrbücher für Psychiatrie, Ed. Drs. Gauster and Meynert, formerly Psychiatrisches Centralsblatt, 1871-8, 1879 (Vienna); Journal de Médecine Mentale. Ed. Dr. Delasiauve, monthly, 1861-1870 (Paris); The Journal of Mental and Nervous Disease, Ed. Dr. Brown 1876, monthly (New York) (formerly Chicago); The Journal of Mental Science (formerly The Asylum Journal, &c.), published by authority of the Medico-Psychological Association of Great Britain and Ireland, Ed. Drs. Hack Tuke and Savage, quarterly, 1853, (London); The Journal of Nervous and Mental Disease, Ed. Dr. Jewell, quarterly, 1874 (Chicago); The Journal of Psychological Medicine and Mental Pathology, Ed. F. Winslow, 1848-60 (London), also ed. F. L. S. Winslow, 1875-82; Il Manicomico Moderno Gior-

Periodical Literature (*continued*)—
nale di Psichiatria. Organo del Manicomio Interp. V. E. II., Ed. Dr. Limoncelli 1885 (Nocera); The Medico-legal Journal, published under the auspices of the Medico-legal Society of New York. Ed. Clark Bell, quarterly, 1883 (New York); Mind, a quarterly review of psychology and philosophy. Ed. G. C. Robertson, quarterly, 1876 (London); Nederlandsch Tijdschrift voor Geneeskunde, tevens Orgaan der Nederlandsche Maatschappij tot Bevordering der Geneeskunst, 1858 (Amsterdam); Neurologisches Centralblatt. Übersicht der Leistungen auf dem Gebiete der Anatomie, Physiologie, Pathologie und Therapie des Nervensystems einschliesslich der Geisteskrankheiten. Ed. Prof. Mendel, monthly, 1882 (Leipzig); Nouvelle Iconographie de la Salpêtrière, Director, Prof. Charcot, bi-monthly (Paris); La Psichiatria, la neuropatologia et le scienze affini, Ed. Dr. Bianchi, quarterly, 1883 (Naples); Psychiatrische Bladen, uitgegeven door de Nederlandsche Vereeniging voor Psychiatrie, Ed. Dr. Tellegen, J. van Deventer, &c., quarterly, 1883 (Amsterdam); The Psychological Journal. Ed. E. Mead, bi-monthly, 1753 only (Cincinnati); The Psychological and Medico-legal Journal. Ed. W. A. Hammond, 2 vols. yearly, 1874–6; also as The Quarterly Journal of Psychological Medicine and Medical Jurisprudence, 1867–9, New York; Rivista frenopatica Barcelonesa, Ed. J. G. y Paratgua, monthly, 1881 (Barcelona); Rivista Sperimentale di Freniatria e di Medicina Legale in relazione con l'antropologia e le Scienze Giuridiche e Sociali, Ed. Prof. Aug. Tamburini and others, monthly, 1875 (Reggio Emilia); Rivista Sperimentale di freniatria e di medicina legale in relazione con l'antropologia, Ed. Dr. Livi and others, monthly, 1875 (Reggio Emilia; Vestnik Sudebnoi Meditsini i obchestvennoi gigien, quarterly, 1882 St. Petersburg); Vierteljahrsschrift für Psychiatrie in ihren Beziehungen zur Morphologie, Pathologie des Central-nervensystems, &c., Ed. Drs. Leidesdorf and Meynert, 1867–9 (Leipzig); West Riding Asylum Medical Reports, Ed. by Sir J. Crichton Browne, yearly, 1871–6 (London); Zeitschrift für die Anthropologie (formerly Z. für psychische Aerzte), Ed. Dr. Nasse, 1816–26; Zeitschrift für Psychologie und Physiologie der Sinnesorgane. Eds. Ebbinghaus und König, bi-monthly (Hamburg).

A. R. U.

TABLE OF LEGAL ABBREVIATIONS.

Abr. Eq. Cas.	Abridgement, Equity Cases.
Add.	Addams' Reports.
A. & E.	Adolphus and Ellis' Reports.
App. Cas.	Appeal Cases.
Atk.	Atkyns' Reports.
Bac. Abr.	Bacon's Abridgement.
B. & Ad.	Barnewall and Adolphus.
B. & C.	Barnewall and Cresswell.
Beav.	Beavan's Reports.
Bing. N. C.	Bingham's New Cases.
Bligh, N. S.	Bligh, New Series.
B. & B.	Broderip and Bingham.
Buller, N. P.	Buller's Nisi Prius.
Camp.	Campbell's Reports.
C. & K.	Carrington and Kirwan.
C. & P.	Carrington and Payne.
Ch. Cas.	Cases in Chancery.
Cas. (temp. Lee)	Cases temp. Lee.
Cl. & F.	Clark and Finnelly.
Co. Litt.	Coke on Littleton.
C. B.	Common Bench.
Com. Dig.	Comyn's Digest.
Cox, C. C.	Cox's Criminal Cases.
Cro. Eliz.	Croke temp. Elizabeth.
C. M. & R.	Crompton, Meeson, and Roscoe.
Curt. E. R.	Curties' Ecclesiastical Reports.
Deane	Deane's Reports.
De Gex	De Gex's Reports in Bankruptcy.
D. M. & G.	DeGex, McNaghten, and Gordon.
Denio	Denio's Reports (U.S.).
Den. C. C.	Denison's Crown Cases.
Dow	Dow's Reports.
Dowl. Rep.	Dowling's Reports.
D. & R.	Dowling and Ryland.
D.	Dunlop's Reports.
East	East's Reports.
Ex.	Exchequer Reports.
F. C.	Faculty Cases (Scotch).
Fonbl.	Fonblanque's Equity.
F. & F.	Foster and Finlason's Reports.
Gray	Gray's Reports (U.S.).
Hagg. C. R.	Haggard's Consistorial Reports.
Hagg. E. R.	Do. Ecclesiastical Reports.
Hale, P. C.	Sir Matthew Hale's Pleas of the Crown.
Hawk. P. C.	Hawkins' Pleas of the Crown.
Hob.	Hobart's Reports.
How. St. Tr.	Howell's State Trials.
H. & N.	Hurlstone and Norman.
Irvine	Irvine's Reports.
Jacob	Jacob's Reports.
J. & Lat.	Jones and Latouch's Reports.
K. & J.	Kay and Johnson.
Kel.	Kelynge's Reports.
L. J., N. S., Ch.	Law Journal, New Series (Chancery).
L. J., N. S., C. P.	Do. (Common Pleas).
L. J., N. S., Ex.	Do. (Exchequer).
L. J., N. S., P. M. & A.	Do. (Probate, Matrimonial, and Admiralty).
L. J., N. S., Q. B.	Do. (Queen's Bench).
L. R., Ch. D.	Law Reports (Chancery Division).
L. R., Eq.	Do. (Equity Cases).
L. R., Ex.	Do. (Exchequer Cases).
L. R., Ir.	Do. (Ireland).
L. R., P. & D. L. R., P. & M.	Do. (Probate and Divorce).
L. R., P. D.	Do. (Probate Division).
L. R., Q. B.	Do. (Queen's Bench Cases).
L. R., Q. B. D.	Do. (Queen's Bench Division).
L. R., Sc. & Div.	Do. (Scotch and Divorce).
L. T.	Law Times (Reports).
Leach	Leach's Reports.
Lew.	Lewin's Crown Cases.
Mac. & G.	McNaghten and Gordon's Reports.
Macph.	Macpherson's Reports (Scotch).
M. & G.	Manning and Granger's Reports.
Mass.	Massachusetts Reports (U.S.).
M. & W.	Meeson and Welsby.
Mod.	Modern Reports.
Moo. P. C.	Moore's Privy Council.
M. & Rob.	Moody and Robinson.
Moor.	Moore's Reports.
Myl. & Cr.	Mylne and Craig.
M. & K.	Mylne and Keen.
N. Y.	New York Reports (U.S.).
Phill., E. R.	Phillimore's Ecclesiastical Reports.
Plowden	Plowden's Reports.
P. (1892)	Probate Reports, 1892.
R.	Rettie's Reports (Scotch).

Rep.	Coke's Reports.
Ridg., P. C.	Ridgway's Pleas of the Crown.
Rob., E. R.	Robertson's Ecclesiastical Reports.
Roberts.	Robertson's Reports.
Russ.	Russell's Reports.
Salk.	Salkeld's Reports.
Sav.	Saville's Reports.
S.	Shaw's Reports (Scotch).
Sid.	Siderfin's Reports.
Sim.	Simons' Reports.
Str.	Strange's Reports.
S. & T.	Swabey and Tristram.
Times L. R.	Times Law Reports.
Ventr.	Ventris's Reports.
Verm.	Vermont Reports (U.S.).
Ves.	Vesey's Reports.
V. & B.	Vesey and Brames.
Ves. Jun.	Reports of Vesey, Junior.
W. N.	Weekly Notes.
W. R.	Weekly Reporter.
Wendell	Wendell's Reports (U.S.).
W. & S.	Wilson and Shaw's Reports (Scotch).
Y. & Coll.	Younge and Collyer's Reports.

TABLE OF LEGAL CASES.

INDEX.*

* This Index, which has been prepared by Dr. Pietersen, omits words which are already given in the Dictionary *sub voc.* For example, only such references are given under "acute delirious mania" as are not found in the article bearing that title.

5 B

PRINTED BY BALLANTYNE, HANSON AND CO.
LONDON AND EDINBURGH.

Lightning Source UK Ltd.
Milton Keynes UK
17 November 2010

163003UK00006B/114/P

9 781174 240232